Wiggs's Veterinary Dentistry

Wiggs's Veterinary Dentistry

Principles and Practice

Second Edition

Edited by

Heidi B. Lobprise, DVM, DAVDC
Main Street Veterinary Hospital and Dental Clinic
Flower Mound
TX, USA

and

Johnathon R. (Bert) Dodd, DVM, FAVD, DAVDC
Veterinary Dentistry
Texas A&M University
College Station
TX, USA

WILEY Blackwell

This edition first published 2019

Edition History
Lippincott (1e, 1997)

Registered Office
John Wiley & Sons, Inc., 111 River Street, Hoboken, NJ 07030, USA

Editorial Office
111 River Street, Hoboken, NJ 07030, USA

For details of our global editorial offices, customer services, and more information about Wiley products visit us at www.wiley.com.

Wiley also publishes its books in a variety of electronic formats and by print-on-demand. Some content that appears in standard print versions of this book may not be available in other formats.

Library of Congress Cataloging-in-Publication Data

Names: Lobprise, Heidi B., editor. | Dodd, Johnathon R., editor.
Title: Wiggs's veterinary dentistry : principles and practice / edited by
Heidi B. Lobprise and Johnathon R. Dodd.
Other titles: Veterinary dentistry
Description: Second edition. | Hoboken, NJ : Wiley-Blackwell, 2018. |
Preceded by Veterinary dentistry / editors, Robert B. Wiggs, Heidi B. Lobprise. c1997. |
Includes bibliographical references and index. |
Identifiers: LCCN 2018026806 (print) | LCCN 2018027769 (ebook) |
ISBN 9781118816165 (Adobe PDF) | ISBN 9781118816080 (ePub) |
ISBN 9781118816127 (hardcover)
Subjects: LCSH: Veterinary dentistry. | MESH: Dentistry–veterinary |
Veterinary Medicine | Stomatognathic Diseases–veterinary
Classification: LCC SF867 (ebook) | LCC SF867 .V47 2019 (print) | NLM SF 867 |
DDC 636.089/76–dc23
LC record available at https://lccn.loc.gov/2018026806

Cover Design: Wiley
Cover Images: © Jo Banyard; © Bonnie Shope; © Roberto Fecchio

Set in 10/12pt Warnock by SPi Global, Pondicherry, India
Printed and bound by CPI Group (UK) Ltd, Croydon, CR0 4YY

C9781118816127_271125

The manufacturer's authorized representative according to the EU General Product Safety Regulation is Wiley-VCH GmbH, Boschstr. 12, 69469 Weinheim, Germany, e-mail: Product_Safety@wiley.com.

Dedication

"Dentistry has emerged over the last twenty years as a distinct and significant part of clinical veterinary medicine. This emergence as a prominent and accepted science has not come easily nor without controversy in the modality of treatments and in organization. The veterinary dental pioneers faced numerous scientific and technical barriers, as well as lack of acceptance on occasion, by colleagues. However, science embraces and accepts science, and as research continues to link oral health with general health, dentistry is becoming more widely appraised and appreciated."

This was the opening paragraph from the first edition of this book published by Robert B. Wiggs and Heidi B. Lobprise twenty years ago. So much of that paragraph is still true today; however, because of the foresight of dental pioneers like Bob Wiggs, Don Ross, Tom Mulligan, Sandy Manfra Maretta, Ben Colmery, Chuck Williams, Colin Harvey, Peter Emily, Steve Holmstrom, and Ed Eisner, the practice of veterinary dentistry today is "widely appraised and appreciated" over these last 40 years.

This book is dedicated to the memory of Robert Bruce (Bob) Wiggs for his vision, his knowledge, his perseverance, and his unending selflessness to advance the level of dentistry in private (and specialty) practice throughout the world. His memory is in the hearts of countless veterinarians whose personal knowledge and skills improved because of Bob's willingness to share with anyone who would ask for help. Bob never asked for anything in return.

Mike Peak had this to say about Bob: "When I started my residency with Dr. Wiggs, I was pretty green and no doubt had a lot to learn. I had been 'doing' dentistry for 4–5 years before beginning the residency and knew 'how' to do procedures, but didn't have the depth of understanding and knowledge 'why' certain procedures were done one way vs. another. I can remember Dr. Wiggs helping me understand certain oral pathologies and treatments, that at the time, in some cases seemed unorthodox. On more than one occasion, I thought for certain he was wrong about what he was telling me. I can remember thinking, 'this just can't be right' or 'there's no way he's right about that'. However, once I researched the literature, or we saw the case through its entirety, it turned out he was right EVERY time. It is amazing, even to this day, I see diseases that have now been more thoroughly investigated and he continues to be right!"

Another colleague, Gregg DuPont, added, "Dr. Bob Wiggs, the lead co-author of the first edition of this book, inspired countless veterinarians to increase their knowledge of dentistry and to improve their level of dental care for their patients. He shared his skills and his wealth of knowledge readily and selflessly with anyone who wanted to learn more about veterinary dentistry. Bob was a good friend who possessed an uncommon combination of knowledge, generosity, and down-to-earth common sense that made time spent together delightful. The field of veterinary dentistry is a better one for his contributions, actions and interactions."

According to Ed Eisner and Steve Holmstrom, Robert Bruce Wiggs was a renaissance man. He was a pioneer of the 1970s dental evolution in veterinary medicine. His closest friends saw many sides of Bob. He was, on the one hand, very proud of his Scottish heritage (Bruce the Fierce), and his Texas roots (1st generation Texas Ranger Ben Wills, known for his integrity as well as his toughness). As a member of one of the "Indian Companies", Ranger Wills helped bring in alive the infamous Commanche renegade, Quantos Parker, in the 1860s.

Bob practiced with a high level of ethics and professional discipline, as well as being known for his dry sense of humor. In the 1980s, before the advent of internet "list serves", Bob organized a dental support group that he nicknamed after one of his favorite comedy groups, The Three Stooges. There were actually five stooges, and this group shared the nuances of all stooges being Presidents of the newly forming American Veterinary Dental College, all were national and international speakers, and all were published authors. The Stooges also boasted a fierce professional football rivalry, Larry championing his Dallas Cowboys, Curly the Denver Broncos, Moe the SF 49ers, Shemp the Philadelphia Eagles, and Curly Joe the Seattle Seahawks. On the occasion of a Cowboys loss, Larry was a good sport. The Stooges were also known for their practical jokes. Among other pranks, they traditionally, at the annual Veterinary Dental Conference, short-sheeted the bed of the incoming Dental College President. When it was Bob's turn, as incoming president, and he was cheerfully asked how he had slept the night before, Bob said "very soundly, thank you". He had slept on top of the covers, innocent of the ongoing shenanigans. There will never be another Bob, or "Larry".

On a more serious note, Dr. Wiggs was a meticulous innovator of dental instruments, hammering out the first set of winged elevators for his small animal dental practice. He also headed up the laboratory animal care unit at the Baylor College of Dentistry in Dallas (now known as the Texas A & M College of Dentistry), and donated his time and expertise in providing dental care for the animals at the Dallas Zoo, the Fort Worth Zoo, and area wild animal sanctuaries. He had gifted hands for oral surgery and the high quality of his procedures were acknowledged both throughout the United States and abroad. Animals of all species benefited by his dental expertise and tireless efforts on their behalf.

Dr. Bob Wiggs' ability to personally share his knowledge of dentistry ceased on November 29, 2009, but his influence on all of us will continue indefinitely.

Heidi B. Lobprise, DVM
Johnathon R. (Bert) Dodd, DVM

Contents

Foreword

Twenty years is a long time to wait on a second edition, and it took nearly four years to organize the contents of this one. The first edition of *Veterinary Dentistry – Principles and Practice* came out in 1997, largely due in part to the tremendous knowledge and dedication of Dr. Robert Bruce Wiggs (1950–2009). Referred to by some as "the bible" of veterinary dentistry, with no irreverence intended, it was probably the most comprehensive book in that field of topic during that time. Not without its shortcomings, such as a lack of adequate figures and illustrations due to publishing restraints, as well as now aged reference listings, it still provided a wealth of information to many a "student".

This edition is a melding of keeping as many of the timeless and true concepts and knowledge, with adding in updated and contemporary viewpoints. Of course, as with any text, by the time the ink dries, there will be newer data published electronically and in journals that will update the information provided. This edition literally rests on the shoulders of giants, from the first edition and stellar human dental resources, to the current knowledge provided by current guest contributors.

In particular, distinct efforts were made to further bolster information about anesthesia and pain management (Chapter 9), to examine traumatic dentoalveolar injuries more closely (Chapter 6), and to dedicate a chapter to Oral and Maxillofacial Tumors (Chapter 7, with a separate chapter on related surgery). Other chapters expand on newer techniques and resources such as restorative endodontic (Chapter 16) and periodontal therapy (Chapter 10) and data related to the application of crowns and prosthodontics for dogs (Chapter 18). Whenever possible, updated terminology (based on the American Veterinary Dental College Nomenclature resources) was integrated, as seen in the feline chapter (Chapter 20), with appropriate abbreviations in tables throughout the book.

There are definitely more images and illustrations than the original edition, but there are still other texts that are known for more complete coverage of specific procedures, such as *Veterinary Dental Techniques* (Holmstrom, Frost, and Eisner) and *Oral and Maxillofacial Surgery in Dogs and Cats* (Verstraete and Lommer). The step-by-step feature of issues of the *Journal of Veterinary Dentistry* is also a good resource for pictoral descriptions, and was utilized in several places in this book as well.

Therefore, as these files are sent to the publisher (interestingly on the day 8 years after Dr. Wiggs' passing), I look back at these four years with plans for when the next edition will be needed (certainly sooner than 20 years), as the future of veterinary dentistry continues to expand. I played a part in that first edition, though it was but a portion of Dr. Wiggs' contribution, which is why, with great respect and fond remembrance, we are pleased to launch the modified name of this text – *Wiggs' Veterinary Dentistry – Principles and Practice*, second edition. I am also pleased and proud to say that the veterinarians involved in this edition have agreed to donate proceeds to the Foundation for Veterinary Dentistry in Dr. Wiggs' name and to the Robert B Wiggs endowed scholarship at Texas A&M University.

Respectfully submitted
Heidi B. Lobprise, DVM, DAVDC

List of Contributors

Jamie G. Anderson, DVM, MS, DAVDC, DACVIM
Sacramento Veterinary Dental Services
Rancho Cordova
CA, USA

Kristin Bannon, DVM, FAVD, DAVDC
Veterinary Dentistry and Oral Surgery of New Mexico, LLC
Algodones
NM, USA

Donald Beebe, DVM, DAVDC
Apex Dog and Cat Dentistry
Englewood
CO, USA

Jan Bellows, DVM, Dipl. AVDC, ABVP (canine and feline)
All Pets Dental
Weston
FL, USA

Robert C. Boyd, DVM, DAVDC
Montgomery
TX, USA

Anthony Caiafa, BVSc, BDSc, MANZCVS
School of Veterinary and Biomedical Sciences
James Cook University
Townsville, Queensland
Australia

Diane Carle, DVM, DAVDC
Animal Medical Center of Seattle
Seattle
WA, USA

Cynthia Charlier, DVM, DAVDC
VDENT Veterinary Dental Education Networking and Training
Elgin
IL, USA

Curt Coffman, DVM, FAVD, DAVDC
Arizona Veterinary Dental Specialists
Scottdale
AZ, USA

Johnathon R. (Bert) Dodd, DVM, FAVD, DAVDC
Veterinary Dentistry
Texas A&M University
College Station
TX, USA

Roberto Fecchio, DVM, MSc., PhD.
Safari Co. – Zoo and Exotic Animals Dental Consultant
São Paulo/SP
Brazil

Marco Antonio Gioso, DVM, DDS, DAVDC
Laboratório de Odontologia Comparada da FMVZ
University of São Paulo
São Paulo, Brazil

Norman Johnston, FRCVS, DAVDC, DEVDC
DentalVets
North Berwick
Scotland, UK

Loïc Legendre, DVM, DAVDC, DEVDC
Northwest Veterinary Dental Services Ltd
North Vancouver
British Columbia, Canada

Matthew Lemmons, DVM, DAVDC
MedVet Medical and Cancer Centers for Pets
Indianapolis
IN, USA

John Lewis, VMD, FAVD, DAVDC
Veterinary Dentistry Specialists
Chadds Ford, PA

Heidi B. Lobprise, DVM, DAVDC
Main Street Veterinary Hospital and Dental Clinic
Flower Mound
TX, USA

Paul Q. Mitchell, DVM, DAVDC
Veterinary Dental Services
North Attleboro
MA, USA

Brook Niemiec, DVM, DAVDC
Veterinary Dental Specialties and Oral Surgery
San Diego
CA, USA

Michael Peak, DVM, DAVDC
Tampa Bay Veterinary Specialists
Largo
FL, USA

Alexander M. Reiter, Dipl. Tzt., Dr. med. vet., DAVDC, DEVDC
School of Veterinary Medicine
University of Pennsylvania
Philadelphia
PA, USA

Bonnie H. Shope, VMD, DAVDC
Veterinary Dental Services, LLC
Boxborough
MA, USA

Christopher Smithson, DVM, DAVDC
The Pet Dentist at Tampa Bay
Wesley Chapel
FL, USA

Christopher Snyder, DVM, DAVDC
School of Veterinary Medicine
University of Wisconsin-Madison
Madison
WI, USA

Lindsey C. Snyder, DVM, MS, DACVAA
School of Veterinary Medicine
University of Wisconsin-Madison
Madison
WI, USA

Maria M. Soltero-Rivera, DVM, DAVDC
School of Veterinary Medicine
University of Pennsylvania
Philadelphia
PA, USA

Jason Soukup, DVM, DAVDC
School of Veterinary Medicine
University of Wisconsin-Madison
Madison
WI, USA

Kevin Stepaniuk, DVM, FAVD, DAVDC
Veterinary Dentistry Education and Consulting
Services, LLC
Ridgefield
WA, USA

Kendall Taney, DVM, DAVDC
Center for Veterinary Dentistry and Oral Surgery
Gaithersburg
MD, USA

Chris Visser, DVM, DAVDC, DEVDC, MRCVS
Arizona Veterinary Dental Specialists
Scottsdale
AZ, USA

Louis Visser, DDS
Arizona Veterinary Dental Specialists
Scottsdale
AZ, USA

1

Oral Anatomy and Physiology

Matthew Lemmons[1] and Donald Beebe[2]

[1] MedVet Medical and Cancer Centers for Pets, Indianapolis, IN, USA
[2] Apex Dog and Cat Dentistry, Englewood, CO, USA

Within this chapter, the dog will be discussed primarily, although some comparative information will be covered. Related anatomy and variations for other species will be discussed within chapters covering those. It is intended that this chapter serve to provide the foundation knowledge for the chapters that follow.

The practice of veterinary dentistry is concerned with the conservation, reestablishment and/or treatment of dental, paradental, and oral structures. In dealing with their associated problems a fundamental awareness of anatomy and physiology is essential for an understanding of the presence or absence of the abnormal or pathologic structure. Anatomy and physiology are acutely interactive, with anatomy considered the study of structure and physiology that of its function. These deal with bones, muscles, vasculature, nerves, teeth, periodontium, general oral functions, and their development.

1.1 General Terms

Dentes decidui – deciduous teeth.
Dentes permanentes – permanent teeth.
Dentes incisivi – incisor teeth.
Dentes canini – canine teeth.
Dentes premolares – premolar teeth.
Dentes molares – molar teeth.

1.1.1 Three Basic Types of Tooth Development

Monophyodont. Only one set of teeth that erupt and remain in function throughout life (no deciduous teeth), such as in most rodents (*heterodont*) and dolphins (*homodont*), as currently accepted.

Polyphyodont. Many sets of teeth that are continually replaced. Most of these are homodonts. In sharks, the replacement is generally of a horizontal nature with new teeth developing caudally and moving rostrally. In reptiles, the replacement is generally of a vertical nature with new teeth developing immediately apical to the teeth in current occlusion and replacing them when lost.

Diphyodont. Two sets of teeth, one designated deciduous and one permanent. Common to most domesticated animals and man.

1.1.2 Common Terms Used with Diphyodont Tooth Development

Deciduous teeth (Dentes decidui). Considered to be the first set of teeth that are shed at some point and replaced by permanent teeth.

Primary teeth (Dentes primarui). Considered to be the first set of teeth that are shed at some point and replaced by permanent teeth. Some distractors feel this term is not totally correct because in some species primary teeth are also their permanent teeth, and even in diphyodonts some permanent teeth (i.e., the dog: first premolar and molars) may theoretically also classify as primary, since all teeth may eventually be exfoliated. The term primary is acceptable when speaking to the layperson, but not acceptable in the professional setting.

Permanent teeth (Dentes permanentes). The final or lasting set of teeth, that are typically of a very durable nature (opposite of deciduous).

Nonsuccessional teeth (Nonsuccedaneous). Permanent teeth that do not succeed a deciduous counterpart. Classically molars of dogs and cats.

Successional teeth (Succedaneous). Permanent teeth that replace or succeed a deciduous counterpart. Typically certain diphyodont incisors, canines, or premolars.

Wiggs's Veterinary Dentistry: Principles and Practice, Second Edition. Edited by Heidi B. Lobprise and Johnathon R. (Bert) Dodd.

Mixed Dentition. The transient complement of teeth present in the mouth after eruption of some of the permanent teeth but before all the deciduous teeth are absent. Commonly seen in diphyodonts during the early stages of permanent tooth eruption, until all deciduous teeth have been exfoliated.

1.1.3 Two Basic Categories of Tooth Types or Shapes

Homodont. All teeth are of the same general shape or type, although size may vary, such as in fish, reptiles, sharks, and some marine mammals.

Heterodont. Functionally different types of teeth are represented in the dentition. The domestic dog and cat have heterodont dentition, characterized by incisors, canines, premolars, and molars.

1.1.4 Three Common Types of Vertebrate Tooth Anchorage

Thecodont. Teeth firmly set in sockets typically using gomphosis, such as dogs, cats, and humans. *Gomphosis.* A type of fibrous joint in which a conical object is inserted into a socket and held.

Acrodont. Teeth are ankylosed directly to the alveolar bone without sockets or true root structure. This type of attachment is not very strong; teeth are lost easily and are replaced by new ones. This formation is common in the order Squamata (lizards and snakes) with the only other teeth formation in this order being pleurodont. Acrodontal tooth attachment is also seen in fish.

Pleurodont. Teeth grow from a pocket on the inner side of the jawbone that brings a larger surface area of tooth in contact with the jawbone and hence attachment is stronger, as in amphibians and some lizards. However, this attachment is also not as strong as thecodont anchorage.

1.1.5 Two Basic Tooth Crown Types

Brachydont. Dentition with a shorter crown to root ratio, as in primates and carnivores. A brachydont tooth has a supragingival crown and a neck just below the gingival margin, and at least one root. An enamel layer covers the crown and extends down to the neck. Cementum is only found below the gingival margin.

Hypsodont. Dentition with a longer crown to root ratio, as in cow, horses, and rodents. These teeth have enamel that extends well beyond the gingival margin, which provides extra material to resist wear and tear from feeding on tough and fibrous diets. Cementum and enamel invaginate into a thick layer of dentin.

Radicular hypsodont (subdivision of hypsodont). Dentition with true roots, sometimes called closed rooted, that erupts additional crown through most of life. These teeth eventually close their root apicies and cease growth. As teeth are worn down new crown emerges from the submerged reserve crown of the teeth, such as in the molars and premolars of the equine and bovine. Known as continually erupting closed rooted teeth.

Aradicular hypsodont (subdivison of hypsodont). Dentition without true roots, sometimes called open rooted, that produces additional crown throughout life. As teeth are worn down new crown emerges from the continually growing teeth, such as in lagomorphs and incisors of rodents. Known as continually growing teeth or open rooted teeth.

1.1.6 General Crown Cusp Terms of Cheek Teeth

Secodont dentition. Having cheek teeth with cutting tubercles or cusps arranged to provide a cutting or shearing interaction, such as premolars in most carnivores, especially the carnassial teeth.

Bunodont dentition. Having cheek teeth with low rounded cusps on the occlusal surface of the crown. Cusps are commonly arranged side by side on the occlusal surface for crushing and grinding, such as molars in primates (including man), bears, and swine.

Lophodont dentition. Having cheek teeth with cusps interconnected by ridges or *lophs* of enamel, such as in the rhinoceros and elephant.

Selenodont dentition. Having cheek teeth with cusps that form a crescent-shaped ridge pattern, such as in the even-toed ungulates, except swine.

1.1.7 Two Types of Jaw Occlusal Overlay

Isognathous. Equal jaw widths, in which the premolars and molars of opposing jaws aligned with the occlusal surfaces facing each other, forming an occlusal plane. Man is an imperfect isognathic, or near equal jaws.

Anisognathous. Unequal jaw widths, in which the mandibular molar occlusal zone is narrower than the maxillary counterpart, such as in the feline, canine, bovine, equine, etc.

1.1.8 The Dog and Cat Dentition

Dogs and cats have diphyodont development, heterodont teeth types, brachyodont crown types, secondont teeth (all premolars, feline mandibular molar and a portion of the canine mandibular first molar), bunodont (feline maxillary molar, canine molars, including a portion of the mandibular first molar), thecodont tooth anchorage and anisognathic jaws.

1.2 Development

Note that the following section will give a brief overview of the embryologic development of the mouth and associated structures. The same tissues in the adult animal will be discussed later in the chapter.

Development of the gastrointestinal tract begins early in embryonic formation. The roof of the entodermal yolk sac enfolds into a tubular tract forming the gut tube, which will become the digestive tract. It is initially a blind tract being closed at both the upper and bottom ends. The bottom ultimately becomes the anal opening and the upper portion connects with the primitive oral cavity known as the stomodeum, or ectodermal mouth. The stomodeum and foregut are at this time separated by a common wall known as the buccopharyngeal membrane. It is located at a level that will become the oropharynx, located between the tonsils and base of the tongue. This pharyngeal membrane eventually disappears, establishing a shared connection between the oral cavity and the digestive tract.

Around day 21 of development, branchial arches I and II are present. By day 23 the paired maxillary and mandibular processes of branchial arch I have become distinct. The mandibular processes grow rostrally, forming the mandible and merging at the mandibular symphysis, which in the dog and cat normally remains a fibrous union throughout life. The paired maxillary processes form most of the maxillae, incisive, and palatine bones.

Initial development of the dental structures occurs during embryonic formation. Rudimentary signs of tooth development occur approximately at the 25th day of development when the embryonic oral (stratified squamous) epithelium begins to thicken. This thickening, known as the dental lamina, forms two U-shaped structures, which eventually become the upper and lower dental arches. The enamel organ, which evenutally is responsible for enamel formation and has a role in induction of tooth formation, arises from a series of invaginations of the dental lamina into the adjacent mesoderm. The oral epithelium, dental lamina, and enamel organ originate from the outer embryonic germ layer known as ectoderm. The dental papilla and sac appear in coordination with the enamel, but originate from mesoderm (ectomesenchyme of the neural crest).

The enamel organ develops through a series of stages known as the bud, cap, and bell (Figure 1.1). The bud stage is the initial budding off from the dental lamina at the areas corresponding to the deciduous dentition. The bud eventually develops a concavity at the deepest portion, noting the start of the cap stage. As the enamel organ enters this stage it is comprised of three parts: the outer enamel epithelium (OEE) on the outer portion of the cap, the inner enamel epithelium (IEE) lining the concavity, and the stellate reticulum within the cap. The onset of the bell stage occurs as a fourth layer to the enamel organ, the stratum intermedium, emerges between the IEE and the stellate reticulum.

Each layer of the enamel organ has specific functions to perform. The OEE acts as a protective layer for the entire organ. Stellate reticulum works as a cushion for protection of the IEE and allows vascular fluids to percolate between cells and reach the stratum intermedium. The stratum intermedium apparently converts the vascular fluids to usable nourishment for the IEE. The IEE goes through numerous changes, ultimately being responsible for actual enamel formation.

The dental lamina buds that form the primary dentition develop lingual extensions referred to as successional

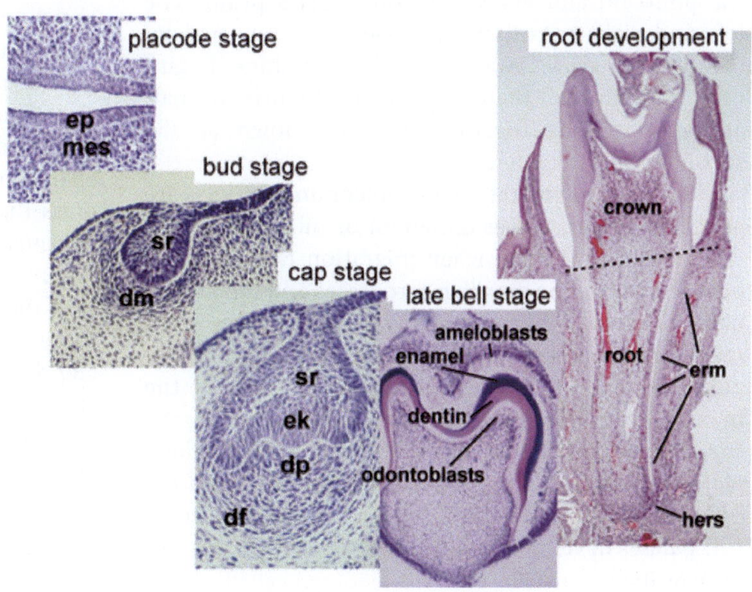

Figure 1.1 Histology of important stages of tooth development. Note that all early development is directed at creating the crown and only then root formation is initiated. Ameloblasts differentiate from the epithelium and odontoblasts from the mesenchyme and they deposit the matrices of enamel and dentin, respectively. Ameloblasts and enamel are missing on the root, which is covered by the softer dentin and cementum. Ep, epithelium; mes, mesenchyme; sr, stellate reticulum; dm, dental mesenchyme; dp, dental papilla; df, dental follicle; ek, enamel knot; erm, epithelial cell rests of malassez; hers, Hertwig's epithelial root sheath. *Source*: from Thesleff, I. and Tummers, M. Tooth organogenesis and regeneration: http://stembook.org/node/551; accessed November 2017.

lamina. The successional laminae progress through bud, cap, and bell stages to eventually form the successional permanent dentition. The non-successional teeth, those permanents not succeeding deciduous counterparts, develop directly from the dental lamina.

During the late bud stage, from an area adjacent to the IEE, mesenchymal cells begin development of the dental papilla and dental sac. The mesodermal cells of the dental papilla form the dentinal and pulpal tissues of the forming tooth. The dental sac is comprised of several rows of flattened mesodermal cells covering the dental papilla and attaching part of the way up the OEE of the bud. It gives rise to cementum, periodontal ligament (PDL), and some alveolar bone.

The frontal prominence, the forehead area of the embryo, occurs in coordination with the stomodeum and mandibular processes. Nasal pits, the beginning of the nasal cavities, are first revealed by two small depressions found low on the frontal prominence. On either side of the nasal pits are the medial and lateral nasal processes. The two medial nasal and two maxillary processes form the upper lip. The groove between the two fills with connective tissue in a process known as migration. If migration fails to occur the tissues will be stretched thin and will tear. This results in a separation between the medial nasal and maxillary process, which causes a cleft lip.

The left and right maxillary processes and the single medial nasal processes also form the palate. The incisal portion (maxilla) of the hard palate is the part from the maxillary incisor teeth back to the incisive foramen. The area of the incisive bone (the premaxilla in some species, and formerly in the dog) is also known as the primary palate and is formed solely by the medial nasal process. The medial nasal process forms the philtrum and helps form the nasal septum. The left and right maxillary processes form two palatal shelves that grow inward toward the midline, beginning rostrally, and then attaching to the primary palate and growing together. This is known as the secondary palate.

Cleft lips and palates are not uncommon. Clefts are generally designated as unilateral or bilateral. A unilateral cleft lip occurs when migration fails to occur between one of the maxillary processes and the medial nasal process. A bilateral cleft lip occurs when both maxillary processes fail to migrate. A unilateral cleft palate occurs when one of the palatal plates of the maxillary processes fails to fuse with the nasal septum. A bilateral cleft palate occurs when both palatal plates of the maxillary processes fail to fuse with the opposite plates at the nasal septum. Clefts of hard or soft palates develop in a wide range of varying degrees of severity.

1.2.1 Enamel, Dentin, and Pulp

These three structures have an intimate relationship during early development, although they do not all develop from the same foundation cells. Enamel is produced by the enamel organ, which is derived from ectoderm. In contrast, the dentin and pulp develop from the dental papilla, which is derived from mesoderm.

During the bell stage, the IEE cells evolve into a taller form and become preameloblasts. The peripheral cells of the dental papilla bordering the preameloblasts transform into low columnar or cuboidal shapes and form odontoblasts. As the newly formed odontoblasts move toward the center of the dental papilla and away from the preameloblasts they leave behind a secreted matrix of mucopolysaccharide ground substance and collagen fibers. This substance appears to stimulate a polarity shift in the preameloblasts of the nucleus from the center of the cell toward the stratum intermedium. It is thought that this shift in polarity is caused by an alteration in the nutritional supply route to the cells. With this shift in polarity, the cells now become ameloblasts and begin secretion of enamel matrix. As this enamel matrix (mucopolysaccharide ground substance and organic fiber) is laid down next to the dentinal matrix, the dentinoenamel junction (DEJ) is formed. As the ameloblasts lay down matrix they move away from the dentin and toward the OEE. Both the dentin and enamel begin to lay down crystal and mineralize at this point into hard tissue.

The enamel matrix is laid down at the end of the bell stage. All of the crystal placed within the rods are laid down at this time. This is known as the mineralization stage of calcification of the enamel rod. The next is the maturation stage of calcification. It is during this stage that the crystals grow in size, becoming tightly packed together within the enamel rod. Should the crystals fail to grow to full size, the rods will be poorly calcified and have less than 96% inorganic composition; this results in a condition known as hypomineralization. As enamel is produced by the ameloblasts, a change occurs in the enamel organ. The ameloblasts gradually begin to compress the two middle layers of the organ, the stratum intermedium and the stellate reticulum. The middle layers are eventually lost and the ameloblasts make contact with the OEE. This activates the final two functions of the ameloblasts to commence. First, a protective layer is laid down on top of the enamel known as the primary enamel cuticle or Nasmyth's membrane. This cuticle remains on the teeth for weeks to months, until it is worn away by abrasion. The cuticle is laid down upon the crown from the tip toward the cementoenamel junction (CEJ). Once the cuticle is formed the ameloblasts merge with the OEE to form the reduced enamel epithelium.

The reduced enamel epithelium is produced on adhesive-like secretion known as the secondary enamel cuticle or epithelial attachment. The epithelial attachment functions to hold the gingiva and tooth together at the bottom of the gingival sulcus. During enamel development, several abnormalities may develop. These are sometimes found on clinical, radiological, or histological examination. Amelogenesis imperfecta is the general term that includes any genetic and/or developmental enamel formation and maturation abnormalities. Enamel hypoplasia refers to inadequate deposition of enamel matrix, i.e., when the density or mineralization is generally normal, but the enamel is thinner than normal. Enamel hypomineralization refers to inadequate mineralization of enamel matrix, resulting in white, yellow, or brown spots in the enamel. This often affects several or all teeth. The crowns of affected teeth may be soft and wear faster than normal teeth.

Mesodermal tissue from the dental papilla forms the pulp. Once developed, it consists of blood vessels, lymphatic vessels, nerves, fibroblasts, collagen fibers, undifferentiated reserve mesenchymal cells, other cells of connective tissue, and odontoblasts. Odontoblasts are an integral part of the dentin, but are also the peripheral cells of the pulp. The pulpal nerves are primarily sensory and transmit only the sensation of pain. There are some motor nerves that innervate the smooth muscles within the blood vessels. These result in constriction of the vessels in response to irritation. Young pulps have a large volume, which is considered primarily cellular, with a small concentration of fibers. The large number of cells allows for repair from trauma. As the pulp ages, it loses volume and reserve cell capacity. This loss of reserve cells is thought to be the reason that older patients are more susceptible to permanent pulpal damage.

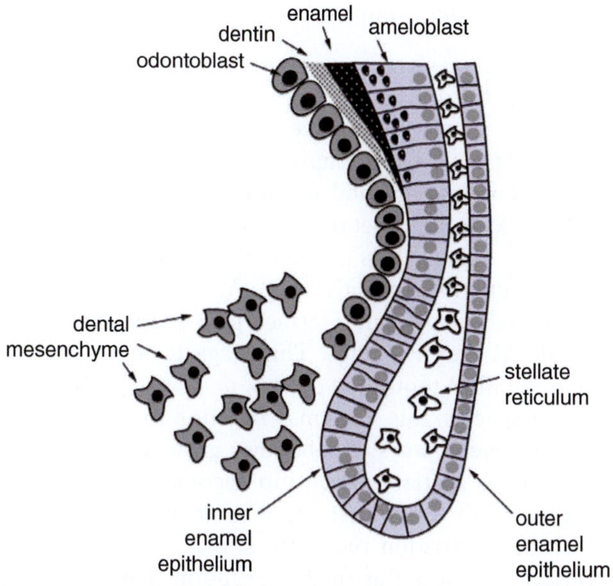

Figure 1.2 Fate of the stem cell progeny in the epithelial stem cell niche of the continuously growing tooth, the cervical loop. Stem cells divide in the stellate reticulum compartment giving rise to cells that will become inserted to the basal layer of epithelium looping around the stellate reticulum. Here the cells proliferate, migrate toward the oral cavity and differentiate into ameloblasts, depositing enamel matrix. *Source:* From Thesleff, I. and Tummers, M. Tooth organogenesis and regeneration: http://stembook.org/node/551 – animation; accessed November 2017.

1.2.2 Root Formation

Formation of the root begins after the general form of the crown has developed, but prior to its complete calcification. At the point where the OEE becomes the IEE, the stellate reticulum and stratum intermedium are missing from the enamel organ at this deepest point, and is referred to as the cervical loop. These two layers of cells become the epithelial root sheath or Hertwig's epithelial root sheath (Figure 1.2). This sheath begins to grow into the underlying connective tissue by rapid mitotic division, initiating root formation. This growth advanced deep into underlying connective tissue, but at some point, angles back toward the center of the forming tooth. The portion of the sheath that turns back in is known as the epithelial diaphragm. The growth pattern of the epithelial diaphragm determines the number of roots a tooth develops. The point at which the epithelial diaphragm meets will be the apex of a single rooted tooth but the furcation in multirooted teeth. As the root sheath makes contact with the dental papilla, it stimulates the peripheral contact cells to differentiate into odontoblasts. Once the odontoblasts begin to produce dentin, the root sheath trapped between the dental sac and the dentin begins to break up. As Hertwig's epithelial root sheath dissolves, the dental sac comes into direct contact with the newly formed dentin. Some of the dental sac cells differentiate into cementoblasts and initiate cementum formation. The cementum that contacts the dentin becomes the dentinocemental junction (DCJ).

The epithelial root sheath cells that move away from the dentin, but fail to dissolve, become entrapped in the PDL and are referred to as epithelial rests or epithelial rests of Malassez. These cell rests are a normal finding, but under the influence of various stimuli, they could proliferate later in life to form epithelial lining of various odontogenic cysts, such as the radicular cyst. When epithelial root sheath cells fail to dissolve and remain in contact with the dentin, they typically convert to ameloblasts. These may secrete enamel on the roots, forming what is known as enamel pearls. If the root sheath's epithelial diaphragm malfunctions, accessory roots may be formed.

1.2.3 Tooth Eruption

The emergence and movement of the crown of the tooth into the oral cavity is typically termed tooth eruption. The eruptive sequence is generally divided into three stages. The pre-eruptive stage commences with crown development and the formation of the dental lamina. With the onset of root development, the eruptive stage begins. This is also sometimes referred to as the pre-functional eruptive stage. When the teeth move into actual occlusion it is termed post-eruptive stage or functional eruptive stage. This stage is considered to continue until tooth loss occurs, or death. In the hypsodont species, this stage may function to serve occlusion in several ways. As the jaws grow, the mandible and maxilla spatial relationship becomes further apart and the teeth continue to erupt to maintain occlusion. With time, attrition results in loss of dental occlusal contacts and it is this further eruption that maintains the occlusal balance. In some cases, this can cause an imbalance in occlusion when teeth are lost and supraeruption of the opposing teeth occurs. Supraeruption is when teeth erupt beyond the normal occlusal line.

Four major theories for eruption have been expounded upon in the literature. Most likely none are totally correct in themselves, but the most accurate picture is probably a combination of them. The theory of root growth is the belief that root growth pushes the crown into the oral cavity. Experiments of removing Hertwig's epithelial root sheath on developing teeth has stopped root formation. However, these rootless teeth still erupt, thus disproving this as a major factor in eruption. The theory of growth of pulpal tissue proposes that continued growth of the pulp tissue while the hard sides of the tooth are forming provides apical propulsion. Yet developing teeth in which the pulp dies or is removed will still erupt, also disproving this as a major factor in eruption. The theory of bone deposition in the alveolar crypt is the precept that bone deposition within the alveolar crypt forces the tooth to erupt. This deposition is not constant and even when the crypt undergoes resorption due to various factors teeth generally still erupt, making this theory a dubious major factor. The theory of PDL force is the hypothesis that it is the PDL's driving force that maintains occlusal contact also thrusts the tooth into the oral cavity. This is the most plausible postulate, although the exact mechanism is unknown. Eruption times are variable not only with size and breed but also within the breeds themselves. Average eruption times of deciduous and permanent teeth can be found in Table 4.1 in Chapter 4 – Developmental Pathology and Pedodontology.

Exfoliation of deciduous dentition is a complex function and not fully understood. It is believed that as the permanent tooth root begins development, the crown makes contact with the deciduous tooth root structure. The pressure of the permanent tooth crown on the deciduous tooth root, and possibly the contact of the permanent tooth's dental sac or the OEE with the deciduous root, stimulates the resorptive process of the deciduous tooth root. Deciduous root resorption occurs in cycles or stages, and is not constant. Once sufficient root support is lost, the crown is shed or exfoliated. Although it is common for deciduous teeth to persist when a permanent successor does not develop, this is not always the case, indicating that other factors may play a part in root resorption.

Persistent deciduous teeth are commonly attributed to four causes. The first is the lack of a permanent successor. The second is ankylosis of the tooth to the alveolus. This may occur during root resorption when holes in Hertwig's root sheath develop and the tooth's cementum makes contact with the alveolar bone and fuses to it. In these cases, it is common to find teeth with almost the entire root structure dissolved, but with the crown still firmly in place. Once the ankylosis is relieved, typically the crown rapidly exfoliates. The third cause for persistent deciduous dentition is failure of the permanent crown to make contact with the deciduous root during eruption. This occurs if either tooth is in an improper position, in comparison to each other. Finally, the fourth reason is hormonal influences, which can affect growth or metabolism.

1.3 Basic Anatomy of the Dental-Periodontal Unit

1.3.1 Directional, Surface, and Ridge Nomenclature

Prior to discussing dental anatomy, a general understanding of directional, surface, and ridge nomenclature is required.

Rostral and caudal are anatomical terms of location applicable to the head in a sagittal plane in non-human vertebrates. Rostral refers to a structure closer to, or a direction toward, the most forward structure of the head. Caudal refers to a structure closer to, or a direction toward, the tail. Anterior and posterior are the synonymous terms used in human dentistry. The term caudal teeth refer to premolars and molars, as opposed to incisors and canines, which are rostral teeth. Incisors, canines, and premolars have four exposed surfaces and a ridge or cusp, making a total of five surfaces. Molars have five exposed surfaces. Sometimes a ridge may be referred to as a surface.

As a general rule, the surfaces of the teeth facing the vestibule or lips are the vestibular surfaces [1] (Figure 1.3). For the incisor and canine teeth, the surface directed toward the lips is commonly called the labial surface. With premolars and molars, the surface facing the cheek is known as the buccal surface. The term "facial" has been used traditionally in human dentistry to refer to the surfaces of the rostral teeth visible from the front. All surfaces facing the tongue are described as lingual, although for the maxillary teeth this surface is often described as the palatal surface. For premolars and molars, the surface making contact with the teeth in the opposite jaw during closure is known as the occlusal surface. The ridge of the premolars that does not make contact with opposing teeth is typically referred to as the occlusal ridge. For the incisors, the ridge along the coronal-most aspect is referred to as the incisal ridge. The cusp is the point or tip of the crown of a tooth. For the canine tooth, the cusp is generally called the cusp surface. Premolars and molars may have multiple cusps. Surfaces facing toward adjoining teeth within the same jaw quadrant or dental arch are collectively called the contact or proximal surfaces. Proximal surfaces may be either distal or mesial. The term distal indicates a proximal surface facing away from the median line of the face. In contrast, the term mesial designates the proximal surface facing toward the median line. The space between two facing proximal surfaces is known as the interproximal space. Apical is a term used to denote a direction toward the root tip. Coronal is a term used to indicate a direction toward the crown tip or occlusal surface. The terms incisal for incisors and occlusal for premolars and molars is also used to indicate the coronal direction. The term cervical either means the juncture of the tooth crown and root or a direction toward that point.

To further break down tooth locations, combinations of the above terms are sometimes used, with one additional term, middle (Figure 1.4). The term middle means at or toward the middle of a designated portion of the tooth and can indicate either a horizontal or vertical middle area.

1.3.2 Crown Line and Point Angles

For the purpose of identifying and classifying distinct areas on teeth in operative dental procedures, the coronal surfaces can be divided and classified by eight line angles and four point angles (see Chapter 17 – Restorative Dentistry). These lines and points are also sometimes used for identification of cavity prep areas.

There are five crown surfaces: vestibular, lingual/palatal, mesial, distal, and occlusal/coronal/incisal. The line angles are simply the dividing lines formed between

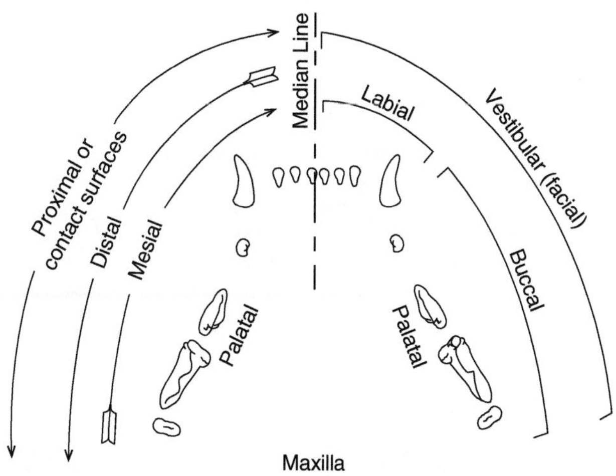

Figure 1.3 Directional nomenclature of the maxillary teeth of the cat. *Source:* Courtesy of Josephine Banyard.

the surface areas. They are named from two of the five surfaces that divide them. Where the surface terms are joined, the "ar" or "al" ending is dropped and "o" is added. The eight line angles are (i) mesiovestibular (mesiolabial, mesiobuccal), (ii) mesiolingual (mesiopalatal), (iii) mesioincisal (mesiocoronal, mesio-occlusal), (iv) distovestibular (distolabial, distobuccal), (v) distolingual (distopalatal), (vi) distoincisal (distocoronal, disto-occlusal), (vii) linguoincisal (linguocoronal, linguo-occlusal), and (viii) vestibuloincisal (vestibulocoronal, vestibulo-occlusal).

The point angles are the junctures of three of the line angles. There are four coronal point angles, each named for the three surfaces that actually make the juncture or point. The four point angles are (i) mesiovestibuloincisal (mesiovestibulocoronal, mesiovestibulo-occlusal, mesiolabioincisal, mesiolabiocoronal, mesiolabio-occlusal, mesiobuccocoronal, mesiobucco-occusal), (ii) mesiolinguoincisal (mesiolinguocoronal, mesiolinguo-occusal, mesiopalatoincisal, mesiopalatocoronal, mesiopalato-occlusal), (iii) distovestibuloincisal (distovestibulocoronal, distovestibulo-occlusal, distolabioincisal, distolabiocoronal, distolabio-occlusal, distobuccocoronal, distobucco-occusal), and (iv) distolinguoincisal (distolinguocoronal, distolinguo-occusal, distopalatoincisal, distopalatocoronal, distopalato-occlusal).

1.3.3 Contact Points and Areas

Contact points and areas are the sites where adjacent or opposing teeth make contact. The term contact area is considered a more correct term than contact point, since an area is typically making contact rather than a specific point. Adjacent teeth have proximal contact areas, where opposing teeth have occlusal contact areas.

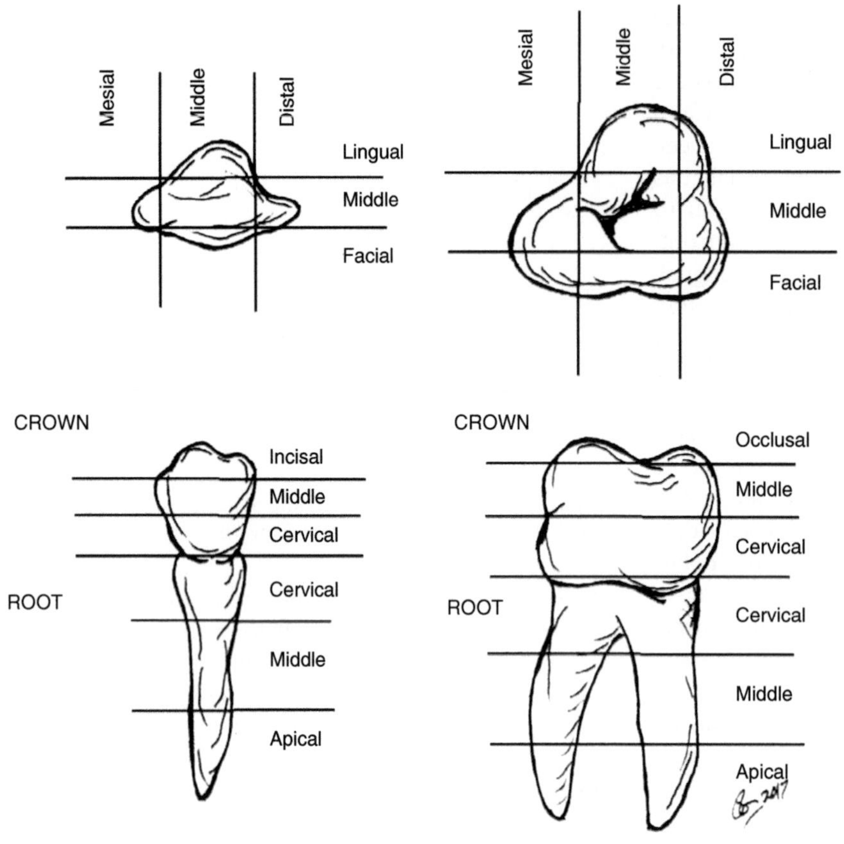

Figure 1.4 Division into thirds. *Source:* Courtesy of Josephine Banyard.

1.3.4 Embrasures

Projecting away from the proximal contact areas are V-shaped areas termed embrasures. They are named for the surface from which they are derived and the direction they radiate toward. There are theoretically four embrasures between each tooth with proximal contacts. The embrasures are the (i) vestibulogingival (labiogingival, buccogingival), (ii) vestibuloincisal (vestibulocoronal, vestibulo-occlusal, labioincisal, labiocoronal, labio-occlusal, buccocoronal, bucco-occlusal), (iii) linguogingival (palatogingival), and (iv) linguoincisal (palatoincisal, palatocoronal, palato-occlusal, linguocoronal, linguo-occlusal).

1.3.5 Tooth Function and Terms

Teeth are multifunctional organs that play an important part in overall animal health and activity. Their shape aids physiologically in protection of the oral mucosa, as well as reduction of stress forces on the teeth and the alveolar process. Teeth are used to catch, hold, carry, cut, shear, crush, and grind sustenance. Besides their masticatory functions, they are used in protection, aggression, and sexual attraction. Sexual dimorphism, such as length of tooth, may play a part in sexual attraction and social behavior for defense.

Each tooth has a crown and a root, except for aradicular hypsodonts (see Chapter 21 – Small Mammal Oral and Dental Diseases). Generally, the brachydont crown is covered with enamel and the root with cementum. Where the enamel of the crown and cementum of root meet is known as the CEJ. The line formed by the CEJ is commonly called the neck, cervix, or cervical line. In many cases, especially during eruption and in hypsodont dentition, not all of the crown may be fully exposed. The entire crown, whether exposed or not, is the anatomical crown. The supragingival portion of the crown is the clinical crown and the subgingival portion is the reserved crown. The reserved crown is occasionally referred to as the clinical root as compared to the anatomical or true root. The incisor teeth are designed to cut, scrape, scoop, pick at or up, and groom. The term incisor means "that which cuts." The actual biting edge of the incisor is the incisal edge or ridge. The incisal edge picks up and cuts food, scrapes meat off bone, grooms the hair, and is used to catch parasites. The concave lingual surface acts as a scoop and, along with the tongue, aids in carrying food into the oral cavity. The canine teeth are designed to pierce and hold a victim. They can also be used to slash and tear when used as weapons in fighting. In the carnivores, canines have the longest crowns and roots. These large roots make them very stable and good anchorage points. Premolars resemble a cross between canine teeth and molars. They are not as long as canine teeth and generally have multiple functional cusps. Being a cross between a canine tooth and a molar, they are designed to function similarly to both. They help to hold and carry, while also helping to break food down into smaller pieces. Molars have an occlusal surface that can be used to grind food or break it down into smaller pieces. The incisors and canine teeth are referred to as rostral teeth, while the premolars and molars are caudal teeth. The carnassial teeth are considered to be the largest shearing teeth in the upper and lower jaws. In the dog and cat these are the maxillary fourth premolars and the mandibular first molars. The term carnassial (commonly used, not an accepted anatomic term) means flesh cutting.

Crown formation generally occurs from four or more growth centers known as lobes. Their fusion, termed coalescence, can result in various depth grooves known as developmental grooves. Most incisors, canine teeth, and premolars develop from four lobes, three vestibular and one lingual. The two developmental grooves on the vestibular surface of the incisors are the coalescence or fusion points of the three vestibular lobes. The three protrusions along the incisal edge formed by the developmental grooves are the mamelons. The deep developmental grooves in many carnivores and some primates appear to help in cutting the flesh as it slides up the tooth and act as bleeding grooves, allowing for blood to escape from the punctures in the victim while still holding them in a firm grasp. The fourth lobe on the lingual surface typically forms the majority of the tooth bulk at the lingual cervical third and is called the cingulum. Just coronal to the incisor cingulum is a slight concavity known as the lingual fossa.

The proximal contacts are the points at which adjacent teeth make contact. These contacts aid in prevention of food being packed between the teeth from above, while the gingival papilla serve the same purpose from the vestibular and lingual surfaces. The contacts of the rostral teeth are located close to the incisal ridge, whereas they are located more apically in the caudal teeth. With the tooth spacings found in the dog and cat, proximal surfaces do not always make contact with the adjacent teeth. The bulge, curvature, or contour of the tooth aids in directing food away from the gingival sulcus, while using frictional movement of the food to clean the gingivae, cheeks, and lips.

1.4 General Anatomy of the Tooth and Periodontium

It is arbitrary to discuss the tooth and periodontium as separate parts as it is one functional unit. However, to more easily understand the anatomy and physiology, it will be separated into the crown, dentin and pulp, root, and periodontium.

The tooth is made up of basically four tissues, three hard and one soft. The hard tissues are enamel, cementum, and dentin; the soft is the pulp. The pulp tissue occupies the cavern within the tooth known as the pulp cavity. This cavity is further divided into pulp chamber, portion in the crown, and root canal, portion within the root. The bottom of the pulp chamber is referred to as the chamber floor and the most coronal part the chamber horns in which the pulp horns reside (Figure 1.5).

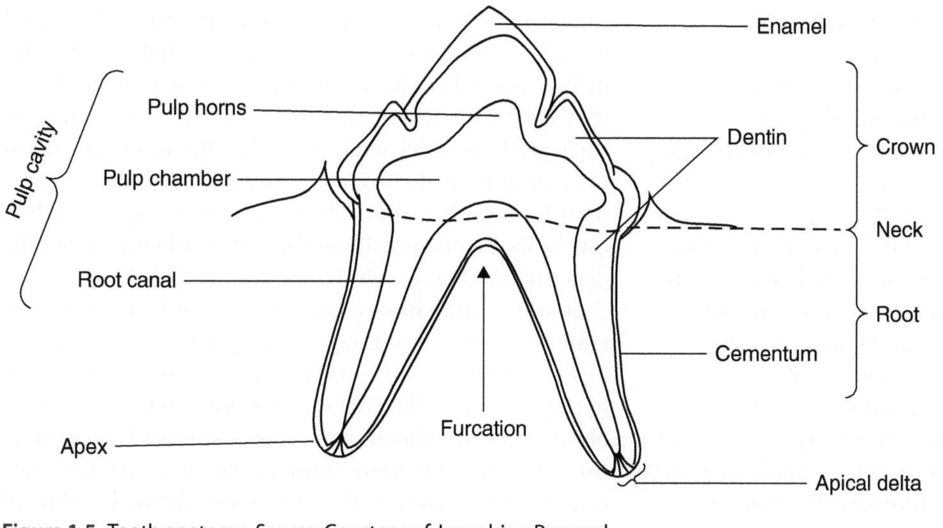

Figure 1.5 Tooth anatomy. *Source:* Courtesy of Josephine Banyard.

1.4.1 Dental Formulas

The currently accepted designations of the dental formula for the dog is as follows:

Deciduous teeth: 2 × (3/3 i, 1/1 c, 3/3 pm) = 28.
Permanent teeth: 2 × (3/3 I, 1/1 C, 4/4 PM, 2/3 M) = 42.

The currently accepted designations of the dental formula for the cat is as follows:

Deciduous teeth: 2 × (3/3 i, 1/1 c, 3/2 pm) = 26.
Permanent teeth: 2 × (3/3 I, 1/1 C, 3/2 PM, 1/1 M) = 30.

(Additional dental formula information for the dog and cat can be found in Chapter 2 – Oral Examination and Diagnosis – and for other species in their related chapters.)

1.4.2 Crown

The crown is the portion of the tooth typically erupted though the gingiva. The brachydont crown is completely covered by enamel. Enamel is the hardest substance in the body and contains the highest percentage of mineral. It has a semi-translucent white color, although it may appear as other colors due to the refraction of the underlying dentin (e.g., intrinsic discoloration). Extrinsic staining and color changes of the enamel can occur with age. Enamel is approximately 96% inorganic in composition. This inorganic portion is calcium phosphate in the form of hydroxyapatite crystals. Fluoride, magnesium, strontium, and lead may also be present [1]. The remaining 4% of enamel composition is principally water and fibrous organic material. Enamel varies in thickness over the surface of the tooth, often thickest at the cusp and thinnest at its border with the cementum at the CEJ [1]. Despite its hardness, enamel is subject to wear attrition from friction of use. Fluorinated enamel has an improved resistance to degradation by acids generated from bacterial activity. Enamel is avascular and has no capability to regenerate itself when damaged; however, it is not a static tissue as it can undergo mineralization changes.

The basic building block of enamel is the enamel rod. Each rod is a column of enamel that extends from the DEJ to the coronal surface of the tooth. These rods are generally perpendicular both to the DEJ and the surface. Each rod is composed of two parts, the rod core and the rod sheath. The rod core is composed of hydroxyapatite crystals. The rod sheath, which surrounds the columnar side of the rod core, is composed mostly of the organic fibrous substance. Crystals are present between rod sheaths called interrod enamel. These crystals are not aligned in the same direction of rod enamel. The rod sheath is incomplete in circumference, allowing contact between the rod and interrod enamel. The shape of the rods in the enamel is round to quad-lobed at the inner layer and hexagonal at the outer layer of enamel. Enamel rods have a round shape in the cat [2].

Three layers of enamel have been described in the cat and dog: a non-prismatic layer at the surface, a regular prismatic layer, and an inner layer with prominent bands of Hunter and Schreger, which may indicate multidirectional orientation of the rods [2]. Bands of Hunter and Schreger are not a true structure but an optical illusion produced by changes in direction between groups of rods [1]. The striae or stripes of Retzius are darker lines in the enamel that radiate out in a curve from the DEJ. These are areas of slight variation in the crystal content of the rods. It appears that approximately every fourth day in the ameloblast cycle, there is a change in the rod development or cycle of rest that results in these lines or striae. As these striae of Retzius are visible on the exposed surface enamel, they cause slight horizontal lines or ripples in the enamel. These are known as imbrication or perikymata lines. These perikymata are not present on the surface of dog or cat teeth, likely due to the angle of the striae of Retzius being nearly parallel to the tooth surface [2].

Enamel tufts are small, branched hypomineralized ribbon-like defects that run longitudinally to the tooth axis and extend from the DEJ one-fifth to one-third the way into enamel toward the enamel surface [3]. They are commonly found on histologic sectioning, especially in bunodont dentition of animals that crush hard materials such as nuts or mollusk shells. Although they have been noted to be a potential source of enamel fractures that arise after extended use or overloading, it appears that they then enable enamel to resist the further progression of these fractures, ultimately preventing mechanical failure [4]. This fracture resistance is one reason why tooth enamel is three times stronger than its constituent hydroxyapatite crystallites that make up its enamel rods [5]. Enamel tufts are frequently confused with enamel lamellae, which are also enamel defects, but which differ in two ways: lamella are linear, and not branched, and they exist primarily extending from the enamel surface, through the enamel and toward the DEJ, whereas enamel tufts project in the opposite direction. The most common form is that caused by trauma resulting in hairline cracks in the enamel. Lamellae can be of clinical significance depending on number and severity [6].

Enamel tufts should also not be confused with the similar enamel spindles. Enamel spindles are also linear defects, similar to tufts and lamellae. They are formed by entrapment of odontoblast processes between ameloblasts prior to and during amelogenesis. Like enamel tufts, spindles are found only at the DEJ; they are typically found histologically and have no known clinical significance.

There is evidence that the enamel of dogs and cats is much thinner than that found in man. In humans, the thickness is reported to be 2–4 mm compared to 0.1–0.3 mm in cats and 0.1–0.6 mm in dogs [7]. Additionally, the cervical bulge often found at the level of the free gingiva does not represent a thickening in the enamel, but a general thickening in the tooth [7].

1.4.3 Root and Periodontium

The tooth root is covered by cementum and anchored to the jaws by the periodontium. The periodontium consists of the cementum, the PDL, the dental alveolus, and the gingiva. The periodontium exists to anchor the tooth, cleanse and protect the tooth, and to serve as sensory tissue.

The root surface is covered by cementum and is located apical to the attached gingiva in health. Teeth may have single or multiple roots. The point at which roots diverge is the furcation; this can be bifurcation, trifurcation, etc. Although there is individual variation, the number of roots is determined by species and type of tooth. In this chapter the dentition of the dog and cat will be the focus.

The incisors and canine teeth of the dog are all single-rooted teeth. The maxillary first and second and all three of the incisors in each mandible have relatively straight roots, which are round to triangular when examined in cross-section. The root of the maxillary third incisor is often triangular to trapezoidal in shape and has a curvature with the greater curvature being mesial to mesiobuccal and the lesser curvature being distal to distobuccal. This curvature may make closed extraction challenging. The root of the maxillary canine tooth is digitally palpable via the jugum. The apices of mandibular canine teeth are positioned lingual to the crowns. This functionally creates more buccal bone at the apical portion of the root and should be kept in mind during exodontia and related surgical procedures. The first premolar of each quadrant has a single root. The second and third premolars have two roots, typically with one root mesial to the other. In brachycephalic dogs the premolars may be rotated 90° such that one root is palatal to the other. Although not typical, a third root of the maxillary third premolar may be found; it is located palatally between the mesial and distal roots. In this case, a palatal cusp of the maxillary third premolar is often present. The maxillary fourth premolar has three roots, two mesial (mesiobuccal and mesiopalatal) and one distal. The maxillary first and second molars have three roots, two buccal (mesiobuccal and distobuccal) and one palatal. The second, third, and fourth premolars of the mandible are two-rooted (one mesial, one distal). The first and second molars are two-rooted (one mesial, one distal). The third molar has a single root. A longitudinal groove may be present on the mesial and distal roots of the mandibular first molar and on the mesial surface of the distal root of the maxillary fourth premolar. These radicular grooves correspond with alveolar ridges in the alveoli and provide extra retentive surfaces and prevent rotation. The grooves may be appreciated radiographically giving the appearance of two PDLs and should be kept in mind during exodontic procedures [8]. Radicular grooves of the mandibular first molar may continue into the furcation, leading to a domed shape of the furcation. This shape should be kept in mind when performing periodontal therapy of this tooth [9]. Similarly, the maxillary fourth premolar has a domed shape at the furcation of the distal root and mesial root trunk as well as a fluted area just coronal to the furcation of the mesial roots [10].

The incisors and canine teeth of the cat are also all single-rooted. The maxillary first premolar is absent. The maxillary second premolar may have a single root, two individual roots, or two fused roots [11]. The maxillary third premolar has two roots and the maxillary fourth premolar has three roots, similar to the dog. The single maxillary molar may have a single root, two individual roots, or two fused roots [11]. The mandibular first and second premolars are absent. The mandibular third and fourth premolars and single mandibular molar each have two roots. The mesial root of the mandibular molar is approximately three times as wide (mesial to distal) as the distal root.

Cementum is an off-white or ivory colored hard substance that covers the root surface. Its composition is approximately 45–50% inorganic and 50–55% organic materials and water. The inorganic portion is primarily hydroxyapatite crystals and the organic part primarily collagen fibers and mucopolysaccharide ground substance.

Cementum formation begins at the neck or cervical circumference of the tooth, forming the CEJ. This junction is generally one of three types formed. These are cementum slightly overlapping the enamel, cementum meeting enamel evenly, or cementum failing to meet the enamel. In this third category, a cervical exposure of dentin occurs, which can result in tooth sensitivity should gingival recession occur.

Cementoblasts secrete cementum as they move away from the DCJ. In the cervical half to two-thirds of the root, the cementoblasts remain on the surface as the cementum is deposited and few if any of these cells become entrapped in the cementum, which is referred to as the acellular cementum. In the apical third, cementoblasts commonly surround themselves with cementum and become trapped. These trapped cells are referred to as cementocytes, and this portion of the cementum is identified as cellular cementum.

The cementoblast on the surface of the cementum deposits cementum around the ends of the PDL, making contact with them, and attaching them to the tooth. These fibers trapped within the cementum are known as Sharpey's fibers. The ends of the fibers entrapped in the alveolar bone are also known as Sharpey's fibers.

The cellular cementum of the root apex typically increases in thickness with time due to occlusal stresses of the tooth. This thickening is known as hypercementosis and is especially common in cats. Should this become excessive, a bulbous apex may form that can increase the difficulty of dental extraction.

Cementum is vital and has the ability to repair itself when injured. The cementoblasts on the surface and the embedded cementocytes receive nourishment from blood vessels of the PDL.

The bone of the jaws that form the socket support for the teeth is known as the alveolar bone. In the mature animal, the bone is approximately 65% inorganic and 35% inorganic in composition, and is mesodermal in origin. The alveolus is composed of three distinct layers. The compact bone on the inside of the socket next to the tooth is known as the cribriform plate and radiographically is termed the lamina dura. It has no periosteal covering, but is covered instead by the PDL. The fibers of the PDL embedded in the cribriform plate are called Sharpey's fibers (as are the Sharpey's fibers that are embedded within cementum). The compact bone rises to the top of the socket and then turns back to form the cortical plates. The top of the compact bone where the cortical and cribriform plates meet is known as the alveolar margin. The cortical plates are covered with periosteum. Between the two plates is spongy, cancellous, or trabecular bone. This is a form of bone marrow. The cribriform plate is constantly undergoing remodeling due to occlusal stresses. This may lead to additional bone being laid down on the plate, referred to as bundle bone.

The PDL is derived from the mesodermal cells of the dental sac. This formation begins after cementum deposition has been initiated. The dental sac on contact with the cementum forms fibroblasts, which produce collagen fibers at the same time other components of the PDL are developing. These are blood vessels, lymphatics, nerves, and various types of connective tissue cells. The nerves of the PDL are quite important in that they provide additional senses to the tooth. It has pain fibers, which the pulp has, but also pressure, heat, and cold fibers, which the pulp does not.

As the fibers of the PDL form, they begin to arrange themselves into three distinct categories, gingival, transseptal, and alveolodental. There are three types of gingival fibers, the dentogingival, alveologingival, and the circular gingival. Dentogingival fibers run from the cementum to either attached or free gingiva, providing a firm support for these tissues. Alveologingival fibers run from the alveolar bone to either attached or free gingiva, providing further support for these tissues. The circular gingival fibers are found in the free gingiva running in a circular pattern around the tooth, providing additional support to hold it firmly against the tooth. Transseptal fibers extend from the cementum of one tooth, across the interproximal area to the cementum of an adjacent tooth. Alveolodental fibers run from the alveolar bone to the cementum and are typically divided into five types: alveolar crest, horizontal, oblique, apical, and interradicular. Alveolar crest fibers run from the crest in an apical-oblique direction to the cementum. These aid in resistance to extrusion and horizontal movement of the tooth. The horizontal fibers also run from the cementum to the alveolar crest, but horizontally, to resist horizontal tooth movements. Oblique fibers extend from the cementum in a coronal-oblique pattern to the alveolar bone and resist occlusal stresses. Apical fibers run from the apex to the alveolar bone and resist extrusional forces. The interradicular fibers are found only in multirooted teeth and go from the interradicular crestal bone to cementum, counteracting various types of movement according to their direction of attachment.

The gingiva is discussed in Section 1.5.1 on oral mucus membrane found below.

1.4.4 Dentin and Pulp

Dentin and pulp should be thought as a single unit as the pulp produces the dentin throughout the life of the tooth and the dentin contains cellular units of the pulp.

Dentin is the hard yellow substance covered by the enamel and cementum. It is approximately 70% inorganic hydroxyapatite crystal (mucopolysaccharide ground substance) and about 30% organic (collagen fibers and water). Dentin grossly appears to be a solid structure, but is perforated by a multitude of openings. In microscopic cross-section, dentin has three distinct areas. The first is the dentinal tubule, which is a tube extending from the DEJ to the pulp. The odontoblastic process or Tomes' fiber is a cellular extension of the odontoblast within the dentinal tubule. The tubule is surrounded by the peritubular dentin. Intertubular dentin comprises the bulk of the dentinal substance and is located between dentinal tubules. The peritubular dentin is more highly mineralized than the intertubular dentin. In the dog the tubule is more ovoid at the periphery and circular toward the pulp. The tubule width has been measured to be 2.2 to 2.5 μm in diameter in the dog and 1–2 μm in the cat [12]. There are approximately 29 000 to 52 000 dentinal tubules per square millimeter of dentin cut in the maxillary canine of the dog [13]. The number increases with patient size and as the cut approaches the pulp.

Primary and secondary dentin are the two normal types of dentin. Primary dentin forms adjacent to the enamel prior to eruption of the tooth and secondary dentin forms after eruption. Primary dentin includes mantle dentin and the granular layer of Tomes. Mantle dentin is found adjacent to enamel and its organization differs from the rest of primary dentin [14]. The granular layer of Tomes is the area of primary dentin adjacent to cementum [14]. This layer is hypomineralized relative to dentin with a higher organic content and it has been hypothesized that the higher organic content may act to dissipate force transmitted through the PDL [15].

Secondary dentin is laid down in layers within the pulp cavity throughout life as long as the pulp is vital, resulting in the pulp cavity gradually decreasing in diameter with age via a process called pulp recession.

Tertiary dentin is formed in response to traumatic stimulation. This type of dentin differs histologically from the normal dentin in that it generally has few if any dentinal tubules present and appears to be very dense and unorganized. It forms immediately below the cause of the irritation and can result in alteration of normal pulp cavity anatomy. The amount of tertiary dentin formation is related to the amount of secondary dentin remaining after injury and the rate of formation appears to be dependent on the type of trauma [16]. Tertiary dentin may be subdivided into reactionary and reparative. Reparative dentin occurs when reserve mesenchymal cells differentiate into new odontoblasts which repair dentin in areas of trauma. Reactionary dentin occurs when existing odontoblasts are involved in the formation of tertiary dentin [1]. As tertiary dentin forms, odontoblasts may become trapped in the dentin, producing osteodentin [1]. Dead tract dentin occurs in an area of dentin in which the dentinal tubules are empty. This typically occurs due to some form of trauma that kills the odontoblasts, leaving the dentinal tubule empty. These open tubules are pathways for bacteria and other substances to make rapid access to the pulp. If the pulp remains viable, reparative dentin may close off the dead tract dentin [1].

Sclerotic dentin is dentin in which the tubule is mineralized. This process increases with age and trauma. This type of dentin increases the transparency of the dentin.

Interglobular dentin is areas of hypocalcified dentin found next to the mantle dentin. It is hypocalcified dentin that occurred during formation. Increased amounts of interglobular dentin occurs in cases of rickets and dental fluorosis [1]. Although Tomes' granular layer and interlobular dentin are both hypomineralized layers adjacent to the outer covering of the tooth, the layers differ more than by location only. The two layers also differ in individual mineral and proteoglycan content [17].

The pulp of the root is contained within the root canal. It consists of blood vessels, nerves, fibroblasts, collagen fibers, undifferentiated reserve mesenchymal cells, other cells of connective tissue, and odontoblasts. The pulp is divided into four zones: odontoblastic, cell-free or zone of Weil, cell-rich, and the pulp core. Odontoblasts are an integral part of the dentin, but are also the peripheral cells of the pulp, which is why pulp and dentin are often thought of as a complex versus individual tissues. As mentioned before, the odontoblastic process is an extension of the odontoblast found within the dentinal tubule. There has been speculation that the process may not typically reach the DEJ [18], but the current accepted theory is that, since components of the process are found through the whole tubule, the process must run the length of the tubule [1]. Odontoblasts do not undergo cell division and must be replaced by undifferentiated ectomesenchymal cells found within the cell-rich zone [1]. The potential for differentiation into new odontoblasts decreases with age and the veterinary dentist should consider this when deciding if vital pulp therapy and direct pulp capping are appropriate for a patient. The nerves are primarily sensory and transmit only the sensation of pain. There are some motor nerves that innervate the smooth muscles within the blood vessels. These result in constriction of the vessels in response to irritation.

The presence of lymphatics within the dental pulp of man and dog is controversial. While most historic studies in man demonstrate the presence of lymphatics, many studies in dogs do not. Recent studies using immunohistochemistry methods did not demonstrate the presence of classic lymphatics in man or the dog [19, 20].

When examined in medium sized dogs, the root canal topography roughly mirrors the external topography of the tooth. The exception is a mesiopalatal root of the maxillary fourth premolar that is compressed buccal to palatal [21]. The endodontist should consider this anatomy as the root canal may appear cylindrical when radiographs are studied, but may be oval, elliptical, or ribbon shaped.

The termination or apical end of the root is the apex. The apex can have a single opening, apical foramen, or multiple openings, the apical delta, through which vessels, nerves, and other structures may pass into the tooth to merge with the pulp. Canine and feline root anatomy is generally in the form of an apical delta. Each opening of the delta is known as an apical ramification. In one study the number of apical ramifications in the dog was found to be 5–20 with a decrease in the number of ramifications with increased age of the patient [22]. When a single apical foramen is present, cementum enters into the foramen. In the case of an apical delta, cementum does not enter into the apical ramifications [22]. The root canal terminus is several millimeters from the surface of the root in the dog and cat and can be up to 6 mm in the cat [23]. This distance increases with age [23].

Non-apical ramifications or accessory canals occur where there is a break in Hertwig's epithelial root sheath during development. This prevents formation of dental hard tissue in a focal area and allows the pulp to communicate with the periodontium. These canals are typically found in the apical 1/3 of the root. Studies of incisors, canines, and maxillary fourth premolars of dogs showed an incidence of lateral canals to only be 2.4%. Of the four teeth that had lateral canals, one was a canine tooth and the other three were maxillary fourth premolar teeth [24]. When examining the maxillary fourth premolar and mandibular first molar, accessory canals were present in 68% of maxillary fourth premolars and 28.4% of mandibular first molars [25]. It has been demonstrated that the canine tooth of the cat has an average of 12.5 apical ramifications [23]. The endodontist should consider the likelihood of accessory canals when performing standard and surgical root canal therapy.

1.5 Mouth

The mouth (*os*) is the entrance or the oral cavity. It is solely the opening between the lips, designating the beginning of the digestive tract. The most rostral extent of the oral cavity is secured by the lips (*labia oris*). The upper lip (*labium superius*) and lower lip (*labium inferius*) converge at the angles of the mouth (*angulus oris*), forming the commissures of the lip.

1.5.1 Oral Mucous Membrane

The stratified squamous epithelium that runs from the margins of the lips to the area of the tonsils and lines the oral cavity is known as the oral mucosa or oral mucous membrane. These oral mucous membranes are divided into three categories. The first is the specialized mucosa, which is found on the dorsum of the tongue. Second is the masticatory mucosa, which undergoes routine masticatory trauma and stress and is generally parakeratinized or keratinized. This is the tissue of the hard palate and gingivae. The third is the general or lining mucosa, which comprises the remaining oral mucosa. It is non-keratinized to parakeratinized with an underlying connective tissue containing fairly well-developed collagen fibers that provide support, but still allow substantial movement of the overlying epithelium.

An interdigitation exists between the epithelium and the underlying connective tissue. The interdigitation of the submucosal connective tissue into the epithelium is termed the dermal papilla. The pegs of epithelium that insert into the connective tissue are known as rete ridges or pegs and cause small dimples in the gingival tissue known as gingival stippling. Stippling can be present or absent in healthy or diseased gingival tissue and therefore is not a reliable indication of gingival health [26–29]. The length of the pegs determines how tight or mobile the epithelium is attached to the underlying connective tissue. The lining mucosa has poorly developed pegs and is therefore fairly movable above the connective tissue. In comparison, the masticatory mucosa has well-developed rete pegs and consequently a tighter attachment.

The gingival masticatory mucosa is one of the most important support structures for the tooth. It is divided into two major parts, the attached gingiva and the free gingiva (marginal gingiva). The attached gingiva is attached to the alveolar bone via periosteum making it relatively immobile. It also has direct attachment to the cementum coronal to the alveolar bone. The width of the attached gingiva is important in planning periodontal treatment. It is widest on the maxilla at the canine teeth and generally thinner at the distal aspect of the fourth premolar and molars. On the mandible it is widest at the region of the first molar. The width of the attached gingiva is measured from the most apical aspect of the sulcus or periodontal pocket to the mucogingival junction.

The free gingiva projects in a coronal direction from the attached gingiva and is not attached to the tooth or alveolar bone. The free gingiva reflects toward the tooth to form shallow groove known as the gingival sulcus. The apical attachment of the sulcus is the epithelial attachment or the junctional epithelium, which directly attaches the gingiva to the tooth. In periodontal disease it is common for the sulcus depth to increase as attachment is lost. A peak of gingiva is found between proximal teeth known as the interdental papilla. The interdental papilla plays an important part in maintenance of gingival health by preventing food and debris from being impacted between the teeth. Between the vestibular and lingual aspects of the interdental papilla may be a peak or a valley of gingiva known as the col. The epithelium lining the sulcus, the col and the junctional epithelium are the very few areas of masticatory mucosa that are typically non-keratinized.

The mucogingival junction is the demarcation between the attached gingiva and alveolar mucosa, which is part of the general or lining mucosa. The mucogingival junction is also referred to as the mucogingival line or margin; it is most distinct on vestibular surfaces and less apparent on lingual and palatal surfaces.

1.5.2 Oral Cavity

The oral cavity (*cavum oris*) is typically considered to be the area extending from the lips to the oral pharynx at the level of the palatine tonsil. Rostrally it is bound by the lips, laterally by the cheeks (*buccae*), dorsally by the hard and soft palates, and ventrally by the floor of the mouth. The oral pharynx is also the location where the digestive and respiratory tracts share a common, intersecting pathway.

The oral cavity is generally subdivided into two parts, the vestibule (*vestibulum oris*) and the oral cavity proper (*cavum oris proprium*). The vestibule is the theoretical space between the lips or cheeks and the teeth, gums, and alveolar ridges. The oral cavity proper extends from the alveolar ridge and teeth to the oral pharynx. It is additionally defined by the roof and floor of the mouth and is generally filled by the tongue.

1.5.2.1 Vestibule

The lips are comprised of three components, one of which is the facial stratified squamous epithelium portion. The vestibular component is covered with oral mucosa that is non-keratinized to parakeratinized squamous epithelium. The juncture where the lips meet the surrounding skin is the vermilion border [30], and the pigmented area within the borders is called the vermilion zone (named after the typical red color in human lips). The transitional zone between facial and vestibular components is the vermilion zone of the lip. The facial or skin part of the upper lip at the midline has an indentation known as the philtrum. Cleft lips are most commonly seen to occur at the lateral board of the philtrum. The point at which the oral mucosa and the top or bottom of the vestibule turn toward the alveolar ridge is known as the mucobuccal or mucolabial fold. The attachment of the mucosa to the alveolar bone is loose and movable, and the point where it becomes tightly attached is the mucogingival junction.

Within the vestibule is also contained the frenula, which are areas where folds of alveolar mucosa form a noticeable ridge of attachment between the lips and the gum. The dog has three primary frenula: one upper and two lower. The upper extends from the midline of the lip to the gingiva immediately below the two central incisors. The lower two extend from the lip to the level of the mandibular canine teeth.

1.5.3 Oral Cavity Proper

Within the oral cavity proper is contained a multitude of structures. Among those are the hard and soft palate, tongue, and floor of the mouth.

1.5.4 Hard Palate

The hard palate (*palatum durum*) is the soft tissue covered, bony vault of the oral cavity proper. It has a median raphe dividing the left and the right sides. The transverse epithelial ridges that radiate out from the median raphe are known as rugae. The rugae should meet symmetrically at the median raphe. Asymmetrical junctures of the rugae at the raphe may be an indication of poor migration of the left and right maxillary processes and a tendency toward cleft palate formation. It is not uncommon to find this asymmetrical rugal pattern in parents of cleft palate puppies. At the beginning of the raphe, immediately caudal to the two central incisor teeth, is a single rounded elevation of tissue known as the incisive papilla (*papilla incisiva*). At each lateral side of the incisive papilla are slit-shaped openings to the incisive ducts (*ductus incisivus*), which pass through the palatine fissure connecting the nasal and oral cavities. From the incisive papilla, the paired incisive ducts travel dorsocaudally to open into each nasal fossa; along their route they also communicate with the paired vomeronasal organs (*organum vomeronasale*). Deep to the incisive papilla is the incisive foramen through which the nasopalatine nerve travels to the soft tissue palatal to the rostral maxillary teeth.

1.5.5 Soft Palate

The soft palate (*palatum molle* or *velum palatinum*) is the unsupported soft tissue that extends caudally from the hard palate, free of the support of the palatine bone. It is relatively thick at its attachment to the hard palate and thins at the margins. In a relaxed state it typically makes contact with the oral surface of the epiglottis, but may also make contact with the respiratory surface of the epiglottis. The hard and soft palates serve to separate the oral cavity from the nasal cavity.

1.6 Osseous Tissue

The head consisting of the skull and mandible support all the teeth. The incisive (formerly premaxillae in the dog and still considered such in some species), maxillary, and mandibular bones have sockets, in which the teeth are seated. This firm attachment of teeth to support is termed *thecodontia*. The alveolar process is that portion of these bones that encompass and support the tooth structure. It is comprised of a cortical plate, trabecular bone, and the cribriform plate. The cortical plate is the outside wall of the process. The cribriform plate, known radiologically as the lamina dura, is the thin layer of bone within the tooth socket. Trabecular bone acts as the support between the cortical plate and the lamina dura. The alveolar crest is the occlusal portion of the alveolar process near the neck of the tooth. The bony partitions between adjacent teeth are referred to as interalveolar septa. Partitions between roots of an individual tooth are known as interradicular septa. The mandibles and maxillae containing the teeth are known as the jaws.

The paired incisive bones accommodate the six maxillary incisor teeth. The bones meet at the mesial line and each articulates with the ipsilateral maxilla at the incisivomaxillary suture. The root of the maxillary canine tooth passes through this suture with the incisive bone housing a portion of the alveolus on the palatal side. The paired palatine fissures are situated in the palatine process of each maxillae directly caudal to the incisor teeth. The main branches of the palatine vessels pass through these fissures. The maxillae act as the mooring for the remainder of the upper dentition. This includes the bulk of the canine, four premolars, and two molars in each maxilla in the dog. The maxillae contain the canine, three premolars, and single molar in the cat. Its lateral wall is relatively thin. This results in prominences in the alveolar bone lateral to many of the tooth roots. These prominences, called alveolar juga, act as landmarks in certain surgical endodontic procedures. The palatine process of each mandible projects medially and along with the paired incisive and palatine bones, serve as the bony support of the hard palate. The mandibles are two bilateral bones attached rostrally at the midline by a strong fibrous joint, referred to as the mandibular symphysis. Each mandible is comprised of two major sections, the body, and ramus (Figure 1.6). The body is composed of the incisive part (*Pars incisiva*) containing the incisors and the molar part (*Pars molaris*), which contains the premolars and molars. On the medial surface of the body at the caudal extent the mandibular foramen is present, located at midpoint between the third molar and angular process in the dog. The mandibular artery, vein, and nerve enter the mandibular canal through this foramen. The artery, vein, and nerve exit the mandibular canal via the rostral, middle, and caudal mental foramina. The rostral mental foramen is located in the incisive part of the mandible between the first and second incisors. The middle mental foramen is located in the molar part at about the level of the apex of the mesial root of the second premolar in the dog and at the level of the labial frenulum in the cat. The caudal mental foramen is located between the two roots of the third premolar.

The ramus constitutes the coronoid process, the condylar process, and the angular process and serves as the majority of insertion for the muscles of mastication. Projecting caudal from the ramus is the neck of the mandible, which supports the head, making the condylar process (http://www.avdc.org/nomenclature.html). The temporomandibular joint (TMJ) is formed by the condylar process of the mandible and the mandibular fossa of the temporal bone. This joint is sometimes referred to as the craniomandibular articulation (CMA). Depending on the species, the joint makes both translation and rotation movement capabilities, which allows for both rostral and lateral movement to a degree, as well as its rotation hinge action. The joint is separated into two compartments, the dorsal (temporal) and ventral (mandibular) by an articular disc. The disc attaches to the temporal bone caudomedially and to the condylar process laterally [31]. Fibrous tissue surrounds the joint capsule, which forms its strong lateral ligament.

A shallow concavity is present on the lateral aspect of the ramus named the masseteric fossa, which is the

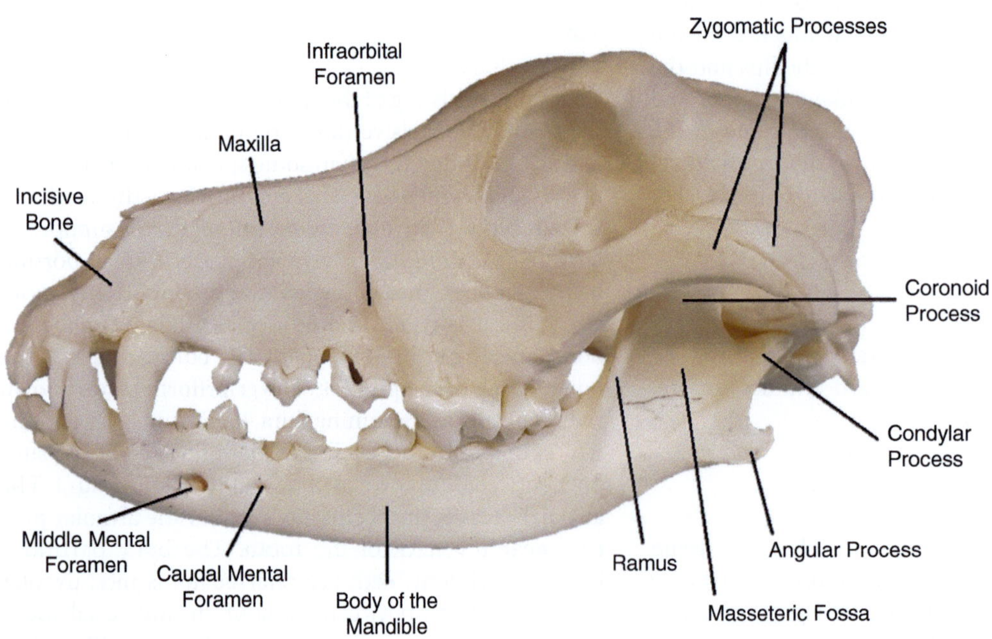

Figure 1.6 Normal skull anatomy of the dog.

insertion for the masseter muscle. Dorsal to the masseteric fossa is the crest of the ramus named the coronoid process. Ventral to the condylar process is a caudally projecting structure, which serves as insertion for the pterygoid and masseter muscles, named the angular process.

The morphology of the mandibular symphysis has been categorized into four types (I, II, III, and IV) [32]. Dogs and domestic cats have type I, meaning the interdigitation between folds of fibrocartilage from each side is shallow, allowing for less rigidity of the joint. Not all Felid species have this type. Many have type III, meaning the interdigitations are deeper and more numerous [32].

Although there is little lateral movement of the canine mandibles due to the strong lateral ligament and occlusion of the Canid dentition, unilateral lateral movement was described by Scapino [31]. This is a two-phase movement beginning with contraction of the zygomaticomandibularis muscle to nearly align the primary cusp of the mandibular first molar with the primary cusp of the maxillary fourth premolar. The caudal aspect of the mandibular symphysis then widens to allow the opposite mandible to move closer to its original position. With this two-phase movement, only one mandible and maxilla are chewing at a time. The zygomaticomandibularis muscle has been described by some as a portion of the masseter and as a separate muscle originating from the medial aspect of the zygomatic bone and inserting in the masseteric fossa of the vertical ramus [33].

The mandible and skull together can form various head types or shapes. Brachycephalic, mesaticephalic, and dolichocephalic are the three most common terms used to describe head shape. Brachycephalic indicates a short, wide head. The shortness of the head commonly results in rotation of premolar teeth. Boxers, Boston Terriers, Chinese Pugs, Bull Dogs, and Pekingese are some of the breeds commonly called brachycephalic. Mesaticephalic designates a head shape of medium portions. Beagles, German Shepard Dogs, Labrador Retrievers, and Poodles are typical examples. Dolichocephalic refers to a long, narrow head shape. The Collie, Borzoi, and Russian Wolf Hound are representative of this head type. Caudal crossbites, where the maxillary fourth premolar is in linguoversion (lingual) relative to the lower first molar, are more common in these breeds.

1.7 Muscles and Related Nerves of Mastication

The majority of the muscles associated with the masticatory action function to close the mandible [34]. Of this group the temporalis muscle is the largest and most powerful in the dog. Its origin is the temporal fossa. It inserts on the lateral and medial surfaces of the coronoid process of the ipsilateral mandible. In the dolichocephalic dog the paired muscles meet dorsally and form a middorsal sulcus where in the brachycephalic dog they do not meet [35]. The masseter muscle consist of three layers: superficial, middle, and deep. The muscle originates from the zygomatic arch (ventrally and medially) and inserts on the ramus of the mandible at the masseteric fossa and at the ventrolateral and ventromedial surfaces of the ramus. The lateral pterygoid muscle arises from the sphenoid bone and medial pterygoid muscles originates from the sphenoid, pterygoid, and palatine bones [35]. The lateral inserts on the medial aspect of the condylar process of the mandible. The medial inserts on the ventromedial aspect of the angular process of the mandible, forming a raphe with the masseter muscle. Identification of this fibrous raphe and elevation the medial pterygoid muscle is useful in the surgical approach to the caudal mandible [36].

The digastric muscle is responsible for opening the jaws, and arises from the paracondylar process of the occipital bone and inserts on the mandible along the ventral border. It has both a rostral and caudal portion (belly) separated by a raphe.

These muscles are all innervated by the mandibular branch of the trigeminal (V) nerve. Only the rostral belly of the digastric muscle is stimulated by the trigeminal nerve, as the caudal belly is innervated by the facial (VII) nerve. Of the muscles innervated by the trigeminal nerve, the masseter, temporal, medial, and lateral pterygoid, tensor tympani, and tensor veli palatine muscles have a unique myosin isoform type 2M, distinguished from the common type 2C fibers of limb muscles [37–39]. Although the rostral belly of the digastric muscle is innervated by the trigeminal nerve, it does not contain type 2M fibers [37]. In the case of masticatory myositis, circulating antibodies are directed specifically to these 2M muscle fibers and inflammation is limited to muscles with this unique myosin component [38]. The etiology of masticatory myositis (MM) is unknown, although it has been speculated that MM may result from antibodies generated in response to an infectious agent cross-reacting with endogenous antigens [39]. These fibers are also found in most carnivores and primates, but masticatory myositis of type 2M fibers has only been reported in the dog.

These muscles, in coordination with the teeth, have a tremendous biting force potential. Biting force is the pressure, typically measured in pounds per square inch (psi), exerted by the teeth when engaged by the muscles of mastication. In man they have been shown to have about 250 to 300 psi of passive biting force [40]. Additionally, with man the abrupt closing or snapping of the jaws shut on the few millimeters of tooth cusp contact can reach a sudden localized biting force of 25 000 to 30 000 psi, which can easily result in tooth fractures or injury to the periodontal structures [41]. In the dog the passive biting force has been indicated to be possibly much greater than that of a human, reaching between the 300 to 800 psi range [42]. This would place the sudden localized biting force potential at 30 000 to 80 000 psi, if correct.

1.8 Neurovascular Structures of Clinical Significance

The arteries of significance in clinical dentistry and oral surgery have a common origin in the common carotid artery. This artery branches into the internal and external carotid arteries. The internal carotid artery blood supply is insignificant in the cat. The external carotid artery continuing as the maxillary artery provides the majority of cerebral blood flow. The maxillary artery lies medial to the angular process of the mandible and branches into the maxillary rete before entering the skull through the orbital fissure. The intracranial portion of the rete forms the cerebral arteries. The extracranial portion is bordered by the pterygoid muscles medially and temporal muscle laterally. It is currently believed that overextension of the mandibles of the cat can lead to compression of the rete and/or compression of the maxillary artery by the angular process of the mandible, leading to cerebral ischemia and resulting in temporary or permanent cortical blindness, loss of hearing, or possibly death [43, 44]. Thus use of spring-loaded speculums is not recommended in feline patients.

The maxillary artery is a branch of the external carotid artery. Just caudal to the maxilla the minor palatine artery branches off the maxillary artery and courses ventral to the palatine bone and maxilla before anastamosing with the major palatine artery. The major palatine artery shares a common trunk with the sphenopalatine artery [34]. The major palatine artery exits the maxilla through the major palatine foramen, located at the level of the distal extent of the fourth premolar and between the corresponding dental arch and palatal midline. The artery travels rostrally through the ipsilateral palatine groove. A branch of the artery travels buccally between the maxillary third incisor and canine [34]. The remainder of the artery passes the palatine fissure and anastamoses with the sphenopalatine artery. The major palatine nerve exits through the same foramen. It is of clinical significance if regional anesthesia for palatal surgery is to be performed. The artery sharing a trunk with the major palatine is the sphenopalatine artery, which courses along the ventral floor of the nasal cavity before anastamosing with the major palatine, as mentioned previously.

The infraorbital artery is the continuation of the maxillary artery after the trunk containing the major palatine and sphenopalatine arteries. It enters the maxilla via the maxillary foramen caudally and travels through the infraorbital canal, giving branches to the zygomatic gland and the alveolar bone of the maxillary teeth [35]. The artery exits the infraorbital foramen just mesial to the mesiobuccal root of the maxillary fourth premolar at the level of the apical half of the root. It begins to branch after exiting the foramen into the dorsal and lateral nasal arteries. The infraorbital nerve follows the same course.

The mandibular arteries and the associated veins are paired structures coursing through the mandibular body, providing the primary blood supply for the teeth and periodontium of the mandibles. The artery is a branch of the maxillary artery. In enters into the mandible via the mandibular foramen. This foramen is located on the medial side of the mandible and between the third molar and angular process in the dog and between the molar and angular process in the cat. The mandibular artery travels through the mandibular canal. The canal is not a medullary canal and treating fractures of the body via an intramedullary pin through this canal will damage the associated neurovascular bundle. When examined in cross-section, the mandibular nerve is located in the dorsolateral portion of the canal with the vein in the ventromedial portion and the artery in the middle [35]. The caudal, middle, and rostral mental arteries are the terminus of the mandibular artery and exit through the same named foramina.

1.9 Tongue

The tongue (*lingua*) is a mobile prehensile structure of the oral cavity used for grooming and the intake of food and fluids. It is formed primarily of skeletal muscle covered by a mucosal membrane. Its actions are controlled by both intrinsic and extrinsic muscles of the tongue (*musculi linguae*). The intrinsic muscle of the tongue is the m. lingualis proprius, which contains superficial longitudinal, deep longitudinal, perpendicular, and transverse muscle fibers. These as a unit produce the complicated protrusion and prehensile movements of the tongue and prevent trauma from teeth. It is innervated by the hypoglossal nerve. The extrinsic muscles are the m. styloglossus, m. hypoglossus, and m. genioglossus. The m. styloglossus draws the tongue caudally, the m. hypoglossus retracts and depresses it, and the m. genioglossus depresses and protrudes the tongue. All three of the extrinsic muscles are also innervated by the hypoglossus nerve. The total innervation of the tongue is by the lingual (V), chorda tympani (VII), glossopharyngeal (IX), and hypoglossal (XII) nerves. The afferent activities of tactile, pain, thermal, and taste, and the efferent activities of tongue gland innervation are controlled by the lingual (V), chorda tympani (VII), and glossopharyngeal (IX) nerves.

The tongue is divided into a tip (*apex linguae*), margin (*margo linguae*), body (*corpus linguae*), and a root (*radix linguae*). It is wide and thin at the two lateral margins that meet at the tip or most rostral portion of the margins, but it becomes thicker toward the body and root. The dorsum is covered with a thick, rough cornified mucous membrane known as the lingual mucosa (*tunica mucosa linguae*). The ventral surface is covered with a smooth, thinner, and less cornified surface. The thicker dorsal mucosa forms into papillae with various shapes and functions. The rostral two-thirds is thickly covered with short, pointed, filiform papillae (*papillae filiformes*) with their tips directed caudally, which may aid in grooming. In the root area are found soft, long, conical papillae (*papillae conicae*) pointing caudally, which probably have a mechanical function. Fungiform papillae (*papillae fungiformes*) are mushroom shaped and scattered along the dorsal sides and the anterior portion of the tongue. Each contains up to eight taste pores, although some have none. A small number of vallate papillae (*papillae vallate*) are found at the posterior border of the tongue where the conical papillae begin. There are three to six vallate papillae in the dog, with four being the most common. These may be simple or complex and contain taste buds. The foliate papillae (*papillae foliatae*) are immediately rostral to the palatoglossal fold located on the dorsolateral aspect of the caudal third of the tongue and contain taste buds. Marginal papillae (*papillae marginales*) are present at birth along the margins of the rostral half of the tongue in the dog. They are mechanical in nature, aiding in nursing by sealing the lips to the nipple for suction and reduce milk spillage around the tongue. These normally disappear as puppies progress to more solid foods. The taste buds (*caliculus gustatorius*) are pear-shaped organs located in the gustatory papillae: fungiform, vallate, and foliate papillae. The filiform, conical, and marginal papillae are mechanical papillae containing no taste buds. There is an extensive number of lingual salivary glands (*glandulae linguales*) in the surface of the tongue. The dorsum of the tongue is divided by a median groove in the anterior portion.

The ventral part of the tongue is covered by smooth mucous membrane. Extending from the floor of the mouth to the anterior ventral base is a fold of tissue known as the lingual frenulum (*frenulum linguae*). Within the ventral portion of the tip, along the midline, is a fusiform cord, composed of fat, muscle, occasionally islands of cartilage, and fibrous sheath tissue known as the lyssa. The lyssa, formerly known as the lytta, is typically about 4 cm in a medium-sized dog and may act as a stretch receptor for the rostral portion of the tongue. Beneath the smooth mucosa of the underside of the tongue is a highly vascular network. The primary blood supply to the tongue is through the paired lingual arteries (*arteria lingualis*) with return via the lingual veins.

The base of the lingual frenulum rests in the floor of the mouth. To either side of this base are small elevations of tissue known as the sublingual caruncles (*caruncula sublingualis*). These serve as the anatomical locations of the duct openings for the sublingual and mandibular salivary glands. A fold of tissue known as the sublingual fold (*plica sublingualis*) extends back from the sublingual caruncle along the floor of the mouth with the side of the tongue. This fold marks the path of numerous structures that run across the floor of the mouth, including the ducts for the sublingual and mandibular salivary glands.

1.10 Salivary Glands

Submerged beneath the mucous membranes of the oral cavity exists a complex system of salivary tissues. These salivary tissues secrete saliva, a serous and mucous fluid, which contains a complex mixture of inorganic and organic substances such as electrolytes, proteins, hormones, minerals, bactericidal substances, vitamins, and, in some species, enzymes. In most animals, a relatively high concentration of amylase is found in saliva from the parotid and slightly lower levels in mandibular secretions. The concentrations of amylase, however, are relatively low in the domestic dog and cat. Fluid formation in the salivary tissue occurs in the acini.

Isotonic water transport is an acinar secretory process in which the main active step is a sodium transport system from the intracellular to the intercellular space. The duct epithelium can secrete and absorb water as well as the basic electrolytes calcium, chloride, bicarbonate, sodium, and potassium. It is also involved with the concentration of iodide and thiocyanate. The concentrations of some salivary constituents such as iodide, calcium, and bicarbonate is dependent upon their blood plasma levels; therefore, the saliva/plasma ratio of these electrolytes remains relatively constant.

Regulation of saliva secretions is controlled by the autonomic nervous system. The centers for saliva secretion are located on the salivary nuclei in the medulla oblongata. The salivary glands are regulated by a double efferent pathway via the parasympathetic and sympathetic portions of the autonomic nervous system. A basal flow of saliva is continuously stimulated by the parasympathetic system's efferent impulses from the salivary nuclei. Sight, taste, and olfactory stimulation initiates afferent impulses to the nuclei, which in turn release efferent impulses to the parasympathetic system to increase salivation. Sympathetic stimulation may increase salivary flow to the mouth due to contraction on the myoepithelial cells by constriction of the lumen of both the acini and the ducts. Sympathetic stimulation actually increases salivary secretion by the acinar cells of some salivary glands in the cat.

Saliva has both qualitative and quantitative aspects. The quantitative properties are twofold, the basal and surge flowrates. The basal production level maintains the protective moist mucoid layer environment for the teeth and mucous membranes. This layer possibly aids in protecting the mucosa from the detrimental effects of bacterial and other toxins, as well as to minor traumas. The flowrate aids to mechanically flush and cleanse the teeth and mucous membranes of the oral cavity, possibly limiting the microbial population in the oral environment. The elevated surge flowrate aids to flush mucoid trapped bacteria and foreign materials from the mouth and into the acidic gastric system for destruction. Additionally, the mucous coats foodstuffs to lubricate while the serous volume acts to carry the material through the tract with the aid of muscular activity.

Qualitatively it is a complex combination of organic and inorganic substances, with a pH component. In broad groups these can be classified as minerals and electrolytes, enzymes and other proteins, low molecular weight compounds, and vitamins. The ultimate composition is generally regulated by the autonomic nervous system, the serum level of systemic counterparts, and humoral activity. The qualitative portion contains a potent antimicrobial component consisting of mucous, pH, lysosomes, antilactobacillus thiocyanate-dependent factors, immunoglobulins, fluoride, and many other possible factors. The teeth are theoretically affected by saliva by reduction of tooth solubility, buffering acids, remineralization, antimicrobial actions, and mechanical cleansing. Enzymes, such as amylase, aid in initiation of digestion while food is still in the mouth. The mixed pH of saliva varies widely, even in individuals. It is affected by numerous factors, but flowrate and duration appear to be the most important. As compared to a slightly acidic average of pH 6.5–7.5 for humans, dogs have shown salivary pH values in a range from 8.5 to 8.65 [45]. Lavy also suggested that the higher salivary pH in dogs compared to humans, while protecting against carious lesions, could lead to precipitation of calcium salts and lead to increased calculus accumulation. Most other domestic animals demonstrate a slight alkaline pH (the horse at 7.5 [46]), except ruminants, which are distinctively alkaline (the cow at 8.53–8.71 [47]).

There is a large assortment of salivary glands and tissue in the oral cavity or that empty into it. The lingual, labial, buccal, and palatine salivary glands represent a large number of very small disseminated glands that secrete minute amounts of serous or mucus fluid into the oral cavity. The lingual salivary glands are located in the submucosa and muscles of the tongue in its caudal third, with numerous small excretory ducts. The labial glands are found scattered throughout in the submucosa of the lips, with numerous small excretory ducts. The buccal glands are situated in the submucosa of the buccal cavity, with numerous small excretory ducts. The palatine glands are located in the submucosa of the ventral surface of the soft palate. There are four or five larger glands more clinically significant in disease and saliva production. In the dog these are the parotid, mandibular, sublingual, and zygomatic (Figure 1.7). In the cat the molar salivary glands are also of clinical importance (Figure 1.8).

The parotid salivary gland (*glandula parotis*) is divided into a superficial portion (*par superficialis*) and a deep portion (*pars profunda*). The gland is generally V-shaped and is located beneath the ear and behind the posterior border of the mandible and the TMJ. Although a part of the gland is superficial in location, its blending with the surrounding anatomy makes it typically difficult to palpate. The parotid lymph nodes usually lie under the rostroventral border of the parotid salivary gland.

The parotid duct (*ductus parotideus*) is formed by the union a few millimeters from the gland of two or three tributaries originating from the ventral third of the rostral border of the gland. It proceeds rostrally and toward the cheek along the lateral surface of the masseter muscle, closely paralleling the muscle fibers. Near the terminal end, the duct generally makes two slight right-angle turns, one medially and one vertically, before passing through the buccal mucosa and opening into the buccal vestibule. The opening is at the parotid papilla located at the rostral end of a blunt ridge of mucosa superficial to the distal root of the upper fourth premolar. For catheterization of the ducts, the terminal angulations can be relatively straightened by lightly retracting the papilla rostrally. The gland produces a primarily serous type saliva.

Accessory parotid glands (*glandulae parotis accessoria*) are typically present in the dog. These are usually located bilaterally above the duct and range from single, small lobules to glandular masses over a centimeter in length. These each have small ducts that empty into the main parotid duct.

The mandibular gland (*glandulas mandibularis*) is an ovoid, compact, yellow to buff colored gland. In the dog, cat, and most domestic animals, the gland is located just caudal to the angle of the jaw and is easily palpable. In most primates, however, it is located beneath the mandible and is referred to as the submandibular salivary gland. The gland shares a connective tissue capsule with a portion of the sublingual gland. In the dog it rests

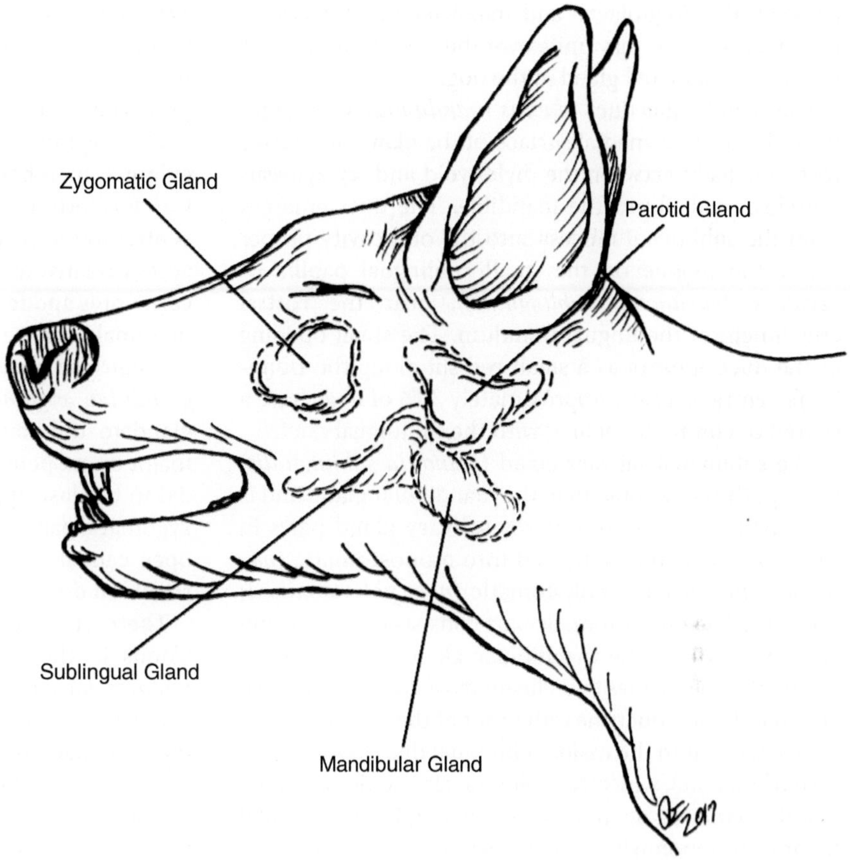

Figure 1.7 Salivary glands of the dog.
Source: Courtesy of Josephine Banyard.

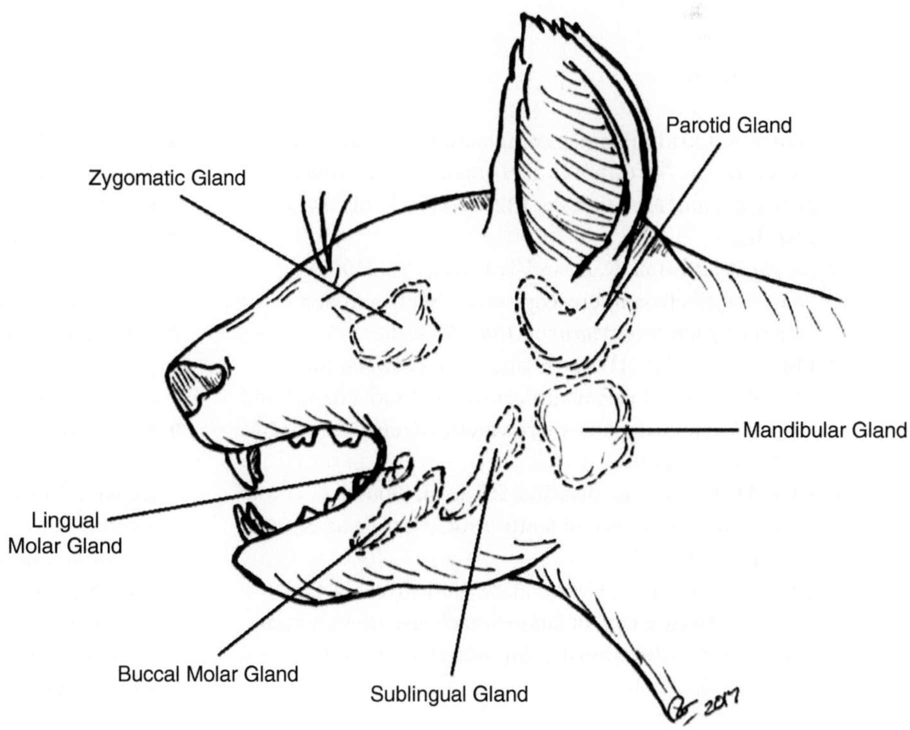

Figure 1.8 Salivary glands of the cat.
Source: Courtesy of Josephine Banyard.

between the linguofacial and maxillary veins, while in the cat these veins may unite over the lateral surface. It is classified as a mixed gland in the dog.

The mandibular duct (*ductus mandibularis*) emerges from the deep or medial surface of the gland. It courses rostromedially between the mylohyoid and styloglossus muscles, medially to the mandible. The duct emerges from the sublingual mucosa into the oral cavity proper below the tongue on the small sublingual papilla or caruncle (*caruncula sublingualis*), near the rostral attachment of the lingual frenulum. The small opening of the duct appears as a small red slit along the frenulum's ventral surface. Approximately 30% of dogs have a shared or common opening with the sublingual duct.

The sublingual salivary gland (*glandula sublingualis*) is a slightly darker pink than the mandibular gland and is the smallest of the four major salivary gland pairs in the dog. The gland is divided into monostomatic (*par monostomatica*) and polystomatic (*pars polystomatica*) portions. The monostomatic part consists of the portion contained within the mandibular gland capsule and a group of loose lobules that cluster close to the sublingual and mandibular ducts near the root of the tongue. These all discharge into the major sublingual duct (*ductus sublingualis major*), which typically travels just dorsal to the mandibular duct, opening one to two millimeters caudal to, or in common with, it on the sublingual caruncle.

The polystomatic portion is a group of 6–12 small scattered lobules of sublingual salivary tissue. These do not communicate with the major sublingual duct, but empty into several minor sublingual ducts (*ductus sublingualis minores*). These empty into the oral cavity between the tongue and mandible in the lateral sublingual recess. The sublingual gland is smaller in the cat with the polystomatic portion sometimes absent.

The zygomatic gland (*glandula zygomatica*) is an enlarged member of the dorsal buccal gland group and was formerly known as the orbital gland. It is located ventral to the rostral end of the zygomatic arch, making access relatively difficult. It is well developed in most carnivores and found only in the dog and cat in domestic mammals. There is one major duct (*ductus glandulae zygomaticae major*) and up to four minor ducts (*ductus glandulae zygomaticae minores*) that travel from the gland to the caudal part of the buccal vestibule. The major duct opens caudal to the parotid papillae and caudal to the last upper molar on a ridge of mucosa at the zygomatic papilla (*papilla zygomatica*). The minor ducts open caudal to the major ducts and appear as a line of small red dots on the mucosa.

There are two paired well-developed molar salivary glands in the cat. The buccal molar gland (*glandula molares buccalis*), also referred to as the labial molar gland, is a modified ventral buccal gland located between the orbicularis oris muscle and the mucous membrane of the lower lip at the angle of the mouth. It empties into the buccal cavity by several small ducts. The second gland is the lingual molar gland (*glandula molars lingualis*), located within a membranous bulge lingual to the mandibular molar tooth. This gland is the tubuloacinar gland with multiple small openings through several small ducts that open on the lingual surface of the membrane [48].

References

1 Nanci, A. (2013). Enamel: composition formation and structure. In: *Ten Cate's Oral Histology: Development, Structure, and Function*, 8e, 122–164. St. Louis, MO: Elsevier.

2 Skobe, Z., Prostak, K. S., and Trombly, P. L. (1985). Scanning electron microscope study of cat and dog enamel structure. *J. Morphol.* 184: 195–203.

3 Osborn, J. W. (1971). The relationship between the optical density of prism borders in dog tooth enamel and the angle from which they are viewed. *Arch. Oral Biol.* 16 (9): 1055–1059.

4 Chai, H., Lee, J. J., Constatino, P. J. et al. (2009). Remarkable resilience of teeth. *Proc. Natl Acad. Sci.* 106 (18): 7289–7293.

5 Bajaj, D., Nazari, A., Eidleman, N., and Arola, D. D. (2008). A comparison of fatigue crack growth in human enamel and hydroxyapatite. *Biomaterials* 29 (36): 4847–4484.

6 Walker, B. N., Makinson, O. F., and Peters, M. C. (1998). Enamel cracks. The role of enamel lamellae in caries initiation. *Aust. Dent. J.* 43 (2): 110–116.

7 Crossley, D. A. (1995). Tooth enamel thickness in the mature dentition of domestic dogs and cats – preliminary study. *J. Vet. Dent.* 12 (3): 111–113.

8 Dupont, G. A. and DeBowes, L. J. (2009). Intraoral radiographic anatomy of the dog. In: *Atlas of Dental Radiography in Dogs and Cats*, 5–80. St. Louis, MO: Saunders.

9 Smith, M. M., Massoudi, L. M., Nunes, J. D. et al. (1992). Furcation anatomy of the first mandibular molar in dogs. *Am. J. Vet. Res.* 53 (2): 242–245.

10 Smith, M. M., Moon, M. L., Callan, M. et al. (1990). Furcation entrance anatomy of the fourth maxillary premolar in dogs. *Am. J. Vet. Res.* 51 (12): 2050–2053.

11 Verstraete, F. J. and Terpak, C. H. (1997). Anatomical variations in the dentition of the domestic cat. *J. Vet. Dent.* 14 (4): 137–140.

12 DeLaurier, A. L., Boyde, A., Horton, M. A., and Price, J. S. (2006). Analysis of the surface characteristics and mineralization status of feline teeth using scanning electron microscopy. *J. Anat.* 209: 655–669.
13 Robb, L., Mark, J., Steenkamp, G. et al. (2007). Scanning electron microscopic study of the dentinal tubules in dog canine teeth. *J. Vet. Dent.* 24 (2): 86–89.
14 Nanci, A. (2013). Enamel: dentin-pulp complex. In: *Ten Cate's Oral Histology: Development, Structure, and Function*, 8e, 165–204. St. Louis, MO: Elsevier.
15 Shackleford, J. M. (1971). The structure of Tomes' granular layer in dog premolar teeth. *Anat. Rec.* 170 (3): 357–363.
16 Ivanovic, V. and Santini, A. (1989). Rate of formation of tertiary dentin in dogs' teeth in response to lining materials. *Oral Surg. Oral Med. Oral Pathol.* 67: 684–688.
17 Tsuchiya, M., Sasano, Y., Kagayam, M. et al. (2001). Characterization of interglobular dentin and Tomes' granular layer in dog dentin using electron probe microanalysis in comparison with predentin. *Calcified Tissue Int.* 68: 172–178.
18 Holland, G. R. (1975). The dentinal tubule and odontoblast process in the cat. *J. Anat.* 120 (1): 169–177.
19 Gerli, R., Secciani, I., Soziio, F. et al. (2010). Absence of lymphatic vessels in human dental pulp: a morphological study. *Eur. J. Oral Sci.* 118 (2): 110–117.
20 Martin, A., Gasse, H., and Staszyk, C. (2010). Absence of lymphatic vessels in the dog dental pulp: an immunohistochemical study. *J. Anat.* 217: 609–615.
21 Rochette, J. (1996). Identification of the endodontic system in carnassial and canine teeth in the dog. *J. Vet. Dent.* 13 (1): 35–37.
22 Masson, E., Hennet, P. R., and Calas, P. L. (1992). Apical root canal anatomy in the dog. *Endod. Dent. Traumatol.* 8: 109–112.
23 Hennet, P. R. and Harvey, C. E. (1996). Apical root canal anatomy of canine teeth in cats. *Am. J. Vet. Res.* 57: 1545–1548.
24 Gioso, M. A., Knobl, T., Venturini, M. A. F. A. et al. (1997). Non-apical root canal ramifications in the teeth of dogs. *J. Vet. Dent.* 14 (3): 89–90.
25 Hernandez, S. Z., Negro, V. B., and Maresca, B. M. (2001). Morphologic features of the root canal system of the maxillary fourth premolar and the mandibular first molar in dogs. *J. Vet. Dent.* 18 (1): 9–13.
26 Greene, A. H. (1962). Study of the characteristics of stippling and its relation to gingival health. *J. Periodontol.* 33: 176.
27 Hurt, W. C. (1976). *Periodontics in General Practice*, 1–65. Springfield, IL: CC Thomas Pub.
28 King, J. D. (1945). Gingival disease in Dundee. *J. Dent. Res.* 65: 9.
29 Orban, B. (1948). Clinical and histological study of surface characteristics of the gingiva. *Oral Surg.* 1: 827.
30 Zwemer, T. J. (1993). *Boucher's Clinical Dental Terminology*, A Glossary of Accepted Terms in all Disciplines of Dentistry, 4e. St. Louis, MO: Mosby.
31 Scapino, R. P. (1965). The third joint of the canine jaw. *J. Morphol.* 116: 23–50.
32 Scapino, R. (1981). Morphological investigation into the functions of the jaw symphysis in carnivorans. *J. Morphol.* 167: 339–375.
33 Yang, H. M., Hu, K. S., Song, W. C. et al. (2010). Innervation patterns of the canine masticatory muscles in comparison to human. *Anat. Rec.* 293: 117–125.
34 Evans, H. E. and deLahunta, A. (2000). The head. In: *Miller's Guide to the Dissection of the Dog*, 5e, 259–276. Philadelphia, PA: Saunders.
35 Evans, H. E. (1993). The heart and arteries. In: *Miller's Anatomy of the Dog*, 3e, 586–681. Philadelphia, PA: Saunders.
36 Verstraete, F. J. M., Arzi, B., and Bezuidenhout, A. J. (2012). Surgical approaches for mandibular and maxillofacial trauma repair. In: *Oral and Maxillofacial Surgery in Dogs and Cats*, 259–264. Philadephia, PA: Saunders.
37 Bubb, W. J. and Sims, M. H. (1985). Fiber type composition of rostral and caudal portions of the digastric muscle in the dog. *Am. J. Vet. Res.* 47 (8): 1834–1842.
38 Shelton, G. D., Bandman, E., and Cardinet, G. H. (1985). Electrophoretic comparison of myosins from masticatory muscles and selected limb muscles in the dog. *Am. J. Vet. Res.* 46 (2): 493–498.
39 Shelton, G. D., Cardinet, G. H., and Bandman, E. (1988). Expression of fiber type specific proteins during ontogeny of canine temporalis muscle. *Muscle Nerve* 11 (2): 124–132.
40 Melmed, C., Shelton, G. D., Bergman, R., and Barton, C. L. (2004). Masticatory muscle myositis: pathogenesis, diagnosis and treatment. *Compend. Cotin Educ. Vet.* 26 (8): 590–605.
41 Fagan, D. A. (1986). Diagnosis and treatment planning. *Veterinary Clinics of North America: Small Animal Practice* (ed. P. Frost) 16 (5): 789.
42 Tholen, M. A. (1983). *Concepts in Veterinary Dentistry*, 135. Edwardsville, KS: Veterinary Medicine Publishing Co.
43 Stiles, J., Weil, A. B., Packer, R. A., and Lantz, G. C. (2012). Post-anesthetic cortical blindness in cats: twenty cases. *Vet. J.* 193 (2): 367–373.
44 Barton-Lamb, A. L., Martin Flores, M., Scrivani, P. V. et al. (2013). Evaluation of maxillary arterial blood flow in anesthetized cats with the mouth closed and open. *Vet. J.* 196: 325–331.

45 Lavy, E., Goldberger, D., Friedman, M., and Steinberg, D. (2012). pH values and mineral content of saliva in different breeds of dogs. *Israel J. Vet. Med.* 67 (4): 244–248.

46 Alexander, F. (1966). A study of parotid salivation in the horse. *J. Physiol.* 184: 646–656.

47 Reid, J. T. and Huffman, C. F. (1949). Some physical and chemical properties of bovine saliva which may affect rumen digestion and synthesis. *J. Dairy Science.* 32 (2): 123–132.

48 Okuda, A., Inouc, E., and Asari, M. (1996). The membranous bulge lingual to the mandibular molar tooth of a cat contains a small salivary gland. *J. Vet. Dent.* 13 (2): 61–64.

2

Oral Examination and Diagnosis

Jan Bellows

All Pets Dental, Weston, FL, USA

2.1 Introduction

Oral and dental pathology is a common finding in companion animals. In many cases, when detected by the owner, the disease will be well advanced and obvious at presentation, while others are more obscure, requiring further diagnostics. Signs and symptoms may indicate oral disease to be primary or secondary in nature [1]. A thorough examination in coordination with a suitable knowledge of anatomy and function is the basis for diagnostic ability. Proper examination and accurate diagnosis is the first step to appropriate treatment and preventative care planning. Clinically, oral diagnosis is a seven-part interactive process of history, whole body physical examination, facial exam, initial oral survey, preanesthesia diagnostic testing, in-depth oral examination, and oral diagnostic testing [2].

2.2 Oral Diagnosis

2.2.1 History

The gathering of history is the foundation of a proper care. It relies on the owner's direct personal involvement and provides information that can be an invaluable aid in directing the full examination. In addition, the history is the link between all other parts of the physical, oral, and laboratory examination. A complete history should provide vaccination status, details of diet, appetite, water consumption, levels of professional and home dental care, past disease problems and treatments, current problems and treatments in progress, exposure to infectious diseases, traumatic incidents, and behavioral changes, all of which may help the clinician fully evaluate every aspect of the animal's general health. Signalment of age, breed, and sex is always the starting point. History encompasses past and present information concerning the individual, family line, other household pets, and breed characteristics. Additionally, medications previously and currently being taken should be recorded, both for general information and avoiding adverse reaction problems [3–5].

Once significant general data are obtained, information more specific to oral and dental pathology should be closely scrutinized. Information of actual oral symptoms should include onset, duration, degree of severity, and recurrence profile [6]. Details of type of diet, water additives, chew toys, and eating habits should be scrutinized. Additionally, history of chronic cough, regurgitation, vomiting, and skin allergies yield important information in that those conditions produce effects on the oral cavity.

Questions with respect to the patient's hesitancy to pick up, chew, or swallow food can provide significant information. Has the animal been observed to drop food, toys, or training articles from the mouth? Has quivering of the jaw or chattering of the teeth been noticed, especially while training articles are in the mouth? What are the training articles and of what are they made? Sensitive teeth more commonly react to metals, from both thermal and galvanic stimulus. Food shifted to or chewed primarily on one side or a preference for soft food may be a sign of periodontal or endodontic disease. Hesitancy in swallowing food can be due to oral inflammations, neoplasia, ulcers, sensitive teeth, tonsillitis, and foreign bodies.

Inappetence and anorexia are associated with general disease processes, as well as signs of oral ulceration, inflammation, and pulp exposure within the oral cavity [6]. True anorexia is uncommon in oral disease, except in cases of severe pain. In such cases, systemic disease should first be ruled out. Oral pain can additionally result in pawing at, tilting, bobbing, shaking, and sliding of the head and mouth along the floor. Differential diagnosis of these signs include pathology of the skin, lips, ears, eyes, salivary glands, and central nervous system.

Wiggs's Veterinary Dentistry: Principles and Practice, Second Edition. Edited by Heidi B. Lobprise and Johnathon R. (Bert) Dodd.

One of the most commonly reported signs of oral disease is simply bad breath or halitosis. This condition is reported more frequently in house pets, probably due to their close contact with owners. Periodontal disease is the most common cause of halitosis [7], which occurs due to the bacterial breakdown of food and other materials in gingival pockets. Other causes of oral malodor are stomatitis, tumors, cleft palates, cleft lips, oronasal and oroantral fistulas, and foreign bodies. Differential diagnosis should include uremia, sinusitis, gastrointestinal problems, respiratory diseases, nasal disorders, diet, lip fold pyoderma, and lesions caused by licking or chewing abscesses or infected anal glands.

Clicking or popping noises noticed during jaw movement is typically associated with problems with the temporomandibular joint (TMJ), or the coronoid process and zygomatic arch [8–10]. Differential diagnoses can be dental, jaw, or palatal fractures.

Acute or chronic oral pain associated with mandibular movement or open mouth behavior can be related to numerous oral problems. Differential diagnoses include dental, jaw or palatal fractures, myositis, foreign bodies, mandibular neuropraxia, salivary gland disease, craniomandibular osteopathy, severe stomatitis, acute necrotizing ulcerative gingivitis (ANUG), contact mucositis (chronic ulcerative paradental stomatitis (CUPS)) or kissing ulcers, tumors, TMJ disease, or coronoid process problems with the zygomatic arch [6, 8–10].

Chronic ptyalism or drooling is most commonly caused by a reluctance or inability to swallow rather than increased salivary flow or production [6]. Acute endodontic exposure, severe inflammatory disease or ulceration of any of the oral mucosae, and foreign bodies are more common oral causes. Other causes can be systemic bacterial infections such as leptospirosis and viral diseases such as rabies and the feline upper respiratory infections. Toxins can also result in acute excessive salivation; examples are man-made organophosphates and animal toxins from the toad *Bufo marinus*. Heat and excitement can also result in ptyalism, but this is generally acute in onset without other obvious symptoms.

Facial swellings, edema, draining tracts, or bleeding from the mouth, nose, or facial area can have oral origins. Endodontic, periodontal, salivary disease, or trauma can result in these symptoms. Differential problems are insect and snake bites, allergic reactions, tumors, hematomas, and subcutaneous air [2, 6].

2.2.2 General Physical Examination

The external physical examination should never be overlooked in the attempt to press on to more obvious oral problems. Flea and skin allergies may lead to hair chewing, resulting in attrition of the incisors with loose hair tangled around teeth, acting to retain debris and to enhance an environment for periodontitis [2]. Excessive panting is often noticed in small breed dogs due to sublingual granulomas (gum chewing lesions). Auscult the heart and lungs for soundness as these are the most common areas to result in complicating factors associated with sedation or anesthesia used in the in-depth oral exam, dental scaling, and oral treatments [2].

2.2.2.1 Facial Exam

Closely observe the face, mandible, and head for swellings that can indicate neoplastic enlargements, cellulitis, or abscesses [2, 7, 11–16]. Cellulitis and abscessation can be due to foreign bodies, fight wounds, periodontal disease, or endodontic disorders (Figure 2.1). Fistulous tracts may be present with or without serous or purulent drainage according to the cycle of disease. Neoplasia and eosinophilic granuloma complexes may result in raised ulcerative lesions of the lip, gingiva, or enlargement of the mandibular lymph nodes [6]. Always palpate the lymph nodes and salivary glands in the head and neck region for enlargement or indications of pain.

Asymmetry of the face or head can be seen in hereditary or congenital abnormalities, inflammatory disease, neoplasia, dislocations, fractures, and nerve damage (Figure 2.2). Some of the more common of these in the cat are dislocation of the TMJ and maxillary or mandibular fractures and in the dog allergic responses and mandibular/maxillary asymmetry [8, 9]. Open mouth disorders are usually a result of trauma to the joint (TMJ), maxillary or mandibular bones (fractures), or nerve damage or disease [8–10].

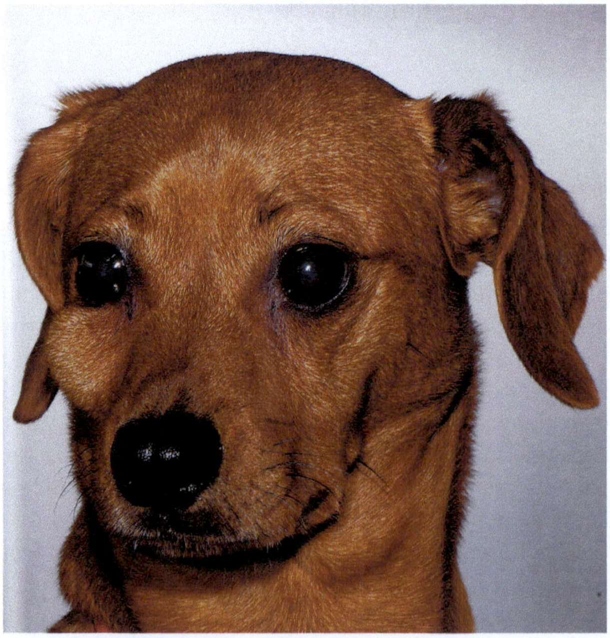

Figure 2.1 Swelling beneath the right eye secondary to endodontic disease.

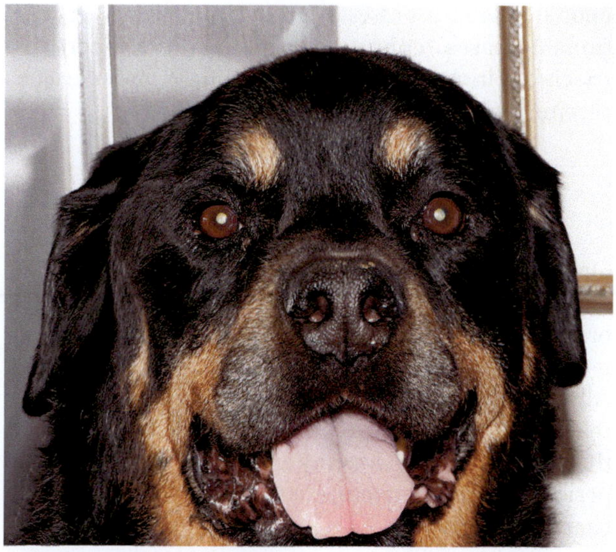

Figure 2.2 Decreased right-sided temporal muscle mass secondary to masticatory myositis.

2.2.3 Initial Oral Survey

The initial oral survey is generally performed in the exam room following the physical examination, but normally without the aid of sedation or anesthesia (Figure 2.3). Correct assessment of an animal's oral and dental health relies on familiarity with normal anatomy. The amount of information that can be obtained varies greatly from individual to individual based upon the animal's temperament and the owner's ability to properly and adequately restrain the pet. A well-trained technician can many times facilitate this process better than the owner, although they will typically need to be present to elaborate on the primary complaint. A detailed systematic approach is necessary for a complete oral examination [17, 18]. Head type and symmetry, swellings, draining lesions, and occlusal evaluation is always the beginning point of the oral examination.

Start with the lips and commissures. Examine for masses, pyoderma, or tumors. Lift the lips with the thumb and forefinger and examine the exposed teeth and mucosae. Note malocclusions (mandibular mesioclusion, mandibular distoclusion, mandibular and maxillary asymmetry) and then progress to an open mouth examination if the patient safely allows.

There are several ways to adequately open and examine the mouth. The most common is an overhand technique with the palm over the bridge of the nose and the thumb behind the canine tooth on one side and the index finger behind the canine tooth on the opposite side. The opposite hand grasps the mandible from below with the forefinger and thumb to either side and the index finger placed on the incisors and used to leverage the mouth open. Care should be exerted in trauma and severe periodontal cases as theses jaws can be easily fractured. Evaluate the mucous membranes for color, perfusion time, petechia, moistness, ulcerations, lacerations, or swellings. Examine the gingivae for color, inflammation, hyperplasia, recession, sulcal exudate, clinical sulcal bleeding, normal architecture, and the presence of swellings or tumors. Inspect the teeth for malposition fractures, discoloration, calculus, plaque, mobility, caries, cervical line lesions, and developmental defects. The buccal surfaces can generally be examined on the alert pet and the lingual surfaces under sedation. The roof of the mouth should be examined for swellings, defects, foreign bodies, rugae symmetry or loss of rugae. The tongue should be mobile and with good strength. Inspection of the

Figure 2.3 Examination of the lips and face.

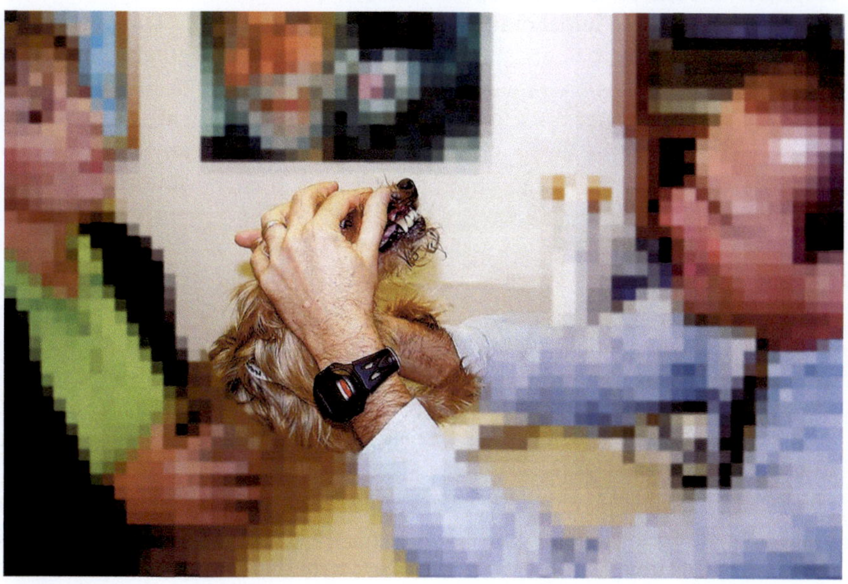

ventral tongue can be facilitated by pushing a finger up into the ventral intermandibular space [6]. Always check under the tongue for tumors, lacerations, ulcerations, and foreign bodies. The salivary papillae should be free of inflammation and patent. Patency can sometimes be difficult to assess without passing a catheter, but in some cases by placing light pressure caudal to the papilla and rolling the finger towards the duct, saliva may be expressed. Observe also for halitosis, oral bleeding, epistaxis, rhinitis, and the condition and strength of the masticatory muscles.

2.2.3.1 Periodontal Disease Test Strips/Thio Levels

Test strips detect changes in gingival health that cannot be seen by visual inspection without anesthetizing the patient. The strips measure the concentration of thiols generated by anaerobic bacteria associated with periodontal disease. Studies have shown that when periodontal health declines, anaerobic bacteria proliferate as periodontal pocket depth increases. The concentration of thiols in gingival crevicular fluid (GCF) increases as periodontal disease increases.

The test strip is rubbed along the gingival margin to collect an oral fluid sample on to a pad located on the end of the strip (Figure 2.4). Once removed, within 10 seconds, the pad will change color if elevated thiol levels are present. The result is compared to a color chart to determine the concentration of thiols, indicating disease activity.

2.2.4 Pre-anesthesia Diagnostic Testing

The pre-anesthesia diagnostic testing is performed in order to reduce the risk of pathological and physiological complications during or following induction [2, 6]. Testing emphasis should be directed by the history, physical examination, and the initial oral survey. Tests are based upon the clinician's assessment of the individual. In questionable cases, consultation with a board-certified specialist in internal medicine and or anesthesia is recommended.

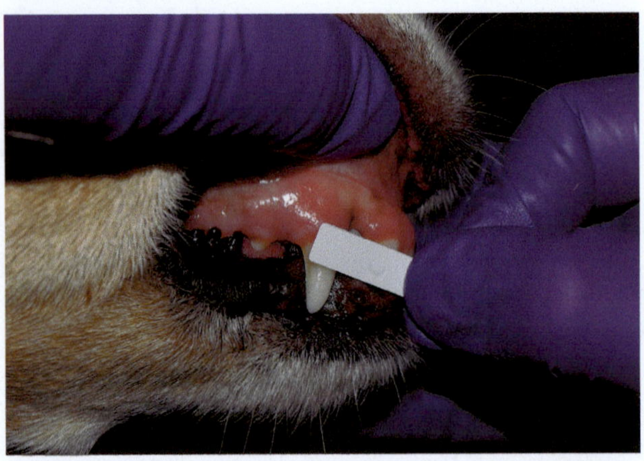

Figure 2.4 The test strip is rubbed along the gingival margin to collect an oral fluid sample on a pad located on the end of the strip.

2.2.5 In-depth Oral Examination and Charting

Once available information has been correlated, the in-depth oral examination can begin. A complete in-depth oral examination can only properly be performed on an intubated patient under general anesthesia (Figure 2.5). All information discussed within the initial oral survey that was not obtained in full detail should be acquired at this time. This should incorporate the oral examination, periodontal examination, dental examination, and the charting process [19].

2.2.5.1 Periodontal Disease

Periodontal disease is initiated when the bacteria in the mouth collects with a matrix of salivary glycoproteins and extracellular polysaccharides to form plaque that adheres to the tooth surface [11]. After a period of time, the plaque will mineralize to form calculus [7, 11–13]. As the plaque contacts the attached gingiva, the bacteria and byproducts, joined later by the body's own immune response, can cause inflammation, infection, and eventually destruction of tissues [20, 21]. At first, the supragingival plaque bacteria are Gram positive, non-motile, aerobic cocci, but as the infection progresses deeper into the sulcus, Gram negative, motile, anaerobic rods predominate. The signs of periodontal disease include edema and inflammation of the gingiva, plaque and calculus deposition, halitosis, gingival bleeding when probed, ulceration, gingival recession, bone loss, mobile teeth, and tooth loss [22, 23].

The gingival sulcus is a groove or space between the gingival margin and the tooth and can be up to 1–3 mm in depth in the normal dog. The gingival margin of a cat is usually so closely associated with the tooth that any sulcus deeper than 0.5 mm may be considered abnormal [24].

The gingival sulcus should be examined with a periodontal probe for abnormal pocket depths and with an explorer for indications of tooth resorption, subgingival plaque, and calculus (Figure 2.6). The sulcus depth should be checked at four to six sites around the tooth, and variations from normal recorded on the animal's chart (see Section 2.3 on Charting). Limited direct observation in the sulcus can be obtained by using a three-way air water syringe. The air can be used to gently blow the sulcus open to look inside. Additionally, thin pieces of calculus may appear as chalky white areas when the air is blown across them.

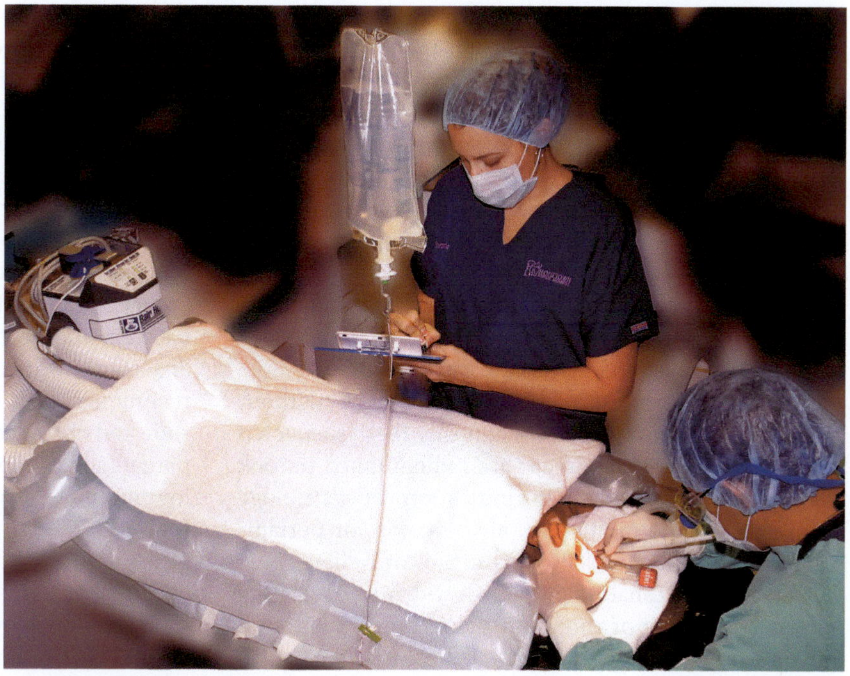

Figure 2.5 General anesthesia is necessary to be able to perform a complete dental examination.

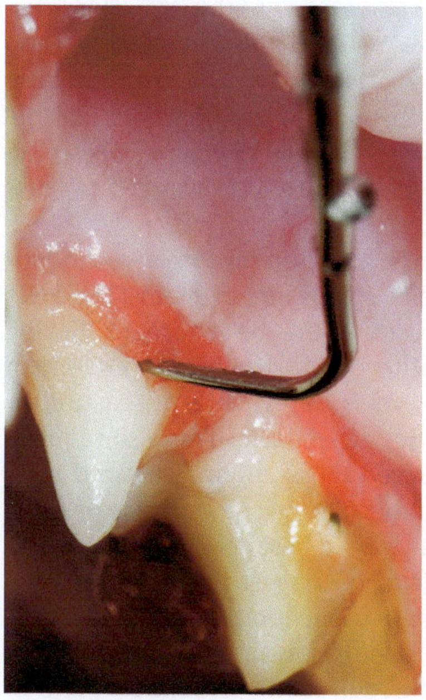

Figure 2.6 Explorer used to identify tooth resorption.

The furcation is the site where two roots separate from the body of the tooth. In multirooted teeth, furcations are common areas of attachment loss and periodontal disease occurrence. Exposure of furcations and degree of exposure should be recorded (see Chapter 5 – Periodontology).

2.2.5.2 Endodontic Disease

Endodontic disease, although not as common as periodontal disease, is common in the dog and cat [14]. While some manifestations are significant indications of pulpal pathology, other endodontically compromised teeth are less obvious in their symptoms. A complete endodontic examination includes visual inspection and radiographic assessment. This assists in the diagnosis of the lesion and its localization to the area of origin [25, 26]. As in all veterinary cases, a thorough medical and dental history is needed to assess both the localized problem and the overall health of the patient. Specifically, any previous indication of oral discomfort, possible dental abscessation or facial trauma may warrant further investigation.

The most obvious sign of endodontic pathology seen by the owner or the veterinarian will be a fractured tooth, whether just a crack or split, or up to partial loss of the crown with exposed canal. If the fracture is recent, the exposed pulp may appear pink or edematous, or hemorrhage may be present. These teeth can be painful, so palpation should be attempted with care. Once the pulp has necrosed and the nerve has died, the tooth should not be acutely sensitive, and a dark spot will indicate the canal opening. Teeth that have sustained enough trauma to disrupt the apical blood supply or cause irreversible pulpitis appear intact but discolored as the inflammatory byproducts leach into the dentinal tubules. An injured tooth that initially appears pink will turn purple to gray or beige later. As the pathology of the infection progresses, various indications of abscessation may become apparent. Mucosal swelling or discoloration, facial swelling, and fistulous tracts may appear, depending on the site of the problem.

Palpating the defect with an endodontic explorer or pathfinder is sometimes possible in the awake patient, but full assessment will require general anesthesia. Checking for mobility of teeth fragments and the tooth proper, as well as gently spreading the cracks to see if they extend vertically, are helpful palpation practices that dictate therapy options. Placing a cold material in contact with various teeth to elicit an exaggerated response is one further test, but is most reliable in a calm, awake patient or one mildly sedated. Water or gelatin from a freezer bag can be frozen in a tuberculin syringe with the tip cut off to make a cold tester.

Endodontic examination is not complete without proper radiographs for valid diagnosis. Teeth suspected of having endodontic disease are radiographed to look for periapical lucency, an indication of pathology including apical granulomas, abscessation, or periapical cysts. The films are also examined for radiographic evidence of root canal/pulp chamber widening, indicating internal resorption or a non-vital pulp. Transillumination of the teeth (shining a bright light through the tooth) can help in the assessment of pulp vitality. If the pulp is non-vital, the light should not transmit well through the tooth. Periodontal support is also indirectly evaluated radiographically to help decide the best treatment option.

2.2.5.3 Temporomandibular Joint

Problems with the TMJ can be difficult to assess at times [8–10]. Radiographs can give much information if the suitable positioning can be attained (see Chapter 3 – Oral Radiology and Imaging). Palpation while manipulating the joint may produce crepitus. A stethoscope can be placed over the TMJ during manipulation to listen for crepitation. Also palpate the zygomatic arch area during manipulation to evaluate if the coronoid process is flaring lateral to the arch that would cause locking, popping, or inflammatory trauma to the area.

2.2.6 Oral Diagnostic Testing

Based upon this information, additional oral diagnostic tests may be considered. Among these are cultures and sensitivities, biopsy and histopathology, transillumination, thermal tests, electronic vitality testing, oral and intraoral radiographs, and GCF tests. Oral and intraoral radiographs and techniques are addressed in the chapter on radiology in detail and will only be lightly addressed here (see Chapter 3 – Oral Radiology and Imaging).

To date, oral culture and sensitivities have not been shown to be of significant importance in the dog and cat [27]. It is rare that sensitivities are called for in endodontic infections as exodontics (extraction) and standard endodontics (root canal therapy) are generally curative. For stomatitis and periodontitis, multiple bacterial isolates are common and expected even in healthy animals, as a large and diverse flora is always present [28–35]. Little research has been performed on the pathogenicity of oral flora in the dog and cat. Bacteria is commonly found on the dorsum of the tongue shortly after birth. As teeth erupt, bacteria will be found colonizing tooth plaque, with the largest populations typically located in the sulcus [36]. It is believed that the most pathogenic bacteria in the oral cavity are motile flagellates and anaerobes, which are rarely detected by routine culture techniques. Small amounts of GCF can be placed on a slide and observed under phase contrast for an estimated percentage of motile bacteria [37]. Typically GCF has a low number of motile bacteria, while in active disease (periodontitis), the GCF typically reveals higher counts. One problem with this is that periodontal disease is cyclic in activity; even in advanced periodontal disease the infection may be inactive at the time of sampling. Oral fungal cultures can be useful in confirmation of *Monilia albicans*, and occasionally disclose the presence of various systemic mycoses contributing to oral lesions. Viral isolate techniques require active viral shedding and can give useful information in some cases, but little data are available on the normal oral viral flora for the dog or cat. A degree of research has been performed on rhinotracheitis and calicivirus infections and oral lesions in cats [38–40].

Thermal tests are typically used for location of sensitive and endodontically compromised teeth [25]. Heat or cold is applied directly to the tooth without making contact with any other oral structures. The main dilemma with these tests is the reliance of reaction by the patient, which is not dependable. This also requires the tests to be performed on an un-anesthetized individual. Reaction to cold may suggest a sensitive or compromised tooth. Sensitivity to heat generally indicates a more serious problem of irreversible pulpitis and impending devitalization of the tooth.

Transillumination is the use of light to examine the reflectivity of the internal tooth structures [41]. In healthy teeth light passes through fairly well, while in devitalized teeth a more opaque effect may be seen. It is best to compare teeth within the same mouth as control guides. Electronic pulp testers have not at this time shown a great deal of reliability in the dog and cat, but new developments in electrical resistance testing may provide precise and reliable instruments in the very near future [42].

GCF tests make use of sulcular fluid samples. Many are currently in use in man and include elastase, AST (aspartate aminotransferase), ALT (alanine aminotransferase), or cellular identification studies [40, 41, 43–48].

Of these tests only GCF/AST has shown any indication to date of being a reliable indicator of periodontitis in the dog and cat [37, 49–51]. Additional research will be necessary to determine the clinical practicality of any of these tests.

Examination of oral lesions microscopically often determines their exact cause, thus dictating further care. Fine needle aspiration and/or touch impression for cytology can be most helpful in determining if an oral lesion is inflammatory or neoplastic. With cytology positive results are diagnostic, where negative results may not be due to sampling errors or poor exfoliation of some lesions.

Incisional biopsy allows for diagnosis prior to complete lesion removal and the determination of the necessity for more radical treatment (maxillectomies, mandibulectomies, radiation therapy, chemotherapy, etc.) before addressing therapy. Such procedures may irritate some lesions, stimulating them to grow, spread, or metastasize [6]. Therefore, incisional biopsy should be selected on those cases where such an occurrence would hopefully not be of serious significance. For this reason, many practitioners will elect to proceed with excisional biopsy. In these cases, the lesion is removed to well beyond the margins in all directions in the hope of total removal. All, or a representative portion, of the tumor is then submitted for histopathology, and determination of the need for additional surgery or therapy.

With most lesions the biopsy should be full depth and include some of the normal margin for reliability. Some lesions such as fibrosarcoma may extend below apparently normal structures, and failure to penetrate these may lead to misdiagnosis. As in all procedures, thought should be given to the tissues, vessels, ducts, canals, nerves, and organs that may run through or deep to lesions, and every precaution taken to avoid unnecessary complications. Biopsy punches are helpful in many cases of incisional biopsy to obtain samples of good depth. Routine tissues collected should be placed in 10% neutral buffered formalin solution once removed for proper fixing. If too large a specimen is placed in the formalin solution, cells deep within the sample may not properly fix.

In lesions suspected of autoimmune involvement, Michel's solution should be used for preservation of the sample rather than formalin. These biopsy samples should be selected from the most active and intact epithelial vesiculation or pocketed serum-like lesions. The margins should also include apparently normal adjacent tissue for comparative histology.

The pathologist can frequently provide a more reliable diagnosis and prognosis when relevant clinical data are provided with the specimen. Standard signalment should be provided, plus location, duration, symptoms, previous biopsy information, and other pertinent history. Most pathologists can be directly contacted for supplementary consultation on cases, which can be informative and educational. Photographic images of the lesions submitted with the tissues is also helpful to the pathologist.

2.3 Oral and Dental Charting

Dental charting provides a graphic report of the patient's teeth and mouth. A blank dental chart depicts anatomically correct maxillary and mandibular teeth with space to note abnormalities. Charting provides a place to record examination findings in order to develop an accurate and comprehensive treatment plan, as well as a thorough record of past treatments.

To evaluate each tooth individually for charting, complete immobilization (general anesthesia) is necessary. The mouth is generally charted before scaling and can be re-charted when a significant amount of calculus has been removed.

Chart formats vary from paperless electronic files incorporated in proprietary veterinary software programs to handwritten paper forms. Whichever system is used, the dental chart should include areas to record the dental history, skull type (brachycephalic, mesaticephalic, dolichocephalic), oral pathology, including the amount and location of plaque and calculus, probing depths, fractured and mobile teeth, oral masses, and radiographic findings. Additionally, therapy provided, recommended therapy but not provided, as well as the future treatment plan and home care instructions should be noted on the dental chart and medical record. Charts should be species specific (Figures 2.7–2.9).

Four-handed (two-person) charting is the fastest and most efficient. One person examines the mouth and the other records information on the chart. For example, the examiner begins by saying "one hundred series" and "101" (which is the maxillary right first incisor according to the modified Triadan system of tooth identification), noting any abnormalities and then moving distally until the right maxillary quadrant is completed. The right mandibular quadrant (four hundred series) follows, the endotracheal tube attachment to the anesthetic machine is detached, the animal's body and head are rotated, the anesthetic machine is reattached to the endotracheal tube, and evaluation and charting of the two and three hundred series is completed. Each tooth is examined completely, including periodontal probing, before the next tooth is viewed. Only abnormalities are noted on the dental chart.

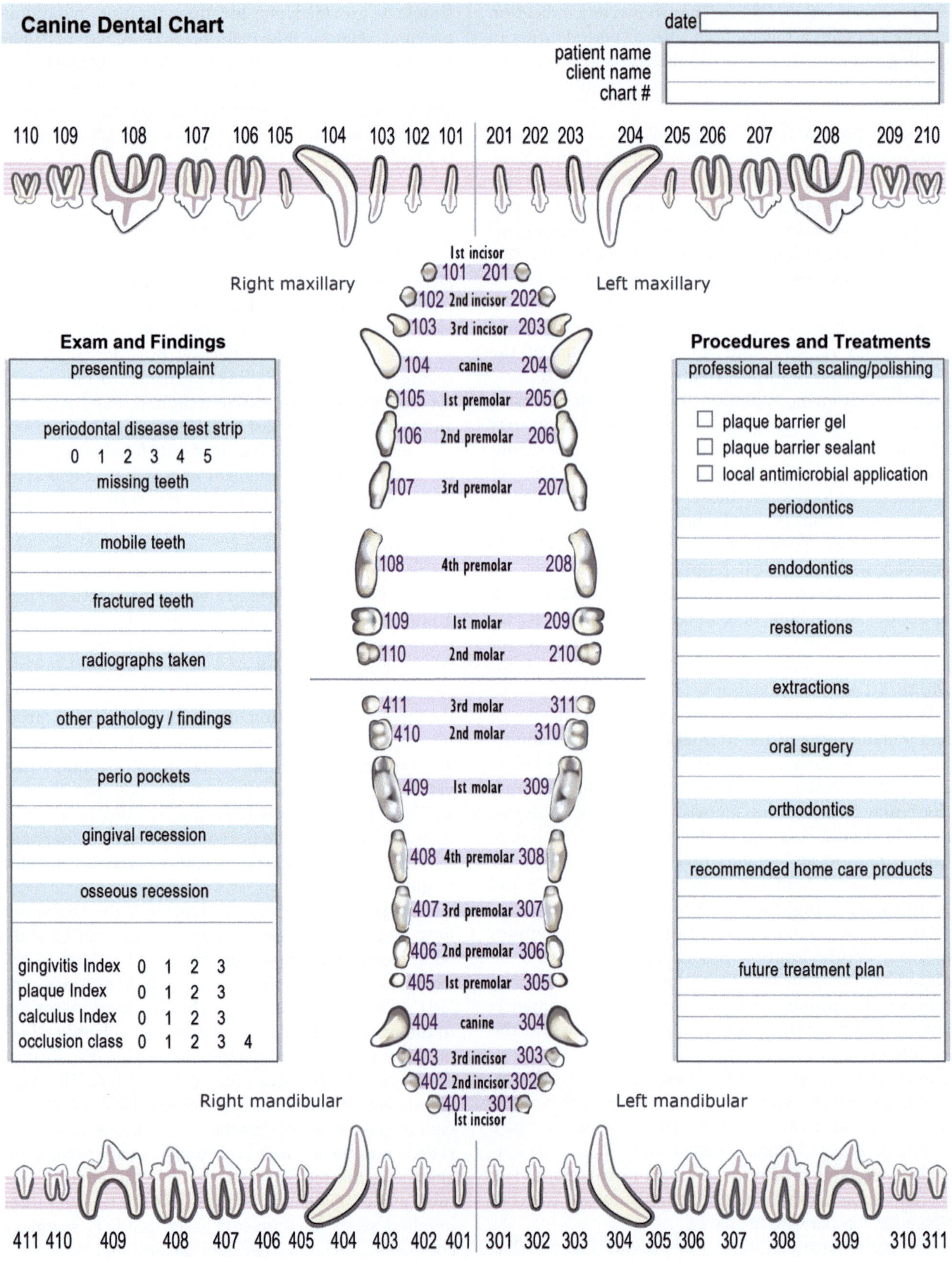

Figure 2.7 Canine Dental Chart example. © Veterinary Information Network/Design by Tamara.

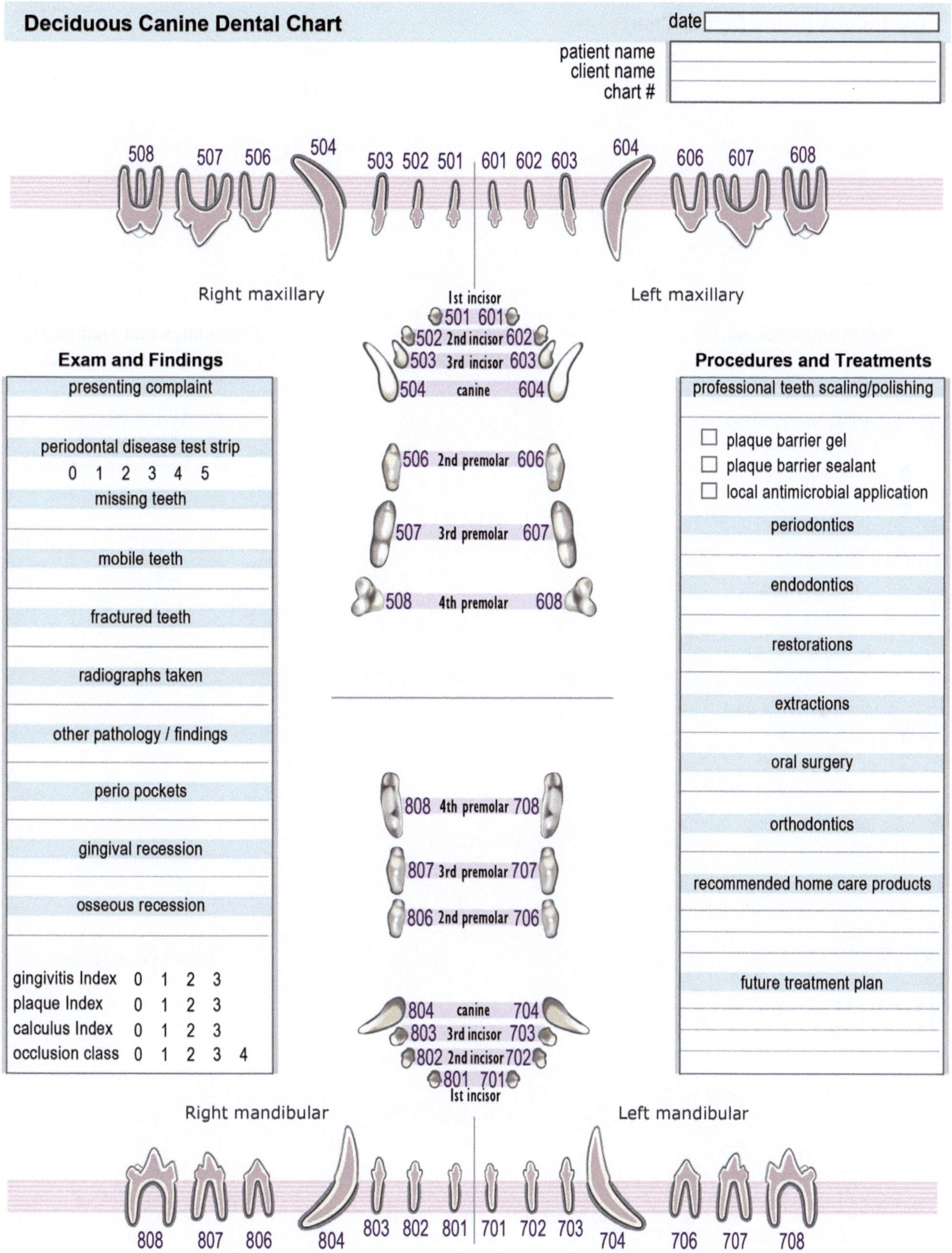

Figure 2.8 Deciduous Canine Dental Chart example. © Veterinary Information Network/Design by Tamara.

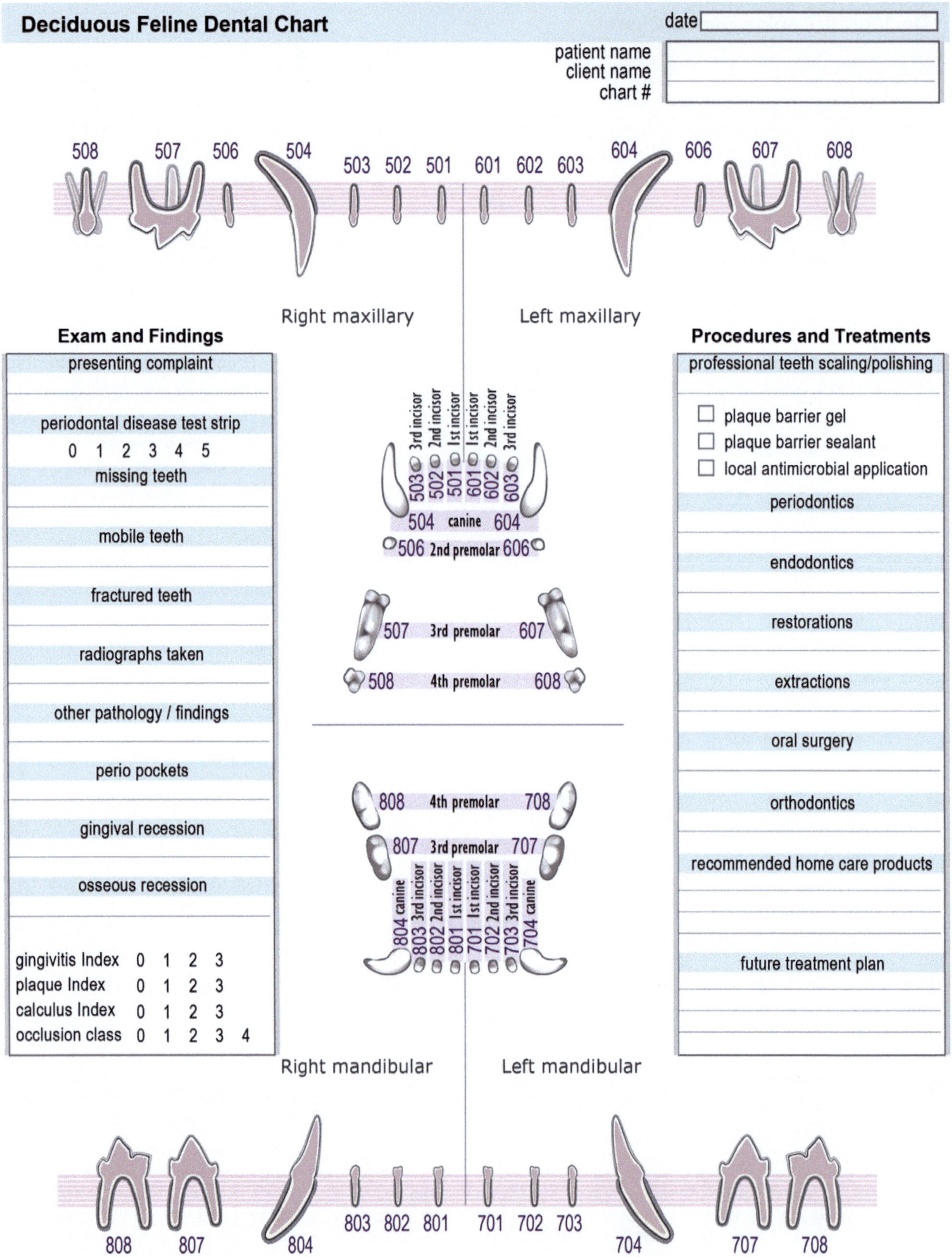

Figure 2.9 Deciduous Feline Dental Chart example. © Veterinary Information Network/Design by Tamara.

2.4 Charting Steps

1) Examine the occlusion rostrally and caudally before intubation and record any abnormalities. Normally the teeth of the opposing arches in cats do not touch.
2) After intubation, examine the mouth for missing teeth and circle all visibly missing teeth on the dental chart. The most commonly missing tooth is the mandibular third premolar.
3) Record obviously fractured teeth.
4) Check for tooth mobility using an instrument handle pressed against the tooth. Record abnormal mobility (M1, M2, M3).
5) Record areas of calculus accumulation.
6) Record abnormal probing depths or attachment levels around each tooth.
7) Expose and process dental radiographs.
8) Scale and polish the teeth.
9) Re-probe if a significant amount of calculus was removed.
10) Formulate a treatment plan through tooth-by-tooth evaluation; draw a diagonal line through teeth that need to be extracted.
11) Calculate fees for the treatment plan and contact the owner for approval while the technician is completing the teeth cleaning process.
12) Once the owner approves, perform needed therapy and record all care on the dental chart.

2.5 Charting Shorthand (www.avdc.org)

The abbreviations (in alphabetical order) following Table 2.1 were adapted from the American Veterinary Dental College. Below the table are extended definitions of some of the terms.

Expanded Definitions of Some Terms

Abrasion (AB). A pathologic wearing-away of dental hard tissue by the friction of a foreign body independent of occlusion. Examples: tennis balls (dirt gets trapped in the fiber, the dog chews or spins the ball in its mouth, and wears down the tooth surface), hair coat, metal furniture.

Carious lesion (CA). Also called a cavity. Most commonly occurs in the molar pits of large dogs. Appears as crater-like lesions.

Enamel hypoplasia (EH). A condition where the enamel is thin or absent. An incomplete or defective development of enamel. In dogs, this is usually caused by a febrile disease some time before the animal was six months old, as the enamel was forming. Initially enamel hypoplasia appears as areas of normal shiny enamel surrounded by opaque areas. Later the opaque areas become stained a brownish color.

Fusion (FU). Union of two teeth buds. The root canals may be separate or joined. Clinically there is one less tooth in the arch. Radiographically there will be two roots with one crown.

FX fractured tooth (T/FX)

- *Enamel infraction (T/FX/EI).* A crack in the enamel that does not enter dentin nor result in loss of tooth substance.
- *Enamel fracture (T/FX/E).* Fracture in which the crown substance is lost, limited to enamel.
- *Uncomplicated crown fracture (T/FX/UCF).* A fracture of the enamel and dentin not involving the pulp. In veterinary species, the types of dental tissue involved in a crown fracture can vary with the species and can include enamel, cementum, and dentin.
- *Complicated crown fracture (T/FX/CCF).* A fracture involving enamel and dentin and exposing the pulp.
- *Uncomplicated crown-root fracture (T/FX/UCRF).* A fracture involving enamel, dentin, and cementum, but not exposing the pulp.
- *Complicated crown-root fracture (T/FX/CCRF).* A fracture involving enamel, dentin, and cementum, and exposing the pulp.
- *Root fracture (T/FX/R).* A fracture involving only the root.

Gemination (G). The division of a single tooth at the time of development, resulting in the incomplete formation of two teeth. On radiographs, there will be one root with a split crown. Clinically there will be an extra tooth in the arch.

Gingival hyperplasia (GH). Proliferation of the attached gingiva. It is an overgrowth of the gingiva above the cementoenamel junction (CEJ).

3D-reparative or sclerotic dentin. Dentin formed as a defense mechanism in reaction to various stimuli. The defect caused by injury, covered by harder dentin than normal. Dental tubules are obliterated by deposits of calcium salts that are harder and denser than normal dentin. Sclerotic dentin appears transparent.

For further terms see Tables 2.2–2.6.

Table 2.1 AVDC abbreviations – oral examination and diagnosis (www.avdc.org).

AB		Abrasion – a pathologic wearing-away of dental hard tissue by the friction of a foreign body independent of occlusion
AT		Attrition – a pathological wearing-away of the tooth caused by an opposing tooth
AV		Avulsion – see T/A
CA		Caries
C		Calculus – see indices
CR	CRD	Crowding
CR/M		Metal crown (full)
D		Discolored tooth – pulpitis
DT		Deciduous tooth
	DT/P	Deciduous tooth: persistent
E		Enamel
	E/D	Enamel defect
	E/H	Enamel hypoplasia – a condition where the enamel is thin or absent
	E/HM	Enamel hypomineralization
FI		Furcation index – see indices
FU		Fusion – see T/FUS
FX		Fractured tooth – see T/F below
G		Gemination – see T/GEM below
GH		Gingival hyperplasia – proliferation of the attached gingiva
GR		Gingival (gum) recession – areas where the gingival margin is below the cementoenamel junction (CEJ)
GV		Gingivectomy/gingivoplasty
I		Impacted – see T/I below
LB		Level bite – the maxillary and mandibular incisors meet at the incisal edges
M		Tooth mobility index – see indices
MAL		Malocclusion – see Chapter 19 – Occlusion and Orthodontics
NE		Near pulp exposure – see T/NE below
O		(Circled) – missing tooth
OM		Oral/maxillofacial mass
ONF		Oronasal fistula – an abnormal communication between the mouth and nasal cavity
PD		Periodontal disease – see indices
PE		Pulpal exposure – see T/PE below – opening of the pulp to the outside environment
PP		Periodontal pocket
PU		Pulpitis – inflammation of the pulp resulting in the discoloration of the tooth
R	ROT	Rotated tooth – usually secondary to tooth crowding; most commonly affected are the maxillary premolars
R		Restoration
	R/C	Restoration – composite
	R/M	Restoration – metallic crown – see CR/M above
RCT		Root canal therapy
RD		Retained deciduous teeth – see DT/P above – primary teeth that have not been shed when the secondary (permanent) teeth erupt
RP		Root planing
	RP/C	Root planing, closed
	RP/O	Root planing, open
RTR		Retained root or reserved crown – areas where the crown is no longer apparent but root(s) remain
S		Supernumerary teeth – see T/SN below – extra teeth, most commonly the first premolars or incisors
3D		Reparative or sclerotic dentin: dentin formed as a defense mechanism

Table 2.1 (Continued)

SE		Supereruption – a condition where teeth have the cementoenamel junction (CEF) erupted above normal
ST		Stomatitis
	ST/CS	Stomatitis – caudal stomatitis
SYM		Symphysis
	SYM/S	Symphyseal separation
T		Tooth
	T/A	Avulsed tooth – separation of a tooth from its alveolus
	T/FX	Fractured tooth
	T/FX/EI	Enamel infraction
	T/FX/EF	Enamel fracture
	T/FX/UCF	Uncomplicated crown fracture
	T/FX/CCF	Complicated crown fracture
	T/FX/UCRF	Uncomplicated crown-root fracture
	T/FX/CCRF	Complicated crown-root fracture
	T/FX/R	Root fracture
	T/FU	Fusion
	T/GEM	Gemination tooth
	T/NE	Near pulp exposure
	T/PE	Pulp exposure
	T/U	Unerupted tooth – tooth that has not perforated the oral mucosa
	T/E	Embedded tooth – unerupted tooth covered in bone whose eruption is compromised by lack of eruptive force
	T/I	Impacted tooth – unerupted or partially erupted tooth whose eruption is prevented by contact with a physical barrier
TMJ		Temporomandibular joint
	TMJ/D	TMJ dysplasia
	TMJ/FX	TMJ fracture
	TMJ/LUX	TMJ luxation
TR		Tooth resorption – see indices
W		Worn tooth – usually secondary to abrasion from grinding or wearing-away of tooth substance from mastication
WF		Wear facet – a flattened, highly polished area on the tooth's surface from sclerotic dentin
X		Closed extraction of a tooth (without sectioning)
XS		Closed extraction of a tooth with sectioning
XSS		Open extraction of a tooth

(Additional abbreviations are available at the AVDC website and in other chapters, including Chapter 8 – General Oral Pathology.)

Table 2.2 Periodontal Disease Index – the degree of severity of periodontal disease relates to a single tooth; a patient may have teeth that have different stages of periodontal disease (www.avdc.org).

Normal	PD 0	Clinically normal – no gingival inflammation or periodontitis clinically evident.
Stage 1	PD 1	Gingivitis only without attachment loss. The height and architecture of the alveolar margin are normal.
Stage 2	PD 2	Early periodontitis – less than 25% of attachment loss or, at most, there is a stage 1 furcation involvement in multirooted teeth. There are early radiologic signs of periodontitis. The loss of periodontal attachment is less than 25% as measured either by probing of the clinical attachment level or radiographic determination of the distance of the alveolar margin from the cementoenamel junction relative to the length of the root.
Stage 3	PD 3	Moderate periodontitis – 25–50% of attachment loss as measured either by probing of the clinical attachment level, radiographic determination of the distance of the alveolar margin from the cementoenamel junction relative to the length of the root, or there is a stage 2 furcation involvement in multirooted teeth.
Stage 4	PD 4	Advanced periodontitis – more than 50% of attachment loss as measured either by probing of the clinical attachment level or radiographic determination of the distance of the alveolar margin from the cementoenamel junction relative to the length of the root, or there is a stage 3 furcation involvement in multirooted teeth.

Table 2.3 Calculus Index (www.avdc.org).

CI 1 – C/sl	Calculus slight	Scattered calculus covering less than one-third of the buccal tooth surface
CI 2 – C/mod	Calculus moderate	Calculus covering between one- and two-thirds of the buccal tooth surface with minimal subgingival deposition
CI 3 – C/h	Calculus heavy	Calculus covering greater than two-thirds of the buccal tooth surface and extending subgingivally

Table 2.4 Furcation Involvement/Exposure Index – FI (www.avdc.org).

Stage 1	F1, furcation involvement	Exists when a periodontal probe extends less than halfway under the crown in any direction of a multirooted tooth with attachment loss.
Stage 2	F2, furcation involvement	Exists when a periodontal probe extends greater than halfway under the crown of a multirooted tooth with attachment loss but not through and through.
Stage 3	F3, furcation involvement	Exists when a periodontal probe extends under the crown of a multirooted tooth, through and through from one side of the furcation out the other.

Table 2.5 Tooth Mobility Index (www.avdc.org).

Stage 0	M0	Physiologic mobility up to 0.2 mm.
Stage 1	M1	The mobility is increased in any direction other than axial over a distance of more than 0.2 mm and up to 0.5 mm.
Stage 2	M2	The mobility is increased in any direction other than axial over a distance of more than 0.5 mm and up to 1.0 mm.
Stage 3	M3	The mobility is increased in any direction than axial over a distance exceeding 1.0 mm or any axial movement.

Table 2.6 Tooth Resorption (TR) Staging Index (www.avdc.org).

TR1	TR Stage 1	Mild dental hard tissue loss (cementum or cementum and enamel).
TR2	TR Stage 2	Moderate dental hard tissue loss (cementum or cementum and enamel with loss of dentin that does not extend to the pulp cavity).
TR3	TR Stage 3	Deep dental hard tissue loss (cementum or cementum and enamel with loss of dentin that extends to the pulp cavity); most of the tooth retains its integrity.
TR4	TR Stage 4	Extensive dental hard tissue loss (cementum or cementum and enamel with loss of dentin that extends to the pulp cavity); most of the tooth has lost its integrity: (TR4a) crown and root are equally affected; (TR4b) crown is more severely affected than the root; (TR4c) root is more severely affected than the crown.
TR5	TR Stage 5	Remnants of dental hard tissue are visible only as irregular radiopacities, and gingival covering is complete.

References

1 Thoma, K. H. and Robinson, H. B. G. (1956). *Oral and Dental Diagnosis*, 3. Philadelphia, PA: WB Saunders Co.

2 Wiggs, R.B. (1993). Oral diagnosis and treatment planning. In *The Friskies Symposium on Veterinary Dentistry*, Kansas City, MO. 32.

3 Torres, H. O. and Ehrlich, A. (1980). *Modern Dental Assisting*, 2e, 481. Philadelphia: WB Saunders Co.

4 (1979). Treatment considerations of dental patients. In: *Accepted Dental Therapeutic*, 38e, 3. Chicago, IL: American Dental Association.

5 Black, G. V. (1936). Operative Dentistry, 7e, vol. 1, 16. Chicago, IL: Medico-Dental Publishing Co.

6 Burrows, C. F. and Harvey, C. E. (1985). Oral examination and diagnostic techniques. In: *Veterinary Dentistry* (ed. C.E. Harvey), 23. Philadelphia, PA: WB Saunders Co.

7 Goodson, J. M., Tanner, A. C., Haffajee, A. D. et al. (1982). Patterns of progression and regression of advanced destructive periodontal disease. *J. Clin. Periodontol.* 9: 472.

8 Lobprise, H. B. and Wiggs, R. B. (1992). Modified surgical treatment of intermittent open-mouth mandibular locking in a cat. *J. Vet. Dent.* 9 (1): 8.

9 Robins, G. and Grandage, J. (1977). Temporomandibular joint dysplasia and open mouthed jaw locking in the dog. *J. Am. Vet. Med. Assoc.* 171 (10): 1072.

10 Lantz, G. C. and Cantwell, H. D. (1986). Intermittent open-mouth lower jaw locking in five dogs. *J. Am. Vet. Med. Assoc.* 188 (12): 1403.

11 Socransky, S. S., Haffajee, A. D., Goodson, J. M., and Lindhe, J. (1984). New concepts of destructive periodontal disease. *J. Clin. Periodontol.* 11: 21.

12 Page, R. C. and Schroeder, H. E. (1976). Pathogenesis of inflammatory periodontal disease. A summary of current work. *Lab. Invest.* 33: 235.

13 Page, R. C. and Schroeder, H. E. (1982). *Periodontitis in Man and Other Animals. A Comparative Review*. Basel, Switzerland: Karger.

14 Wiggs, R. B. (1995). Is periodontal disease a measurement of a pet's general health? *Vet. Forum.* 66.

15 Floyd, M. R. (1991). The modified Triadan system: nomenclature for veterinary dentistry. *J. Vet. Dent.* 8 (4): 18.

16 Schumacher, C. B. (1993). Charting and the oral examination. *J. Vet. Dent.* 10 (3): 9.

17 Gruffydd-Jones, T. J., Evans, R. J., and Gaskell, C. J. (1983). The alimentary system. In: *Feline Medicine* (ed. P.W. Pratt), 202. Santa Barbara, CA: American Veterinary Publishers.

18 Holzworth, J. and Stein, B. S. (1987). The sick cat. In: *Diseases of the Cat* (ed. J. Holzworth), 4. Philadelphia, PA: WB Saunders Co.

19 Eversole, L. R. (1978). *Clinical Outline of Oral Pathology: Diagnosis and Treatment*, 20. Philadelphia, PA: Lea & Febiger.

20 Ranney, R. R. (1993). Classification of periodontal diseases. *Periodontology 2000* 2 (13).

21 Page, R. C. (1986). Gingivitis. *J. Clin. Periodontol.* 13 (5): 345.

22 Theilade, E. (1986). The non-specific theory in microbial etiology of inflammatory periodontal disease. *J. Clin. Periodontol.* 13: 905.

23 Rateitschak, K. H. (1989). *Periodontology*, 2e, 130. New York, NY: Thieme Medical Publishers.

24 Wiggs, R. B. and Lobprise, H. B. (1993). Dental disease. In: *Feline Practice* (ed. G.D. Norsworthy), 290. Philadelphia PA: JB Lippincott Co.

25 Cohen, S. (1991). Diagnostic Procedures. In: *Pathways to the Pulp*, 5e (ed. S. Cohen and R. Burns), 2. Baltimore, MD: Mosby Year Book.

26 Chambers, I. G. (1982). The role and method of pulp testing: a review. *Int. Endod. J.* 15: 10.

27 Kaufman, A. Y. (1989). An enigmatic sinus tract origin. *Endod. Dent. Trau.* 5: 159.

28 Harvey, C. E. and Emily, P. P. (1993). *Small Animal Dentistry*, 35. Philadelphia, PA: Mosby-Year Book Inc.

29 Saphir, D. A. and Carter, C. R. (1976). Gingival flora of the dog with special reference to bacteria associated with bites. *J. Clin. Microbiol.* 3: 344.

30 Clapper, W. E. and Meade, G. H. (1963). Normal flora of the nose, throat, and lower intestine of dogs. *J. Bacteriol.* 85: 643.

31 Smith, J. E. (1961). The aerobic flora of the nose and tonsils of healthy dogs. *J. Comp. Pathol.* 71: 428.

32 Keyhani, M. (1977). Characteristics of coagulase-positive staphylococci from the nose and tonsils of apparently healthy dogs. *J. Comp. Pathol.* 87 (2): 311.

33 Syed, S. A., Svanberg, M., and Svanberg, G. (1980). The predominant cultivable dental plaque flora of beagle dogs with gingivitis. *J. Periodont. Res.* 15: 123.

34 Syed, S. A., Svanberg, M., and Svanberg, G. (1981). The predominant cultivable dental plaque flora of beagle dogs with periodontitis. *J. Periodont. Res.* 8: 45.

35 Theilade, E., Wright, W. H., Jensen, S. D., and Loe, H. (1966). Experimental gingivitis in man. *J. Periodont. Res.* 1: 13.

36 Burrows, C. F. and Harvey, C. E. (1985). Oral examination and diagnostic techniques. In: *Veterinary Dentistry* (ed. C.E. Harvey), 27. Philadelphia, PA: WB Saunders Co.

37 Armitage, G. C. (1993). Periodontal diagnostic aids. *Calif. Dent. Assoc. J.* 21 (11): 35.

38 Johnson, R. P. and Povey, R. C. (1982). Effect of diet on oral lesions of feline calicivirus infection. *Vet. Rec.* 110: 106.

39 Gaskell, R. M. and Wardley, R. C. (1978). Feline viral respiratory disease: a review with particular references to its epizoology and control. *J. Small Anim. Pract.* 19: 1.

40 Thompson, R. R., Wilcox, G. E., Clark, W. T., and Jansen, K. L. (1984). Association of calicivirus infection with chronic gingivitis and pharyngitis in cats. *J. Small Anim. Pract.* 25: 207.

41 Goerig, A. C. (1991). Endodontic Emergencies. In: *Pathways to the Pulp*, 5e (ed. S. Cohen and R. Burns), 31. Baltimore, MD: Mosby Year Book.

42 Samulson, M. H. (1984). Classification and diagnosis of pulp pathosis. *Dent. Clin. North Am.* 28: 699.

43 Wiggs, R.B., and Lobprise, H.B. (1993). Assessment of GCF/ALT (SGPT) in fifteen dogs as a marker of active periodontal disease and response to therapy. DDS AC Clinical Study, performed.

44 Lamster, I. B., Vogel, R. J., Hartley, L. J. et al. (1985). Lactate dehydrogenase, beta-glucuronidase and arylsulfatase in gingival crevicular fluid associated with experimental gingivitis in man. *J. Periodontol.* 56: 130.

45 Last, K. S., Stanbury, J. B., and Emberg, G. (1985). Glycosaminoglycans in human crevicular fluid as indicators of active periodontal disease. *Archs. Oral Biol.* 30: 275.

46 Golub, L. M., Siegal, K., Ramamurthy, N. S., and Mandel, I. D. (1976). Some characteristics of collagenase activity in gingival crevicular fluid and its relationship to gingival diseases in humans. *J. Dent. Res.* 55: 1049.

47 Offenbacher, S., Odle, B. M., and Van Dyke, T. E. (1986). The use of crevicular fluid prostaglandin E_2 levels as predictor of periodontal attachment loss. *J. Periodont. Res.* 21: 101.

48 Palcanis, K. G., Larjava, I. K., Wells, B. R. et al. (1992). Elastase as an indicator of periodontal disease progression. *J. Periodontol.* 63: 237.

49 Chambers, D. A., Crawford, J. M., Mukherjee, S., and Cohen, R. L. (1984). Aspartate aminotransferase increases in crevicular fluid during experimental periodontitis in beagle dogs. *J. Periodontol.* 55 (9): 526.

50 Chambers, D. A., Imrey, P. B., Cohen, R. L. et al. (1991). A longitudinal study of aspartate aminotransferase in human gingival crevicular fluid. *J. Periodont. Res.* 26: 65.

51 Imrey, P. B., Crawford, J. M., Cohen, R. L. et al. (1991). A cross-sectional analysis of aspartate aminotransferase in human crevicular fluid. *J. Periodont. Res.* 26: 75.

3

Oral Radiology and Imaging

Brook Niemiec

Veterinary Dental Specialties and Oral Surgery, San Diego, CA, USA

3.1 Importance of Dental Radiology

Numerous oral/dental lesions exist that can only be properly diagnosed and treated with the information provided by dental radiographs. These conditions are present in many of our patients and are seen in veterinary practice on a daily basis. Not radiographing these conditions often means leaving painful and/or infectious disease behind.

The knowledge obtained from dental radiographs not only improves patient care, it increases acceptance of treatment recommendations. This leads to increased numbers of dental procedures performed. This information can smooth and speed dental procedures as well as decrease complications.

Finally, numerous studies and papers have demonstrated that dental radiographs are almost always indicated and that they are often critical for proper diagnosis and treatment of oral and dental disease [1–3].

3.1.1 Periodontal Disease

Periodontal disease is by far the most common problem in small animal veterinary medicine. While periodontal probing is a critical first step in the evaluation of periodontal disease, there are several reasons that dental radiographs are required for a comprehensive evaluation [4].

1) Periodontal pockets can easily be missed due to a narrow pocket, tight interproximal space (particularly in the molar region), or a ledge of calculus.
2) Dental radiographs serve as a visual (objective) baseline to evaluate the progression of disease.
3) Radiographs are absolutely critical in cases of mandibular periodontal disease in small/toy breed dogs as well as in the mandibular canine area of cats. In these patients, periodontal disease can markedly weaken the mandible [5], significantly increasing the chance of iatrogenic fracture during extraction [6] (Figure 3.1).

3.1.2 Feline Tooth Resorption (TR)

Because these lesions initiate at or below the gingival margin, clinical evidence may not occur until late in the disease course. Consequently, severe root and painful cervical crown resorption may be present undetected for a significant time. Therefore, most veterinary dentists recommend full mouth dental radiographs for all feline patients.

Dental radiographs are also critical for appropriate therapeutic decisions. There are two commonly recognized types of tooth resorption (TR) [7, 8]. Type 2 lesions, the most common form encountered, demonstrate replacement resorption (the lost tooth structure is replaced by bone) of the roots, making extraction very difficult [8]. Resorption may continue until no recognizable tooth structure remains (ghost roots). In cases of advanced replacement resorption, endodontic infection is not known to occur [9]. This finding has resulted in the accepted (although still somewhat controversial) therapy of crown amputation for advanced type 2 TRs [9, 10].

Conversely, type 1 TRs do not undergo replacement resorption [7, 8]. These teeth typically retain sufficient normal root and pulp structure to result in pain and infection following incomplete extraction. If the dental radiograph reveals intact root structure or, worse, evidence of active infection, complete extraction of the root is required [7, 10].

Crown amputation is indicated *only* if there is significant ankylosis and root resorption (no evidence of periodontal ligaments or endodontic system), as well as no evidence of infection [7, 10]. In addition, patients with caudal stomatitis should not receive crown amputation [7].

3.1.3 Endodontic Disease

Endodontic disease is very common in veterinary patients. However, due to the fact that there are rarely

Wiggs's Veterinary Dentistry: Principles and Practice, Second Edition. Edited by Heidi B. Lobprise and Johnathon R. (Bert) Dodd.

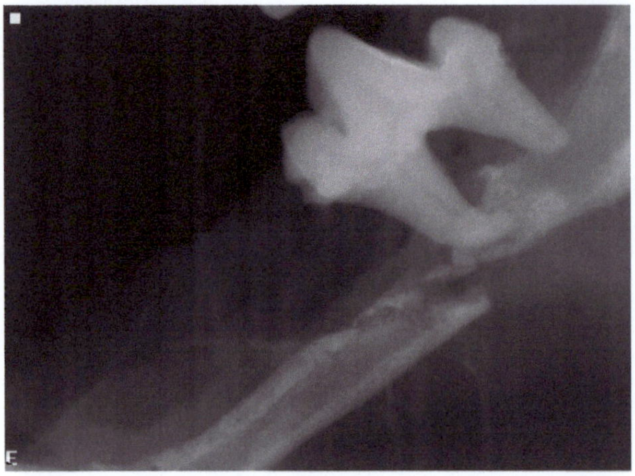

Figure 3.1 Pathologic fracture of mandible.

outward clinical signs, animal patients often suffer for an extensive period prior to diagnosis and treatment. This is because cats and dogs very rarely show any obvious signs of oral pain or infection [7, 11].

By far the most common cause of endodontic disease that is uncovered by dental radiology are uncomplicated crown fractures. The dentinal exposure may allow the endodontic system to be infected via the dentinal tubules [7, 12, 13]. This painful infection cannot be diagnosed without dental radiographs. Therefore, every tooth with direct dentin exposure should be radiographed to rule out endodontic disease [13, 14] (Figure 3.2a,b). In addition, worn teeth (with attrition and/or abrasion) can also be endodontically infected, even if the pulp chamber is not directly exposed [15, 16]. Finally, clinically normal teeth can also be endodontically infected [2–4, 16].

3.1.4 Persistent Deciduous Teeth

If the root of the deciduous tooth is normal and is held in by the periodontal ligament, extraction is straightforward and root fracture should not occur if the extraction is performed carefully and correctly [17]. These roots may undergo resorption due to the pressure placed on them by the erupting permanent dentition (among other things); however, an intact root canal is often still present [16]. The resorption makes extraction very difficult. Regardless, if an identifiable root canal is present, complete extraction is necessary to avoid pain and infection. A surgical approach is advised in these cases.

Finally, the root structure of the deciduous tooth may have been completely resorbed and the crown is only being held in by the gingival tissues. Proper therapy for this requires that only the crown and the remaining root segment be removed.

3.1.5 "Missing" Teeth

Incomplete dental arches are quite common in veterinary patients. In some cases, the tooth is truly missing, but often the tooth/root is actually present and may create a disease state. Do not assume that the tooth is not present just because it is missing or previously extracted if radiographs have not been taken of the area.

Possible etiologies for "missing" teeth include [17]:

1) *Congenitally missing* [18]. This is most common in small, toy, and brachycephalic breeds [19].
2) *Previously extracted or exfoliated.* The most common reason for this is previous extraction, but periodontal disease and trauma are also possible.

(a) (b)

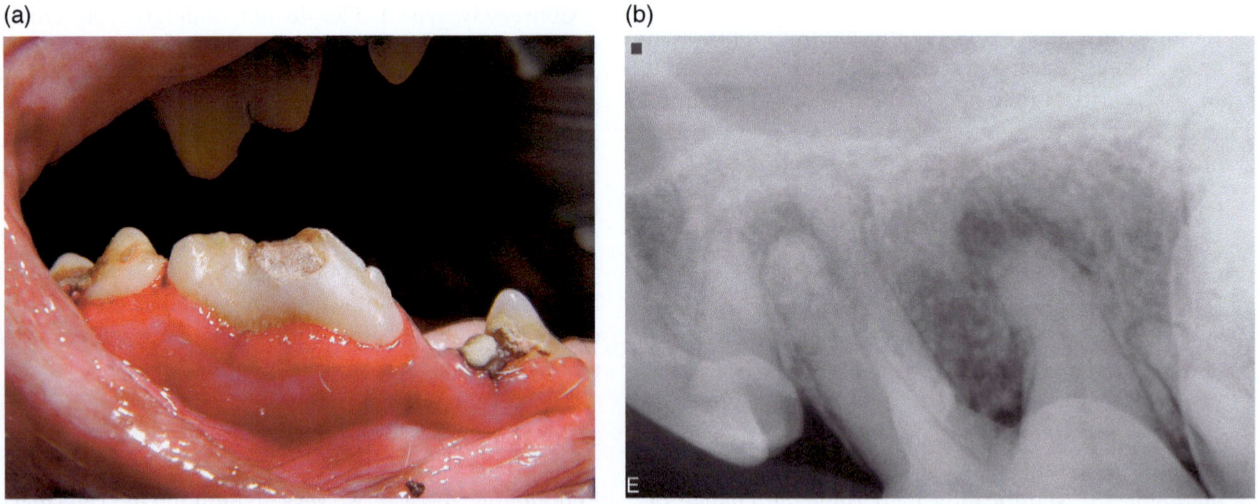

Figure 3.2 (a) and (b) Endodontic disease discovered by dental radiology caused by uncomplicated crown fractures with dentinal tubule exposure.

3) *Fractured below the gingival margin.* This may also occur secondary to trauma or an incomplete extraction attempt. Retained roots following extraction attempts are quite common. One study on the success rate of carnassial teeth extractions in dogs and cats revealed retained roots in almost 90% of cases [20]. Dental radiographs will confirm a retained root and often an infectious/inflammatory lesion. If there is any evidence of infection, or if the root appears relatively normal (i.e., not significantly resorbed), surgical extraction is generally recommended.
4) *Impacted or embedded.* This condition is most common in the first and second premolars of brachycephalic breeds.

The biggest concern with unerupted or impacted teeth is the development of dentigerous cysts. These cysts arise from the enamel-forming organ of the unerupted tooth. It has been reported that the incidence of cystic formation on impacted teeth in dogs is 29% [21]; however, pathologic changes were associated with 32.9% of impacted teeth in one human study [22]. These cysts can grow quite large, thus resulting in weakened bone. This may necessitate an extensive surgery or even result in a pathologic fracture. In addition, they can become infected and create significant swelling and pain. Finally, malignant transformation has occurred [18]. It is critical to note that two of the causes for "missing" teeth require no therapy and the other two can lead to significant pathologic changes. Therefore, all "missing" teeth should be radiographed to ensure that they are truly missing (Figure 3.3).

3.1.6 Mandibular Fractures

Mandibular fractures are generally traumatic in nature, but in small and toy breed dogs there is an emerging problem known as a "pathologic" fracture [5]. Chronic periodontal loss decreases the tooth support and can eventually result in exfoliation. In most pets, this occurs prior to severe bone weakening. However, in several situations significant bone thinning will occur prior to tooth exfoliation.

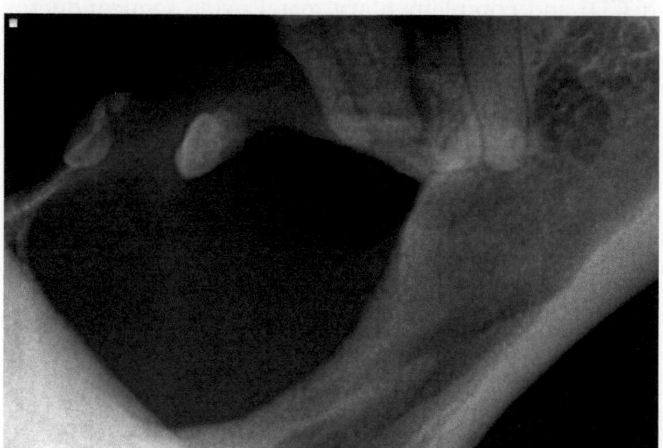

Figure 3.3 Dentigerous cyst.

"Pathologic" fractures are most common in small and toy breed dogs for several reasons, but mostly because they have proportionally larger teeth than do larger breeds. This results in the apices of the mandibular first molar being very close to the ventral cortex of the mandible [23]. In addition, the mandibular canines comprise 60–70% of the strength of the rostral mandible of all small animal veterinary patients, with minimal bone surrounding the apex [4].

Pathologic fractures typically occur due to mild trauma or during extraction procedures [6]. Diagnosis of a pathologic fracture is generally only possible with dental radiographs, as skull films typically provide insufficient detail. The classic appearance of a pathologic fracture is bone loss around the tooth and/or periapical rarefaction in the area of the fracture or other root of a multirooted tooth [16]. The fracture will not heal no matter how perfect the fixation is if the diseased tooth root is not extracted [5].

3.1.7 Oral Masses

Dental radiology is an important piece of diagnostic information in the treatment of oral masses. Various types of growths generally have different radiographic appearances. Therefore, noting the type and extent of bony involvement (if any) on the histopathology request form will aid the pathologist. Conversely, it is critical to interpret the histopathology in the light of the radiographic findings. A diagnosis of a malignancy without bony involvement should be questioned. Conversely, a benign tumor diagnosis with significant bony reaction should be further investigated.

Regardless, histopathological testing is necessary for accurate diagnosis of oral masses since a variety of benign or malignant tumors appear radiographically similar. In addition, osteomyelitis can create the same radiographic findings as malignant tumors. Finally, aggressive tumors may show no bone involvement early in the course of disease.

3.1.8 Extractions

Pre- and post-operative dental radiographs should be exposed for all extraction procedures [24–26]. Pre-extraction radiographs allow the practitioner to determine the amount of disease present as well as any root abnormalities (e.g., extra, fused, or curved). Fully 10% of maxillary third premolars in cats have a third root [26]. One of the more important findings on pre-operative dental radiographs is the presence and degree of ankylosis [4]. In addition, for mandibular canine and first molar extractions, knowing the amount of remaining mandibular bone can help avoid an iatrogenic fracture. Finally, the radiographs will serve as legal evidence of the need for extraction.

Post-extraction dental radiographs are equally important [27]. Regardless of the appearance of complete extraction, there is still a possibility of retained roots or other problems, making post-operative radiographs critical in all cases. A recent study on the success rate of carnassial tooth extraction in dogs and cats revealed that 86.4% had retained roots and that two-thirds of these roots had radiographic evidence of infection [20].

3.1.9 Conclusions

Considering that *nearly* every veterinary dental patient has some form of oral disease and that dental radiographs are indicated for all oral disease, virtually all patients will benefit from the information provided by dental radiographs.

3.2 Dental Radiography Equipment

3.2.1 Dental Radiograph Generators [28–30]

Radiographic exposure is controlled by three components: kVp (kilovolt peak), mA (milliamperage), and exposure time. KVp controls the power of each particular X-ray particle, which controls the penetration of the beam through tissues. This equates to the "quality" of the X-ray beam. The "quantity" of the exposure is determined by the combination of mA and time of exposure. The higher the mA, the more X-rays produced over a given time period.

Since there is minimal variation of tissues within the oral cavity, the kVp and mA are constant on most dental radiology units; the only variable factor is time. Exposure is typically measured in seconds (or parts thereof), but some units use pulses. Most dental radiology units have a digital control for the exposure, which is set by the operator. Recently, however, veterinary specific machines have become available that have a computer that sets the exposure based on the size of the patient, the type of film used (or digital system), and the object tooth/teeth.

Finally, hand-held devices are currently available. These are particularly valuable in practices with minimal space as well as mobile practices. The reader should note that they are not approved in all states/countries and the reader is directed to their local government for direction.

3.2.2 Dental Radiographic Film [8, 29–31]

There are three speeds of dental film in common use: "D," "E," and "F." The speed is dependent on the size of the silver halide crystals and therefore the amount of radiation required. "E" speed film requires approximately ½ the amount of radiation for exposure than "D" speed film, and "F" speed is ¼–½ of "E" [33, 34]. There is a slight decrease in resolution with faster films due to the larger crystal size, but according to most experts, the difference is negligible [34, 35]. It is critical to note that different speed films require different safe light colors (see below).

There are different sizes of dental film available (4, 3, 2, 1, and 0). The most common sizes used in veterinary medicine are 4, 2, and 1. Size 4 film is the largest available and is generally used for full mouth radiographs and major maxillofacial surgery. Size 2 is the most commonly used film size for single tooth radiographs. It should be noted, however, that the canines of large breed dogs cannot be completely imaged on a size 2 film. Size 1 or 0 are used for small dogs and cats, especially for mandibular views.

3.2.3 Digital Dental Radiography [36]

3.2.3.1 Semi-direct Systems – Computed Radiography (CR)

These systems utilize a photo-stimulable phosphor (PSP) plate, which is covered with phosphor crystals that (temporarily) store the X-ray photon energy. Following exposure, the plate is scanned with a near-red wavelength laser beam. This creates an electronic "message" of the image, which is then sent to a computer for processing and image creation. Once the image has been scanned, it can be "erased" by exposure to a bright visible light.

3.2.3.2 Direct Systems – Digital Radiography (DR)

These systems employ solid-state sensors. The two major types of solid-state sensors are the charge-coupled device (CCD) and complementary metal oxide semiconductor (CMOS). These systems convert the energy from X-ray photons into electronic signals. A scintillation layer is placed on top of the sensor in order to turn X-ray photons into light photons, which are subsequently absorbed by the chip.

3.2.3.3 Creation of the Digital Image

Regardless of the digital system, the images are created in a similar fashion. The plates/sensors measure the intensity of the photons following passage through the oral tissues, typically on a 256 unit gray scale. Zero corresponds to the maximum measurable radiation (or black) and 255 corresponds to no exposure (or white).

Intensity measurements are performed over a number of very small regions of the sensor called pixels (which stands for picture element). Resolution of a digital dental image is determined by the pixels, specifically the size, number, and color depth. Each pixel is 15–40 square micrometers (μm) in size, equating to thousands of pixels on a size 2 sensor. After the intensity is measured, the score of each individual pixel is transferred to the computer for image creation. The computer assigns a gray-scale value to each pixel and places it in the correct location. The computer then generates the "raw" image one pixel at a time.

All digital dental software programs have the ability to manipulate this numerical information, thus changing the appearance of the image. This is performed by subjecting the information to mathematical equations called *algorithms*. A simple algorithm is reversing the gray scale (white becomes black) to create a "negative." However, there are numerous highly complicated algorithms that can improve contours and/or contrast, and can even adjust an image that is over- or underexposed. These changes can be done manually, although all systems have the ability to either "optimize" the image automatically or provide the user with a group of pre-set settings to choose from. This is responsible for much of the differences in the appearance of the images between manufacturers.

3.2.3.4 CR versus DR

Numerous studies have compared DR to CR produced images. The majority of these studies report that DR systems may have a higher resolution [37, 38]. These same studies report, however, that PSP systems will produce quality images over a wider exposure range (see below) [37–39]. In contrast, one study reported that PSP plates had superior image quality to solid-state (DR) images [39]. The 2008 and 2010 sensor shootouts showed that the PSP system compared favorably to the sensor systems. Finally, a good technique to determine the quality of the digital system is to compare line pairs.

3.2.3.5 Advantages of Digital Radiography [36, 40–44]

The main advantage of digital radiography is decreased radiation exposure and anesthesia time. With DR technology, the image is available in seconds. Additionally, since the image is produced while the sensor and tubehead are still in place, minor technique adjustments can be performed without starting again. The scanning of the CR phosphor plates takes about 10 seconds, and the plate must be removed from the patient's mouth. This negates some of the speed advantage; however, the larger plates that are available (size 4 and even larger) can make up for this time shortcoming. Experienced practitioners can actually be faster with CR systems, but for the novice, the ease of retakes with DR improves the learning curve. In addition, CR plates have increased latitude of exposure than either DR or standard film, which limits retakes.

Digital images have other advantages over analog films, including [45]:

- Large size of the image projected on the computer screen combined with the ability to manipulate the image allows for easier interpretation.
- The ability to "mark" the images facilitates client communication.
- Digital images are permanent (if properly stored) and therefore do not degrade over time.
- The use of toxic chemicals is avoided, as well as the hassle of proper disposal.
- Digital images save storage space in the clinic and staff time searching for previous films.
- Digital images can be quickly uploaded to telemedicine sites or e-mailed to specialists for consultation.
- DR sensors have an additional advantage of creating far less radiographic exposure than standard film.

It should be noted, however, that one study (admittedly older) actually showed an increase in exposure with a digital system using a dosimeter [46]. These properties can make dental radiographs a very effective marketing tool.

3.2.3.6 Disadvantages of Digital Radiography

The main argument against digital radiographs was that they provided less detail than standard radiographic film [47–51]. This is controversial at this time as other studies report similar quality, with the difference depending on several factors [43, 52–55]. When image quality in general is studied, digital radiographs are typically rated inferior to standard film. However, some studies report that digital images are overall superior to standard film [56]. Additionally, when particular pathology or procedural aspects are studied, digital images can be superior to plain film. At this point they are at least equal to and in some instances superior to standard film [57–60]. The one point of agreement in almost every study was that enhanced images were superior to the raw images [55, 60, 61]. Further, when digital systems are compared to analog film, less exposure errors were created [60, 61]. The biggest drawback to DR systems is the lack of a size 4 sensor plate [36]. This is mostly a problem in large breed dogs as some teeth cannot be completely imaged on one film. In addition, exposing full-mouth radiographs in large and giant breed dogs requires significantly more exposures.

Most DR sensors have a very narrow exposure range to create an acceptable image, and consequently this may increase retakes. There is one exception that has a wide latitude of exposure (Sopix Digital Dental Sensor, Dental FocusTM, LLC, Neshanic Station, NHJ), but it is recommended that the lowest possible exposure setting should be used.

The CR system negates many of the above issues. First, it has a size 4 plate and the individual plates are generally under $100. Therefore, replacement of damaged plates is not a huge expense. However, these plates reach "wear out" faster than direct digital systems and can easily be scratched, therefore requiring more frequent replacement.

The major concern with CR systems is that their optimum radiographic exposure is higher than Ektaspeed film. In addition, the wide latitude of dose levels allows a diagnostic radiograph to be created with exceedingly high exposure. Practitioners must be very careful and use the lowest possible setting.

The additional disadvantage with digital radiography is the initial setup cost. However, over time the savings in film and development costs (not to mention time) will more than pay for the system. The only other disadvantage to digital systems is the need for consistent backup of the computer information. If a computer fails, the information will be lost. Backup to a mirrored hard drive, CDS, or preferably a web-based storage location is mandatory.

3.2.4 Recommendations [36]

Standard (analog) film is certainly still acceptable for intraoral dental radiography. It is of similar quality to digital and is initially much less expensive. Therefore, it is certainly a great first step. However, over time, the cost of film and chemicals will negate this. This does not count the decreased time enjoyed with dental systems.

For most general practices, a size 2 DR sensor is the best choice. This is because in general it is faster than CR or standard film systems. This is especially true when inexperienced technicians are taking images, as retakes are much faster. For technicians who are confident in their sills, the size 4 phosphor plate can make full mouth radiographs faster (especially in large breed dogs). Feline-only practices would benefit from a size 1 sensor, as its smaller size better fits the feline anatomy, but this size would not be useful for extra oral radiography of the temporomandibular joint (TMJ).

Any practice can benefit from the variations in size offered by CR systems. However, those practices performing major maxillofacial surgery greatly benefit from the larger images available from these systems. Further mixed practices who may see equine patients should consider a CR system, especially one that can take even larger films than a size 4. Finally, PSP plates are excellent for small mammal and reptile radiographs. If you are still confused as to which system is best for your practice, a pre-purchase consult can be extremely valuable.

A final thought to consider when purchasing a digital dental system is your monitor. The fine resolution, depth of color, and algorithms in high-end digital dental systems are not likely to be appreciated on inexpensive monitors. This is particularly true of laptop computer screens, which are what the majority of clinics use. Make sure to purchase a monitor that justifies your investment.

3.3 Dental Radiograph Positioning

3.3.1 Step 1: Patient Positioning

Position the patient so that the area of interest is convenient to the radiographic beam. In general, this is where the arcade to be imaged is "up." When imaging the mandibular canines and incisors the patient should be in dorsal recumbency. For mandibular cheek teeth, the patient can stay in dorsal, or be placed in lateral recumbency with the affected side "up."

Positioning for maxillary teeth is controversial, with some dentists recommending ventral and others lateral recumbency. While it is easier to visualize angles in ventral recumbency, rolling patients into this position for intra- and/or post-op images is arduous and time consuming. In addition, this typically displaces the monitoring leads, adding time to the procedure. Finally, it can be traumatic to the spine of older pets as well as the hips of large breed dogs. For these reasons, in our practice virtually all maxillary radiographs are exposed in lateral recumbency (Figure 3.4a,b).

3.3.2 Step 2: Film Placement [11, 29, 62–64]

When utilizing standard film, there is an embossed dot on the film packet that should be placed toward the X-ray beam. In most films, this side is pure white and the opposite or "back" side of the film is colored. The dot should also be positioned away from the structures to be imaged to avoid interference.

For DR sensors, the cord will exit on the "back" side of the sensor and this side goes away from the tube head. For PSP plates, the side with writing goes away from the tube head.

The film should be placed as near as possible to the teeth and oral mucosa to minimize distortion. Position the film/sensor in the mouth so that the entire tooth (crown and entire root surface) is covered by the film/sensor (if possible). If the target tooth is larger than the size 2 sensor (which is common in large breed dogs), it is recommended to:

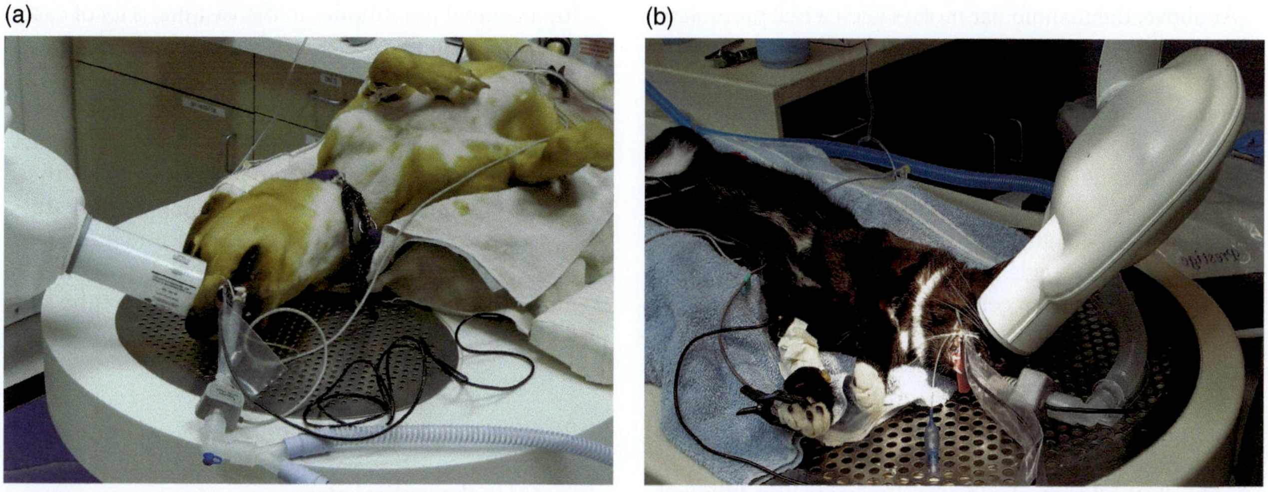

Figure 3.4 (a) and (b) Maxillary radiographs taken with patient in lateral recumbency.

- Position the sensor apically enough to expose the apex of the tooth and 3 mm beyond. This will not expose the crown, but in many cases the crown is not a critical piece of information.
- Expose two images (one of the root and one of the crown).

3.3.3 Step 3: Positioning the Beam Head [11, 28–30, 32, 63–66]

There are two major techniques for positioning the beam head in veterinary patients, both of which are used on a daily basis.

3.3.3.1 Parallel Technique

This is where the film is placed parallel to the object being radiographed and the beam placed perpendicular to both the film/sensor and the tooth/root. This provides the most accurate image, but is only useful in the mandibular molars and caudal premolar teeth. The maxillary teeth cannot be imaged due to the fact that dogs and cats do not have an arched palate, which interferes with parallel placement. Similarly, the symphysis interferes with parallel placement for the rostral mandibular teeth (including the first and second premolar in dogs and occasionally third premolar in cats).

3.3.3.2 Bisecting Angle Technique

This is the most common type of dental radiograph taken in veterinary patients. This is the most scientifically correct way to image veterinary patients, but is very cumbersome and time consuming. This technique utilizes the theory of equilateral triangles to create an image that accurately represents the tooth and roots.

1) Place the film/sensor as parallel as possible to the tooth root.
2) Measure the angle between the tooth root and film.
3) Cut the measure angle in half.
4) Place the beam placed to the bisected angle.
5) This gives the most accurate representation of the root.

If this angle is incorrect, the radiographic image will be distorted. This is because the X-ray beam will create an image that is longer or shorter than the object imaged.

The best way to conceptualize this technique is to imagine a building and the sun. The building creates a 90° (right) angle to the ground. The bisecting angle in this case is 45°.

Early and late in the day, the sun is at an acute angle to the ground and casts a long shadow. In radiography, this occurs when the angle of the beam to the sensor/film is too small and is known as elongation. At some point in the late morning and early afternoon, the sun is at a 45° angle to the building, which is the bisecting angle, which gives an accurate representation of the building height. As the sun continues up, the shadow shortens. This occurs in veterinary radiography when the angle of the beam to the sensor/film is too great and is known as foreshortening. Finally, at noon, the sun is straight up from the building, which gives no shadow.

3.3.3.3 Simplified Technique

This technique [28], developed by Dr. Tony Woodward, does not utilize direct measurement of any angle, instead relying on approximate angles to create diagnostic images. There are only three angles used for all radiographs in this system, 20, 45, and 90.

As above, the mandibular molars and caudal premolars are exposed at a 90° angle (parallel technique).

Maxillary premolars and molars have their roots straight up from the crowns, with the sensor essentially flat across the palate. This creates a 90° angle and thus a 45° bisecting angle is used.

Canines and incisors curve backward significantly (approaching a 40° angle to the palate) and therefore are imaged with a 20° angle rostrocaudally.

There are only four conditions where this technique may not be sufficient.

1) *Maxillary canines* [67]. The roots of the maxillary canines are directly dorsal to the maxillary first and second premolars in dogs and the second and occasionally third premolar in cats. Therefore, an additional rotation to 20° lateral is necessary to avoid superimposition of the canine and these teeth. This will image the root over the nasal cavity.
2) *Mesial mandibular premolars* [32, 65]. The apices of these teeth are often not imaged on films using the parallel technique. This is because the symphysis interferes with the ventral placement of the film/sensor. On occasion this can be alleviated by simply slightly rotating the PID ventrally to foreshorten the radiograph. If this is insufficient, the bisecting angle technique is utilized. To perform the bisecting angle technique for these roots, place the film/sensor in position for the canines/incisors and place the PID 45° laterally.
3) *Maxillary cheek teeth in cats* [32, 65]. When using the standard intraoral bisecting angle technique, the zygomatic arch may interfere with good visualization of the maxillary fourth premolar/first molar as well as the distal root of the maxillary third premolar. This author does not feel that this significantly affects interpretation with digital systems. However, if the practitioner wishes to view these teeth without interference, the extraoral technique can be utilized.
   a) Place the film/sensor on the table.
   b) Position the cat on the sensor with the arcade to be imaged down.
   c) Gently hold the jaws apart with a radiolucent mouth gag.
   d) Angle the beam through the mouth to create the bisecting angle (approximately 30°).
      **Since this image was created extraorally, it will be opposite the arcade determined by the techniques presented later in this chapter.
4) *Mesial roots of the maxillary fourth premolar* [66]. The straight lateral 45° bisecting angle gives a good representation of the mesial roots but they will be overlapped. In this author's opinion, this is sufficient for a general practitioner in the vast majority of cases. It is exceedingly rare to see a periapical lucency on only one root of this tooth and periodontal disease can be easily seen on the straight lateral. Therefore, in most cases extra images are not necessary. However, if the practitioner desires to view these roots separately, an additional angle is necessary. The PID is angled in both the vertical and horizontal planes. The horizontal shift can either be in the mesial or distal direction and is called the tube shift technique [63].

To perform this technique:

1) Position the PID in position for the straight lateral image:
   a) 45° in the vertical plane.
2) Rotate the PID approximately 30° in the horizontal plane. This can either be done distally or mesially.

Once the roots are split, it is imperative to know which root is which. The classic way of determining the mesiobuccal from the mesiopalatal root is to determine it via the SLOB (same lingual/opposite buccal) technique [30, 63]. This means that the root that is more lingual (or palatal) will be imaged in the same direction the tube is shifted and the buccal root will be imaged in the opposite direction. Therefore, with a distal tube shift, the palatal root will move distally in comparison to the buccal root. With a mesial tube shift, the palatal root will move mesial in relation to the buccal.

However, there is a much simpler way to determine which root is which. If the PID has been shifted mesially, the distal root of the fourth premolar will be imaged over the first molar. In this case, the buccal root is in the middle. When the PID is shifted distally, the distal root is well visualized, away from the first molar and the palatal root is in the middle. Since the whole tooth cannot be effectively evaluated with the mesial tube shift technique, this author recommends that only the distal tube shift technique be used, thus creating a quality image of the entire tooth. If the distal root is imaged well, the palatal root is in the middle.

3.3.4 Step 4: Setting the Exposure [29]

If your machine has manual settings, you will need to determine the correct exposure time. In general, cats require only two settings, one for the maxilla and one for the mandible. For dogs, there will be about five settings regardless of size of tooth or patient.

If you are utilizing the computer-controlled system, set the buttons for the species, film/digital system, and tooth to be imaged. These settings will probably not perfect, so minor adjustments will still be necessary.

3.3.5 Step 5: Exposing the Radiograph [29]

Dental radiograph machines have a hand-held switch to expose the radiograph. Stay at least 6 ft away from the tube-head and at a 90° to 130° angle to the primary beam to minimize radiation exposure. Make sure you hold the button down until the machine stops beeping. These switches are "dead man's," which means if you let up during the exposure, it will stop the production of X-ray beams and you will need to start again.

3.4 Developing Dental Radiographs

Dental radiographs can be developed via hand or automatic dental film processors. This author strongly recommends against using standard radiograph automatic processors for developing dental films. This is because the chemistry for standard films is different form dental films, which negatively affects the images [29, 64]. For automatic dental processing, refer to the operating manual. However, since the cost of digital systems has dropped, an investment in an automatic dental film developer is unjustified.

3.4.1 Hand Developing

Step 1. Create a light safe environment [28, 30, 68, 69].

This can be performed in a dark room using household cups or bowls; however, developing in the operatory utilizing a chairside developer is recommended. The film and solutions are visualized through a colored filter, while the hands are placed through a light-safe aperture. Advantages of chairside developing include: not needing a dark room, time efficiency, and allowing for continual patient monitoring by the technician during the development process. Amber filters are used for "D" speed films and red is correct for "E" and "F" speeds.

Step 2. Removal of film from the protective packet [68].

Carefully open the package by grasping the supplied tag. Once opened, the three components will be exposed: film, black paper, and a lead sheet. Carefully remove the contents and separate the film from the other pieces. Grasp only the corner of the film to avoid "fingerprint artifacts" [6]. Place the film clip on the film prior to separation as a help to avoid touching the film. The clip should be placed on the edge of the film and ideally in the embossed dot to decrease artifacts.

Step 3. Development and fixing [30, 64, 68].

Hand developing can be performed by two different techniques to correctly produce an image: time/temperature or "sight." Regardless, both techniques are best performed when the chemicals are at room temperature (between 60 and 75 °F with 70 being ideal) [69, 70]. Both methods ideally employ a two-step rapid development solution. The solutions designed for standard radiographs are a poor substitute since time of development will be greatly increased and the quality film will be inferior [30, 64, 68].

Time/temperature development is performed by continually monitoring the temperature of the developing solution and determining the required development time by consulting the manufacturers chart [30]. This is the most scientifically correct method of development, but can be cumbersome. In addition, it does not take chemistry exhaustion into account.

Sight development is accomplished by dipping the film in the developer for a short time and then examining the film with a safe light or through the filter [68]. This process is repeated until the very first hint of an image appears, which indicates that the film is properly developed [68]. Sight development has several significant advantages over the time/temperature technique:

- Continuous temperature monitoring is unnecessary.
  - Solution temperatures typically rise during the day, speeding development, possibly resulting in overdeveloped films.
- The time measurement becomes inaccurate as the chemicals become exhausted, leading to underdeveloped films.
- The biggest advantage of sight developing is that minor technique errors can be corrected by slightly over- or underdeveloping the film.
  - This will not compensate for major errors, but will avoid some retakes.

3.4.2 Sight Development Technique

a) Remove the film from the packet and place in the developer solution.
   Some authors recommend an initial short placement in water [29].
b) To ensure full development, ensure that the entire film is submerged.
   This is most important when using size 4 dental films as these will barely fit in the supplied cups.
c) Following complete development, the film is rinsed by agitating in distilled water for one minute.
d) Place the film in the fixer for one full minute. At this point, it can be removed from the darkroom and quickly interpreted [68], although dry films are ideal for interpretation. To archive the film for later viewing, it should be replaced in the fixer for a minimum of 10 to 30 minutes depending on the condition of the fixer.
e) Rinse the film completely.

Water rinse for a minimum of 10 minutes. However, if true archival quality is desired, a 30 minute rinse is recommended.

f) The radiograph must be dried completely prior to storage or the films will stick together, resulting in significant film damage.
   Drying can be accomplished with a dental film dryer or hair dryer. Alternatively, the radiographs may be hung to air dry for 24 hours.
g) Following complete drying, the radiographs are stored in an envelope labeled with the patients name and date. This can be kept in an indexable box or in the individual patients chart.

When using small cups, the chemicals used in hand development must be replaced frequently [69]. Six ounces of developer will generally develop 10–15 size 4 films, or a larger number of smaller size 2 films, before replenishment is necessary [11].

Regardless of the quality of development, some degradation of the film quality is expected over time. Therefore, it is recommended to take high-quality digital photos of the radiographs and store them in a folder on a computer that is routinely backed-up. This is a permanent copy of the film and will also facilitate telemedicine consultations with specialists or other veterinarians.

3.4.3 Errors of Development [30, 68, 69, 71]

There are numerous opportunities for errors in the development of dental radiographs, which include:

- Under- or overdeveloping
- Underfixing
- Underrinsing
- Light exposure.

Washed out or "light" radiographs are either underdeveloped or underexposed. However, this can also occur due to exhausted developer solution. This issue can be corrected by either increasing development time or exposure. If this does not resolve the issue, the solutions should be replaced.

Overdeveloping (or overexposing) film results in a radiograph that is "dark." This problem is ideally corrected by decreasing exposure time, but occasionally decreasing the development time may be effective.

Extreme underfixing will cause the film to blacken immediately. This can be avoided by leaving the film in the fixer for at least one full minute. Slight underfixing will cause the radiograph to yellow over time.

Initially, the radiograph will not be adversely affected by insufficient rinsing. However, over time, the fixer that remains on the film will turn it brown, resulting in unreadable films.

Unfortunately, errors of underfixing and rinsing are not discovered at the time of the procedure and are therefore irreplaceable.

Fogged or unclear radiographs occur secondary to a variety of problems including:

- Old/exhausted solutions
- Old film
- Poor radiographic technique
- Light exposure
- Improper light filter or developer type.

Light fogging (due to leakage) in a darkroom can be confirmed by placing a coin on an opened film for a few minutes and then developing the film [69]. If the coin is visible, there is a light leak. Finally, if you are using the wrong color safelight, overexposure and non-diagnostic films can result [72].

3.5 Dental Radiograph Interpretation

Dental radiograph interpretation can appear daunting; however, it is very similar to interpreting a standard bony radiograph. In addition, most dental lesions are fairly obvious. However, there are pathologic states that are unique to the oral cavity and several normal anatomic structures exist that may mimic pathological changes.

This section concentrates on the most common pathological lesions. In practice, these lesions may be more subtle. The reader is directed to additional continuing education meetings to further their expertise.

3.5.1 Identifying Teeth [73–75]

The first step in radiographic interpretation is to determine which teeth have been imaged. This requires a firm knowledge of oral anatomy and the architecture of dental films/digital systems. Digital systems with veterinary templates do not require this step as long as the images are properly placed. However, do not assume that this was done correctly.

The key to properly identifying the imaged teeth on standard (analog) film is the embossed dot. When exposing a radiograph, the convex surface must point toward the radiographic tube head. This is the same with DR digital systems where the cord needs to be on the side opposite the tube head.

1) Place the dot toward you, which means you are looking at the teeth as if your eyes are the tube head.
   a) This is done for you on most digital systems.

2) Determine maxillary from mandibular views.
   a) Maxillary films will have nasal turbinates visible, may have a three-rooted tooth (fourth premolar), and will have a radiodense white line running across the canine and just dorsal to the premolars and molar.
   b) Mandibular films will have a large two-rooted molar and may have a mandibular symphysis, canal, or ventral cortex visible.
3) Rotate (do not flip) the film so that the roots are in their natural position.
   a) Roots point up on maxillary and down on mandibular views.
   b) This orients the image as if the pet is standing in front of you.
4) Molars and premolars: ascertain mesial from distal.
   a) Teeth generally get larger as they go distal.
   b) In dogs, the premolars are sharp and the molars blunt.
   c) If the mesial side is on the left side of the film, it is a radiograph of the left side of the patient and vice versa for the right.
5) Canines and incisors: this orients the film so the right side of the mouth is on the left and left side is on the right.
   a) Like a VD abdominal radiograph.

3.5.2 Normal Radiographic Anatomy [30, 32, 36, 75–77]

There are numerous structures within the oral cavity that can mimic pathologic states. A firm grasp of normal radiographic anatomy helps avoid overinterpretation.

Normal alveolar bone appears gray and relatively uniform throughout the arcade. It is slightly more radiopaque "darker" than tooth roots and is slightly but regularly mottled. The alveolar bone completely fills the area between the roots (the furcation) and ends within 2 mm of the cementoenamel junction (CEJ) [78]. There should be no radiolucent areas in the teeth or bone. A regular thin dark line is visualized around the roots (periodontal ligament).

The root canals should all be the same width in relation to the size of the tooth. Suspicious changes in the diameter of the root canal of a tooth should be compared against surrounding as well as contralateral teeth. It is important to note that root canals are not exact cylinders (especially in canine teeth). A lateral view may have a much different canal width than a V/D view.

Additional normal radiographic findings include [67]:

- A radiodense line running across the root of the maxillary canine and then just above the roots of the maxillary premolars is where the nasal surface merges with the palatine process.
- The radiodense line on the midline of the palate is the vomer bone.
- The radiodense structure running over the maxillary third and fourth premolars in cats is the zygomatic arch.

There are several normal anatomic findings that are commonly misinterpreted in dental images as being pathologic:

- On radiographs of the mandibular cheek teeth, the mandibular canal is seen as a thick, horizontal radiolucent line coursing parallel to and just coronal to the ventral cortex of the mandible.
- Circular radiolucent areas are seen in the area of the apices of the rostral mandibular premolars, which are the mental foramina (middle and caudal).
- On rostral mandibular views for the canines and incisors, a radiolucent line will be present between the central incisors, extending to the ventral cortex. This is the fibrocartilagenous mandibular symphysis. This can be quite thick, especially in young and brachycephalic patients.
- In the rostral maxillary area, there are paired radiolucent areas distal to the intermediate incisors, which are the palatine fissures.

3.5.3 Periodontal Disease [78–80]

Alveolar bone loss from periodontal disease occurs due to osteoclastic activity induced by plaque bacteria. The first sign is blunting of the alveolar crest. The bone can be lost across the arcade (horizontal) or down the tooth (vertical) [80].

Horizontal bone loss is the most common pattern of bone loss in veterinary patients [81]. This is seen when the bony defect is at approximately the same level across the arcade (or a portion of it). Exceptions to this are the palatine surface of the maxillary canines and the distal root of the mandibular first molars, where vertical pockets are common.

Vertical (or angular) bone loss is diagnosed when there is an area of bone that is significantly apical to the surrounding bone on a particular tooth [80, 81]. This is the most common type of bone loss in human patients, but is not often seen in veterinary patients, other than in the places mentioned above.

It is common to have a combination of the two types in the same arcade. In addition, both can actually occur on the same tooth.

3.5.4 Endodontic Disease [4, 7, 12, 16, 30, 32, 72, 82–85]

Endodontic disease may be diagnosed radiographically in several ways. An affected tooth may have one, some, or all of the various signs listed below, but only one of these changes needs to be present to establish a presumptive diagnosis of endodontic disease. These radiographic changes may be broken into two broad classifications:

1) Changes in the surrounding bone.
2) Changes within the tooth (typically endodontic system) itself.

3.5.4.1 Osseous Changes

The classic radiographic finding is periradicular rarefaction, which appears as a radiolucent area surrounding the apex. There may occasionally be a midroot lucency, but these will virtually always be seen in conjunction with periapical disease. Other changes include a widened periodontal ligament, a thickened or discontinuous lamina dura, or even periradicular opacities.

It is critical to be cognizant of the possibility of superimposed lucencies that could be artifacts. Normal anatomic structures (i.e., mental foramina) can be imaged over an apex and falsely appear as periapical rarefaction. There are several clues that these lucencies are not real periapical rarefaction.

- Superimposed artifacts are typically seen on only one root, whereas it is very rare to find a true periapical lesion on only one root of a multirooted tooth.
- Artifacts tend to be regular in appearance, whereas true periapical lesions are ragged.

If any area is in question, it is best to expose an additional film with a slightly different angle. If the lucency is still centered over the apex, it is likely to be real and not an artifact.

Another common radiographic finding that is misdiagnosed as endodontic disease is a slight widening of the periodontal ligament space. This is most common on the maxillary canines and carnassial teeth (particularly mandibular) in dogs [86]. It has been postulated that this improves the "shock-absorber" function of the periodontal ligament [87]. This presentation is even wider when the apex resides within the mandibular canal. When it occurs in canines, it is called the "chevron effect." These changes may be differentiated from pathologic lesions due to the fact that they are regular and bilateral. In addition, on canines, the radiolucent area is V-shaped, as opposed to irregular and round. Also, compare the apex to the contralateral tooth. If the lucency is bilateral, it is likely to be anatomic as opposed to pathologic. Finally, if there are no other clinical signs of non-vitality (fracture/intrinsic staining), these teeth should be monitored.

3.5.4.2 Tooth Changes

The most common change within the tooth itself is a root canal with a different width/diameter. As a tooth matures, secondary dentin production causes a decrease in canal width/diameter. When a tooth dies, this development stops and the size of the canal remains the same. Width discrepancy can be compared to any tooth (taking the size of tooth into consideration) but it is most accurate to compare it to the contralateral tooth.

However, pulpitis may result in increased dentin production (dystrophic calcification), resulting in an endodontically diseased tooth with a smaller root canal. This finding is especially common in teeth that are also periodontally diseased or discolored. This could potentially lead to a misdiagnosis of which tooth is endodontically diseased. Therefore, evaluating the adjacent teeth as well as the contralateral teeth is important.

As stated above, the endodontic system in canine teeth is not perfectly cylindrical [88]. It is oblong and wider in the rostrocaudal direction than in the lateral. Therefore, the projection will affect the size of the canal, particularly in young, large breed dogs. Therefore, it is important to image the contralateral control images at the same angle.

Finally, root resorption can be a sign of endodontic disease. Internal resorption results from odontoclastic activity within the root canal system, creating an irregular, enlarged region within an area of the root canal system. External root resorption can also be seen, which appears as a defect of the external surface of the root, generally accompanied by a loss of bone in the area. External resorption most commonly occurs at the apex in companion animals and is common in cats with longstanding endodontic disease.

3.5.5 Tooth Resorption (TR) [7, 10, 72, 79, 89]

This is often the result of odontoclastic destruction of feline teeth, classified as type 2 TR with replacement of the lost root structure by bone. Determining type 1 from type 2 tooth resorption is critical for proper treatment of tooth resorption. Tooth resorption may also be identified in dog teeth.

Type 1 TRs have normal root density in some areas and a well-defined periodontal space. In addition, there is often a definable root canal in the intact part of the tooth. This type may have significant root resorption which is *not* replaced by bone. These teeth *must* be completely extracted.

The radiographic appearance of type 2 TRs are teeth that have a different radiographic density compared to normal teeth. This is because they have undergone significant replacement resorption. Findings will include areas with no discernable periodontal ligament space (dentoalveolar ankylosis) or root canal. In the late stages, there will be little to no discernable root structure. These teeth may be properly treated with crown amputation.

3.5.6 Neoplasia [90, 91]

3.5.6.1 Benign Masses and Cysts

Most benign neoplastic growths will have no bony involvement. If bone involvement does occur with a benign growth it will typically be expansive, resulting in the bone "pulling away" from the advancing tumor. This will leave a distinct, decalcified, soft tissue filled space. Benign growths with bony involvement will typically cause tooth movement.

3.5.6.2 Malignant Neoplasia

Malignant oral neoplasms typically invade bone early in the course of the disease, resulting in irregular, ragged bone destruction. The bone will initially have a mottled "moth eaten" appearance, but radiographs late in the disease course will reveal a complete loss of bone. If the cortex is involved, an irregular periosteal reaction will be seen. In general, the teeth remain in their normal position. Histopathologic testing is always necessary for accurate diagnosis of oral masses since different tumors may still appear radiographically similar and aggressive tumors have no bone involvement early in the course of the disease.

3.6 Alternate Imaging Technologies

3.6.1 Magnetic Resonance Imaging (MRI)

This technology *does not* utilize radiation; rather, it uses a very strong magnetic field and radiofrequency pulses [92]. The image signal of tissues is based on hydrogen ion concentration [93]. Like computed tomography (CT) below, it examines very small "slices" of the patient and puts them together via computer processing. Magnetic resonance imaging (MRI) technology creates the best soft tissue detail and has some oral indications due to its ability to separate cortical from cancellous bone [93–96]. In addition, MRI can be quite effective in imaging the TMJ [97–99]. This soft tissue resolution makes this valuable in imaging the salivary glands and may even be useful for differentiating benign from malignant growths [99–102].

However, the lack of good bone resolution significantly limits its application in oral surgery [103]. MR studies have significant artifacts from metallic objects (albeit less that CT) [93]. The other imaging modalities presented are far superior for oral and maxillofacial surgery.

3.6.2 Ultrasound (US)

These images are created by ultra high-frequency sound waves [93]. Although US is not generally used for oral conditions, it is actually quite effective at evaluating the oral soft tissues (e.g., tissue cancers, salivary glands, and lymph node metastasis) [101, 104–106]. It is also effective in finding non-metallic foreign bodies [107].

3.6.3 Panoramic Radiographs

This modality is quite common and useful in human dentistry because they are readily available for a relatively low cost, low relative radiation risk, and post-processing algorithms are available. These are particularly valuable in orthodontic and implant dentistry; however, it is less effective for oral surgical cases [108]. Panoramics provide a view of the entire arch on one image, allowing for effective evaluation of tooth relationships. However, there is reduced spatial resolution compared to intraoral radiology, a relatively thick image layer, some ghost images, and minor image distortion [109]. In addition, this technology is not currently available for veterinary patients. The main reason for this is the great variability in head size and shape in veterinary patients [110].

3.6.4 Computed Tomography (CT)

These images are produced by making multiple radiographs of the object which are then digitized. Then, a computer processes the numerical information and reconstructs the object's three-dimensional (3D) structure [111]. It has been shown to be the best modality for surgical treatment planning in maxillofacial surgery cases [112–117]. It is also highly accurate in determining surgical margins in oncologic surgery [118]. The three-dimensional reconstruction and good detail provided allow for excellent surgical planning and have shown excellent results [119]. The ability to utilize intravenous (IV) contrast agents markedly increases the soft tissue visualization and diagnostic quality [93]. CT is most appropriate for the diagnosis and extent of many oral lesions and for surgical planning including [120]:

- Fracture repair
- Diagnosis and extent of infections
- Neoplastic and cystic resection and reconstruction
- TMJ surgery.

This technology represents a quantum leap forward in maxillofacial surgery. All practices providing advanced oral surgery should have access to at least a fairly recent unit. CT imaging can provide crucial information that may not be appreciated with skull films or dental radiographs.

CT may also be superior to dental radiographs at determining alveolar bone height [121, 122]. In addition, high-res CT appears to be more effective than dental radiology at finding and mapping furcational defects from periodontal disease [123].

Despite the obvious advantages, there are several limitations to this diagnostic modality when it comes to general dental practice. Chief of these is decreased resolution compared to dental radiographs and cone beam CT, which is necessary for endodontic and restorative diagnosis/therapy [124]. Other limitations include: cost and inconvenience (intra and post-op imaging would be difficult to impossible). In most instances, a CT must be performed at a place distant to the surgery site and oftentimes this requires additional anesthesia.

3.6.5 Cone Beam Computed Tomography (CBCT) [125]

This modality provides the benefits of traditional cat scans such as 3D imaging and computerized treatment planning with a lower cost and decreased radiation [93]. It is most effective for imaging osseous lesions. It is superior to dental radiographs in the detection of small areas of bone loss as well as endodontically involved teeth [126–134]. In addition, it appears to be best for mapping root canal morphology and finding extra roots/canals [135–141] (Figure 3.5). Finally, the 3D imaging capability is useful when planning the approach for surgical endodontics [142]. Cone beam computed tomography (CBCT) has also been shown to be more effective than standard radiographs in the diagnosis and mapping of internal and external resorptive lesions [143, 144] and in evaluating periodontal loss [145–148]. It also has been shown to be valuable for orthodontic therapy planning and follow-up [149, 150]. This has been shown to be invaluable for surgical treatment planning and provides fairly accurate bone measurements [124, 151–155]. It has exceedingly high resolution and is less affected by metal artifacts. It has easy accessibility and handling, a small footprint, and can be used intraoperatively. In addition, it has proven superior in the diagnosis of most pathologic conditions [156].

While these positive attributes are significant, especially for evaluation of small areas of diseased bone as well as infected teeth, there are limitations to this technology. Chief among these is the small detector size creating a limited field of view and low scan volume. Therefore, the entire traumatized area may not be imaged, which can make treatment planning challenging. The increased scatter from significantly radiodense materials (e.g., endodontic filling materials and metallic implants such as bone plates and wires) and "noise" can further reduce contrast [157]. In addition, CBCT may require a higher radiation dose than digital dental radiographs [127, 158]. Finally, one veterinary study revealed that this technology did not appear to provide the same resolution in veterinary patients [110].

When compared to intraoral radiography, CBCT provided faster image acquisition (40 seconds versus 10 minutes) with high image quality, was associated with low ionizing radiation levels, enabled image editing, and reduced the exam duration [159]. In addition, patient repositioning is not required for CBCT.

However, the increased dose of radiation that some studies reported in comparison to intraoral radiography as well as its other limitations has led to less than enthusiastic recommendations for its use in general [160–163]. However, recent studies have reported that there is minimal increase in radiation exposure over standard periapical radiography and significantly less than standard CT [164]. Finally, it appears this technology may not be as applicable for veterinary dentistry as compared to that of humans [110].

In summary, CBCT appears to be excellent for the diagnosis and treatment of endodontic disease, cysts, and periodontal disease. CBCT is of particular use for three rooted teeth (maxillary P4 and M1 in dogs) due to the ability to achieve a 3D image quickly and is not as technique sensitive as dental radiography [66, 159]. This technology is becoming the standard of care for human endodontics and will likely be economically feasible on the veterinary side in the near future [165].

3.6.6 Recommendation

Dental radiographs are the current minimum standard of practice for dental treatment and oral surgery. It has excellent resolution and the ability to be used within the operatory. Cone beam CT has similar positives to dental radiographs with better resolution and the possibility of three-dimensional rendering. If financially feasible, this modality should be considered.

At present, standard CT is the modality of choice for oral and maxillofacial trauma and oncologic surgery. This technology allows for an overall view of the entire surgical area, good resolution, and three-dimensional reconstruction of the area. The major limitations to this technology are its cost, lack of great

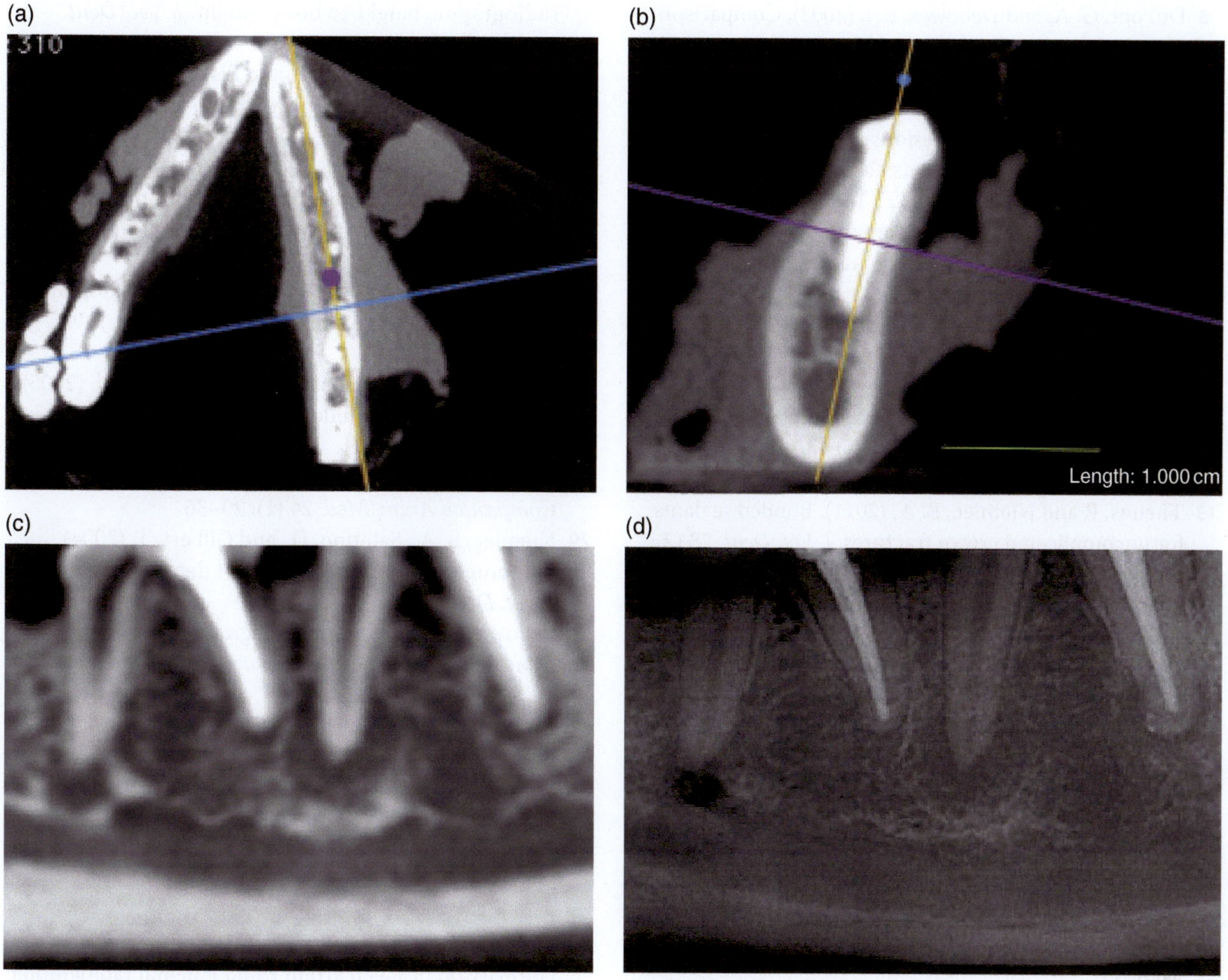

Figure 3.5 CBCT for root canal morphology.

evaluation of the periapical structures, and distance from the operatory.

Panoramic radiography is very valuable in human dentistry, but due to variation in skull size and shape it is not currently effective in veterinary medicine. Similarly, MRI is not generally indicated for oral conditions. Finally, skull films are generally considered insufficient for proper diagnosis and therapy of dental and oral conditions.

References

1 Tsugawa, A. J. and Verstraete, F. J. (2000). How to obtain and interpret periodontal radiographs in dogs. *Clin. Tech. Small Anim. Pract.* 15 (4): 204–210.

2 Verstraete, F. J., Kass, P. H., and Terpak, C. H. (1998). Diagnostic value of full-mouth radiography in cats. *Am. J. Vet. Res.* 59 (6): 692–695.

3 Verstraete, F. J., Kass, P. H., and Terpak, C. H. (1998). Diagnostic value of full-mouth radiography in dogs. *Am. J. Vet. Res.* 59 (6): 686.

4 Niemiec, B. A. (2011). The importance of dental radiology. *Eur. J. Comp. Anim. Pract.* 20 (3): 219–229.

5 Taney, K. G. and Smith, M. M. (2010). Problems with the bones, muscles and joints. In: *Dental, Oral, and Maxillofacial Disease, a Color Handbook* (ed. B.A. Niemiec), 199–224. London: Manson.

6 Mulligan, T., Aller, S., and Williams, C. (1998). *Atlas of Canine and Feline Dental Radiography*, 176–183. Trenton, NJ: Veterinary Learning Systems.

7 Dupont, G. A. (2010). Pathologies of the dental hard tissue. In: *Dental, Oral, and Maxillofacial Disease, A Color Handbook* (ed. B.A. Niemiec), 127–157. London: Manson.

8 DuPont, G. A. and Debowes, L. J. (2002). Comparison of periodontitis and root replacement in cat teeth with resorptive lesions. *J. Vet. Dent.* 19 (2): 71–76.

9 Lommer, M. J. and Verstraete, F. J. (2000). Prevalence of odontoclastic resorption lesions and periapical radiographic lucencies in cats: 265 cases (1995–1998). *J. Am. Vet. Med. Assoc.* 217 (12): 1866–1869.

10 DuPont, G. A. (2002). Crown amputation with intentional root retention for dental resorptive lesions in cats. *J. Vet. Dent.* 19 (2): 107–110.

11 Holmstrolm, S., Frost, P., and Eisner, E. (1998). *Veterinary Dental Techniques*, 2e, 493. Philadelphia, PA: Saunders.

12 Startup, S. (2011). Tooth response to injury. In: *Veterinary Endodontics* (ed. B.A. Niemiec). Tustin, CA: Practical Veterinary Publishing.

13 Theuns, P. and Niemiec, B. A. (2011). Bonded sealants for uncomplicated crown fractures. *J. Vet. Dent.* 28 (2): 130–132.

14 Woodward, T. M. (2008). Bonded sealants for fractured teeth. *Top Companion Anim. Med.* 23 (2): 91–96.

15 Trowbridge, H., Kim, S., and Suda, H. (MO 2002). Structure and functions of the dentin and pulp complex. In: *Pathways of the Pulp*, 8e (ed. S. Cohen and R.C. Burns), 441–456. Mosby: St. Louis.

16 Niemiec, B. A. (2008). Case based dental radiology. *Top Companion Anim. Med.* 24 (1): 4–19.

17 Niemiec, B. A. (2010). Pathology in the pediatric patient. In: *Dental, Oral, and Maxillofacial Disease, a Color Handbook* (ed. B.A. Niemiec), 89–126. London: Manson.

18 Neville, B. W., Damm, D. D., Allen, C. M., and Bouquot, J. E. (2002). Abnormalities of teeth. In: *Oral and Maxillofacial Pathology*, 2e, vol. 2001, 49–106. Philadelphia, PA: Saunders.

19 Harvey, C. E. and Emily, P. P. (1993). Occlusion, occlusive abnormalities, and orthodontic treatment. In: *Small Animal Dentistry*, 266–296. St. Louis, MO: Mosby.

20 Moore, J. I. and Niemiec, B. A. (2014). Evaluation of extraction sites for retained roots in dogs and cats. *JAAHA*.

21 Babbitt, S. G., Krakowski Volker, M., and Luskin, I. R. (2016). Incidence of Radiographic Cystic Lesions Associated with Unerupted Teeth in Dogs. *Journal of Veterinary Dentistry* 33 (4): 226–233.

22 Raghoebar, G. M., Boering, G., and Vissink, A. (1991). Clinical, radiographic, and histological characteristics of secondary retention of permanent molars. *J. Dent.* 19: 164–170.

23 Gioso, M. A., Shofer, F., Barros, P. S., and Harvey, C. E. (2001). Mandible and mandibular first molar tooth measurements in dogs: relationship of radiographic height to body weight. *J. Vet. Dent.* 18 (2): 65–68.

24 Holmstrolm, S. E., Frost, P., and Eisner, E. R. (1998). Exodontics. In: *Veterinary Dental Techniques*, 2e, 238–242. Philadelphia, PA: Saunders.

25 Blazejewski, S., Lewis, J. R., and Reiter, A. M. (2006). Mucoperiosteal flap for extraction of multiple teeth in the maxillary quadrant of the cat. *J. Vet. Dent.* 23 (3): 200–305.

26 Verstraete, F. J. and Terpak, C. H. (1997). Anatomical variation in the dentition of the domestic cat. *J. Vet. Dent.* 14 (4): 137–140.

27 Holmstrolm, S. E., Bellows, J., Colmrey, B. et al. (2005). AAHA dental care guidelines for dogs and cats. *J. Am. Anim. Hosp. Assoc.* 41.

28 Woodward, T. M. (2009). Dental radiology. *Top Companion Anim. Med.* 24 (1): 20–36.

29 Niemiec, B. A., Sabitino, D., and Gilbert, T. (2004). Equipment and basic geometry of dental radiography. *J. Vet. Dent.* 21 (1): 48–52.

30 Bellows, J. (2004). Dental radiography. In: *Small Animal Dental Equipment, Materials, and Techniques, a Primer*, 63–104. Blackwell.

31 Mulligan, T. W., Aller, M. S., and Williams, C. A. (1998). Basic equipment needs. In: *Atlas of Canine and Feline Dental Radiology*, 7–14. NJ, Veterinary Learning Systems: Trenton.

32 Bellows, J. (2010). Radiology. In: *Feline Dentistry Oral Assessment, Treatment, and Preventative Care*, 39–83. Ames: IA,Wiley Blackwell.

33 Geist, J. R. and Brand, J. W. (2001). Sensitometric comparison of speed group E and F dental radiographic films. *Dentomaxillofac. Radiol.* 30 (3): 147–152.

34 Farman, T. T. and Farman, A. G. (2000). Evaluation of a new F speed dental X-ray film. The effect of processing solutions and a comparison with D and E speed films. *Dentomaxillofac. Radiol.* 29 (1): 41–45.

35 Ludlow, J. B. and Platin, E. (1995). Densitometric comparisons of ultra-speed, Ektaspeed, and Ektaspeed plus intraoral films for two processing conditions. *Oral. Surg. Oral. Med. Oral. Pathol. Oral. Radiol. Endod.* 79 (1): 105–113.

36 Niemiec, B. A. (2007). Digital dental radiography. *J. Vet. Dent.* 24 (3): 192–197.

37 Borg, E. (1999). Some characteristics of solid-state and photo-stimulable phosphor detectors for intra-oral radiography. *Swed. Dent. J. Suppl.* 139 (i-viii): 1–67.

38 Bóscolo, F. N., Oliveira, A. E., Almeida, S. M. et al. (2001). Clinical study of the sensitivity and dynamic range of three digital systems, E-speed film and digitized film. *Braz. Dent J.* 12 (3): 191–195.

39 Farrier, S. L., Drage, N. A., Newcombe, R. G. et al. (2009). A comparative study of image quality and radiation exposure for dental radiographs produced

using a charge-coupled device and a phosphor plate system. *Int. Endod. J.* 42 (10): 900–907.
40 van der Stelt, P. F. (2005). Filmless imaging: the uses of digital radiography in dental practice. *J. Am. Dent. Assoc.* 136 (10): 1379–1387.
41 van der Stelt, P. F. (2008). Better imaging: the advantages of digital radiography. *J. Am. Dent. Assoc.* 139 (Suppl): 7S–13S.
42 van der Stelt, P. F. (1992). Improved diagnosis with digital radiography. *Curr. Opin. Dent.* 2: 1–6.
43 Farman, A. G. and Farman, T. T. (1999). RVG-ui: a sensor to rival direct-exposure intra-oral x-ray film. *Int. J. Comput. Dent.* 2 (3): 183–196.
44 Hayakawa, Y., Shibuya, H., Ota, Y., and Kuroyanagi, K. (1997). Radiation dosage reduction in general dental practice using digital intraoral radiographic systems. *Bull. Tokyo Dent. Coll.* 38 (1): 21–25.
45 Gröndahl, K. (1987). Computer-assisted subtraction radiography in periodontal diagnosis. *Swed. Dent. J. Suppl.* 50: 1–44.
46 Jones, G. A., Schuman, N. J., and Woods, M. A. (1998). Estimated skin exposure as an indicator for comparing radiovisiography (RVG) versus conventional Ektaspeed plus dental radiography. *J. Clin. Pediatr. Dent.* 22 (2): 121–123.
47 Versteeg, K. H., Sanderink, G. C., Velders, X. L. et al. (1997). *In vivo* study of approximal caries depth on storage phosphor plate images compared with dental X-ray film. *Oral. Surg. Oral. Med. Oral. Pathol. Oral. Radiol. Endod.* 84 (2): 210–213.
48 Hintze, H., Wenzel, A., and Frydenberg, M. (2002). Accuracy of caries detection with four storage phosphor systems and E-speed radiographs. *Dentomaxillofac. Radiol.* 31 (3): 170–175.
49 Bhaskaran, V., Qualtrough, A. J., Rushton, V. E. et al. (2005). A laboratory comparison of three imaging systems for image quality and radiation exposure characteristics. *Int. Endod. J.* 38 (9): 645–652.
50 Ludlow, J. and Mol, A. (2001). Image-receptor performance: a comparison of trophy RVG UI sensor and Kodak Ektaspeed Plus film. *Oral. Surg. Oral. Med. Oral. Pathol. Oral. Radiol. Endod.* 91 (1): 109–119.
51 Sanderink, G. C., Huiskens, R., van der Stelt, P. F. et al. (1994). Image quality of direct digital intraoral X-ray sensors in assessing root canal length. The RadioVisioGraphy, Visualix/VIXA, Sens-A-Ray, and Flash Dent systems compared with Ektaspeed films. *Oral. Surg. Oral Med. Oral Pathol.* 78 (1): 125–132.
52 Wenzel, A. (2000). Digital imaging for dental caries. *Dent. Clin. North Am.* 44 (2): 319–313.
53 Vandre, R. H., Pajak, J. C., Abdel-Nabi, H. et al. (2000). Comparison of observer performance in determining the position of endodontic files with physical measures in the evaluation of dental X-ray imaging systems. *Dentomaxillofac. Radiol.* 29 (4): 216–222.
54 Eikenberg, S. and Vandre, R. (2000). Comparison of digital dental X-ray systems with self-developing film and manual processing for endodontic file length determination. *J. Endod.* 6 (2): 65–70.
55 Woolhiser, G. A., Brand, J. W., Hoen, M. M. et al. (2005). Accuracy of film-based, digital, and enhanced digital images for endodontic length determination. *Oral. Surg. Oral. Med. Oral. Pathol. Oral. Radiol. Endod.* 99 (4): 499–504.
56 Kondylidou-Sidira, A., Fardi, A., Giannopoulou, M., and Parisis, N. (2013). Detection of experimentally induced root fractures on digital and conventional radiographs: an in vitro study. *Odontology* 101 (1): 89–95.
57 Crombie, K., Parker, M. E., Nortje, C. J., and Sanderink, G. C. (2009). Comparing the performance of storage phosphor plate and insight film images for the detection of proximal caries depth. *SADJ* 64 (10): 452, 454–456, 458, 459.
58 Shokri, A., Mortazavi, H., Salemi, F. et al. (2013). Diagnosis of simulated external root resorption using conventional intraoral film radiography, CCD, PSP, and CBCT: a comparison study. *Biomed. J.* 36 (1): 18–22.
59 Shintaku, W. H., Venturin, J. S., Noujeim, M., and Dove, S. B. (2013). Comparison between intraoral indirect and conventional film-based imaging for the detection of dental root fractures: an *ex vivo* study. *Dent. Traumatol.* 29 (6): 445–449.
60 Yoshiura, K., Kawazu, T., Chikui, T. et al. (1999). Assessment of image quality in dental radiography, part 2: optimum exposure conditions for detection of small mass changes in 6 intraoral radiography systems. *Oral. Surg. Oral. Med. Oral. Pathol. Oral. Radiol. Endod.* 87 (1): 123–129.
61 de Oliveira, M. L., Pinto, G. C., Ambrosano, G. M., and Tosoni, G. M. (2012). Effect of combined digital imaging parameters on endodontic file measurements. *J. Endod.* 38 (10): 1404–1407.
62 Zhang, W., Huynh, C. P., Abramovitch, K. et al. (2012). Comparison of technique errors of intraoral radiographs taken on film v. photostimulable phosphor (PSP) plates. *Tex Dent. J.* 129 (6): 589–596.
63 Mulligan, T. W., Aller, M. S., and Williams, C. A. (1998). Intraoral imaging techniques. In: *Atlas of Canine and Feline Dental Radiology*, 27–44. Trenton, NJ: Veterinary Learning Systems.
64 Oakes, A. (2000). Introduction: radiology techniques. In: *An Atlas of Veterinary Dental Radiology* (ed. D.H. Deforge and B.H. Colmery), xxi–xxiv. Ames, IA: Iowa State University Press.

65 Niemiec, B. A. and Furman, R. (2004). Feline dental radiology. *J. Vet. Dent.* 21 (4): 252–257.
66 Niemiec, B. A. and Furman, R. (2004). Canine dental radiography. *J. Vet. Dent.* 21 (3): 186–190.
67 Gracis, M. (1999). Radiographic study of the maxillary canine tooth of four mesaticephalic cats. *J. Vet. Dent.* 16 (3): 115–128.
68 Niemiec, B. A., Sabitino, D., and Gilbert, T. (2004). Developing dental radiographs. *J. Vet. Dent.* 21 (2): 116–121.
69 Mulligan, T. W., Aller, M. S., and Williams, C. A. (1998). Technical errors and troubleshooting. In: *Atlas of Canine and Feline Dental Radiography*, 45–64. Veterinary Learning Systems: Trenton, NJ.
70 Langland, O. E., Langlais, R. P., and Preece, J. W. (2002). Processing and film mounting procedures. In: *Principals of dental imaging. Lippincott*, 139–154. Baltimore, MD: Williams, and Wilkens.
71 Tutt, C. (2006). *Small Animal Dentistry a Manual of Techniques*, 97–98. Ames: IA, Wiley-Blackwell.
72 Niemiec, B. A. (2005). Dental radiographic interpretation. *J. Vet. Dent.* 22 (1): 53–59.
73 Verstraete, F. J. (1999). *Self-Assessment Color Review of Veterinary Dentistry*. Ames: IA, Iowa State University Press.
74 Woodward, T. M. (2009). Interpretation of dental radiographs. *Top Companion Anim. Med.* 24 (1): 37–43.
75 Aller, M. S. (2000). Normal feline oral radiographic anatomy. In: *An Atlas of Veterinary Dental Radiology* (ed. D.H. Deforge and B.H. Colmery), 117–134. Ames, IA: Iowa State University Press.
76 DeBowes, L. J., DeForge, D. H., Kesel, M. L., and Hawkins, B. J. (2000). Normal canine intraoral radiographic anatomy. In: *An Atlas of Veterinary Dental Radiology* (ed. D.H. Deforge and B.H. Colmery), 3–14. Ames: IA, Iowa State University Press.
77 Mulligan, T. W., Aller, M. S., and Williams, C. A. (1998). Normal radiographic anatomy. In: *Atlas of Canine and Feline Dental Radiography* (ed. D.H. Deforge and B.H. Colmery), 68–90. Trenton, NJ: Veterinary Learning Systems.
78 Gawor, J. (2013). Dental radiology for periodontal disease. In: *Veterinary Periodontology* (ed. B.A. Niemiec), 107–128. WileyBlackwell.
79 Lyon, K. F., Visser, C. J., Okuda, A., and Anthony, J. M. G. (2000). Feline stomatitis syndrome, periodontal disease, and feline odontoclastic resorptive lesions. In: *An Atlas of Veterinary Dental Radiology* (ed. D.H. Deforge and B.H. Colmery), 177–198. Ames, IA: Iowa State University Press.
80 Bellows, J. (2004). Periodontal equipment, materials, and techniques. In: *Small Animal Dental Equipment, Materials, and Techniques, a Primer*, 115–173. Blackwell.
81 Carranza, F. A. and Takei, H. H. (2006). Bone loss and patterns of bone destruction. In: *Carranza's Clinical Periodontology*, 452–466. St. Louis, MO: WB Saunders.
82 Niemiec, B. A. (2005). Endodontics. *Vet. Clin. N. Am. Small Anim. Pract*, Holmstrom SE, ed. 35 (4): 837–868.
83 Anthony, J. M. G., Marretta, S. M., and Okuda, A. (2000). Feline Endodontics. In: *An Atlas of Veterinary Dental Radiology* (ed. D.H. Deforge and B.H. Colmery), 149–158. Ames: IA, Iowa State University Press.
84 Marretta, S. M. and Anthony, J. M. G. (2000). Canine Endodontics. In: *An Atlas of Veterinary Dental Radiology* (ed. D.H. Deforge and B.H. Colmery), 35–58. Ames: IA, Iowa State University Press.
85 Mulligan, T. W., Aller, M. S., and Williams, C. A. (1998). Interpretation of endodontic disease. In: *Atlas of Canine and Feline Dental Radiography*, 124–152. Trenton, NJ: Veterinary Learning Systems.
86 Matsuo, M. and Takahashi, K. (2002). Scanning electron microscopic observation of microvasculature in periodontium. *Microsc. Res. Tech.* 56 (1): 3–14.
87 Stepaniuk, K. and Hinrichs, J. E. (2013). The structure and function of the periodontium. In: *Veterinary Periodontology* (ed. B.A. Niemiec), 3–17. Ames: IA, Wiley Blackwell.
88 Rochette, J. (1995). Identification of the endodontic system in carnassial teeth in the dog. *J. Vet. Dent.* 13 (1): 35–37.
89 DuPont, G. A. (2005). Radiographic evaluation and treatment of feline dental resorptive lesions. *Vet. Clin. North Am. Small Anim. Pract.* 35 (4): 943–962.
90 Sarkiala-Kessel, A. M. and Revenaugh, A. F. (2000). Feline oral neoplasia. In: *An Atlas of Veterinary Dental Radiology* (ed. D.H. Deforge and B.H. Colmery), 159–170. Ames: IA, Iowa State University Press.
91 Dhaliwal, R. (2010). Malignant oral neoplasia. In: *Small Animal Dental, Oral and Maxillofacial Disease – A Color Handbook* (ed. B.A. Niemiec), 225–235. London: Manson.
92 Dennis, R. (1993). Magnetic resonance imaging and its application to veterinary medicine. *Vet. Int.* 6 (2): 3–10.
93 Benson, B. W., Flint, D. J., Liang, H., and Opatowsky, M. J. (2014). Advances in diagnostic imaging for pathologic conditions of the jaws. *Head Neck Pathol.* 8: 383–391.
94 Gray, C. F., Redpath, T. W., and Smith, F. W. (1996). Pre-surgical dental implant assessment by magnetic resonance imaging. *J. Oral Implantol.* 22 (2): 147–153.
95 Revenaugh, A. F. (2000). Computed tomography and magnetic resonance imaging in veterinary dentistry and oral surgery diagnostics. In: *An Atlas of Veterinary Dental Radiology* (ed. D.H. Deforge and B.H. Colmery), 261–263. Ames: IA, Iowa State University Press.
96 White, S. C. and Pharoah, M. J. (2008). The evolution and application of dental maxillofacial imaging modalities. *Dent. Clin. N. Am.* 52: 689–705.

97 Harms, S. E. and Wilk, R. M. (1987). Magnetic resonance imaging of the temporomandibular joint. *Radiographics* 7 (3): 521–542.

98 Yang, Z. J., Song, D. H., Dong, L. L. et al. (2015). Magnetic resonance imaging of temporomandibular joint: morphometric study of asymptomatic volunteers. *J. Craniofac. Surg.* 26 (2): 425–429.

99 Kendi, A. T., Khariwala, S. S., Zhang, J. et al. (2011). Transformation in mandibular imaging with sweep imaging with Fourier transforms magnetic resonance imaging. *Arch. Orolaryngol. Head Neck Surg.* 137 (9): 916.

100 Liu, Y., Li, J., Tan, Y. R. et al. (2015). Accuracy of diagnosis of salivary gland tumors with the use of ultrasonography, computed tomography, and magnetic resonance imaging: a meta-analysis. *Oral Surg. Oral Med. Oral Pathol. Oral Radiol.* 119 (2): 238–245.

101 Davachi, B., Imanimoghaddam, M., Majidi, M. R. et al. (2014). The efficacy of magnetic resonance imaging and color Doppler ultrasonography in diagnosis of salivary gland tumors. *J. Dent. Res. Dent. Clin. Dent. Prospects* 8 (4): 246–251.

102 Probst, F. A., Probst, M., Pautke, C. et al. Magnetic resonance imaging: a useful tool to distinguish between keratocystic odontogenic tumours and odontogenic cysts. *Br. J. Oral. Maxillofac. Surg.* 52015 3 (3): 217–222.

103 Adams, W. H., Daniel, G. B., Pardo, A. D., and Selcer, R. R. (1995). Magnetic resonance imaging of the caudal lumbar and lumbosacral spine in 13 dogs (1990–1993). *Vet. Rad. Ultrasound* 36 (1): 3–13.

104 Joshi, P. S., Pol, J., and Sudesh, A. S. (2014). Ultrasonography – a diagnostic modality for oral and maxillofacial diseases. *Contemp. Clin. Dent.* 5 (3): 345–351.

105 Wakasugi-Sato, N., Kodama, M., Matsuo, K. et al. (2010). Advanced clinical usefulness of ultrasonography for diseases in oral and maxillofacial regions. *Int. J. Dent.*

106 Dayanand, S. M., Desai, R., and Reddy, P. B. (2010). Efficiency of ultrasonography in assessing cervical lymph node metastasis in oral carcinoma. *Natl. J. Maxillofac Surg.* 1 (2): 117–122.

107 Javadrashid, R., Fouladi, D. F., Golamian, M. et al. (2015). Visibility of different foreign bodies in the maxillofacial region using plain radiography, CT, MRI and ultrasonography: an in vitro study. *Dentomaxillofac. Radiol.* 44 (4): 20140229.

108 Huang, G., Zheng, J., Zhang, S., and Yang, C. (2014). The value of panoramic radiograph, CT and MRI for the diagnosis of condylar fracture. *Zhonghua Kou Qiang Yi Xue Za Zhi.* 49 (7): 434–439.

109 White, S. C. and Pharoah, M. J. (2014). Other imaging modalities. In: *Oral Radiology—Principles and Interpretation*, 7e (ed. S.C. White and M.J. Pharoah), 229–249. Philadelphia: PA, Elsevier.

110 Van Thielen, B., Siguenza, F., and Hassan, B. (2012). Cone beam computed tomography in veterinary dentistry. *J. Vet. Dent.* 29 (1): 27–34.

111 Feeney, D. A., Fletcher, T. F., and Hardy, R. M. (1991). *Atlas of Correlative Imaging Anatomy of the Normal Dog*. Philadelphia, PA: WB Saunders.

112 Yu, H., Shen, S. G., Wang, X. et al. (2013). The indication and application of computer-assisted navigation in oral and maxillofacial surgery-Shanghai's experience based on 104 cases. *J. Craniomaxillofac. Surg.*

113 Yu, H. B., Shen, G. F., Zhang, S. L. et al. (2008). Application of computer assisted navigation in the treatment of temporomandibular joint ankylosis. *Shanghai Kou Qiang Yi Xue* 17 (5): 452–456.

114 Foley, B. D., Thayer, W. P., Honeybrook, A. et al. (2013). Mandibular reconstruction using computer-aided design and computer-aided manufacturing: an analysis of surgical results. *J. Oral. Maxillofac. Surg.* 71 (2): e111–e119.

115 Markiewicz, M. R. and Bell, R. B. (2011). Modern concepts in computer-assisted craniomaxillofacial reconstruction. *Curr. Opin Otolaryngol. Head Neck Surg.* 19 (4): 295–301.

116 Hirsch, D. L., Garfein, E. S., Christensen, A. M. et al. (2009). Use of computer-aided design and computer-aided manufacturing to produce orthognathically ideal surgical outcomes: a paradigm shift in head and neck reconstruction. *J. Oral. Maxillofac. Surg.* 67 (10): 2115–2122.

117 Bar-Am, Y., Pollard, R. E., Kass, P. H., and Verstraete, F. J. (2008). The diagnostic yield of conventional radiographs and computed tomography in dogs and cats with maxillofacial trauma. *Vet. Surg.* 37 (3): 294–299.

118 Gendler, A., Lewis, J. R., Reetz, J. A., and Schwarz, T. (2010). Computed tomographic features of oral squamous cell carcinoma in cats: 18 cases (2002–2008). *J. Am. Vet. Med. Assoc.* 236 (3): 319–325.

119 Abboud, M., Guirado, J. L., Orentlicher, G., and Wahl, G. (2013). Comparison of the accuracy of cone beam computed tomography and medical computed tomography: implications for clinical diagnostics with guided surgery. *Int. J. Oral Maxillofac. Implants* 28 (2): 536–542.

120 Bononmo, L., Foley, D., Imhof, H. et al. *Multidetector Computed Tomography Technology: Advances in Imaging techniques*. London: Royal Society of Medicine.

121 Fuhrmann, R. A., Bücker, A., and Diedrich, P. R. (1995). Assessment of alveolar bone loss with high

resolution computed tomography. *J. Periodontal. Res.* 30 (4): 258–263.

122 Langen, H. J., Fuhrmann, R., Diedrich, P., and Günther, R. W. (1995). Diagnosis of infra-alveolar bony lesions in the dentate alveolar process with high-resolution computed tomography. Experimental results. *Invest. Radiol.* 30 (7): 421–426.

123 Fuhrmann, R. A., Bücker, A., and Diedrich, P. R. (1997). Furcation involvement: comparison of dental radiographs and HR-CT-slices in human specimens. *J. Periodontal. Res.* 32 (5): 409–418.

124 Loubele, M., Guerrero, M. E., Jacobs, R. et al. (2007). A comparison of jaw dimensional and quality assessments of bone characteristics with cone-beam CT, spiral tomography, and multi-slice spiral CT. *Int. J. Oral Maxillofac. Implants* 22 (3): 446–454.

125 Ahmad, M., Jenny, J., and Downie, M. (2012). Application of cone beam computed tomography in oral and maxillofacial surgery. *Aust. Dent. J.* 57 (Suppl. 1): 82–94.

126 Garcia de Paula-Silva, F. W., Hassan, B., Bezerra da Silva, L. A. et al. (2009). Outcome of root canal treatment in dogs determined by periapical radiography and cone-beam computed tomography scans. *J. Endod.* 35 (5): 723–726.

127 Patel, S., Dawood, A., Pitt-Ford, T., and Whaites, E. (2007). The potential applications of cone beam computed tomography in the management of endodontic problems. *Int. Endod. J.* 40: 818–830.

128 Wu, M. K., Shemesh, H., and Wesselink, P. R. (2009). Limitations of previously published systematic reviews evaluating the outcome of endodontic treatment. *Int. Endod. J.* http://onlinelibrary.wiley.com/doi/10.1111/j.1365-2591.2009.01600.x/abstract;jsessionid=B7AECEEE2034A7452EC8E2C083AF2E80.f01t03.

129 de Paula-Silva, F. W., Wu, M. K., Leonardo, M. R. et al. (2009). Accuracy of periapical radiography and cone-beam computed tomography scans in diagnosing apical periodontitis using histopathological findings as a gold standard. *J. Endod.* 35 (7): 1009–1012.

130 Estrela, C., Bueno, M. R., Leles, C. R. et al. (2008). Accuracy of cone beam computed tomography and panoramic and periapical radiography for detection of apical periodontitis. *J. Endod.* 34 (3): 273–279.

131 Patel, S., Wilson, R., Dawood, A. et al. (2012). The detection of periapical pathosis using digital periapical radiography and cone beam computed tomography-part 2: a 1-year post-treatment follow-up. *Int. Endod. J.* 45 (8): 711–723.

132 de Paula-Silva, F. W., Santamaria, M. Jr., Leonardo, M. R. et al. (2009). Cone-beam computerized tomographic, radiographic, and histologic evaluation of periapical repair in dogs' post-endodontic treatment. *Oral. Surg. Oral. Med. Oral. Pathol. Oral. Radiol. Endod.* 108 (5): 796–805.

133 Velvart, P., Hecker, H., and Tillinger, G. (2001). Detection of the apical lesion and the mandibular canal in conventional radiography and computed tomography. *Oral. Surg. Oral. Med. Oral. Pathol. Oral. Radiol. Endod.* 92 (6): 682–688.

134 Ordinola-Zapata, R., Bramante, C. M., Duarte, M. H. et al. (2011). The influence of cone-beam computed tomography and periapical radiographic evaluation on the assessment of periapical bone destruction in dog's teeth. *Oral. Surg. Oral. Med. Oral. Pathol. Oral. Radiol. Endod.* 112 (2): 272–279.

135 Baziar, H., Daneshvar, F., Mohammadi, A., and Jafarzadeh, H. (2014). Endodontic management of amandibular first molar with four canals in a distal root by using cone-beam computed tomography: a case report. *J. Oral. Maxillofac. Res.* 5 (1): e5.

136 Zhang, R., Wang, H., Tian, Y. Y. et al. (2011). Use of cone-beam computed tomography to evaluate root and canal morphology of mandibular molars in Chinese individuals. *Int. Endod. J.* 44 (11): 990–999.

137 Silva, E. J., Nejaim, Y., Silva, A. V. et al. (2013). Evaluation of root canal configuration of mandibular molars in a Brazilian population by using cone-beam computed tomography: an in vivo study. *J. Endod.* 39 (7): 849–852.

138 Kumar, R. (2014). Report of a rare case: a maxillary first molar with seven canals confirmed with cone-beam computed tomography. *Iran Endod. J.* 9 (2): 153–157.

139 Almeida, G., Machado, R., Sanches Cunha, R. et al. (2015). Maxillary first molar with 8 root canals detected by CBCT scanning: a case report. *Gen. Dent.* 63 (2): 68–70.

140 Raghavendra, S. S., Hindlekar, A. N., Desai, N. N. et al. (2014). Endodontic management of maxillary first molar with seven root canals diagnosed using cone beam computed tomography scanning. *Indian J. Dent.* 5 (3): 152–156.

141 La, S. H., Jung, D. H., Kim, E. C., and Min, K. S. (2010). Identification of independent middle mesial canal in mandibular first molar using cone-beam computed tomography imaging. *J. Endod.* 36 (3): 542–545.

142 Rigolone, M., Pasqualini, D., Bianchi, L. et al. (2003). Vestibular surgical access to the palatine root of the superior first molar: "low-dose cone-beam" CT analysis of the pathway and its anatomic variations. *J. Endod.* 29 (11): 773–775.

143 Maini, A., Durning, P., and Drage, N. (2008). Resorption: within or without? The benefit of cone-beam computed tomography when diagnosing a

case of an internal/external resorption defect. *Br. Dent. J.* 204 (3): 135–137.

144 Cohenca, N., Simon, J. H., Mathur, A., and Malfaz, J. M. (2007). Clinical indications for digital imaging in dento-alveolar trauma. Part 2: root resorption. *Dent. Traumatol.* 23 (2): 105–113.

145 Grimard, B. A., Hoidal, M. J., and Mills, M. P. (2009). Comparison of clinical, periapical radiograph, and cone-beam volume tomography measurement techniques for assessing bone level changes following regenerative periodontal therapy. *J. Periodontol.* 80 (1): 48–55.

146 Vandenberghe, B., Jacobs, R., and Yang, J. (2008). Detection of periodontal bone loss using digital intraoral and cone beam computed tomography images: an in vitro assessment of bony and/or infrabony defects. *Dentomaxillofac. Radiol.* 37 (5): 252–260.

147 Misch, K. A., Yi, E. S., and Sarment, D. P. (2006). Accuracy of cone beam computed tomography for periodontal defect measurements. *J. Periodontol.* 77 (7): 1261–1266.

148 Mol, A. and Balasundaram, A. (2008). In vitro cone beam computed tomography imaging of periodontal bone. *Dentomaxillofac. Radiol.* 37 (6): 319–324.

149 Merrett, S. J., Drage, N. A., and Durning, P. (2009). Cone beam computed tomography: a useful tool in orthodontic diagnosis and treatment planning. *J. Orthod.* 36 (3): 202–210.

150 Dudic, A., Giannopoulou, C., Martinez, M. et al. (2008). Diagnostic accuracy of digitized periapical radiographs validated against micro-computed tomography scanning in evaluating orthodontically induced apical root resorption. *Eur. J. Oral Sci.* 116 (5): 467–472.

151 de Oliveira-Santos, C., Souza, P. H., de Azambuja Berti-Couto, S. et al. (2012). Assessment of variations of the mandibular canal through cone beam computed tomography. *Clin. Oral Investig.* 16 (2): 387–393.

152 Ghaeminia, H., Meijer, G. J., Soehardi, A. et al. (2009). Position of the impacted third molar in relation to the mandibular canal. Diagnostic accuracy of cone beam computed tomography compared with panoramic radiography. *Int. J. Oral. Maxillofac. Surg.* 38 (9): 964–971.

153 Ghaeminia, H., Meijer, G. J., Soehardi, A. et al. (2011). The use of cone beam CT for the removal of wisdom teeth changes the surgical approach compared with panoramic radiography: a pilot study. *Int. J. Oral. Maxillofac. Surg.* 40 (8): 834–839.

154 Umar, G., Obisesan, O., Bryant, C., and Rood, J. P. (2013). Elimination of permanent injuries to the inferior alveolar nerve following surgical intervention of the "high risk" third molar. *Br. J. Oral Maxillofac. Surg.* 51 (4): 353–357.

155 Halperin-Sternfeld, M., Machtei, E. E., and Horwitz, J. (2014). Diagnostic accuracy of cone beam computed tomography for dimensional linear measurements in the mandible. *Int. J. Oral Maxillofac. Implants* 29 (3): 593–599.

156 Ahmad, M. and Freymiller, E. (2010). Cone beam computed tomography: evaluation of maxillofacial pathology. *J. Calif. Dent. Assoc.* 38 (1): 41–47.

157 Makins, S. R. (2014). Artifacts interfering with interpretation of cone beam computed tomography images. *Dent. Clin. North Am.* 58: 485–495.

158 Bechara, B., McMahan, C. A., Noujeim, M. et al. (2013). Comparison of cone beam CT scans with enhanced photostimulated phosphor plate images in the detection of root fracture of endodontically treated teeth. *Dentomaxillofac. Radiol.* 42 (7): 201–204.

159 Roza, M. R., Silva, L. A., Barriviera, M. et al. (2011). Cone beam computed tomography and intraoral radiography for diagnosis of dental abnormalities in dogs and cats. *J. Vet. Sci.* 12 (4): 387–392.

160 Patel, S., Durack, C., Abella, F. et al. (2014). European Society of Endodontology position statement: the use of CBCT in Endodontics. *Int. Endod. J.* 47 (6): 502–504.

161 (2013). American Academy of Oral and Maxillofacial Radiology: clinical recommendations regarding use of cone beam computed tomography in orthodontics. Position statement by the American Academy of Oral and Maxillofacial Radiology. *Oral Surg. Oral Med. Oral Pathol. Oral Radiol.* 116 (2): 238–257.

162 Silva, M. A., Wolf, U., Heinicke, F. et al. (2008). Cone-beam computed tomography for routine orthodontic treatment planning: a radiation dose evaluation. *Am. J. Orthod. Dentofacial. Orthop.* 133 (5): 640. e1–5.

163 Grünheid, T., Kolbeck Schieck, J. R., Pliska, B. T. et al. (2012). Dosimetry of a cone-beam computed tomography machine compared with a digital x-ray machine in orthodontic imaging. *Am. J. Orthod. Dentofacial. Orthop.* 141 (4): 436–443.

164 Scarfe, W. C., Farman, A. G., and Sukovic, P. (2006). Clinical applications of cone-beam computed tomography in dental practice. *J. Can. Dent. Assoc.* 72 (1): 75–80.

165 Mao, T. and Neelakantan, P. (2014). Three-dimensional imaging modalities in endodontics. *Imaging Sci. Dent.* 44 (3): 177–183.

4

Developmental Pathology and Pedodontology

Bonnie H. Shope[1], Paul Q. Mitchell[2], and Diane Carle[3]

[1] Veterinary Dental Services, LLC, Boxborough, MA, USA
[2] Veterinary Dental Services, North Attleboro, MA, USA
[3] Animal Medical Center of Seattle, Seattle, WA, USA

4.1 Introduction

Small animal veterinary pedodontics is the branch of veterinary dentistry that provides dental care to young dogs and cats. Young dogs and cats can present with many dental conditions, including developmental abnormalities, traumatic injury, neoplasia, and oral diseases.

4.2 Dentition of Puppies and Kittens

Puppies and kittens are born with fully developed, but unerupted, deciduous dentition. Permanent dentition is present in the mandible in the bell stage, with the mandibular first molar teeth beginning to calcify [1]. The dog's deciduous canine and incisor teeth begin erupting at three weeks and the second through third premolars erupt at 4–12 weeks, ending with a total of 28 deciduous teeth. There are no deciduous precursors to first premolar teeth in the dog or to molar teeth in the dog or the cat. Deciduous teeth begin erupting at two to three weeks in the cat, beginning with the incisor teeth, followed by the canines at three to four weeks and the premolars at three to six weeks until the cat's full 26 deciduous teeth have erupted. Table 4.1 shows the eruption schedule of deciduous teeth. Missing deciduous teeth at six weeks of age in the cat or 12 weeks of age in the dog are significant as the associated permanent tooth is unlikely to develop [2].

When identifying deciduous cheek teeth, it is important to remember that the crown of the deciduous tooth resembles the crown of the next caudal-most permanent tooth. For example, the deciduous mandibular fourth premolar tooth has three cusps and resembles the permanent mandibular first molar tooth, rather than the single-crowned permanent fourth premolar tooth that succeeds it (Figure 4.1). Also, the maxillary deciduous third and fourth premolar teeth closely resemble the permanent fourth premolar and first molar teeth.

At about three months of age in the cat and the dog, the deciduous incisor teeth begin to shed and are replaced by their permanent counterparts. Permanent tooth eruption continues until five to seven months of age in the dog and four to six months of age in the cat. Table 4.1 shows the eruption schedule of the permanent teeth. Eruption schedules for permanent teeth can vary by weeks or even months. Teeth in large breed dogs erupt sooner than those in small breed dogs [3]. For the most part, permanent teeth erupt lingually to the deciduous teeth, except for the maxillary canine teeth, which erupt mesial to their deciduous counterparts. Occasionally, a persistent deciduous fourth premolar may be found palatal to the erupting permanent fourth premolar.

A normal dog has 42 teeth by seven months of age and cats have 30 teeth by about six months of age.

Table 4.1 Eruption schedule of deciduous teeth.[a]

	Deciduous teeth (weeks)		**Permanent teeth (months)**	
	Dog	Cat	Dog	Cat
Incisors	3–4	2–3	3–5	3–4
Canines	3	3–4	4–6	4–5
Premolars	4–12	3–6	4–6	4–6
Molars	—	—	5–7	4–5

Source: From reference [56].
[a] Eruption varies with breed and size of animals. Gingival eruption continues to full crown height over a period of weeks.

Wiggs's Veterinary Dentistry: Principles and Practice, Second Edition. Edited by Heidi B. Lobprise and Johnathon R. (Bert) Dodd.

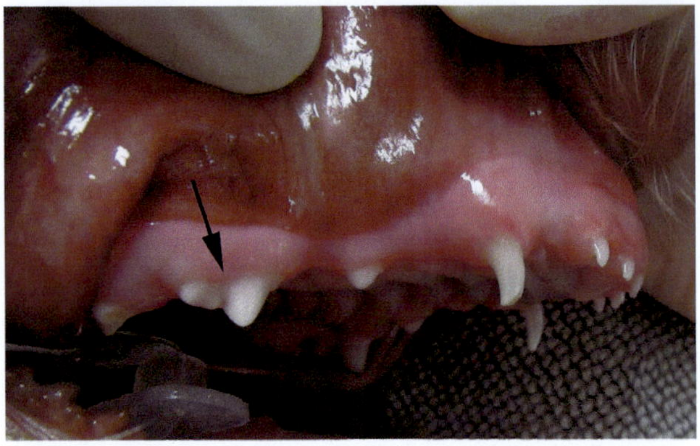

Figure 4.1 Deciduous dentition in a dog. The deciduous maxillary third premolar tooth (arrow) resembles the adult maxillary fourth premolar tooth.

4.3 Developmental Abnormalities of the Mouth

4.3.1 Developmental Abnormalities of the Tongue

Macroglossia, or a congenitally enlarged tongue, is an uncommon condition in dogs. Brachycephalic breeds have a relatively large tongue for their oral cavity, but do not have true macroglossia. Dogs with true macroglossia will have decreased function of the tongue with reduced range of motion and increased susceptibility to lingual trauma [4]. Macroglossia has been found in seven Dachshunds with a nasopharyngeal dysgenesis resulting in abnormally thickened palatopharyngeal muscles and hypertrophic geniohyoid and genioglossus muscles. The combined effect of the enlarged tongue and thickened pharyngeal muscles resulted in coughing, retching, and progressive dysphagia. Dogs in the study appeared to have impaired ability to push a food bolus caudodorsally. Outcomes for the dogs were generally poor, even with surgery to remove excess pharyngeal tissue. No attempt was made to resect tongue tissue in any of the dogs [5]. Macroglossia was also found in a family of Giant Schnauzers with congenital hypothyroid dwarfism. Four out of five Giant Schnauzers treated with thyroid supplement had complete resolution of clinical signs [6]. In humans, macroglossia is usually treated surgically and reduction efforts aim to preserve the tip of the tongue when possible, in order to preserve aesthetic, speech, and taste capabilities [7]. Resection of the traumatized portion of the tongue has been reported to produce good clinical results in dogs [8].

Microglossia is a recessive autosomal defect that results in a short, narrow, pointed, upward curled tongue. This condition is also known as "bird tongue" and has been reported in a litter of Miniature Schnauzers [9]. The condition was also reported in one or more puppies in 12 different related Basset Hound litters [10]. The condition initially presents as an inability to suckle properly. Dogs affected with this defect may initially be diagnosed with "fading puppy" syndrome until the malformed tongue is identified [9]. The condition in the Schnauzer dogs was associated with other serious congenital syndromes and euthanasia was recommended as the puppies failed to thrive even with intensive nursing care [9]. The condition in the Basset Hound litter was not associated with any other abnormalities [10]. There is no known treatment for microglossia in dogs [4, 9, 10].

Ankyloglossia, or "tongue-tie" is characterized by a congenitally short and thick lingual frenulum. This abnormality is often accompanied by a notched or "W" shaped tip of the tongue [11]. In most cases, there are no other craniofacial abnormalities, although a single case of concurrent lingual bifida has been reported [11, 12]. Individuals affected by ankyloglossia often have difficulty suckling, licking, swallowing, and vocalizing. Dogs can also have difficulty with thermoregulation due to a reduced ability to cool themselves through the tongue. Difficulty with prehension of food and excessive drooling have also been reported [13]. The condition is very rare in dogs and has only been reported in Anatolian Shepherd dogs (Kangal dog). Ankyloglossia is believed to arise from failure of breakdown of the cranial 2/3 of the membrane that adheres the tongue to the floor of the mouth in early development [11]. Successful treatment has been achieved by freeing the abnormally attached portion of the tongue with frenuloplasty [13, 14].

Heterotrophic hair shafts, also known as "hairy tongue," is a condition where hairs are found along the median sulcus of the tongue (Figure 4.2). This condition has been attributed to hair becoming embedded in the tongue's dorsal surface as a result of grooming. However, post mortem histology has shown that hairs found on tongues of at least some dogs were actually heterotrophic hair shafts and this has been attributed to normal surface ectoderm-neural crest mesenchyme interaction, which normally results in hair formation, occurring in an inappropriate location [15, 16]. This condition is usually not treated unless the hairs cause glossitis. Treatment is removal of the hairs and flushing with an antibacterial solution; however, the hairs frequently grow back [4].

4.3.2 Abnormalities in Teeth

4.3.2.1 Variations in Number of Teeth

Variations in the number of teeth that develop are common in animals. Hyperdontia (HYP) is the development of extra, or supernumerary, teeth in the mouth. Supernumerary teeth (T/SN) are thought to develop from continued proliferation of the permanent or deciduous

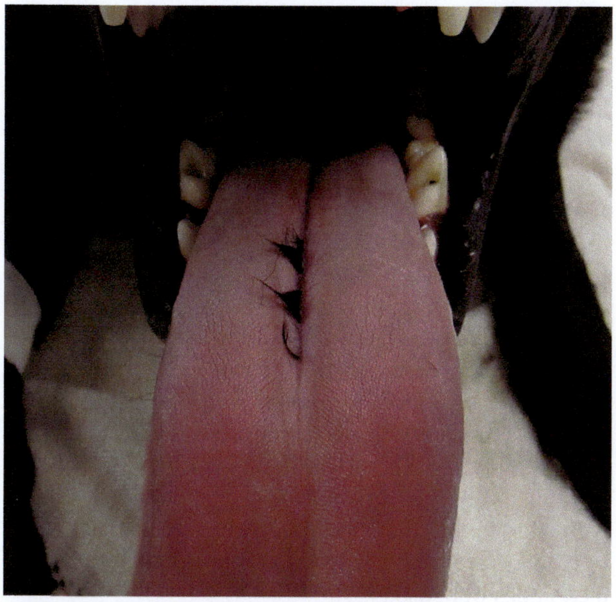

Figure 4.2 Heterotrophic hair shafts along the median raphe of a Labrador Retriever's tongue.

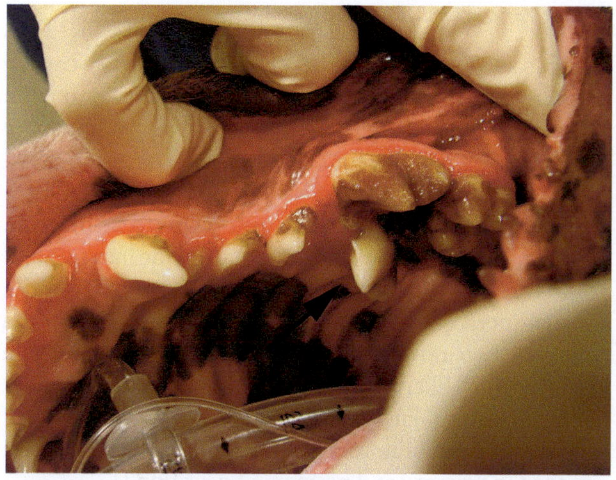

Figure 4.3 A supernumerary maxillary left fourth premolar tooth at the palatal aspect of the fourth premolar tooth.

dental lamina to form a third tooth germ, or from disturbances during tooth development. They can be found in either primary or permanent dentition, but are most commonly found in permanent dentition [17, 18]. Supernumerary teeth are common in the Greyhound, Boxer, Bulldog, and Rottweiler dogs but are rarely found in cats [17, 19]. Supernumerary teeth are more commonly found in the maxilla than the mandible. One study found more than one-third of Greyhounds had supernumerary teeth, most frequently the first premolar tooth. Supernumerary incisor teeth have been noted in Boxers and Bulldogs [18, 20]. Extra teeth can cause crowding and increased risk of periodontal disease, although in dolichocephalic breeds they do not commonly cause crowding [18]. If supernumerary teeth cause crowding or a malocclusion, they should be extracted to prevent periodontal or occlusal complications. A supernumerary maxillary fourth premolar tooth is shown in Figure 4.3. This has been associated with facial swelling in a dog and was attributed to food impaction and occlusal trauma resulting in periodontitis [21].

Tooth agenesis is failure of one or more teeth to develop. Hypodontia (HYP) describes the absence of one to six teeth, while oligodontia is used to refer to the absence of more than six teeth. Anodontia is the complete lack of tooth development [2]. Hypodontia and oligodontia are more commonly seen in humans in the permanent dentition than in the deciduous dentition [22]. When a deciduous tooth is missing, the permanent successor is more likely to be missing as well [2]. Tooth agenesis is believed to result from a failure of the dental lamina and neural crest mesenchyme to interact. Hypodontia, oligodontia, and anodontia have been reported in dogs and cats and are associated with hairless breeds as well as a variety of syndromes including ectodermal dysplasia [17]. Oligodontia of the deciduous teeth and anodontia of permanent dentition has been reported in an otherwise normal cat and anodontia has been reported in an adult cat whose dentition as a kitten was unknown [23, 24]. Complete anodontia has also been reported in a dog [3]. In cats, the maxillary second premolar is frequently absent, and the prevalence of this varies widely with location, ranging from 3 to 28% [19]. Tooth agenesis has been associated with the Affenpinscher, the Kerry Blue Terrier, hairless breed dogs, large dolichocephalic breed dogs, and small breed dogs including the Miniature Poodle, [17, 20, 25]. In humans, non-syndromic tooth agenesis has been demonstrated to be inherited as an autosomal dominant, autosomal recessive, or sex-linked trait, but this has not been researched in dogs and cats [2].

4.3.2.2 Variation in Size of Teeth

Variations of normal tooth size can occur in animals. These disorders can be generalized or localized in the mouth. Microdontia (T/MIC) and macrodontia (T/MAC) refer to teeth that are smaller than normal or larger than normal, respectively. In humans, macrodontia is a rare dental anomaly where a tooth is larger than average [26]. In veterinary medicine this has been reported to occur with tooth germination [17]. Microdontia describes teeth with crowns, roots, and nerves that are normal in shape yet smaller than usual. This commonly occurs in the third incisors in the dog. One form of microdontia is a "peg tooth" where the crown of the tooth has an abnormal conical shape in a tooth that normally has a more complex crown shape [27].

4.3.3 Variation in Structure of the Tooth

Teeth can vary greatly in shape, and often this can be attributed to morphological anomalies of developmental origin. The term "double teeth" refers to two teeth that are partially joined by dentin or even pulp. These abnormal looking teeth are either the result of gemination (T/GEM) or fusion (T/FUS). Gemination is thought to result from the failed attempt of one tooth germ to divide into two and should be suspected when there is a large tooth and a normal tooth count. Fusion is believed to arise from the union of two normally separated tooth germs. Double teeth are most likely the result of fusion when the adjacent tooth is missing. Fusion may involve the entire length of the tooth or only the roots. Both gemination and fusion are seen in primary and permanent dentition [17].

A condition known as dens invaginatus (T/DENS) or dens-en-dente is found in dogs and humans [28, 29] (Figure 4.4). This condition develops during tooth development from an in-folding of the dental papilla prior to calcification of the dental tissues [30]. It has been reported in dogs in the maxillary canine tooth and in the mandibular first and second molar teeth [29, 31, 32]. The etiology of this condition is unknown, but there is some evidence in humans that it may be genetic in origin [33]. These teeth may be incompletely lined by enamel [31]. Teeth with suspected dens invaginatus should be radiographed. If no periapical pathology is noted and no obvious opening in the invagination is seen, the teeth can be treated conservatively with periodic radiographs. However, invaginations can predispose the tooth to endodontic disease as well as periodontal disease and these teeth frequently require extraction. There are numerous reports of successful endodontic treatment of these teeth in humans [34]. A report of a dog treated successfully with endodontic treatment recommends extensive irrigation and chemical debridement, but standard obturation techniques were used [29].

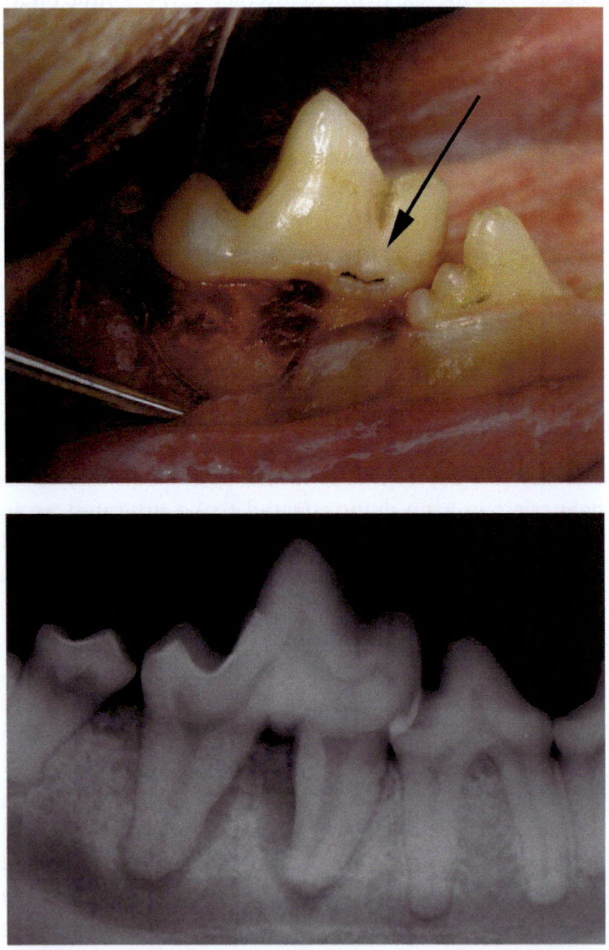

Figure 4.4 Mandibular right first molar tooth in a dog with dens invaginatus. The dark linear defect between the mesial and central cusps is an infolding of the enamel. The radiograph shows marked periapical bone loss at both roots, the result of endodontic disease from the infolded enamel.

Root hypoplasia, also called dentin hypoplasia, has been found in dogs, and often accompanies other disorders such as enamel hypoplasia (Figure 4.5). The root begins developing after the crown shape has formed, but before calcification, so developmental insults affecting enamel can also affect the developing root. Root hypoplasia has been documented in dogs with histories of distemper as well as a dog with unknown history, but the condition appears to be often accompanied by enamel dysplasia [35–37]. In humans, root hypoplasia is attributed to disruption in the development of Hertwig's root sheath [38]. Nutritional factors such as deficiency in vitamin D or phosphorus, infectious factors, and traumatic factors have been implicated in root hypoplasia. Hypoplastic roots often are not mobile and are functional for several years [35]. These teeth can be left in place unless they have radiographic signs of disease or are mobile.

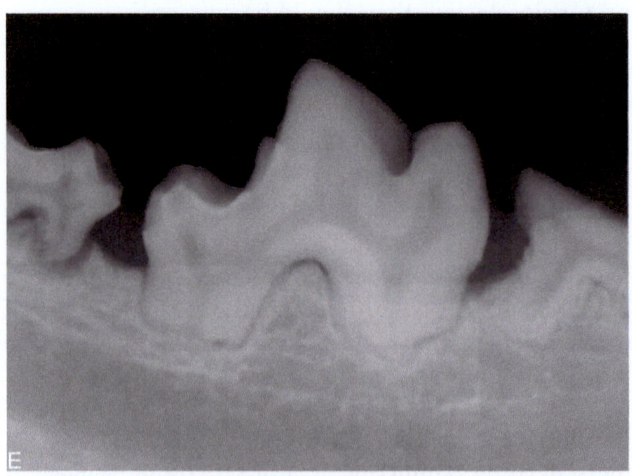

Figure 4.5 Root hypoplasia in a 10-month-old hound dog mix.

Dilaceration refers to an abnormal bend in the root or crown of a tooth. It occurs most frequently in the root of the tooth, but can appear anywhere along the length of the tooth. The condition is thought to occur due to trauma or infection during tooth formation [17]. In humans, dilacerated teeth have been associated with non-eruption, prolonged retention of the deciduous predecessor teeth, and apical fenestration of the labial cortical plate [39]. In dogs and cats, these teeth are usually asymptomatic, although they can be more difficult to extract and more difficult to treat with endodontic therapy.

Supernumerary roots are common in dogs in the upper second and third premolar teeth, and in cats in the upper third premolar tooth [19, 40, 41]. Convergent roots, where two normally shaped roots are fused, can be found in dogs and cats [27]. Concrescence is a form of fusion when two neighboring teeth are joined by cementum. This process, which is thought to be related to trauma or crowding, can take place before or after eruption [17]. Teeth with these types of variations in root structures are not usually clinically significant, but are important to recognize when extracting teeth.

4.3.4 Regional Odontodysplasia

Regional odontodysplasia, or odontoblastic dysplasia, is a condition where all the components of the tooth that derive from the dental organ in the affected teeth are abnormal. This includes the enamel, dentin, and cementum. However, unlike other similar conditions, only one or a few teeth are affected, as opposed to conditions such as amelogenesis imperfecta, where all the teeth are involved. Patients with regional odontodysplasia often present for delayed eruption or failure of eruption of teeth. Teeth can have non-inflammatory gingival swellings near the affected teeth due to caries, or bacterial infection of the pulp through defective enamel or dentin [42]. Histologically, the pulp chamber and canals of a tooth are filled with abnormal dentin and collagenous stroma [43]. This condition has been reported in a maxillary canine tooth in a Beagle and in multiple teeth in a Boerboel dog [42, 43].

4.3.5 Enamel Defects

During enamel development, several abnormalities may occur. These are sometimes found on clinical, radiological, or histological examination. Enamel formation starts before the eruption of the first teeth and involves many different genes. Defects in any one of these genes can result in defects in the formation of deciduous and permanent teeth. Amelogenesis imperfecta is the general term that includes any genetic and/or developmental enamel formation and maturation abnormalities [44]. This condition results from a disturbance in the ectodermal layers of developing teeth. It is often a hereditary abnormality that includes genetic and/or developmental enamel formation and maturation abnormalities such as enamel hypoplasia (E/H) and enamel hypomineralization (E/M). This condition is inherited in the Standard Poodle, Italian Greyhound, and the Samoyed [45–47]. In the Italian Greyhound and the Samoyed, this disease is known to have an autosomal recessive inheritance pattern, although different genetic mutations are involved. Normal enamel functions to seal the tooth from bacteria, protect and insulate the tooth, provide strength to the tooth, and create a smooth surface, which helps prevent plaque from accumulating on the surface of the tooth. The crowns of affected teeth are pitted, rough, and are chalky or discolored brown. The teeth readily stain and attract plaque. Dogs affected with enamel defects, regardless of the cause, are prone to abrasion and fracture of teeth, periodontal disease, dentin sensitivity, and possibly pulpitis and pulp death. Restoration of teeth can be performed to protect the pulp from thermal and mechanical stress and from bacterial infection, to decrease sensitivity, plaque adhesion, susceptibility to abrasion and fracture, and to improve cosmetic appearance [48–50]. Fastidious oral hygiene is also important to keep the periodontium healthy.

Enamel hypoplasia refers to inadequate deposition of enamel matrix (Figure 4.6). This results in normal density or mineralization but enamel that is thinner than normal. This can affect one or several teeth and may be focal or multifocal. The crowns of affected teeth can have areas of normal enamel next to areas of hypoplastic or missing enamel [44]. The thin enamel often gives view to the yellowish-brown dentin underneath. Enamel hypoplasia can be found in dogs that have a history of distemper while in utero or during formation of permanent dentition. Enamel hypomineralization refers to inadequate mineralization of enamel matrix, resulting in white, yellow, or brown spots in the enamel. This often affects several or all teeth. The crowns of affected teeth may be soft and wear faster than normal teeth. The enamel can be difficult to distinguish from dentin radiographically in these teeth, as it has the same radiopacity as the dentin.

Dentinogenesis imperfecta is a hereditary abnormality in the formation of dentin. The clinical appearance of affected teeth varies from gray to brownish violet to a yellowish-brown color, but the teeth can also exhibit a characteristic unusual translucent or opalescent hue. The enamel frequently can be separated from the dentin quite easily, and the exposed dentin demonstrates rapid attrition. Radiographically, the teeth exhibit thin roots, cervical constrictions, and pulp chambers and root

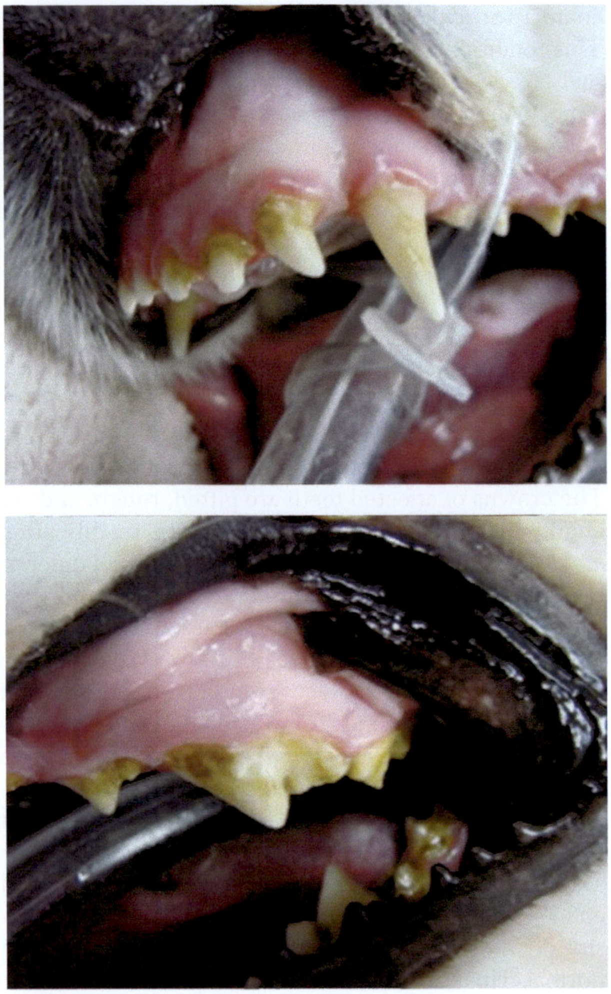

Figure 4.6 Enamel dysplasia in the Samoyed dog.

canals may be partially or completely obliterated [51]. Dental hypomineralization has also been documented as a recessive genetic condition in related Border Collies, causing abnormal abrasion and exposure of teeth [52].

4.3.6 Congenital Porphyria

Congenital porphyria is a rare hereditary defect of hemoglobin formation resulting in anemia and discolored teeth and bones. It is an autosomal recessive trait. The congenital form has not been reported in dogs, but has been seen in cats. Affected teeth emit a red fluorescence, which can distinguish the condition from tetracycline-associated staining that emits a more orange or yellow green color and teeth stained by fluoride toxicosis that will not fluoresce at all. Urine of affected cats will contain porphyrin. There are no published reports of treatment outcomes or prognosis for affected cats, but milder forms may permit reasonable quality of life for more than 10 years [53].

4.4 Abnormalities in Tooth Eruption

4.4.1 Persistent Deciduous Teeth (DT/P)

In human dentistry, a deciduous premolar tooth is considered persistent if the tooth remains when more than three-fourths of the replacing tooth has erupted [54]. In veterinary dentistry, there is no precise definition of when a tooth is considered persistent, but deciduous teeth that persist (DT/P) for more than a few days after eruption of the permanent teeth should be removed to prevent displacement of the adult teeth (Figure 4.7). Deciduous teeth that persist without a corresponding permanent tooth must be radiographed to rule out an unerupted permanent tooth. If no permanent tooth is present and the deciduous tooth is clinically and radiographically healthy, the tooth can be left in place. However, the tooth should be monitored, because deciduous teeth are smaller and more delicate than permanent teeth and may be more prone to fracture. Furthermore, the roots of these teeth can eventually resorb and become mobile and must be extracted at that point. Studies in persistent deciduous human teeth with no permanent successor have found that the deciduous teeth can remain healthy for prolonged periods of time, although ankylosis of the root is an occasional complication [54].

Persistent deciduous teeth (DT/P) are rare in the cat, but have been noted in the maxillary canine teeth and maxillary third premolar teeth. Persistent deciduous canine teeth in cats are found distal to the permanent canines [55, 56].

Extraction is often necessary to treat persistent deciduous teeth, but may also be helpful in treating traumatic fractures to deciduous teeth and in treating various malocclusions of puppies and kittens. Whenever performing extractions of these delicate teeth, extreme care and finesse should be exercised to avoid fracturing their

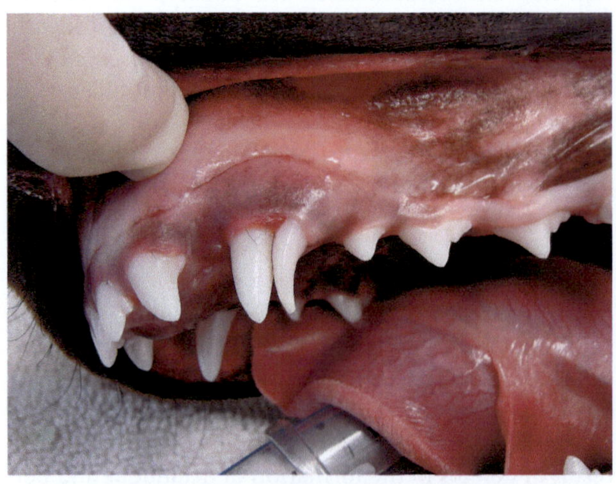

Figure 4.7 Photograph of a persistent left maxillary deciduous canine tooth.

roots and to avoid damage to the surrounding permanent teeth. The adjacent permanent tooth may be in vulnerable stages of development and can be damaged as a result of the extraction process, even with the greatest of care. Pet owners should always be informed of the possibility of adult tooth damage during deciduous tooth extraction.

The first step in the extraction process is to obtain an intraoral radiograph of the tooth in question and the surrounding area. This radiograph will provide invaluable information about the anatomy of the tooth to be extracted, as well as the positioning of the adjacent permanent teeth, so that the operator can plan the best approach for a safe and successful extraction. A post-operative radiograph should also be obtained after the deciduous tooth is removed.

The use of sharp root elevators/luxators, ergonomic comfort for the operator, and patience cannot be overemphasized. The key to success is taking the necessary time to methodically sever the periodontal ligament fibers that attach the tooth to the alveolar bone. Stretching the periodontal ligament fibers through the twisting and holding of the root elevator/luxator should be performed gently, as this may lead to fracturing of these delicate roots. It is equally important to avoid the use of the root elevator/luxator between the deciduous tooth and the adjacent adult tooth.

Horizontal release incisions in the gingiva along the alveolar crest may help to provide more room for an easier insertion of the root elevator/luxator. These incisions are made with either a number 11 or 15C scalpel and may also extend around the circumference of the tooth to be extracted.

Should the root fracture during extraction, an intraoral radiograph should be obtained before proceeding. When compared to the preoperative radiograph, the intraoperative image can aid in guiding the best path for root removal. Every reasonable effort should be made to cautiously remove the remaining root fragment(s) from the alveolus. Some authors have suggested that retained root material of a persistent deciduous tooth may cause many potential problems, including difficulty with complete eruption of the adult tooth [57]. An enlarged mucoperiosteal flap may be helpful to gain more exposure and directly visualize the root fragment.

Some authors have also suggested a more surgical approach to the extraction of persistent deciduous teeth [58, 59]. This involves creating and elevating a mucoperiosteal flap to facilitate exposure and direct visualization of the root and overlying alveolar bone. With the flap held safely out of the way, some of the buccal bone is carefully removed over the root. Just as in surgical extraction of permanent teeth, this bone removal can greatly reduce the force and effort required to completely remove the deciduous tooth root. After removal of the tooth, the mucoperiosteal flap is apposed with absorbable suture material.

One of the most important concerns following the extraction of persistent deciduous teeth is the occlusion of the permanent teeth. An immediate post-operative assessment should be made and follow-up oral examinations should be performed to monitor the bite and detect any malocclusions early.

4.4.2 Unerupted Teeth (T/U)

Failure of teeth to erupt can be due to impaction or primary retention. Impaction (T/I) is prevention of eruption due to a physical barrier such as adjacent teeth, overlying bone, or tissue. Primary retention occurs when a normally placed and developed tooth germ fails to emerge despite the absence of any identifiable barrier to eruption [60].

Soft tissue impaction describes teeth that have emerged from the jaw, but have failed to penetrate the overlying gingiva (Figure 4.8). This has been attributed

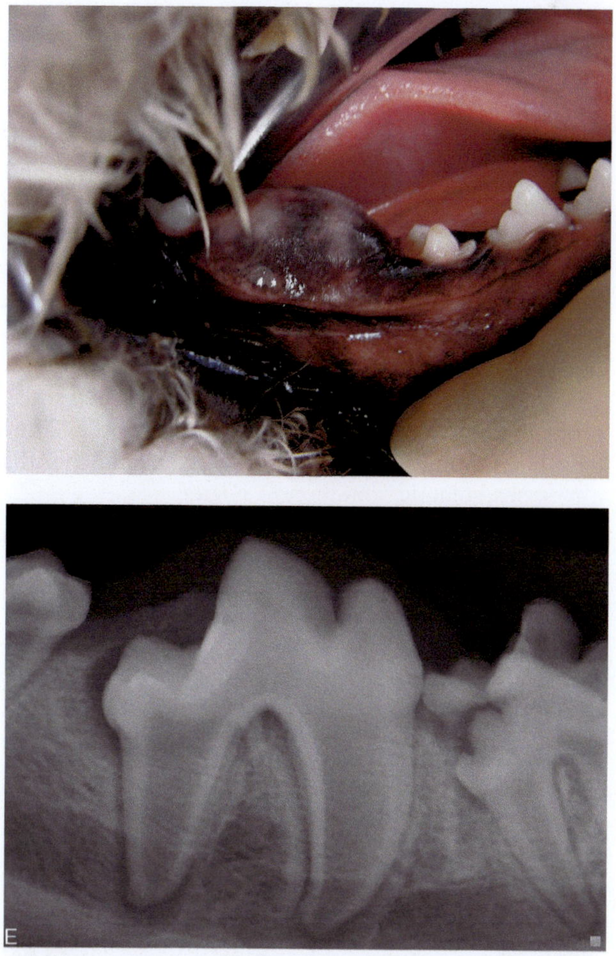

Figure 4.8 Soft tissue impaction of the mandibular right first molar tooth in an eight-month-old Bedlington Terrier. There is also a small amount of bone remaining at the distal aspect of the tooth.

to tough overlying gingiva or a failure of the normal breakdown of overlying tissue [61]. If this condition is treated while the teeth still have eruption potential, indicated by open apices, they can be treated with operculectomy and usually erupt normally.

Bony impaction, or impaction by adjacent teeth, can also be treated if the cause of impaction can be removed and the teeth still have eruption potential. Strategic removal of less critical teeth can be performed if the impacted tooth is a major functional tooth.

Canine distemper has been associated with unerupted teeth, possibly due to damage to the enamel epithelium, preventing resorption of the connective tissue between the crown and the enamel epithelium [35, 37].

If the eruption potential has been lost, or if no reason for failure of the tooth to erupt is identified, the tooth must be extracted or treated with orthodontic forced extrusion because impacted teeth can form dentigerous cysts (DTCs) [62]. Other consequences of impacted teeth include nasal discharge, facial swelling, osteomyelitis, bone loss, loss of adjacent teeth, and malignant transformation of impacted teeth [63, 64].

4.4.3 Dentigerous Cysts (DTC)

Dentigerous cysts (DTCs) are the most common type of odontogenic cyst found in dogs and have been found associated with unerupted canine and first premolar teeth. They have occasionally have been found bilaterally [65, 66] (Figure 4.9). They have also been found in cats associated with unerupted maxillary canine teeth [67, 68]. Radiographically, these lesions present as well-defined, radiolucent areas surrounding an unerupted tooth. Histologically, these cysts are lined with stratified squamous epithelium with a few inflammatory cells. They have been found in dogs ranging in age from 6 months to 10 years, but are most commonly diagnosed in dogs between two and three years of age. Some breeds, including Boxers, Pugs, and Shih Tzus, develop DTCs more commonly than other breeds [65]. Treatment consists of surgical debridement of the cystic lining, but pre-emptive extraction of impacted teeth is recommended to prevent potential destruction of bone and teeth adjacent to DTCs.

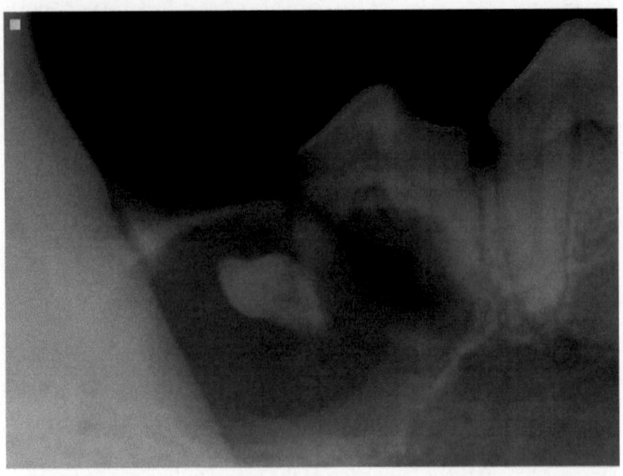

Figure 4.9 Radiograph of a dentigerous cyst in a Bull Mastiff. Note the unerupted first premolar tooth.

Extracting unerupted teeth can require non-standard approaches to avoid damaging adjacent erupted teeth. For example, in one report, extracting an unerupted maxillary canine tooth required partial ostectomy of the maxilla [64]. Orthodontic treatment by forced extrusion is also possible [68].

4.4.4 Abnormalities of the Mandible and Maxilla

4.4.4.1 Cleft Palate (CFP)

Clefts are defects of development that result in failure of palatal tissues to fuse normally. Clefts may occur to primary (cleft lip) and/or secondary (cleft palate) palates. Primary clefts occur rostral to the maxillary processes and may be either unilateral or bilateral. Cleft lips (CFLs) may or may not communicate with the nasal cavity and often surgical repair can be delayed in uncomplicated cases [62].

Clefts of the secondary palate occur caudal to the incisive bone and result in oronasal fistulation, thus allowing milk and other oral contents into the nasal passages when nursing. Patients with CFPs may develop significant medical problems, such as upper respiratory infection, malnutrition, and pneumonia. If these patients can be supported during the early development process, it is typically advisable to delay surgical repair as long as possible. Surgery has been recommended to be delayed until at least three to four months of age, or even six months of age [57, 69]. While surgical repair is demanding and complications are common, chances for success seem to improve if the patient is able to grow and develop more tissue for closure.

4.5 Diseases of the Jaws in Puppies and Kittens

4.5.1 Mandibular Periostitis Ossificans (MPO)

Mandibular periostitis ossificans (MPO) is a pathologic syndrome of immature large breed dogs, first reported in 2010 in a case report of five dogs. It has similarities to the inflammatory condition periostitis ossificans in humans [70]. Patients present with a unilateral, non-painful, caudal mandibular swelling, which centers on the erupting first molar tooth. While some mandibular enlargement may be permanent, most cases spontaneously resolve. The lesions extend from either the third/fourth premolar or the fourth premolar/first molar to beyond the third molar teeth. The swelling is firm ventrally but fluctuant intraorally. Biopsy demonstrates that the outer cortex forms a pseudocystic wall of excessive periosteal new bone, with areas of well-differentiated lamellar bone. The core of the swelling contains necrotic bone, sterile fluid, fibrin, marked proliferation of immature granulation tissue, and new blood vessels, and demonstrates acute inflammation. Lateral radiographs reveal a two-layered or double ventral mandibular cortex, with a space between the two cortices. Occlusal radiographs reveal a double cortex lingually and buccally, with a space between the two cortices. Reported breeds affected include the Labrador Retriever, Dogue de Bordeaux, Great Dane, and Great Pyrenees. Symptoms present at three to five months of age; the median age is 4.1 months. Four of the dogs in the five-dog study were affected on the left mandible, and all dogs were male. Diagnosis is based on incisional biopsy and radiographic appearance. The authors present the theory that in large breed puppies MPO results from an inflamed or infected dental follicle, developing an unerupted tooth and/or secondary to pericoronitis [70].

4.5.2 Craniomandibular Osteopathy (CMO)

Craniomandibular osteopathy (CMO), also known as "lion jaw," "Westie Jaw," or "Scottie jaw," is a self-limiting, developmental orthopedic disease of young animals, ages three to eight months of age. The disease is characterized by a non-neoplastic proliferation of the parietal bone, occipital bone, tympanic bulla, mandibular rami, or the bones of the temporomandibular joint (TMJ) [71] (Figure 4.10). Occasionally, long bones are involved [72, 73]. Presenting symptoms may include pain on opening the mouth, pain on palpation of the jaw, intermittent fever, excessive salivation, bilateral firm painful mandibular swellings, restricted jaw movement, and atrophy of the muscles of mastication [71, 74]. Most cases are self-limiting and are treated with supportive care including nutritional support, fluid therapy, and pain medication, including non-steroidal anti-inflammatories and, in some cases, steroids. In cases where symptoms resolve, boney enlargement remains. However, in certain cases, severe pain and extensive boney changes involving the TMJ can progress to an inability to open the mouth, coinciding with malnourishment and a guarded prognosis [75, 76].

Diagnosis is based on radiographic and/or computed tomography (CT) findings and clinical symptoms, and confirmed with histopathology [77]. Histopathology in a case report exhibited "interconnected trabeculae of

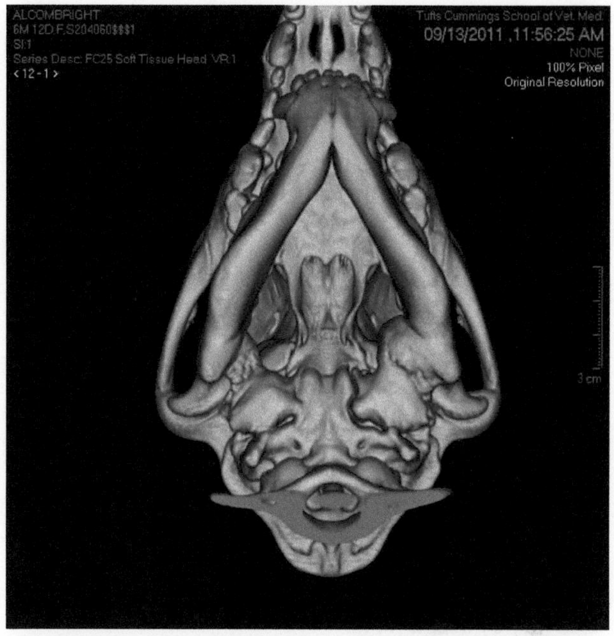

Figure 4.10 Craniomandibular osteopathy. 3D reconstruction of CT of a seven-month-old female Pitbull mix, showing proliferation of mandibular bone and fusion of the TMJ bilaterally. *Source:* Credit Randy Boudrieau.

woven bone, proliferative endosteal new bone, and abundant osteoclasts on the bone surface. The marrow spaces were filled with loose connective tissue and few foci of dense infiltrations of inflammatory cells" [75]. CMO predominately affects young West Highland White Terriers and was initially thought to have an autosomal recessive mode of inheritance [78]. Recent research shows that the inheritance pattern in the West Highland White Terrier, Cairn Terrier, and the Scottish Terrier is more complex, and that this disease is caused by a monogenic mutation in chromosome 5, which is autosomal dominant and has incomplete penetrance. The CMO associated gene is SLC7A2, which is a glucose-phosphate transporter in osteoclasts, and its defect suggests an impaired glucose homeostasis in developing bone, leading to hyperostosis. The disease has varying expression depending on whether the mutation is heterozygous, which confers a lower risk of CMO, or homozygous, which confers a higher risk of CMO. The actual risk of penetrance is unknown and environmental factors or other genetic modifiers may affect expression of the phenotype. Incomplete penetrance and varying expression of disease mean that many unaffected carrier dogs exist. In one study of 303 West Highland White Terriers, 36% carried the mutation. Additional research is needed to investigate other genetic and potentially non-genetic influences on this disease. There is no indication, so far, that this genetic mutation is involved in CMO in other breeds. A genetic test is available to determine the genotype of these three breeds, with regard to the mutation shown to cause CMO. An analogous disease in humans is Caffey's disease [52].

CMO has also been reported with much less frequency in several other breeds including the Boston Terrier, Pit Bull Terrier, other terrier breeds, Doberman Pinscher, Labrador Retriever, Great Dane, Boxer, Shetland Sheepdog, Pyrenean Mountain Breeds, English Bulldog, Bull Mastiff, and the Akita [71, 73, 75–77, 79–84]. The patterns of inheritance and the underlying mutations are unknown in these cases.

Calvarial hyperostosis presents as a firm swelling of the cranium in the region of the frontal sinus and appears histologically as periosteal new bone formation, with thick trabeculae of immature woven and mature lamellar bone separated by cementing lines. Idiopathic canine juvenile cranial hyperostosis is a proposed new term for cranial mandibular osteopathy and calvarial hyperostosis, theorized to be one disorder with predilection sites that vary by breed [77].

4.6 Oral Masses in Young Dogs and Cats

4.6.1 Papillary Squamous Cell Carcinoma (PSCC)

Papillary squamous cell carcinoma (PSCC) is an oral tumor most commonly found in young animals (Figure 4.11). It is malignant and potentially metastatic, but is generally only invasive locally [85]. There are no known reports of PSCC metastasizing. New studies have found that the tumor has a wider age range than previously thought, with multiple cases of PSCC in dogs as old as nine years of age [86, 87]. This tumor has been initially diagnosed as an acanthomatous ameloblastoma in several cases, but on further investigation is identified as PSCC [88, 89]. It is unknown whether the tumor is the result of malignant transformation of a papilloma, but there is some evidence that it is associated with persistent oral trauma [89]. A PSCC was found in an 18-month-old dog eight months following extraction of an impacted maxillary canine tooth [88]. There is some debate as to whether it is a histologic variant of squamous cell carcinoma similar to verrucous carcinoma or is a distinct neoplasm. It appears that surgical excision with 1-cm margins is curative and one case of palliative piroxicam therapy has resulted in a stable disease for 26 months [89].

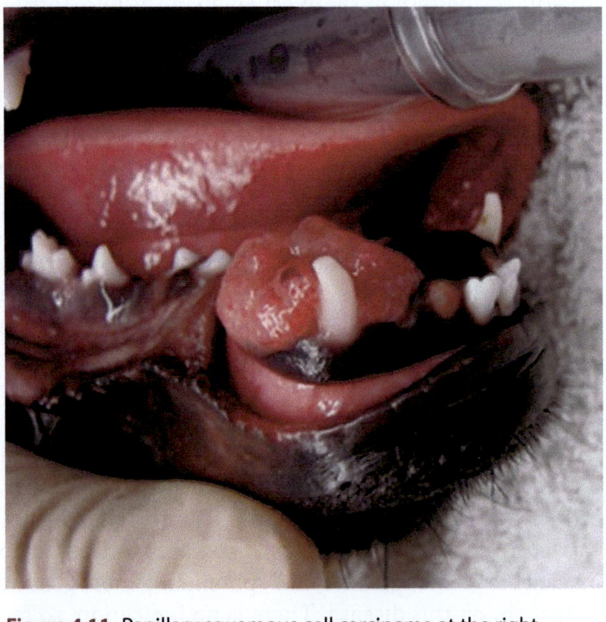

Figure 4.11 Papillary squamous cell carcinoma at the right deciduous mandibular canine tooth of a three-month-old Labrador Retriever puppy.

4.6.2 Feline Inductive Odontogenic Tumor (OM/FIO)

Feline inductive odontogenic tumor (OM/FIO) is a rare tumor that has been found in cats less than three years of age, with most occurring in cats less than 18 months of age [90] (Figure 4.12). The tumor is benign but rapidly expansive and locally destructive, and occurs most frequently in the maxilla [91]. Males and females are equally affected and most occur in domestic short haired cats [90]. This tumor has also been called an adamantinoma, ameloblastoma, ameloblastic fibroma, and inductive fibroameloblastoma [91]. The tumor is classified as inductive because odontogenic epithelium induces mesenchymal cells to form aggregated foci of dental pulp-like cells [92]. Radiographically the tumor can present as radiolucent bone with or without radiodense deposits [90–92].

Complete excision is recommended as the tumor has been shown to recur rapidly if excision is incomplete, although a 1-year-old cat with only 90% excision of the visible portion of the mass remained alive and well 44 months after surgery, despite some early regrowth of the mass [90, 92].

4.6.3 Odontomas

Odontomas are mixed odontogenic tumors that have been found in young dogs. Compound odontomas consist of small tooth structures, or denticles, with an orderly pattern of dental tissues similar to normal teeth, while complex odontomas are disorganized arrangements of dental tissue [93]. They are benign tumors and often associated with an unerupted tooth and alveolar bone swelling. The prognosis for these tumors is good with marginal excision or enucleation and thorough debridement [94].

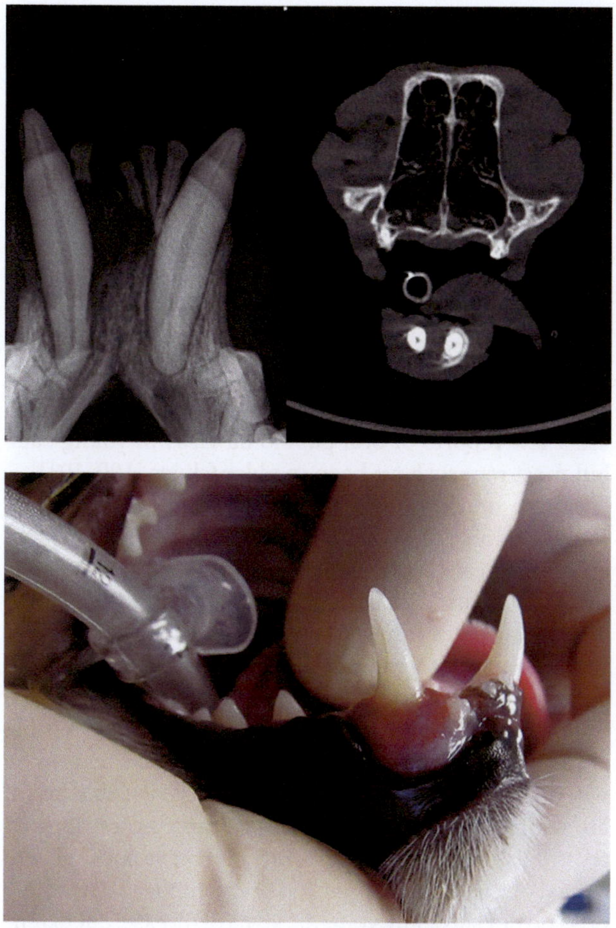

Figure 4.12 Feline inductive odontogenic tumor in the rostral mandible of a cat. Radiograph and CT scan showing extensive bone lysis at the site.

4.7 Other Oral Diseases Found in Young Dogs and Cats

4.7.1 Juvenile Periodontitis/Gingivitis in Cats

Juvenile feline hyperplastic gingivitis is an inflammatory condition of the attached gingiva in the young cat, which occurs around the time of tooth eruption [95, 96] (Figure 4.13). The etiology is unknown and the incidence has not been reported. Susceptibility decreases by around two years of age. Affected cats develop marked gingival inflammation, with erythema, edema, and gums that bleed readily during mastication and oral examination, as well as gingival enlargement and formation of pseudopockets where enlarged gum tissue covers the crowns of teeth. Affected cats do not appear to be in pain and the caudal oral mucosa is not inflamed [95]. While any breed can be affected, there is a genetic predisposition in the Siamese, Somali, Maine Coon, Persian, and Abyssinian [94]. Treatment involves early dental prophylactic cleaning, diligent daily

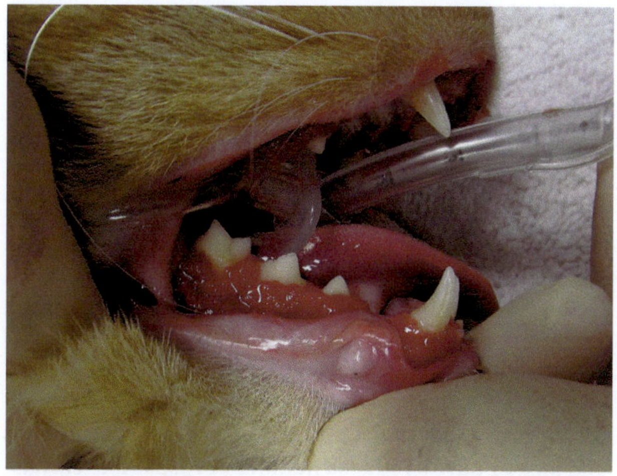

Figure 4.13 Marked inflammation in a nine-month-old cat with juvenile stomatitis.

home care, and gingivectomy to eliminate pseudopockets and inflammation [95]. Some patients require frequent dental cleanings every three to six months [96]. With treatment, symptoms can resolve, however without treatment, rapid progression of periodontal disease typically ensues, with loss of teeth [95]. Additionally, some cases develop chronic oropharyngeal inflammation [96].

Juvenile onset periodontitis is seen in young cats less than nine months of age. The Siamese, Maine Coon, and Domestic Short Haired cats are predisposed [96]. Affected cats have a rapid accumulation of plaque and calculus, with subsequent gingivitis, significant early bone loss, periodontal pocket formation, gum recession, and furcation exposure [96, 97]. Periodontitis is worse around the mandibular first molar teeth and the mandibular incisor teeth, which are often mobile [97]. Halitosis is typical at the time of tooth eruption [96]. Treatment and effective management is difficult and extraction of significantly diseased teeth is indicated [95]. Management of the disease requires early dental cleanings around nine months of age and frequent dental cleanings every six to nine months, as well as diligent home care to control plaque. Radiographic assessment is valuable to examine for loss of alveolar bone, and to diagnose early tooth resorption often seen at sites of periodontal inflammation [96].

4.7.2 Ectodermal Dysplasia

Ectodermal dysplasia is a congenital condition seen in dogs, humans, mice, and cattle, which affects structures of ectodermal origin, including the skin, lacrimal glands, and teeth. Complete alopecia, or partial alopecia on top of the head, ventral chest, and abdomen, the absence of eccrine sweat glands, and severe dental and craniofacial abnormalities are hallmarks of this condition in the dog. Histologically, alopecic regions lack piloglandular units.

Chinese Crested and Mexican Hairless dogs have an autosomal dominant form. Other reported breeds include the Miniature Poodle, Belgian Shepherd, Labrador Retriever, Bichon Frise, German Shepherd, Whippet, Cocker Spaniel, Miniature Pinscher, and Pekingese mixed breeds.

An X-linked recessive mutation in the ectodysplasin (EDA) ligand has been documented in a colony of mixed breed dogs with X-linked hypohidrotic ectodermal dysplasia [97]. Affected dogs are generally male and rarely female. In one published study, dental abnormalities are common, including hypodontia (HYP) and oligodontia (Figure 4.14). Premolars are the most absent tooth. Many rostral and caudal teeth have conical-shaped crowns and lack or have a reduced number of cusps. The carnassial teeth are especially affected. Roots are frequently dilacerated, fused, smaller than normal, or have a reduction in the number of roots. Persistent deciduous teeth and mixed dentition of adult dogs with this condition is common. Immature dogs with deciduous dentition often lack the successional permanent teeth and 94.1% of dogs had a malocclusion, with 15/17 dogs having a class 1 malocclusion with mesioversion of maxillary and/or mandibular canine teeth. Deciduous and permanent canine teeth were often mesioverted. The authors observed the appearance of a narrow muzzle in affected dogs [98].

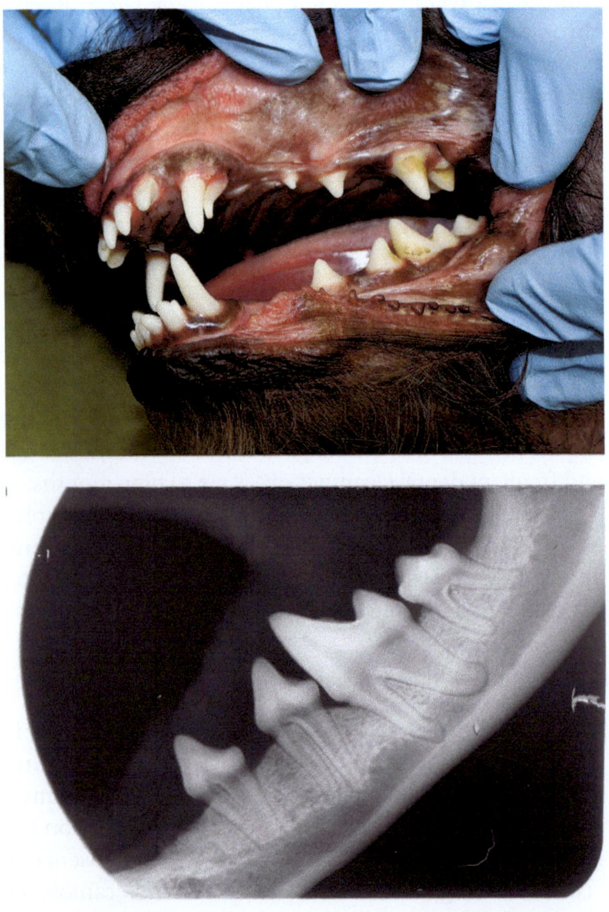

Figure 4.14 Image and radiographs of a dog with X-linked ectodermal hypohidrotic dysplasia. Note the conical shape of the crowns of teeth and several missing teeth. *Source:* Credit John Lewis.

4.8 Papillomaviruses (PV)

Papillomaviruses (PV) occur in mammalian, avian, and reptile species. Oral papillomatosis is common in young dogs and presents as multiple exophytic vegetative warts involving the lips and oral cavity [99] (Figure 4.15). Although rare, oral papillomas also occur in cats. There are a few reports of oral papilloma virus in young cats, but most reports have been in older felines [100, 101].

PV are small non-enveloped, icosahedral viruses that infect the stratified squamous epithelium through microabrasions in the mucocutaneous epithelium [101]. PV is primarily spread by direct contact, but can survive in the environment, so can also be spread indirectly. Most PV infections are inapparent because the immune system prevents the PV from changing normal epithelial cell regulation. However, some infections result in visible epithelial hyperplasia. The host factors that determine whether or not a PV infection will cause a visible lesion are poorly understood, but immunosuppression appears to predispose to development of the lesions. There appears to be a breed predisposition in dogs [101]. Most dogs do not show any systemic signs of disease, but extensive disease can interfere with eating or breathing [101]. There is accumulating evidence that PVs may cause cancer in dogs and cats, but there is little direct evidence from *in vitro* experiments [99, 101].

Virus transmission is reduced by preventing contact between animals that have not been exposed and infected

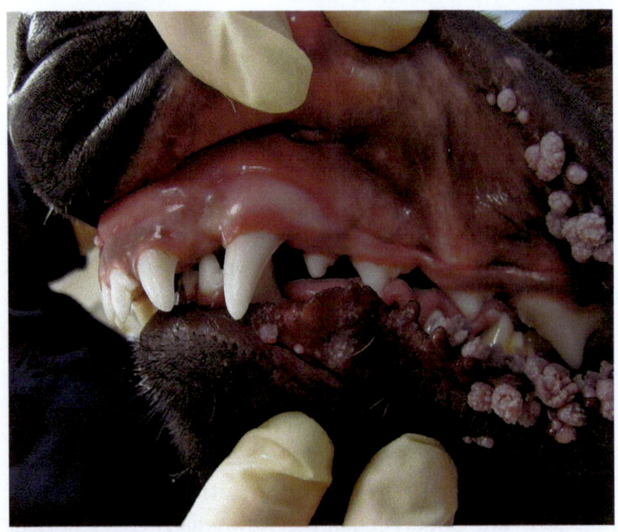

Figure 4.15 Papillomatosis in an eight-month-old Rhodesian Ridgeback dog.

animals, but PVs are resistant within the environment and infection may be possible even without contact with an affected animal [99]. Crude wart extract has been used as a prophylactic vaccine in preventing oral papillomatosis and has been used to protect large dog populations [99].

Most naturally occurring oral canine papilloma lesions regress before three months, but regression can take up to a year [102]. Some oral canine papillomas interfere with the ability to eat, bleed frequently, or otherwise interfere with the dog's quality of life. If the papillomas persist they require treatment. Treatments for persistent canine papilloma lesions are mostly anecdotal and it is hard to discriminate between spontaneous regression and therapeutic effect [100]. Surgical excision and laser ablation are frequently used in veterinary medicine, but there are no published reports of the success rate for this treatment [103]. There is some evidence that surgical excision of oral papillomas is associated with latent infection and increased recurrence [100]. Other anecdotally reported treatments include imiquimod, interferon-alpha2a, autologous, or recombinant papilloma virus vaccine and homeopathic tarantula venom [103]. Azithromycin had a 100% success rate in a placebo-controlled trial in 17 dogs [104]. A case study of persistent oral PV-induced lesions that persisted for 14 weeks despite treatment with oral interferon-alpha2a reported permanent regression of the lesions with one treatment by cryotherapy. Lesions were treated with liquid nitrogen to selectively freeze and destroy abnormal tissue. Five to six freeze–thaw cycles were used. However, regression occurred within the 1-year period that natural regression usually occurs, so it was not possible to determine if regression was due to treatment or the result of natural regression [103]. Another case study using a series of six vaccinations with recombinant canine vaccine prepared using a technique described in Suzich et al. apparently resulted in regression of oral papillomas in 15 weeks [105]. The patient was a 16-month-old Siberian Husky with oral PV that had not responded to two previous treatments of laser surgery [106]. Another study with a dog that received both viral capsid and autologous vaccines stimulated antibody production; however, it did not result in regression [107]. Dogs that have contracted oral PV appear to be protected from reinfection [99].

4.9 Oral Examination and Preventative Care of the Young Dog and Cat

The initial oral examination in a young dog and cat offers an opportunity to avoid many future complications. A juvenile oral examination should include careful examination of occlusion, dentition, tooth surfaces, tongue, mucosal surfaces, and oropharynx. Malocclusions detected early in development and addressed can prevent long-term trauma to periodontium from maloccluded teeth closing on soft tissue or opposing teeth. Dentition should be assessed to determine if the appropriate number of deciduous and/or permanent teeth are present. Persistent deciduous teeth can be extracted to prevent long-term changes to adult dentition such as labioverted maxillary canine teeth. Missing permanent teeth can be radiographed to detect and remove unerupted teeth (T/U) to prevent DTC formation. Tooth surfaces should be examined for enamel defects and crown fractures. Oral masses such as PSCC can be detected and removed as early as possible before extensive destruction can occur.

The initial oral examination is also an important opportunity to address preventative care with the owner. Owners should be encouraged to begin tooth brushing early, using training techniques including gradual buildup to brushing the full mouth, with rewards following brushing to establish a lifetime habit of daily brushing. Clients can also be educated to avoid giving pets marrow bones, nylon bones, and other hard toys to prevent broken teeth. Safe alternatives such as rubber toys and non-abrasive soft toys can be recommended.

4.10 AVDC Abbreviations

Abbreviations for some terms in this chapter can be found in Table 4.2.

Table 4.2 AVDC abbreviation listing [44].

CFL		Cleft lip
CFP		Cleft palate
CMO		Craniomandibular osteopathy
DT		Deciduous tooth
	DT/P	Persistent deciduous tooth
DTC		Dentigerous cyst
E		Enamel
	E/H	Enamel hypoplasia
	E/HM	Enamel hypomineralization
HYP		Hypodontia
OM	OM/FIO	Feline inductive odontogenic tumor
T		Tooth
	T/DEN	Dens invaginatus
	T/FUS	Fusion
	T/GEM	Gemination
	T/I	Impacted tooth
	T/MAC	Macrodontia
	T/MIC	Microdontia
	T/SN	Supernumerary tooth
	T/U	Unerupted tooth

References

1 Williams, R.C. and Evans, H.E. (1978). Prenatal development in the dog, *Canis familiaris*: chronology of tooth germ formation and calcification of deciduous teeth. *Zbl. Ved. Med. C Anat. Histol. Embryol.* 7: 152–163.

2 Klein, O.D., Oberoi, S., Huysseune, A. et al. (2013). Developmental disorders of the dentition: an update. *Am. J. Med. Genet. Part C Semin. Med. Genet.* 163C: 318–332.

3 Evans, H.E. (2012). The digestive apparatus and abdomen. In: *Miller's Anatomy of the Dog*, 4e (ed. N.S. Evans), 281–299. Elsevier.

4 Buelow, M. (2011). Lingual lesions in the dog and cat: recognition, diagnosis, and treatment. *J. Vet. Dent.* 28: 151–162.

5 Kirberger, R.M., Steenkamp, G., Spotswood, T.C. et al. (2006). Stenotic nasopharyngeal dysgenesis in the dachshund: seven cases (2002-2004). *J. Am. Anim. Hosp. Assoc.* 42: 290–297.

6 Greco, D.S., Feldman, E.C., Peterson, M.E. et al. (1991). Congenital hypothyroid dwarfism in a family of Giant Schnauzers. *J. Vet. Int. Med.* 5: 57–65.

7 Balaji, S.M. (2013). Reduction glossectomy for large tongues. *Ann. Maxillofac. Surg.* 3: 167–172.

8 Lobprise, H.B. and Wiggs, R.B. (1993). Anatomy, diagnosis and management of disorders of the tongue. *J. Vet. Dent.* 10: 16–23.

9 Wiggs, R.B., Lobprise, H.B., and DeLahunta, A. (1994). Microglossia in three littermate puppies. *J. Vet. Dent.* 11: 129–133.

10 Hutt, F.B. and DeLahunta, A. (1971). A lethal glossopharyngeal defect in the dog. *J. Hered.* 2: 291.

11 Karahan, S. and Cinar Kul, B. (2009). Ankyloglossia in dogs: a morphological and immunohistochemical study. *Anat. Histol. Embryol.* 38: 118–121.

12 Ozaydin, I., Demirkan, I., and Ozba, B. (2000). A case of congenital permanent frenulum linguae and lingua bifida (bifid tongue) in an Anatolian shepherd (Kangal) dog. *J. Fac. Med. Uni. Kafkas* 6: 107–109.

13 Temizsoylu, M.D. and Avki, S. (2003). Complete ventral ankyloglossia in three related dogs. *J. Am. Vet. Med. Assoc.* 223: 1443–1445.

14 Grundman, S. and Hoffman, A. (2006). Ankyloglossia in an Anatolian Shepherd Dog. *Schwier arc. tierheilkd.* 148: 417–420.

15 Swanson, E.A. (1981). Hair follicles in the canine tongue. *Oral. Surg. Oral. Med. Oral Path.* 51: 277–280.

16 Teifke, J.P. and Lohr, C.V. (1997). Heterotrophic hairs in the tongue of two dogs. *J. Comp. Path.* 117: 267–270.

17 Pavlica, Z., Erjavec, M., and Petelin, M. (2001). Teeth abnormalities in the dog. *Acta Vet. Brno.* 70: 65–72.

18 Dole, R.S. and Spurgeon, T.L. (1998). Frequency of supernumerary teeth in a dolichocephalic canine breed, the Greyhound. *Am. J. Vet. Res.* 59: 16–17.

19 Verstraete, F.J., van Aarde, R.J., Nieuwoudt, B.A. et al. (1996). Dental pathology of feral cats on Marion Island, part I: congenital, developmental, and traumatic abnormalities. *J. Comp. Path.* 115: 265–282.

20 Andrews, A.H. (1972). A case of partial anodontia in the dog. *Vet. Rec.* 90: 144–145.

21 Skrabalak, D.S. and Looney, A.L. (1993). Supernumerary tooth associated with facial swelling in a dog. *J. Am. Vet. Med. Assoc.* 203: 266.

22 Jorgeoson, R.J. (1980). Clinicians view of hypodontia. *J. Am. Dental Assoc.* 101: 283–286.

23 Vieira, A.L.S., Ocoarino, N.M., Boeloni, J.N. et al. (2009). Congenital oligodontia of the deciduous teeth and anodontia of the permanent teeth in a cat. *J. Feline Med. Surg.* 11: 156–158.

24 Elzay, R.P. and Hughes, R.D. (1969). Complete anodontia in a cat. *J. Am. Vet. Med. Assoc.* 154: 667–670.

25 Aksenovich, T.I., Sorkalsov, I.V., Aulchenko, Y.S. et al. (2004). Inheritance of hypodontia in Kerry Blue Terrier Dogs. *Genetika* 40: 658–666.

26 Pereira, L., Assincao, P.A., Salazar, A. et al. (2014). Uncommon true isolated developmental macrodontia of a maxillary tooth. *J. Contemp. Dent. Pract.* 15: 116–118.

27 Dupont, G.A. and DeBowes, L.J. (2009). Developmental dental abnormalities. In: *Atlas of Dental Radiography in Dogs and Cats* (ed. G.A. Dupont and L.J. DeBowes), 195–207. St. Louis, MO: Saunders/Elsevier.

28 Deforge, D. (1992). Dens-en-dente in a six-year-old Doberman pinscher. *J. Vet. Dent.* 9: 9.

29 Coffman, C., Visser, C., and Visser, L. (2009). Endodontic treatment of dens invaginatus in a dog. *J. Vet. Dent.* 26: 220–225.

30 Hulsmann, M. (1997). Dens invaginatus: aetiology, classification, prevalence, diagnosis and treatment considerations. *Int. End. J.* 30: 79–90.

31 Stein, K.E., Marretta, S.M., and Eurell, J.A. (2005). Dens invaginatus of the mandibular first molars in a dog. *J. Vet. Dent.* 22: 21–25.

32 Duncan, H.L. (2010). Diagnostic imaging in veterinary dental practice. Dens invaginatus leading to arrested maturation of the right and left mandibular first molar teeth. *J. Am. Vet. Med. Assoc.* 237: 1251–1253.

33 Alani, A. and Bishop, K. (2008). Dens invaginatus: part 1, classification, prevalence, and aetiology. *Int. End. J.* 41: 1123–1136.

34 Alani, A. and Bishop, K. (2008). Dens invaginatus: part 2, clinical radiographic features and management options. *Int. End. J.* 41: 1137–1154.

35 Bittegeko, S., Arnbjerg, J., Nkya, R., and Tevik, A. (1995). Multiple dental developmental anomalies following canine distemper infection. *J. Am. Anim. Hosp. Assoc.* 31: 42–45.

36 Fiani, N. and Arzi, B. (2009). Diagnostic imaging in veterinary dental practice. *J. Am. Vet. Med. Assoc.* 235: 271–273.

37 Boutoille, F.F. (2011). Diagnostic imaging in veterinary dental practice. *J. Am. Vet. Med. Assoc.* 238: 1251–1253.

38 Kumakami-Sakano, M., Otsu, K., Fujiwara, N., and Harada, H. (2014). Regulatory mechanisms of Hertwig's epithelial root sheath formation and anomaly correlated with root length. *Exp. Cell Res.* doi: 10.1016/j.yexcr.2014.02.005.

39 Jafarzadeh, H. and Abbott, P.V. (2007). Dilaceration: review of endodontic challenge. *J. Endod.* 33: 1025–1030.

40 Verstraete, F.J. and Terpak, C.H. (1997). Anatomical variations in the dentition of the domestic cat. *J. Vet. Dent.* 14: 137–140.

41 Verstraete, F.J. and Terpak, C.H. (1998). Diagnostic value of full-mouth radiography in dogs. *Am. Vet. Res.* 59: 686–691.

42 Schamberger, G., Manfra Maretta, S., Dubielzig, R. et al. (2010). Regional odontodysplasia in a juvenile dog. *J. Vet. Dent.* 27: 98–103.

43 Smithson, C.W., Smith, M.M., and Gamble, D.A. (2010). Multifocal odontoblastic dysplasia in a dog. *J. Vet. Dent.* 27: 242–247.

44 AVDC. Nomenclature: https://www.avdc.org/Nomenclature/Nomen-Teeth.html#enamel

45 Mannerfelt, T. and Lindgren, I. (2009). Enamel defects in Standard Poodle Dogs in Sweden. *J. Vet. Dent.* 26: 213–215.

46 Gandolfi, B., Liu, H., Griffioen, L. et al. (2013). Simple recessive mutation in ENAM is associated with amelogenesis imperfecta in Italian Greyhounds. *Anim. Genet.* 44: 569–578.

47 Pedersen, N., Shope, B., and Liu, H. (2017). An autosomal recessive mutation in SCL24A4 causing enamel hypoplasia in Samoyed and its relationship to breed-wide genetic diversity. *J. Canine Genet. Epidemiol.* 4: 11.

48 Kaplan, B. and Marx, S.G. (1967). Restoration of the maxillary canine teeth of a dog with enamel and dentin hypoplasia. *J. Am. Vet. Med. Assoc.* 150: 603–607.

49 Greenfield, B.A. (2012). Enamel defect restoration of the left mandibular first molar tooth. *J. Vet. Dent.* 29: 36–43.

50 Holmstrom, S.E., Fitch, P.F., and Eisner, E.R. (2004). Restorative dentistry. In: *Veterinary Dental Techniques*, 425–462. Philadelphia, PA: Elsevier.

51 Allen, C., Bouquot, J., Damm, D. et al. (2002). Abnormalities of teeth. In: *Oral and Maxillofacial Pathology*, 2e (ed. B.W. Neville), 50–100. Philadelphia, PA: WB Saunders.

52 Hytönen, M.K., Arumilli, M., Lappalainen, A.K. et al. (2016). Molecular characterization of three canine models of human rare bone diseases: Caffey, van den Ende-Gupta, and Raine syndrome. *PLoS Genet.* 12: e1006037.

53 Aeffner, F., O'Brien, M., and Birkhold, A. (2013). Pathology in practice. *J. Am. Vet. Med. Assoc.* 243: 217–219.

54 Sabri, R. (2008). Management of the over-retained mandibular deciduous second molars with and without permanent successors. *World J. Orthod.* 9: 209–220.

55 Wissdorf, H. and Hermanns, W. Persistierende Milchhakenzahne (Cd) in Oberkiefer einer Hauskatze. *Kleinterpraxis* 19: 14.

56 Harvey, C.E. and Emily, P.P. (1993). *Small Animal Dentistry*, 294–295. St. Louis, MO: Mosby Year-Book.

57 Fulton, A.J., Fiani, N., and Verstraete, J.M. (2014). Canine pediatric dentistry. *Vet. Clin. North Am. Small Anim. Pract.* 44: 569–578.

58 H.P. (2005). Extraction of retained primary canine teeth in a dog. *J. Vet. Dent.* 22: 132–137.

59 Lewis, J.R. (2014). The problematic deciduous canine tooth. *Veterinary Practice News.* http://veterinarypracticenews.com/May-2012/the-problematic-deciduous-canine-tooth. accessed 10 October 2014.

60 Suri, L., Gagari, E., and Vastardis, H. (2004). Delayed tooth eruption pathogenesis, diagnosis, and treatment: a literature review. *Am. J. Orthod. Dentofacial Orthrop.* 126: 432–445.

61 Carle, D.S. and Shope, B.S. (2014). Soft tissue impaction in a 7-month old Bedlington Terrier. *J. Vet. Dent.* 31: 96–105.

62 Hale, F.A. (2005). Juvenile veterinary dentistry. *Vet. Clin. North Am. Small Anim. Pract.* 35: 794–810.

63 Kramek, B.A., O'Brien, T.D., and Smith, F.O. (1996). Diagnosis and removal of a dentigerous cyst complicated by ameloblastic fibro-odontoma in a dog. *J. Vet. Dent.* 13: 9–11.

64 Taney, K.G. and Smith, M.M. (2006). Surgical extraction of impacted teeth in a dog. *J. Vet. Dent.* 23: 168–177.

65 Verstraete, F.J., Zin, B.P., Kass, P.H., and Cox, D.P. (2011). Clinical signs and histologic findings in dogs with odontogenic cysts: 41 cases (1995-2010). *J. Am. Vet. Med. Assoc.* 239: 1470–1476.

66 Baxter, C.J. (2004). Bilateral mandibular dentigerous cysts in a dog. *J. Small Anim. Pract.* 45: 210–211.

67 Gioso, M.A. and Carvalho, V.G. (2003). Maxillary dentigerous cyst in a cat. *J. Vet. Dent.* 20: 28–30.

68 Surgeon, T.W. (2000). Surgical exposure and orthodontic extrusion of an impacted canine tooth in a cat: a case report. *J. Vet. Dent.* 17: 81–85.

69 Taney, K.G. (2008). Secondary cleft palate repair. *J. Vet. Dent.* 25: 150–153.

70 Blazjewski, S.W. III, Lewis, J.R., Gracis, M. et al. (2010). Mandibular periostitis ossificans in immature large breed dogs: 5 cases (1999 – 2006). *J. Vet. Dent.* 27: 148–159.
71 Watson, A.D.J., Adams, W.M., and Thomas, C.B. (1995). Craniomandibular osteopathy in dogs. *Comp. Cont. Ed. Pract. Vet.* 11: 37–43.
72 Pettitt, R., Fox, R., Comerford, E.J. et al. (2012). Bilateral angular limb deformity in a dog with craniomandibular osteopathy. *Vet. Comp. Orthop. Traumatol.* 25: 149–154.
73 Riser, W.H., Parkes, L.J., and Shirer, J.F. (1967). Canine craniomandibular osteopathy. *Am. Vet. Radiol. Soc.* 8: 23–30.
74 Alexander, J.W. (1983). Selected skeletal dysplasias: craniomandibular osteopathy, multiple cartilaginous exostoses, and hypertrophic osteodystrophy. *Vet. Clin. North Am. Small Anim. Pract.* 13: 55–70.
75 Huchkowski, S.L. (2002). Craniomandibular osteopathy in a bullmastiff. *Can. Vet. J.* 43: 883–885.
76 Schultz, S. (1978). A case of craniomandibular osteopathy in a Boxer. *J. Small Anim. Pract.* 19: 749–757.
77 Thompson, D.J., Rogers, W., Owen, M.C., and Thompson, K.G. (2011). Idiopathic canine juvenile cranial hyperostosis in a Pit Bull Terrier. *N.Z. Vet. J.* 59: 201–205.
78 Padgett, G.A. and Mostosky, U.V. (1986). The mode of inheritance of craniomandibular osteopathy in West Highland White Terrier Dogs. *Am. J. Med. Genet.* 25: 9–13.
79 Alexander, J.W. and Kallfelz, F.A. (1975). A case of craniomandibular osteopathy in a Labrador Retriever. *Vet. Med. Small Anim. Clin.* 70: 560–563.
80 Burk, R.L. and Broadhurst, J.J. (1976). Craniomandibular osteopathy in a Great Dane. *J. Am. Vet. Med. Assoc.* 169: 635–636.
81 Taylor, S.M., Remedios, A., and Myers, S. (1995). Craniomandibular osteopathy in a Shetland Sheepdog. *Can. Vet. J.* 36: 437–439.
82 Franch, J., Cesari, J.R., and Font, J. (1998). Craniomandibular osteopathy in two Pyrenean Mountain Dogs. *Vet. Res.* 142: 455–459.
83 Hathcock, J.T. (1982). Craniomandibular osteopathy in an English Bulldog. *J. Am. Vet. Med. Assoc.* 181: 389.
84 Ratterree, W.O., Glassman, M.M., Driskell, E.A. et al. (2011). Craniomandibular osteopathy with a unique neurological manifestation in a young Akita. *J. Am. Anim. Hosp. Assoc.* 47: 7–12.
85 Stapleton, B.L. and Barrus, J.M. (1996). Papillary squamous cell carcinoma in a young dog. *J. Vet. Dent.* 13: 66–68.
86 Nemec, A., Murphy, B.G., Kass, P.H., and Verstraete, F.J. (2011). Histological subtypes of oral non-tonsillar squamous cell carcinoma in dogs. *J. Comp. Path.* 147: 111–120.
87 Nemec, A., Murphy, B.G., Jordan, R.C. et al. (2013). Oral papillary squamous cell carcinoma in twelve dogs. *J. Comp. Path.* 150: 155–161.
88 Smith, M.M. and Mask, C.S. (2001). Squamous cell carcinoma associated with extraction of a maxillary canine tooth in a dog. *J. Vet. Dent.* 18: 193–196.
89 Soukup, J., Snyder, C.J., Simmons, B.T. et al. (2014). Clinical, histological, and computed tomographic features of oral papillary squamous cell carcinoma in dogs: 9 cases (2008–2011). *J. Vet. Dent.* 30: 18–24.
90 Beatty, J.A., Charles, J.A., Malik, R. et al. (2000). Feline inductive odontogenic tumour in a Burmese cat. *Aust. Vet. J.* 78: 452–455.
91 Gardner, D.G. and Dubielzig, R.R. (1995). Feline inductive odontogenic tumor (inductive fibroblastoma) – a tumour unique to cats. *J. Oral. Pathol. Med.* 24: 185–190.
92 Sakai, H., Mori, T., Lida, T. et al. (2008). Immunohistochemical features of proliferative marker and basement membrane components of two feline inductive odontogenic tumors. *J. Fel. Med. Surg.* 10: 296–299.
93 Poulet, F.M., Valentine, B.A., and Summers, B.A. (1992). A survey of epithelial odontogenic tumors and cysts in dogs and cats. *Vet. Pathol.* 29: 369–380.
94 Walker, K.S., Lewis, J.R. et al. (2009). Diagnostic imaging in veterinary dental practice. *J. Am. Vet. Med. Assoc.* 235: 1279–1281.
95 Niemiec, B.A. (2010). Pathology in the pediatric patient. In: *Small Animal Dental, Oral and Maxillofacial Disease, a Color Handbook* (ed. B.A. Niemiec), 189–226. London: Manson.
96 Bellows, J. (2010). Oral assessment, treatment, and preventive care. In: *Feline Dentistry* (ed. J. Bellows), 109–110. Ames, IA: Wiley-Blackwell.
97 Casal, M.L., Jezyk, P.F., Greek, J.M. et al. (1997). X-linked ectodermal dysplasia in the dog. *J. Hered.* 88: 513–517.
98 Lewis, J.R., Reiter, A.M., Mauldin, E.A. et al. (2010). Dental abnormalities associated with X-linked hypohidrotic ectodermal dysplasia in dogs. *Orthod. Craniofac. Res.* 13: 40–47.
99 Lange, C. and Favrot, C. (2011). Canine papillomaviruses. *Vet. Clin. North Am. Small Anim. Pract.* 41: 1183–1195.
100 Sundberg, J.P., Van Ranst, M., Montall, R. et al. (2000). Feline papillomas and papillomaviruses. *Vet. Pathol.* 37: 1–10.
101 Munday, J., Thomason, N., and Luff, J. (2017). Papillomaviruses in dogs and cats. *Vet. J.* 225: 23–31.
102 Sancak, A., Favrot, C., Geisseler, M.D. et al. (2015). Antibody titers against canine papillomavirus 1 peak

around clinical regression in naturally occurring oral papillomatosis. *Vet. Dermatol.* 26: 57–59. e19–20.

103 Richman, A., Kirby, A., Rosenkrantz, W., and Muse, R. (2017). Persistent papilloma treated with cryotherapy in three dogs. *Vet. Dermatol.* 28: 1–4.

104 Yagci, B.B., Ural, K., Ocal, N., and Haydardedeoğlu, A.E. (2008). Azithromycin therapy of papillomatosis in dogs: a prospective, randomized, double-blinded, placebo controlled clinical trial. *Vet. Dermatol.* 19: 194–198.

105 Suzich, H.A., Ghim, S.J., Palmer-Hill, F.J. et al. Systemic immunization with papillomavirus L1 protein completely prevents the development of viral mucosal papillomas. *Proc. Natl. Acad. Sci. U.S.A.* 92: 11553–11537.

106 Kuntsi-Vaattovaara, H., Verstraete, F.J.M., Newsome, J.T., and Yuan, H. (2003). Resolution of persistent oral papillomatosis in a dog after treatment with a recombinant canine oral papillomavirus vaccine. *Vet. Comp. Oncol.* 1: 57–63.

107 Nichols, P.K., Klaunberg, B.A., Moore, R.A. et al. (1999). Naturally occurring, nonregressing canine oral papillomavirus infection: host immunity, virus characterization, and experimental infection. *Virology* 265 (3): 65–374.

5

Periodontology

Kevin Stepaniuk

Veterinary Dentistry Education and Consulting Services, LLC, Ridgefield, WA, USA

5.1 Introduction

Oral and periodontal health is an important component of overall patient health. Similar to the neglect of global oral and periodontal health of human beings' worldwide, periodontal health and disease is a neglected area of veterinary medicine and the veterinary college curriculums [1]. It should not be inevitable that veterinary patients will suffer with periodontal infections, pain, inflammation, lose teeth as they age, and suffer local and systemic ramifications of periodontal disease (PD). Understanding periodontal disease and implementation of periodontal and oral health wellness programs is necessary in order to help veterinary patients, prevent periodontal disease, advocate for their comfort and well-being, educate pet owners, and become comprehensive in patient care.

Periodontal disease is the most common disease in companion dogs and cats. An aggregate review of the literature suggests the prevalence of the disease is 80–85% in the canine and feline patient over two to three years of age [2–12]. Periodontology is the study of the periodontium (i.e., gingiva, periodontal ligament (PDL), cementum, and alveolar bone) in health and disease, and the study of its treatment to maintain or reestablish periodontal health. The pathological process of progressive attachment loss around the tooth is termed periodontal disease. This can occur in periods of active destruction (periodontitis) and periods of quiescence. Gingivitis (i.e., inflammation of the gingiva) begins along the free gingival margin and is the first stage of periodontal disease. Periodontitis (i.e., inflammation of the periodontium) is defined as an *active* disease state of the periodontium. Periodontal disease is a subgingival disease. Subgingival refers to the region apical to the free gingival margin and in the sulcus or periodontal pocket. Supragingival is the opposite and refers to the tooth coronal to the free gingival margin.

Periodontal disease is an insidious, progressive, subgingival disease requiring anesthetized oral examinations and intraoral radiographs to assess, diagnose, and develop comprehensive treatment plans. Periodontitis causes attachment loss of the periodontium at variable rates. Contributing factors include, but are not limited to, systemic health, preventive dental home care (or lack thereof), crowding and rotation of teeth, occlusal abnormalities, professional dental care, genetics, and nutrition (Figure 5.1). It is important to note that the animal's immune system and inflammatory response to the plaque biofilm contributes to the periodontal attachment loss. Periodontitis begins with gingivitis, but not all untreated gingivitis develops into periodontitis, and nor does all periodontitis progress to initiate attachment loss [13]. However, eventual loss of attachment occurs if the insult is not eliminated and the inflammatory response persists.

5.2 Periodontal Anatomy and Physiology

To recognize and understand periodontal disease and its treatment requires a familiarity with the normal anatomy and physiology of the periodontium. The alveolar mucosa is separated from the gingival mucosa by the mucogingival junction. The gingiva is divided by the free gingival groove into the free gingiva and the attached gingiva [14]. The free gingival margin has a flat knife-edge or more curved edge in young and old dogs, respectively [14]. The attached gingiva is not mobile and is firmly attached to underlying structures. It is thickest in the regions of the canine teeth, maxillary fourth premolars, and mandibular first molars [15, 16]. Likewise, the entire gingival width from the free gingival margin to the mucogingival margin is widest at the canine teeth

Wiggs's Veterinary Dentistry: Principles and Practice, Second Edition. Edited by Heidi B. Lobprise and Johnathon R. (Bert) Dodd.

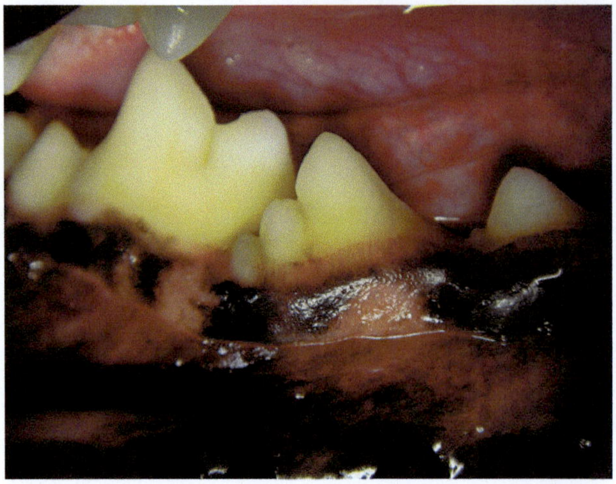

Figure 5.1 Crowding of dentition, as seen in this right mandibular first molar (409) and fourth premolar (408), can be a contributing factor to development of periodontitis.

compared to the premolars [17]. The interdental papilla is formed by gingiva between adjacent teeth. Where the buccal and lingual gingival papilla meet, a non-visible col is formed. Most the gingival epithelium is parakeratinized stratified squamous epithelium although the col and gingival sulcus are lined by non-keratinized stratified squamous epithelium. This epithelium can be easily irritated, leading to gingivitis [18]. The normal space between the free gingiva and the tooth is the sulcus. The sulcular epithelium continues to the junctional epithelium (JE) at the apical portion of the sulcus. The junctional epithelium attaches the gingiva to the tooth, acts as a barrier to the apical periodontal structures, allows passage of gingival crevicular fluid, and allows diapedesis of inflammatory cells. Every 4–6 days and 9–12 days the junctional epithelium and gingival epithelium are replaced, respectively [19, 20]. In healthy periodontal tissues the apical boundary of the junctional epithelium ends at the cementoenamel junction (CEJ). Once the cells reach the bottom of the gingival sulcus, they are sloughed. Replacement of the sulcular epithelium is at a rate between junctional and gingival epithelium replacement rates.

The extensions of the gingival epithelium (rete pegs) and the connective tissue extensions (dermal papilla) interdigitate in order to form a strong attachment. The resulting clinical appearance is gingival stippling in some animals. However, the interdigitation may not correlate in stippling in dog gingiva [14, 21]. The most prominent stippling may be found in the same regions of the widest and thickest gingiva (i.e., the strategic canine teeth, mandibular first molars, and maxillary fourth premolars) [21]. Stippling can be present or absent in healthy or diseased gingival tissue.

The cementum is both a mineralized portion of the tooth and the periodontium. It is approximately 45–50% mineralized and 55–50% connective tissue receiving blood supply from the PDL [22–24]. This avascular tissue lacks innervation and the organic tissue is composed of primarily Type I collagen. The cellular layers of cementum are thickest apically and thinnest coronally [14]. Cementum is divided into acellular (referred to as primary) and cellular (referred to as secondary). Cementum is further divided into six types by the origin of the collagen fibers from fibroblasts (extrinsic fiber cementum) and cementoblasts (intrinsic fiber cementum) [19]. The densely packed Sharpey's fibers inserting into cementum function to anchor the PDL to the tooth.

The PDL anchors the tooth to the alveolar bone, is actively involved in periodontal maintenance, and dampens occlusal forces. The PDL contains Sharpey's fibers primarily of type I collagen [22]. Alveolodental fibers that anchor the cementum to the alveolar bone are divided into six groups [19]. The PDL has a good supply and the polygonal mesh vascular network and unique oxytalan fibers provide shock absorption for occlusal forces [25, 26]. The rete venosum in alveolar bone may act as the reservoir of displaced blood during occlusal loading forces [25]. Connective tissue cells of the PDL include fibroblasts, osteoblasts, cementoblasts, and undifferentiated cells that can uniquely differentiate into any of those cells [19, 27, 28]. The fibroblast is the most abundant cell and can synthesize and phagocytize collagen of the PDL for normal physiological maintenance and attachment to alveolar bone [19, 26]. In some species (e.g., aradicular hypsodont and radicular hypsodont teeth), immature teeth, an interdigitating fiber arrangement called the intermediate plexus, have been demonstrated traversing the periodontal space allowing for continual growth and/or eruption [27].

Alveolar bone serves as the anchor for Sharpey's fibers holding the teeth in the maxillofacial skeleton. The bone is continuously remodeled as it distributes occlusal forces of mastication. Plates of cortical bone (compact bone), with spongy cancellous bone (trabecular bone) in between, compose alveolar bone [29]. Bundle bone, produced by osteoblasts, is the location of Sharpey's fiber insertion [30]. The inner cortical bone is denser, compared to trabecular bone, and appears radiographically as the lamina dura. The marginal alveolar bone is the thinnest portion of the alveolar process, especially facially, as there is no underlying trabecular bone supporting it. In the maxilla of the dog, this facial surface closely follows the contour of the roots, forming palpably distinct juga over the roots.

The alveolar bone is under constant remodeling by osteoclasts and osteoblasts [30]. The coordinated removal of bone by osteoclasts is regulated by the RANK (receptor-activated nuclear factor κβ)/RANKL (receptor-activated nuclear factor κβ ligand)/OPG (osteoprotegrin) [28]. The macrophage-colony stimulating factor must be present in addition to osteoblasts to regulate osteoclasts. RANK is found on osteoclast precursor cell membranes and RANKL on osteoblasts. OPG is produced by osteoblasts to bind the RANKL in order to prevent activation of osteoclasts and balance bone removal, by osteoclasts, and bone production, by osteoblasts. However, inflammatory cytokines in periodontitis change the balance and allow induction of osteoclasts and associated bone resorptive activity.

5.3 Etiology and Pathophysiology of Periodontal Disease

The pathophysiology of periodontal disease is similar between veterinary patients and humans [11, 31, 32]. Periodontitis is active inflammation of the periodontium. It begins with the accumulation of the dental pellicle (0.1–0.8 mm) (e.g., salivary glycoproteins) that occurs within seconds of a tooth being cleaned. Within hours, Gram positive oral bacterial first colonize the pellicle and the plaque biofilm is formed. With the addition of extracellular polysaccharides (i.e., bacterial byproducts), plaque takes on its classic ivory to yellow to grayish appearance. The plaque biofilm is established in 24 hours and matures within days. Maturation of the plaque biofilm to a stage where anaerobic organisms are supported is within 24 hours [33, 34]. Mineralization of the plaque biofilm results in calculus (Figure 5.2). Periodontitis is caused by the bacterial biofilm (plaque) and the associated inflammatory response. Significant periodontal disease can be present without calculus. Likewise, some patients can have significant calculus with minimal periodontal disease. Additionally, periodontal disease may be quiescent or have periods of active inflammation (i.e., periodontitis).

The *plaque* is an organic matrix of salivary glycoproteins, oral bacteria, lipids, cellular debris, and extracellular polysaccharides that adhere to the tooth surface. The glycoproteins and polysaccharides provide the adherence for the bacteria [35]. Dental plaque is not a food residue. It forms more readily during sleep when there is no food taken in and has been shown to form in humans when parenteral feeding is being utilized for nutrition [36]. The mechanical action of food and stimulated saliva deters and slows plaque formation. Plaque is a biofilm [37, 38].

The plaque biofilm is a complex, cooperative community of bacteria that can resist host defenses and is shaped by the local environmental and host factors in the oral cavity [39]. The biofilm inhibits antimicrobial penetration, prevents desiccation, and limits the host immune system [40, 41]. Additionally, the biofilm bacteria benefit from cooperation and altered gene expressions, adding to the tenacity of the protective biofilm. Furthermore, there is no host blood supply to the tooth surface to deliver oxygen and inflammatory cells to directly target the biofilm. The inflammatory cells must first move into the gingival crevicular fluid or periodontal exudate in order to reach the outer surface of the biofilm. Biofilms in medicine and surgery cannot be seen visually, require disruption in order to treat, and require a robust blood supply to heal [42]. Mechanical removal and disruption of the plaque biofilm professionally and with tooth brushing is necessary in order to treat and prevent periodontal disease, respectively.

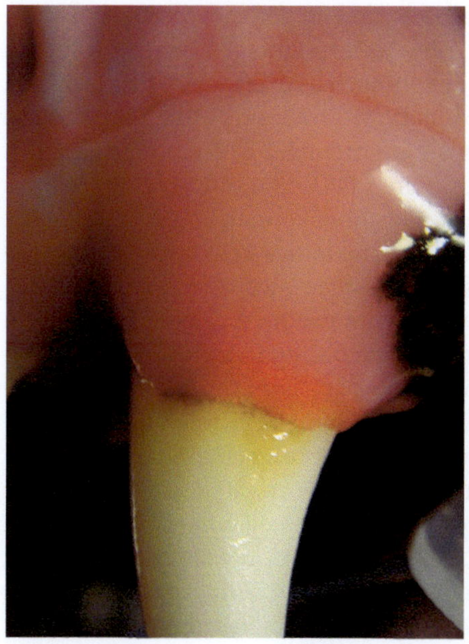

Figure 5.2 The plaque biofilm is the inciting cause of periodontal disease. As the plaque biofilm matures it is mineralized to form calculus that can be visualized on the tooth surface of the left maxillary canine tooth (204). The layman term for calculus is tartar.

Supragingival plaque influences the growth accumulation and pathogenicity of subgingival plaque in the early stages of periodontal disease. The plaque biofilm protects the subgingival plaque and reduces the oxygen available deeper in the plaque matrix, thereby allowing Gram negative anaerobes to proliferate. Although the supragingival and subgingival bacterial communities are a continuum, during maturation delineation occurs, separating the two different communities [43]. The oral bacteria and those bacteria in the biofilm community may be aerobic bacteria (e.g., require oxygen), facultative bacteria (e.g., survive in aerobic or anaerobic conditions), and anaerobic bacteria (e.g., require oxygen-free environments). Bacteria can also be found in the gingival crevicular fluid (i.e., planktonic bacteria) and some can actively invade gingival tissue. The black pigmented anaerobic bacilli have virulence factors such as direct epithelial invasion, collagenase production, protease production, release endotoxins, impair neutrophils, and activate the host inflammatory cytokines [44]. The activated neutrophils release cytokines and produce metalloproteinases that recruit additional inflammatory cells and destroy the periodontal tissues while fighting the bacteria. The pathogenic bacteria in primate, canine, and feline periodontal disease arise from similar bacterial families and although some genus and species are found in the comparative species, specific bacteria have been identified in carnivores with cultures and molecular cloning and sequencing. Black-pigmented Gram negative anaerobes and spirochetes have been incriminated in canine periodontal disease [45, 46]. Oral bacteria incriminated in periodontal disease in the dog and cat include, at this time, *Bacteroides* sp., *Porphorymonas* sp., *Prevotella intermedia*, *Tannerella forsythensia*, *Campylobacter rectus*, *Peptostreptococcus* sp., *Treponema denticola*, *Fusebacterium canifelinum*, *Pseudomonas* sp., *Capnocytophaga* sp., and *Desulfomicrobium* sp. [45–57]. As the biofilm matures the population of the anaerobic bacteria and spirochetes increases, changing the ratio of anaerobic and aerobic bacteria in the biofilm.

As the plaque biofilm matures, early bacterial colonizers, Gram positive aerobic cocci, become less predominant as the biofilm switches to Gram negative anaerobes and spirochetes located more apical in the periodontal pockets. Bacterial products such as ammonia, volatile sulfur compounds, and proteolytic enzymes contribute to the destruction of the periodontium. The host inflammatory response, matrix metalloproteinases that degrade collagen of the PDL, elastase, and prostaglandins (PGE_2) are directly responsible for tissue damage and/or stimulate osteoclastic bone resorption (PGE_2, IL-1β, IL-6, TNF-α). Cytokines affect immune cells and resident cells of the periodontium, integrating aspects of the innate and adaptive immune response to plaque pathogens [58]. This host inflammatory response substantially contributes to destruction of the periodontium.

The theories of periodontal disease continue to evolve [59]. The "specific plaque hypothesis" explains that periodontitis is caused by specific strains of virulent bacteria. This type of hypothesis could explain the nature of certain forms of aggressive periodontitis. When reduced host resistance allows facultative pathogens found in the normal oral flora to proliferate, periodontitis results. The "non-specific plaque hypothesis" best explains chronic periodontitis. This mixed bacterial population in the plaque biofilm, with lack of professional and home care, proliferates and induces an inflammatory response resulting in periodontitis and attachment loss.

Calcium carbonate and calcium phosphate, with small amounts of magnesium, potassium, and sodium in the saliva mineralize the plaque biofilm to form calculus [44]. Accumulation begins hours after plaque formation and is clinically detectable in 48–72 hours. Calculus is mineralized dental plaque adhering to the tooth root and crown. Plaque and calculus accumulation appears to be more severe on the buccal surface of the maxillary teeth, with the carnassial being the worst affected. Calculus increases the surface area for further plaque biofilm accumulation and can mechanically irritate the gingiva [34]. Calculus adheres supragingivally and subgingivally and is not easily removed with home care and dentifrices. Therefore, professional dental cleanings are necessary to remove the deposits.

5.4 Histological Changes in Periodontal Disease

Inflammation of the gingiva (i.e., gingivitis) is considered reversible with treatment. However, periodontal attachment loss from periodontitis is not reversible with the exception of added osseous surgery such as guided tissue regeneration. It is normal to have small numbers of neutrophils in relatively healthy gingiva and gingival crevicular fluid. As inflammation begins the junctional epithelium will have lateral proliferation in the coronal region and more neutrophils, plasma cells, and other inflammatory cells accumulate. An increase exudate in the sulcus occurs and connective tissue loss begins. Edematous gingivitis is common. However, fibrous gingival response to plaque occurs in some breeds (Figure 5.3).

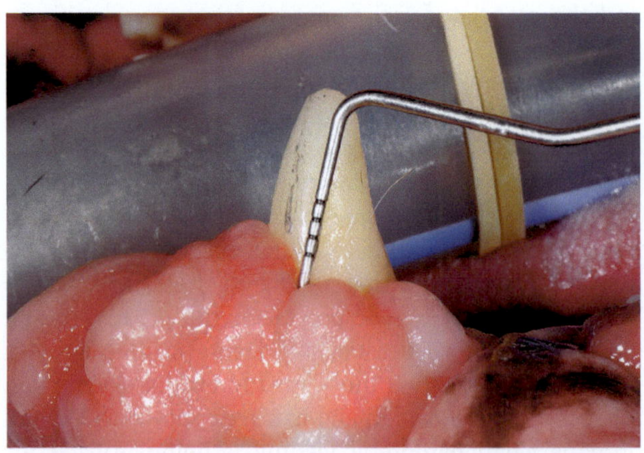

Figure 5.3 In some breeds of dogs, rather than an edematous gingivitis response to plaque, a fibrous gingival enlargement will result. Note the deep periodontal probing depth on the buccal aspect of the left mandibular canine tooth (304) identifying the initial pseudopocket. The pseudopockets can progress to suprabony and infrabony pockets. *Source:* Photograph used with permission, courtesy of Wade Gingerich, DVM, DAVDC.

The time frame for initial gingivitis is two to four days once the plaque starts to accumulate. The earliest clinically observable gingivitis is considered to be an established gingivitis. Within one to three weeks the junctional epithelium continues to proliferate, inflammatory cells and exudate accumulate, and collagen loss increases. Early in gingivitis, the migration of neutrophils and exudate flow moves parallel to the tooth surface, similar to the movement and sloughing of junctional epithelial cells, providing the host with another defense against bacteria by moving bacteria and exudate out of the sulcus. However, bacteria move through the large spaces in the JE and into the connective tissue of the PDL, resulting in bacterial colonization of the PDL and related cementum and bone. With periodontal pocket formation exudate flow changes to a perpendicular flow in relation to the tooth surface, diminishing the normal cleansing flow. Pocket formation and attachment loss occurs and spontaneous healing is no longer possible.

5.5 Cofactors in Periodontal Disease Pathophysiology

Many of the smaller breeds of dogs and purebred breeds have been subjectively and anecdotally been associated with an increased predilection toward crowding of the teeth and malocclusions, both of which predispose for the development of periodontal disease [5]. The thinner gingiva and alveolar bone in toy breed dogs contributes to the likelihood of a poor periodontal stage [16]. In the cat, the Somalis and Abyssinian both are well known for their predilection for aggressive forms of periodontal disease. Additionally, many lines of Miniature Schnauzers, Maltese, and Sight Hounds have a similar propensity for aggressive periodontitis. Genetics can also predispose to oral disease by affecting structure size, immune system, organ health, and numerous other body systems. The overall patient general health is important. Animals in poor health are more susceptible to infections and disease. Animals with underlying systemic problems, such as diabetes mellitus, immunosuppressant diseases, or those that are receiving commonly used immunosuppressive medications for various dermatological and systemic diseases (e.g., cyclosporine, corticosteroids) have an altered immune response and can be expected to have more periodontal health problems. With improved diets and medical care, animals are living longer, healthier lives. Unfortunately, it has also been demonstrated that as animals age, dental and periodontal disease increases [5, 60]. As pet owners take better care of dogs and cats, the pets have longer life spans and increases in age-related chronic diseases such as periodontal disease occur. Without professional dental care and daily home care, the pets, clients, and veterinarians are reacting and extracting teeth rather than focusing on prevention and wellness. Additionally, awareness of dental disease and oral pathology in companion pets is a relatively recent evolution in veterinary medicine, making owners and veterinarians aware of the health issues that were ignored generations before.

Home dental care can dramatically affect the development and control of periodontal disease. Home care encompasses diet, chew toys, chemicals, oral solutions and gels, and brushing [61–88]. Chewing behavior affects the oral cavity, teeth, and periodontium. Pet food nutrients and food components have been involved with the changes in general health and longer life expectancies [89]. These have generally required less chewing, thereby reducing the need for a functional dentition.

However, appropriate chewing is beneficial for the gingiva and teeth. Some dental chews help reduce calculus and plaque that can lead to periodontal disease. However, inappropriate chewing of various hard chew toys such as bones, antlers, hard nylon bones, cow hooves, and other devices frequently can cause tooth fractures resulting in endodontic disease and/or endodontic-periodontal disease [3, 90, 91]. Finally, many dental chews may make no difference in controlling plaque and calculus.

Abnormal chewing from behavioral or dermatological problems may cause damage to the periodontium. With dermatologic problems, animals may chew excessively, resulting in abrasion, at times exposing the pulp canal. This can result in endodontic disease. Second, hair wrapped around teeth or even small pieces caught in the gingival sulcus act as local irritants, leading to gingivitis and periodontitis. Separation and storm anxiety may cause a pet to chew various articles, or attempt to chew out of confining areas, causing damage to the teeth and periodontium.

Textures of diets may influence chewing if the pet has dentition and dentition that is pain free. Chewing can help with the natural cleaning effects of the teeth. Textures deal not only with the coarseness of a food, but its compressibility and resistance to tearing. Soft diets compared to hard diets have been debated. However, at this time there is no strong evidence that either soft diets or hard diets preferentially lead to greater plaque accumulation in dogs and cats [61, 92].

The nutritional components of a diet (e.g., vitamins, minerals, carbohydrates, sugars, fats, proteins) and variation can produce numerous tooth, alveolar bone, and periodontium problems. Vitamin C and the mineral selenium deficiencies have both been shown to result in a weak PDL that is easily damaged. Increases in sugars, decreased minerals, and increased pH can all have effects on the development of caries.

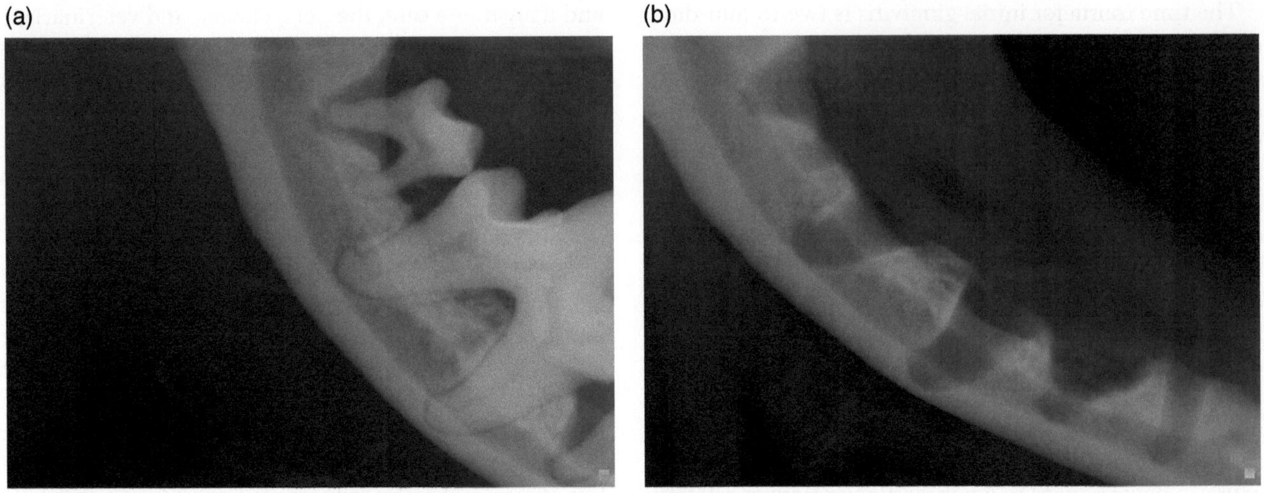

Figure 5.4 The tooth-to-bone ratio has not remained proportional, as dogs have been bred smaller. (a) The dentition of the right mandible of this young toy breed dog has stage 4 periodontal disease. The digital radiographic software measured the ventral cortical mandibular bone apical to the mesial root of the right mandibular first molar (409) as 1 mm. (b) Severe periodontal disease in this region of the mandible predisposes the mandible to fracture. Post-extraction radiographs document the empty alveoli and intact ventral mandibular cortex.

Saliva quality and quantity have an influence on supragingival plaque formation in humans. Individuals with reduced salivary flow or "dry mouth" have a higher rate of supragingival plaque development. Anatomically and histologically the salivary glands in dogs and cats have been characterized [93, 94]. However, very little is known about the constituents (e.g., proteonome, hormone, transcriptome) of saliva in dogs and cats.

Local trauma such as trauma of occlusion, bruxism, and foreign bodies influence periodontal disease. Hair in the gingival sulcus is a foreign body, stimulating inflammation, ulceration, and profuse exudation. Likewise, small fragments from chew toys can break off and lodge between teeth and/or in the gingival sulcus.

5.6 Periodontal Disease and Local Sequelae

Periodontal disease and the associated periodontal pockets can cause oronasal fistulas (ONFs). The ONF may not be apparent and only identified with an anesthetized examination, periodontal probing, and intraoral radiographs. Furthermore, these hidden ONFs are a cause for chronic inflammatory rhinitis [95, 96].

The juxtaposition of the maxillary molars to the incomplete orbit in the dog and cat allows periodontal disease to contribute to periocular/ocular diseases such as retrobulbar cellulitis and ophthalmic inflammation [97–99]. The proximity of the teeth (e.g. canine tooth) to the nasolacrimal canal can be a contributing factor to nasolacrimal disease and epiphora [100–105]. These conditions are more pronounced in brachycephalic dogs and cats.

The tooth-to-jaw ratio has not remained proportional as dogs have been bred smaller (Figure 5.4a and b) [106]. Not only are these crowded teeth more predisposed to periodontal disease but when attachment loss occurs it predisposes the mandible to "pathological" fractures [107]. A relatively normal force may lead to mandibular fractures in small and toy breed dogs.

5.7 Periodontal Disease and Systemic Health

Periodontal disease in humans has shifted from the Focal Infection Theory to Periodontal Medicine, where there is a two-way relationship between the periodontium and the rest of the body. It is accepted that infection and inflammation of periodontal disease in humans leads to systemic ramifications such as premature and low birthweight babies, cardiovascular disease, systemic inflammatory disease, cerebrovascular events, neurological disease, pulmonary disease, and male reproductive disorders. Diabetes mellitus (DM) is a complicated bidirectional relationship with glycosylation of the microvasculature and inhibition of the local immune response in the oral cavity. Oral infection is a factor in systemic resistance to insulin in diabetic patients. In the opposite direction from oral inflammation leading to systemic disease, systemic disease can lead to oral disease. It is known that systemic neutrophil disorders, connective tissue disorders, genetic diseases, and calcium phosphate disorders can lead to aggressive periodontitis in humans [108].

Dogs have been used as models for human periodontal disease for many decades [109, 110]. Since the pathophysiology of periodontal disease and these conditions are similar in dogs and cats, systemic ramifications are possible in these species. Evidence of distant organ changes, systemic inflammation, and bacteremia associated with periodontal bacteria has been documented in dogs and cats [111–121]. Both human literature and veterinary literature conclude associations between dental infection and systemic disease. However, a direct causal relationship cannot necessarily be drawn. Caution is necessary as the pathophysiology of some systemic diseases in humans (i.e., cardiovascular disease) is different when comparing dogs and cats. The veterinary profession needs to be cautious in evaluation of the evidence in animals. Although in some cases human associations can be extrapolated.

Mechanisms of distant systemic changes include (i) direct spread of bacterial pathogens, (ii) systemic spread of bacterial endotoxin, and (iii) systemic inflammatory cytokines. Periodontal bacterial pathogens migrate through the sulcular epithelium and into the periodontal connective tissues, thereby gaining access to the pets' vascular system. The regional tissues and reticuloendothelial system are then continuously challenged. A local and systemic inflammatory response occurs and continues until the source of infection/inflammation is controlled. Inflammatory cytokines (e.g., Interleukin-1β, Interleukin-6, Interleukin-10, Prostaglandin E_2, Tumor Necrosis Factor-α) and lymphocytes accumulate in the periodontal pocket and increase in the systemic system. Furthermore, Gram negative bacteria produce endotoxin (i.e., Lipopolysaccharide), which will induce a systemic inflammatory response and acute phase proteins from the liver [117, 118]. Although bacteria may be a contributing factor to distant organ effects, the chronic inflammatory mediators associated with periodontal disease are known to cause histological changes in organs and are as, or more, important in distant effects compared to the bacteria [116–118].

Chronic systemic inflammation associated with periodontal disease has been documented in dogs and cats with c-reactive protein [111, 119, 121]. Hepatic parenchymal inflammation, changes in renal interstitial and glomerular tissue, and some cardiac tissue have been associated with periodontal disease in dogs [116–118]. Cardiovascular changes in dogs are more controversial at this time, due to a single case report, flawed retrospective studies, and the pathophysiology of canine heart disease [112–115]. Different methods for assessment of "periodontal disease," "tooth abscess," etc., question the accurate assessment of dental/periodontal disease whereas accepted American Veterinary Dental College (AVDC) staging methods with intraoral radiographs would be more accurate. Furthermore, different methods of "assessment" do not lend themselves for future meta-analysis.

It will be difficult to find direct large causal relationships between dental infection and inflammation and distant systemic disease in dogs and cats. Veterinary medicine does not lend itself to prospective large studies (i.e., thousands to tens of thousands of patients). When the numbers are attempted it is retrospective with poorly controlled definitions and criteria written in medical records [112, 113, 120]. Small conflicting studies and case reports blur potential associations [113]. Confounding factors in small clinical veterinary studies makes interpretation of data challenging. Financial costs for a well-designed clinical study with large numbers of patients seems almost unrealistic unless comparative translational medical research grants or industry partnerships are achieved in which human health care and/or businesses have a potential return on investment. Furthermore, periodontal disease has a complex pathophysiology with periods of quiescence and active periodontitis, and establishing research during the active phase is necessary. Nevertheless, the current human and veterinary literature does support the contention that dental infection *is associated* with many current systemic diseases and organ changes.

5.8 Clinical Signs Associated with Periodontal Disease

The clinical signs of periodontal disease are often hidden and insidious. Halitosis, gingivitis, supragingival plaque and calculus, reluctance to chew, head shyness, pawing at the mouth, dropping food, sneezing, nasal discharge, exaggerated jaw movements while eating, food and water bowl aversion, are clinical signs. The complaint of halitosis is the result of volatile sulfur compounds (e.g., hydrogen sulfide, methyl-mercaptans, dimethyl sulfide, volatile fatty acids) produced by oral bacteria [120–126]. Unfortunately, many of these clinical signs require astute client observation and/or careful questioning from the clinician. Other clinical signs occur late in the disease course after the patient has suffered silently for months or years with chronic pain and infection. Commonly, there may be no obvious clinical signs to the owner and untrained veterinarian. Almost all the patients are still eating and many pet owners are unaware their pets have significant infection, inflammation, and pain in the oral cavity.

The American Animal Hospital Association (AAHA) Dental Guidelines and Canine and Feline Life Stages

Guidelines recommend annual evaluations of the oral cavity [127–129]. The recommended time to start professional evaluations and cleanings, in order to prevent disease, is in the first to second year of life. Veterinary medicine needs to focus on prevention and wellness and not sickness when treating pets [129]. Periodontal disease is a preventable disease!

5.9 Clinical Examination Findings Associated With Periodontal Disease

5.9.1 Conscious Oral Examination

Periodontal assessment begins in the examination room with the client and the conscious patient. A complete medical and oral history, general physical examination, and conscious oral examination are necessary. Questions such as, but not limited to, onset, duration, environment, chew toys, oral health care, current medications, diet, past illness, past anesthetic episodes, and behavioral changes are explored. Many patients with oral disease do not have obvious clinical signs.

The maxillofacial skeletal structures are palpated and the eyes retropulsed for pain or resistance. The basic skull type is noted. The regional lymph nodes and salivary glands are palpated for enlargement. Facial symmetry and occlusion are noted. The range of motion of the temporomandibular joints should be palpated and the patient observed for pain and/or difficulty in opening and closing the mouth. The lips and mucocutaneous junctions should be observed for ulcerations that might indicate an autoimmune disease or pyoderma from ptyalism. Finally, the dentition is evaluated and the teeth counted to determine if all teeth are present. Discolored teeth, persistent deciduous teeth, root and furcation exposure, crowded teeth, rotated teeth, oral mucosal lesions, sinus tracts, tongue abnormalities, oral masses, plaque and calculus, etc., are noted.

The owner is counseled that, although we do our best to estimate the extent of disease, anesthesia, anesthetized oral exam, periodontal probing, and intraoral radiographs [130–133] will often identify hidden disease subgingivally; thus, the conscious exam and plan is our best good faith estimate for a treatment plan.

5.9.2 Anesthetized Periodontal Examination

A periodontal examination can never be complete without full probing of all periodontal pockets, which requires general anesthesia [134]. A systematic and methodical examination is necessary to assess all the oral structures. All information gathered from the owner during the history gathering should be coupled with any oral examination physical clues.

The most important diagnostic instruments in periodontal therapy are the explorer/probe and intraoral radiographs. The probe end is marked in millimeters, which is gently inserted into the sulcus to measure its depth. Pocket depth, gingival recession, and root exposure should be assessed and combined to determine the total percentage of attachment loss. Dental radiographs are crucial in this evaluation. *Attachment loss* refers to the tissues of the periodontium. This attachment loss data can then be converted into the staging of periodontal disease. Deeper periodontal probing depths greater than 5 mm may require periodontal surgery to correct and home care to maintain the newly established smaller pocket depth.

The explorer is the sharp pointed end of the explorer/probe, which may be hooked, angled, or straight. It can be gently drawn against the tooth in the sulcus (avoiding soft tissue damage) to help detect hidden calculus, resorptive lesions, or cavities in the subgingival area. The explorer can also be used to aid in the detection of open pulp canals (endodontic disease) due to tooth fractures or caries.

During the anesthetized oral examination, the gingival indices, calculus indices, furcation exposure, and tooth mobility, in association with the periodontal disease stages, can help determine not only the extent of disease but whether active periodontal disease or a period of quiescence is present. It must be noted that there can be different stages of periodontal disease present in the same oral cavity, and even different levels of involvement of different areas of the same tooth. All abnormalities should be properly recorded.

5.10 Periodontal Charting

Knowledge of the dental formula of the permanent teeth will help in recognition of abnormalities. There are 42 and 30 teeth, in the adult canine and feline mouth, respectively. Many methods for charting are available; consistency in charting is the key. With general anesthesia the patient can receive a full oral examination, periodontal probing, intraoral radiographs, and dental charting.

The normal gingival sulcus depth in a dog is less than 3 mm and less than 0.5 mm in a cat. The edema, inflammation, and bleeding of the gums are noted (gingivitis). Purulent debris around the teeth, buccal mucositis, glossitis, palatitis, and caudal mucositis are investigated and recorded in the patient record.

While attachment loss and its measurement are the focal aspect of evaluating periodontal disease, there are many other indices and stages that may be used to quantify the extent of inflammation and disease. It is virtually impossible to cover every index available, that could be adapted from human periodontology, and some assessments may have numerous evaluation schematics to choose from. Current AVDC nomenclature is presented below with other periodontal indices [135].

When assessing and recording disease various categorical criteria can be applied. It is important to understand the assignment of the disease description [135] (reprinted with permission, AVDC).

> "A stage is the assessment of the extent of pathological lesions in the course of a disease that is likely to be progressive (e.g. stages of periodontal disease, staging of oral tumors) A grade is the quantitative assessment of the degree of severity of a disease or abnormal condition at the time of diagnosis, irrespective of whether the disease is progressive (e.g. grading mast cell tumors based on mitotic figures). An index (indice) is a quantitative expression of predefined diagnostic criteria whereby the presence and/or severity of pathological conditions are recorded by assessing a numerical value (e.g. gingival index, plaque index, calculus index)."

Gingival inflammation is assessed. Gingival index (Loe and Silness) [136]:

Gingival indice of 1. Inflammation and swelling of the gingiva with no bleeding during periodontal probing.
Gingival indice of 2. Inflammation and swelling of the gingiva with bleeding during periodontal probing.
Gingival indice of 3. Inflammation and swelling of the gingiva with spontaneously bleeding of the inflamed gingiva prior to periodontal probing.

Swelling of the gingiva will increase pocket depth. After resolution of gingivitis, either spontaneous or after therapy, the acute inflammation in the gingiva will resolve, and gingival shrinkage may occur, returning the probing depth to a measurement consistent with a normal sulcus. Shrinkage and resolution of the gingival edema should be differentiated from true gingival recession, which is measured from the level of the CEJ.

Furcation exposure (involvement) occurs when a periodontal probe can extend between the roots, under the crown, of multirooted teeth as a result of attachment loss (Figure 5.5) [135–138]. Extensive problems can occur with attachment loss in these areas, including increasing food and plaque retention, rapid attachment loss, and external inflammatory resorptive lesions. Pathologic invasion of a furcation is best determined by careful probing with a curved explorer, although radiographs finalize the diagnosis.

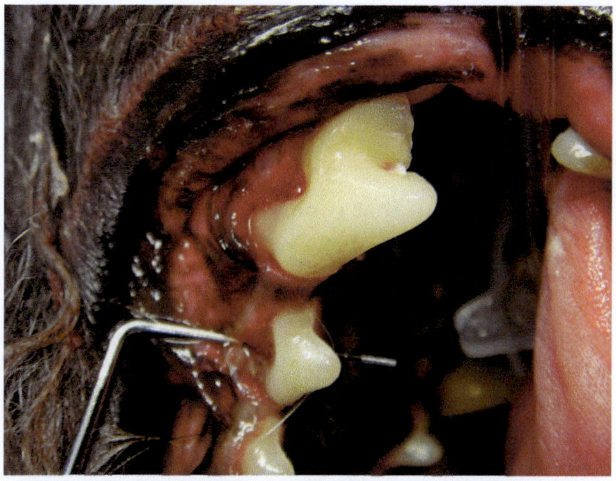

Figure 5.5 The left third premolar (207) has a furcation 3 exposure diagnosed by the probe passing completely through the furcation region. Note that the gingiva is displaced slightly apical to the furcation in order to find this defect. During periodontal probing it is necessary to carefully identify furcation exposures as they may be hidden by swollen gingiva. Also note the severe gingival recession on the mesial buccal root of the left maxillary fourth premolar (208) and the visible furcation.

The following is the AVDC furcation staging system used in veterinary dentistry [135] (reprinted with permission, AVDC):

"*Stage 1 furcation (F1).* The periodontal probe extends less than halfway under the crown in any direction of a multirooted tooth with attachment loss.
Stage 2 furcation (F2). The periodontal probe extends greater than halfway under the crown of a multirooted tooth with attachment loss but not through and through.
Stage 3 furcation (F3). The periodontal probe extends under the crown of a multirooted tooth, through and through from one side of the furcation to the other."

The presence of furcation involvement generally results in a poor prognosis. It is difficult to clean the furcation area clinically and with daily home care. If these problems can be reasonably resolved and daily home care with tooth brushing can be administered, some teeth with furcation exposure can be treated and maintained with a client committed to daily brushing and semi-annual and annual periodontal cleanings, as indicated. However, most teeth with furcation 3 exposure require extraction.

Mobility of the tooth refers to the movement of the tooth within the alveolus. Mobility of teeth is a critical diagnostic and prognostic tool. As mobility increases, so does the proportional chance of tooth loss. Some degree of tooth movement is considered normal and is termed physiologic mobility. The physiologic mobility of a tooth is limited to the width of the PDL and the elasticity of the periodontal support. Pathologic mobility is defined as the displacement of a tooth, either vertically or horizontally, beyond its physiologic movement [139]. However, a tooth that is mobile does not necessarily denote the presence of periodontal disease. Mobility can be present in a clinically normal periodontium as the result of previously applied stress, such as orthodontics, or due to a fibrous alveolus, such as seen in mandibular first incisors in the fibrous connective tissue symphysis. In addition, some transient mobility may occur following traumatic injuries, endodontic treatment, and periodontal therapy.

The following is a classification for stages of mobility used in veterinary dentistry [135] (reprinted with permission, AVDC):

"Stages of Tooth Mobility:

Stage 0 (M0). Physiologic mobility up to 0.2 mm.

Stage 1 (M1). The mobility is increased in any direction other than axial over a distance of more than 0.2 mm and up to 0.5 mm.

Stage 2 (M2). The mobility is increased in any direction other than axial over a distance of more than 0.5 mm and up to 1.0 mm.

Stage 3 (M3). The mobility is increased in any direction than axial over a distance exceeding 1.0 mm or any axial movement."

While mobility of a tooth is primarily influenced by the degree of bone loss associated with periodontal disease, occlusal forces can also contribute to progressive mobility [140, 141]. Parafunctional occlusal habits such as bruxism and cage biting can result in mobility problems. The mobility itself can be detrimental and perpetuate periodontal disease and inhibit healing [141]. Periodontal splinting may be required in addition to periodontal treatments to control the inflammation and mobility. Severe mobility nearly always results in tooth loss while the patient has been suffering months or years with chronic infection, inflammation, and pain. The elimination or even control of pathologic tooth mobility can only be gained by the interference with the causative pathology. In the majority of cases, once the tooth is actually lost, the inflammation around the region lessens or even resolves, as the plaque retentive surface is no longer present. Too little too late!

Gingival recession (root exposure) is measured from the location of the CEJ to the free gingival margin (Figure 5.6). Any probing depths, whether normal or not, are recorded because an additional probing depth is additive to periodontal attachment loss. For example, if there is 3 mm of gingival recession and a 2 mm probing depth (normally,

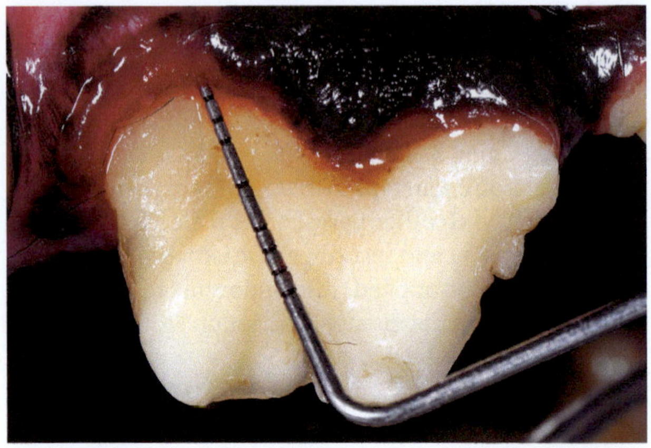

Figure 5.6 A right maxillary fourth premolar (108) with severe gingival recession is presented. The root exposure is measured from the cementoenamel junction (noted at the 5 mm mark on the periodontal probe in this case) to the free gingival margin. When the periodontal probe was gently inserted into the periodontal pocket a probing depth of 2 mm was measured. Therefore, the attachment loss measured with periodontal probing, and confirmed with intraoral radiography, was 7 mm on the distal root. *Source:* Photograph used with permission, courtesy of Wade Gingerich, DVM, DAVDC.

2 mm would be considered within the normal probing depth of a dog), then total attachment loss is 5 mm. Generalized recession does occur, but more commonly one to several teeth are often involved. Periodontitis, labial frenulum tension (e.g., brachycephalic breeds), improper tooth brushing techniques, orthodontic therapy, breed (e.g., Greyhound), and even overall aggressive scaling can contribute to the recession.

At times, gingival recession can start by the formation of a small groove, or Stillman cleft [142]. A fibrotic, noninflammatory response can result in a thickening of the remaining attached gingiva, rolling into a lesion known as McCall's festoons. Inflammation can become part of the picture if inadequate hygiene is provided or if the recession extends beyond the mucogingival junction. Recession is typically found on the buccal/labial surfaces of teeth.

Periodontal pockets are clinical periodontal probing measurements greater than the normal sulcus. The normal gingival sulcus depth of the dog is less than 3 mm with slightly accepted larger measurements for giant breeds and slightly less measurements for toy breeds. The normal gingival sulcus in a cat is less than 0.5 mm. The periodontal probe is gently walked 360° around each tooth; a minimum of six probing locations are measured (mesial, buccal, distal, mesial-palatal/lingual, palatal/lingual, distal-palatal/lingual). Even in a normal healthy gingiva the periodontal probe can still easily penetrate the junctional epithelium, resulting in readings of up to 2–3 mm depending on patient size. For this reason, all probing should be done with an appropriate sized instrument and with minimal pressure. It is difficult to probe healthy domestic feline gingiva. Therefore, if the periodontal probe measures any depth in a cat, significant attachment loss is occurring/occurred. Intraoral radiographs in conjunction with probing are necessary to accurately assess attachment loss and develop an individual treatment plan.

Attachment loss expresses itself as some form of tissue recession. This recession generally shows as either root exposure, suprabony pockets, infrabony (intrabony) pockets or a combination of root exposure and pocket formation [143, 144]. Periodontal pockets can be a combination of various types of pockets created by periodontal bone loss and gingival enlargements. Periodontal pockets are a haven for Gram negative anaerobic bacteria and spirochetes in the subgingival plaque biofilm and planktonic bacteria in the pocket gingival crevicular fluid. There are often combinations of periodontal pocket types as they are not mutually exclusive. However, they may be simplified for clinical practice.

Pseudopockets are created when the gingiva enlarges (gingival enlargement) and the marginal bone remains at the appropriate level (Figure 5.7a). Though sometimes quite focal, often these lesions are well generalized, particularly in breeds that show a familial tendency, such as Boxers, Bulldogs, and Collies. Gingival enlargement can also be caused by hormonal changes, different drug administration (e.g., cyclosporine, amlodipine, phenytoin) [145, 146]. Specific gingival growths or tumors may initially present as an inflammatory or hyperplastic appearance, and all should be biopsied.

Suprabony pockets occur when marginal bone loss exceeds gingival recession (the marginal bone is lost horizontally below the tissue). A suprabony pocket has its base, or bottom of the pocket, coronal to the alveolar marginal bone. It is usually associated with early pocket formation, gingival hyperplasia, or an underlying horizontal bone loss pattern (Figure 5.7b and c).

Infra(intra)bony pockets occur when bone is lost vertically around a tooth. Infrabony pockets can be classified as one-wall, two-wall, three-wall, and four-wall (cup or crater) defects. The number of infrabony pocket walls surrounding the tooth root classifies infrabony pockets. An infrabony pocket has its base apical to the marginal bone (Figure 5.7d and e). This means that the pocket, at its depth, is between the tooth and bone.

Common locations for infrabony pockets in dog patients include the distal aspect of the mandibular first molars, the furcation of the mesial roots of the maxillary fourth premolars (Figure 5.8), the mesial aspects of the mandibular canine teeth, particularly after the third incisors are lost or are extracted without proper technique, and the palatal aspect of the maxillary canine teeth. Without osseous surgery (i.e., osseous additive or osseous resective surgery) to treat these bone defects, they will simply continue to cause periodontium destruction and chronic inflammation and infection in the patient.

Three-wall infrabony pocket. The defect is formed by the root acting as one wall and three osseous surfaces as the other walls.

Two-wall infrabony pocket. Extends interdentally to communicate with the root of an adjacent tooth; the two tooth surfaces make up two walls and the other two walls are formed by bone on the labial and lingual surfaces.

One-wall infrabony pocket. The two-wall infrabony extends to include destruction of the labial or lingual osseous wall, resulting in replacement by connective and inflammatory tissue and leaving only one bony surface.

Cup defect or four-wall infrabony pocket. A defect surrounding the tooth like a moat.

The buccal cortical bone is thin and can be compromised, resulting in fenestration and dehiscence but still being covered by connective tissue (i.e., gingiva, alveolar mucosa). Isolated areas of buccal bone loss on the buccal and lingual root surfaces where only periosteum and gingiva remain is termed fenestration. If the fenestration extends to, and includes, the marginal bone it is termed dehiscence. The thin buccal and lingual cortical bone can be lost rapidly due to periodontitis. Often these lesions are not easily demonstrated radiographically. The superimposition of mineralized tooth structure, alveolar bone, and cortical bone on the opposing tooth surfaces makes identification very challenging. Cone beam computed tomography (CBCT) is being utilized in human periodontology to aid in the diagnosis.

5.11 Roentgen Signs of Periodontal Disease

It takes approximately 30–50% mineral loss of tooth and bone structures before radiographic changes can be visualized on the dental film or digital dental radiographic system. Therefore, radiographs underestimate the extent of bone loss and pathology and may not always correlate with acute clinical signs. Radiographs are a snapshot in time and recheck radiographs 6–12 months following the initial radiographic image are often necessary to evaluate the progression of disease and/or healing of bone and tooth structures. Finally, radiographs are two-dimensional representations of three-dimensional structures. Therefore, overlying structures causing summation and superimposition frequently create artifacts that obscure or mimic pathology. The value of intraoral

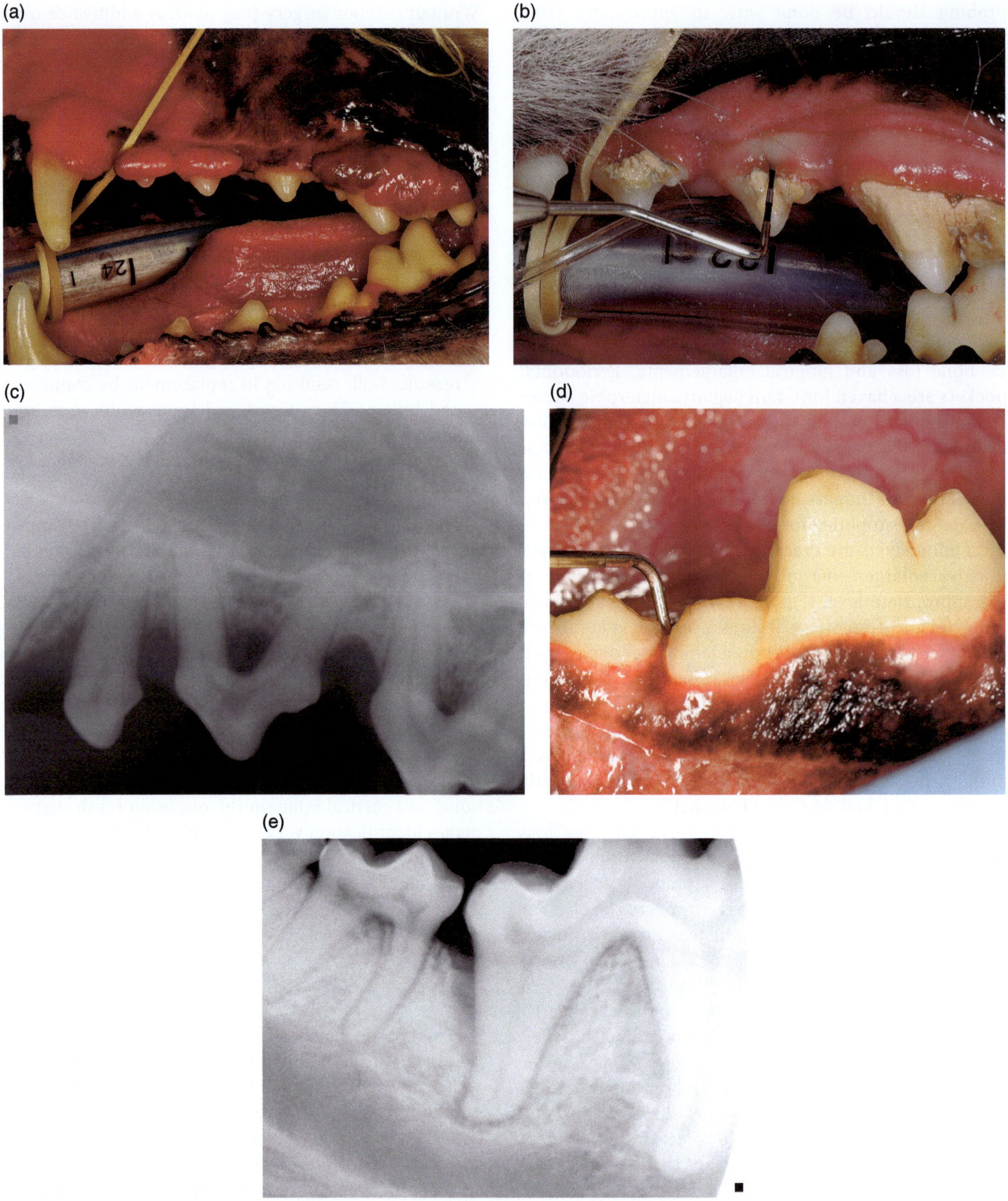

Figure 5.7 Periodontal pockets can be classified into pseudopockets, suprabony pockets, and infra(intra)bony pockets. (a) All the dentition in the left maxilla of this dog has pseudopockets that resulted when the gingiva enlarged and the marginal bone remained at the appropriate level. Gingival enlargement can occur secondary to drugs such as amlodipine, as in this case, and cyclosporine. (b and c) A left maxillary dental arch and corresponding intraoral dental radiograph in a dog is presented. There are suprabony pockets of the first, second, and third left maxillary premolars (205, 206, 207) diagnosed by periodontal probing and identified horizontal bone loss on the intraoral radiograph. A suprabony pocket has its base, or bottom of the pocket, coronal to the alveolar marginal bone. (d and e) An infrabony pocket has its base apical to the marginal bone. Note the lack of significant supragingival plaque and calculus, emphasizing that periodontal disease is caused by the subgingival plaque biofilm. However, with periodontal probing and intraoral radiographs during an anesthetized examination and cleaning an infrabony pocket with periodontal disease stage 4 was diagnosed in the right maxillary first molar (409). *Source:* Photographs used with permission, courtesy of Wade Gingerich, DVM, DAVDC.

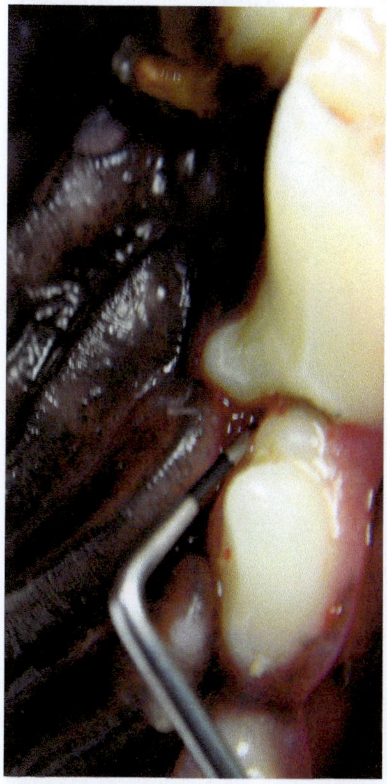

Figure 5.8 Infrabony pockets can be found in the furcation region of the mesial palatal and mesial buccal roots of the maxillary fourth premolar as seen in this left maxillary fourth premolar (208). It is important to note that summation of the bone and roots during intraoral radiography can hide the periodontal pocket on radiographs. In this patient the crowded third and fourth premolars (207, 208) led to a 13 mm periodontal pocket (periodontal isease s 4) that was best identified with periodontal probing. Intraoral radiographs helped confirm the findings.

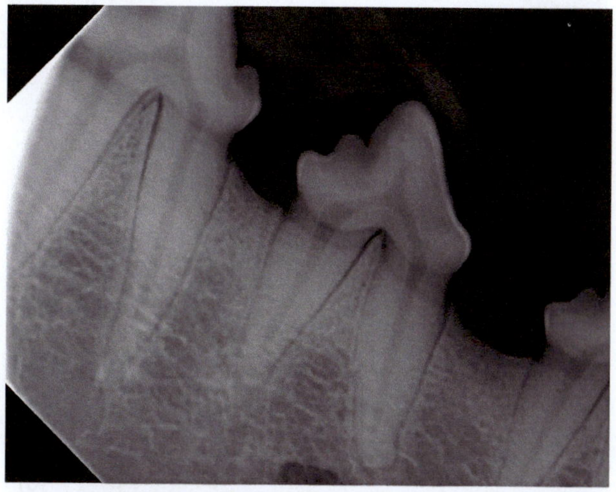

Figure 5.9 When cortical and alveolar bone is lost around a tooth at a similar rate, horizontal bone loss can be seen on the intraoral radiograph. The percentage of bone loss (i.e., attachment loss) can be measured from the region of the cementoenamel junction to the apex of the tooth. The mandibular right third premolar (407) has less than 25% attachment loss with a diagnosis of periodontal disease stage 2.

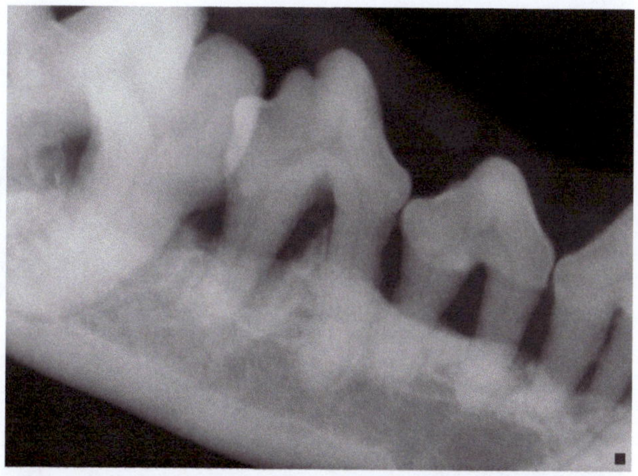

Figure 5.10 In many cases of moderate to severe periodontal disease a pattern of mixed horizontal and vertical bone loss will often be identified with intraoral radiography. Note the horizontal bone loss of the right mandibular cheek teeth (409, 408, 407, and 406) and the combined vertical bone loss on the distal root of the right fourth mandibular premolar (408).

radiographs has been documented in all aspects of veterinary dentistry including periodontal disease [130–132, 147, 148].

With periodontal disease, radiographically there will be loss of the marginal bone, loss of the lamina dura, widening of the lamina lucida (i.e., PDL space), and horizontal and vertical bone loss due to the resorption of bone. Horizontal bone loss occurs when the cortical supporting bone around the tooth and adjacent teeth is lost at a similar rate (Figure 5.9). If the soft tissue does not recess at a similar rate as the bone, a suprabony periodontal pocket will be formed. Vertical bone loss occurs when there is one area of bone loss around a tooth with adjacent supporting bone and mineralized tooth structures remaining more coronal. Vertical bone loss results in infrabony pockets (single wall defect, two wall defect, three wall defect, and four wall defect). In many cases there may be a combination of both horizontal and vertical bone loss (Figure 5.10).

5.12 Periodontal Stages

AVDC veterinary dental nomenclature allows us to classify periodontal disease into stages. Treatment plans can be designed based on the individual tooth stage as well as the overall periodontal stage of the oral cavity. With periodontal probing and intraoral radiographs various diagnostic stages of periodontal disease can be assigned (Figure 5.11a to e) [135] (reprinted with permission, AVDC).

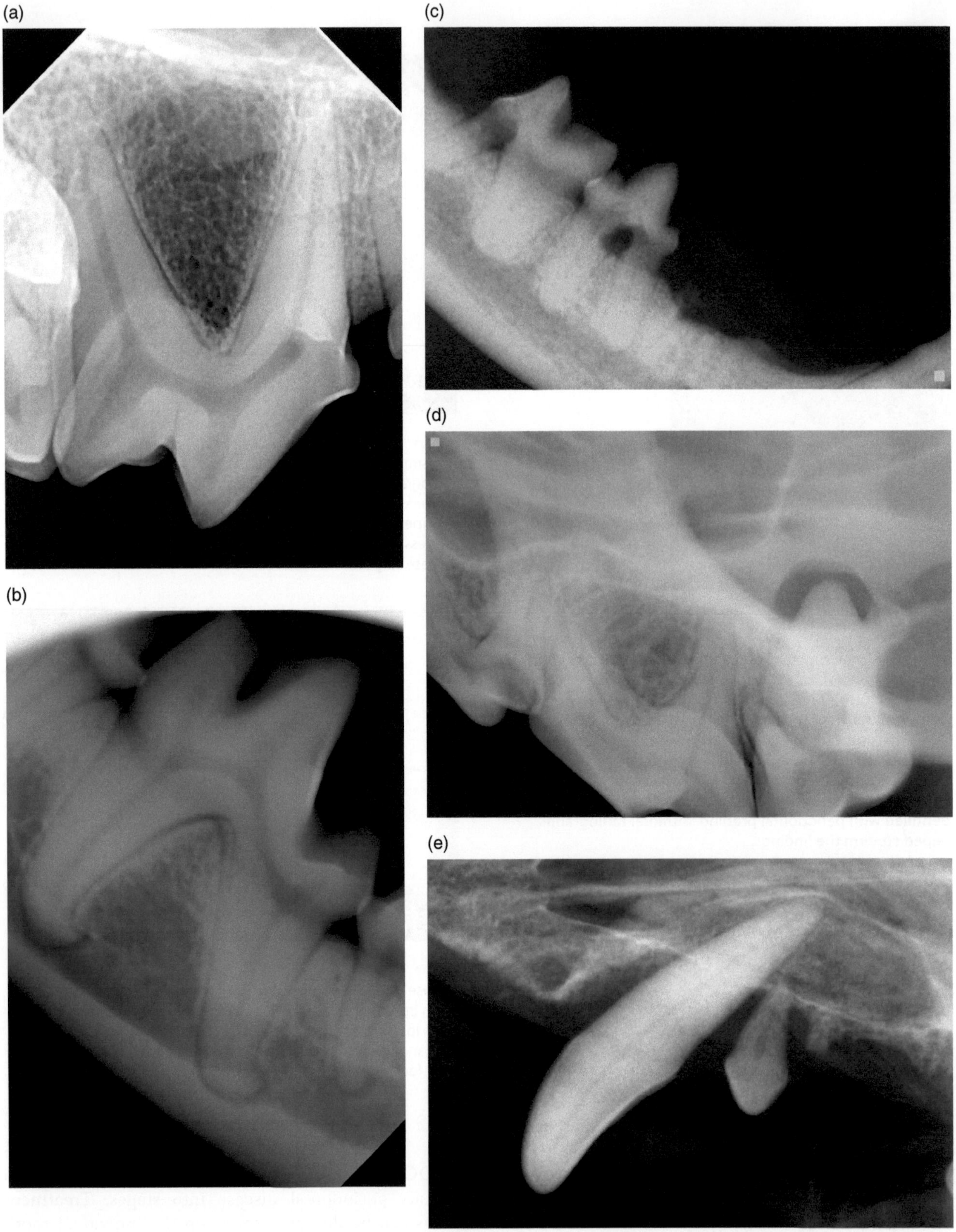

Figure 5.11 Stages of periodontal disease are based on percentage of attachment loss and furcation exposure: (a) periodontal disease stage 1 (gingivitis with no attachment loss); (b) periodontal disease stage 2 (<25% attachment loss); (c) periodontal disease Stage 3 (25–50% attachment loss); (d and e) and periodontal disease stage 4 (>50% attachment loss) are identified on intraoral radiographs. Note the marginal bone to the level of the mesial marginal bone of tooth 108 A (PD1) and the distal root of tooth 309 B (PD2). The right mandibular feline molar (409) and fourth premolar (408) had 25–50% bone loss in C (PD3). The left maxillary first molar (209) has 100% bone loss of the palatal root and > 50% bone loss of the mesial buccal root in D (PD4). The maxillary left canine (204), first premolar (205), and retained mesial tooth root (206) have greater than 50% attachment loss E (PD4).

"Normal (PD 0): clinically normal – no gingival inflammation or periodontitis clinically evident.

Stage 1 (PD 1). Gingivitis only without attachment loss. The height and architecture of the alveolar margin are normal.

Stage 2 (PD 2). Early periodontitis – less than 25% of attachment loss or, at most, there is a stage 1 furcation involvement in multirooted teeth. There are early radiologic signs of periodontitis. The loss of periodontal attachment is less than 25% as measured either by probing of the clinical attachment level, or radiographic determination of the distance of the alveolar margin from the cemento-enamel junction relative to the length of the root.

Stage 3 (PD 3). Moderate periodontitis – 25–50% of attachment loss as measured either by probing of the clinical attachment level, radiographic determination of the distance of the alveolar margin from the cemento-enamel junction relative to the length of the root, or there is a stage 2 furcation involvement in multirooted teeth.

Stage 4 (PD 4). Advanced periodontitis – more than 50% of attachment loss as measured either by probing of the clinical attachment level, or radiographic determination of the distance of the alveolar margin from the cemento-enamel junction relative to the length of the root, or there is a stage 3 furcation involvement in multirooted teeth."

5.13 Chronic and Aggressive Periodontitis

Chronic periodontitis related to age and progression of the disease over time is the most common form of periodontitis in pets. However, an aggressive form of periodontitis characterized by early age onset, a high rate of disease progression, and involvement of multiple teeth without a systemic cause are the diagnostic criteria in humans [149, 150]. Certain bacterial pathogens may be involved in human and canine aggressive periodontitis [151, 152]. Earlier classification systems of periodontitis categorized adult onset periodontitis, juvenile onset periodontitis, pre-pubertal periodontitis, and rapidly progressive and refractory periodontitis. However, based on current scientific information, nomenclature changed in 1999 to chronic periodontitis and aggressive periodontitis [149, 153]. These human classifications may be extrapolated to veterinary species but the veterinary profession must be cautious in overextrapolating and assigning aggressive periodontitis etiology until individual breed differences, bacterial pathogens, and other risk factors are worked out in various dog and cat breeds.

Chronic periodontitis is a slow progressing form more commonly seen in adult patients, but may have had its beginning when the animal was relatively young. It is the most common form of periodontal disease seen, typically experienced as a slow, chronic gradual development with an irregular distribution. Although it can be generalized, there may be some areas more predisposed than others to more extensive forms of the disease. The community of bacteria in the plaque biofilm and the associated inflammatory response are responsible. Initially, treatment is typically professional periodontal cleanings and good home care. It is seen in all breeds and species.

Aggressive periodontitis is a rapidly progressive form seen mostly in young adults and is commonly generalized. In some cases, cyclic episodes of acute infections of Gram negative anaerobes may be followed by quiet periods. It may have normal looking gingiva, but with areas of bone loss radiographically. In other cases, there may be significant gingival inflammation and bleeding present. Uncontrolled cases will usually have continued attachment loss at the time of diagnosis. Breeds such as the Miniature Schnauzer, Greyhound, Maltese, Abyssinian, Siamese, and Somali may be overrepresented. Certain aspects of human populations are known to be at increased risks [153, 154]. In some cases pericoronitis associated with erupting deciduous teeth can aggressively continue once the adult dentition has fully erupted. Unfortunately, many of these cases progress, become refractory to treatment, and may be associated with buccal mucositis (see further in the chapter).

5.14 Periodontal-Related Oral Pathology

There are many conditions and diseases that can affect the periodontal tissues. A more complete listing of periodontal-related diseases can be found elsewhere in this textbook. Some oral inflammatory conditions may be related to an underlying immunological pathology [155]. Autoimmune disease such as pemphigus vulgaris, bullous pemphigoid, mucous membrane pemphigoid, and systemic lupus erythematosus may manifest early in the oral cavity and be associated with gingivitis and mucositis. It is often difficult to clinically identify true vesicles and bulla associated with some of the diseases. Evaluation of the entire patient is necessary. Abnormalities in an animal's immune system (e.g., immunosuppression, immune dysregulation) can have varying effects on the periodontal tissues. Infection, stress, or drugs may lead to alterations in the pets' immune response, which may predispose an individual to opportunistic infections. This may be a decrease in response or, at times, an exaggerated response to relatively normal stimuli. Exaggerated immune responses result in buccal mucositis and ulcerative stomatitis (e.g., Maltese dogs). In severe buccal mucositis (formerly known as chronic ulcerative paradental stomatitis (CUPS)) there may be a marked ulceration of buccal mucosa that contacts a tooth surface. This condition appears to develop as a result of plaque intolerance, with the consequence of an excessive immune response to plaque biofilm deposition. Initially, the condition is primarily localized to areas adjacent to the canine and distal maxillary fourth premolars and molars, but may rapidly progress to a more generalized stage. Plaque control is crucial but may be difficult in some patients. The use of antibiotics and anti-inflammatories are only temporarily helpful and not a long-term treatment strategy. If effective plaque control cannot be maintained, often extractions are necessary as medical therapy only provides temporary relief. Selective extractions of compromised teeth in addition to home care and medical therapy can help many patients. Each patient may respond differently and require additional extractions. Extractions, daily brushing, semi-annual to annual periodontal cleanings, and, in some cases, medical therapy are necessary to control the painful condition.

Most cases of periodontal disease are hidden and insidious. However, in some cases a true periodontal abscess with purulent debris may develop. If necrotic tissue or debris gets trapped within the confines of the sulcus and is not removed, expelled, or resorbed, an abscess may result. A parulis may develop, which is a raised nodule at the opening of a draining sinus tract (Figure 5.12a and b). If the parulis is located apical to the mucogingival junction it is often associated with endodontic disease. If the parulis is located at, or coronal to, the mucogingival junction it is often associated with periodontal disease. In some cases, a periodontal abscess will present as firm or soft swellings on the mandible and maxilla with or without purulent drainage. These may also occur with endodontic infections.

Generally periodontal abscesses can be divided into three categories: acute, chronic, and chronic/acute. Acute periodontal abscesses may be accompanied by pain, swelling, tenderness of the gingiva, tooth sensitivity on percussion, and possibly systemic signs such as malaise, fever, and leukocytosis. These early lesions may present without notable clinical lesions or radiographic changes. Acute lesions, when improperly or untreated, may eventually subside, but persist in a chronic state of infection and inflammation. Chronic periodontal abscesses appear asymptomatic. However, chronic, dull pain often occurs and is hidden by the pet. Chronic lesions may develop without ever having experienced an acute state, but a chronic state may flare up periodically into an acute condition. Acute on chronic periodontal abscesses are acute exacerbations of chronic lesions that, anecdotally, appear to be the most common in our dogs and cats.

Maxillary and mandibular draining tracts should be investigated for odontogenic infections such as periodontal disease or endodontic disease prior to extensive dermatological or neoplastic workups. Teeth should be the primary differential for the maxillofacial swellings and draining tracts. The pathology is easily diagnosed with an appropriate anesthetized examination and intraoral radiographs if the veterinarian has knowledge of the dental pathophysiology. If an odontogenic infection is not the cause, then evaluation for neoplasia, etc.,

(a) (b)

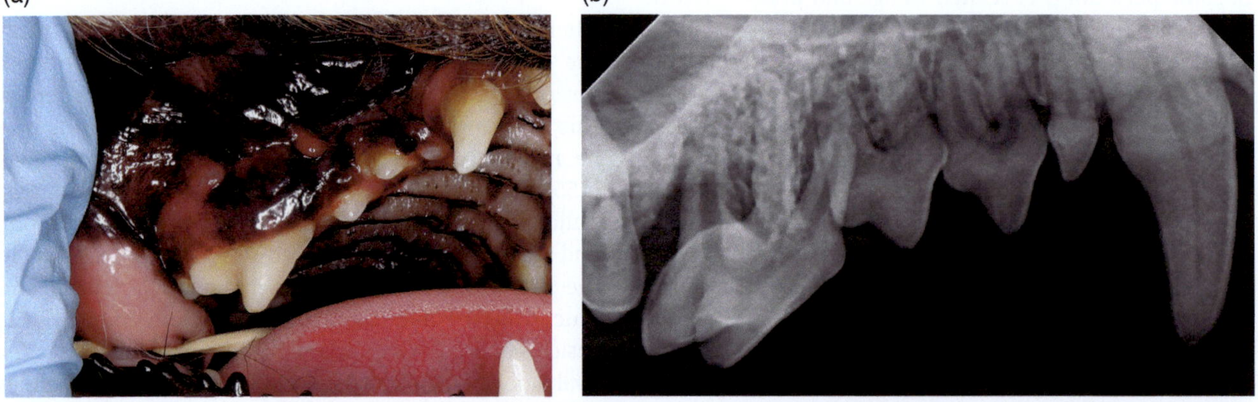

Figure 5.12 (a) The right maxillary arcade in this small breed dog shows crowded maxillary premolars (105, 106, 107, and 108), with only mild plaque and calculus, minimal gingivitis of tooth 108, no identifiable tooth fractures, but two parulides at the mucogingival junction. (b) Intraoral radiographs identified 100% bone loss of tooth 108 distal and mesial buccal roots. Periodontal disease stage 4 was diagnosed with a presumptive periodontal-endodontic lesion. Despite the minimal supragingival plaque and calculus, this case demonstrates the requirement for general anesthesia, oral examination, periodontal probing, and intraoral radiographs in order to properly diagnose and treat periodontal disease. *Source:* Photographs used with permission, from K. Stepaniuk, Top 5 Oral and Dental Lesions (Figures 3 and 4), Clinician's Brief, October 2014, pp. 31–34.

can be pursued with imaging and biopsy. Often if it is neoplasia, a tooth is near the lesion and surgical extraction and deep biopsy via the extraction site will provide a histological diagnosis in some cases.

Brachycephalic cats often have a scissors occlusion or level bite of the incisors. However, the mandibles may have bowed laterally during growth. As a result, the central cusp of the maxillary fourth premolars contact the mesial and buccal tooth surfaces and periodontium of the mandibular first molars, resulting in periodontal dehiscence and disease. Also, some cats may have a tight occlusion resulting in periodontal trauma of occlusion – of the maxillary teeth to the mandibular region. The veterinarian may extract the lower first molar or identify a mass pre- or post-extraction that has a histological description of pyogenic granuloma or lymphoplasmacytic gingivitis. Often these lesions are secondary to the trauma created by the maxillary fourth premolars. Surgical extraction of a periodontally expired mandibular first molar is necessary. The maxillary fourth premolar requires surgical extraction, appropriate crown reduction, and endodontic and restorative treatment or odontoplasty and restorative treatment to remove the offending cusp(s).

5.15 Endodontic Periodontic Relationship

Infection from periodontal disease may have adverse effects upon the pulp [156]. Generally, the involvement occurs from the spread of infection along the root surface, gaining entrance to the endodontic system through lateral or accessory canals, or through the apical delta (see Chapter 15 – Basic Endodontic Therapy). There may be periodontal-endodontic pathology, endodontic-periodontal pathology, or true combined periodontal-endodontic pathology.

5.16 Periodontal Therapy/Treatment

Since the cause of periodontal disease is the plaque biofilm of microorganisms, the primary goal of periodontal disease is to control the subgingival plaque biofilm. However, failure to control secondary causes and contributing factors can result in failure to attain the primary goal. Therefore, address all known possible contributing factors. Therapy can be divided into six basic categories:

1) Professional periodontal cleaning (teeth cleaning).
2) Periodontal surgeries.
3) Dental and oral surgery (e.g., extraction).
4) Restorative dentistry.
5) Adjunctive medical therapy if indicated.
6) Home dental hygiene.

5.17 Treatment of Periodontal Disease

Veterinary patients should be scheduled for a periodontal cleaning when there is gingivitis and before irreversible periodontal disease and attachment loss has occurred. Supragingival scaling and subgingival scaling is performed. Subgingival scaling separates a professional dental cleaning from a purely cosmetic procedure. Correct subgingival cleaning is impossible in the non-anesthetized patient [134]. As far back as 1975, it has been demonstrated in dogs that daily tooth brushing and dental cleanings can establish and maintain normal periodontium over several years [157]. Depending on patient signalment, AAHA guidelines recommend a professional dental cleaning in the first to second year of a patient's life [127]. However, even at the time of this chapter, the collective veterinary profession continues to struggle with promoting wellness and preventive veterinary dentistry. Both real and perceived challenges implementing preventive periodontal programs exist. The collective profession should advocate for the oral health of veterinary patients based on historical and current literature in order to eliminate pain, infection, and systemic ramifications of periodontal disease.

A professional dental (periodontal) cleaning takes time to assess the oral cavity, obtain intraoral radiographs, and professionally clean the oral cavity. Additional periodontal treatments, periodontal surgery and extractions, as indicated, can easily increase the anesthetic treatment time. Therefore, appropriate time must be scheduled in the surgical schedule to allow unrushed assessment and execution of treatment plans.

5.17.1 Professional Dental Cleaning

A professional dental cleaning *requires general anesthesia* and must be differentiated from a "non-professional dental scaling" (NPDS) and "anesthesia free dentistry" in dogs and cats. It is impossible to assess and treat the subgingival plaque biofilm and the associated periodontal disease without general anesthesia. Clients may falsely believe that their pets are receiving medical care when only the supragingival crowns are cleaned in the NPDS practices. Their pets continue to suffer from chronic subgingival inflammation, infection, and pain. An American Veterinary Dental College position statement supports the need for general anesthesia to professionally diagnose and treat subgingival periodontal disease [134]. The safety of the pet, the safety of the veterinary professional, protection of the airways from inhalation, appropriate exam and diagnosis, and necessary subgingival cleaning require general anesthesia.

During a dental cleaning bacteremia from the oral pathogens will occur within at least 40 minutes [158, 159]. However, in most cases and with some exceptions, perioperative antibiotics are not necessary. A dental "*prophylaxis*" is a dental cleaning to prevent periodontal disease. Therefore, the term periodontal cleaning, periodontal treatment, and/or dental cleaning are more appropriate terms when a veterinary patient is treated. The benefits of performing a complete and proper prophylaxis to aid in control of early periodontal disease or a periodontal cleaning to help salvage more advanced cases cannot be overemphasized.

Equipment necessary for a complete, professional periodontal cleaning includes, but is not limited to, ultrasonic scalers (piezoelectric and magnetostrictive (ferromagnetic stacks and ferrite rods)), hand scalers, universal curettes, gracey curettes, a slow-speed handpiece, polishing heads and cups for polishing, a means of irrigation, dental probes and explorers, and dental charts.

5.17.2 Periodontal Cleaning Steps

Client consent is required prior to the initiation of treatment. Masks, caps, gloves, and protective eyewear are worn. (i) General anesthesia *is required.* (ii) The oral cavity is rinsed with a 0.12% chlorhexidine gluconate oral rinse to decrease aerosolization of bacteria [160]. (iii) Supragingival scaling involves removing the calculus and plaque from above the gumline (using hand scalers and water-cooled ultrasonic scalers – no more than five to seven seconds per tooth to prevent thermal and concussive injury) [161]. (iv) Subgingival scaling (root planing and subgingival curettage) is crucial for the treatment and prevention of periodontal disease. Hand curettes and some water-cooled ultrasonic scalers, with periodontal or universal tips, are used to clean subgingivally. (v) Polishing involves using a pumice (i.e., fine) to smooth out roughness created in the enamel during the periodontal cleaning. Polishing should be minimized to less than three seconds per tooth. The polishing cup should flare 1–2 mm subgingivally to polish the subgingival tooth surface cleaned during the subgingival scaling. (vi) The air–water syringe is used to irrigate the sulcus and remove debris, plaque, and polishing paste. (vii) Full mouth intraoral radiographs are obtained. (viii) Client education and home care are planned and discussed with the client.

Supragingival scaling can be done in several ways, with numerous different instruments. Gross removal of supragingival calculus and plaque is accomplished initially by removing larger pieces manually with hand dental scalers or ultrasonic scalers, being careful not to injure the soft tissue. A detailed scaling with hand instruments and/or ultrasonic scalers is performed. Hand scaling, although slow, can be gentle to the tooth yet very effective [162–164]. However, hand scalers should be kept sharp, maintained, and replaced, as indicated, to prevent crushing of calculus and burnishing plaque into the tooth surface [165]. Hand scalers are made for use above the gumline, and with a pull stroke away from the soft tissues. If used below the gumline, laceration of the epithelial attachment occurs, allowing bacteria to more freely enter the periodontal tissues.

Subgingival scaling can be done with ultrasonic instruments, when proper tips and irrigation are used. However, hand curettes are still needed to remove any remaining areas of hidden subgingival plaque and calculus. Subgingival deposits of plaque and calculus (up to 5 mm pocket depth) can be removed using a curette below the gingiva. Curettes have a rounded toe and heal that can reduce damage to the epithelial attachment in the bottom of the sulcus. Curette selection must adapt to the root anatomy to be effective. In cases where the root surface is still firm and reasonably smooth, simple subgingival debridement with a periodontal tip on an appropriate ultrasonic instrument may suffice for treatment, or the light use of a curette. However, as the root surface becomes more diseased as well as the cementum, root planing is necessary. Rough root surface areas will irritate the gingiva and allow for ease in reaccumulation of plaque and calculus. The instrument is adapted with shank parallelism and the curette is drawn across the root in several different directions, with multiple strokes, to completely remove all debris and smooth the root surface. A subgingival curettage (or the more appropriate term, gingival curettage) may also be employed to gently debride diseased tissue and bacteria from the inside of the gingival pocket or sulcus. However, in most cases this procedure is performed inadvertently (i.e., inadvertent curettage) during subgingival debridement and root planing.

The angle of the curette shank dictates areas of best use. The way in which the instrument contacts the intended surface is known as instrument adaptation. The distal shank of the instrument is parallel to the long axis of the tooth – shank parallelism. A modified pen grasp is used on the instrument. The motion of activation is the way in which scalers and curettes are used in the hand to effect proficient work. Rotary, wrist, or digital motion can be used. However, digital motion can cause repetitive motion injuries and is not recommended [166]. The contours of the dental curette allow it to be introduced gently into the sulcus with the face "closed," so the cutting edge does not yet engage the tooth surface. Once reaching the depth of the sulcus, the curette is angled to bring the working edge into contact with the surface, and a pull stroke is used to dislodge the calculus and debris and bring it out of the canal. These pull strokes can be combined in vertical, horizontal, and oblique directions to provide a smooth, clean surface, in a procedure called root planing. The instrument may also be slightly angled, bringing the other working edge against the soft tissue, with gentle digital pressure on the external gingival surface to debride any diseased tissue, bacteria, or debris, known as subgingival curettage.

Any type of ultrasonic or hand scaling causes defects in the enamel surface, thus increasing the surface for the plaque biofilm to rapidly colonize; polishing is then necessary to smooth the tooth surface. Polishing has been under some scrutiny in human dentistry for its gradual abrasive reduction of the enamel over the life of a human patient with annual or semi-annual treatments. This has not been documented in the life span of the dog and cat. However, excessive polishing should be avoided to prevent enamel loss and dentin tubule exposure in addition to hyperthermic pulpitis. Polishing is performed with a slow-speed hand piece, a hygienic disposable prophylaxis angle and cup, and a fine textured polishing paste. The use of light circular strokes up to three seconds per tooth with a fine pumice slurry and taking care not to exceed 1–3000 rpm will help to avoid hyperthermia and avoid tooth damage. Pressure must be applied to the cup in order to splay and flare the cup margin subgingivally. Pumice must always be between the polishing cup and the tooth. Pumice is an abrasive formed from a mixture of complex aluminum, potassium, and sodium silicates. Many prophylaxis pastes have included fluoride and other products.

Polishing as well as minor cleaning of the teeth can also be performed with an air-powder prophylaxis unit. These units use an air power source to spray a water and abrasive powder across the teeth to polish. The abrasive is usually a finely ground sodium bicarbonate powder. They create a sandblasting effect. However, the sodium load created by the abrasive may be contraindicated in some cases. Barotrauma can occur if used incorrectly.

Polishing is followed by sulcus irrigation or lavage using water, saline, or a 0.12% oral chlorhexidine solution. This is done to flush all remaining pumice and debris out of the sulcus, to prevent foreign body irritations that might lead to periodontal inflammation and/or abscessation. A blunt-tipped irrigation needle and syringe can be used or a periodontal irrigating device if an air–water syringe is not available on the dental unit. The air–water syringe can be used to gently dry the tooth surface to identify any remaining calculus that will appear "chalky" on the tooth surface.

The periodontal cleaning is not complete until client education is presented. If the procedure was a periodontal cleaning without surgery, then the client should be educated on home care at discharge. If surgery was performed, education may be delayed until the recheck appointment to verify the surgical sites are healed prior to instituting a plaque control home care program. A recall for the next periodontal cleaning and oral exam is set for 6–12 months depending on the stage of periodontal disease, client commitment to home care, and signalment of the patient.

A thorough periodontal cleaning will lead to reversal of gingivitis and shrinkage and healing of some suprabony pockets with long junctional epithelium. In some cases of suprabony pockets, periceuticals may be used in order to medically treat the suprabony pocket following the mechanical treatment [167–169]. Pseudopockets, infrabony pockets, mobile teeth, and some furcation defects will require additional periodontal surgery.

Treatment of periodontal disease is not a once in a lifetime event for the patient but rather an ongoing treatment program throughout continued life stages of the patient. Gingivitis is reversible. However, once periodontium attachment destruction occurs, the process is not reversible. The goal with periodontitis is to stop the disease, minimize further attachment loss, and treat compromised teeth (e.g., periodontal surgery, guided tissue regeneration, and extraction as indicated). Therefore, education and prevention of disease (daily brushing, dentifrices, and frequent professional dental care) are the best defenses. A professional dental cleaning, to return the tooth to a clean surface, followed by daily home care, to remove the plaque biofilm, is the gold standard to prevent and control periodontal disease. If pockets are eliminated and the plaque biofilm removed on a daily basis, then the maturation of plaque and further pocket formation can be controlled and minimized.

5.17.3 Disclosing Agents

Rarely, disclosing agents are used to identify plaque and calculus during a dental cleaning and as a client educational tool. Disclosing agents are solutions or wafers that are effective in staining plaque, calculus, and bacterial deposits on the teeth, tongue, and gingiva. However, these products can cause staining to hair, oral tissues, hands, clothing, sinks, tables, etc., and must be used cautiously, as they can be a client irritator rather than a motivator.

5.18 Home Dental Care and Dentifrices

Home care is a veterinary team approach involving the doctor, technician, assistant, and entire staff. Client education about the proper methods and materials for dental hygiene is crucial to the entire process. Staff members should be well trained and knowledgeable about home care techniques, so they can demonstrate home care to the pet owners. More than just showing a step-by-step process, the staff should understand the concepts to the point that they truly believe in the tremendous benefits available, and should exuberantly try to instill this commitment in clients. The enthusiasm should be contagious! All-in clinic efforts may be worth little if there is no client compliance (e.g., home care and reevaluations). Be accustomed to utilizing the products for educating clients. Start pets out slowly with home care, allowing healing time for the gingiva following professional prophylaxis or other periodontal treatments. If periodontal disease or other painful oral conditions are present (e.g., fractured teeth) it is necessary to first anesthetize the patient, assess the oral cavity, obtain intraoral radiographs, treat disease, and establish the oral cavity to a new normal baseline. Then a home care plan can be developed for the individual patient.

A way to determine if a product or diet meets its label claims is to look for the veterinary oral health council (VOHC) seal. The VOHC recognizes home care products that the make claims of plaque and "tartar" retardation [170]. The submitted products need to meet pre-met standards and protocols of research, which will then be evaluated by the VOHC. The VOHC does not test products but awards the VOHC seal if the product research meets a claim, in one of two categories, that the product helps control plaque or helps control "tartar." Various diets, chews, and additives have been awarded the VOHC seal [170].

No home care product is a monotherapy to treat periodontal disease caused by the plaque biofilm. Home care products are not a substitution for a professional periodontal cleaning. General anesthesia, complete oral examination and assessment, and professional periodontal cleaning are necessary to treat the oral cavity. Home care products help prevent and slow the return of plaque and calculus. Even with meticulous home care, anesthesia for complete oral examinations and subgingival scaling is necessary throughout the life of the patient.

The list of home care products and over-the-counter products is extensive. Some products make unsubstantiated claims and exacerbate clients' fears of general anesthesia that is required for veterinary dentistry. Many products simply control/mask halitosis and do not address the cause of periodontal disease – the subgingival plaque biofilm. Dental and oral surgical patients can be safely anesthetized with proper pre-anesthetic planning, multimodal anesthesia, patient monitoring and support, and/or referral to a veterinary dentist and veterinary anesthesiologist when indicated in order to establish a clean tooth surface [171, 172]. The following list is fairly general, due to the numerous products available in the market and the number of products that enter and leave the consumer market.

5.18.1 Tooth Brushing

Tooth brushing is the most effective home care plaque control method. Tooth brushing should be started prior to the establishment of periodontal disease. Tooth brushing has been demonstrated to be effective in dogs to prevent and control gingivitis if performed on a daily basis [65, 66]. Care should be taken in attempting home care on certain individuals; some pets may be difficult to treat and the risk of injury to the owner needs to be assessed. Likewise, a painful mouth may cause the patient to become averse to dental brushing. As in any training method, it is best to start out slow and easy, trying to make it a fun and rewarding experience for all participants. Daily brushing with a soft-bristled nylon toothbrush is the most effective method of plaque control and is the gold standard. The soft bristles mechanically remove the plaque biofilm. However, it should be noted it is often difficult for owners to reach all areas of the mouth. Particularly, the distal maxillary and mandibular molars and the lingual/palatal sides of the dentition may be missed. The bristles may help remove plaque 1–2 mm into the gingival sulcus with appropriate techniques. Therefore, active periodontal disease and periodontal pockets require professional treatment to eliminate periodontal pockets and reestablish normal sulcular measurements. Additives to pet toothpastes are used to increase palatability, augment the normal salivary protective systems, and provide chemical control of plaque. Do not use human toothpaste as the fluoride and detergents can be toxic to the pet. Likewise, sodium bicarbonate toothpastes when swallowed can increase the patients' sodium load and be detrimental in heart disease. The toothbrush should be held at a 45–60 angle to the tooth and used in a coronally directed stroke. Ultrasonic toothbrushes are a great alternative for effective daily brushing when the pets are trained to accept them.

5.18.2 Mechanical Cleansing (e.g., Diets, Chews)

There are a variety of dental chews that help control plaque and calculus [72–81]. They are often designed to encourage chewing so the tooth can be mechanically scrubbed. Additionally, some products have the addition of different chemical antiplaque compounds and chemicals to bind the volatile compounds causing halitosis. Extremely hard chew toys (e.g., cow hooves, nylon style bones, butcher bones, ice cubes, antlers) commonly fracture teeth, leading to endodontic disease and hidden periapical infections.

Some veterinary prescription dental diets control plaque through fiber arrangement. The tooth is mechanically cleaned as the pet chews through the kibble. If chewing teeth are absent, occluding teeth are absent, or the pet does not chew the food, then diets or chews will not be effective dentifrices. There are diets and chews with the addition of polyphosphates that control calculus accumulation by binding the salivary calcium carbonate in the saliva and thereby prevent some mineralized deposits (calculus) on the teeth.

5.18.3 Chemical Treatments

There are 0.1–0.12% chlorhexidine gluconate and acetate oral rinses that can be used on a daily basis. It has shown abilities to inhibit the development of plaque and the development of periodontal disease in the dog [68–70]. Chlorhexidine is a cationic bis-biguanide that disrupts bacterial cell wall lipoproteins and precipitates the bacterial cytoplasm. It can bind to the pellicle and have a prolonged effect. It can be inactivated when interacting with other oral product compounds. It is available in solutions, gels, and dentifrices. It does have a bitter taste and has been reported to cause severe skin and mucosal irritations on occasions when used in high concentration or if left on tissues for too long a period of time.

Zinc-containing products (zinc ascorbate, zinc gluconate) may help control plaque [88]. The mechanism has an antibacterial effect and supports collagen synthesis. Also, binding of volatile sulfur compounds that cause halitosis occurs.

Xylitol is a sugar alcohol incorporated in many human dental products and gum for its anticaries effects. It has been incorporated into various drinking water additives for pets. It should be noted that acute life-threatening hypoglycemic episodes and hepatic necrosis has been reported in dogs consuming *human* products containing xylitol [173]. Careful review of manufacturer safety studies, peer reviewed literature, efficacy studies, poison control center data, and individual patient susceptibility should be investigated prior to using these products.

Fluoride is present in many different formulations for use in human dentistry [174]. Fluoride in treated water is absorbed from the gastrointestinal tract and is distributed throughout the body to exert a systemic effect. This systemically absorbed fluoride is recycled to the saliva to provide low-level topical delivery that can effectively repair acidic demineralized tooth surfaces [174]. Since fluoride is readily absorbed, there is the potential for toxicity from both dietary and topical fluoride preparations. Excessive fluoride ingestion can be fatal. Any professionally or owner applied topical fluoride has the potential to exert systemic toxicity, since animals will not normally expectorate the fluoride. For this reason, if a veterinary professional chooses to use fluoride, it is important to apply the higher concentration of fluoride directly to isolated teeth, thereby minimizing soft tissue absorption. Application with a small brush or cotton swab and cotton roll isolation can minimize oral soft tissue contact and thus absorption. For initial treatments, the teeth are cleaned, dried, isolated with cotton rolls, and the teeth coated with the fluoride by brush or in trays for three to five minutes. The material is then removed by vacuum, blown free with air, or gently wiped clean, but not rinsed off with water.

Fluoride has an antibacterial affect and reduces dental sensitivity. Application of fluoride (gels, foams, or varnishes) to the tooth surfaces may be of some value. However, it must be recognized that although canine patients do develop caries they do not suffer the prevalence of caries in the human population [175]. Clients should understand that targeted fluoride use in pets is different from humans. Fluoride use in dogs and cats is used mainly for the antibacterial effects of fluoride and the potential desensitizing effects for the dental tubules.

5.18.4 Enzyme Systems

Enzyme systems are often added to pet toothpastes and dental products. Common enzymes are glucose oxidase and lactoperoxidase that react with oxygen and water in the oral cavity to form hypothiocyanite (an endogenous salivary product shown to have antibacterial effects).

5.18.5 Dental Surface Barrier Sealants/Treatments

Inert polymer sealants applied to teeth following a periodontal cleaning, and at home, are designed to form an electrostatic bond to the tooth enamel. Once bound, they are designed to provide a hydrophobic barrier that diminishes attachment of plaque and stain [83, 84, 86]. Other products are designed to be applied following a professional cleaning and provide a six month barrier [85].

5.18.6 Water Additives

Both chemical and natural water additives are available. The veterinarian and client should read all labels and instructions to be certain products are used correctly. A natural water additive for dogs to help control plaque received VOHC approval. A combination of natural antibacterial products, antioxidants, and natural preservatives are included in the formulation.

5.18.7 Host Modulation

Host modulation is an emerging treatment for human periodontal disease. Once again, it is *not* a substitute for professional subgingival periodontal cleanings and treatment. Rather, it helps address the inflammatory response to the plaque biofilm. Subtherapeutic doxycycline and azithromycin have been shown to exert anti-inflammatory effects in periodontal disease and diseases associated with periodontal disease [176–179]. Likewise, in select cases of aggressive periodontitis the use of non-steroidal anti-inflammatories may be beneficial with a comprehensive treatment plan that includes periodontal cleanings and daily home care. Host modulation must only be used with a complete treatment planning that includes periodontal cleanings, treatments, rechecks, and daily home care.

5.19 Pet Owners and Non-professional Dental Scalers (NDPSs)

Some owners, groomers, lay people, and poorly educated veterinary health professionals will use dental scalers to remove hard calculus deposits from the supragingival areas. They require education about the subgingival plaque biofilm. The pet and/or client may be injured during the hand scaling by the sharp instrument, resulting in trauma and infection to both. As with all scaling the tooth surface is roughened, making polishing necessary to smooth the rough surfaces. The roughened surface allows plaque to adhere even more quickly. Again, as with all areas, client education makes the difference.

5.20 Antibiotic Use in Periodontal Disease

Monotherapy with antibiotics is not a treatment for periodontal disease. There are two basic forms of antimicrobial treatment, local and systemic. Systemic antibiotics are not needed in most professional periodontal cleanings involving gingivitis or mild periodontal disease. Periodontal infection is treated by removal of the plaque biofilm, periodontal surgery, and/or extraction of the tooth with end stage periodontal disease. The use of antibiotics by itself is not a treatment. Antibiotics should never be used as a monotherapy for periodontal disease. Systemic antibiotic use is not indicated in routine dental prophylactic procedures. Perioperative antibiotic recommendations in more moderate and severe periodontal infections, immunocompromised individuals, patients with implants (e.g., pacemakers, total hip replacements, metallic implants within the last 12 months), and uncontrolled systemic disease should be considered when indicated. The selection of antibiotics should be chosen based on pathogens causing disease (Gram negative anaerobes) [180–183]. Therefore, clindamycin, amoxicillin/clavulanic acid, and tetracyclines/doxycyclines (in appropriate aged animals and certain conditions) and metronidazole are reasonable choices. Remember that oral bacteria are constantly released into the bloodstream during chewing and eating and the normal reticuloendothelial system manages the transient bacteremia. Worldwide antibacterial resistance is a global problem for human and veterinary health care. Overuse of antibiotics in pets and people leads to bacterial resistance and we have a professional responsibility to use antibiotics correctly and judiciously.

Local applications of doxycycline and clindamycin periceuticals have been used in suprabony pockets identified with periodontal probing and intraoral radiographs. Inappropriate use within infrabony pockets, suprabony periodontal pockets requiring periodontal surgery, or in cats with periodontal pockets must be avoided. Local applications are not a substitute for a proper subgingival scaling.

5.21 Periodontal Surgery

Periodontal surgery occurs with, and after, the oral cavity has had a thorough assessment, intraoral radiographs, and professional periodontal cleaning. Often, it is best to stage the procedures so that the periodontal surgery is performed several weeks after a periodontal cleaning if periodontal flaps or guided tissue regeneration are being utilized. Soft tissue resection and some osseous subtractive surgeries may be performed during the periodontal cleaning (see Chapter 10 – Oral Surgery – Periodontal Surgery).

References

1 Jin, L. J., Armitage, G. C., Klinge, B. et al. (2011). Global oral health inequalities: task-group-periodontal disease. *Adv. Dent. Res.* 23: 221–226.

2 Lund, E. M., Armstrong, P. J., Kirk, C. A. et al. (1999). Health status and population characteristics of dogs and cats examined at private veterinary practices in the United States. *J. Am. Vet. Med.* 9: 1336–1341.

3 Golden, A. L., Stoller, N., and Harvey, C. E. (1982). A survey of oral and dental diseases in dogs anesthetized at a veterinary hospital. *J. Am. Hosp. Assoc.* 18: 891–899.

4 Sorensen, W. P., Löe, H., and Ramfjord, S. P. (1980). Periodontal disease in the beagle dog. A cross sectional clinical study. *J. Periodontal. Res.* 15: 380–389.

5 Harvey, C. E., Shofer, F. S., and Laster, L. (1994). Association of age and body weight with periodontal disease in North American dogs. *J. Vet. Dent.* 11: 94–105. Erratum in: *J. Vet. Dent.* 1994; 11: 133.
6 Harvey, C. E. (1998). Periodontal disease in dogs. Etiopathogenesis, prevalence, and significance. *Vet. Clin. North Am. Small Anim. Pract.* 28: 1165–1188.
7 Hoffmann, T. and Gaengler, P. (1996). Clinical and patholomorphological investigation of spontaneously occurring periodontal disease in dogs. *J. Small Anim. Pract.* 37: 471–479.
8 Page, R. C. and Schroeder, H. E. (1981). Spontaneous chronic periodontitis in adult dogs. *J. Periodontol.* 52: 60–73.
9 Kortegaard, H. E., Eriksen, T., and Baelum, V. (2008). Periodontal disease in research beagle dogs – an epidemiological study. *J. Small Anim. Pract.* 49: 610–616.
10 Gad, T. (1968). Periodontal disease in dogs. *J. Periodontal. Res.* 3: 268–272.
11 Rosenberg, H. M., Rehfeld, C. E., and Emmering, T. E. (1966). A method for the epidemiologic assessment of periodontal health-disease state in a beagle hound colony. *J. Periodontol.* 37: 208–213.
12 Hull, P. S., Soames, J. V., and Davies, R. M. (1974). Periodontal disease in a beagle dog colony. *J. Comp. Pathol.* 84: 143–150.
13 Page, R. C. (1986). Gingivitis. *J. Clin. Periodontol.* 13 (5): 345–355.
14 Berglundh, T., Lindhe, J., and Sterrett, J. D. (1991). Clinical and structural characteristics of periodontal tissues in young and old dogs. *J. Clin. Periodontol.* 18: 616–623.
15 Kyllar, M. and Witter, K. (2008). Gingival thickness in dogs: association with age, gender, and dental arch location. *J. Vet. Dent.* 25: 106–109.
16 Kyllar, M., Doskarova, B., and Paral, V. (2013). Morphometric assessment of periodontal tissues in relation to periodontal disease in dogs. *J. Vet. Dent.* 30: 146–149.
17 Muller, H. P., Schaller, N., Eger, T. et al. (2000). Thickness of masticatory mucosa. *J. Clin. Periodontol.* 27: 431–436.
18 McHugh, W. D. (1971). The interdental gingivae. *J. Periodont. Res.* 6: 227–236.
19 Cho, M. I. and Garant, P. R. (2003). Development and general structure of the periodontium. *Periodontol. 2000* 31: 12–31.
20 Pöllänen, M. T., Salonen, J. I., and Uitto, V. J. (2000). Structure and function of the tooth-epithelial interface in health and disease. *Periodontol. 2000* (24): 9–27.
21 Kyllar, M., Witter, K., and Tichy, F. (2010). Gingival stippling in dogs: clinical and structural characteristics. *Res. Vet. Sci.* 88: 195–202.
22 Bartold, P. M. and Narayanan, A. S. (2006). Molecular and cellular biology of healthy and diseased periodontal tissues. *Periodontol. 2000* 40: 29–49.
23 Dale, B. A. (2002). Periodontol epithelium: a newly recognized role in health and disease. *Periodontol. 2000* 30: 70–78.
24 Diekwisch, T. G. (2001). The developmental biology of the cementum. *Int. J. Dev. Biol.* 45: 695–706.
25 Matsuo, M. and Takahashi, K. (2002). Scanning electron microscopic observations of microvasculature of the periodontium. *Microsc. Res. Tech.* 56: 3–14.
26 Beertsen, W., McCulloch, C. A., and Sodek, J. (1997). The periodontal ligament: a unique, multifunctional connective tissue. *Periodontol. 2000* 13: 20–40.
27 Zwarych, P. D. and Quigley, M. B. (1965). The intermediate plexus of the periodontal ligament: history and further observations. *J. Dent. Res.* 44: 383–391.
28 Bosshardt, D. D. (2005). Are cementoblasts a subpopulation of osteoblasts or a unique phenotype? *J. Dent. Res.* 84: 390–406.
29 Saffar, J. L. and Lasfargues JJ Cherruau, M. (1997). Alveolar bone and the alveolar process: the socket that is never stable. *Periodontol. 2000* 13: 76–90.
30 Sodek, J. and McKee, M. D. (2000). Molecular and cellular biology of alveolar bone. *Periodontol. 2000* 24: 99–126.
31 Saxe, S. R., Bohannon, H. M., Greene, J. et al. (1967). Oral debris, calculus, and periodontal disease in the beagle dog. *Periodontics* 5: 217–225.
32 Lindhe, J., Hamp, S. E., and Loe, H. (1973). Experimental periodontitis in the beagle dog. *J. Periodont. Res.* 3: 1–10.
33 Harvey, C. E., Thornsberry, C., and Miller, B. R. (1995). Subgingival bacteria--comparison of culture results in dogs and cats with gingivitis. *J. Vet. Dent.* 12: 147–150.
34 Harvey, C. E. (2005). Management of periodontal disease: understanding the options. *Vet. Clin. Small Anim.* 31: 819–836.
35 Lindhe, J., Hamp, S. E., and Loe, H. (1975). Plaque induced periodontal disease in beagle dogs: a four-year study. *J. Periodontol. Res.* 10: 243–255.
36 Egelbery, J. (1965). Local effect of diet on plaque formation and development of gingivitis in dogs, III: effect of frequency of meals and tube feeding. *Odont. Revy.* 16: 50–60.
37 DuPont, G. A. (1997). Understanding dental plaque; biofilm dynamics. *J. Vet. Dent.* 14: 91–94.
38 DuPont, G. A. (1998). Prevention of periodontal disease. *Vet. Clin. Small. Anim.* 28: 1129–1145.
39 Pöllänen, M. T., Paino, A., and Ihalin, R. (2013). Environmental stimuli shape biofilm formation and the virulence of periodontal pathogens. *Int. J. Mol. Sci.* 14: 17221–17237.

40 ten Cate, J. M. and Zaura, E. (2012). The numerous microbial species in oral biofilms: how could antibacterial therapy be effective? *Adv. Dent. Res.* 24: 108–111.
41 Marsh, P. D. (2010). Controlling the oral biofilm with antimicrobials. *J. Dent.* 38: S11–S15.
42 Swanson, E. A., Freeman, L. J., Seleem, M. N. et al. (2014). Biofilm-infected wounds in a dog. *J. Am. Vet. Med. Assoc.* 244: 699–707.
43 Teles, R., Teles, F., Frias-Lopez, J. et al. (2103). Lessons learned and unlearned in periodontal microbiology. *Periodontol. 2000* (62): 95–162.
44 Harvey, C. E. (1998). Periodontal disease in dogs: etiopathogenesis, prevalence, and significance. *Vet. Clin. Small Anim.* 28: 1111–1128.
45 Boyce, E. N., Ching, R. J. W., Logan, E. I. et al. (1995). Occurrence of gram-negative black-pigmented anaerobes in subgingival plaque during the development of canine periodontal disease. *Clin. Infect. Dis.* 20: S317–S319.
46 Hardham, J., Dreier, K., Wong, J. et al. (2005). Pigmented-anaerobic bacteria associated with canine periodontitis. *Vet. Microbiol.* 106: 119–128.
47 Dahlén, G., Charalampakis, G., Abrahamsson, I. et al. (2012). Predominant bacterial species in subgingival plaque in dogs. *J. Periodont. Res.* 47: 354–364.
48 Nordhoff, M., Rühe, B., Kellermeier, C. et al. (2008). Association of *Treponema spp.* with canine periodontitis. *Vet. Microbiol.* 127: 334–342.
49 Riggio, M. P., Lennon, A., Taylor, D. J. et al. (2011). Molecular identification of bacteria associated with canine periodontal disease. *Vet. Microbiol.* 150: 394–400.
50 Rober, M., Quirynen, M., Haffajee, A. D. et al. (2008). Intra-oral microbial profiles of beagle dogs assessed by checkerboard DNA-DNA hybridization using human probes. *Vet. Microbiol.* 127: 79–88.
51 Di Bello, A., Buonavoglia, A., Franchini, D. et al. (2014). Periodontal disease associated with red complex bacteria in dogs. *J. Small Anim. Pract.* 55: 160–163.
52 Pérez-Salcedo, L., Herrera, D., Esteban-Saltiveri, D. et al. (2013). Isolation and identification of *Porphyromonas spp.* and other putative pathogens from cats with periodontal disease. *J. Vet. Dent.* 30: 208–213.
53 Valdez, M., Haines, R., Riviere, K. H. et al. (2000). Isolation of oral spirochetes from dogs and cats and provisional identification using polymerase chain reaction (PCR) analysis specific for human plaque *Treponema* spp. *J. Vet. Dent.* 17: 23–26.
54 Riviere, G. R., Thompson, A. J., Brannan, R. D. et al. (1996). Detection of pathogen-related oral spirochetes, *Treponema denticola*, and *Treponema socranskii* in dental plaque from dogs. *J. Vet. Dent.* 13: 135–138.
55 Hennet, P. R. and Harvey, C. E. (1991). Spirochetes in periodontal disease in the dog: a review. *J. Vet. Dent.* 8: 16–17.
56 Hennet, P. R. and Harvey, C. E. (1991). Anaerobes in periodontal disease in the dog: a review. *J. Vet. Dent.* 8: 18–21.
57 Hennet, P. R. and Harvey, C. E. (1991). Aerobes in periodontal disease in the dog: a review. *J. Vet. Dent.* 8: 9–11.
58 Preshaw, P. M. and Taylor, J. J. (2011). How has research in cytokine interactions and their role in driving the immune responses impacted our understanding of periodontitis? *J. Clin. Periodontol.* 38: 60–84.
59 Bartold, P. M. and Van Dyke, T. E. (2013). Periodontitis: a host-mediated disruption of microbial homeostasis. Unlearning learned concepts. *Periodontol. 2000* (62): 203–217.
60 Berglundh, T. and Lindhe, J. (1993). Gingivitis in young and old dogs. *J. Clin. Periodontol.* 20: 179–185.
61 Roudebush, P., Logan, E., and Hale, F. A. (2005). Evidence-based veterinary dentistry: a systematic review of homecare for prevention of periodontal disease in dogs and cats. *J. Vet. Dent.* 22: 6–15.
62 Hale, F. A. (2003). The owner-animal-environment triad in the treatment of canine periodontal disease. *J. Vet. Dent.* 20: 118–122.
63 Hale, F. A. (2003). Home care for the veterinary dental patient. *J. Vet. Dent.* 20: 52–54.
64 JM, G. C. and Markwell, P. J. (1998). Effect on canine oral health of adding chlorhexidine to a dental hygiene chew. *J. Vet. Dent.* 15: 129–134.
65 Tromp, J. A. H., Jansen, J., and Pilot, T. (1986). Gingival health and frequency of tooth brushing in the beagle dog model. *J. Clin. Periodontol.* 13: 164–168.
66 Tromp, J. A. H., van Rijn, L. J., and Jansen, J. (1986). Experimental gingivitis and frequency of tooth brushing in the beagle dog. *J. Clin. Periodontol.* 13: 190–194.
67 Gorrel, C. and Rawlings, J. M. (1996). The role of tooth-brushing and diet in the maintenance of periodontal health in dogs. *J. Vet. Dent.* 13: 139–143.
68 Tepe, J. H., Leonard, G. J., Singer, R. E. et al. (1983). The long-term effect of chlorhexidine on the plaque, gingivitis, sulcus depth, gingival recession, and loss of attachment in beagle dogs. *J. Periodontal. Res.* 18: 452–458.
69 Briner, W. W., Gibberman, B. P., Leonard, G. J. et al. (1980). Effects of chlorhexidine on plaque, gingivitis and alveolar bone loss in beagle dogs after seven years of treatment. *J. Periodontal. Res.* 15: 390–394.
70 Robinson, J. G. (1995). Chlorhexidine gluconate--the solution for dental problems. *J. Vet. Dent.* 12: 29–31.
71 Harvey, C. E., Shofer, F. S., and Laster, L. (1996). Correlation of diet, other chewing activities and periodontal disease in North American client-owned dogs. *J. Vet. Dent.* 13: 101–105.

72 Gorrel, C., Inskeep, G., and Inskeep, T. (1998). Benefits of a 'dental hygiene chew' on the periodontal health of cats. *J. Vet. Dent.* 15: 135–138.

73 Quest, B. W. (2013). Oral health benefits of a daily dental chew in dogs. *J. Vet. Dent.* 30: 84–87.

74 Clarke, D. E., Kelman, M., and Perkins, N. (2011). Effectiveness of a vegetable dental chew on periodontal disease parameters in toy breed dogs. *J. Vet. Dent.* 28: 230–235.

75 Stookey, G. K. (2009). Soft rawhide reduces calculus formation in dogs. *J. Vet. Dent.* 26: 82–85.

76 Hennet, P., Servet, E., and Venet, C. (2006). Effectiveness of an oral hygiene chew to reduce dental deposits in small breed dogs. *J. Vet. Dent.* 23: 6–12.

77 Brown, W. Y. and McGenity, P. (2005). Effective periodontal disease control using dental hygiene chews. *J. Vet. Dent.* 22: 16–19.

78 Ingham, K. E., Gorrel, C., and Bierer, T. L. (2002). Effect of a dental chew on dental substrates and gingivitis in cats. *J. Vet. Dent.* 19: 201–204. Erratum in: *J. Vet. Dent.* 2003; 20: 136.

79 Logan, E. I., Finney, O., and Hefferren, J. J. (2002). Effects of a dental food on plaque accumulation and gingival health in dogs. *J. Vet. Dent.* 19: 15–18.

80 Gorrel, C. and Bierer, T. L. (1999). Long-term effects of a dental hygiene chew on the periodontal health of dogs. *J. Vet. Dent.* 16: 109–113.

81 Hennet, P. (2001). Effectiveness of an enzymatic rawhide dental chew to reduce plaque in beagle dogs. *J. Vet. Dent.* 18: 61–64.

82 Clarke, D. E. (2006). Drinking water additive decreases plaque and calculus accumulation in cats. *J. Vet. Dent.* 23: 79–82.

83 Smith, M. M. and Smithson, C. W. (2014). Dental wax decreases calculus accumulation in small dogs. *J. Vet. Dent.* 31: 26–29.

84 Bellows, J., Carithers, D. S., and Gross, S. J. (2012). Efficacy of a barrier gel for reducing the development of plaque, calculus, and gingivitis in cats. *J. Vet. Dent* 29: 89–94. Erratum in: *J. Vet. Dent.* 2012; 29: 196.

85 Sitzman, C. (2013). Evaluation of a hydrophilic gingival dental sealant in beagle dogs. *J. Vet. Dent.* 30: 150–155.

86 Gengler, W. R., Kunkle, B. N., Romano, D. et al. (2005). Evaluation of a barrier dental sealant in dogs. *J. Vet. Dent.* 22: 157–159.

87 Hennet, P. (2002). Effectiveness of a dental gel to reduce plaque in beagle dogs. *J. Vet. Dent.* 19: 11–14.

88 Clarke, D. E. (2001). Clinical and microbiological effects of oral zinc ascorbate gel in cats. *J. Vet. Dent.* 18: 177–183.

89 Watson, A. D. J. (1994). Diet and periodontal disease in dogs and cats. *Aust. Vet. J.* 71: 313–318.

90 Niemiec, B. A. (2005). Fundamentals of Endodontics. *Vet. Clin. North Am. Small Anim. Pract.* 35: 837–868.

91 United States Food and Drug Administration. (2014). No bones about it: bones are unsafe for your dog. http://www.fda.gov/downloads/ForConsumers/ConsumerUpdates/UCM209196.pdf. accessed 12 June 2014.

92 Logan, E. I. (2006). Dietary influences on periodontal health in dogs and cats. *Vet. Clin. North Am. Small Anim. Pract.* 36: 1385–1401.

93 Eubanks, D. L. and Woodruff, K. A. (2010). The basics of saliva. *J. Vet. Dent.* 27: 266–267.

94 Okuda, A., Inouc, E., and Asari, M. (1996). The membranous bulge lingual to the mandibular molar tooth of a cat contains a small salivary gland. *J. Vet. Dent.* 13: 61–64.

95 Marretta, S. M. (1992). Chronic rhinitis and dental disease. *Vet. Clin. North Am. Small Anim. Pract.* 22: 1101–1117.

96 Stepaniuk, K. S. and Gingerich, W. (2015). Suspected odontogenic infection etiology for canine lymphoplasmacytic rhinitis. *J. Vet. Dent.* 32 (1): 22–29.

97 Ramsey, D. T., Marretta, S. M., Hamor, R. E. et al. (1996). Ophthalmic manifestations and complications of dental disease in dogs and cats. *J. Am. Anim. Hosp. Assoc.* 32: 215–224.

98 Paiva, S. C., Froes, T. R., Lange, R. R. et al. (2013). Iatrogenic nasolacrimal duct obstruction following tooth extraction in a cat. *J. Vet. Dent.* 30: 90–94.

99 Negro, V. B. and Hernandez, S. Z. (2003). Odontogenic periorbital fistula in a cat. *J. Vet. Dent.* 20: 31–33.

100 Anthony, J. M. G., Sandmeyer, L. S., and Laycock, A. R. (2010). Nasolacrimal obstruction caused by root abscess of the upper canine in a cat. *Vet. Ophthalmol.* 13: 106–109.

101 Losonsky, J. M., Abbott, L. C., and Kuriashkin, I. V. (1997). Computed tomography of the normal feline nasal cavity and paranasal sinuses. *Vet. Radiol. Ultrasound.* 38: 251–258.

102 Noller, C., Henninger, W., Grönemeyer, D. H. et al. (2006). Computed tomography-anatomy of the normal feline nasolacrimal drainage system. *Vet. Radiol. Ultrasound.* 47: 53–60.

103 Schlueter, C., Budras, K. D., Ludewig, E. et al. (2009). Brachycephalic feline noses: CT and anatomical study of the relationship between head conformation and the nasolacrimal drainage system. *J. Feline Med. Surg.* 11: 891–900.

104 George, T. F. and Smallwood, J. E. (1992). Anatomic atlas for computed tomography in the mesaticephalic dog: head and neck. *Vet. Radiol. Ultrasound.* 33: 217–240.

105 Burk, R. L. (1992). Computed tomographic anatomy of the canine nasal passages. *Vet. Radiol. Ultrasound.* 33: 170–176.

106 Gioso, M. A., Shofer, F., Barros, P. S. et al. (2001). Mandible and mandibular first molar tooth measurements in dogs: relationship of radiographic height to body weight. *J. Vet. Dent.* 18: 65–68.
107 Hale, F. A. (2002). Management of bilateral, pathologic, mandibular fractures in a dog. *J. Vet. Dent.* 19: 22–24.
108 Khocht, A. and Albandar, J. M. (2014). Aggressive forms of periodontitis secondary to systemic disorders. *Periodontol. 2000* 65: 134–148.
109 Lindhe, J., Hamp, S. E., and Löe, H. (1973). Experimental periodontitis in the beagle dog. *J. Periodontol. Res.* 8: 1–10.
110 Albuquerque, C., Morinha, F., Requicha, J. et al. (2012). Canine periodontitis: the dog as an important model for periodontal studies. *Vet. J.* 191: 299–305.
111 Cave, N. J., Bridges, J. P., and Thomas, D. G. (2012). Systemic effects of periodontal disease in cats. *Vet. Q.* 32: 131–144.
112 Sykes, J. E., Kittleson, M. D., Pesavento, P. A. et al. (2006). Evaluation of the relationship between causative organisms and clinical characteristics of infective endocarditis in dogs: 71 cases (1992–2005). *J. Am. Vet. Med. Assoc.* 228: 1723–1734.
113 Tou, S. P., Adin, D. B., Castleman, W. L. et al. (2005). Mitral valve endocarditis after dental prophylaxis in a dog. *J. Vet. Intern. Med.* 19: 268–270.
114 Peddle, G. D., Drobatz, K. J., Harvey, C. E. et al. (2009). Association of periodontal disease, oral procedures, and other clinical findings with bacterial endocarditis in dogs. *J. Am. Vet. Med. Assoc.* 234: 100–107.
115 Glickman, L. T., Glickman, N. W., Moore, G. E. et al. (2009). Evaluation of the risk of endocarditis and other cardiovascular events on the basis of the severity of periodontal disease in dogs. *J. Am. Vet. Med. Assoc.* 234: 486–494.
116 DeBowes, L. J. (1998). The effects of dental disease on systemic disease. *Vet. Clin. North Am. Small Anim. Pract.* 28: 1057–1062.
117 DeBowes, L. J., Mosier, D., Logan, E. et al. (1996). Association of periodontal disease and histological lesions in multiple organs from 45 dogs. *J. Vet. Dent.* 13: 57–60.
118 Pavlica, Z., Petelin, M., Juntes, P. et al. (2008). Periodontal disease burden and pathological changes in organs of dogs. *J. Vet. Dent* 25: 97–105.
119 Rawlings, J. E., Goldstein, R. E., Reiter, A. M. et al. (2011). Association of periodontal disease with systemic health indices in dogs and the systemic response to treatment of periodontal disease. *J. Am. Vet. Med. Assoc.* 238: 601–609.
120 Glickman, L. T., Glickman, N. W., Moore, G. E. et al. (2011). Association between chronic azotemic kidney disease and the severity of periodontal disease in dogs. *Prev. Vet. Med.* 99: 103–200.
121 Kouki, M. I., Papadimitriou, S. A., Kazakos, G. M. et al. (2013). Periodontal disease as a potential factor for systemic inflammatory response in the dog. *J. Vet. Dent.* 30: 26–29.
122 Simone, A., Jensen, L., Setser, C. et al. (1994). Assessment of oral malodor in dogs. *J. Vet. Dent.* 11: 71–74.
123 Eubanks, D. L. (2009). "Doggy breath": what causes it, how do I evaluate it, and what can I do about it? *J. Vet. Dent.* 26: 192–193.
124 Culham, N. and Rawlings, J. M. (1998). Oral malodor and its relevance to periodontal disease in the dog. *J. Vet. Dent.* 15: 165–168.
125 Rawlings, J. M. and Culham, N. (1998). Studies of oral malodor in the dog. *J. Vet. Dent.* 15: 169–173.
126 Clarke, D. E. (1999). The crystalline components of dental calculus in the domestic cat. *J. Vet. Dent.* 16: 165–168.
127 Holmstrom, S. E., Bellows, J., and Juriga, S. (2013). 2013 AAHA Dental Care Guidelines for Dogs and Cats. *J. Am. Anim. Hosp. Assoc.* 49: 75–82.
128 Vogt, A. H., Rodan, I., Brown, M. et al. (2010). AAFP-AAHA Feline Life Stage Guidelines. *J. Feline Med. Surg.* 12: 43–54.
129 Bartges, J., Boynton, B., Vogt, A. et al. (2012). AAHA Canine Life Stage Guidelines. *J. Am. Hosp. Assoc.* 48: 1–11.
130 Verstraete, F. J., Kass, P. H., and Terpak, C. H. (1998). Diagnostic value of full-mouth radiography in cats. *Am. J. Vet. Res.* 59: 692–695.
131 Verstraete, F. J., Kass, P. H., and Terpak, C. H. (1998). Diagnostic value of full-mouth radiography in dogs. *Am. J. Vet. Res.* 59: 686–691.
132 Tsugawa, A. J., Verstraete, F. J. et al. (2003). Diagnostic value of the use of lateral and occlusal radiographic views in comparison with periodontal probing for the assessment of periodontal attachment of the canine teeth in dogs. *Am. J. Vet. Res.* 6: 255–261.
133 Lommer, M. J. and Verstraete, F. J. (2001). Radiographic patterns of periodontitis in cats: 147 cases (1998–1999). *J. Am. Vet. Med. Assoc.* 218: 230–234.
134 American Veterinary Dental College. (2014). AVDC Position Statements. http://www.avdc.org/statements.html. accessed 12 June 2014.
135 American Veterinary Dental College. (2014). Nomenclature. http://www.avdc.org/nomenclature.html#top. accessed 15 May 2014.
136 Loe, H. and Silness, J. (1963). Periodontal disease in pregnancy. I. Prevalence and severity. *Acta. Odont. Scand.* 21: 533–551.

137 Herr, Y., Matsuura, M., Lin, W. et al. (1995). The origin of fibroblasts and their role in the early stages of horizontal furcation defect healing in the beagle dog. *J. Periodontol.* 66: 716–730.
138 Klinge, B., Nilveus, R., and Egelberg, J. (1985). Bone regeneration pattern and ankylosis in experimental furcation defects in dogs. *J. Clin. Periodontol.* 12: 456–464.
139 Greenstein, G. and Polson, A. (1988). Understanding tooth mobility. *Compendium* 9: 473–479.
140 Svanberg, G. (1974). Influence of trauma from occlusion on the periodontium of dogs with normal or inflamed gingivae. *Odontol. Revy.* 25: 165–178.
141 Nyman, S., Linde, J., and Ericcson, I. (1978). The effect of progressive tooth mobility on destructive periodontitis in the dog. *J. Clin. Periodontol.* 5: 213–225.
142 Rawlinson, J. E. and Reiter, A. M. (2005). Repair of a gingival cleft associated with a maxillary canine tooth in a dog. *J. Vet. Dent.* 22: 234–242.
143 Gingerich, W. and Stepaniuk, K. (2011). Guided tissue regeneration for infrabony pocket treatment in dogs. *J. Vet. Dent.* 28: 282–288. Erratum in: *J. Vet. Dent.* 2012; 29: 9.
144 Greenfield, B. A. (2010). Open root planing for a periodontal pocket of a maxillary canine tooth. *J. Vet. Dent.* 27: 34–39.
145 Lindhe, J., Attstrom, R., and Bjorn, A. L. (1968). Influence of sex hormones on gingival exudate in dogs with chronic gingivitis. *J. Periodontol. Res.* 3: 279–283.
146 Lewis, J. R. and Reiter, A. M. (2005). Management of gingival enlargement in the dog – case report and literature review. *J. Vet. Dent.* 22: 160–169.
147 DeHaven, W. (2014). Are we really doing enough to provide the best veterinary care for our pets? *J. Am. Vet. Med. Assoc.* 244: 1017–1018.
148 Kim, C. G., Lee, S. Y., Kim, J. W. et al. (2013). Assessment of dental abnormalities by full-mouth radiography in small breed dogs. *J. Am. Hosp. Assoc.* 49: 23–90.
149 Albandar, J. M. (2014). Aggressive periodontitis: case definition and diagnostic criteria. *Periodontol. 2000* 65: 13–26.
150 Albander, J. M. (2014). Aggressive and acute periodontal diseases. *Periodontol. 2000* 65: 7–12.
151 Mikx, F. H. and van Campen, G. J. (1982). Microscopical evaluation of the microflora in relation to necrotizing ulcerative gingivitis in the beagle dog. *J. Periodontal. Res.* 17: 576–584.
152 Könönen, E. and Müller, H. P. (2014). Microbiology of aggressive periodontitis. *Periodontol. 2000* 65: 46–78.
153 Susin, C., Haas, A. N., and Albandar, J. M. (2014). Epidemiology and demographics of aggressive periodontitis. *Periodontol. 2000* 65: 27–45.
154 Kulkarni, C. and Kinane, D. F. (2014). Host response in aggressive periodontitis. *Periodontol. 2000* 65: 79–91.
155 Lommer, M. J. (2013). Oral inflammation in small animals. *Vet. Clin. North Am. Small Anim. Pract.* 43: 555–571.
156 Nemec, A., Pavlica, Z., Stiblar-Martincic, D. et al. (2007). Histological evaluation of the pulp in teeth from dogs with naturally occurring periodontal disease. *J. Vet. Dent.* 24: 212–223.
157 Lindhe, J., Hamp, S. E., and Löe, H. (1975). Plaque induced periodontal disease in beagle dogs. A 4-year clinical, roentgenographical and histometrical sudy. *J. Periodontal. Res.* 10: 243–255.
158 Nieves, M. A., Hartwig, P., Kinyon, J. M. et al. (1997). Bacterial isolates from plaque and from blood during and after routine dental procedures in dog. *Vet. Surg.* 26: 26–32.
159 Harari, J., Besser, T. E., Gustafson, S. B. et al. (1993). Bacterial isolates from blood cultures of dogs undergoing dentistry. *Vet. Surg.* 22: 27–30.
160 Bowersock, T. L., Wu, C. C., Inskeep, G. A. et al. (2000). Prevention of bacteremia in dogs undergoing dental scaling by prior administration of oral clindamycin or chlorhexidine oral rinse. *J. Vet. Dent.* 17: 11–16.
161 Vérez-Fraguela, J. L., Vives Vallés, M. A., and Ezquerra Calvo, L. J. (2000). Effects of ultrasonic dental scaling on pulp vitality in dogs: an experimental study. *J. Vet. Dent.* 17: 75–79.
162 Fichtel, T., Crha, M., Langerová, E. et al. (2008). Observations on the effects of scaling and polishing methods on enamel. *J. Vet. Dent.* 25: 231–235.
163 Brine, E. J., Marretta, S. M., Pijanowski, G. J. et al. (2000). Comparison of the effects of four different power scalers on enamel tooth surface in the dog. *J. Vet. Dent.* 17: 17–21.
164 Yonkers, T. D. (2000). Ultrasonic debridement and proper home care. *J. Vet. Dent.* 17: 96–97.
165 Angel, M. (2014). Sharpening periodontal instruments. *J. Vet. Dent.* 31: 58–64.
166 Aller, S. M. (2005). Personal safety and ergonomics in the dental operatory. *J. Vet. Dent.* 22: 124–130.
167 Dennis, M., Wilson, T., and Woodward, T. (2012). Retention of antimicrobial activity after reconstitution of doxycycline gel. *J. Vet. Dent.* 29: 84–87.
168 Polson, A. M., Southard, G. L., Dunn, R. L. et al. (1996). Periodontal pocket treatment in beagle dogs using subgingival doxycycline from a biodegradable system. Initial clinical responses. *J. Periodontol.* 67: 1176–1184.
169 Johnston, T. P., Mondal, P., Pal, D. et al. (2011). Canine periodontal disease control using a clindamycin hydrochloride gel. *J. Vet. Dent.* 28: 224–229.

170 Veterinary Oral Health Council. http://www.vohc.org/all_accepted_products.html. accessed 13 June 2014.

171 Stepaniuk, K. and Brock, N. (2008). Hypothermia and thermoregulation during anesthesia for the dental and oral surgery patient. *J. Vet. Dent.* 25: 279–283. Erratum in: *J. Vet. Dent.* 2009; 26: 8.

172 Stepaniuk, K. and Brock, N. (2008). Anesthesia monitoring in the dental and oral surgery patient. *J. Vet. Dent.* 25: 143–499.

173 Dunayer, E. K. and Gwaltney-Brant, S. M. (2006). Acute hepatic failure and coagulopathy associated with xylitol ingestion in eight dogs. *J. Am. Vet. Med. Assoc.* 229: 1113–1117.

174 Gunn, A. R. and Bánóczy, J. (2013). Fluoride toothpastes and fluoride mouthrinses for home use. *Acta Medica. Academia.* 42: 168–178.

175 Hale, F. A. (1998). Dental caries in the dog. *J. Vet. Dent.* 15: 79–83.

176 Bartold, P. M., du Bois, A. H., Gannon, S. et al. (2013). Antibacterial and immunomodulatory properties of azithromycin treatment implications for periodontitis. *Inflammopharmacology* 21: 321–338.

177 Rosenberg, A., Rosenkrantz, W., Griffin, C. et al. (2013). Evaluation of azithromycin in systemic and toothpaste forms for the treatment of ciclosporin-associated gingival overgrowth in dogs. *Vet. Dermatol.* 24: 337–345.

178 Ramalho, V. L. C. and Ramalho, H. J. (2007). Comparison of azithromycin and oral hygiene program in treatment of cyclosporine-induced gingival hyperplasia. *Ren. Fail.* 29: 265–270.

179 Kim, S. E., Kim, S., Jeong, M. et al. (2013). Experimental determination of a subantimicrobial dosage of doxycycline hyclate for treatment of periodontitis in beagles. *Am. J. Vet. Res.* 74: 130–135.

180 Radice, M., Martino, P. A., and Reiter, A. M. (2006). Evaluation of subgingival bacteria in the dog and susceptibility to commonly used antibiotics. *J. Vet. Dent.* 23: 219–224.

181 Harvey, C. E., Thornsberry, C., Miller, B. R. et al. (1995). Antimicrobial susceptibility of subgingival bacterial flora in cats with gingivitis. *J. Vet. Dent.* 12: 157–160.

182 Harvey, C. E., Thornsberry, C., Miller, B. R. et al. (1995). Antimicrobial susceptibility of subgingival bacterial flora in dogs with gingivitis. *J. Vet. Dent.* 12: 151–155.

183 Zetner, K. and Thiemann, G. (1993). The antimicrobial effectiveness of clindamycin in diseases of the oral cavity. *J. Vet. Dent.* 10: 6–9.

6

Traumatic Dentoalveolar Injuries

Jason Soukup

School of Veterinary Medicine, University of Wisconsin-Madison, Madison, WI, USA

6.1 Introduction

Traumatic dentoalveolar injuries (TDI) are a collection of specific injuries to the tooth (crown/root) and/or the tooth supporting structures (periodontal ligament (PDL)/alveolar bone) sustained as a result of a traumatic force. TDI affect one in four patients [1, 2], making it one of the most prevalent oral diseases in animals, second only to periodontal disease in dogs. In addition, patients that are affected by TDI typically have more than one injury at the time of diagnosis [1, 3]. The consequences of traumatized teeth contribute substantially to a negative quality of life and may include periodontal pain and infection, endodontic pain and infection, osteomyelitis, systemic dissemination of inflammatory mediators and chronic bacteremia, which may contribute to systemic disease [4–6]. In addition, the perceived functional and cosmetic value of the canine and feline dentition from the pet owner's point of view is higher today than ever. Considered in this light, TDI should be seen as a serious health threat to dogs and cats and, as such, justifies in-depth study.

6.2 Classification

There are several systems that have been utilized to classify TDI [7–10]. However, in veterinary dentistry, two systems seem to have the most value and are worth discussing here. The American Veterinary Dental College (AVDC) has adopted a classification of dental crown fractures, which includes enamel infraction (T/FX/EI), enamel fracture (T/FX/EF), uncomplicated crown fracture (T/FX/UCF), complicated crown fracture (T/FX/CCF), and crown-root fracture, of which the pulp may (complicated – T/FX/CCRF) or may not (uncomplicated – T/FX/UCCRF) be involved [11] (Table 6.1 includes other nomenclature abbreviations). However, this system fails to account for root fractures and luxation injuries (concussion, subluxation, luxation, and avulsion). In a recent study, these injuries were found to be quite prevalent and, thus, should be included in any useful classification system [1]. The use of a more inclusive classification system, which includes dental fractures (enamel infraction, enamel fracture, enamel-dentin fracture, enamel-dentin-pulp fracture, crown-root fracture (with or without pulpal involvement), root fracture); luxation injuries (concussion, subluxation, luxation (lateral, intrusive, and extrusive), avulsion) and a special category of alveolar fracture has been successfully used in both human and veterinary dental traumatology studies and is recommended by this author [12] (Table 6.2) [13].

6.3 Epidemiology

6.3.1 Prevalence

Historically, the epidemiology of TDI has been poorly studied. As a result, very little data on the prevalence of TDI in dogs and cats are available. Only a few studies have fully investigated the topic [1, 3]. Most available studies have focused solely on dental fractures and have generally ignored luxation injuries [2, 14]. In addition, the few available studies have not utilized a standardized classification system. As a result the reported prevalence of TDI varies considerably. The prevalence of dental fractures in dogs has been reported between 2.6% and 27% [2, 14]. The prevalence of TDI in dogs and cats with concurrent maxillofacial fractures increases dramatically to just over 70% [3, 15]. A recent study in the United States has shown a high prevalence of TDI in dogs and cats that is consistent with the prevalence of human TDI. In the study, 26.2% of dogs and cats had at least one TDI with a mean of 1.45 TDI per patient [1]. The worldwide

Wiggs's Veterinary Dentistry: Principles and Practice, Second Edition. Edited by Heidi B. Lobprise and Johnathon R. (Bert) Dodd.

Table 6.1 AVDC nomenclature abbreviations.

AB		Abrasion
AT		Attrition
CT		Computed tomography
	CT/CB	Cone-beam CT
	FX/R/IDS	Interdental splinting (between teeth within a dental arch)
T		Tooth
	T/A	Avulsed tooth
	T/FX	Fractured tooth (see next seven listings for fracture types)
	T/FX/EI	Enamel infraction
	T/FX/EF	Enamel fracture
	T/FX/UCF	Uncomplicated crown fracture
	T/FX/CCF	Complicated crown fracture
	T/FX/UCRF	Uncomplicated crown-root facture
	T/FX/CCRF	Complicated crown-root fracture
	T/FX/RF	Root fracture
	T/NE	Near pulp exposure
	T/NV	Non-vital tooth
	T/PE	Pulp exposure
	T/RI	Tooth reimplantation (for an avulsed tooth)
	T/RP	Tooth repositioning (for a luxated tooth)

prevalence may vary due to socioeconomic, behavioral, and cultural diversity. Several injuries (e.g., concussion, subluxation, root fracture) are likely to go undiagnosed due to lack of acceptable diagnostic ability and/or skill, which varies between veterinarians and veterinary practices.

6.3.2 Distribution by Sex, Age, and Breed

Within the general population, there appears to be no obvious sex predilection as males and females have a similar frequency of TDI [1]. However, when TDI associated with concurrent maxillofacial fractures is considered, young male animals are overrepresented, which may be related to the stereotypical young male behaviors [3, 16]. Although juveniles tend to have more TDI associated with maxillofacial fractures, within the general population TDI prevalence tends to increase throughout adolescence and peaks between three and six years of age [1] (Figure 6.1). After six years of age, the prevalence tends to drop off [1]. This may be explained either by the more docile nature of older animals; by an increase in dentin thickness from continued dentinogenesis, which makes the tooth more fracture resistant; or by a combination of both (and possibly other) factors. No obvious breed predilection has been reported. However, in one study, German Shepherd Dogs were the second most common breed affected with TDI [1].

Table 6.2 Classification system of traumatic dentoalveolar injuries recommended by this author.

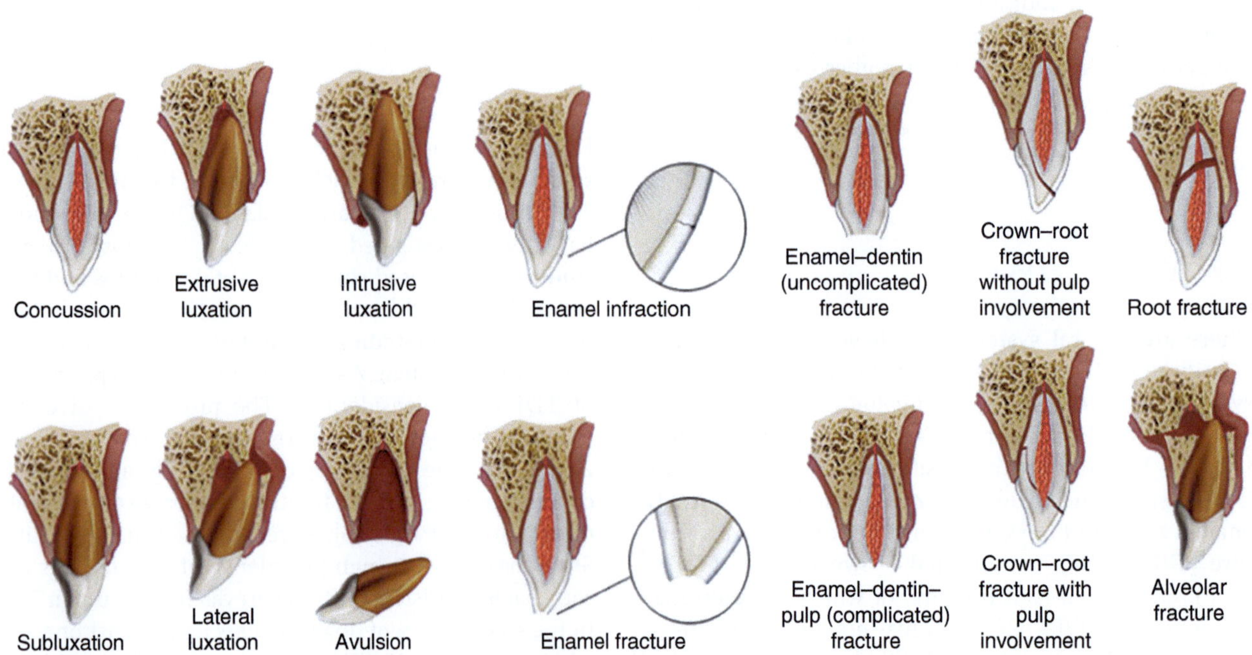

Source: Modified and reprinted with permission from reference [13].

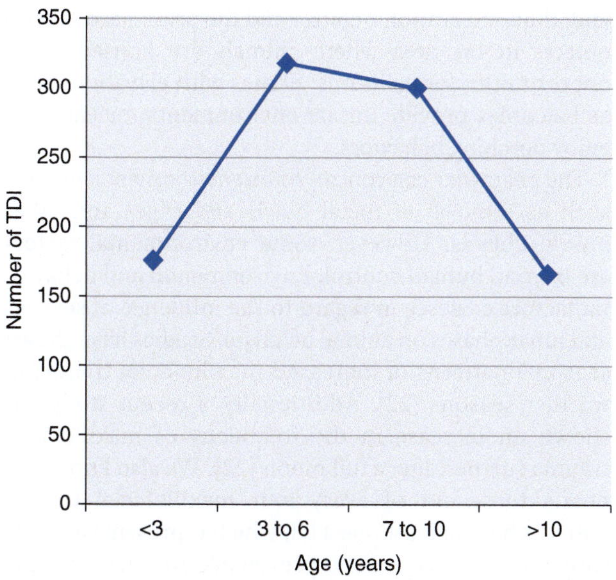

Figure 6.1 Association between age and frequency of TDI. *Source:* Reprinted with permission from reference [1].

6.3.3 Teeth Involved

Studies have shown that the majority of TDI occur in the upper jaw and most affect the rostral oral cavity (incisors and canines) [1–3, 14]. The most commonly injured teeth are, in order of decreasing frequency, the canine teeth, the premolar teeth, the incisor teeth, and the molar teeth [1, 14]. Considering only luxation injuries, the teeth most commonly affected are the canine and incisor teeth and are most often concussion injuries [1, 3]. Of the fracture injuries the premolar teeth have the highest frequency followed by the canine teeth, incisor teeth, and, lastly, molar teeth [1, 14]. The majority of TDI occur in strategic (canine and carnassial) teeth. Of the carnassial teeth injured, the vast majority of TDI are sustained by the maxillary fourth premolar teeth [1, 14]. Most injuries affect single teeth. However, luxation injuries and alveolar fractures often involve several sequential teeth.

Some distinct patterns of TDI are seen with specific mechanisms. A very good example of a typical TDI pattern is that seen in cats, which have sustained trauma associated with high-rise syndrome. In addition to typical soft tissue and maxillofacial fracture patterns, specific teeth are usually traumatized. The initial impact of the cat hitting the surface is to the ventral mandible. The energy is then distributed into the maxilla causing mandibular molar and maxillary fourth premolar fractures [15]. Additionally, after the chin makes contact, one or both maxillary canines will make contact with the substrate, leading to maxillary canine fractures [15]. These maxillary canine fractures are also seen in cats that have presumably jumped off elevations within the home and have hit the teeth on the ground. In addition, it has been shown that the direction from which the traumatic force comes has a significant influence on the fracture pattern of dog canine teeth [17]. This information may give the clinician and owner some clue as to possible mechanisms of injury.

6.3.4 Types of Injuries

TDI are broadly categorized as either dental fractures or luxation injuries. Dental fractures are the most common injury at 82.3% of all TDI [1]. Enamel-dentin-pulp fractures were reported to be the most common TDI in one study followed by concussion and enamel-dentin fractures [1]. However, enamel-dentin fractures may be much more common than reported as they often go undiagnosed and untreated. Luxation injuries are much less common than dental fractures. However, they may also be more prevalent than reported because many concussion and subluxation injuries ultimately go undiagnosed. Most of the luxation injuries reported in a recent study were concussion injuries [1]. Most (66.8%) TDI are considered severe injuries that result in significant consequences if not treated in a timely fashion [1, 3]. For the purposes of discussion in this chapter, we will group TDI into four major categories: crown fractures, crown-root fractures, root fractures, and luxation injuries.

6.4 Etiology

6.4.1 Mechanisms

TDI may be caused by any collision with sufficient force to overcome the natural resistance of the dentoalveolar apparatus, such as altercations with other animals, motor vehicle accidents, falls from height, contact with a moving object, or simply sustained during playful activity, collision with another animal or object, or even during chewing/mastication. However, as these injuries often occur during unsupervised activities, the mechanism of injury is often unknown [1–3, 14], which increases the challenge of conducting highly fruitful epidemiological studies. In one study, German Shepherd dogs were found to be the second most common breed affected by TDI [1]. The duties in which this breed and other similar military and working breeds are often engaged may be considered a predisposing mechanistic factor for TDI. Some teeth may be biomechanically compromised and more susceptible to fracture under normal oral loads. Many dogs, especially military and police dogs, sustain distal abrasion (AB) of the canine teeth (i.e., cage chewer syndrome) through oral parafunctional habits [18] (Figure 6.2). This particular abrasion pattern creates a stress concentration point that decreases the fracture resistance of the tooth [19, 20].

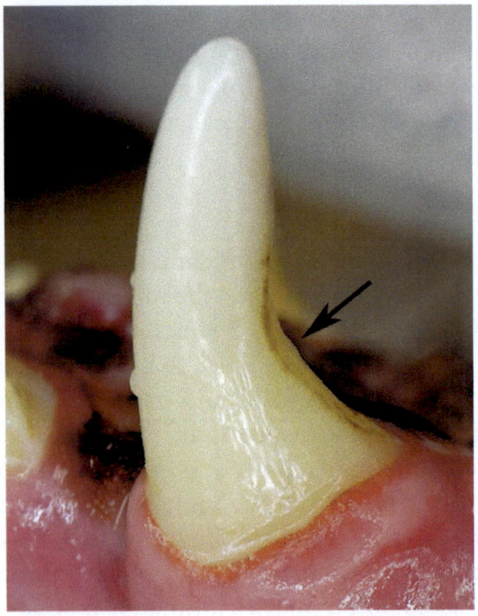

Figure 6.2 Abrasion on the distal surface of a canine tooth (black arrow) often seen in working dogs and secondary to parafunctional habits.

6.4.2 Behavior

Numerous studies have shown an association between age-related behavior and trauma [3, 16]. Young animals are known to be more exuberant, curious, and playful, which increases the likelihood of roaming, engagement in risky activities, and engagement in altercations with other animals, which in turn increases the risk of sustaining TDI.

Innate behavioral traits may also put certain animals at risk for acquiring TDI. For example, curiosity is a behavior innate to most cats. This curiosity often puts them into situations (e.g., perching and walking on elevations) where the risk of obtaining TDI is increased.

A probable causative factor in cage chewer syndrome discussed above is hyperactive behavior and anxiety disorders. In some working dogs, hyperactive behavior may be selected as a desirable trait that aids in their job performance. Hyperactivity is known to be an etiologic factor in the prevalence of TDI in children [21]. However, these behavioral traits alone do not cause the abrasion pattern that makes the teeth biomechanically weak. In the previously described scenario, the animal must have an abrasive object, such as a metal bowl or cage, to chew on in order for the behavior to manifest in dental abrasion, which brings us to a discussion of the animal's environment as an etiologic factor.

6.4.3 Environment

Often the animal's surrounding environment may contribute to the risk of acquiring TDI. Some examples of how the environment influences the risk of TDI include: multipet households may increase the level of competition and, thus, altercations; clutter and the presence of unsafe objects in the area where animals are housed invite opportunities for collisions; homes with elevations such as balconies provide unsafe environments for cats that enjoy perching behaviors.

The pet owner can control some environmental factors, such as removal of metal bowls and cages and other unsafe objects. However, some environmental factors are beyond human control. Environmental and behavioral factors coalesce in regard to the influence of seasons and lunar phases on animal behavior. Studies have shown seasonal patterns of increased maxillofacial trauma in warmer seasons [22]. Additionally, a recent study has shown an increase in the frequency of maxillofacial trauma surrounding a full moon [22]. We also know that nearly three out of every four maxillofacial trauma patients have at least one TDI, which represents a nearly threefold increase in the prevalence of TDI over the general population [3]. Therefore, any etiologic factor contributing to maxillofacial trauma should be considered to have a similar impact on TDI.

Likewise, environmental factors are important when considering "high-rise syndrome" in cats, which, concurrent with a typical pattern of maxillofacial fracture, presents with a typical TDI pattern [15]. Cats that are placed in a risky environment (e.g., access to elevated patio/balconies) are at an increased risk of elevated falls and are much more likely to sustain TDI than cats that do not have similar access to elevations.

6.5 Examination and Diagnosis of TDI

Today's pet owner appreciates the importance of maintaining the dentition when possible. The dog and cat dentition functions as a unit but each tooth also has a singular and important purpose. Within the confines of veterinary ethics, evidence-based medicine, and the priorities of our clients, veterinarians are ethically, morally, and legally bound to offer treatments to preserve these teeth. We are also similarly obliged to refer the patient for such treatments when a client requests or when we do not possess the necessary knowledge and skill to not only deliver the treatment but also to successfully negotiate any complications encountered. Therefore, any dental injury should be considered an emergency and should be treated as soon as possible in order to control pain and provide the best possible prognosis for tooth maintenance.

The focus of the remainder of this chapter is on the preservation of the dentition. Therefore, recommendations regarding diagnosis and treatment of TDI in this chapter will be offered with endodontic and periodontal maintenance as the primary goal. However, when evidence-based medicine and/or our client priorities require the extraction of a tooth, we can be comforted by the knowledge that domestic animals can and do live happy, healthy, and fruitful lives with missing teeth.

Additionally, TDI are discussed as isolated, individual injuries keeping in mind that in many cases several injuries will affect a tooth concurrently. However, the treatment usually stays the same for the injury. For example, for a patient with a concurrent luxation and an enamel-dentin-pulp fracture, the recommended treatment would be endodontic therapy for the fracture and tooth splinting for the luxation. In addition, TDI often occur concurrently with more serious fractures of the maxillofacial bones and/or head trauma, which may have a higher priority status for management. It is assumed that proper triage of more serious or even life-threatening injuries has already occurred.

6.5.1 History

While information related to the timing and nature of the injury is incredibly beneficial in determining the most appropriate treatment method, this information is typically absent in veterinary patients. TDI more often occur in the absence of a witness who can speak to the mechanism and the exact timing of the injury. As a result, TDI are often incidental findings of the owner or veterinarian, which can negatively impact the prognosis for endodontic therapy. However, an effort should still be made to gather as much information as possible from the owner. Historical information regarding when, where and how the injury occurred and any previous injury or treatment may be useful in determining the most appropriate diagnostic and/or treatment method as well as future prevention.

6.5.2 Clinical Examination

6.5.2.1 Oral Examination

A thorough oral and maxillofacial examination is the first step in the proper management of any trauma to the oral and maxillofacial region. Use of a standardized examination chart is recommended. All oral and extraoral soft tissue wounds should be noted as they may be telling as to the nature of the injury or the likely dental and maxillofacial manifestations. Additionally, soft tissue wounds may have foreign material and/or dental fragments imbedded within (Figure 6.3).

Prior to fully examining the dentition for possible TDI, the oral cavity should be gently cleansed of dried blood and debris as this material may make injuries undetectable. Evaluation of the full extent and direction of the dental injury, as well as the magnitude when dealing with a luxation injury, is important information for determining an injury classification. If possible the patient's occlusion should be assessed prior to intubating as this may provide revealing information for subtle luxation injuries or jaw fractures.

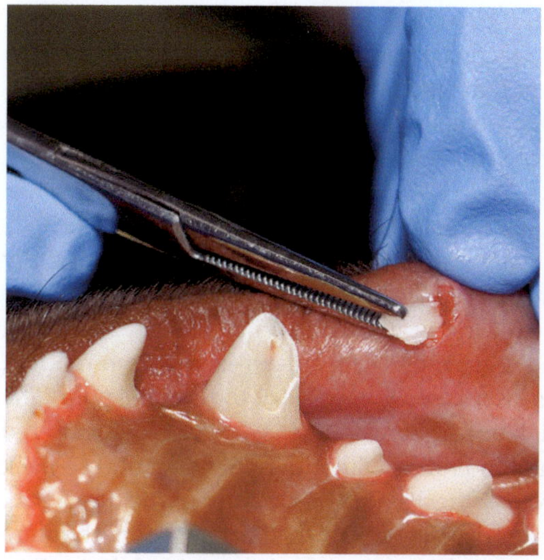

Figure 6.3 Clinical image depicting tooth fragments being removed from the lip.

The clinical examination of individual teeth makes up a substantial contribution to the clinical decision-making process in TDI. Because of the lack of objective and consistent feedback from dogs and cats, evaluation is a challenge that is unique to the practice of veterinary dentistry.

6.5.2.2 Percussion

Because some TDI, such as concussion or subluxation, may only cause periodontal inflammation, the diagnosis is based primarily on patient feedback to percussion. Percussion, by lightly tapping a tooth with a minor PDL injury with a solid object (such as mirror handle), will result in pain. This pain response is likely to be unreliable or may even be absent in the dog or cat. Therefore, the results of percussion testing should not be relied upon.

6.5.2.3 Thermal Pulp Testing

Various methods for thermal pulp testing have been advocated and utilized with success for many years in human dentistry. Standardized methods for use of heated gutta percha, ice, frozen carbon dioxide, dichlorodifluoromethane, and ethyl chloride have been developed [23–27]. These methods also rely upon patient feedback and, thus, are unreliable in animals. Not only are these tests unreliable in animals, the application of extremely cold items such as frozen carbon dioxide and dichlorodifluoromethane have been shown to cause enamel infraction (enamel cracks) due to thermal shock [28].

6.5.2.4 Electric Pulp Testing

Electric pulp testing is commonly utilized in humans and has been advocated in animals [29–31]. However, because the test evaluates nerve function, it does not directly evaluate pulp vitality [32]. In addition, like other testing methods, electric pulp testing relies on the cooperation of the animal, the ability of the animal to provide feedback, and the ability of the veterinarian to interpret that feedback. False positive and false negative results are also quite possible due to variations in patient stoicism.

6.5.2.5 Laser Doppler Flowmetry

Any clinically useful diagnostic tool for successfully evaluating pulpal vitality in animals must rely on objective data collection rather than on patient feedback to a stimulus. Laser Doppler flowmetry is one such method in which a laser beam is directed at the coronal pulp. The light, which undergoes a frequency shift as it is scattered by moving blood cells within the pulp, is reflected back to the probe, detected, and processed to yield a signal. Sensitivity and specificity of this diagnostic method are very high [33, 34]. However, there are several limitations that reduce the practicality of its clinical use. Teeth discolored by blood pigments may interfere with the laser light transmission and confound results. The equipment is largely unrefined and takes 15–20 minutes to test a single tooth [35]. Several studies have reported test times of up to one hour [36]. Finally, the cost of the equipment may be prohibitive for most veterinarians [35].

6.5.2.6 Pulse Oximetry

A much more clinically practical objective test for evaluating pulp vitality may be pulse oximetry. Studies evaluating pulse oximetry in humans have reported mixed success [37–39]. One human study has shown pulse oximetry to be very useful and accurate in primary and immature permanent teeth [40]. Because pulse oximetry measures the amount of light absorbed as it passes through the tissue, the thickness of the dentin is likely to be a factor that may decrease the sensitivity and specificity of the test in older patients.

6.5.3 Diagnostic Imaging

6.5.3.1 Dental Radiography

Dental radiography is considered the mainstay imaging modality in dental traumatology and is the modality to which all other modalities are compared. A more in-depth discussion of intraoral dental radiography can be found elsewhere in this text. In addition, details regarding the specific radiological features found with individual types of TDI are discussed later in this chapter. However, there are a few general points worth making here. To begin with, every traumatized tooth should be examined radiographically in order to visualize the degree of development and condition of the root and pulp. It is typically beneficial, and often crucial, to acquire three images of each traumatized tooth at differing angulations. Additionally, fracture tooth fragments may be found in the soft tissues of the lip and/or cheek. Any soft tissue laceration or puncture near the site of a fractured tooth should be investigated with imaging.

6.5.3.2 Computed Tomography

While computed tomography (CT) has shown to be a crucial tool in the accurate diagnosis of maxillofacial trauma, the spatial resolution is generally considered suboptimal when evaluating the dentition [41]. However, given the prevalence of this imaging modality in veterinary medicine, it may prove beneficial in the diagnosis of some specific TDI. This author has successfully utilized CT for the diagnosis of vertical root fractures where traditional intraoral radiography has proven ineffective. When utilizing CT for imaging the dentition, utilizing an optimal CT protocol is crucial. In a recent study the optimal CT conditions in which to image the canine dentition was shown to be a sequential mode with slice thickness and interval no larger than 1 mm with a high-frequency image reconstruction algorithm and an additional moderate edge enhancement [42] (Figure 6.4).

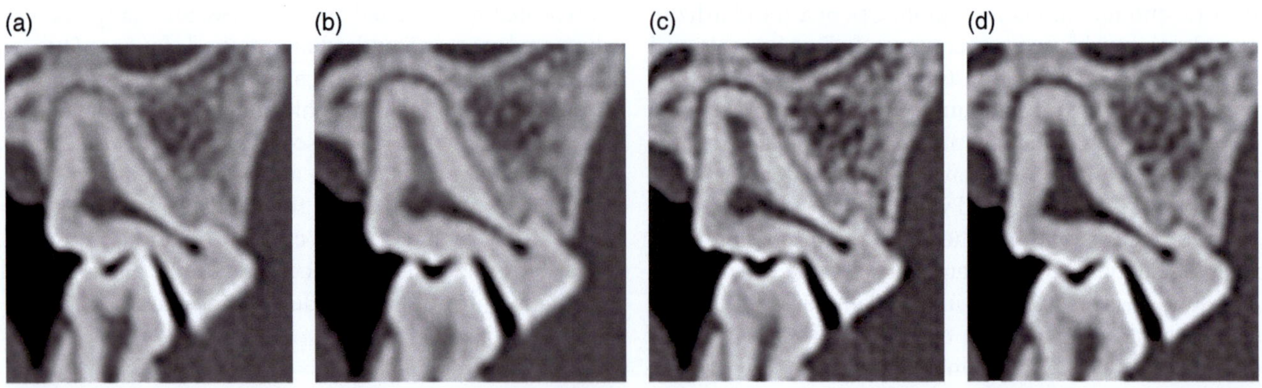

Figure 6.4 Four-detector row CT images generated with a high-frequency image reconstruction algorithm without edge enhancement of the left maxillary first molar (209) (a) with helical 1 mm slice thickness, (b) with sequential 1 mm slice thickness, (c) with helical 0.5 mm slice thickness, (d) and with sequential 0.5 mm slice thickness. The image quality improves from (a) to (d). *Source:* Reprinted with permission from reference [42].

6.5.3.3 Cone Beam Computed Tomography

Cone beam computed tomography (CBCT), however, has been shown to provide superior image quality for trabecular bone, enamel, dentin, pulp cavity, PDL space, lamina dura, and overall evaluator impression when compared to traditional CT in humans and dogs [41]. Combined with the ability to quickly and efficiently acquire three-dimensional reconstructions, this imaging modality may in the future prove to be the standard of care in veterinary maxillofacial and dental traumatology. However, at this time, there are very few machines designed for animal use. In addition, the technology requires additional refinement for veterinary patients before its use in veterinary practice becomes widespread.

6.6 Response of Oral Tissue to Trauma

6.6.1 Dentin–Pulp Complex Response

Dentin is a complex mineralized structure that makes up the bulk of the tooth structure of a mature tooth. Dentin is a permeable structure composed of tubules, which traverse the dentin from the dental pulp to the dentinoenamel junction. These dentinal tubules create a highly permeable tissue that serves as a potential pathway for bacterial contamination of the dental pulp. In the healthy tooth, the dentinal tubule contains an odontoblastic process (see below), collagen fibers, and nerve fibers.

The dental pulp consists of four organized and named layers. The outermost stratum of the healthy pulp is the odontoblast layer, which lies immediately subjacent to the dentin. The odontoblast is the cell responsible for dentin production and possesses a process that extends into the dentinal tubules. Disturbances to dentin result in pulpal consequences. In turn, disturbances in the dental pulp impact the quantity and quality of dentin produced. For this reason it is useful to consider the dentin and pulp as an integrated, dynamic unit known as the dentin–pulp complex.

In the event of a peripheral insult, such as an enamel–dentin fracture, the odontoblasts within the region of insult have the potential to respond in a reparative way. The earliest response of the pulp is to decrease dentin permeability. Through a process known as dentin sclerosis, mineral crystals are deposited within the dentinal tubules. In addition, the surviving primary odontoblasts can be stimulated to produce a type of tertiary dentin often referred to as reactionary dentin (Figure 6.5). If the primary odontoblasts do not survive, newly differentiated odontoblasts can be recruited to the site of injury and produce a second type of tertiary dentin called reparative dentin (Figure 6.5). Dentin sclerosis and tertiary dentin often give a clinical appearance to the tooth of a central brown spot, particularly in areas of abrasion/attrition (Figure 6.6). If the process is slowly progressive, the dentin–pulp complex may be able to effectively protect itself and prevent pulpitis via dentin sclerosis and/or tertiary dentin. However, if the insult is prolonged, more rapid, or more severe, the pulp undergoes an inflammatory/immune reaction, which can become irreversible and result in a non-vital/necrotic pulp. In addition, if the insult is rapid enough, the pulp cannot respond quickly enough to effectively decrease dentin permeability, which can lead to direct pulp exposure.

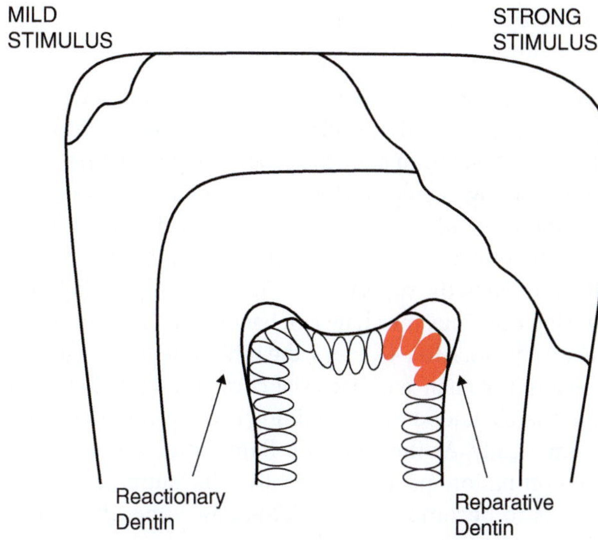

Figure 6.5 Drawing depicting the difference between reactionary and reparative dentin. Reparative dentin is formed by new odontoblasts (red) recruited to the site of injury after the primary odontoblasts have died. *Source:* Reprinted with permission from reference [43].

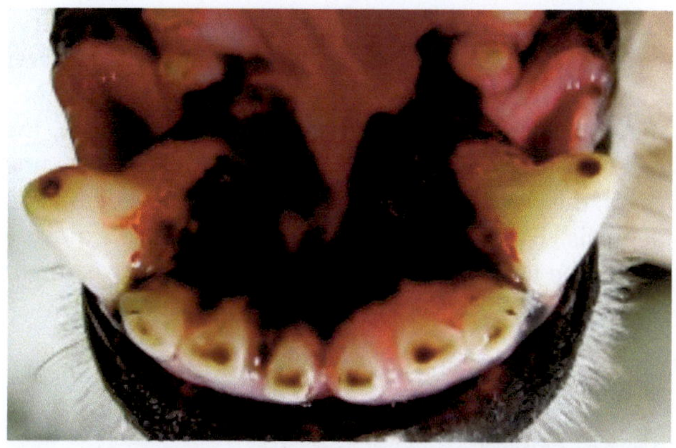

Figure 6.6 Clinical image depicting centralized brown dental discolorations consistent with tertiary dentin formation secondary to dental wear.

6.6.2 Pulp Response to Full and Near Pulp Exposure

Pulpal exposure, if left untreated, will result in pulpal necrosis and apical periodontitis (Figure 6.7). Although the patient will be in pain, the process of pulpal inflammation resulting in pulpal death and necrosis may take weeks to months. Within the first 24–48 hours after pulp exposure the inflammation (pulpitis) is primarily proliferative and limited to the superficial 2–5 mm of the pulp [44–47]. During this time, the chance of bacterial contamination is relatively low. After 48 hours, the inflammation progresses apically, the chance of bacterial contamination increases, and the likelihood of maintaining a vital tooth decreases dramatically. As the zone of inflammation and bacterial contamination progress apically, the superficial pulp begins to become necrotic. This new zone of necrosis also rapidly advances apically.

A dental fracture that comes near, but does not reach, the pulp can still result in a profound pulpal response. The dentinal tubules exposed by the trauma are vulnerable to bacteria and their byproducts, which can lead to death of the odontoblasts near the trauma. In addition, the trauma often severs odontoblastic processes, which can also result in odontoblast death. The exposed nerve fibers result in pain, which can be substantial. The nearer the fracture is to the pulp (when a pinkish hue is visible, there is approximately only 0.5 mm of dentin left), the more profound the pulpal response (Figure 6.8). In some cases, the pulpal response may even be pulpal death and necrosis. For these reasons, even near pulp exposure should be taken seriously and the sooner the treatment rendered the better the prognosis for the tooth.

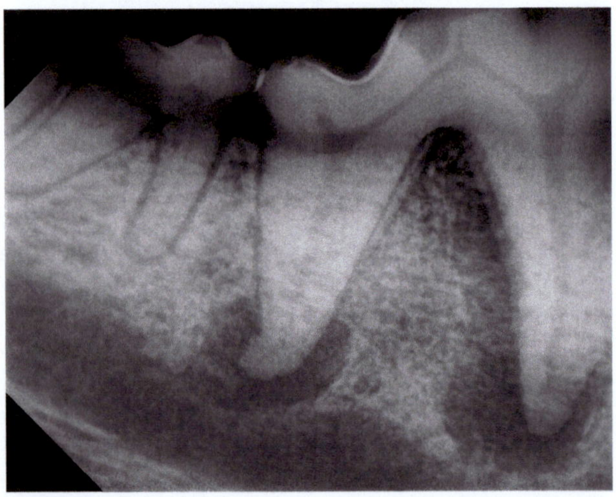

Figure 6.7 Intraoral radiograph of a right mandibular molar tooth with a comparatively wide root canal and periapical lucency consistent with halted dentinogenesis, pulpal necrosis, and apical periodontitis.

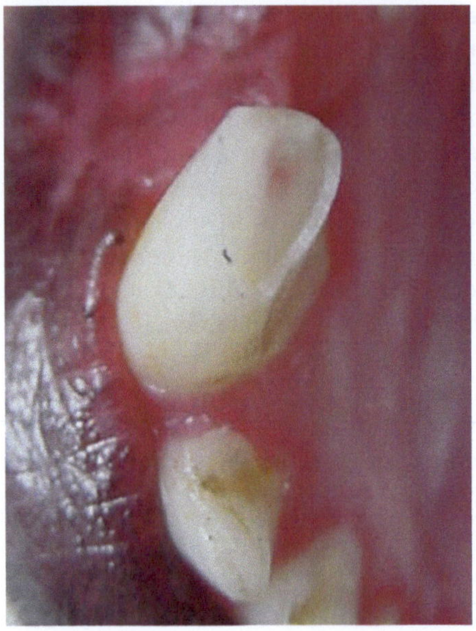

Figure 6.8 Clinical image of a right mandibular canine tooth depicting an enamel–dentin fracture with a centralized pinkish hue indicative of near pulp exposure. *Source:* Image courtesy of Dr. Stephen Juriga, Veterinary Dental Center, Oswego, IL.

6.6.3 Influence of Age on Pulpal Repair and Dentin Production

The unyielding environment of the tooth that encases the pulp can significantly limit the pulps reparative potential. Age has an impact on the effectiveness of that response. An immature tooth has an open apex, thin dentinal walls and a very robust blood supply, which has incredible potential to recover from significant injury and even regenerate. However, during normal tooth maturation, two events occur that negatively influence the healing potential. As the tooth matures, the apex closes and the root canal narrows. Subsequently, the blood supply and the healing potential of the pulp diminish with age.

A young tooth with thin dentinal walls is biomechanically weak. As the tooth ages and more secondary dentin is produced by a healthy vital pulp, the dentinal walls get thicker and the tooth gets stronger. These are important considerations when determining the most appropriate endodontic therapy, as discussed near the end of this chapter.

6.6.4 Periodontal Tissue Response

6.6.4.1 Gingival and Periosteal Complex

TDI are often accompanied by trauma to the gingival and periosteal complex (Figure 6.9). Luxations and avulsions always result in some degree of disruption of the gingival attachment. Any laceration of the gingiva will

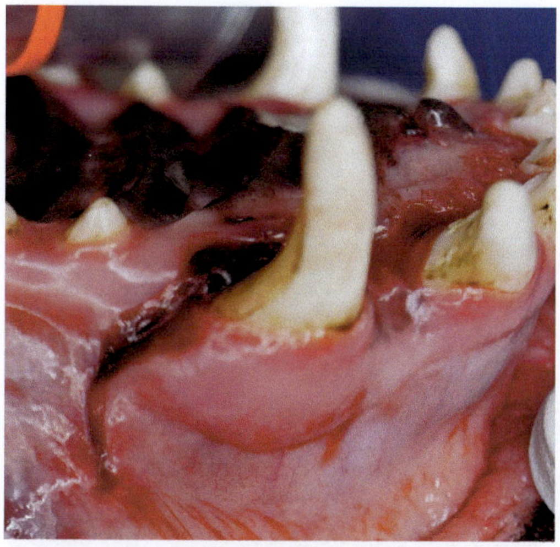

Figure 6.9 Clinical image revealing a gingival and mucosal laceration accompanying a lateral luxation of a maxillary canine tooth.

result in disruption in the continuity of the gingival periodontal fibers. Fortunately, the healing potential of the gingiva is tremendous. The junctional epithelium and gingival periodontal fibers are able to reestablish normal architecture with seven days of injury [48–51]. In addition, the periosteum may be traumatically separated from the underlying alveolar bone, which results in an inflammatory resorption of the osseous surface [52–54]. In the young patient, this bone loss is quickly recovered due to their high osteogenic potential [55, 56].

6.6.4.2 Periodontal Ligament-Cementum Complex

In crown fractures, most of the energy from a traumatic force is absorbed in the crown. If the crown is not fractured, the energy is transferred into the tooth root and PDL. However, all TDI result in at least some injury to the PDL–cementum complex. Depending on the severity of the injury, which is related to the degree of energy transferred into the periodontal space, there is a magnitude-dependent degree of periodontal compression, tension, and/or shear, which results in an inflammatory response [57]. In minor injuries, such as subluxation, minor compression and hemorrhage occurs that typically resolves within seven days. However, more severe injuries, such as luxation and avulsion, may result in severe influx of inflammatory cells, PDL necrosis, and surface root and alveolar bone resorption [57] (Figure 6.10).

6.7 Crown Fractures

Comprising nearly four-fifths of all TDI, crown fractures in dogs and cats are very common [1]. Most of these fractures (near 75%) are sustained by the canine and

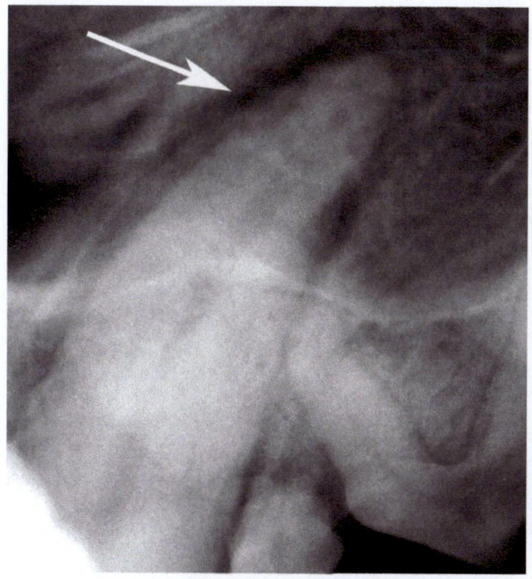

Figure 6.10 Intra-oral radiograph depicting severe alveolar bone resorption (white arrow) in an avulsed canine tooth occurring 10 days after replantation and splinting.

premolar teeth with incisor fractures accounting for about 20% of all fractures [1]. Enamel infraction, enamel fractures, enamel-dentin (uncomplicated) fractures and enamel-dentin-pulp (complicated) fractures are all recognized types of crown fractures. Additionally, within this chapter we will discuss the vertical enamel-dentin crack as a distinct entity.

The use of the terms "complicated" and "uncomplicated" to indicate involvement and lack of involvement of the pulp, respectively, deserves some discussion. The so-called "uncomplicated" crown fracture involves the porous, tubular dentin, the exposure of which may lead to significant pulpal consequences. The term "uncomplicated" implies that the injury does not carry the potential for significant consequences, which may lead to under treatment [7]. The terms "complicated" and "uncomplicated" were introduced in an attempt to universalize the classification of dental trauma to improve the evaluation of epidemiologic data and were not meant to guide clinicians in making therapeutic decisions [8]. The use of subjective terms, such as "uncomplicated" and "complicated," may not be prudent and should be avoided when possible [7]. In their place, the terms enamel–dentin fracture (when referring to a dental crown fracture that does not involve the pulp) and enamel–dentin–pulp fracture (when the fracture does involve the pulp) may then be used.

6.7.1 Enamel Infraction

Enamel infractions are incomplete fractures (cracks) of the enamel (Figure 6.11). This condition is sometimes

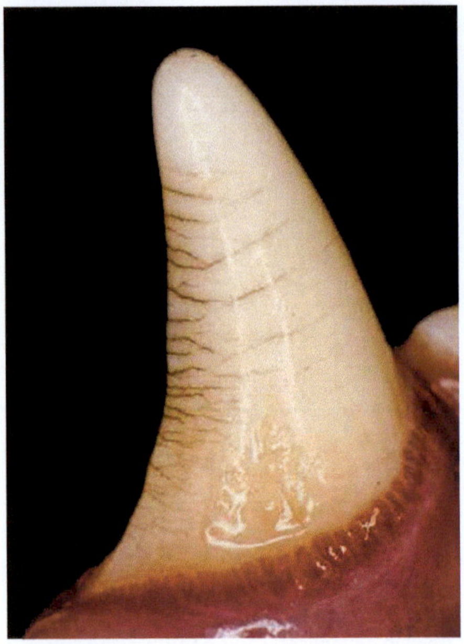

Figure 6.11 Photograph of enamel infraction in a mandibular canine tooth. *Source:* Copyright AVDC®, used with permission.

referred to as crazing. No tooth structure is lost and often, unless absorbing stain, the cracks are quite subtle. Hence, enamel infractions are often overlooked. Enamel infractions are reportedly uncommon, asymptomatic, and typically found incidentally; thus, they do not usually require treatment. However, it has been proposed that these cracks may propagate over time and make the tooth less resistant to fracture [58]. In addition, the trauma that caused the infraction may have also caused other injuries to the tooth, such as a concussion. If so, it may be, or may become, intrinsically stained. For this reason, radiographic assessment of the pulp and root structure should be performed at the time of diagnosis and the tooth should be monitored for progression.

6.7.2 Enamel Fracture

Defined as a fracture with loss of tooth structure but confined to the enamel, the enamel fracture can be difficult to appreciate (Figure 6.12). The enamel in dogs and cats is very thin [59]. Thus, most fractures will not be confined to the enamel. Consequently, enamel fractures are the fifth most common TDI, as reported in one study [1]. When they do occur, they more commonly are sustained by the incisor and premolar teeth [1]. Because no dentin tubules are exposed, this injury should not cause pain or compromise the pulp. Radiographic examination of the pulp and periodontium will be normal. However, radiographic examination should always be performed to rule out concurrent injuries (e.g., root fracture).

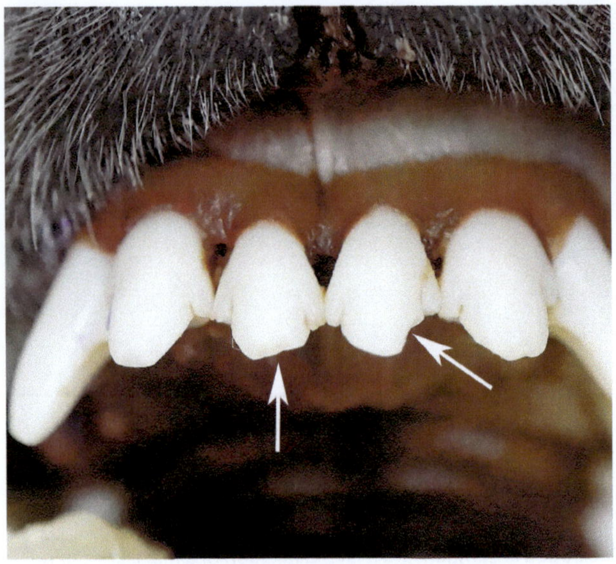

Figure 6.12 Photograph depicting minor enamel fractures of maxillary central incisors (white arrows).

Treatment should include odontoplasty to remove any sharp or jagged areas of enamel, either with or without application of a bonded restoration. The trauma that caused the enamel fracture may also have been strong enough to cause a concussion to the pulp and subsequent pulp necrosis. Therefore, a tooth diagnosed with an enamel fracture should, at the very least, be visually inspected for intrinsic staining for a period of at least one year.

6.7.3 Vertical Enamel–Dentin Cracks

Trauma to a tooth does not always result in a transverse crack/fracture or the obvious loss of tooth structure. In some cases a vertical crack through enamel and into the crown dentin can occur (Figure 6.13). If this crack is not protected from normal masticatory forces, the patient can experience pain (the so-called "cracked tooth syndrome") from deflection of the portions of crown on either side of the crack [58]. In addition, the crack will propagate and eventually involve the pulp and/or root, at which time extraction of the tooth is the only viable treatment option [58]. Vertical cracks present a diagnostic dilemma. The crucial clinical question when presented with a vertical crown crack is whether the crack extends into the root or into the pulp. Dental radiography and clinical examination is unlikely to provide the necessary information [60]. Advanced imaging such as CT or CBCT, however, has been shown to be superior to dental radiography for imaging vertical cracks and fractures [61]. This author has used CT to determine the presence or absence of pulpal involvement in vertical crown cracks. Placement of a full metal

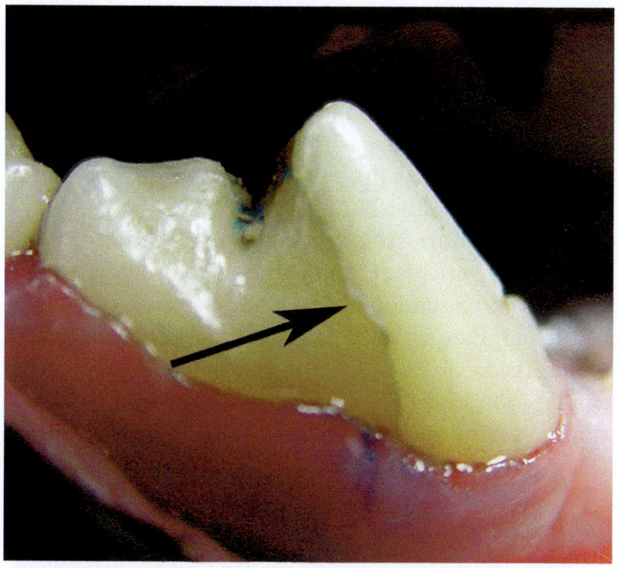

Figure 6.13 Clinical image depicting a vertical enamel–dentin crack (black arrow) on the buccal surface of a maxillary fourth premolar tooth.

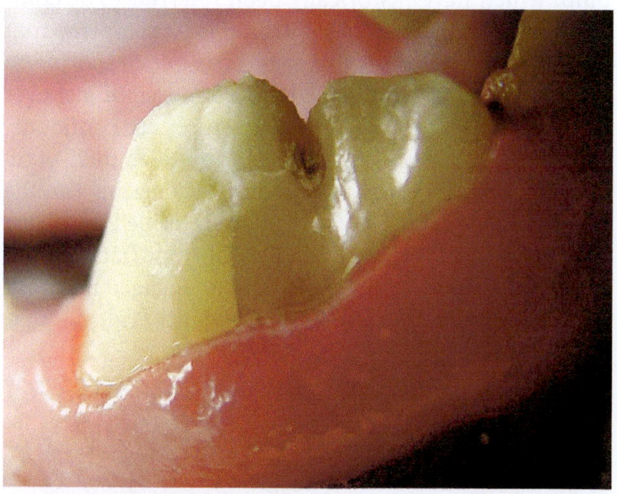

Figure 6.14 Photograph of an enamel–dentin fracture in a maxillary fourth premolar tooth.

crown will help distribute the occlusal load, stop the pain, and prevent progression of the crack into the pulp or into the root [62].

6.7.4 Enamel–Dentin (Uncomplicated) Fracture

An enamel–dentin fracture is a fracture confined to the enamel and dentin, with loss of tooth structure (Figure 6.14). It does not directly involve the pulp. However, as discussed above, it may be useful to consider the presence of "microscopic" pulpal exposure because, although the pulp cannot be clinically visualized, a direct communication from the oral cavity to the pulp exists via the dentinal tubules. For each 1 mm^2 of dentin exposed, as many as 5200 dentinal tubules are exposed, each one with a diameter just large enough for bacteria to penetrate [63].

One study found enamel–dentin fractures to be the fourth most common TDI in dogs and cats and the premolar tooth is the most common site [1]. However, the authors suggested that the injury may not always be assigned the level of importance deserved and thus the injury is likely to be underdiagnosed.

The clinical presentation, diagnosis, and treatment of enamel–dentin fractures vary depending on the interval of time that has passed between the injury and the assessment. In the acute injury, direct exposure of the nerve fiber within the tubule causes pain, in particular when the tooth is touched or when hot or cold liquids come into contact. Aside from the missing tooth structure, there should not be any significant findings on radiography. Treatment of an acute case would consist of odontoplasty and sealing the exposed dentin with a restoration in order to avoid bacterial ingress and allow for pulpal recovery. The type and degree of restoration may be anything from a bonded dentinal sealant to a full metal crown and depends on the amount of tooth lost, the location of structure tooth loss, and the tooth affected. The tooth should continue to be monitored for signs of concussion.

Most enamel–dentin fractures are not diagnosed or treated in the acute phase. Most injuries have been present for months to years before diagnosis. If the tooth is not restored soon after the injury, the pulpitis that is present in the acute injury may progress and lead to death of the local odontoblasts. At this point, one of two results is possible. Undifferentiated mesenchymal cells within the cell-rich zone of the pulp may migrate to the odontoblastic layer, differentiate, and replace the dead odontoblasts. Once there, they will produce tertiary dentin that will fill the exposed dentinal tubules and protect the pulp so that the inflammation can resolve. In this scenario, treatment is as described above for an acute injury.

However, if no reserve odontoblasts are able to replace the dead odontoblasts near the injury, the pulpitis will become irreversible and lead to pulp necrosis. The bacteria from the oral cavity can gain access to the necrotic pulp through the open dentinal tubules and, subsequently, lead to apical periodontitis. Radiographically, this may be visualized as a widened root canal with periapical rarefaction. In this scenario, the recommended treatment is endodontic therapy with restoration of the crown fracture.

6.7.5 Enamel–Dentin–Pulp (Complicated) Fracture

When a crown fracture is extensive enough to create visible exposure of the pulp it is referred to as an enamel–dentin–pulp fracture (Figure 6.15). This injury is reportedly the most common TDI in dogs and cats and is most often sustained by the strategic teeth, canine teeth in particular [1, 2, 14].

The exposure of pulp is extremely painful and, if left untreated, will lead to pulp necrosis and periapical periodontitis. If diagnosed in the acute phase, pulpal hemorrhage may be present. Radiographic abnormalities will be absent. Pulpal proliferation (pulp polyp) may be seen in younger patients (Figure 6.16). In the chronic lesion, as these often are because of delayed diagnosis, hemorrhage at the pulpal exposure site will be absent. In its place will, most often, be a darkly discolored pulp filled with hair and miscellaneous debris. Radiographs of teeth with chronic exposure may reveal a widened root canal space (pulp death), either with or without periapical rarefaction (periapical lucency).

Crown fractures that directly expose the pulp must be treated with endodontic therapy or, alternatively, extraction. The endodontic therapy chosen is dependent on the age of the patient and the duration of pulp exposure. A discussion on endodontic treatment decision-making can be found later in this chapter. An in-depth discussion regarding endodontic therapy can also be found in Chapter 15 – Basic Endodontic Therapy.

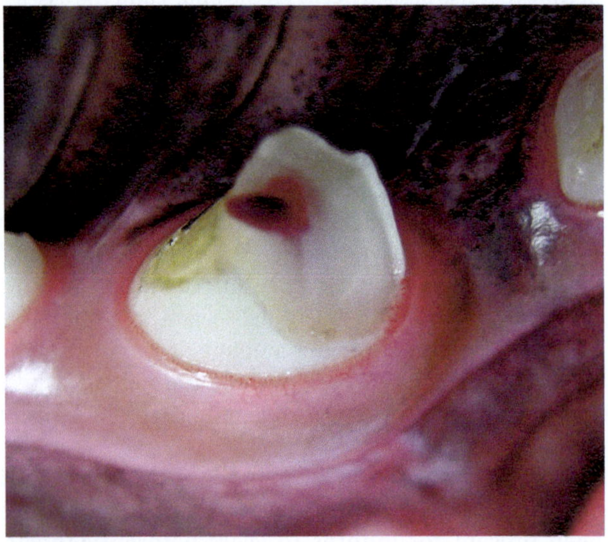

Figure 6.15 Clinical photograph of an enamel–dentin–pulp fracture in a maxillary canine tooth.

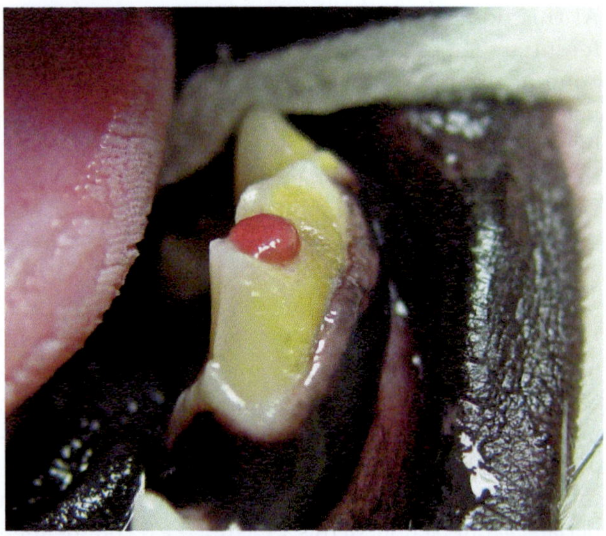

Figure 6.16 Image depicting a proliferative pulpal response often seen in younger patients.

6.8 Crown-Root Fractures

Dental fractures are not always isolated to the crown. Often the root is also involved, creating a crown–root fracture (Figure 6.17) that may or may not involve the pulp, which have historically been referred to as complicated crown–root and uncomplicated crown–root fractures, respectively. This injury has been reported to be the third most common TDI, accounting for just over 10% of all TDI [1]. Crown–root fractures are commonly sustained by the maxillary fourth premolar (half of all crown–root fractures) and, when occurring on the buccal aspect of the tooth, is often described as a "slab fracture" [1, 64] (Figure 6.18). Crown–root fractures are also often seen on canine teeth of dogs engaged in apprehension training and competition activitiy [19].

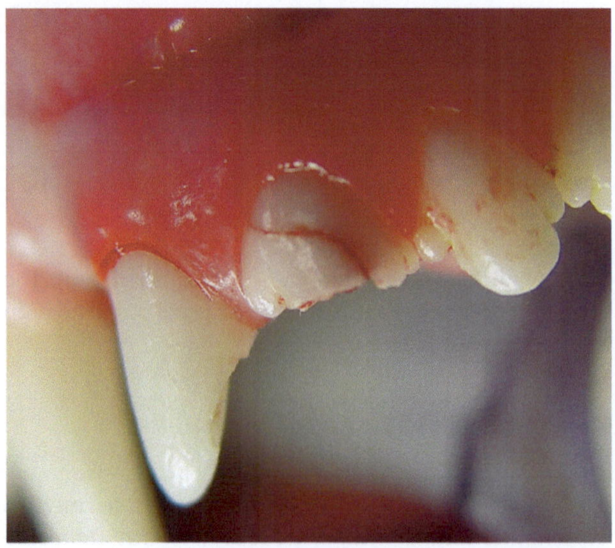

Figure 6.17 Crown–root fracture in a maxillary incisor tooth. Note that the fracture line extends subgingivally to involve the crown and root.

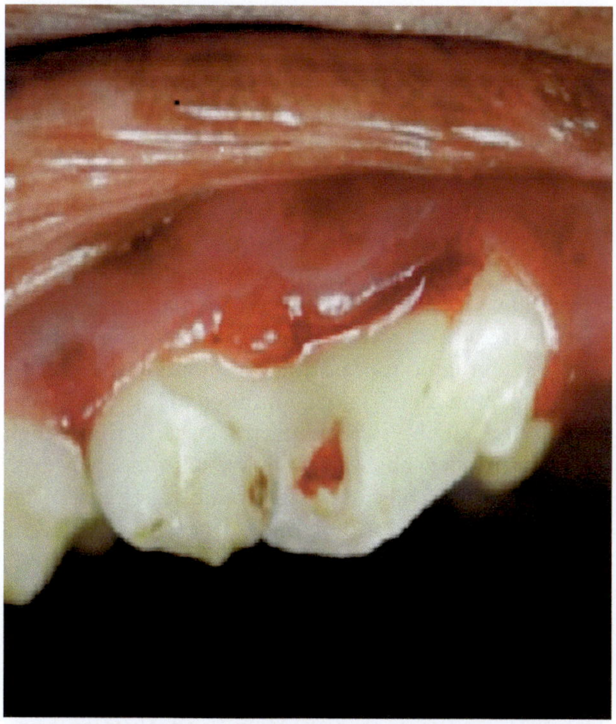

Figure 6.18 Crown–root fracture affecting the buccal wall of a maxillary fourth premolar tooth. This injury is often referred to as a "slab fracture." In this case there is pulpal exposure.

The coronal (fractured) segment is often retained by the attached gingival fibers, particularly with the maxillary fourth premolar. However, the segment is likely to be mobile. If the injury is chronic, the coronal segment may have become detached. Retention of the fractured segment is less common in the canine tooth. The apical extent of the fracture is typically not visible clinically. In addition, radiography may prove ineffective because the fracture line is often perpendicular to the central beam and the close approximation of the two fracture fragments at the root level. Therefore, determination of the apical extent of the fracture may require surgical exploration (Figure 6.19).

The endodontic consequences, and thus the endodontic management, of crown–root fractures are the same as for enamel–dentin and enamel–dentin–pulp fractures. However, additional management of the root component is more complex and requires addition consideration. Specifically, in order to have long-term success, the fracture needs to be restored in a way that does not compromise the health of the periodontium. First, the apical extent of the root fracture must be determined. Because the periodontium cannot heal to a restoration, the bone and gingival margin has to be reestablished apical to the fracture line via type 2 crown lengthening or orthodontic extrusion in order to reestablish biologic width. In some cases, this is too far apically for the long-term maintenance of the tooth and extraction of the traumatized tooth may be more practical.

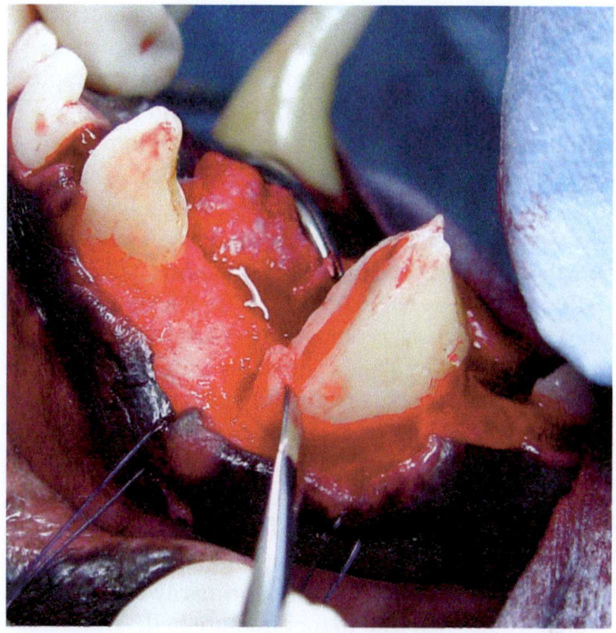

Figure 6.19 Photograph depicting surgical exploration of the apical extent of a crown–root fracture in a maxillary canine tooth.

6.9 Root Fractures

A fracture confined to the root (involving cementum, dentin, and pulp) of a tooth is a root fracture (Figure 6.20). The lesion can be further classified if the coronal

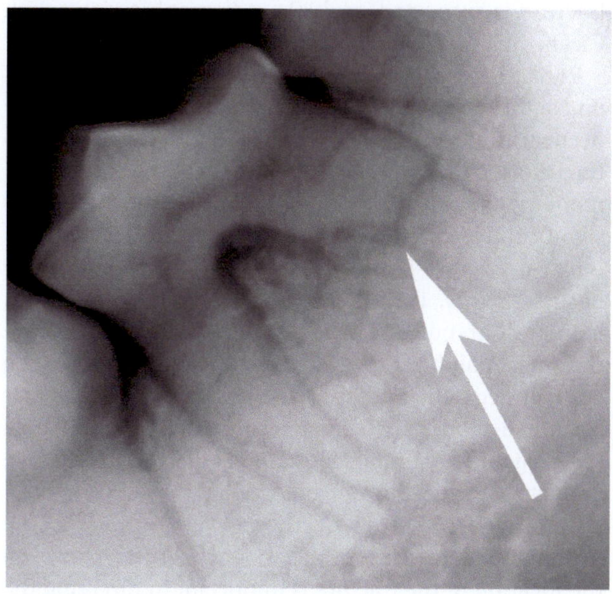

Figure 6.20 Intraoral radiograph of mandibular second molar tooth depicting a horizontal root fracture (white arrow).

segment is displaced (see luxation injury descriptions above). In addition, root fractures can be further classified according to the location of the fracture (apical, middle, cervical). The fracture location and the degree of displacement of the coronal segment are important in determining treatment and prognosis. For example, if the coronal segment is displaced significantly, the pulp may be significantly stretched if not completely severed, which will negatively impact the prognosis.

Root fractures have a reported frequency of 3.5% of all TDI and most commonly are found in the incisor region [1]. The frequency increases with increasing age and almost invariably are found in patients > three years of age [1]. This may be intuitive when dental biomechanics are considered. The flexibility of the PDL and alveolar bone decreases with increasing age [65]. Therefore, the energy transfer from a traumatized tooth to surrounding structures may be partly inhibited in older patients and may remain primarily in the tooth, which would then lead to root fracture [65].

Given that veterinary patients are typically quite stoic, root fractures are often incidental findings. Upon oral examination the affected tooth may be slightly extruded and mobile. The magnitude of mobility is dependent on the location of the fracture along the length of the root. Cervical root fractures are usually more mobile than apical root fractures. Differential diagnoses for mobile teeth are periodontal disease and luxation injuries. Periodontal disease can usually be ruled out by observing normal sulcus depths. Radiographs will reveal a transverse radiolucent line through the tooth root but may only be seen if the central beam is directed within a maximum range of 15–20° of the fracture plane [66, 67]. Thus, if a root fracture is suspected, multiple radiographic views with varying angulations should be acquired.

Root fractures can undergo the healing process with one of three outcomes [68]. True hard tissue healing may occur with formation of a hard tissue union between the fracture segments under ideal conditions (i.e., minimal mobility and pulp not severed). However, if the pulp is significantly stretched or severed, influx of PDL between the two fracture segments results in connective tissue healing. Lastly, if the coronal pulp becomes necrotic, ingress of granulation tissue into the fracture site from the apical pulp occurs, which results in loosening of the coronal segment and localized resorption of alveolar bone and tooth. The degree of mobility of the coronal segment and the timing of treatment delivery has a large impact on the healing outcome [69].

Treatment of a root fracture is very similar to the principles of treating a long bone fracture. However, the location of the fracture is important in directing the treatment. Treatment is best rendered within 48 hours of the injury. However, as mentioned above, this rarely occurs in veterinary dentistry because these injuries may go unrecognized for prolonged periods of time. Fractures in the apical third are typically non-mobile and may not require splinting (the periodontal attachment provides a natural splint). The pulpitis that occurs from the injury may resolve without endodontic treatment. However, radiographic monitoring for pulpal death should be performed every three to six months for at least one year. Fractures in the middle third of the root may or may not be mobile. However, even if non-mobile, splinting for four to six weeks provides the best chance of healing [70]. Radiographic monitoring for endodontic health is required. If the client is not committed to this, extraction may be indicated. Fractures in the cervical third (high root fracture) will absolutely require splinting. However, even with rigid splinting, the prognosis for healing is guarded [69]. In this author's experience, most high root fractures are extracted.

6.10 Luxation Injuries

The PDL, tooth root cementum, and alveolar bone comprise the dentoalveolar, a type of gomphosis, joint. As such, the dentoalveolar joint can be luxated to varying degrees. Concussion, subluxation, lateral luxation, intrusive luxation, extrusive luxation, and avulsion are all possible types of luxation injuries. Luxation injuries are considered to be far less common in animals than dental fractures. One study reported a frequency of 17.3% of all TDI [1]. Nearly half of all luxation injuries occur in animals < three years of age [1]. It has been proposed that at this age the more flexible PDL and low mineralization of the supporting alveolar bone are more conducive to luxation injuries than tooth fractures [69]. In dogs and cats, involvement of the canine and incisor teeth represent nearly 80% of all luxation injuries, most of which are concussions and lateral luxations [1, 71]. Avulsions are reportedly quite rare.

6.10.1 Concussion and Subluxations

A concussion is a blunt injury to the tooth that may or may not cause visible trauma to the tooth. Other concurrent injuries (crown fracture, root fracture, luxation, etc.) may or may not be present. A concussion invariably leads to some degree of pulpitis and acute traumatic periodontitis, both of which may resolve without intervention [72]. Severely concussed teeth may take on a blue/pink/purple/gray discoloration, often referred to as intrinsic (endogenous) staining [73] (Figure 6.21). This discoloration is caused by hemorrhage of the pulp into the confined space of the pulp chamber. The breakdown products of the hemolyzed blood enter the dentinal

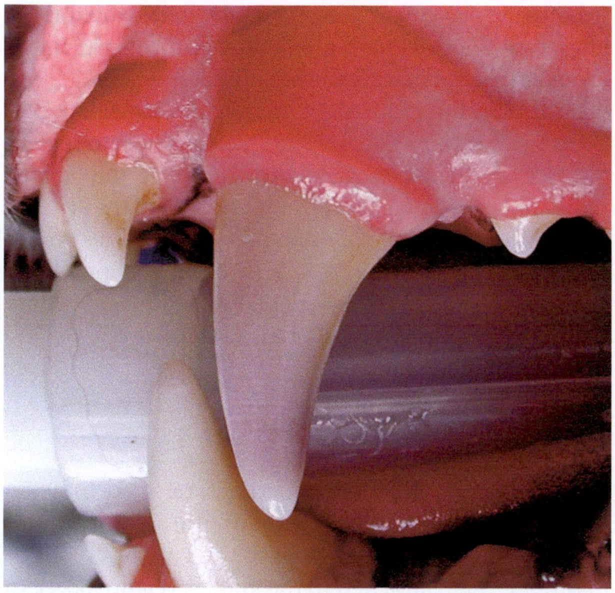

Figure 6.21 Purple-pink discoloration of a maxillary canine tooth consistent with intrinsic staining secondary to a concussion injury.

tubules and lead to what is essentially a contusion. Crown discoloration secondary to a concussion injury appears to be quite common in animals with a reported frequency of 14.4% of all TDI, most often involving the canine and incisor teeth [1]. Given that not all concussion injuries will lead to crown discoloration, and thus will go undiagnosed, the true prevalence of concussion injuries in dogs and cats is likely higher than that reported. The prevalence of pulp necrosis following a concussion injury in humans is <5% [72]. If this is also true for dogs, that would indicate that the true prevalence of concussion injuries is very high. It has been reported that in most cases (~92%) an intrinsically stained tooth is non-vital [73]. A non-vital tooth will almost invariably become painful and necrotic. Therefore, endodontic therapy is the recommended treatment for most, if not all, intrinsically stained teeth. Concussions that do not cause discoloration will likely recover without treatment. However, a suspected concussed tooth should be monitored via visual inspection for intrinsic staining and via dental radiography for pulpal health. The acute periodontitis that accompanies a concussion injury is caused by the compression of the PDL and is likely to be painful. However, outward clinical signs of this pain would be quite subtle. Fortunately, as long as the pulp recovers, the acute periodontitis and pain should be transient. No clinical or radiographic signs will be present.

A subluxated tooth is one that has received a traumatic force, which has led to increased mobility of the tooth. Other than slight mobility of the tooth, which would be likely to go unappreciated, there are no other outward clinical signs. As such, subluxations present a sizeable challenge in diagnosis. Thus, despite the low reported frequency (0.1% of all TDI) [1], subluxations may be more common than reported. Differential diagnoses for a mobile tooth should include attachment loss from periodontitis and root fracture. Attachment loss can be ruled out by the lack of periodontal pocketing on oral examination. A radiograph is necessary to rule out a root fracture and confirm the diagnosis of subluxation. In most cases a subluxation will not require treatment. The mobility will likely resolve within 7–10 days [70]. During the healing period, the patient should be fed a soft diet.

6.10.2 Extrusive, Intrusive, and Lateral Luxations

An extrusive luxation is a condition where the tooth is partially dislocated out of the alveolus in an axial direction and is characterized by partial or total separation of the PDL. The tooth will appear elongated on visual inspection and some degree of root exposure will be present. Gingival hemorrhage, pain, and mobility will be present in the acute injury. In addition, the gingiva may or may not be lacerated. These clinical findings may be similar to a root fracture. The diagnosis can be confirmed by the presence of a widened periapical space and the absence of a root fracture on radiographs.

As for any luxation, the appropriate treatment is digital replacement of the tooth within the alveolus and splinting (details regarding tooth splinting can be found later in this chapter). Any gingival lacerations should be sutured. Because the neurovascular supply to the pulp is invariably severed, the pulp will be compromised and become non-vital. In the immature permanent tooth (open apex) revascularization may occur. However, in a mature tooth (closed apex), root canal therapy is required and should be performed within seven days of splinting.

When a tooth is dislocated axially in an apical direction (into the alveolus) it is called an intrusive luxation. It will present clinically with a short or completely absent clinical crown and usually has some indication of gingival hemorrhage and mobility. Because the traumatic force is concentrated in the small surface area of the apical PDL, the location of the vascular origin of the pulp, this injury invariably leads to irreversible pulpitis and subsequently a non-vital tooth [72]. In addition, because of the severe periapical periodontitis that accompanies this injury root resorption and/or root ankylosis may ensue.

In minor intrusive luxations, the recommended treatment is repositioning of the tooth (either orthodontically or surgically) and splinting. Endodontic therapy is also likely to be necessary. If the injury is chronic the best treatment option may be surgical extraction due to a poor prognosis. In this author's experience, most intrusive luxations involve severe luxation of the maxillary canine tooth into the nasal cavity. In such cases, surgical removal of the tooth via a buccal rhinotomy approach is typically recommended.

A lateral luxation is characterized by luxation of the tooth in any direction other than axially (i.e., facial, buccal, labial, lingual, palatal, mesial, distal). In dogs most lateral luxations are labially directed luxations of the canine tooth [71, 74] (Figure 6.22) and may clinically and radiologically appear similar to an extrusive luxation. However, it is almost invariably accompanied by a fracture of one of the alveolar plates [71] (Figure 6.23).

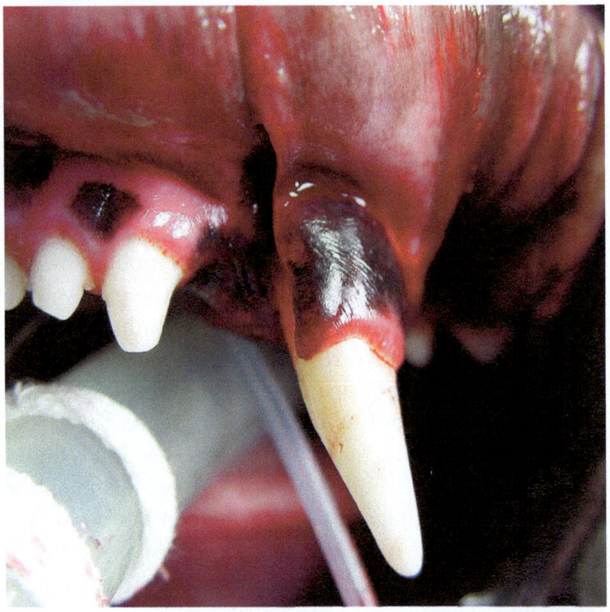

Figure 6.22 Clinical photograph of a lateral luxation of a maxillary canine luxated in a labial direction.

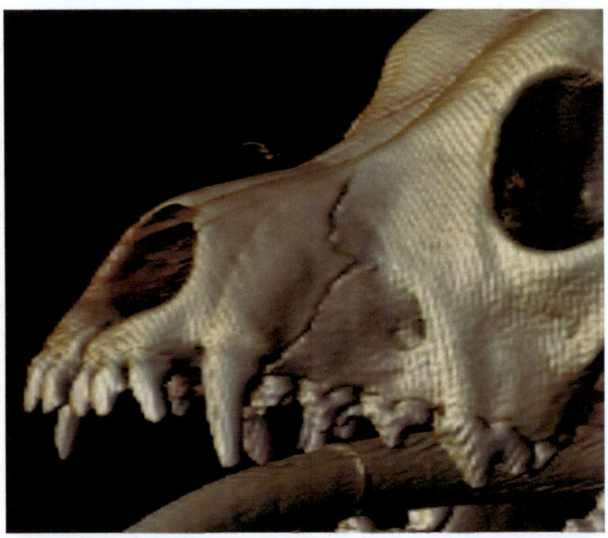

Figure 6.23 Computed tomographic image of an alveolar process fracture seen in conjunction with lateral luxation of a maxillary canine tooth.

If both alveolar plates are fractured, which would more often be associated with a mandibular tooth, the injury should be classified as an alveolar fracture.

Treatment for a lateral luxation is the same as for an extrusive luxation. The only additional step is to replace the fractured alveolar plate after replacing the luxated tooth. In addition, to allow proper healing of the alveolar process fracture, the splint should stay in place for an additional one to two weeks. Root canal therapy should be performed within one week of the splinting procedure and not delayed until the splint is removed.

6.11 Avulsions

An avulsion injury, also sometimes referred to as an ex-articulation, implies that the tooth has been completely displaced out of the alveolus. The tooth may or may not remain attached to the gingiva (Figure 6.24). In the process of being avulsed, the neurovascular supply to the pulp is completely severed, the PDL is also completely severed, and the entire root surface becomes exposed to the external environment. In addition, the injury may be accompanied by alveolar process fractures and gingival lacerations. Although avulsion injuries may be more common than has been reported in the veterinary literature (0.3% of all TDI), it is likely that their prevalence is still quite low and similar to what has been reported in humans (<3%) [1].

The response of the dentoalveolar apparatus to avulsion injuries can be broken down into the response of the pulpal tissues and the response of the periodontal tissues. The damage to these tissues is extensive and the healing potential is significantly dependent on the extra-oral period and the extra-alveolar handling.

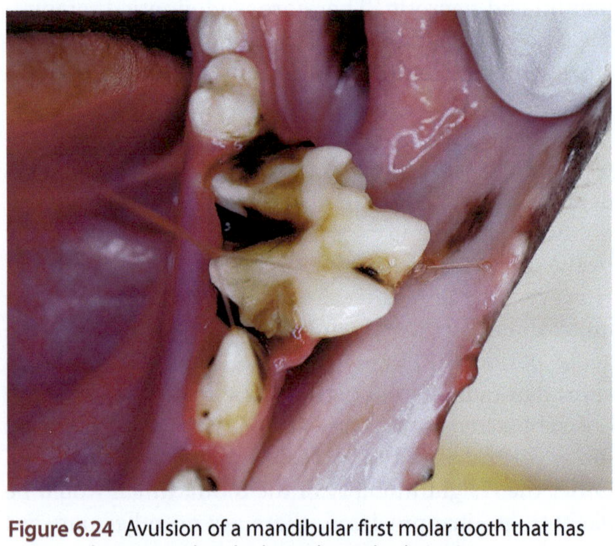

Figure 6.24 Avulsion of a mandibular first molar tooth that has remained connected to the buccal attached gingiva.

Pulpodentinal healing in immediately replanted teeth in animals can be broadly broken down into healing via influx of seven different tissues into the pulp [75–82]:

1) Regular tubular reparative dentin
2) Irregular reparative dentin
3) Osteodentin
4) Immature bone
5) Mature bone
6) Internal resorption
7) Pulp necrosis.

The healing outcome of the pulp is directly proportional to the stage of tooth development, with mature teeth being more likely to suffer pulp necrosis [83]. Studies of immediately replanted avulsed teeth in dogs have shown that revascularization begins within four days and is complete after 30 days [78, 79]. Revascularization of pulp may be possible in immature permanent teeth in dogs if the avulsed tooth is replanted within three hours and stored in the appropriate storage media. However, replantation rarely if ever occurs this quickly. Thus, root canal therapy is almost always indicated and should be pursued one week after being replanted [84, 85]. Endodontic therapy should not be performed during the extra-oral period as studies have shown excessive tooth handling to damage any surviving periodontal fibroblasts, leading to increased root resorption [84, 85].

Perhaps a more pressing concern for avulsed teeth is the response of the periodontal tissues. If the root surface of an avulsed tooth is exposed to the external environment for prolonged periods of time, the remaining fibroblasts attached to the tooth root become desiccated, which leads to an inflammatory response that may result in root resorption, making successful replantation impossible (see Figure 6.10). While some experimentally avulsed teeth in dogs that have immediately been replanted have undergone complete healing with normal PDL, most replanted teeth will eventually suffer from some degree of root resorption. Healing with root resorption can take on three forms [86, 87], the type and degree of which is dependent primarily on the extra-oral dry time [88–91]:

1) Healing with surface resorption (repair-related resorption)
2) Healing with replacement resorption (ankylosis)
3) Healing with inflammatory resorption (infection-related resorption).

The treatment decision-making process is complex and depends on the extra-alveolar time, the extra-alveolar storage media and the age of the patient (open apex versus closed apex) [88–95]. The most important thing to remember is that the tooth needs to be replanted as soon as possible, ideally within five minutes of exarticulation [96]. If the owner witnessed the injury and has the tooth, he/she should be advised to replant the tooth and immediately travel to a veterinary dentist. If the tooth cannot be replanted, the tooth should be stored in an appropriate media (milk, saline, saliva) while they drive to the nearest veterinary dentist. Prior to implantation, the tooth and the empty alveolus should be gently rinsed with saline, being careful not to debride the root surface in any way that may remove any remaining viable PDL cells. If the apex is closed the tooth should then be replanted. However, if the apex is open, pretreatment with a tetracycline may improve the outcome [96]. Pretreatment protocols have been advocated for immature teeth. The details of these protocols are beyond the scope of this chapter and the reader is referred to recent protocol guidelines for the management of tooth avulsion in humans for more information [96].

Once the tooth has been replanted, it should be splinted. Endodontic treatment is usually automatically delivered within seven days after replantation and before splint removal in all mature teeth [96]. Delay in delivery of endodontic treatment will negatively impact the treatment outcome [97]. Immature teeth, on the other hand, have the potential to revascularize if implanted within three hours. Therefore, it is reasonable to consider delaying endodontic therapy for immature teeth. However, follow-up monitoring of pulpal health with serial radiography for several years after reimplantation is critical. Additionally, the prophylactic delivery of systemic tetracyclines has been shown to decrease the degree of root resorption in non-human primates but does not improve the chance of pulpal healing [82, 98].

In this author's experience avulsions and other luxation injuries in cats are most often secondary to significant attachment loss from periodontal disease. In such cases, replantation is contraindicated.

6.12 The Use of Splints in Dentoalveolar Trauma

Several TDI, such as root fractures, luxation, and avulsions, require the application of a splint for healing. A splint that closely approximates the physiologic movement of the natural dentoalveolar structure provides the optimal biomechanics for healing. A non-physiologic (i.e., non-flexible) splint applied for prolonged periods of time can delay periodontal and pulpal healing and increase the chance of permanent ankylosis [99–103]. In fact, experimental animal studies have shown that optimal PDL healing was obtained when a replanted tooth was not splinted at all [100–106]. In addition, splinting decreases the degree of pulpal revascularization and increases pulpal necrosis and inflammatory resorption in non-human primate studies [97]. However, a splint must be used to keep the replanted tooth in an appropriate position during the healing period. Therefore, care must be taken when choosing the type and duration of a trauma splint. The ideal splint in animals would meet the following requirements [107, 108]:

1) Direct intraoral application
2) Easily constructed from common dentistry materials
3) Does not increase periodontal injury
4) Does not irritate oral soft tissues
5) Does not exert orthodontic force
6) Versatile in providing a rigid, semi-rigid, or flexible splint
7) Easy and safe to remove
8) Allows for endodontic access
9) Hygienic.

Splints can be considered as either flexible (more mobility than a normal tooth), semi-rigid (equal mobility to a normal tooth), and rigid (less mobility than a normal tooth) [108]. Several splints have been used in human dentistry that are either contraindicated or not particularly practical in animals (i.e., arch bar splints and orthodontic appliances) [109–112]. Wire-composite splints, resin splints, and titanium trauma splints are among the most versatile splints and have been employed in animals [71, 74, 107].

Wire-composite splints are semi-rigid splints that are easily employed with materials typically present in a dentistry practice. A properly constructed wire-composite splint incorporates 0.3–0.4 mm diameter soft round steel wire and small blebs of composite over the center of the tooth crown [108]. By avoiding the incorporation of composite into the interdental spaces the splint allows for normal physiologic mobility between teeth.

The most commonly employed splint in dogs is a figure-of-eight wire-reinforced composite or resin splint used for lateral luxation of maxillary canine teeth [71, 74, 107] (Figure 6.25). Because the figure-of-eight splint described in dogs incorporates composite or resin over the entire wire surface area, when composite is used it may be considered a composite splint. Composite splints are considered rigid splints and are generally considered to be undesirable when considering the ideal splinting scenario. However, if resin is used in a figure-of-eight splint, rather than composite, some flexibility can occur. Additionally, the use of wire with a diameter larger than 0.5 mm may result in a rigid splint [108]. Therefore, in order to maintain a flexible figure-of-eight splint, fabricated with resin, an appropriate diameter wire is essential.

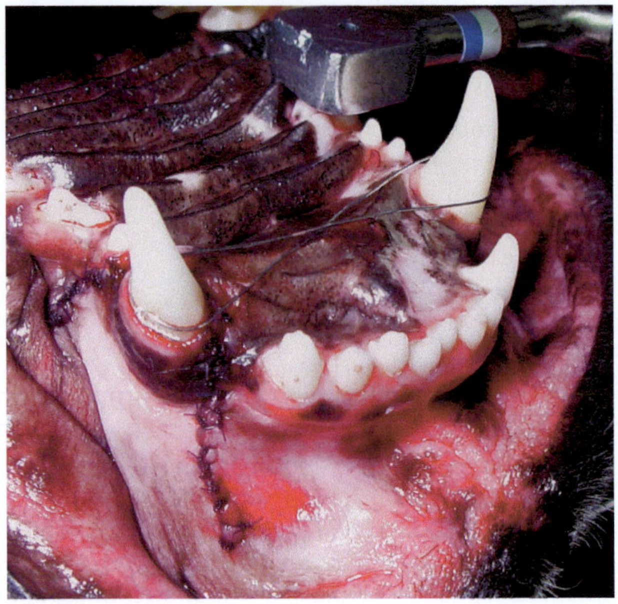

Figure 6.25 Figure-of-eight wire-reinforced composite splint immediately prior to placement of the composite on the maxillary canine teeth.

Prefabricated metal splinting materials are also commercially available. This author has successfully utilized the prefabricated titanium trauma splint for lateral luxations. The material is 0.2 mm thick and can easily be adapted to the dental arch by bending with fingers. The titanium trauma splint is applied similarly to wire-composite splints.

The degree of rigidity and the duration of immobilization a splint should provide are dictated primarily by the type of TDI. Generally speaking, a fixation period of two to three weeks is recommended for luxation injuries. However, for avulsions, where ankylosis is a concern, the fixation period should be reduced to about 7–10 days. When the injury is accompanied by an alveolar process fracture (i.e., lateral luxation with an alveolar process fracture), one to two weeks should be added to the recommended fixation period. Intrusive luxations may also need additional healing time. The principles of splinting root fractures may be considered very similar to the principles of long bone fracture. A rigid or semi-rigid splint can be utilized for a period of four to six weeks.

References

1 Soukup, J.W., Hetzel, S., and Paul, A. (2015). Classification and epidemiology of traumatic dentoalveolar injuries in dogs and cats: 959 injuries in 660 patient visits (2004–2012). *J. Vet. Dent.* 32: 6.

2 Golden, A.L., Stoller, M., and Harvey, C.E. (1982). A survey of oral and dental diseases in dogs anesthetized at a veterinary hospital. *J. Am. Anim. Hosp. Assoc.* 18: 891–899.

3 Soukup, J.W., Mulherin, B.L., and Snyder, C.J. (2013). Prevalence and nature of dentoalveolar injuries among patients with maxillofacial fractures. *J. Small Anim. Pract.* 54: 9–14.

4 DeBowes, L.J., Mosier, D., Logan, E. et al. (1996). Association of periodontal disease and histologic lesions in multiple organs from 45 dogs. *J. Vet. Dent.* 13: 57–60.

5 Rawlinson, J.E., Goldstein, R.E., Reiter, A.M. et al. (2011). Association of periodontal disease with systemic health indices in dogs and the systemic response to treatment of periodontal disease. *J. Am. Vet. Med. Assoc.* 238: 601–209.

6 Kouki, M.I., Papadimitriou, S.A., Kazakos, G.M. et al. (2013). Periodontal disease as a potential factor for systemic inflammatory response in the dog. *J. Vet. Dent.* 30: 26–29.

7 Feliciano, K.M.P.C. and de Franca Caldas, A. Jr. (2006). A systemic review of the classification of traumatic dental injuries. *Dent. Traumatol.* 22: 71–76.

8 World Health Organization (1978). *Application of the International Classification of Diseases to Dentistry and Stomatology, ICD-DA*, 2e, 88–89. Geneva, Switzerland: WHO.

9 Johnson, R. (1981). Descriptive classification of traumatic injuries to the teeth and supporting structures. *J. Am. Dent. Assoc.* 102: 195–197.

10 Garcia-Godoy, F. (1981). A classification for traumatic injuries to primary and permanent teeth. *J. Pedodont.* 5: 295–297.

11 AVDC Nomenclature Committee. Dental fracture classification. AVDC, May 2012. Web. accessed 18 August 2013.

12 Andreasen, J.O. (1972). *Traumatic Injuries of the Teeth.* Copenhagen, Denmark: Munksgaard.

13 Andreasen, J.O., Lauridsen, E., and Gerds, T.A. (2012). Dental Trauma Guide: a source of evidence-based treatment guidelines for dental trauma. *Dent. Traumatol.* 28: 345–350.

14 Capik, I., Ledecky, V., and Sevcik, A. (2000). Tooth fracture evaluation and endodontic treatment in dogs. *Acta Vet. BRNO* 69: 115–122.

15 Bonner, S.E., Reiter, A.M., and Lewis, J.R. (2012). Orofacial manifestations of high-rise syndrome in cats: a retrospective study of 84 cases. *J. Vet. Dent.* 29: 10–18.

16 Mulherin, B.L., Snyder, D.J., Soukup, J.W. et al. (2014). Retrospective evaluation of canine and feline maxillomandibular trauma cases. A comparison of signalment with non-maxillomandibular traumatic injuries (2003–2012). *Vet. Comp. Orthop. Traumatol.* 27: 192–197.

17 Goldschmidt, S., Zimmerman, C., Collins, C. et al. (2017). The influence of force direction on the fracture pattern and fracture resistance of canine teeth in dogs. *J. Vet. Dent.* 34 (1): 8–17.

18 Le Brech, C., Hamel, L., Le Nihouannen, J.C. et al. (1997). Epidemiological study of canine teeth fractures in military dogs. *J. Vet. Dent.* 14: 51–55.

19 Pilkey, W.D. and Pilkey, D.F. (2008). Shoulder fillets. In: *Pilkey's Stress Concentration Factors*, 3e (ed. W.D. Pilkey and D.F. Pilkey), 135–175. Hoboken, NJ: Wiley.

20 Anusavice, K.J. (2003). Mechanical properties of dental materials. In: *Phillips' Science of Dental Materials*, 11e (ed. K.J. Anusavice), 73–101. St. Louis, MO: Elsevier.

21 Lalloo, R. (2003). Risk factors for major injuries to the face and teeth. *Dent. Traumatol.* 19: 12–14.

22 Mulherin, B.L., Snyder, D.J., Soukup, J.W. et al. (2014). Retrospective evaluation of canine and feline maxillomandibular trauma cases. Comparison of lunar cycle and seasonality with non-maxillomandibular traumatic injuries (2003–2012). *Vet. Comp. Orthop. Traumatol.* 27: 198–203.

23 Mumford, J.M. (1964). Evaluation of gutta-percha and ethyl chloride in pulp-testing. *Br. Dent. J.* 116: 338–342.

24 Dacht, S.F., Haley, J.V., and Sanders, J.E. (1967). Standardization of a test for dental sensitivity to cold. *Oral Surg. Oral Med. Oral Pathol.* 24: 687–692.

25 Fulling, H.-J. and Andreasen, J.O. (1976). Influence of maturation status and tooth type of permanent teeth upon electrometric and thermal pulp testing. *Scan. J. Dent. Res.* 84: 286–290.

26 Kopel, H.M. and Johnson, R. (1985). Examination and neurologic assessment of children with oro-facial trauma. *Endod. Dent. Traumatol.* 1: 155–159.

27 Rowe, A.H.R. and Pitt Ford, T.R. (1990). The assessment of pulpal vitality. *Int. Endod. J.* 23: 77–83.

28 Bachmann, A. and Lutz, F. (1976). Schmelzsprunge durch die Sensibilitatsprufung mit CO_2_ Schnee und Dichlor-difluormethan – eine vergleichende in-vivo-Untersuchung. *Schheiz. Monatsschr. Zahnheilk.* 86: 1042–1059.

29 Newton, A.V. and Mumford, J.M. (1968). Transduction of square wave stimuli through human teeth. *Arch. Oral Biol.* 13: 831–832.

30 Mumford, J.M. (1966). Drying of enamel under rubber dam. *Br. Dent. J.* 121: 178–179.

31 Remeeus, P. and Verbeek, M. (1997). Use of the dental pulp tester in veterinary dentistry. *J. Vet. Dent.* 14: 23–28.

32 Seltzer, S., Bender, I.B., and Ziontz, M. (1963). The dynamics of pulp inflammation: correlations between diagnostic data and actual histologic findings in the pulp. Part I. *Oral Surg.* 16: 846–871.

33 Olgart, L., Gazelius, B., and Lindh-Stromberg, U. (1988). Laser Doppler flowmetry in assessing vitality in luxated permanent teeth. *Int. Endod. J.* 21: 300–306.

34 Gazelius, B., Olgart, L., and Edwall, B. (1988). Restored vitality in luxated teeth assessed by laser Doppler flowmetry. *Endod. Dent. Traumatol.* 4: 265–268.

35 Andreasen, F.M., Andreasen, J.O., and Tsukiboshi, M. (2007). Examination and diagnosis of dental injuries. In: *Textbook and Color Atlas of Traumatic Injuries to the Teeth*, 255–279. Copenhagen: Blackwell Munksgaard.

36 Evans, D., Reid, J., Strang, R. et al. (1999). A comparison of laser Doppler flowmetry with other methods of assessing the vitality of traumatized anterior teeth. *Endod. Dent. Traumatol.* 15: 284–290.

37 Schnettler, J.M. and Wallace, J.A. (1991). Pulse oximetry as a diagnostic tool of pulp vitality. *J. Endod.* 17: 488–490.

38 Dastmalchi, N., Jafarzadeh, H., and Moradi, S. (2012). Comparison of the efficacy of a custom-made pulse oximeter probe with digital electric pulp tester, cold spray, and rubber cup for assessing pulp vitality. *J. Endod.* 38: 1182–1186.

39 Gopikrishna, V., Tinagupta, K., and Kandaswamy, D. (2007). Evaluation of efficacy of a new custom-made pulse oximeter dental probe in comparison with electrical and thermal tests for assessing pulp vitality. *J. Endod.* 33: 411–414.

40 Pozzobon, M.H., de Sousa Vieira, R., Alves, A.M. et al. (2011). Assessment of pulp blood flow in primary and permanent teeth using pulse oximetry. *Dent. Traumatol.* 27: 184–188.

41 Soukup, J.W., Drees, R., and Koenig, L.J. (2015). Comparison of the diagnostic image quality of the canine maxillary dentoalveolar structures obtained by cone beam computed tomography and 64-multidetector row computed tomography. *J. Vet. Dent.* 32 (2): 80–86.

42 Esmans, M.C., Soukup, J.W., and Schwarz, T. (2014). Optimized canine dental computed tomographic protocol in medium-sized mesaticephalic dogs. *Vet. Radiol. Ultrasound* 55 (5): 506–510. doi: 10.1111/vru.12158 [Epub ahead of print].

43 Lovschall, H., Giannobile, W.V., Somerman, M.J. et al. (2007). Stem cells and regeneration of injured dental tissue. In: *Textbook and Color Atlas of Traumatic Injuries to the Teeth*, 4e (ed. J.O. Andreasen, F.M. Andreasen and L. Andersson). Copenhagen, Denmark: Blackwell Munksgaard.

44 Harran-Ponce, E., Holland, R., Barreiro-Lois, A. et al. (2002). Consequences of crown fractures with pulpal exposure: histopathological evaluation in dogs. *Dent. Traumatol.* 18: 196–205.

45 Cvek, M. (1978). A clinical report on partial pulpotomy and capping with calcium hydroxide in permanent incisors with complicated crown fractures. *J. Endod.* 4: 232–237.

46 Cvek, M., Cleaton-Jones, P.E., Austin, J.C. et al. (1982). Pulp reactions to exposure after experimental crown fractures or grinding in adult monkeys. *J. Endod.* 8: 391–397.

47 Heide, S. and Mijor, I.A. (1983). Pulp reactions to experimental exposures in young permanent monkey teeth. *Int. Endod. J.* 16: 11–19.

48 Nasjleti, C.E., Cafesse, R.G., Castelli, W.A. et al. (1975). Healing after tooth reimplantation in monkeys. A radioautographic study. *Oral Surg. Oral Med. Oral Pathol.* 39: 361–375.

49 Hurst, R.W. (1972). Regeneration of periodontal and transseptal fibres after autografts in Rhesus monkeys. A qualitative approach. *J. Dent. Res.* 51: 1182–1192.

50 Andreasen, J.O. (1980). A time-related study of periodontal healing and root resorption activity after replantation of mature permanent incisors in monkeys. *Swed. Dent. J.* 4: 101–110.

51 Prove, M.P. and Polson, A.M. (1982). Repair in different zones of the periodontium after tooth reimplanation. *J. Periodontol.* 53: 379–389.

52 Borden, S.M. (1948). Histological study of healing following detachment of tissue as is commonly carried out in the vertical incision for the surgical removal of teeth. *Can. Dent. Assoc.* 14: 510–515.

53 Dedolph, T. and Clark, H.B. (1958). A histological study of mucoperiosteal flap healing. *J. Oral Surg.* 16: 367–376.

54 Kohler, C.A. and Ramfjord, S.P. (1960). Healing of gingival mucoperiosteal flaps. *Oral Surg. Oral Med. Oral Pathol.* 13: 89–103.

55 Nwoku, A.L. (1980). Unusually rapid bone regeneration following mandibular resection. *J. Maxillofac. Surg.* 8: 309–315.

56 Shuker, S. (1985). Spontaneous regeneration of the mandible in a child. A sequel to partial avulsion as a result of a war injury. *J. Maxillofac. Surg.* 13: 70–73.

57 Skoglund, A. (1981). Vascular changes in replanted and autotransplanted apicoectomized mature teeth of dogs. *Int. J. Oral Surg.* 10: 100–110.

58 Clark, D.J., Sheets, C.G., and Paquette, J.M. (2003). Definitive diagnosis of early enamel and dentin cracks based on microscopic evaluation. *J. Esthet. Restor. Dent.* 15: 391–401.

59 Crossley, D.A. (1995). Tooth enamel thickness in the mature dentition of domestic dogs and cats: preliminary study. *J. Vet. Dent.* 12 (3): 111–113.

60 Rud, J. and Omnell, K.A. (1970). Root fractures due to corrosion: diagnostic aspects. *Scand. J. Dent. Res.* 78: 397–403.

61 Youssefzadeh, S., Gahleitner, A., Dorffner, R. et al. (1999). Dental vertical root fractures: value of CT in detection. *Radiology* 210: 545–549.

62 Wolcott, J., Rossman, L.E., and Hasselgren, G. (2011). Management of endodontic emergencies. In: *Cohen' Pathways of the Pulp*, vol. 2011, 40–48. St. Louis, MO: Mosby Elsevier.

63 Robb, L., Marx, J., Steenkamp, G. et al. (2007). Scanning electron microscopic study of the dentinal tubules in dog canine teeth. *J. Vet. Dent.* 24: 86–89.
64 Reiter, A.M. and Lewis, J.R. (2008). Dental bulge restoration and gingival collar expansion after endodontic treatment of a maxillary fourth premolar crown-root fracture in a dog. *J. Vet. Dent.* 25: 34–45.
65 Lauridsen, E., Hermann, N.V., Gerds, T.A. et al. (2012). Pattern of traumatic dental injuries in the permanent dentition among children, adolescents, and adults. *Dent. Traumatol.* 28: 358–363.
66 Bender, I.B. and Freedland, J.B. (1983). Clinical considerations in the diagnosis and treatment of intra-alveolar root fractures. *J. Am. Dent. Assoc.* 107: 595–600.
67 Andreasen, F.M. and Andreasen, J.O. (1988). Resorption and mineralization processes following root fracture of permanent incisors. *Endod. Dent. Traumatol.* 4: 202–214.
68 Andreasen, F.M., Andreasen, J.O., and Cvek, M. (2007). Root fractures. In: *Textbook and Color Atlas of Traumatic Injuries to the Teeth*, 337–371. Copenhagen, Denmark: Blackwell Munksgaard.
69 Andreasen, J.O., Andreasen, F.M., Mejare, I. et al. (2004). Healing of 400 intra-alveolar root fractures. 1. Effect of pre-injury and injury factors such as sex, age, stage of root development, fracture type, location of fracture and severity of dislocation. *Dent. Traumatol.* 20: 192–202.
70 Diangelis, A.J., Andreasen, J.O., Ebeleseder, K.A. et al. (2012). International Association of Dental Traumatology Guidelines for the management of traumatic dental injuries: 1. Fractures and luxations of permanent teeth. *Dent. Traumatol.* 28: 2–12.
71 Gracis, M. and Orsini, P. (1998). Treatment of traumatic dental displacement in dogs: six cases of lateral luxation. *J. Vet. Dent.* 15: 65–72.
72 Andreasen, F.M. and Pedersen, B.V. (1985). Prognosis of luxated permanent teeth – the development of pulp necrosis. *Endod. Dent. Traumatol.* 1: 207–220.
73 Hale, F.A. (2001). Localized intrinsic staining of teeth due to pulpitis and pulp necrosis in dogs. *J. Vet. Dent.* 18: 14–20.
74 Ulbricht, R.D., Manfra Marretta, S., and Klippert, L.S. (2004). Mandibular canine tooth luxation injury in a dog. *J. Vet. Dent.* 21: 77–83.
75 Anderson, A.W., Sharav, Y., and Massler, M. (1968). Reparative dentine formation and pulp morphology. *Oral Surg. Oral Med. Oral Pathol.* 26: 837–847.
76 Kvinnsland, I. and Hyeraas, K.J. (1989). Dentin and ostedodentin matrix formation in apicoectomized replainted incisors in cats. *Acta Odontol. Scand.* 47: 41–52.
77 Kvinssland, I. and Heyeraas, K.J. (1990). Cell renewal and ground substance formation in replanted cat teeth. *Acta Odontol. Scand.* 48: 203–215.
78 Skoglund, A. and Tronstad, L. (1978). A morphologic and enzyme histochemical study on the pulp of replanted and autotransplanted teeth in young dogs. *J. Dent. Res.* 57. IADR Abstract no. 478.
79 Skoglund, A., Tronstad, L., and Wallenius, K. (1978). A microangiographic study of vascular changes in replanted and autotransplanted teeth of young dogs. *Oral Surg. Oral Med. Oral Pathol.* 45: 17–28.
80 Skoglund, A., Hasselgren, G., and Tronstad, L. (1981). Oxidoreductase activity in the pulp of replanted and autortransplanted teeth in young dogs. *Oral Surg. Oral Med. Oral Pathol.* 52: 205–209.
81 Cvek, M., Cleaton-Jones, P., Austin, J. et al. (1990). Pulp revascularization in reimplanted immature mondey incisors – predictability and the effect of antiobiotic systemic prophylaxis. *Endod. Dent. Traumatol.* 6: 157–169.
82 Cvek, M., Cleaton-Jones, P., Austin, J. et al. (1990). Effect of topical application of doxycycline on pulp revascularization and periodontal healing in reimplanted monkey incisors. *Endod. Dent. Traumatol.* 6: 170–176.
83 Andreasen, J.O. and Andreasen, F.M. (2007). Avulsions. In: *Textbook and Color Atlas of Traumatic Injuries to the Teeth*, 255–279. Copenhagen, Denmark: Blackwell Munksgaard.
84 Andreasen, J.O. (1981). The effect of pulp extirpation or root canal treatment on periodontal healing after replantation of mature permanent incisors in monkeys. *J. Endod.* 7: 245–252.
85 Andreasen, J.O. (1981). Interrelation between alveolar bone and periodontal ligament repair after replantation of mature permanent incisors in monkeys. *J. Periodontal. Res.* 16: 228–235.
86 Andreasen, J.O. and Hjorting-Hansen, E. (1966). Replantation of teeth. II. Histological study of 22 replanted anterior teeth in humans. *Acta Odont. Scand.* 24: 287–306.
87 Andreasen, J.O. (1971). Treatment of fractured and avulsed teeth. *ASDC J. Dent. Child.* 38: 29–48.
88 Andreasen, J.O. and Schwartz, O. (1986). The effect of saline storage before replantation upon dry damage of the periodontal ligament. *Endod. Dent. Traumatol.* 2: 67–70.
89 Matsson, L., Andreasen, J.O., Cvek, M., and Granath, L. (1982). Ankylosis of experimentally reimplanted teeth related to extra-alveolar period and storage environment. *Pediatr. Dent.* 4: 327–329.
90 Andersson, L., Bodin, I., and Sorensen, S. (1989). Progression of root resorption following replantation of human teeth after extended extraoral storage. *Endod. Dent. Traumatol.* 5: 38–47.

91 Andersson, L. and Bodin, I. (1990). Avulsed human teeth replanted within 15 minutes – a long-term clinical follow-up study. *Endod. Dent. Traumatol.* 6: 37–42.

92 Andreasen, J.O., Borum, M., Jacobsen, H.L. et al. (1995). Replantation of 400 avulsed permanent incisors. IV. Factors related to periodontal ligament healing. *Endod. Dent. Traumatol.* 11: 76–89.

93 Andreasen, J.O. (1987). Experimental dental traumatology: development of a model for external root resorption. *Endod. Dent. Traumatol.* 3: 269–287.

94 Andreasen, J.O., Borum, M., Jacobsen, H.L. et al. (1995). Replantation of 400 avulsed permanent incisors. II. Factors related to pulp healing. *Endod. Dent. Traumatol.* 11: 59–68.

95 Kling, M., Cvek, M., and Mejare, I. (1986). Rate and predictability of pulp revascularization in therapeutically reimplanted permanent incisors. *Endod. Dent. Traumatol.* 2: 83–89.

96 Andersson, L., Andreasen, J.O., Day, P. et al. (2012). International Association of Dental Traumatology guidelines for the management of traumatic dental injuries: 2. Avulsion of permanent teeth. *Dent. Traumatol.* 28: 88–96.

97 Kinirons, M.J., Boyd, D.H., and Gregg, T.A. (1999). Inflammatory and replacement resorption in reimplanted permanent incisor teeth: a study of the characteristics of 84 teeth. *Endod. Dent. Traumatol.* 15: 269–272.

98 Hammarstrom, L., Blomlof, L., Feiglin, B. et al. (1986). Replantation of teeth and antibiotic treatment. *Endod. Dent. Traumatol.* 2: 51–57.

99 Mandel, U. and Vidik, A. (1989). Effect of splinting on the mechanical and histological properties of the healing periodontal ligament in the vervet monkey (*Cercopithecus aethiops*). *Arch. Oral Biol.* 34: 209–217.

100 Andreasen, J.O. (1974). The effect of splinting upon periodontal healing after replantation of permanent incisors in monkeys. *Acta Odontol. Scand.* 33: 313–323.

101 Nasjleti, C.E., Castelli, W.A., and Caffesse, R.G. (1982). The effects of different splinting times on replantation of teeth in monkeys. *Oral Surg. Oral Med. Oral Pathol.* 53: 557–566.

102 Kristerson, L. and Andreasen, J.O. (1983). The effect of splinting upon periodontal and pulpal healing after auto-transplantation of mature and immature permanent incisors in monkeys. *Int. J. Oral Surg.* 12: 239–249.

103 Andersson, L., Lindskog, S., Blomlof, L. et al. (1985). Effect of masticatory stimulation on dentoalveolar ankylosis after experimental tooth replantation. *Endod. Dent. Traumatol.* 1: 13–16.

104 Bauss, O., Schilke, R., Fenske, C. et al. (2002). Auto-transplantation of immature third molars: influence of different splinting methods and fixation periods. *Dent. Traumatol.* 18: 322–328.

105 Andreasen, J.O., Paulsen, H.U., Yu, Z. et al. (1990). A long-term study of 370 auto-transplanted premolars. Part II. Tooth survival and pulp healing subsequent to transplantation. *Eur. J. Orthod.* 12: 14–24.

106 Wesselink, P.R. and Beertsen, W. (1994). Repair processes in the periodontium following dento-alveoloar ankylosis: the effect of masticatory function. *J. Clin. Periodontol.* 21: 472–478.

107 Startup, S. (2010). Wire-composite splint for luxation of the maxillary canine tooth. *J. Vet. Dent.* 27: 198–202.

108 Oikarinen, K.S. (2007). Splinting of traumatized teeth. In: *Textbook and Color Atlas of Traumatic Injuries to the Teeth*, 842–851. Copenhagen: Blackwell Munksgaard.

109 Ngassapa, D.N., Freihofer, H.P., and Maltha, J.C. (1986). The reaction of the periodontium to different types of splints. (I). Clinical aspects. *Int. J. Oral Maxillofac. Surg.* 15: 240–249.

110 Croll, T.P. and Helpin, M.L. (2002). The use of self-etching adhesive system and compomer for splinting traumatized incisors. *Pediatr. Dent.* 24: 53–56.

111 Filippi, A., Von Arx, T., and Lussi, A. (2002). Comfort and discomfort of dental trauma splints – a comparison of a new device (TTS) with three commonly used splinting techniques. *Dent. Traumatol.* 18: 275–280.

112 Prevost, J., Louis, J.P., Vadot, J. et al. (1994). A study of forces originating from orthodontic appliances for splinting teeth. *Endod. Dent. Traumatol.* 10: 179–184.

7

Oral and Maxillofacial Tumors, Cysts, and Tumor-Like Lesions

Jason Soukup[1] *and John Lewis*[2]

[1] *School of Veterinary Medicine, University of Wisconsin-Madison, Madison, WI, USA*
[2] *Veterinary Dentistry Specialists, Chadds Ford, PA*

Knowledge of clinical appearance and biological behavior of maxillofacial tumors is an important component of everyday veterinary practice. This chapter reviews the important clinical information of maxillofacial tumors, cysts, and tumor-like lesions of dogs and cats, including odontogenic tumors, non-odontogenic tumors, odontogenic cysts, bone-associated lesions, and tumor-like lesions of the gingiva and oral mucosa. Staging and incisional biopsy techniques will also be discussed.

7.1 Introduction: Terminology

The term "tumor" is derived from the Latin *tumere*, "to swell." The term has evolved to describe benign or malignant neoplastic disease. Tumors are generally considered to be either benign or malignant. Benign tumors may be locally invasive but do not metastasize to distant sites. Malignant tumors are not only locally invasive but also have the potential to metastasize to other sites in the body. In this chapter we will broadly define tumors and similar lesions of the maxillofacial region as non-odontogenic or odontogenic and then describe their biological nature as either benign or malignant. Odontogenic tumors are defined by the World Health Organization (WHO) as "lesions derived from epithelial, ectomesenchymal, and/or mesenchymal elements that still are, or have been, part of the tooth-forming apparatus." Odontogenic tumors comprise a large portion of oral tumors seen in dogs and are less common in cats than non-odontogenic tumors. Some odontogenic tumors, such as odontomas, are not true tumors. They are hamartomas, which are disorganized accumulations of histologically normal tissues. Any tumor that does not arise from odontogenic tissues is considered to be non-odontogenic. Cysts, on the other hand, are not tumors but rather epithelium lined potential spaces, which, in the maxillofacial region, are generally of odontogenic origin.

"Epulis" is a non-specific, clinical term used to describe tumors and tumor-like masses of the gingiva. The term is derived from the Greek *epi-oulon* meaning "on the gum." In the human literature, the term is used to describe any focal growth of the gingiva. Within the veterinary literature, this term has been used indiscriminately in various contexts and it is the authors' opinion that the term "epulis" should be avoided in lieu of more specific descriptions.

7.2 Maxillofacial Oncological Principles

7.2.1 Clinical Presentation

Oral tumors account for approximately 5% of all canine tumors and approximately 6–10% of feline tumors [1, 2]. In dogs, the oral cavity is the fourth most common site of neoplasia. There is not a definitive gender or breed predilection, but many purebred dogs have been reported to have a higher risk of developing oral tumors, including Cocker Spaniels, Chow Chows, Retrievers, and Poodles.

Dogs and cats are presented once an oral mass is noticed by the pet owner or by its veterinarian during routine physical examination. Some patients have a history of mobile teeth in the area of the tumor, and the cause of tooth mobility may have originally been presumed to be due to periodontal disease. Animals having neoplasia of the caudal oral cavity or tonsils are usually diagnosed later in the course of the disease. Clinical signs of oral tumors include halitosis, oral hemorrhage (spontaneous or after eating, drinking, chewing, or playing with objects), drooling, maxillofacial deformity, difficulty or pain upon opening the mouth, weight loss, or exophthalmos. With advanced maxillary tumors, there

Wiggs's Veterinary Dentistry: Principles and Practice, Second Edition. Edited by Heidi B. Lobprise and Johnathon R. (Bert) Dodd.

is invasion of the nasal cavity with subsequent sneezing, nasal discharge/hemorrhage. Some patients are diagnosed during a professional dental cleaning procedure or are presented for an enlarged mandibular lymph node.

7.2.2 Principles of Tumor Staging

The TNM (Tumor-Node-Metastasis) System devised by the WHO is the standard system for most tumors in veterinary medicine. Currently the TNM is developed and maintained by the Union for International Cancer Control (UICC) to achieve consensus on one globally recognized standard for classifying the extent of spread of cancer. The TNM classification is also used by the American Joint Committee on Cancer (AJCC) and the International Federation of Gynecology and Obstetrics (FIGO). In 1987, the UICC and AJCC staging systems were unified into a single staging system (http://www.uicc.org/resources/tnm). The system is used to assess the extent of tumor involvement based upon primary tumor (T), regional nodes (N), and metastasis (M). Information about the primary tumor, regional lymph nodes, and distant metastasis are used to provide a stage of I, II, III, or IV (Table 7.1).

Table 7.1 Clinical staging (TNM) of oral tumors in dogs and cats. TX or NX can be used initially if the tumor or node cannot be assessed at the time of diagnosis. T0 or N0 can be used if there is no sign of tumor (T0) or if tumor cells are absent from lymph nodes (N0).

T			Tumor
	Tis		Tumor in situ (pre-invasive carcinoma)
	T1		Tumor 2 cm or less at maximum diameter
		T1a	Without bone involvement
		T1b	With bone involvement
	T2		Tumor 2–4 cm maximum diameter
		T2a	Without bone involvement
		T2b	With bone involvement
	T3		Tumor more than 4 cm maximum diameter
		T3a	Without bone involvement
		T3b	With bone involvement
N			Regional lymph nodes (*mandibular, retropharyngeal,* and *parotid*)
	N0		Regional lymph nodes not palpable
	N1		Movable ipsilateral lymph nodes
		N1a	No evidence of lymph node metastasis
		N1b	Evidence of lymph node metastasis
	N2		Movable contralateral lymph nodes
		N2a	No evidence of lymph node metastasis
		N2b	Evidence of lymph node metastasis
	N3		Fixed lymph nodes
M			Distant metastasis
		M0	No evidence of distant metastases
		M1	Distant metastases present

Stage grouping

Stage grouping	T	N	M
I	T1	N0, N1a or N2a	M0
II	T2	N0, N1a or N2a	M0
III	T3	N0, N1a or N2a	
	Any T	N1b	M0
IV	Any T	N2b or N3	M0
	Any T	Any N	M1

TX or NX can be used initially if the tumor or node cannot be assessed at the time of diagnosis.
T0 or N0 can be used if there is no sign of tumor (T0) or if tumor cells are absent from lymph nodes (N0).

Dogs and cats with an oral or maxillofacial tumor should be thoroughly evaluated. A thorough examination and staging can be done under general anesthesia at the time of incisional biopsy. The tumor is palpated and measurements are taken in three dimensions. The tumor's attachment to adjacent tissues can be assessed and categorized as pedunculated or broad-based. The teeth are assessed for mobility and the bone is assessed radiographically. Regional lymph nodes are palpated to assess size and mobility. Mandibular lymph node enlargement may be associated with an oral mass, especially in cases of tonsillar squamous cell carcinoma (SCC) and melanoma. Medial retropharyngeal lymph node enlargement can be difficult to discern because this lymph node is deep in the neck. The parotid lymph node is located at the rostral aspect of the parotid salivary gland and is typically not palpable. Assessment of the retropharyngeal lymph nodes is important, since both the parotid and mandibular nodes drain to the medial retropharyngeal lymph node and anastomotic connections exist from the medial retropharyngeal lymph node to the contralateral medial retropharyngeal node in the dog [3].

Depending on tumor location, the full extent of tumors may be difficult to assess with dental radiography. Computed tomography (CT) is particularly helpful for maxillary, caudal mandibular, and pharyngeal masses. Head and neck CT may diagnose enlargement of the medial retropharyngeal lymph nodes, which may not be evident on clinical examination. CT provides a more sensitive evaluation than three-view thoracic radiographs for detection of small nodule pulmonary metastasis [4]. Three-dimensional CT reconstructions of the primary tumor can be very helpful for surgical planning. Magnetic resonance imaging (MRI) provides assessment of various soft tissues, but is limited in its usefulness in evaluating bone. Since evaluation of bony structures is often important with oral and maxillofacial tumors, CT is often the test of choice for advanced imaging of the mouth, face, and head.

7.2.3 Principles of Diagnostic Imaging

Intraoral radiography is essential in evaluating oral tumors. Malignant tumors often show a combination of bone lysis and periosteal proliferation. Teeth in the area of a malignant tumor often show evidence of root resorption by the encroaching tumor. In contrast, benign tumors may show no lysis or central mineralization (e.g., peripheral odontogenic fibromas (POFs)), or focal lysis (e.g., acanthomatous ameloblastoma), little or no periosteal proliferation, and displacement of teeth rather than root resorption. Radiographic evidence of demineralization may not be evident until greater than 40% of bone becomes demineralized [5]. Since obtaining surgical margins around a tumor may require removal of radiographically normal bone, ostectomy may still be necessary in the absence of significant bony changes, if tumor type dictates aggressive treatment. Intraoral dental radiographs are most helpful when performed with a size 4 or larger phosphor plate or conventional size 4 dental radiographic films.

7.2.4 Principles of Biopsy Acquisition

Incisional biopsy is an important first step to discern the biological behavior of an oral tumor and treatment options. Even when excisional surgery is expected to be the best option, an initial incisional biopsy will help to determine appropriate surgical margins. The goal of incisional biopsy is to obtain a representative sample without increasing morbidity and without making definitive treatment of the tumor more difficult. For most oral tumors, an incisional biopsy is best taken through the oral mucosa rather than through the skin. A variety of instruments may be used, including a number 15 blade, a biopsy punch, a Tru-cut™ biopsy instrument, and in some cases rongeurs. The authors prefer use of a number 15 blade to obtain one or more deep but narrow wedges that may be easily sutured with 4-0 or 5-0 absorbable monofilament on a tapered needle. If the tumor is too friable to hold suture, a variety of hemostatic agents may be used at the biopsy site in lieu of suturing the site. The pet owner should be warned of potential for postoperative bleeding. Some oral masses may exhibit necrotic or severely ulcerated areas: these sites should be avoided in favor of sites without necrosis or infection. If the mass is small and pedunculated, such as in cases of suspected POFs, removal at the level of the normal gingiva is appropriate with careful documentation of where the mass arose from on the dental record to ensure no confusion of the original site when/if further surgery is necessary. When performing regional nerve blocks prior to biopsy, it is important to avoid seeding of the tumor into the deeper tissues via travel of the needle. For example, if a suspected melanoma is centered over the infraorbital foramen, then a maxillary nerve block may be more appropriate than a deep infraorbital block.

The anesthetic event for the incisional biopsy is an opportunity to perform a thorough examination of the patient. Regional lymph node aspirates and photos of the primary tumor site can be obtained for planning of future curative-intent surgery. Debulking of aggressive oral masses is generally unrewarding. In fact, in some cases, debulking may actually cause more morbidity than doing nothing, due to lack of normal healing of tumor tissue and increased bleeding from the debulked site. One exception where debulking may be helpful is with pedunculated tumors: this may provide the opportunity to exchange a large area of tumor ulceration for a smaller area of ulceration at the pedunculated incision site.

7.3 Non-odontogenic Tumors

7.3.1 Malignant Oral and Maxillofacial Tumors

The most common malignant oral tumor in the dog is malignant melanoma (MM), followed by SCC and fibrosarcoma (FSA). In the cat, SCC is the most common oral tumor, accounting for 60–70% of cases, followed by FSA.

7.3.1.1 Malignant Melanoma

MM is the most common oral and maxillofacial tumor in dogs, but oral MM is rare in cats. Breeds with pigmented oral mucosa appear to be predisposed to MM. Melanoma is usually ulcerated and friable, readily bleeding and often pigmented. However, it is not uncommon for MM to be amelanotic (Figure 7.1). Necrosis is common in larger tumors.

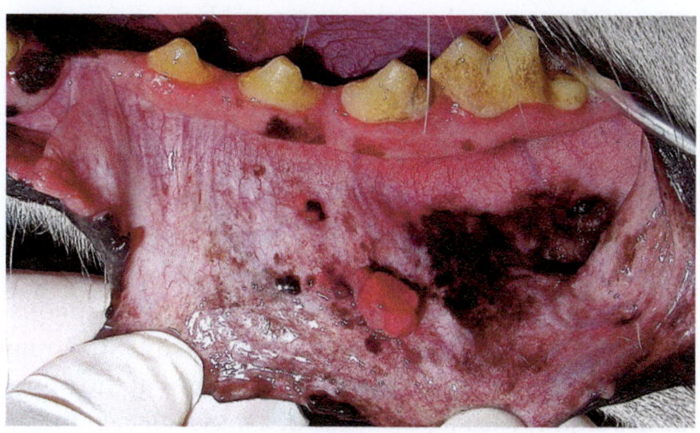

Figure 7.1 Amelanotic melanoma of the left mandibular labial mucosa of a 12-year-old Coonhound. The amelanotic melanoma is surrounded by smaller satellites of melanotic and amelanotic melanoma.

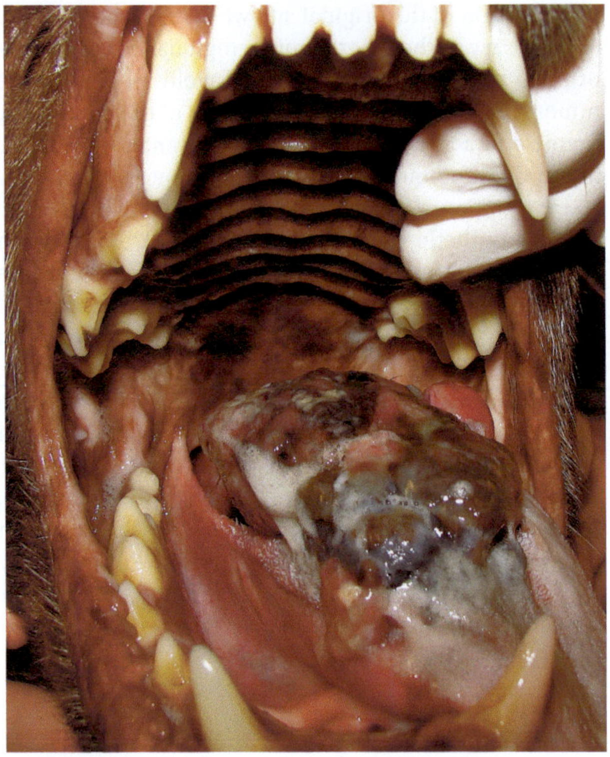

Figure 7.2 Large malignant melanoma of the tongue in a large mixed breed dog.

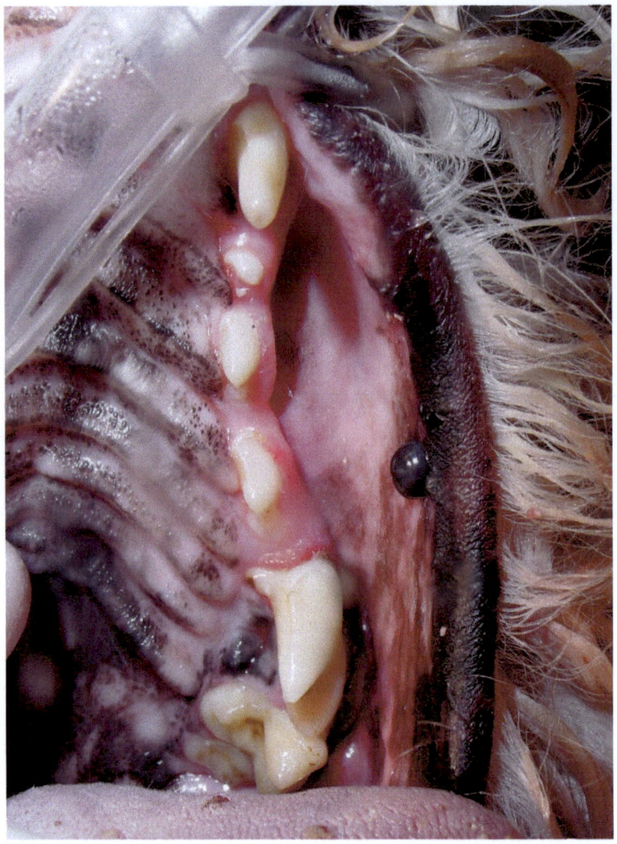

Figure 7.3 Melanocytoma (benign melanocytic tumor) upper lip margin in a dog.

Melanoma is usually located on the tongue, gingiva, and mucosa (alveolar, labial, or buccal mucosa). Large pigmented tumors are likely to be MM (Figure 7.2). Histologically, MM may show a lack of differentiation and be diagnosed as undifferentiated malignant tumor or anaplastic sarcoma. A benign variant of oral melanoma, often referred to as oral melanocytoma, has been described. Melanocytomas tend to be very well circumscribed and less than 1 cm in diameter at the time of diagnosis (Figure 7.3). They respond well to marginal or wide excision rather than radical mandibulectomy or maxillectomy [6]. Oral MM has a variable metastatic rate, with metastasis to the nodes and lungs being common with progressed tumors. There seems to be a great degree of variation in the survival time in dogs treated for MM.

7.3.1.2 Squamous Cell Carcinoma

SCC is the most common oral tumor in cats and the second most common malignant oral tumor in dogs. It usually has the appearance of a pink or red, verrucous, ulcerated mass that may bleed very easily. SCC may be evident as ulceration of the soft tissues of the upper or lower jaw, with no evidence of a mass. Occasionally, cats or dogs with SCC will present with the clinical finding of a loose tooth or teeth, which may be mistaken for periodontal disease. Risk factors in cats may include use of flea collars, eating canned tuna, and canned cat food. Exposure to environmental tobacco smoke increased risk of SCC by two times but was not found to be statistically significant [7]. Tumor biopsy samples from cats exposed to environmental tobacco smoke were 4.5 times more likely to overexpress p53 than were tumors from unexposed cats [8]. SCC rapidly infiltrates bone, especially in the cat. In dogs, the metastatic rate is considered to be low for rostral tumors and high for lingual and tonsillar tumors. Lingual SCC, if small at the time of diagnosis, may be cured by radical glossectomy, but micrometastasis to regional lymph nodes may become apparent after surgery. Though glossectomy may cause significant functional issues in both canine and feline patients, dogs appear to adapt better than cats to radical glossectomy. A multicenter study of 44 dogs with tonsillar SCC showed a median survival time of 179 days (Figure 7.4). Clinical signs of anorexia and lethargy were significantly associated with a poor prognosis [9]. Metastasis rates in feline SCC has historically been considered to be low, but more recent studies suggest a metastatic rate of 31% to the mandibular lymph nodes [10, 11].

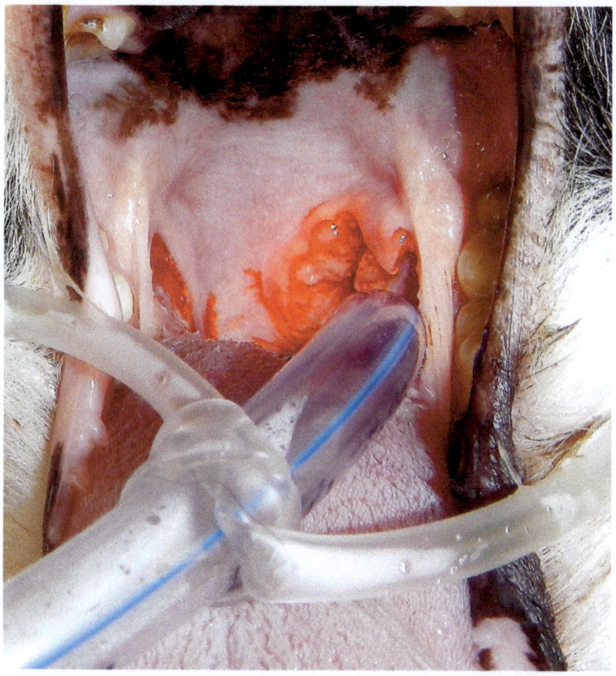

Figure 7.4 Tonsillar squamous cell carcinoma of the left tonsil in a dog.

7.3.1.3 Fibrosarcoma

FSA is the second most common malignant oral and maxillofacial tumor in cats and the third most common in dogs. It occurs more commonly in large breed dogs than in small breed dogs. FSA usually presents as a broad based mass causing a diffuse firm swelling. In some cases, FSA can appear benign histologically and may be misdiagnosed as a fibroma or a low-grade FSA, even with large incisional biopsies, since it may not show typical histopathological criteria of malignancy [12]. Pathologists with an interest in the manifestations of oral neoplasia will often provide the best chance for a correct diagnosis. Treatment of histologically low-grade, biologically high-grade FSA (also called "high-low FSA") must be very aggressive. FSA is infiltrative, and even with advanced diagnostics, it is challenging to discern the full extent of the tumor in dogs and cats. Radical surgery, sometimes in conjunction with post-surgical radiation therapy, provides the best chance for a cure. In one study, prevalence of pulmonary metastasis in dogs with high–low FSA was 12% (3/25 dogs) and regional lymph node metastasis was 20% [12].

7.3.1.4 Malignant Peripheral Nerve Sheath Tumor

Malignant peripheral nerve sheath tumor (MPNST) is an uncommon tumor of the oral cavity, but when it occurs it manifests as a diffuse, poorly delineated mass involving a large portion of the mandible or maxilla. The authors have seen MPNST arising in the area rostral to the infraorbital foramen and as a fleshy mass arising from the mandibular neurovascular bundle, as seen on dental radiographs as bone loss in the area of the mandibular canal. MPNST may be the most challenging oral tumor to prevent local recurrence due to tracking of the tumor along nerve sheaths. Therefore, radical surgery is necessary (2 cm or greater margins) for a possible cure. Prevalence of regional and distant metastasis for MPNST has not been determined.

7.3.1.5 Osteosarcoma

Osteosarcoma (OSA) of the oral cavity often presents as a soft tissue mass, red, and friable, with surrounding bone lysis rather than hard tissue proliferation. Mandibular OSA appears to have a better prognosis than appendicular OSA [13]. In a recent study of canine mandibular OSA, median survival time was 525 days and 58% of dogs developed metastatic disease [14].

7.3.1.6 Hemangiosarcoma

Hemangiosarcoma (HSA) often presents similarly to OSA: a rapidly growing, red, vascular mass with or without bone lysis seen on dental radiographs. In the authors' experience, maxillary and mandibular HSA has been locally invasive with the potential for regional and distant metastasis. However, a study of 20 cases of lingual HSA showed a median overall survival time of 553 days. This suggests lingual HSA may be less aggressive that those arising in other areas of the oral cavity [15]. The authors have rarely seen a case where an HSA in the mouth appeared to be a metastatic lesion from a primary HSA elsewhere in the body. Therefore, staging of oral HSA patients is important prior to performing oral surgery.

7.3.1.7 Multilobular Tumor of Bone

Osteochondrosarcoma (multilobular tumor of bone, chondroma rodens) is a hard, nonulcerated mass, occurring preferentially on the caudal mandible, hard palate, zygomatic arch, base of the skull, and calvarium. The radiographic appearance is a characteristic combination of well-circumscribed mineralized and non-mineralized tissue, which has been referred to as a "popcorn ball" appearance. One study of 39 dogs showed a metastatic rate of 56% and 47% of treated dogs had local recurrence. However, median survival times were good at 797 days [16].

7.3.1.8 Mast Cell Tumor

A mast cell tumor (MCT) occurs rarely in the oral cavity, though the authors have seen MCT arising from the gingiva, the skin lateral to the nasal planum, lips, and tongue. There appears to be a predilection for older male cats to develop cutaneous MCTs, especially in the head and neck region [17]. Cutaneous MCT that occur in the head and neck region of cats tend not to metastasize or show local recurrence after excision. However, aggressive cutaneous MCTs in cats are possible. MCT should be considered as a differential with any waxing and waning oral/perioral mass. A retrospective study of 44 cases of canine oral and perioral MCTs showed 59% of dogs had metastasis at the time of presentation. Overall median survival time was 52 months, which dropped to 14 months for dogs with the presence of lymph node metastasis. Median survival time in dogs without lymph node metastasis was not achieved during the study period [18].

7.3.1.9 Lymphosarcoma

When lymphosarcoma occurs in the oral cavity, it often manifests as a diffuse process referred to as epitheliotropic lymphoma, also called cutaneous T-cell lymphoma. In earlier literature, it was referred to as mycosis fungoides. Clinically, epitheliotropic lymphoma shows diffuse depigmentary changes of the mucosa, adjacent skin, and nasal planum. Gingiva may also be affected and may be diffusely red with punctate areas of increased redness/petechiation [19] (Figure 7.5). Survival times, even with chemotherapy, rarely exceed six months with epitheliotropic lymphoma. Low-grade (indolent) T-cell lymphoma (T-zone lymphoma) may also occur in the oral cavity, which has a much better prognosis, with an overall mean survival time of 4.4 years in one study [20] (Figure 7.6).

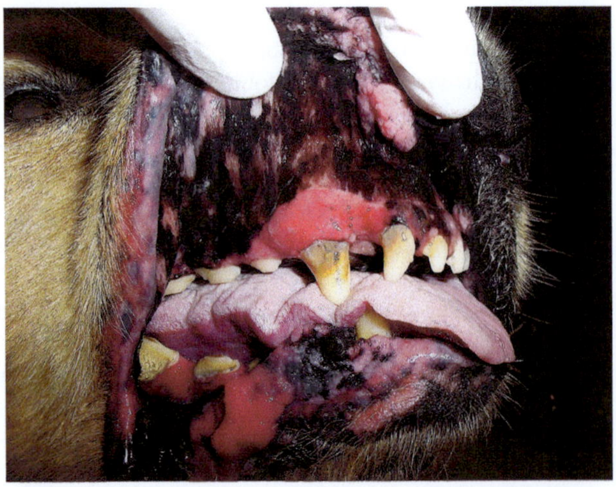

Figure 7.5 Cutaneous T-cell lymphoma in a 10-year-old Golden Retriever. Note the depigmentation of pigmented mucosa and severe hyperemia of the full height of the gingiva.

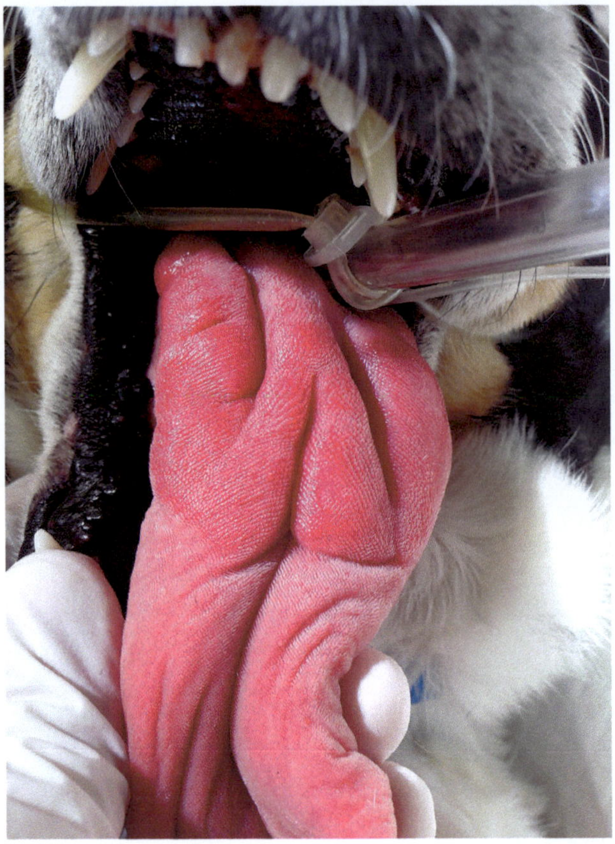

Figure 7.6 T-zone lymphoma of the tongue. In contrast to T-cell lymphoma, T-zone lymphoma is an indolent lymphoma with a good long-term prognosis.

7.3.2 Benign Non-odontogenic Oral Tumors

7.3.2.1 Osteoma

Osteomas may occur in dogs or cats. They have been reported on the hard palate, zygomatic arch, or caudal mandible. Osteomas tend to be very well-circumscribed. Biopsy results may not show obvious characteristics of neoplasia and may show a histopathological diagnosis of normal woven bone. Of four cats treated in one study, surgical treatment of mandibulectomy, maxillectomy, or debulking resulted in greater than one-year survival in all cats [21].

7.3.2.2 Plasmacytoma

Plasmacytomas may arise at various locations, but common locations include the dorsal surface of the tongue and the mucosa of the lips, which manifests as a well-circumscribed, red mass, often less than 1 cm in diameter (Figure 7.7). Surgical margins of 1 cm or slightly less have been curative in cases treated by the authors.

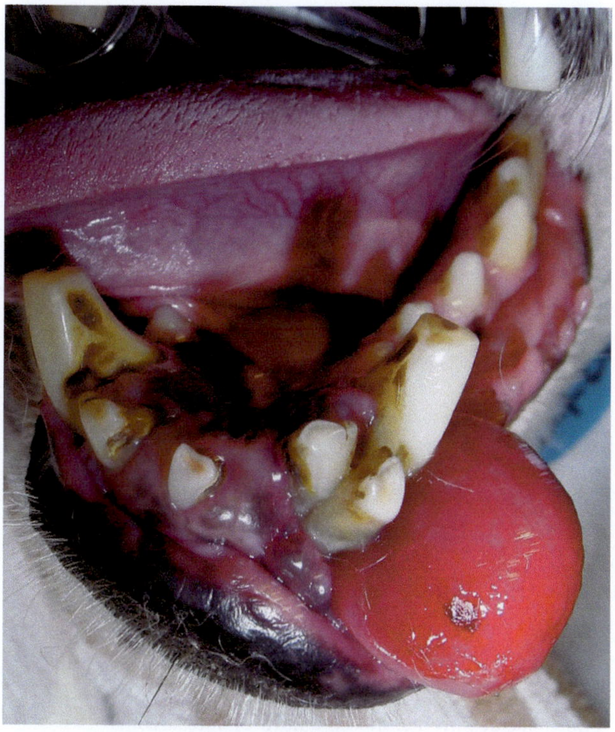

Figure 7.7 Plasmacytoma of the gingiva lateral to the left mandibular canine tooth in a Parson Russell Terrier. Unilateral rostral mandibulectomy was curative in this case.

7.3.2.3 Papilloma

Papillomas are often seen in young dogs as multiple verrucous lesions on the tongue, lips, and cheeks. The untraumatized lesions have a characteristic "sea anemone" appearance. These lesions often regress on their own once young dogs' immune response allows for clearance. Severe refractory cases of oral papillomas may be seen in elderly dogs with concurrent illnesses such as lymphoma or other immunocompromising disease. A recombinant canine oral papillomavirus vaccine has been described for use in refractory cases [22].

7.4 Odontogenic Tumors

7.4.1 Pathogenesis

Possession of a clear understanding of the embryological development of odontogenic structures aids in the understanding of odontogenic tumors in dogs and cats. This process is described in detail in Chapter 1 – Oral Anatomy and Physiology. However, for the purposes of this chapter, there are some important concepts in understanding the development of odontogenic tumors worth discussing here.

The first concept relates to the continued presence of epithelial rests from the degenerating dental lamina and epithelial root sheath upon completion of odontogenesis and tooth eruption. These epithelial rests normally remain quiescent. However, if some carcinogenic or inflammatory mechanism stimulates their proliferation they can develop into an odontogenic tumor or cyst.

The second concept relates to the reciprocal inductive interaction between neural crest-derived ectomesenchymal cells and epithelium that lines the oral cavity. Odontogenic potential depends upon the continued interaction between differentiating odontogenic epithelium and differentiating ectomesenchyme. The degree of interaction, and thus differentiation, of these cell lines to a large degree determines the type of odontogenic tumor that may develop. This process is particularly underscored when considering the histogenesis of ameloblastic fibromas described later in this chapter.

7.4.2 Classification of Odontogenic Tumors

Advances in our understanding of animal odontogenic tumors have transpired since the most recent veterinary classification system was created more than a decade ago [23]. Veterinary pathologists and clinicians have successfully implemented the more inclusive WHO classification system, utilized to classify human odontogenic tumors, to classify most odontogenic tumors in dogs and cats [24–26]. However, the current human classification system does not accommodate a few odontogenic tumors that are described as unique to animals. For the purposes of this chapter, a modification of the 2005 WHO classification system is utilized [27] (Table 7.2).

7.4.3 Odontogenic Tumors

7.4.3.1 Tumors of Odontogenic Epithelium with Mature Fibrous Stroma, Without Odontogenic Ectomesenchyme

7.4.3.1.1 Ameloblastomas

Ameloblastomas are a group of slowly growing, locally invasive tumors of odontogenic epithelial origin. The WHO currently recognizes four distinct biologic subtypes of ameloblastoma based on their clinical behavior in humans: solid/multicystic ameloblastoma, unicystic ameloblastoma, desmoplastic ameloblastoma, and peripheral ameloblastoma [27]. In dogs there is a distinct biologic subtype known as canine acanthomatous ameloblastoma (CAA). The unicystic ameloblastoma has not been reported in animals and it is debatable whether the peripheral ameloblastoma exists in animals [28].

Table 7.2 Comparison between the WHO 2005 classification of odontogenic tumors in man and the author's modified classification of odontogenic tumors in animals.

2005 WHO classification – Human	Author's modified classification – Animals
Malignant Tumors	*Malignant Tumors*
Odontogenic carcinomas	Odontogenic carcinomas
Metastasizing (malignant) ameloblastoma	
Ameloblastic carcinoma – primary type	Ameloblastic carcinoma[a]
Ameloblastic carcinoma – secondary type (dedifferentiated), intraosseous	
Ameloblastic carcinoma – secondary type (dedifferentiated), peripheral	
Primary intraosseous squamous cell carcinoma – solid type	Primary intraosseous squamous cell carcinoma[a]
Primary intraosseous squamous cell carcinoma derived from keratocystic odontogenic tumor	
Clear cell odontogenic carcinoma	
Ghost cell odontogenic carcinoma	
Odontogenic Sarcomas	Odontogenic Sarcomas
Ameloblastic fibrosarcoma	Ameloblastic fibrosarcoma
Ameloblastic fibrodentino- and fibro-odontosarcoma	Ameloblastic fibrodentino- and fibro-odontosarcoma
Benign Tumors	*Benign Tumors*
Odontogenic epithelium with mature, fibrous stroma without odontongenic ectomesenchyme	Odontogenic epithelium with mature, fibrous stroma without odontongenic ectomesenchyme
Ameloblastoma, solid/multicystic type	Ameloblastoma, solid/multicystic type
Ameloblastoma, extraosseous/peripheral type	
Ameloblastoma, desmoplastic type	Ameloblastoma, desmoplastic type
Ameloblastoma, unicystic type	
Squamous odontogenic tumor	
Calcifying epithelial odontogenic tumor	Calcifying epithelial odontogenic tumor
Adenomatoid odontogenic tumor	
Keratocystic odontogenic tumor	
	Amyloid producing odontogenic tumor
Odontogenic epithelium with odontogenic ectomesenchyme, with or without hard tissue formation	Odontogenic epithelium with odontogenic ectomesenchyme, with or without hard tissue formation
Ameloblastic fibroma	Ameloblastic fibroma
Ameloblastic fibrodentinoma	Ameloblastic fibrodentinoma
Ameloblastic fibro-odontoma	Ameloblastic fibro-odontoma
Odontoma	Odontoma
Odontoma, complex type	Odontoma, complex type
Odontoma, compound type	Odontoma, compound type
Odontoameloblastoma	
Calcifying cystic odontogenic tumor	Calcifying cystic odontogenic tumor
Dentinogenic ghost cell tumor	
	Feline inductive odontogenic tumor
Mesenchyme and/or odontogenic ectomesenchyme with or without odontogenic epithelium	Mesenchyme and/or odontogenic ectomesenchyme with or without odontogenic epithelium

Table 7.2 (Continued)

2005 WHO classification – Human	Author's modified classification – Animals
Odontogenic fibroma	Peripheral odontogenic fibroma
Odontogenic myxoma/myxofibroma	Odontogenic myxoma/myxofibroma
Cementoblastoma	
Bone-related lesions	Bone-related lesions
Ossifying fibroma	Ossifying fibroma
Fibrous dysplasia	Fibrous dysplasia
Osseous dysplasia	
Central giant cell lesion (granuloma)	Central giant cell lesion (granuloma)
Cherubism	
Aneurysmal bone cyst	Aneurysmal bone cyst
Simple bone cyst	

[a] Due to lack of appropriate documentation, no distinction between PIOSCC variants is made.

7.4.3.1.2 Solid/Multicystic Ameloblastoma

The solid/multicystic ameloblastoma is also recognized as the central ameloblastoma, classical intraosseous ameloblastoma, and conventional ameloblastoma [27]. There are two histologic patterns – follicular and plexiform. The follicular pattern includes four recognized histologic variants. When the central cells of the epithelial islands are spindle-shaped, basaloid, granular, or show squamous differentiation, they are referred to as spindle cell ameloblastoma, basal cell ameloblastoma, granular ameloblastoma, and acanthomatous ameloblastoma, respectively [27]. The histologic variants are believed to represent only variation in histological presentation and not variation in biological behavior or prognosis. Note that the acanthomatous ameloblastoma described here is not considered analogous to the CAA described in more detail below.

7.4.3.1.3 Desmoplastic Ameloblastoma

The desmoplastic ameloblastoma is a rare biologic subtype of the ameloblastoma in humans marked by a dominant accumulation of dense connective tissue/stroma (desmoplasia) [27]. It is also very rare in dogs and cats. A thorough literature search only reveals one reported case in a dog [26]. One author of the current chapter (JS) has seen several additional cases.

7.4.3.1.4 Canine Acanthomatous Ameloblastoma

The CAA is one of the more common oral tumors in dogs, with one study reporting a prevalence of 45% of all odontogenic tumors biopsied [26]. However, other studies have reported a lower prevalence [29, 30]. While it may share some histological features, the biological behavior and radiological features of the CAA are not completely analogous to any of the histologic variants of the solid/multicystic ameloblastoma recognized in humans. Some have equated the CAA to the human peripheral ameloblastoma due to its apparent origin within the gingival epithelium [29, 31]. However, the CAA may arise either peripherally or intraosseously in dogs, whereas in humans the peripheral ameloblastoma always occurs peripherally and never invades bone [32].

7.4.3.2 Clinical Presentation of Ameloblastomas in Animals

The clinical presentation, biological behavior, and radiological features of ameloblastomas are dependent on the biologic subtype. For example, the solid/multicystic ameloblastoma generally presents as a slow-growing, expansile lesion of the jaw with no (or minimal) gingival involvement and uni- to multilocular radiolucency on radiographs or imaging (Figure 7.8). A recent study in dogs reported ameloblastomas to present as either primarily intraosseous lesions or as primarily extraosseous lesions, which could be appreciated on computed tomographic imaging [33]. The intraosseous presentation will be more often seen in solid/multicystic ameloblastomas. The CAA is the most common type of ameloblastoma in animals and more commonly presents as an extraosseous lesion with an irregular surface that arises within the gingiva [33] (Figure 7.9). Enlargement of ameloblastomas may displace teeth and invade the underlying bone [32]. The CAA is often reported to be more common in the mandible, particularly the rostral mandible, than the maxilla and typically affects middle-aged dogs [26, 30, 32, 34, 35]. One study reported the mean age of 68 dogs

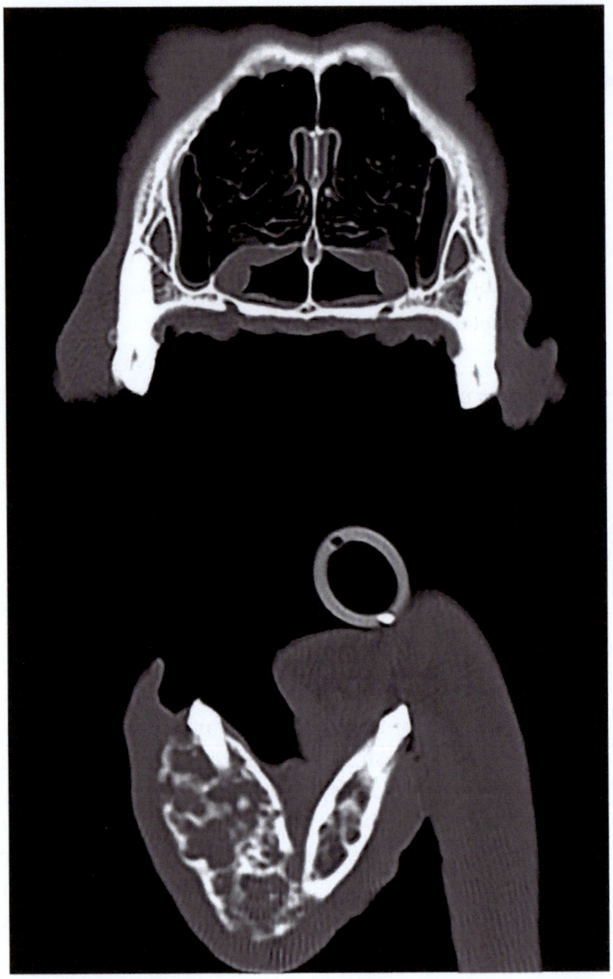

Figure 7.8 Computed tomographic (CT) image of a solid/multicystic ameloblastoma of the right rostral mandible. Note the multi-locular appearance.

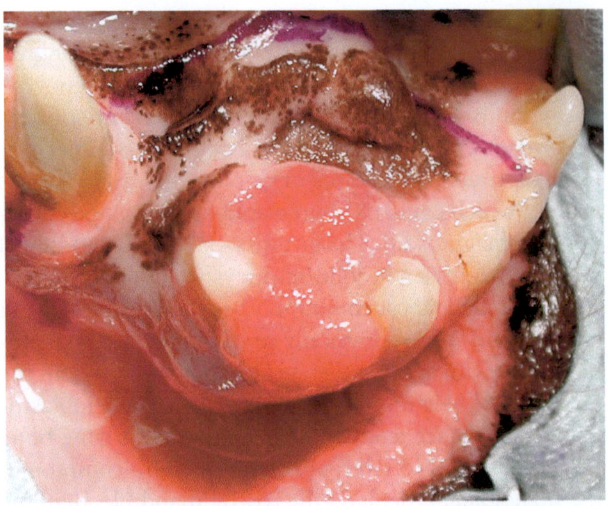

Figure 7.9 Photograph of a left maxillary canine acanthomatous ameloblastoma.

diagnosed with CAA to be 8.8 ± 2.6 years of age at the time of presentation [26]. Golden Retrievers, Akitas, Cocker Spaniels, and Shetland Sheepdogs may be overrepresented; however, no clearly documented sex predilection is apparent [26].

7.4.3.3 Treatment of Ameloblastomas in Animals

Given that the most common location of ameloblastomas in animals is the rostral mandible, complete surgical excision is realistic and prognosis with clean margins is good to excellent, making wide surgical excision the treatment of choice [26, 36, 37] (see Chapter 14 – Oral Surgery – Oral and Maxillofacial Tumors, for more detail on surgical management). However, non-surgical alternatives have been described. Radiation therapy has been utilized in dogs and cats with variable results [35, 38–41]. This variability is likely to be due to the fact that the biologic subtypes of ameloblastomas may possess different biological behaviors. Some ameloblastomas are located primarily within bone and are, as such, more radioresistant [42]. However, radiation therapy may remain a viable treatment option for those tumors that are too large to resect completely. Additionally, intralesional bleomycin has been used with some success in small populations of dogs [43, 44].

7.4.3.4 Amyloid Producing Odontogenic Tumor and Calcifying Epithelial Odontogenic Tumor

The amyloid producing odontogenic tumor (APOT) and calcifying epithelial odontogenic tumor (CEOT) are very similar (if not essentially the same) variants of a locally invasive epithelial odontogenic neoplasm that have been reported in several species. The CEOT was first described in humans by Pindborg in 1955; therefore CEOTs are often referred to as Pindborg tumors in the literature. Most CEOT cases that were described in the earlier veterinary literature [31, 45–49] have subsequently been designated as APOT by more contemporary authors [50]. However, a few published reports of CEOTs in animals do seem to fit the criteria for CEOT described in humans [45, 46, 48, 49]. While amyloid deposits are the distinguishing histologic feature described for APOT, amyloid deposits are often found in CEOTs as well. For this reason, the authors support the argument that the APOT and CEOT are the same type of tumor only that the CEOT undergoes a process in which the amyloid deposits become mineralized. More recently, biochemical and immunohistochemical evidence has been provided to support the contention that the amyloid in APOT is derived from ameloblasts [51, 52]. Thus, the APOT and CEOT may simply be additional histologic variants of a biologic subtype of ameloblastoma.

Clinically, CEOT and APOT present as a slow-growing, expansile mass, similar to the ameloblastoma, in middle-aged to older animals with radiologic features of a uni- to multilocular radiolucency (Figure 7.10). When the amyloid deposits become mineralized, as in the CEOT, there is typically a mixed radiolucent–radiopaque appearance. They do not appear to metastasize and can be successfully treated with surgical resection. However, too few cases have been reported, most with little to no detail of the clinical aspects of the case, to fully appreciate the biologic behavior of these tumors. Upon review of the cases reported in the literature, these tumors appear to have a high recurrence rate. However, the surgical method employed (enucleation and curettage versus surgical resection with margins) is poorly described and caution must be used when evaluating the available data. In the authors' experience, the chance of recurrence with 1 cm surgical margins is low.

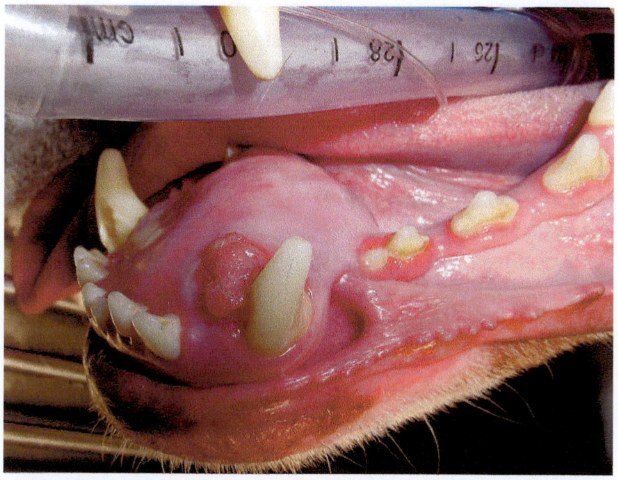

Figure 7.10 Amyloid-producing odontogenic tumor (APOT) in a six-year-old Pit Bulldog.

7.4.3.5 Tumors of Odontogenic Epithelium with Odontogenic Ectomesenchyme, with or without Hard Tissue Formation

7.4.3.5.1 Ameloblastic Fibroma, Ameloblastic Fibro-dentinoma, and Ameloblastic Fibro-odontoma

The WHO defines the ameloblastic fibroma as a mixed odontogenic neoplasm consisting of "odontogenic mesenchyme resembling the dental papilla and epithelial strands and nests resembling dental lamina and enamel organ" [27]. When dentin is present the lesion is known as ameloblastic fibro-dentinoma. When both enamel and dentin are present the lesion is known as ameloblastic fibro-odontoma. As such, these entities simply represent differing points along a spectrum of differentiation.

The ameloblastic fibroma, ameloblastic fibro-dentinoma, and ameloblastic fibro-odontoma have been reported in dogs and cats [23, 25, 53–62]. Although very little information regarding the biologic behavior of these tumors is available in the literature, they are generally considered to be benign and slow-growing tumors that tend not to infiltrate bone [55]. Radiographically, they often present as unilocular expansile lesions of the jaws with a central radiolucency [55]. Ameloblastic fibro-dentinomas and fibro-odontomas may also contain numerous small, calcified densities within the radiolucent center depending on the degree of organization of the enamel and dentin (Figure 7.11a,b).

Due to the paucity of literature regarding treatment, appropriate surgical management is based primarily on

(a) (b)

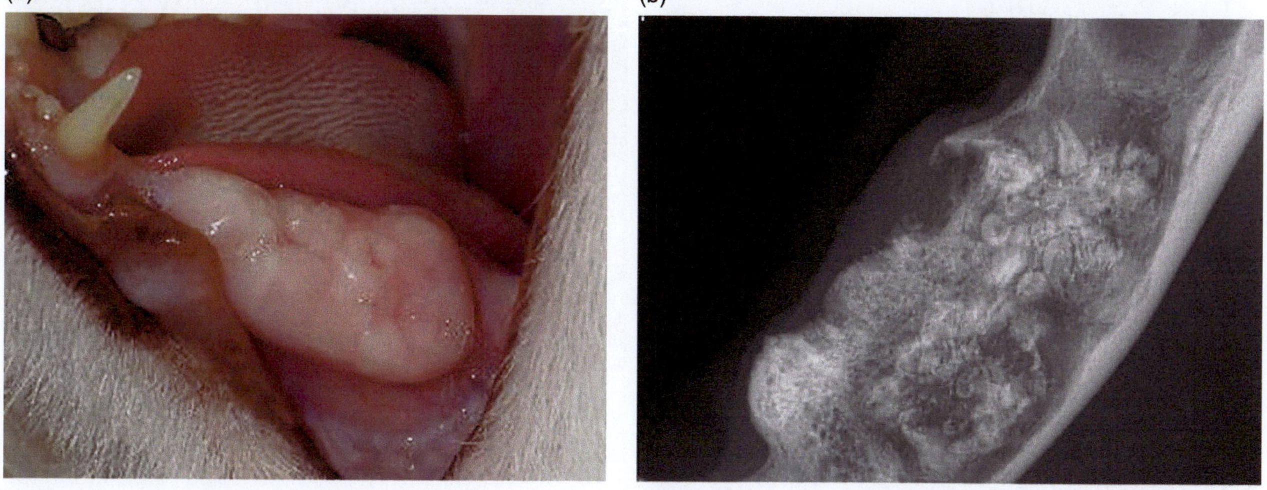

Figure 7.11 (a) Photograph and (b) intraoral radiograph (b) of an ameloblastic fibro-odontoma of the left mandible of a cat. *Source:* Photograph courtesy of Dr. Don Otten.

the human literature. Although the treatment method was not clearly stated, one report found no recurrence after treatment of an ameloblastic fibroma in a 14 year old cat [53]. Available literature on the management of ameloblastic fibromas in humans and animals supports an en bloc resection (ameloblastic fibroma) or surgical enucleation (ameloblastic fibro-dentinoma and -odontoma) and a good to excellent prognosis. In general, the more well differentiated the lesion, the more conservative the surgical approach can be.

7.4.3.5.2 Feline Inductive Odontogenic Tumor

The feline inductive odontogenic tumor (FIOT) is a rare mixed odontogenic tumor of cats that has also been referred to as inductive fibroameloblastoma. While the FIOT is currently recognized as a distinct histologic entity, initially described by Gardner and Dubielzig [63], many consider the FIOT to simply be a histologic variant (albeit unique to cats) of the more common ameloblastic fibroma described above [53, 54, 64, 65]. In fact, its typical biological behavior is identical to that of the ameloblastic fibroma. As the name implies, it is noted for its inductive behavior. However, many odontogenic tumors have the same inductive potential. The FIOT classically is considered a central tumor typically presenting as a large swelling of the rostral maxilla in young cats. Radiologic evaluation of the rostral maxilla reveals an expansile osteolytic lesion with variable amounts of periosteal proliferation with or without impacted teeth (Figure 7.12a,b). The FIOT is locally infiltrative with no known metastatic potential.

Similar to most odontogenic tumors, no case controlled studies have been performed to evaluate the appropriate treatment for FIOTs. However, if one considers it to be a variant of the ameloblastic fibroma, reliance on the treatment recommendations for ameloblastic fibromas becomes more appropriate. In this regard, the tumor does not appear to be radioresponsive and it appears that if the tumor is surgically resected in its entirety, similar to the ameloblastic fibroma, the tumor is unlikely to recur and the prognosis is good to excellent.

7.4.3.5.3 Odontoma

Often regarded as hamartomas rather than neoplasias, odontomas are characterized by their high degree of odontogenic differentiation and morphogenesis [27]. The *compound odontoma* is distinguished from the *complex odontoma* based on its high degree of differentiation, which allows for the arrangement of dental tissues into discrete tooth-like structures known colloquially as denticles.

Both variants typically present as asymptomatic alveolar swellings in the maxilla or mandible of young dogs. A deviation from the normal quantity of teeth either in the form of a mixed dentition, supernumerary teeth, or clinically absent (impacted) teeth is a common presentation. The radiologic appearance is often described as near pathognomonic and consists of an invasive, osteolytic, expansile lesion of mixed central radiopacity with a corticated border adjacent to a thin radiolucent margin [66]. The presence of denticles within a central radiolucent zone is a pathognomonic feature of the compound odontoma. Odontomas have tremendous growth potential, which allows them to reach particularly large sizes in the maxilla. The prognosis of odontomas is excellent with appropriate surgical treatment, which typically is conservative enucleation and curettage [67].

(a) (b)

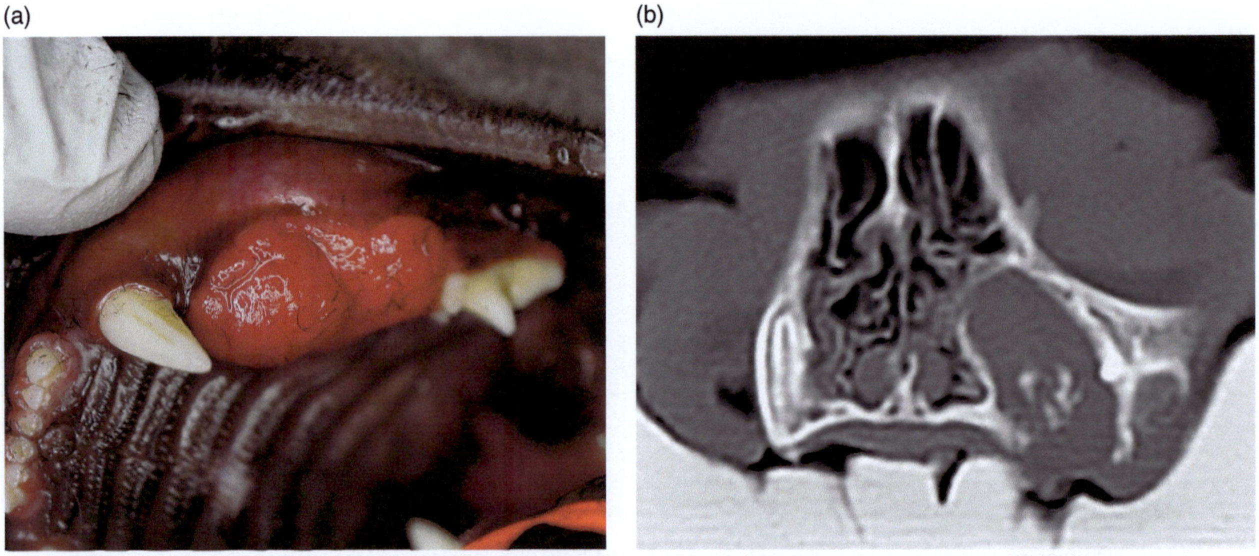

Figure 7.12 (a) Photograph and (b) CT of a left maxillary feline inductive odontogenic tumor.

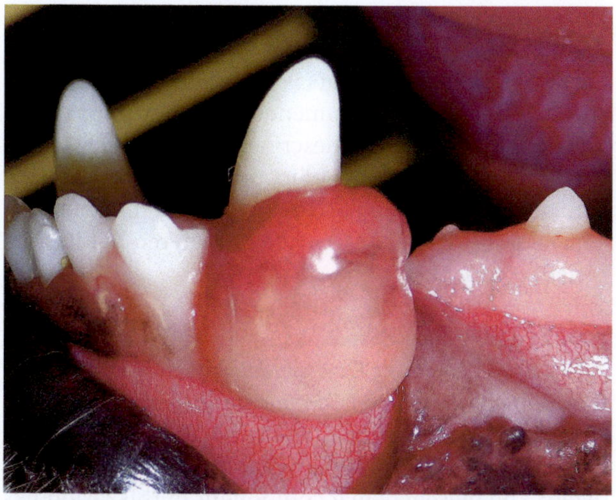

Figure 7.13 Photograph of a peripheral odontogenic fibroma affecting the labial gingival of the left mandibular canine tooth. *Source:* Photograph courtesy of Dr. Don Otten.

7.4.3.6 Tumors of Mesenchyme and/or Odontogenic Ectomesenchyme with or without Odontogenic Epithelium

7.4.3.6.1 Peripheral Odontogenic Fibroma

In the dog, the POF is typically a firm, sessile to pedunculated, non-ulcerated lesion that is most often associated with the free gingiva of a tooth [23, 26, 27, 34, 68] (Figure 7.13). However, infrequently, it is seen primarily in the attached gingiva rather than the free gingiva. Additionally, some cases may be seen in which the lesion is broad-based, spanning the distance of several teeth with no clear delineation between normal and abnormal tissue. There is no clear predilection for age, sex, breed, or jaw location [26]. Although the POF does not possess invasive features, as it enlarges it may lead to secondary periodontitis and may become traumatized during mastication. The radiographic appearance is usually that of only a soft tissue swelling. Because the POF is not an invasive lesion, underlying alveolar bone involvement is only present in the face of secondary periodontitis. However, due to the propensity of the lesion to undergo osseous metaplasia, mineralization is sometimes seen within the center of the lesion (ossifying type, described below) and may be continuous with the underlying alveolar bone in larger lesions.

There are two variants of the POF historically described in the dog: fibromatous and ossifying types, which are analogous to the historical identifiers fibromatous epulis and ossifying epulis [69], respectively. The only difference between the two variants is the presence of osseous metaplasia within the ossifying type, which has minimal impact on the treatment or prognosis.

Although some have suggested that the lesion is of periodontal ligament origin, others argue that POFs arise from the gingiva or underlying periosteum at or near the cementoenamel junction rather than within the periodontal ligament proper. Histologic evaluation of numerous en bloc sections of POF have shown that the base of the proliferative neoplastic fibrous tissue is almost exclusively anchored to the periosteal surface of the alveolar crestal bone near the cementoenamel junction with no involvement of the periodontal ligament proper (JS, personal observation). Therefore, although tooth extraction, or even *en bloc* resection of the tumor and associated teeth, has been historically advocated by many, a conservative approach may be appropriate. Local conservative excision of the tumor with particular attention paid to removing the entire lesion, excising down to and including the affected periosteum, should be anticipated to be curative. Such an approach may, however, require reconstruction of the gingiva surrounding the remaining tooth. Recurrence is likely if the entire lesion is not excised. More aggressive treatments may be reserved for recurrent lesions or those that have a more regional broad-based presentation.

7.4.3.6.2 Feline "Epulides"

Although we have previously stated that the term epulis (plural – epulides) should be avoided whenever possible, it is quite difficult to avoid the use of the term as it pertains to gingival masses in the cat. While some state that the feline epulis is analogous to the POF in dogs, it is not clear whether clinicopathologic features of POF in dogs and CAA can be extrapolated to this similar entity in the cat. The veterinary literature describes the fibromatous, ossifying, and acanthomatous epulis in the cat [70, 71]. A unique feature common to most feline epulides is the presence of a combination of fibromatous, ossifying, and acanthomatous features within the same lesion. This clearly makes classification a challenge.

It is clear that surgical management of feline epulides, while recommended, is not as straightforward as is the case with canine POF. This is due to the fact that most cats are presented with multifocal lesions, making local surgical excision alone challenging. Recurrence with such a conservative approach is likely and some cases require multiple extractions and gingivectomy to achieve complete resolution.

7.4.3.6.3 Odontogenic Myxoma/Myxofibroma

Odontogenic myxomas are mesenchymal tumors that arise from the developing dental papilla, occasionally found in conjunction with a large amount of collagen present. When the latter is the case, the more appropriate designation is odontogenic myxofibroma [27].

Due to their rarity, few generalities can be made regarding their clinical behavior other than to say that metastasis has not been reported in animals. In dogs and cats the tumor has been described as a slow-growing, mandibular swelling typically with a uni- to multilocular radiolucency described as a honeycomb (aka soap-bubble) pattern [72, 73]. Displacement or resorption of adjacent tooth roots and cortical expansion may also be seen.

Odontogenic myxomas are highly infiltrative necessitating surgical resection with at least 1 cm margins. The expression of antiapoptotic proteins has been associated with a high recurrence rate in humans [66].

7.4.4 Malignant Odontogenic Tumors

Malignant odontogenic tumors (MOTs) may be presumed to be extremely rare in dogs and cats. Most of the MOTs are defined by histologic criteria of malignancy rather than documented metastasis [27]. The few available reports in animals describe tumors with infiltrative behavior and cytologic features of malignancy. A single published report describes metastasis of a malignant ameloblastic fibro-odontoma [74]. The rarity of MOT and the minimal degree of information regarding their biological behavior warrants some degree of caution when considering the diagnosis of MOT in animals. Local surgical control remains the primary treatment objective for MOT and recommendations for margins follow those of their benign counterparts [66]. However, the potential for regional and systemic spread must be considered. Adjunct chemotherapy may be instituted but true effectiveness in unknown at this time. MOTs may be broadly described as either odontogenic carcinomas or odontogenic sarcomas.

7.4.4.1 Odontogenic Carcinomas

7.4.4.1.1 Ameloblastic Carcinoma

Ameloblastic carcinomas are one of the few MOTs that have been reported in dogs [25, 26, 29, 75, 76]. According to the diagnostic criteria established by the WHO [27], and as followed in most animal reports, the diagnosis of ameloblastic carcinoma is made based on histologic signs of malignancy (cellular atypia) and aggressive behavior of the tumor rather than documented evidence of metastatic spread.

7.4.4.1.2 Primary Intraosseous Squamous Cell Carcinoma

Odontogenic rests and the epithelial lining of odontogenic cysts may give rise to SCC [27]. In such an occurrence the term primary intraosseous squamous cell carcinoma (PIOSCC) is appropriately used. PIOSCC is a rare central jaw carcinoma derived from odontogenic epithelial remnants that is described in humans and dogs [27, 53]. Given the central nature of the neoplasia, they may be discovered incidentally on routine radiography. However, they may also lead to cortical bone expansion. Only two cases fitting this criterion have been described in dogs [53]. However, the authors has seen canine and feline cases that fit the features of this tumor. The biological behavior of PIOSCC in dogs and cats is unknown. However, wide surgical excision is recommended. From a comparative aspect, these tumors are described as moderately differentiated, but possess the ability to spread locoregionally and distantly in people. Based on this information, adjuvant chemotherapy may be considered but its true benefit is unknown.

7.4.4.2 Odontogenic Sarcomas

7.4.4.2.1 Ameloblastic Fibrosarcoma, Ameloblastic Fibrodentinosarcoma, and Fibroodontosarcoma

A malignant variant of the ameloblastic fibroma discussed above, known as the ameloblastic FSA, is recognized. The mesenchymal component in this lesion has the appearance of an FSA. Rare cases of ameloblastic FSA, ameloblastic fibrodentinosarcoma, and ameloblastic fibroodontosarcoma have been reported in dogs and cattle [25, 29, 34, 74]. Generally speaking, too little evidence exists to clearly understand the biologic behavior or metastatic potential in dogs at this time. However, surgical management recommendations remain similar to those recommendations made for their benign counterparts.

7.5 Benign Tumor-Like Lesions

7.5.1 Focal Fibrous Hyperplasia

Focal fibrous hyperplasia (FFH) is an overexuberant repair of fibrous connective tissue that in dogs and cats is likely to be secondary to chronic gingival trauma and/or irritation [34, 77]. Histologically, exuberant stromal collagen, with or without osseous metaplasia, underlies mucosal epithelium that is often hyperplastic and/or hyperkeratotic. FFH is one of the most common oral masses seen in dogs, representing between 16% and 57% of all oral lesions [26, 29, 30]. This lesion presents as a broad-based, painless swelling that is most often found in the rostral maxilla. The lesion is easily treated by surgical excision and removal of the inciting trauma/source of inflammation, which is often periodontal disease.

7.5.2 Pyogenic Granuloma

The pyogenic granuloma represents a reactive lesion of the gingiva or mucosa characterized by exuberant connective tissue proliferation in response to an injury [77, 78]. The clinical lesion is a raised, broad-based or pedunculated, red lesion with an ulcerated surface (Figure 7.14). The ulcerated surface is often covered by a yellow,

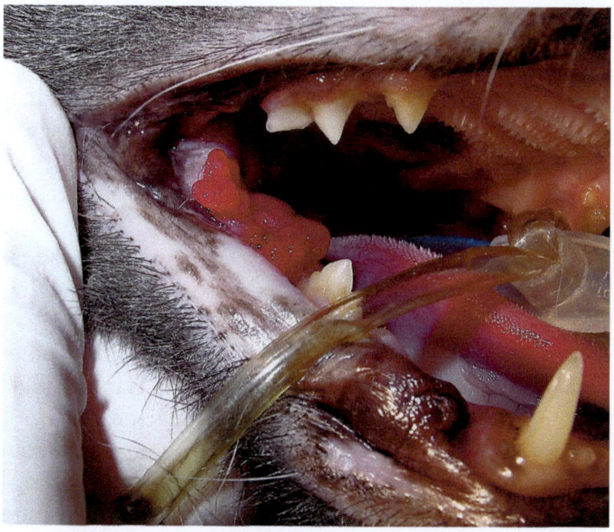

Figure 7.14 Pyogenic granuloma in the area of a missing right mandibular first molar tooth in a cat.

fibrinous membrane. Differential diagnosis includes FFH, plasmacytic gingivostomatitis, SCC (particularly in cats), and chronic proliferative gingivitis. Two recent publications characterize this entity as it occurs in cats in the buccal mucosa of the mandibular first molar [79, 80]. The etiology of pyogenic granuloma in this particular location in cats appears to be caused by trauma to the mucosa from the maxillary fourth premolar secondary to an as yet undefined malocclusion. Previous surgical extraction of the mandibular molar may be a predisposing factor [79]. Additionally, pyogenic granuloma may be seen in association with severe proliferative inflammation of the palatoglossal arches that typically accompanies feline chronic gingivostomatitis. Surgical excision combined with removal of etiologic factors is curative. In cases of the maxillary fourth premolar contacting the mandibular vestibular mucosa, crown reduction and odontoplasty, or extraction, of the maxillary fourth premolar and surgical excision of the lesion most often results in resolution of the lesion in the authors' experience.

7.5.3 Peripheral Giant Cell Granuloma

Peripheral giant cell granuloma (PGCG) is a hyperplastic response to an injury, rather than a neoplasm [81]. With a prevalence of 0.99% of all gingival "epulides," as reported in one canine study, it is a rare lesion [82]. However, in cats the reported prevalence is as high as 28.8% of all feline "epulides" [70]. Although it is an uncommon lesion, it has been described in man, dogs, and cats [70, 81–83]. In the veterinary literature it is sometimes referred to as the giant cell epulis. The presence of abundant multinucleated giant cells (possibly related to osteoclasts) within a background of vascular, fibroblastic connective tissue is the characterizing histologic feature. PGCG most often affects middle-aged dogs and cats and may have a propensity to occur in the maxilla rather than the mandible [70, 82]. Marginal surgical excision of the lesion should be curative [82]. The incidence of recurrence is low and cases of recurrence are believed to be a result of incomplete excision [82].

7.6 Non-neoplastic Bone-Related Maxillofacial Lesions

7.6.1 Aneurysmal Bone Cyst

The aneurysmal bone cyst is a reactive pseudocyst of the maxillofacial region that has not previously been described in small animals. However, it has been described in horses and a bull [84–86]. The etiology is uncertain and has been ascribed to trauma, vascular malformation, or disruption of normal osseous hemodynamics. They generally occur as a rapidly developing and progressive swelling of the jaws. Radiographic studies most often reveal a uni- to multilocular radiolucency of the affected jaw with cortical expansion and thinning. Cortical perforation may occur but, in humans, spread into the adjacent soft tissues has not been reported. In general, treatment by enucleation and curettage is effective and recurrence is dependent upon complete removal. In larger cases, surgical resection may be required.

7.6.2 Central Giant Cell Granuloma (Giant Cell Lesion)

The central giant cell lesion is another bone-related lesion that, like many others, is quite rare in animals [87, 88]. Although some have suggested that the lesion is a reparative response to trauma or intraosseous hemorrhage, in most cases there is no evidence to support this reasoning. Therefore, the lesion should be considered to have an idiopathic etiology.

Central giant cell lesions present as asymptomatic expansile swelling of the jaws that are seen as uni- to multilocular radiolucent defects on radiological examination. Lesions may or may not have an aggressive behavior. Aggressive lesions typically are characterized by pain, rapid progression, and cortical perforation.

Non-aggressive lesions may be treated with curettage of the central lesion. However, more aggressive and recurrent lesions may require more radical surgical excision to achieve a cure [66].

7.7 Benign Fibro-osseous Lesions

7.7.1 Ossifying (Cementifying) Fibroma

The ossifying fibroma is a benign non-odontogenic, fibro-osseous lesion composed of fibrous, osseous, and sometimes cementum-like tissue [23]. While some suggest that this lesion is of odontogenic origin, lesions have also been reported in non-oral locations such as the cranium [89].

Ossifying fibromas present as local asympotomatic swellings of the jaw generally with distinct margins [90, 91]. Radiographically, the lesion may present with a completely radiolucent center (when composed primarily of fibrous tissue) or with a mixed radiopaque center (when composed of fibrous and mineralized tissue). Ossifying fibromas may exhibit some degree of bony lysis on imaging [92] (Figure 7.15a,b). A predilection for the mandible appears to be present in dogs and humans. The treatment recommendation is dependent on the biological behavior of the lesion as determined by CT. Well-defined, unilocular lesions may be managed with enucleation. However, less defined, invasive lesions or recurrent lesions may require wide (1 cm) surgical resection. These lesions do not metastasize and prognosis with complete resection is good to excellent.

7.7.2 Fibrous Dysplasia

Fibrous dysplasia is a benign nonodontogenic, developmental, tumor-like condition characterized by gradual replacement of the bones of the maxillofacial region with proliferating fibrous connective tissue [93, 94]. Although quite rare, a few cases have been reported in dogs [95, 96]. In humans it is understood to be a genetic defect, which is present at birth. However, the gradual nature of the condition results in some lesions going unnoticed even into adulthood.

The superimposition of poorly mineralized bone trabeculae within the lesion provides the classic radiographic feature of a "ground glass" opacification [66] (Figure 7.16a,b). The lesion is typically not well demarcated and the margin is difficult to determine on radiography. Small lesions may be resected completely. In some cases the condition takes on a slow clinical course and may not require specific therapy. In many cases, however, it leads to significant expansion and disfigurement, trauma, or even pathologic fracture of the jaws. In such cases surgical debridement/recontouring may be indicated. Attempts to surgically remove all affected tissue via resection are often impractical because the lesions are poorly delineated and typically recur. Otherwise conservative monitoring may be sufficient. Clinically, fibrous

(a) (b)

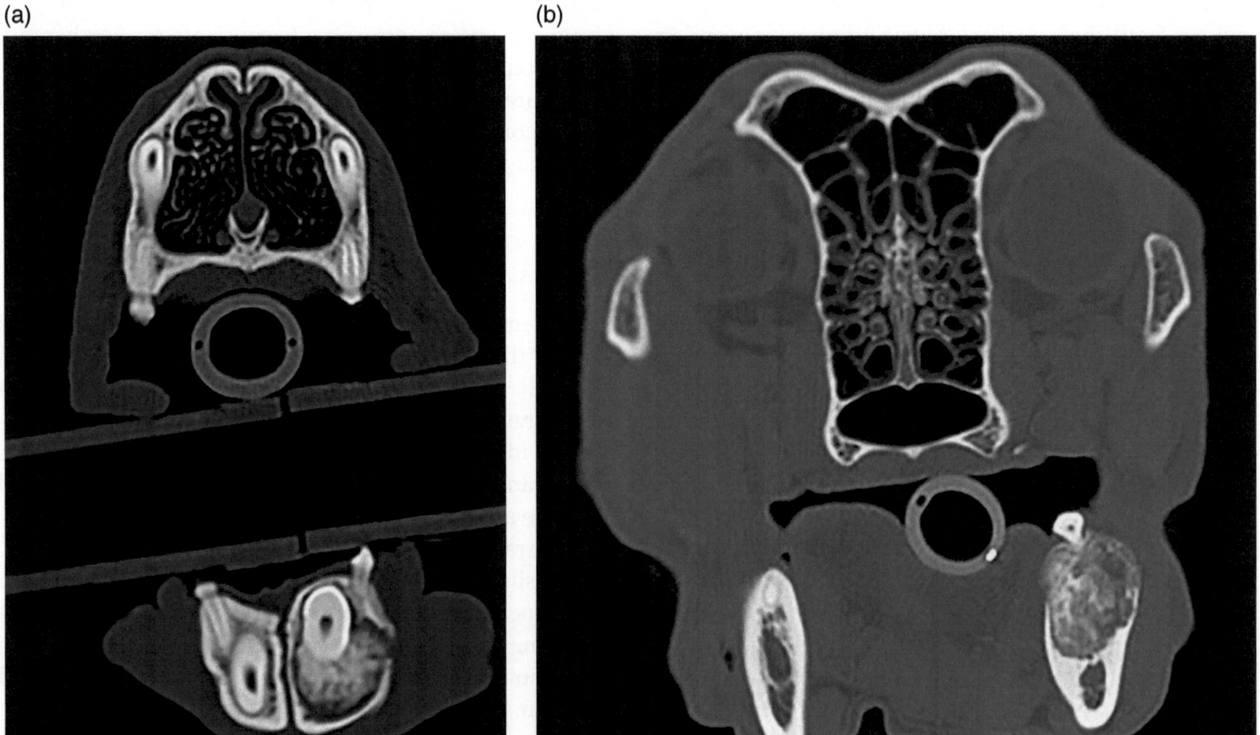

Figure 7.15 (a) Computed tomographic image of an ossifying fibroma in the rostral mandible (b) and the caudal mandible in two separate dogs.

(a) (b)

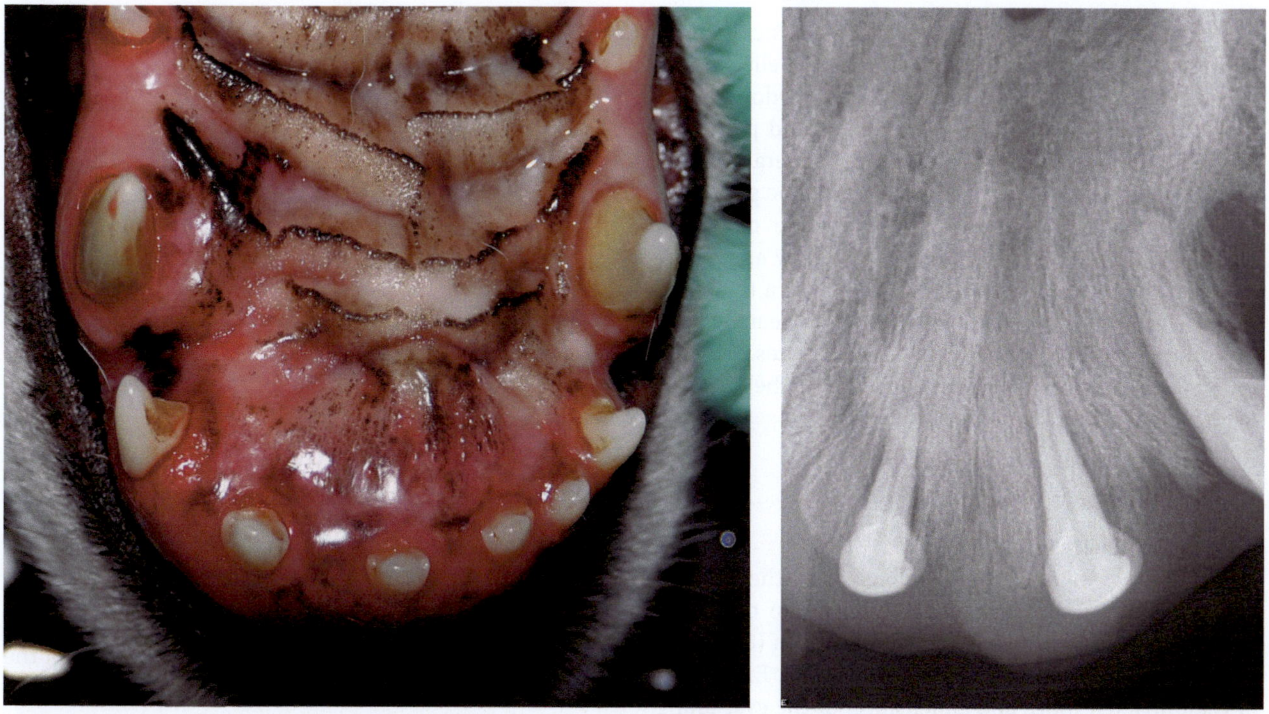

Figure 7.16 (a) Photograph and (b) intraoral radiograph of a 10-year-old Husky affected with fibrous dysplasia of the rostral maxilla. Note the generalized expansion and disfigurement of the rostral maxilla and the "ground glass" appearance of the trabecular bone. *Source:* Photograph courtesy of Dr. Debra Nossaman.

osteodystrophy due to renal or nutritional etiologies (often referred to as "rubber jaw") can mimic the developmental fibrous dysplasia [97]. Nutritional or renal secondary hyperparathyroidism may be obvious in the maxilla and mandible before other bones in the body due to the frequent use of these bones, resulting in more rapid remodeling and changes in appearance that may occur when the maxilla and/or mandible are affected.

7.8 Odontogenic Cysts

7.8.1 Classification

Odontogenic cysts are broadly classified as developmental or inflammatory cysts [66]. Developmental cysts include dentigerous (follicular) cysts and, less common, lateral periodontal cysts and gingival cysts. In humans, the class of developmental cysts also includes a small number of cysts that typically have very distinctive features including odontogenic keratocyst (keratocystic odontogenic tumor), calcifying odontogenic cyst, and glandular odontogenic cyst. Most of these distinctive cysts have not been reported in dogs, with the exception of odontogenic keratocysts [53, 98] and the uniquely named canine odontogenic parakeratinized cyst [99]. Inflammatory cysts include the periapical (radicular) cyst and the less common inflammatory paradental cyst (IPC). These are acquired cysts that originate in the context of inflammatory disease and the epithelium of origin is not clear, but is likely to be reduced enamel epithelium, odontogenic cell rests, and/or remnants of the dental lamina.

7.8.2 Notes on the Histological Features of Odontogenic Cysts

Histopathology can confirm a cystic lesion as a true cyst (i.e., the cavitated space is lined by epithelium). However, the histologic criteria for classification of odontogenic cysts overlap from class to class, vary within each class, and are rarely distinctive. Although widely described, the number of epithelial layers observed in the cyst lining has no significance. Inflammatory cells infiltrate the cyst wall of developmental cysts nearly as frequently as inflammatory cysts. Conversely, some inflammatory cysts have sparse inflammatory cell infiltrates. These limitations of histopathology are generally not acknowledged and inaccurate diagnostic criteria remain widely used by veterinary surgical pathologists.

7.8.3 Radiological Features of Odontogenic Cysts

Odontogenic cysts share many of the same general radiographic features, all having an epithelial lining surrounded by fibrous tissue and bone. Odontogenic cysts are found in tooth-bearing regions and possess a well-defined, corticated border. They are generally round to oval (balloon-like) and may occasionally be scalloped with internal septa (multiloculated). The center is usually completely radiolucent. Because they are generally slow growing, as they enlarge they have a tendency to displace (but may also resorb) teeth and create expansion, rather than destruction, of cortical plates. Specific radiological features are discussed below as they pertain to particular types of odontogenic cyst.

7.8.4 Developmental Cysts

7.8.4.1 Dentigerous Cysts

Dentigerous cysts are thought to derive from the reduced enamel epithelium of an impacted tooth. In dogs, the first premolar is the most common location (83%) followed by the canine tooth [99] (Figure 7.17). Extraction of the impacted tooth and enucleation of the cyst lining is important for definitive treatment. Histopathology of the epithelium is also important as ameloblastomas can develop within the cyst lining.

7.8.4.2 Odontogenic Keratocyst (Keratocystic Odontogenic Tumor; Canine Odontogenic Parakeratinized Cyst)

In order to better reflect its aggressive nature, the WHO Working Group recommended the traditional designation of odontogenic keratocyst be replaced with keratocystic odontogenic tumor in man [27]. The lesion historically referred to as odontogenic keratocyst has been reported in the veterinary literature [53, 98]. More recently, it has been proposed that the term canine odontogenic parakeratinized cyst may be a more appropriate designation, as the histologic features of the lesion in dogs is not completely analogous to the keratocystic odontogenic tumor of man [99]. In addition, it is not known if the lesion in dogs is as aggressive as the keratocystic odontogenic tumor in humans. However, in the authors' experience, the lesion margins are less well defined compared to other odontogenic cysts. Therefore, en bloc resection may be prudent, particularly in cases of recurrence.

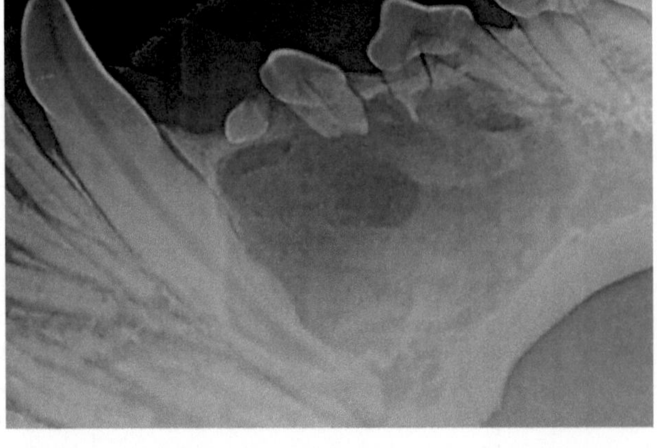

Figure 7.17 Intraoral radiograph of a dentigerous cyst around an unerupted left mandibular first premolar tooth. *Source:* Radiograph courtesy of Dr. Rebecca Martin.

7.8.4.3 Lateral Periodontal Cyst

The lateral periodontal cyst is an uncommon developmental odontogenic cyst that occurs along the lateral root surface [66, 99, 100] (Figure 7.18). Like any odontogenic cyst, complete enucleation of the cyst lining is required for resolution. Since the cyst is not associated with endodontic or periodontal disease, the involved teeth do not necessarily need to be extracted. However, if the cyst has caused enough bone resorption to compromise the integrity of the teeth or has caused root resorption, extraction of the associated tooth may be indicated.

7.8.5 Inflammatory Cysts

7.8.5.1 Periapical Cyst (Radicular Cyst)

Epithelial rests at the apex of a non-vital tooth may be stimulated by inflammation to form a periapical cyst [101]. As the epithelium desquamates into the lumen of

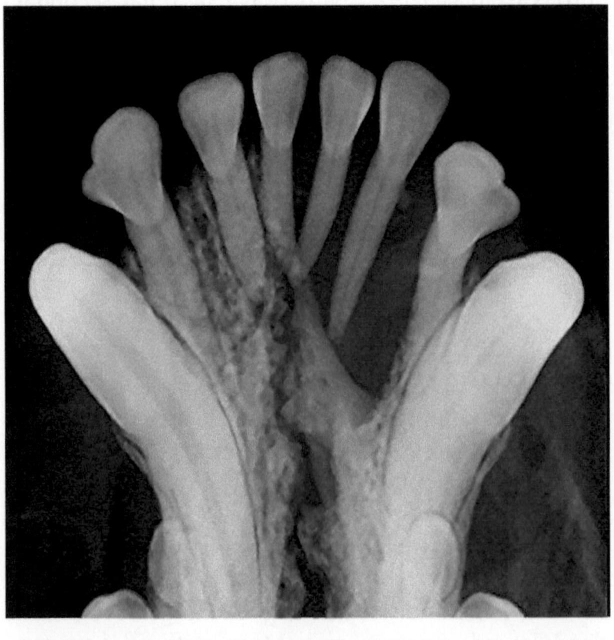

Figure 7.18 Intraoral radiograph of a lateral periodontal cyst associated with the left mandibular second incisor tooth. *Source:* Radiograph courtesy of Dr. Jennifer Martin.

the cyst, an osmotic gradient is established that promotes fluid accumulation within the cyst, contributing to growth of the cyst [100]. Additionally, molecular activity may also play a role in cyst expansion [101].

Periapical cysts appear radiologically similar to other odontogenic cysts but are most often found at the apex of a non-vital tooth (Figure 7.19). Occasionally, the cyst is found along the lateral aspect of a root (lateral radicular cyst) and appears radiologically identical to the lateral periodontal cyst. However, in the latter, the tooth remains vital.

Although periapical cysts have often been reported as uncommon to rare in animals, determining the true prevalence is challenging for two major reasons. The radiologic appearance often resembles that of a periapical granuloma and thus may be treated as such and not biopsied. A potential remedy for this issue is to always submit removed periapical tissue for histological analysis. The second issue is that definitively determining whether a pulp is vital or not is often challenging due to the lack of sensitive and specific techniques to measure pulpal blood flow.

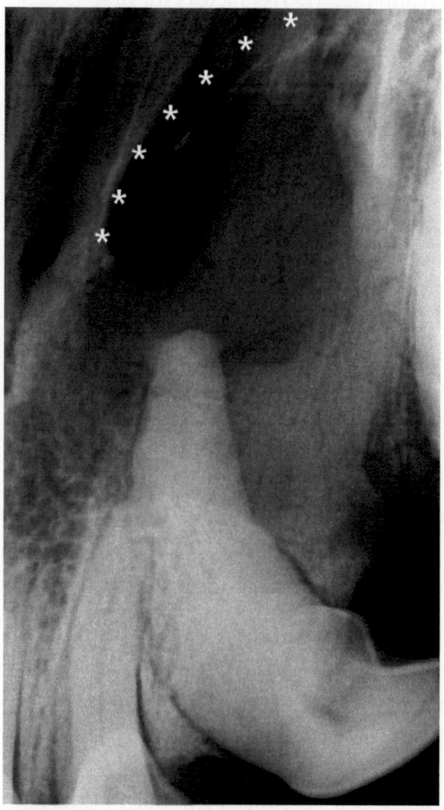

Figure 7.19 Intraoral radiograph of a periapical (radicular) cyst at the apex of the left maxillary third incisor tooth. *Source:* Radiograph courtesy of Dr. Charles Schor. Note the corticated border of the cyst (white asterisks).

Appropriate treatment entails enucleation of the cyst lining along with root canal therapy to treat the pulpal necrosis. An alternative to root canal therapy would be extraction of the tooth. However, when extraction is performed it is important to enucleate the entire cyst lining to avoid the development of a residual periapical cyst.

7.8.5.2 Canine Furcation Cyst/Inflammatory Paradental Cyst

The inflammatory paradental cyst (IPC) is defined as a cyst occurring lateral to the root and near the cervical margin of a vital tooth that affects human teeth. The histological features are indistinguishable from other inflammatory cysts. In humans, the IPC most often arises at a mandibular molar affected by superficial periodontal inflammation (pericoronitis) [102].

This entity has not been described in the veterinary literature. However, this author has seen a similar cyst in dogs striking similarity to cases of IPC in humans. In dogs, the cyst currently being referred to as the Canine Furcation Cyst, has been seen in the furcation region of the maxillary fourth premolar tooth. A clear cause is not apparent. However, in all cases, the tooth has been vital as determined by histologic evaluation. The recommended treatment is enucleation of the cyst ± extraction of the tooth depending on the degree of attachment loss/tooth resorption. Like other odontogenic cysts, the recurrence rate is dependent on the ability to remove the entire cyst lining.

7.8.6 Treatment Principles for Odontogenic Cysts

Generally speaking, odontogenic cysts can be enucleated while the affected tooth is maintained. However, extraction often provides better visualization of the cyst lining and improved visualization may decrease the chances of recurrence. In order to prevent recurrence, the entire cyst lining must be removed. The tooth associated with a radicular cyst requires root canal therapy. It is generally recommended that an unerupted tooth be extracted when associated with a dentigerous cyst. Larger cysts often require additional considerations, such as when associated with root resorption of the associated or nearby teeth. In this scenario, the radiologic information must be used to determine whether the associated tooth and/or adjacent teeth require extraction. Larger cysts may be marsupialized for a period of time in order to reduce the size of the cyst prior to definitive enucleation. However, in the authors' experience this is rarely necessary.

7.9 American Veterinary Dental College (AVDC) Abbreviation List (https://www.avdc.org/traineeinfo.html; accessed 3 March 2018)

See Table 7.3.

Table 7.3 AVDC Nomenclature Abbreviations.

B	Biopsy
B/B	Bite biopsy
B/CN	Core needle biopsy
B/E	Excisional biopsy
B/I	Incisional biopsy
B/NA	Needle aspiration
B/NB	Needle biopsy
B/P	Punch biopsy
B/S	Surface biopsy
DTC	Dentigerous cyst
DTC/R	Dentigerous cyst removal
EM	Erythema multiforme
ENO	Enophthalmos
EOG	Eosinophilic granuloma
EOG/L	Eosinophilic granuloma (lip)
EOG/P	Eosinophilic granuloma (palate)
EOG/T	Eosinophilic granuloma (tongue)
OM	Oral/maxillofacial mass
OM/AA	Acanthomatous ameloblastoma
OM/AD	Adenoma
OM/ADC	Adenocarcinoma
OM/APN	Anaplastic neoplasm
OM/APO	Amyloid-producing odontogenic tumor
OM/CE	Cementoma
OM/FIO	Feline inductive odontogenic tumor
OM/FS	Fibrosarcoma
OM/GCG	Giant cell granuloma
OM/GCT	Granular cell tumor
OM/HS	Hemangiosarcoma
OM/LI	Lipoma
OM/LS	Lymphosarcoma
OM/MCT	Mast cell tumor
OM/MM	Malignant melanoma
OM/OO	Osteoma
OM/OS	Osteosarcoma
OM/MTB	Multilobular tumor of bone
OM/PAP	Papilloma
OM/PCT	Plasma cell tumor
OM/PNT	Peripheral nerve sheath tumor
OM/POF	Peripheral odontogenic fibroma
OM/RBM	Rhabdomyosarcoma
OM/SCC	Squamous cell carcinoma
OM/UDN	Undifferentiated neoplasm

References

1 Tholen, M.J. and Hoft, R.F. (1990). Oral pathology. In: *Small Animal Oral Medicine and Surgery* (ed. M.J. Bojrab and M.T. Tholen), 42. Philadelphia, PA: Lea and Febiger.

2 Stebbins, K.E., Morse, C.C., and Goldschmidt, M.H. (1989). Feline oral neoplasia: a ten-year survey. *Vet. Pathol.* 26: 121–128.

3 Belz, G.T. and Heath, T.J. (1995). Lymph pathways of the medial retropharyngeal lymph node in dogs. *J. Anat.* 186: 517–526.

4 Nemanic, S., London, C.A., and Wisner, E.R. (2006). Comparison of thoracic radiographs and single breath-hold helical CT for detection of pulmonary nodules in dogs with metastatic neoplasia. *JVIM* 20: 508–515.

5 Bender, I.B. (1982). Factors influencing the radiographic appearance of bony lesions. *J. Endod.* 8: 161–170.

6 Esplin, D.G. (2008). Survival of dogs following surgical excision of histologically well-differentiated melanocytic neoplasms of the mucous membranes of the lips and oral cavity. *Vet. Pathol.* 45: 889–896.

7 Bertone, E.R., Snyder, L.A., and Moore, A.S. (2003). Environmental and lifestyle risk factors for oral squamous cell carcinoma in domestic cats. *JVIM* 17: 557–562.

8 Snyder, L.A., Bertone, E.R., Jakowski, R.M. et al. (2004). p53 expression and environmental tobacco smoke exposure in feline oral squamous cell carcinoma. *Vet. Pathol.* 41: 209–214.

9 Mas, A., Blackwood, L., Cripps, P. et al. (2011). Canine tonsillar squamous cell carcinoma - a multi-centre retrospective review of 44 clinical cases. *J. Small Anim. Pract.* 52: 359–364.

10 Gendler, A., Lewis, J.R., Reetz, J.A., and Schwarz, T. (2010). Computed tomographic features of oral squamous cell carcinoma in cats: 18 cases (2002–2008). *J. Am. Vet. Med. Assoc.* 236: 319–325.

11 Soltero-Rivera, M.M., Krick, E.L., Reiter, A.M. et al. (2014). Prevalence of regional and distant metastasis in cats with advanced oral squamous cell carcinoma: 49 cases (2005–2011). *J. Feline Med. Surg.* 16: 164–169.

12 Ciekot, P.A., Powers, B.E., Withrow, S.J. et al. (1994). Histologically low-grade, yet biologically high-grade, fibrosarcomas of the mandible and maxilla in dogs: 25 cases (1982–1991). *J. Am. Vet. Med. Assoc.* 204: 610–615.

13 Farcas, N., Arzi, B., and Verstraete, F.J. (2014). Oral and maxillofacial osteosarcoma in dogs: a review. *Vet. Comp. Oncol.* 12: 169–180.

14 Coyle, V.J., Rassnick, K.M., Borst, L.B. et al. (2015). Biological behavior of canine mandibular

osteosarcoma. A retrospective study of 50 cases (1999–2007). *Vet. Comp. Oncol.* 13 (2): 89–97.

15 Burton, J.H., Powers, B.E., and Biller, B.J. (2014). Clinical outcome in 20 cases of lingual hemangiosarcoma in dogs: 1996–2011. *Vet. Comp. Oncol.* 12: 198–204.

16 Dernell, W.S., Straw, R.C., Cooper, M.F. et al. (1998). Multilobular osteochondrosarcoma in 39 dogs: 1979–1993. *J. Am. Anim. Hosp. Assoc.* 34: 11–18.

17 Buerger, R.G. and Scott, D.W. (1987). Cutaneous mast cell neoplasia in cats: 14 cases (1975–1985). *J. Am. Vet. Med. Assoc.* 190 (11): 1440–1444.

18 Hillman, L.A., Garrett, L.D., de Lorimier, L.P. et al. (2010). Biological behavior of oral and perioral mast cell tumors in dogs: 44 cases (1996–2006). *J. Am. Vet. Med. Assoc.* 237: 936–942.

19 Fontaine, J., Heimann, M., and Day, M.J. (2010). Canine cutaneous epitheliotropic T-cell lymphoma: a review of 30 cases. *Vet. Dermatol.* 21: 267–275.

20 Flood-Knapik, K.E., Durham, A.C., Gregor, T.P. et al. (2013). Clinical, histopathological and immunohistochemical characterization of canine indolent lymphoma. *Vet Comp. Oncol.* 11 (4): 272–286.

21 Fiani, N., Arzi, B., Johnson, E.G. et al. (2011). Osteoma of the oral and maxillofacial regions in cats: 7 cases (1999–2009). *J. Am. Vet. Med. Assoc.* 238: 1470–1475.

22 Kuntsi-Vaattovaara, H., Verstraete, F.J., Newsome, J.T., and Yuan, H. (2003). Resolution of persistent oral papillomatosis in a dog after treatment with a recombinant canine oral papillomavirus vaccine. *Vet. Comp. Oncol.* 1: 57–63.

23 Dubielzig, R.R. (2003). Histologic classification of tumors of odontogenic origin of domestic animals. In: *WHO Histological Classification of Tumors of the Alimentary System of Domestic Animals*, second series, vol. X (ed. K.W. Head, J.M. Cullen, et al.), 46–57. Washington, DC: Armed Forces Institute of Pathology.

24 Svendenius, L. and Warfvinge, G. (2010). Oral pathology in Swedish dogs: a retrospective study of 280 biopsies. *J. Vet. Dent.* 27: 91–97.

25 Boehm, B., Breuer, W., and Hermanns, W. (2011). Odontogenic tumours in the dog and cat. *Tierarztl. Prax. Ausg. K Kleintiere Heimtiere* 39: 305–312.

26 Fiani, N., Verstraete, F.J. et al. (2011). Clinicopathologic characterization of odontogenic tumors and focal fibrous hyperplasia in dogs: 152 cases (1995–2005). *J. Am. Vet. Med. Assoc.* 238: 495–500.

27 Barnes, L., Eveson, J.W. et al. (2005). Odontogenic tumours. In: *World Health Organization Classification of Tumours – Pathology of Head and Neck Tumours* (ed. L. Barnes, J.W. Eveson, P. Reichart, et al.), 283–327. Lyon, France: IARC Press.

28 Gardner, D.G. and Baker, D.C. (1993). The relationship of the canine acanthomatous epulis to ameloblastoma. *J. Comp. Pathol.* 108: 47–55.

29 Verstraete, F.J., Ligthelm, A.J., and Weber, A. (1992). The histological nature of epulides in dogs. *J. Comp. Pathol.* 106: 169–182.

30 Yoshida, K., Yanai, T. et al. (1999). Clinicopathological study of canine oral epulides. *J. Vet. Med. Sci.* 61: 897–902.

31 Ohmachi, T., Taniyam, H. et al. (1996). Calcifying epithelial odontogenic tumours in small domesticated carnivores: histological, immunohistochemical and electron microscopical studies. *J. Comp. Pathol.* 114: 305–314.

32 Gardner, D.G. (1995). Canine acanthomatous epulis. The only common spontaneous ameloblastoma in animals. *Oral Surg. Oral Med. Oral Pathol. Oral Radiol. Endod.* 79: 612–615.

33 Amory, J.T., Reetz, J.A. et al. (2014). Computed tomographic characteristics of odontogenic neoplasms in dogs. *Vet. Radiol. Ultrasound.* 55: 147–158.

34 Gardner, D.G. (1996). Epulides in the dog: a review. *J. Oral Pathol. Med.* 25: 32–37.

35 Thrall, D.E. (1984). Orthovoltage radiotherapy of acanthomatous epulis in 39 dogs. *J. Am. Vet. Med. Assoc.* 184: 826–829.

36 Bjorling, D.E., Chambers, J.N., and Mahaffey, E.A. (1987). Surgical treatment of epulides in dogs: 25 cases (1974–1984). *J. Am. Vet. Med. Assoc.* 190: 1315–1318.

37 White, R.A.S. and Gorman, T. (1989). Wide local excision of acanthomatous epulides in the dog. *Vet. Surg.* 18: 12–14.

38 Langham, R.F., Motosky, U.V., and Schirmer, R.G. (1977). X-ray therapy of selected odontogenic neoplasms in the dog. *J. Am. Vet. Med. Assoc.* 170: 820–822.

39 Dubielzig, R.R. and Thrall, D.E. (1982). Ameloblastoma and keratinizing ameloblastoma in dogs. *Vet. Pathol.* 19: 596–607.

40 Theon, A.P., Rodgriguez, C. et al. (1997). Analysis of prognostic factors and patterns of failure in dogs with periodontal tumors treated with megavoltage irradiation. *J. Am. Vet. Med. Assoc.* 210: 785–788.

41 Moore, A.S., Wood, C.A. et al. (2000). Radiation therapy for long-term control of odontogenic tumours and epulis in three cats. *J. Feline Med. Surg.* 2: 57–60.

42 Gardner, D.G. (1996). Some current concepts on the pathology of ameloblastomas. *Oral Surg. Oral Med. Oral Pathol. Oral Radiol. Endod.* 82: 660–669.

43 Yoshida, K., Watarai, Y. et al. (1998). The effect of intralesional bleomycin on canine acathomatous epulis. *J. Am. Anim. Hosp. Assoc.* 34: 457–461.

44 Kelly, J.M., Belding, B.A. et al. (2010). Acanthomatous ameloblastoma in dogs treated with intralesional bleomycin. *Vet. Comp. Oncol.* 8: 81–86.
45 Head, K.W. (1976). Tumours of the upper alimentary tract. *Bull. World Health Organ.* 53: 145–166.
46 Vos, J.H., Goedegebuure, S.A., and Bron-Dietz, G.M. (1985). A feline dental tumor resembling calcifying epithelial odontogenic tumor in man. *Vet. Pathol.* 22: 508–510.
47 Bruer, W., Geisel, O. et al. (1994). Light microscopic, ultrastructural, and immunohistochemical examinations of two calcifying epithelial odontogenic tumors (CEOT) in a dog and a cat. *Vet. Pathol.* 31: 415–420.
48 Ishikawa, T. and Yamamoto, H. (1996). Case of calcifying epithelial odontogenic tumour in a dog. *J. Small Anim. Pract.* 37: 597–599.
49 Calvo, I., Castejón, A. et al. (2004). Calcifying epithelial odontogenic tumor in a dog. *J. Vet. Dent.* 21: 26–28.
50 Gardner, D.G., Dubielzig, R.R., and McGee, E.V. (1994). The so-called calcifying epithelial odontogenic tumour in dogs and cats (amyloid-producing odontogenic tumour). *J. Comp. Pathol.* 111: 221–230.
51 Hirayama, K., Miyasho, T. et al. (2010). Biochemical and immunohistochemical characterization of the amyloid in canine amyloid-producing odontogenic tumor. *Vet. Pathol.* 47: 915–922.
52 Delaney, M.A., Singh, K. et al. (2012). Immunohistochemical and biochemical evidence of ameloblastic origin of feline amyloid-producing odontogenic tumors in cats. *Vet. Pathol.* 50: 238–242.
53 Poulet, F.M., Valentine, B.A., and Summers, B.A. (1992). A survey of epithelial odontogenic tumors and cysts in dogs and cats. *Vet. Pathol.* 29: 369–380.
54 Head, K.W. (1990). Tumors of the alimentary tract. In: *Tumors in Domestic Animals*, 3e (ed. J.E. Moulton), 357–362. Berkeley, CA: University of California Press.
55 Miles, C.R., Bell, C.M. et al. (2011). Maxillary ameloblastic fibroma in a dog. *Vet. Pathol.* 48: 823–826.
56 Nold, J.B., Powers, B.E. et al. (1984). Ameloblastic odontoma in a dog. *J. Am. Vet. Med. Assoc.* 185: 996–998.
57 Langham, R.F., Mostosky, U.V., and Schirmer, R.G. (1969). Ameloblastic odontoma in the dog. *Am. J. Vet. Res.* 30: 1873–1876.
58 Boyd, R.C. (2002). Ameloblastic fibro-odontoma in a German shepherd dog. *J. Vet. Dent.* 19: 148–150.
59 Kramek, B.A., O, Brien, T.D., and Smith, F.O. (1996). Diagnosis and removal of a dentigerous cyst complicated by ameloblastic fibro-odontoma in a dog. *J. Vet. Dent.* 13: 9–11.
60 Walsh, K.M., Denholm, W.L., and Cooper, B.J. (1987). Epithelial odontogenic tumours in domestic animals. *J. Comp. Pathol.* 97: 503–521.
61 Gorlin, R.J., Meskin, L.H., and Brodey, R. (1963). Odontogenic tumors in man and animals: pathologic classification and clinical behavior – a review. *Ann. N.Y. Acad. Sci.* 108: 722–771.
62 Nyska, A. and Dayan, D. (1995). Ameloblastic fibroma in a young cat. *J. Oral Pathol. Med.* 24: 233–236.
63 Gardner, D.G. and Dubielzig, R.R. (1995). Feline inductive odontogenic tumor (inductive fibroameloblastoma) – a tumor unique to cats. *J. Oral Pathol. Med.* 24: 185–190.
64 Andrews, L.K. Tumors of the alimentary system. In: *Diseases of the Cat*, vol. 198 (ed. J. Holzworth), 486–507. Philadelphia, PA: WB Saunders.
65 Bell, C.M. and Soukup, J.W. (2014). Nomenclature and classification of odontogenic tumors – Part II: clarification of specific nomenclature. *J. Vet. Dent.* 31: 234–243.
66 Neville, B.W., Damm, D.D. et al. (2009). Odontogenic cysts and tumors. In: *Oral and Maxillofacial Pathology*, 3e (ed. B.W. Neville, D.D. Damm, et al.), 678–731. St. Louis, MO: Saunders Elsevier.
67 Carlson, E.R. (2004). Odontogenic cysts and tumors. In: *Peterson's Principles of Oral and Maxillofacial Surgery*, 2e (ed. M. Miloro, G.E. Ghali, et al.), 576–596. Hamilton, Ontario, BC: Decker Inc.
68 Gardner, D.G. and Baker, D.C. (1991). Fibromatous epulis in dogs and peripheral odontogenic fibroma in human beings: two equivalent lesions. *Oral Surg. Oral Med. Oral Pathol.* 71: 317–321.
69 Dubielzig, R.R., Goldschmidt, M.H., and Brodey, R.S. (1979). The nomenclature of periodontal epulides in dogs. *Vet. Pathol.* 16: 209–214.
70 De Bruijn, N.D., Kirpensteijn, J. et al. (2007). A clinicopathological study of 52 feline epulides. *Vet. Pathol.* 44: 161–169.
71 Colgin, L.M., Schulman, F.Y., and Dubielzig, R.R. (2001). Multiple epulides in 13 cats. *Vet. Pathol.* 38: 227–229.
72 Meyers, B., Boy, S.C., and Steenkamp, G. (2007). Diagnosis and management of odontogenic myxoma in a dog. *J. Vet. Dent.* 24: 166–171.
73 Gupta, K., Singh, A. et al. (2005). A rare case of odontogenic myxoma in a dog. *J. Vet. Med. A Physiol. Pathol. Clin. Med.* 52: 401–402.
74 Ueki, H., Sumi, A. et al. (2004). Malignant ameloblastic fibro-odontoma in a dog. *Vet. Pathol.* 41: 183–185.
75 Sakai, H., Yanai, T. et al. (1996). Ameloblastoma with prominent ossification in the mandible of a dog. *J. Vet. Med. Sci.* 58: 1113–1115.
76 Jimenez, M.A., Castejon, A. et al. (2007). Maxillary ameloblastic carcinoma in an Alaskan malamute. *Vet. Pathol.* 44: 84–87.
77 Regezi, J.A., Sciubba, J.J., and Jordan, R.C.K. (2008). Connective tissue lesions. In: *Oral Pathology: Clinical Pathologic Correlations*, 5e (ed. J.A. Regezi, J.J.

Sciubba and R.C.K. Jordan), 155–177. St. Louis, MO: Saunders Elsevier.

78 Regezi, J.A., Sciubba, J.J., and Jordan, R.C.K. (2008). Red-blue lesions. In: *Oral Pathology: Clinical Pathologic Correlations*, 5e (ed. J.A. Regezi, J.J. Sciubba and R.C.K. Jordan), 107–125. St. Louis, MO: Saunders Elsevier.

79 Riehl, J., Constantaras, M. et al. (2014). Clinicopathologic characterization of pyogenic granuloma in 8 cats. *J. Vet. Dent.* 31: 80–86.

80 Gracis, M., Molinari, E., and Ferro, S. (2015). Caudal mucogingival lesions secondary to traumatic dental occlusion in 27 cats: macroscopic and microscopic description, treatment and follow-up. *J. Feline Med. Surg.* 17: 318–328.

81 Valentine, B.A. and Eckhaus, M.A. (1986). Peripheral giant cell granuloma (giant cell epulis) in two dogs. *Vet. Pathol.* 23: 340–341.

82 Desoutter, A.V., Goldschmidt, M.H., and Sanchez, M.D. (2012). Clinical and histologic features of 26 canine peripheral giant cell granulomas (formerly giant cell epulis). *Vet. Pathol.* 49: 1018–1023.

83 Rothwell, J.T. and Valentine, B.A. (1988). Peripheral giant cell granuloma in a cat. *J. Am. Vet. Med. Assoc.* 192: 1105–1106.

84 Lamb, C.R. and Schelling, S.H. (1989). Congenital aneurysmal bone cyst in the mandible of a foal. *Equine Vet. J.* 21: 130–132.

85 Stenberg, T., Dowling, B.A., and Dart, A.J. (2004). Mandibular bone cysts in two horses. *Aust. Vet. J.* 82: 417–418.

86 Belknap, E.B., Brodie, S. et al. (1992). Aneurysmal bone cyst in a Holstein bull. *J. Am. Vet. Med. Assoc.* 201: 1413–1415.

87 Valentine, B.A., Flanders, J.A. et al. (1988). Central giant cell granuloma in the mandible of a dog. *J. Am. Vet. Med. Assoc.* 192: 657–658.

88 Trigo, F.J., Leathers, C.W., and Brobst, D.F. (1983). A comparison of canine giant cell tumor and giant cell reparative granuloma of bone. *Vet. Pathol.* 20: 215–222.

89 Bordelon, J.T. and Rochat, M.C. (2007). Use of a titanium mesh for cranioplasty following radical rostrotentorial craniectomy to remove an ossifying fibroma in a dog. *J. Am. Vet. Med. Assoc.* 231: 1692–1695.

90 Miller, M.A., Towle, A.M., Heng, H.G. et al. (2008). Mandibular ossifying fibroma in a dog. *Vet. Pathol.* 45: 203–206.

91 Speltz, M.C., Pool, R.R., and Hayden, D.W. (2009). Pathology in practice. Ossifying fibroma of the right mandible. *J. Am. Vet. Med. Assoc.* 235: 1283–1295.

92 Soltero-Rivera, M., Engiles, J.B., Reiter, A.M. et al. (2015). Benign and malignant proliferative fibro-osseous and osseous lesions of the oral cavity. *Vet. Pathol.* 52 (5): 894–902.

93 Alawi, F. (2002). Benign fibro-osseous diseases of the maxillofacial bone. A review and differential diagnosis. *Am. J. Clin. Pathol.* 118: S50–S70.

94 DeCaprio, M.R. and Enneking, W.F. (2005). Fibrous dysplasia. Pathophysiology, evaluation and treatment. *J. Bone Joint Surg. Am.* 87: 1848–1864.

95 Carrig, C.B. and Seawright, A.A. (1969). A familial canine polyostotic fibrous dysplasia with subperiosteal cortical defects. *J. Small Anim. Pract.* 10: 397–405.

96 Fitzgerald, W., Slocombe, R., and Caiafa, A. (2001). Fibrous dysplasia of mandibular bone in a dog. *J. Vet. Dent.* 9: 77–81.

97 Carmichael, D.T., Williams, C.A., and Aller, M.S. (1995). Renal dysplasia with secondary hyperparathyroidism and loose teeth in a young dog. *J. Vet. Dent.* 12 (4): 143–146.

98 Watanabe, K., Kadosawa, T. et al. (2004). Odontogenic cysts in three dogs: one odontogenic keratocyst and two dentigerous cysts. *J. Vet. Med. Sci.* 66: 1167–1170.

99 Verstraete, F.J.M., Zin, B.P. et al. (2011). Clinical signs and histologic findings in dogs with odontogenic cysts: 41 cases (1995–2010). *J. Am. Vet. Med. Assoc.* 239: 1470–1476.

100 Regezi, J.A., Sciubba, J.J., and Jordan, R.C.K. (2008). Cysts of the jaws and neck. In: *Oral Pathology. Clinical Pathologic Correlations*, 5e (ed. J.A. Regezi, J.J. Sciubba and R.C.K. Jordan), 237–259. Saunders Elsevier: St. Louis, MO.

101 Lin, L.M. and Huang, G.T.-J. (2011). Pathobiology of the periapex. In: *Cohen's Pathways of the Pulp*, 10th ed. (eds. Hargreaves, K.M., Cohen, S., and Berman, L.H.), 529–558. St. Louis: Mosby Elsevier.

102 Philipsen, H.P., Reichart, P.A. et al. (2004). The inflammatory paradental cyst: a critical review of 342 cases from a literature survey, including 17 new cases from the author's files. *J. Oral Pathol. Med.* 33: 147–155.

8

General Oral Pathology

Heidi B. Lobprise

Main Street Veterinary Dental Clinic, Flower Mound, TX, USA

8.1 Introduction

Oral pathology is considered present when a departure from normal occurs that is sufficient to cause signs or symptoms. Symptoms are the abnormalities detected by the patient or owner, while signs are those noted by the clinician. A syndrome is a defined group of signs or symptoms, but not always resulting from the same specifically defined cause. Etiology is the theory of the cause of the disease, though when there is no acceptable theory as to the etiology available, it is called idiopathic. This chapter will cover those conditions of the oral cavity other than certain dental lesions, congenital and developmental issues, traumatic lesions, and tumors/cysts, which are covered in other chapters. Each specific region/category will be addressed, with those conditions, lesions, and diseases that affect them.

8.2 Oral Cavity – General

While some lesions in the oral cavity will affect multiple surfaces and tissues, some affect distinct or focal regions. Though the diagnosis of inflammation should be determined histopathologically, physical exam findings (swelling, redness, ulceration) can often lead to a reasonable description, based on the tissue involved (seeTable 8.1). The American Veterinary Dental College (AVDC) is an excellent resource for terminology and nomenclature (https://www.avdc.org/Nomenclature). Diseases and conditions that affect the oral cavity in general will first be discussed and then distinct regions/tissues will be covered.

8.2.1 Infectious Diseases

Though an inflammatory response is expected in the typical pathogenesis of periodontal disease, there are many factors that can contribute to excessive levels of inflammation. Infectious agents, such as bacteria, viruses, protozoans, and fungi can elicit tremendous response from healthy individuals, and in hyperresponsive or immunosuppressed animals, even normally innocuous agents may elicit substantial soft tissue changes.

8.2.1.1 Bacterial

Necrotizing ulcerative gingivitis (NUG) in people occurs when spirochetes and *Prevotella intermedia,* normally opportunistic oral flora, synergistically act in the presence of physical or emotional stress as well as a decreased resistance to infection, nutritional defects, or debilitating disease [1]. The classic initial lesion is ulceration of the interdental papillae or marginal gingiva with spirochetes that may be found in the exudates and epithelium, but seldom penetrating into the connective tissue [2]. As the process continues, the surface epithelium is replaced by fibrin, necrotic epithelial cells, and neutrophils, termed a pseudomembrane [1]. In immunocompromised patients, NUG can progress to a more aggressive course and lead to necrotizing ulcerative periodontitis (NUP), with destruction of underlying periodontium, including bone [1]. Vincent's angina affects the throat, larynx, and even the middle ear with a fusospirochetal infection. Treatment with metronidazole can be optimal to help avoid yeast overgrowth (candidiasis).

Systemic bacterial infections, which are considered to be more of an exogenous type of infection as related to the oral cavity, may also exhibit lesions. Oral lesions from *Leptospira* spp. infections are likely to be secondary to more generalized conditions such as vasculitis, which can result in injected mucous membranes, petechiae, and ecchymosis. Severe renal involvement due to leptospirosis may result in oral ulceration secondary to uremia [3]. In cats, infection with *Mycobacterium lepraemurium,* or feline leprosy, can cause one or more raised, plaque-like

Wiggs's Veterinary Dentistry: Principles and Practice, Second Edition. Edited by Heidi B. Lobprise and Johnathon R. (Bert) Dodd.

Table 8.1 Terms – oral and oropharyngeal inflammation.

Gingivitis	Inflammation of gingiva
Gingival enlargement	A clinical term, referring to overgrowth or thickening of gingiva in the absence of a histological diagnosis
Gingival hyperplasia	A histological term, referring to an abnormal increase in the number of normal cells in a normal arrangement and resulting clinically in gingival enlargement
Periodontitis	Inflammation of non-gingival periodontal tissues (i.e., the periodontal ligament and alveolar bone)
Alveolar mucositis	Inflammation of alveolar mucosa (i.e., mucosa overlying the alveolar process and extending from the mucogingival junction without obvious demarcation to the vestibular sulcus and to the floor of the mouth)
Sublingual mucositis	Inflammation of mucosa on the floor of the mouth
Labial/buccal mucositis	Inflammation of lip/cheek mucosa
Caudal mucositis	Inflammation of mucosa of the caudal oral cavity, bordered medially by the palatoglossal folds and fauces, dorsally by the hard and soft palate, and rostrally by alveolar and buccal mucosa
Contact mucositis and contact mucosal ulceration	Lesions in susceptible individuals that are secondary to mucosal contact with a tooth surface bearing the responsible irritant, allergen, or antigen. They have also been called "contact ulcers" and "kissing ulcers"
Palatitis	Inflammation of mucosa covering the hard and/or soft palate
Glossitis	Inflammation of mucosa of the dorsal and/or ventral tongue surface
Cheilitis	Inflammation of the lip (including the mucocutaneous junction area and skin of the lip)
Osteomyelitis	Inflammation of the bone and bone marrow
Stomatitis	Inflammation of the mucous lining of any of the structures in the mouth; in clinical use the term should be reserved to describe widespread oral inflammation (beyond gingivitis and periodontitis) that may also extend into submucosal tissues (e.g., marked caudal mucositis extending into submucosal tissues may be termed caudal stomatitis)
Tonsillitis	Inflammation of the palatine tonsil
Pharyngitis	Inflammation of the pharynx

lesions on the lips and/or the tongue, but are generally not painful. Granulomatous lesions on the mucous membrane of the tongue [4] and oral cavity [5] may be an uncommon presentation of canine visceral leishmaniasis that often must be biopsied to be differentiated from other oral lesions [6].

8.2.1.2 Fungal-Mycotic Yeast

In atopic dogs, *Malassezia pachydermatis* has been isolated in 33% of the oral cavities of patients studied, though no oral lesions were mentioned. Its presence is likely to be due more to cross-contamination of a secondary overgrowth with an alteration of the cutaneous microhabitat [7].

In 34 dogs with symptoms of gingivostomatitis, 11.8% had *Candida albicans*, an opportunistic yeast, cultured from their mouths [8]. While considered a normal part of the microbiota, if cultured repeatedly, as a result of overgrowth in immunocompromised patients or those treated extensively with antibiotics, this should be treated with the appropriate medication, systemically or topically. Mycotic stomatitis may be initiated in the presence of immunodeficiency (thrush mouth in HIV patients), systemic disease, or antibiotic administration [9]. Primarily seen on the tongue and at the mucocutaneous margins, the ulcers can also be seen throughout the oropharynx, coated with a white plaque. Occasionally, extension of a nasal aspergillosis infection through the nasopalatine ducts may lead to hyperemia or ulceration at the incisive papilla [10]. The tongue or even mucosa and underlying bone can rarely be the site of lesions related to a systemic histoplasmosis [11] or blastomycosis infection.

8.2.1.3 Viral

Feline Calicivirus (FCV) replicates primarily in the oropharynx, and it is likely that it has a role in chronic gingivostomatitis and caudal mucositis [12]. Lingual ulceration, in combination with nasal discharge and rhinitis is a common oral sign. Feline herpes virus (FHV) typically affects the respiratory system and eyes, with less frequent oral lesions [13]. Calicivirus in the dog presents primarily as an enteric disease, though glossitis has been described [14]. Other viruses in the cat that are more systemic and affect the immune system, such as feline leukemia virus (FeLV) and feline immunodeficiency virus (FIV) may predispose the individual to secondary oral infections (see Chapter 20 – Domestic Feline Oral and Dental Diseases). Distinct, wart-like growths on the buccal mucosa, lips, and tongue are generally a self-limiting lesion in dogs caused by exposure to the papillomavirus.

8.2.2 Immune System

There are many means by which an abnormality in the body's immune system can have an effect on the oral cavity. While certain viruses, stress, and corticosteroids may lead to a decreased immune response that predisposes an individual to opportunistic infections, in other individuals the immune response may be an exaggerated one to relatively normal stimuli.

8.2.2.1 Contact Mucositis

An increase in IgG and immune complex deposition in a syndrome of ulcerative stomatitis in Maltese dogs, particularly males, may explain an excessive host response (increased gingival index) in the presence of minimal stimuli (low plaque and calculus indices). Other breeds may show similar syndromes, such as Cavalier King Charles Spaniels (CKCS) [15]. There may be marked ulceration of buccal mucosa that contact a tooth/calculus surface, known as contact mucositis or contact mucosal ulceration ("kissing lesions"). These animals appear to develop a plaque intolerance with the consequence of an excessive immune response to any accumulation. The condition is typically in localized areas of the canine and carnassial teeth initially, but may progress to a more general condition throughout the mouth. If effective plaque control cannot be maintained, and as anti-inflammatory medications provide only a transitory relief, often extractions are necessary. Additionally, selective extractions customarily only provide temporary relief as the condition tends to recur at new sites, adjacent to other teeth.

8.2.2.2 Pemphigoid and Blistering Syndromes

While distinct autoimmune syndromes such as pemphigus foliaceous have dermal lesions primarily (with rare oral lesions), up to 90% of patients with pemphigus vulgaris (PV) will have oral lesions, frequently at the mucocutaneous junctions, with some mucous membrane ulceration [16]. With early detection in the oral cavity, some patients with PV can be treated before the disease becomes generalized [17]. Pemphigus vegitans (PVeg) has been described as a proliferative variation of PV in humans, with one similar case in a dog [18], though other cases do not exhibit oral involvement. A newer identification of mucous membrane pemphigoid (MMP) as part of a group of AISBD (autoimmune subepidermal blistering disease) includes cases that were likely to be previously classified as bullous pemphigoid (BP) [19]. Immunohistochemistry may be needed to distinguish BP and MMP from the more severe, ulcerative epidermolysis bullosa acquista, described most frequently in Great Danes, characterized with epithelial sloughing and a poor prognosis [19, 20]. With any vesiculobulbous disorder, it is best to biopsy a fresh "blister," which often occurs first on oral mucous membranes.

Even less common in the dog, oral sequelae of systemic lupus erythematosus (SLE) may appear as ulceration of mucocutaneous junctions and oral mucosa [21]. Discoid lupus erythematosus (DLE), considered a benign variant of SLE, primarily affects the nasal planum, face, and ears, but the lips can be involved with depigmentation [21].

Another blistering and ulcerative syndrome, erythema multiforme (EM), is uncommon and self-limiting if mild, with likely immune-mediated factors involved [22]. Oral lesions have been seen in up to 31.8% of the cases, but oral-only presentations have not been described [23]. Apoptosis of keratinocytes have been attributed to EM lesions associated with everything from canine parvovirus infection [24], a moderate form of drug-induced reactions [25], and even a paraneoplastic disorder associated with thymoma in a dog [26]. Immunohistochemistry and clonality testing may be necessary to distinguish EM from epitheliotropic T-cell lymphoma (ETCL) [22].

8.2.2.3 Hypersensitivity

The immune system also plays a part in acute hypersensitivity reactions to drugs (adverse drug reaction – ADR) such as trimethoprim sulfonamides and others [27]. What can be a simple dermal lesion (fixed drug eruption) may also present as ulceration with dermal and oral lesions (drug-induced EM) or even a severe, life-threatening syndrome with full thickness epidermal peeling and necrosis (toxic epidermal necrolysis – TEN) [25, 28].

8.2.3 Oral Manifestation of Systemic Diseases

With the tremendous vascularity, high cell turnover, and potential for external exposure, examination of the soft tissue of the oral cavity will often reveal things about the entire patient. A change in mucosal color may indicate anemia (pale), shock (white), cyanosis (blue), bleeding disorders (petechiation), or uremic ulcers. There are many systemic conditions that will manifest themselves in the oral cavity. With uremic ulceration, as ammonia levels in the saliva rise, it can cause irritation and dehydration [29]. Clotting abnormalities can occur and the hemorrhagic ulceration of the dorsum of the tongue can lead to necrosis and sloughing. Vasculitis and xerostomia seen with diabetes mellitus can enhance the progression of periodontitis if untreated. The decreased calcium in hypoparathyroidism can contribute to ectodermal disorders, including enamel calcification, delayed eruption, and disruption in root development if severe [30]. In people, hypothyroidism can hinder the development and eruption of teeth, as well as causing macroglossia and thick lips (cretinism) [31].

Although not caused by any known systemic problem, the idiopathic deposition of amorphous calcified tissue, or calcinosis circumscripta may be identified by the white, chalky, gritty nodules in the tongue and buccal mucosa. These are typically found in young, large breed dogs and can progress to shallow ulceration.

8.2.3.1 Hematology

Hematological disorders also may have oral symptoms, such as anemia due to blood loss, shock or an iron deficiency causing pale mucous membranes that are slow to heal. If the pallor is accompanied by gingival bleeding, petechiae, purpura, or ulcers with a surrounding erythema, thrombocyte irregularities should be considered. Neutropenia, in addition to other systemic signs, may include large, deep, irregular mucosal irritation that can be painful and become necrotic. There are many things that can contribute to a neutropenia, including viral diseases, chemotherapy or radiation treatment, estrogens, chloramphenicol, or phenylbutazone toxicity. Dogs with cyclic neutropenia, or Gray Collie Syndrome, a simple recessive autosomal problem, present with lethargy, fever, joint swelling and many systemic issues, as well as gingivitis, ulceration, and malocclusions of permanent teeth [32]. Leukemia and other myeloproliferative disease can cause non-specific signs. Petechial or ecchymotic hemorrhage, gingival bleeding, or ulceration can be some of the initial manifestations of the disease [33]. In myelocytic leukemia, gingival enlargement, bleeding, and ulcerations are the most common oral symptoms [33].

8.2.4 Systemic Therapy Adverse Reactions

Systemic treatments may give rise to oral lesions, as stated previously. Chemotherapy may result in ulcers that are large, irregular and foul smelling, at times with concurrent anemia, as evident with the pale mucous membranes. The most common sequela to radiation therapy, mucositis, can be minimized with advanced therapy systems [34]. With radiation treatment, there may also be a reduction in salivary flow, an increase in its viscosity, or xerostomia, which can contribute to periodontal disease and caries formation [35]. Severe damage by radiation may lead to a later osteoradionecrosis (ORN), particularly with post-treatment trauma or infection [34].

Chrysotherapy may result in a secondary stomatitis with a peripheral eosinophilia, especially during the initial treatment [36]. Ingestion of warfarin and indandione may lead to various degrees of clotting abnormalities, while doses of thallium can cause erythema and inflammation of the oral epithelium and lips, as well as other tissues. Horseshoe or linear ulcers on the tongue and/or palate can be seen after ingestion of caustic chemicals.

8.2.5 Nutrition

Nutritional deficiencies or excesses should be fairly uncommon, given the opportunities for well formulated pet diets. However, clients may try less traditional options without realizing that their pet's nutritional needs may not be well served. Since the oral cavity has a high rate of cell turnover, initial signs may occur there [37]. A protein-calorie malnutrition, as can be seen in a protein-losing enteropathy or a nephropathy, contributes to a decrease in cell-mediated immunity and can result in a linear ulceration on the dorsum of the tongue [38]. Chronic niacin deficiency has been associated with pellagra in humans and "black tongue" in dogs [39]. Biotin deficiency, while rare, can lead to skin lesion, anorexia, and glossitis [39], and riboflavin deficiency may cause an angular stomatitis (CDC, riboflavin: http://www.cdc.gov/mmwr/preview/mmwrhtml/mm5714a3.htm).

Deficiencies of vitamin C lead to scurvy lesions in animals unable to store the nutrient, mainly humans and guinea pigs. Vitamin C is an important component in maintaining the health of the gingiva and mucous membranes.

Low calcium intake can directly affect the periodontium and all calcified tissues during formative stages. More importantly, if a decreased calcium intake leads to a secondary hyperparathyroidism (or due to renal causes), there will be resorption of calcium from alveolar bone, leaving it soft and contributing to tooth mobility and "rubber jaw" [40].

One nutrient in particular that should be avoided in excessive amounts is vitamin A, found in large amounts in organ meats such as liver. Most signs of excess vitamin A are related to a deforming cervical spondylosis, but it can depress bone growth at very high levels [41]. Moderate increases have not been shown to impact bone growth in the dog [42].

8.3 Palate/Soft Palate/Oropharynx/Tonsils

Many conditions previously described in the general oral pathology portion of this chapter apply to the palate and palatal mucosa (infectious, immune-mediated, metabolic, nutrition, etc.) A significant consideration for the palate (hard and soft) involves cleft defects in the developing dog or cat (see Chapter 4 – Developmental

Pathology and Pedodontology) Another topic with prevalent palatal involvement is that of oral trauma (see Chapter 6 – Traumatic Dentoalveolar Injuries – and Chapter 13 – Oral Surgery – Fracture and Trauma Repair). Particular attention is paid to the palate in specific diseases or cases, such as that of infiltrative aspergillosis [10] or acute corrosion of the palatal mucosa due to the ingestion of Multicolored Asian Lady Beetles (*Harmonia axyridis*) that embed in the soft tissue, causing a chemical-like burn [43]. In cats, hemorrhage from the oral cavity should always instigate a thorough evaluation of the palatal mucosa, particularly in the region of the palatal arteries. It is thought that cats with atopy or other dermatological conditions can damage the mucosa covering this vasculature and while the source may be sometimes difficult to identify, the amount of hemorrhage can be significant.

As a primary divider of the oral and nasal cavities, the palate's integrity is important to maintain their separation. Any cause, from trauma to extension of periodontal disease, can contribute to oronasal or oroantral fistulation that requires repair, to keep the cavities from communicating. The pharynx is described as the region where the digestive and respiratory systems share a common, intersecting pathway, and is divided into the nasopharyngeal, oropharyngeal, and laryngopharyngeal regions [44]. The oropharynx is that section located between the tonsils and the base of the tongue, and while the oral mucosal epithelium lining the region extends beyond the tonsils into the laryngopharynx and further, the oral cavity is considered to extend only to the level of the tonsils. The close association of this region, and even the hard and soft palates that separate the oral and nasal cavities, with the respiratory tract and associated structures, results in syndromes that may affect each other. In a study of 67 dogs with pharyngeal disorders, 7 of those involved the oropharynx (10.5%) with 20 having soft palate disorders that affected the laryngopharynx. Of the oropharyngeal lesions, there were four soft palate granulomas with fistulation, one tonsillar abscess, one soft/hard palate neoplasia, and one mucocele [44]. In a study of 53 cats with nasopharyngeal disorders, classification included 49% with lymphosarcoma and 28% with polyps [45].

Swallowing disorders may include diseases impacting the oropharyngeal phase of swallowing, related to the voluntary prehension and mastication of food and passage of the formed bolus into the pharynx, followed by the involuntary phase of swallowing [46]. The patient can at times adjust to oral dysphagia, while intervention may be needed with pharyngeal and cricopharyngeal dysphagia [46].

8.4 Soft Palate

With brachycephalic airway obstruction syndrome (BAOS), up to 94% of affected dogs have an elongated soft palate, along with stenotic nares, everted laryngeal saccules, and even everted tonsils (56%) [47]. Another study showed an increase in the thickness of the soft palate (not an increase in length), but this was in anesthetized, intubated dogs, and in humans, inspiratory efforts increase the length of the soft palate [48]. Dysplasia of the soft palate has also been associated with nasopharyngeal stenosis [49, 50]. Though less common in cats, an enlongated soft palate in a brachycephalic individual that was overlying the epiglottis and causing airway obstruction resulted in pulmonary edema [51]. Several Dachshunds have been diagnosed with a congenital nasopharyngeal stenosis with thickened palatopharyngeal muscles, dyspnea (expiratory cheek puff), dysphagia, and even macroglossia [52]. The brachycephalic conformation of CKCS with increased soft palate thickness, decreased nasopharyngeal aperture, and possible auditory tube dysfunction may be associated with the high incidence of otitis media with effusion (OME) in the breed [41]. Whether determined radiographically or by clinical signs, there are numerous reports of the association of palatal defects, both cleft palates [53, 54] and soft palate hypoplasia [55, 56], with middle ear disease. The palatal dysfunction is probably just one of multiple predisposing factors to the otitis, as the palate abnormalities are likely to be congenital with the otitis occurring more often later in life [56].

Ventral displacement of the caudal soft palate may result from the presence of a retropharyngeal abscess, tumor, large retained developmental cyst [57], or even a nasopharyngeal polyp. The latter, seen usually in young cats that demonstrate dysphagia and nasal discharge, are protruding, pedunculated growths from the mucous membranes of the auditory canal caused by a response to chronic inflammation. While not a distinct oral process, it is part of a differential diagnoses list, a factor to be ruled out. Often the soft palate must be gently retracted to visualize a polyp, and its treatment sometimes requires a ventral tympanic bullae osteotomy in addition to the polyp removal [58, 59].

Infectious components such as blastomycosis [60] can be found in the pharyngeal region, as well as other agents described in the general oral cavity portion of this chapter. The pharynx can often be involved with foreign body ingestion or injury, and the severity of the lesion may depend on the extent of damage to the respiratory tract, which may include cervical emphysema [61, 62]. Distinct objects such as teeth with intrusion back into the pharynx due to periodontal disease [63] or trichobezoars [64] may be successfully removed when identified. Detection of non-radiopaque objects may be challenging with standard radiography, but may be more likely to be successful with magnetic resonance imaging (MRI) [65].

8.5 Tonsils

Located at the back of the pharynx on either side, the tonsils will often not be visible in their crypts, though the presence of everted tonsils is a frequent observation in brachycephalic airway obstruction syndrome (BAOS) [47]. As a component of the lymphatic system (MALT – mucosa associated lymphoid tissue), enlargement may be due to any type of immune response, such as inflammatory or infective processes (Figure 8.1). Any lesion that does not respond well to conservative therapy such as antibiotics should be biopsied, as both primary and secondary neoplastic cells may be present. A biopsy can help distinguish neoplasia from lesions of cystic formation, lymphangiomatous polyp [66], or an enlargement of the tonsils as part of a non-specific respiratory syndrome seen in racing Greyhounds [67] (see Chapter 7 – Oral and Maxillofacial Tumors, Cysts, and Tumor-Like Lesions – for further discussion).

8.6 Tongue

Like the palate, many problems of the tongue are extensions of generalized oral problems such as ulcerative stomatitis. Due to the high cell turnover rate of the lingual mucosa, the tongue may exhibit changes more quickly than elsewhere in the oral cavity, especially with nutritional causes. In a study looking at histopathology samples of tongue biopsies (0.8% of all biopsies submitted), 54% were neoplastic (64% malignant but only 2–4% of all oral neoplasia), 33.2% were due to glossitis (pyogranolomatous, foreign body 10%, etc.), and 12.2% other, including 3% calcinosis circumscripta and 3% eosinophilic granuloma complex [68].

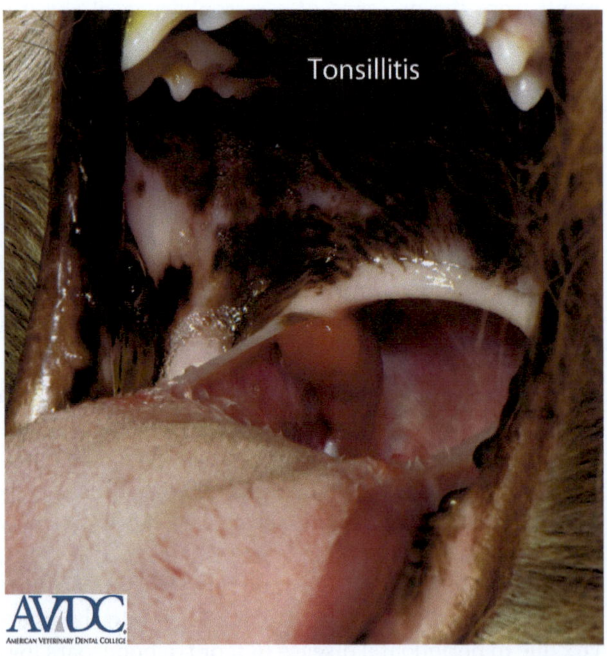

Figure 8.1 Inflamed tonsil visible beyond the crypt edges. *Source:* Copyright® AVDC®, used with permission.

8.6.1 Infectious Agents

Infectious agents that have a particular predilection for the tongue include calicivirus, herpes virus, and rhinotracheitis virus in the cat with ulceration, and a vesicular glossitis associated with calicivirus in the dog [69]. *Leptospira canicola* leads to severe congestion with a glossitis related to uremia that can eventually necrose the tongue tip. Opportunistic infections of acute necrotizing ulcerative gingivitis (ANUG) may exhibit necrotic bleeding ulcers, while candidiasis stimulates a diffuse inflammation with a whitish plaque coating of the surface. Leishmaniasis, while usually manifested by fever, lymphadenopathy, weight loss, lameness, and skin lesions, can also cause the formation of nodular lesions on the tongue. Caused by a flagellate protozoa transmitted by sand flies, diagnosis of one case was confirmed by identifying the presence of amastigotes in a biopsy of the lingual lesion [4].

8.6.2 Lingual Masses

In canine oral papillomatosis, single to multiple or coalescing white to tan hyperkeratotic, pedunculated nodules are virally induced and often spontaneously regress [70]. If extensive, surgical removal can be utilized to debulk the masses, while interferon with or without azithromycin have also been suggested as treatment options [71]. Other tumors and masses are covered in Chapter 7 – Oral and Maxillofacial Tumors, Cysts, and Tumor-Like Lesions.

8.6.3 Metabolic

Metabolic uremia as described earlier demonstrates distinct lingual signs, including hemorrhagic, brownish ulcers of the dorsal tongue with potential necrosis and sloughing. Hypothyroidism in earlier stages of development may result in a macroglossia, while hypoparathyroidism can contribute to ulceration and necrosis of the tongue tip. In an adult Dalmatian, acromegaly and insulin resistance due to growth hormone hypersecretion (somatroph adenoma of the pituitary gland) had signs of enlargement of the tongue and thickening of the skin noticed by the owner [72]. A case of atypical mucosal xanthoma associated with hyperlipidemia has been reported, characterized by granular plaques and nodules with a foamy cell, where the lipid content is similar to oral verruciform xanthomas in humans [73].

Calcinosis circumscripta refers to the idiopathic deposition of calcified (hydroxyapatite or amorphous calcium phosphate), chalky nodules on the surface of the tongue or in the sublingual area. The etiology is unknown and is not due to the degeneration of an apocrine gland, as once thought [74]. Young (74% < 2 year, 88% < 4 year), large breed dogs (28.6% German Shepherd dog (GSD), 13% Rottweiler, 9% Labrador) are most commonly affected, and dermal lesions may also be present [75]. Three types have been identified with the dystrophic or idiopathic being most common in animals and the metastatic form being more common in humans [75]. The use of von Kossa or Alizarin red stains on cytological smears from fine needle aspiration can confirm the calcified nature of the lesion without biopsy [76]. If clinical signs are present, the lesions may be resected, but they are benign and not locally progressive. One report of an atypical case described lesions found in a 10 month old Shih Tzu, where whitish masses with amorphous calcium salts were accompanied by a slight nutritional myopathy, possibly due to vitamin E and/or selenium deficiency [77].

8.6.4 Immune Mediated

Most of the immune-mediated diseases described for the general oral cavity can have lingual lesions. An uncommon finding, reactive histiocytosis of the sublingual region, was described in an eight year old Miniature Pinscher that responded to tetracycline and niacinamide administration over a period of eight months [78].

8.6.5 Trauma

Traumatic lesions to the tongue may be related to the primary damage or secondary insult due to infection, such as a glossitis secondary to bite wounds contaminated with *Pasteurella multocida* [79].

The sublingual area can be swollen or distended due to a number of reasons. Unilaterally, a soft, fluctuant swelling may be indicative of a leakage of saliva into the area, also known as a ranula [70]. Sublingual edema may be secondary to venous obstruction in the pharyngeal region due to abscessation or surgery. Proliferative or hyperplastic tissue in the sublingual region or buccal mucosa can be seen due to chronic, recurrent self-trauma of the tissues. These "gum-chewers" lesions should be biopsied for a definitive diagnosis, and excess tissue can be surgically removed if trauma is severe or tissue is severely hyperplastic.

8.6.6 Miscellaneous

Other lingual lesions may include a condition called "hairy tongue," where filiform papillae are elongated to resemble hairs and are often stained darkly. This is typically an incidental finding during oral examination. Rarely will a glossitis be present and debridement of impacted material is seldom necessary.

Tongue atrophy as a part of an atypical polymyositis has been described in Pembroke Welsh Corgis in Japan, with marked myofiber loss and mixed mononuclear infiltrate on histopathology [80, 81]. Dysphagia and hypersalivation were the presenting signs of one case that progressed to aspiration pneumonia and eventual death.

8.7 Salivary Glands

8.7.1 Congenital

A congenital atresion of a salivary duct or absence of one gland is unlikely to make a difference due to the presence of the other glands. Ptyalism, (excessive drooling) has been seen in cases with congenitally enlarged parotid ducts, but these are rare primary salivary gland abnormalities and can be managed well by ligating the duct. Sialadenitis, of probable immune- mediated causes, was described in a young Golden Retriever presented for epiphora and facial swelling extending from the inflamed submucosal glands. The condition responded to anti-inflammatory treatment [82].

8.7.2 Acquired

The overall incidence of salivary gland disease in dogs and cats has been reported as very low (0.3%) [83]. Malignancies accounted for only 30% of this overall low rate and epithelial malignancies accounted for approximately 85% of salivary gland tumors, but lymphoma, fibrosarcoma, and mast cell tumors have involved the salivary glands through invasion or direct extension from surrounding tissues [84] (see Chapter 7 – Oral and Maxillofacial Tumors, Cysts, and Tumor-Like Lesions).

8.7.2.1 Sialadenitis

Sialadenitis composed 26% of the overall incidence rate of salivary disease, both as primary and secondary disease (Figure 8.2a–c). It presents as inflammation and enlargement of the salivary gland, often with formation of a sialocele. Possible causes include injury, infection (local, systemic, or secondary to regional), or immune-mediated disease. One study of 11 dogs with zygomatic sialadenitis compared clinical signs and diagnostic imaging with 20 control dogs [85]. Most were medium to

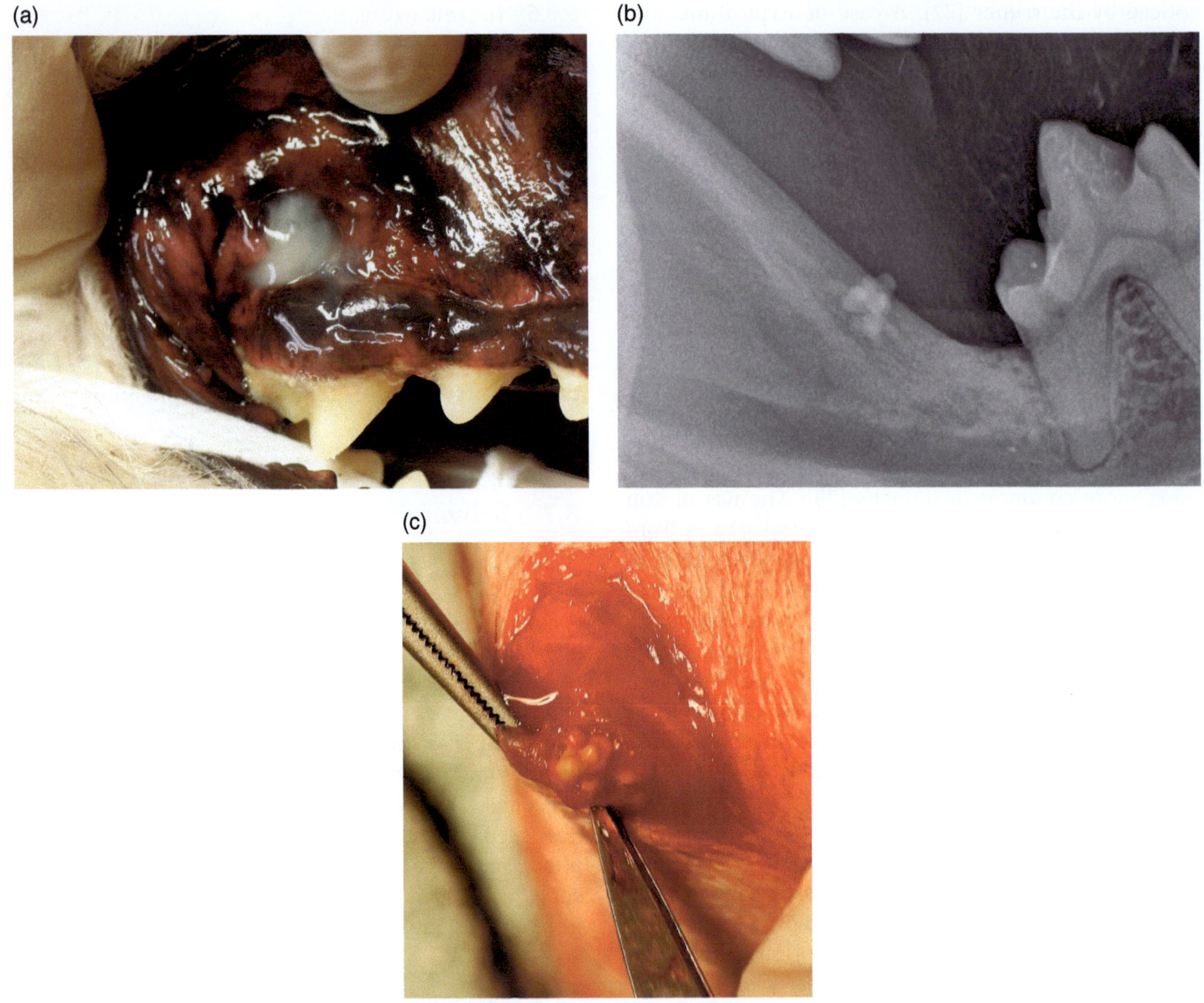

Figure 8.2 (a) Suppurative discharge from parotid duct. (b) Radiograph revealing radiopaque sialolith in parotid duct. (c) Multilobular sialolith surgically removed from parotid duct; resolution of sialadenitis.

large breed dogs with unilateral disease, and signs of retrobulbar disease and sialoceles were present in seven cases. Visualization of the lesion and adjacent structures was excellent with MRI and computed tomography (CT), while ultrasonography was useful for sample collection [85]. Another reported case described necrotizing sialadenitis of the mandibular salivary glands, likely due to immune-mediated cause (responded to corticosteroids), with zygomatic gland enlargement and sialoceles [86]. Hypersalivation in the absence of gastrointestinal signs, exophthalmus, and pain on opening the mouth were some presenting symptoms, with possible epileptic activity.

Another case reported episodic acute facial swelling ventral to the right eye that would resolve the next day, with eventual progression leading to swelling of the hard and soft palate due to suppurative sialadenitis of the palatal submucosal salivary tissue [82]. The pain on opening the mouth and inability to close the mouth resolved with antibiotics and corticosteroids, but recurred when the latter was discontinued, leading to suspicion of possible bacterial and/or immune etiologies.

In two reported feline cases, necrotizing sialometaplasia was differentiated from neoplasia by the presence of lobular necrosis with squamous metaplasia conforming to the duct and/or acinar outlines, with preservation of lobular morphology [87]. In humans, this is an ischemic disease, and salivary gland infarction has been reported to be associated with 13% of feline salivary gland disease [83]. Surgical removal was performed successfully.

8.7.2.2 Sialadenosis

Enlargement of salivary glands with ptyalism and dysphagia that is responsive to phenobarbital has been described in cats [88], a 10 week old GSD [89] and others, consistent with a diagnosis of sialadenosis, with no abnormalities noted on histopathology [90]. This may represent peripheral autonomic dysfunction or a form of limbic epilepsy [89].

On the other extreme, a case of xerostomia and xerophthalmia in a cat (similar to Sjogren's syndrome in humans) has been reported in a cat [91]. This was likely to be due to lymphocytic-mediated destruction of exocrine glands that responded to symptomatic therapy for the eyes, as well as regular application of pilocarpine to the tongue to stimulate salivation to a small degree [91].

8.7.2.3 Sialocele

Sialoceles (mucoceles) are accumulations of saliva in soft tissue surrounding the glands that may make up to 9% of all salivary gland disease [83]. These are not cysts as they lack a fluid-producing cellular lining. Possible causes include trauma to the gland and/or duct, foreign material, infection, sialoliths or anything that can inflame or damage the salivary tissue, allowing the saliva to leak out, causing further inflammation. While most specific causes are unknown [92], cases report zygomatic mucocele (sialocele) secondary to caudal hemimaxillectomy [93], parotid duct obstruction after caudal maxillectomy [94], fight trauma to a parotid gland [95], penetrating stick [96], tooth extraction [97], and even post-enucleation mucocele formation at a previously transposed parotid duct (that was then repositioned to the oral cavity) [98]. Metaplastic ossifications of a cervical sialocele has also been seen [99].

Sialocele presentation can be variable, depending on the gland affected (see Table 8.2) [100]. Sublingual and cervical mucoceles are most common, while pharyngeal and zygomatic mucoceles are rare [101]. Fine needle aspirates of the area are likely to reveal a viscous, yellowish, clear, or blood-tinged fluid with a low cell count [100]. Pink to violet staining clumps of mucin (periodic acid-Schiff for definitive diagnosis) may be accompanied by large phagocytic cells with foamy cytoplasm and epithelial cells. Sialography can be used to further confirm diagnosis and identify the affected gland, but this is generally reserved for trauma patients or draining tracts [100]. Histopathological examination of the excised tissue will confirm diagnosis. Sialoceles are not cysts as they lack a fluid-producing cellular lining.

Radiography is often not rewarding with most salivary disease, unless sialoliths or ossification is present. Sialography with contrast media can help locate duct rupture or obstructions, such as sialoliths [102]. Ultrasonography is a non-invasive means of initial assessment of any suspected salivary enlargement or inflammation, particularly those lesions smaller than 3 cm [103], and can begin the differentiation process. Ultrasonographic appearances of mucoceles vary depending on the chronological stage of the disease [103]. Advanced imaging with MRI and CT provide superior diagnostics, which can be very helpful, particularly with zygomatic mucoceles to rule out other causes of retrobulbar disease, including neoplasia [104–106].

While chemical treatment of mucoceles has been described [107] and marsupialization may be selected for sublingual mucoceles, surgical removal of the lesion and the corresponding salivary gland is the most frequent treatment recommended [108]. Surgical removal of both the mandibular and sublingual salivary glands is recommended for treating cervical, pharyngeal, and sublingual mucoceles (see Chapter 12 – Oral Surgery – General). For cats, there have been reports of sialocele caused by ruptured ducts being successfully managed by ligating the duct, resulting in gland atrophy [109], but variable response in duct ligation studies reveals that the innervations of the gland must also be dealt with (chorda tympani) [110].

8.7.2.4 Sialoliths

Salivary stones (sialoliths) are uncommon in the dog (0.4% incidence [83]), with most reports being in the parotid duct, though many are likely to go undiagnosed [111].

Table 8.2 Siaolocele characteristics.

Location	Gland	Type	Features	Comments
Intermandibular space, jaw angle, upper cervical region	Sublingual	Cervical mucocele	Soft, fluctuant, pain only in acute phase	
Sublingual tissues	Mandibular or sublingual	Ranula	Soft swelling, blood-tinged saliva while eating	
Pharyngeal wall	Sublingual	Pharyngeal mucocele	Respiratory distress, dysphagia	Miniature and toy poodles
Ventral to the globe	Zygomatic	Zygomatic mucocele	Periorbital facial swelling, exophthalmus, pain	
Angle of the jaw, ventral to ear	Parotid	Parotid mucocele	Swelling ventral to ear	

Composition of the sialoliths can include calcium carbonate, magnesium carbonate, and magnesium ammonium phosphate. Chronic inflammation with desquamated cells and exudates may be the nidus for sialolith formation within a sialocele or associated with sialadenitis. In one report of a sublingual swelling identified as a sialocele (with histological signs of inflammation – sialadenitis), mineralized structures within the gland or sialocele were seen radiographically [111]. Surgical removal of the affected glands and drainage of the sialocele resolved this lesion, but a ductal sialolith on the other side one month later required surgical removal of those glands. Other reported cases include the removal of a single parotid duct sialolith that was only partially obstructing the duct, with the incision left to heal by second intention [102], and parotid duct sialocele with glandular duct stenosis in a cat, treated by the removal of the duct and gland [109].

Salivary glands may also be affected by radiation therapy of the head and neck. While some saliva will still be produced, it will tend to be more viscous in nature, causing a "dry mouth." This can predispose the patient to oral infections, even leading to post-irradiation caries in humans in 2–10 months if quality oral hygiene is not maintained. The patient's teeth may also be more sensitive to hot and cold.

8.8 Cheeks/Lips

Congenital or developmental lesions of the lips may include cleft defects or a tight lip in Shar Pei dogs (see Chapter 4 – Developmental Pathology and Pedodontology) (see Figure 8.3a and b). Particularly in fractious patients, lesions on the lips may be the only oral-related problems that some owners will ever notice. Cheilitis, or inflammation of the lip(s), may occur as a secondary bacterial infection after some irritant (plastic bowl) or trauma (electric cord) has injured the lips. Severe trauma may cause the avulsion of the soft tissue of the lower lip from the mandible. Spaniels and other breeds with pendulous lips can get lip fold dermatitis as saliva drains into the folds, keeping them moist and readily susceptible to infection. Any inflammatory lesion that does not respond to routine treatment should always be biopsied.

Since the mucocutaneous regions of the lips include both mucosal surfaces and tissues of the skin, processes that can involve either type may be present in the lips, from neoplasia to autoimmune disorders. While neoplasia is fairly uncommon at this site, reports of a variety of tumors have been published, including primary intraoral leiomyosarcoma [112], melanocytic tumors [113–115], mast cell tumors [116–118], squamous cell carcinoma [119], canine cutaneous clear cell adnexal carcinoma [120], and even cutaneous epitheliotropic lymphoma [121], which should be differentiated from cutaneous lymphoid hyperplasia [122]. Xanthoma formation [73], leishmaniasis lesions [123, 124], and eosinophilic granuloma complex lesions may also be found.

8.9 Skeletomuscular

8.9.1 Myopathy

Without the proper action of the muscles of mastication, all oral function would cease. In a review of 200 canine inflammatory myopathies, 45 (22.5%) were identified as canine masticatory muscle myositis (CMMM) [125]. Characterized by an inability to open the jaws (trismus),

(a) (b)

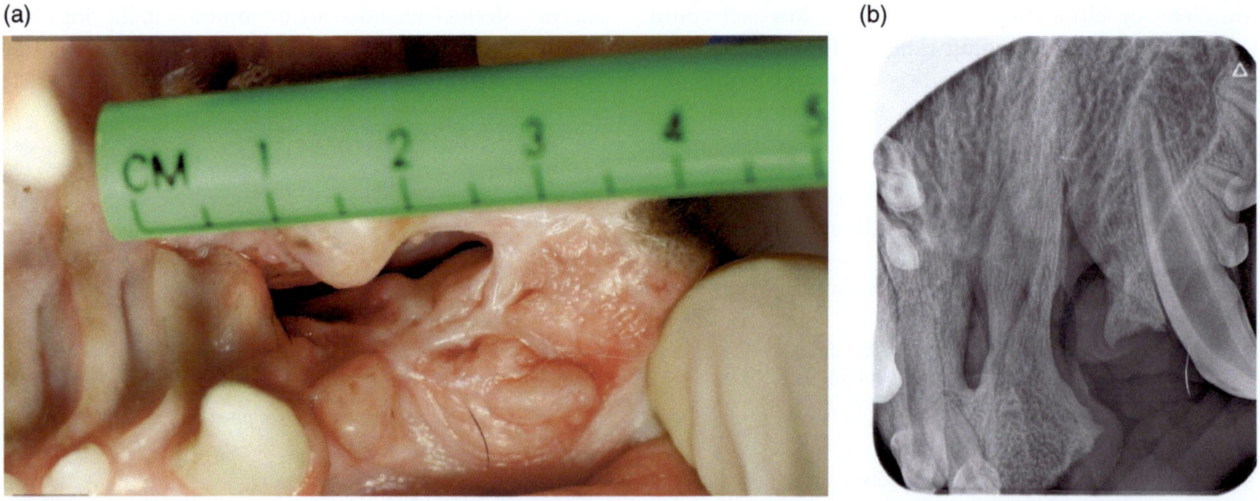

Figure 8.3 (a) Left unilateral primary cleft lip still present after three surgical attempts at closure; palatal portion of the cleft was repaired. (b) Radiograph of left unilateral primary cleft.

jaw pain and masticatory muscle atrophy, with occasional exophthalmos, this immune-mediated syndrome impacts those muscles innervated by the mandibular branch of the trigeminal nerve (masseter, temporalis, pterygoids). While the gold standard for diagnosis is Type 2M fiber (muscle fiber unique to masticatory muscles) antibody detection, these autoantibodies are more likely to be found in the active phase of the disease [126]. More chronic presentations will show the atrophy with or without restricted jaw mobility [127]. Elevated CK and ALT levels may be present, but typically not as elevated as in generalized polymyositis conditions, and eosinophilia was found in 30% of CMMM [125]. Other imaging modalities can be helpful adjuncts, with MRI being able to reflect the stage [128, 129] and CT helping to guide biopsy collection [130]. Biopsies of affected muscles often reveal a collection of lymphocytes and macrophages, and immunohistochemical assays may be helpful.

Some unusual presentations of MMM include a group of three out of four CKCS that demonstrated signs starting at 12 weeks of age [131], or a case with concurrent myasthenia gravis [132]. Care should be taken during diagnostic procedures, even with a temporary tracheostomy or laryngeal mask, as tongue protrusion and subsequent venous congestion during one surgical case was not resolved even with digastricus and masseter muscle attachment removal [133]. A mandibular symphysiotomy was needed to finally reduce the entrapment pressure.

Other muscular disorders may include atrophy of the masticatory muscles as a sequel of leishmaniasis [6, 134], polymyositis conditions that can affect the tongue [80] and diseases of the trigeminal nerve that can result in atrophy [135–137]. The inability to open the mouth may also be present with a tetanus infection, but this is primarily due to the spasms of the masticatory and facial muscles. While dogs may be less susceptible to *Clostridium tetani* than other species (horse, man), the characteristic "grimace" of the lips being pulled back and overall weakness may lead a clinician to suspect this.

8.9.2 Trigeminal Neuropathy

Trigeminal neuropathy (mandibular neuropraxia) may be suspected if a dog is presented with an open mouth that can be closed passively with little effort. In a retrospective study of 29 dogs with flaccid paralysis or paresis of the masticatory muscles innervated by the trigeminal nerve, 26 were determined to be idiopathic, based on resolution of clinical signs and lack on long-term neuropathy [138]. If the animal has a history of carrying heavy or large objects in its mouth, it is possible that the branches of the nerves supplying the masticatory muscles have been stressed or stretched, though one case presented signs secondary to a nervous system lymphosarcoma [139]. Recovery in idiopathic cases usually occurs in two to four weeks with rest and conservative support, as use of corticosteroids had no effect on the clinical course of the disease [138].

8.10 Temporomandibular Joint

The temporomandibular joint (articulation temporomandibularis) (TMJ) can be impacted by trauma, skeletal abnormalities, dysplasia, inflammation, and tumors. Many of the issues concerning the TMJ are trauma-related, either immediately due to acute damage to specific components of the joint or chronic changes such as osteoarthritis or ankylosis (characterized as a formation by osseous or fibrous elements at an articulation) [140].

Problems or perception of pain in opening or closing the mouth, while sometimes due to other diseases (MMM, trigeminal neuropraxia), should always include a complete evaluation of the bilateral TMJs. Palpation for swelling, enlargements, detecting the range of motion (ROM), eliciting pain, and auscultating for crepitus are important steps in evaluation. Imaging with radiographs can be challenging due to superimposition of maxillofacial/cranial structures, requiring some rotation in either the lateral (10–30°) or long axis (10–30°) to isolate the individual structures [141]. Using the "nose-up" projection of about 20° or a lateral 20° oblique has also been described [142]. Advanced imaging provided additional benefits, from CT [143, 144] to MRI [145].

8.10.1 Dysplasia

Other than traumatic lesions, dysplasia of the temporomandibular joint can predispose patients to a myriad of issues. With radiographic evidence of the flattening of the condylar process of the mandible and mandibular fossa, hyperplastic or misshapened retroarticular process, the widened irregular joint space may also be associated with osteophytosis and rotation or obliquity of the articular surface [146]. In younger dogs, the joint spaces may appear wider and slightly less curved, due to the fact that the cartilage is incompletely ossified [146]. In certain breeds, such as Dachshunds [147] and CKCS [141] apparent dysplasia can be fairly widespread and asymptomatic, and should be regarded as a normal morphological variation. While there is some transverse motion possible in dogs, even with the lateral and caudal ligaments providing support (and a thickening of the lateral capsule in cats), dysplastic changes in the TMJs can provide sufficient laxity to contribute to conditions such as subluxation, luxation, and abnormal positioning, particularly if the mandibular symphysis has laxity as well.

The wider angle between the mandibles of cats may allow unilateral luxation without concurrent mandibular fracture or symphyseal separation [148]. Most luxations are traumatic in nature [149].

8.10.2 Open-Mouth Locking

The combination of joint and symphyseal laxity had been considered contributing factors to the development of an open-mouth locking syndrome where the dorsal edge of the coronoid process moves laterally to the zygomatic arch when the mouth is opened widely [150–155]. While this condition can be quickly reduced by opening the mouth further and pressing on the coronoid process bulge to move it back into position, it will recur with some frequency until the mode of interlocking can be corrected. Treatments have included bilateral condylectomies [151], approaches for partial excision (rostroventral) of the zygomatic arch, partial excision (dorsal) of the coronoid process [155], a portion of both [150, 153], and even combining these with an intermandibular arthrodesis of the symphysis [154]. Surgical intervention is typically successful unilaterally, though bilateral disease may require bilateral resection [152].

8.10.3 Closed-Mouth Locking

Closed-mouth locking has been described in a Bulldog that required fluoroscopy during TMJ manipulation to demonstrate the dynamic interference of the rostrodorsal aspect of the coronoid process with the medial surface of the zygomatic bone and orbital ligament [156]. Resection of the coronoid process removed the mechanical interference in that case. Proliferative diseases that impact the bones in the region can also disrupt the ROM of the joints, including skull osteomyelitis [157], ossification of adjacent soft tissues (bilateral lateral pterygoid muscles) [158], tumors [159], and trauma [160, 161]. Pathological changes in the middle ear (cholesteatomas) [162, 163] and tympanic bullae (squamous cell carcinoma) [164] can have extensions into the TMJ region that cause a range of symptoms from pain when opening the mouth to complete ankylosis of the joint.

8.10.4 Ankylosis

True or articular ankylosis occurs rarely, most often due to traumatic damage to some part of the joint, and surgery (gap arthroplasty) [165] is often the treatment of choice [140, 165–167] (see Chapter 13 – Oral Surgery – Fracture and Trauma Repair). When osseous or fibrous callous of structures outside of the joint result in its immobilization, it is termed a false ankylosis, or pseudoankylosis, a more common presentation than true ankylosis, and typically due to trauma [140]. Resection of the offending tissue can be challenging, but often may be sufficient to ameliorate the TMJ signs.

8.11 Osteomyelitis

There are many routes for an infection to start in the bones of the oral cavity. Extensions from periodontal and periapical infections, retained roots, as well as exposure to pathogens from trauma, bite wounds, or penetrating foreign objects can set up an active infection, as can a hematogenous or systemic source, including fungal infections [168]. In one study of cats and dogs with anaerobic osteomyelitis, the mandible was the third most common site, outranked by the radius and ulna [169]. The swelling associated with the lesion can become large and firm, and is often painful on palpation. Radiographically there may be a zone of bony destruction surrounded by a region of increased density or sclerosis. Additionally, periosteal reaction may be present and sequestration may be noted. Osteomyelitis of the jaws is typically seen as a proliferative reaction of the periosteum at the periphery of the lesion with lysis of the associated cortical and alveolar bone. The bone lysis may give the appearance that teeth are supported primarily by soft tissue, but seldom are the teeth displaced (such as seen with many cysts and tumors). In the oral region, fractures and tooth infections are commonly an initiating force. Any lesion that does not respond to treatment of curettage and appropriate antibiotic therapy (sometimes extensive) should be biopsied. In a CT study of four young dogs with skull osteomyelitis, all were due to trauma or bite wounds and showed a variety of signs from osteolysis and osteoproliferation to even bony sequestrum [157].

8.12 Hyperostosis

Proliferation of bone can be seen in a number of syndromes that have been identified in young dogs in a variety of breeds, and the term "idiopathic canine juvenile cranial hyperostosis" has been used to group these together [170]. These syndromes are covered in Chapter 4 – Developmental Pathology and Pedodontology.

8.12.1 Osteodystrophia Fibrosa

The jaws may also appear swollen in cases of hyperparathyroidism, whether primary or secondary to dietary calcium deficiency or renal failure [29, 31, 171]. The resulting resorption of calcium from calcified tissues generally begins with the mandible, progressing to the maxilla, skull, axial, and then long bones. The areas of resorption are replaced with fibro-osseous tissue – osteodystrophia fibrosa ("rubber jaw") – with radiographic densities affected first with the loss of definition of the lamina dura and then of the trabecular and cortical bone regions. Tooth loss will be accelerated due to loss of bony support. Since the mandible may be the first indication of a problem, it is very important to investigate the primary cause, and if this is dietary or renal, make steps for correction where possible.

8.13 Acquired Dental Lesions

A variety of dental lesions are covered in other chapters of this book, including:

- Congenital and developmental lesions in Chapter 4 – Developmental Pathology and Pedodontology
- Traumatic fractures and injuries in Chapter 6 – Traumatic Dentoalveolar Injuries
- Dental defense mechanism and pulp response in Chapter 17 – Restorative Dentistry
- Tooth resorptions (TRs) in cats (in greater detail) in Chapter 20 – Domestic Feline Oral and Dental Diseases

The remaining miscellaneous lesions are covered here.

8.13.1 Enamel–Dentinal Lesions

There can be an expected level of physiological attrition or wear seen as a gradual loss of tooth substance and if the process is gradual enough, once the enamel is gone, reparative dentin, often brown in color, will be deposited to help protect the pulp from being exposed. With slow, chronic wear, the crown may become level with the gingiva, yet the canal may still be closed, the "retreating" pulp being protected by the dentinal deposition. Dental attrition, or increased wear of a tooth, is due to mastication or grinding between teeth. People who grind their teeth (bruxism) is a classic example, while animals with malocclusions causing tooth-to-tooth contact is another. Abrasion is caused by mechanical actions other than mastication (including eating roughage or deliberate chewing on ingestible objects) or tooth-to-tooth contacts, such an incorrect tooth-brushing or teeth being used as a tool – to groom or catch balls. Erosion is the progressive loss of tooth substance by chemical or acid dissolution, without bacterial action, probably due to acidic compounds in contact with the tooth, either ingested or from regurgitated or vomited stomach fluids. If these acids are retained in the gingival sulci, the erosion can be localized in that area. Any loss of enamel can expose dentinal tubules and considerations for placing a dentinal bonding agent on these tubules may be considered.

Abfraction lesions are non-carious cervical lesions thought to be caused by biomechanical loading forces (flexing and stress) so that the enamel separates from the inner dentin layer, as described in people, though the theory is not yet proven. Further abrasion from aggressive brushing could put teeth with cervical hard-tissue loss at risk for fracture, as could forceful manipulation of hand instruments to clean teeth during anesthesia-free dental cleanings (in this author's opinion). Crazing of a tooth refers to the fine cracks in the outermost layer of enamel caused by stress placed on a tooth, though the tooth is structurally sound.

More vigorous or extensive chewing, or traumatic events, can cause a more precipitous loss of enamel and dentin – or dental fractures. Specific descriptions and classifications are covered in Chapter 6 – Traumatic Dentoalveolar Injuries – and treatment, from extraction (Chapter 11 – Oral Surgery – Extraction) to endodontic therapy (Chapter 15 – Basic Endodontic Therapy), are also covered elsewhere in this book.

8.13.2 Caries

Hard tissue loss of a tooth due to the effects of oral bacteria or caries can result in the decay of the enamel, with potential progression into the dentin and even the pulp. This first begins as a decalcification of inorganic material by acids formed when bacterial enzymes ferment carbohydrates [171], often in sheltered areas between teeth or in pits and fissures. These lesions are not common in most animals up to a 5.2% incidence in one study [176]. The most prevalent area for carious formation is on the occlusal surface of first maxillary molars in dogs, though smooth surface caries can be seen on teeth with close interproximal contacts, or even on roots (root caries).

A chalky white spot known as an incipient caries is the first indication of enamel demineralization which progresses relatively slowly, and may be reversible through remineralization by use of a fluoride varnish or pit and fissure sealant [172]. Once the protein matrix has been compromised, the now irreversible lesion will be seen as a structural defect filled with dark dentinal material. The sharp tip of an explorer can easily sink into this softened dentin, and it can be debrided with hand instruments initially. The demineralization process proceeds more rapidly in the dentin, sometimes mushrooming underneath the enamel, potentially undermining it. Without intervention, the decay can extend into the pulp cavity itself, resulting in infection and eventual pulp necrosis. These lesions are classically staged by the G.V. Black classification (see Chapter 17 – Restorative Dentistry).

8.13.3 Tooth Resorption (TR)

Tooth resorption may occur as either internal or external resorption. Tooth resorption has been frequently reported in cats and more recently described in the literature in dogs [172]. The AVDC classifications for tooth resorption are applicable to both dogs and cats and will be discussed in more detail in Chapter 20 – Domestic Feline Oral and Dental Disease.

Briefly, in relation to tooth resorption in dogs, external lesions are more commonly seen, including external surface resorption, external replacement resorption, external cervical root surface resorption and external inflammatory (Type 1) resorption [173]. These lesions are diagnosed radiographically, frequently involving multiple teeth, yet with few coronal lesions, unless significantly progressed. A variety of factors from mastication forces, orthodontic forces, and even the presence of oral tumors at distant sites have been implicated [174], but often the cause is not fully known. Internal resorption is less common, and might be detected initially due to a pinkish hue in the crown of the affected tooth. Pulpal inflammation is the most likely factor and continued vitality of the pulp should be monitored if the tooth is to be treated and retained [175]. Further discussion of the pathogenesis of pulpitis can be found in Chapter 15 – Basic Endodontic Therapy.

8.13.4 Tooth Discoloration

Whether due to external or internal causes, any discoloration of a tooth requires its full assessment, including radiographs and transillumination. Teeth with dentinogenesis imperfecta may be grayish to bluish in color and seem more translucent than a normal tooth (see Chapter 4 – Developmental Pathology and Pedodontology) (Figure 8.4a,b).

In a study looking at discolored teeth, most due to localized intrinsic staining due to pulpitis or pulpal necrosis, 59 of 64 of the affected teeth had either partial or total pulp necrosis (the remaining 20 pulps were not examined of the 84 teeth total) [176]. Radiographically, 36 of the 84 teeth had no radiographic indications of pulpal compromise such as wider pulp canals or periapical changes, though all but two of the teeth treated endodontically ($n = 54$) had radiographic changes.

Stains on the surface of teeth that can be polished away with abrasives are known as extrinsic stains. The color changes in the teeth are often due to pigments in dietary substances, habits such as cage biting, or the byproducts of bacteria in dental plaque and tartar. Regular use of chlorhexidine products can result in a dark staining of the tooth surfaces, though the use of a monoperoxyphthalic acid (MPA) rinse prior to CHX has been shown to decrease the amount of staining, and even the extent of plaque accumulation and gingivitis [177].

Intrinsic stains result from the deposition of systemically circulating substances during tooth development or from byproducts from within the tooth. Tetracycline staining can be found when pregnant mothers, or young animals, are administered tetracycline for the treatment of infections. The use of tetracycline can produce a permanent yellow or gray-brown discoloration of the affected teeth, enamel hypoplasia, and disorders of dentin deposition. The severity of stains depends on the time and duration of the drug administration and the dosage.

A grayish black discoloration of teeth may occur with both pulpal necrosis and intrapulpal hemorrhage. When the nerve of the tooth undergoes necrosis, tissue disintegration byproducts are released. These byproducts penetrate dentinal tubules and cause discoloration of the surrounding dentin. After traumatic injury to a tooth

(a) (b)

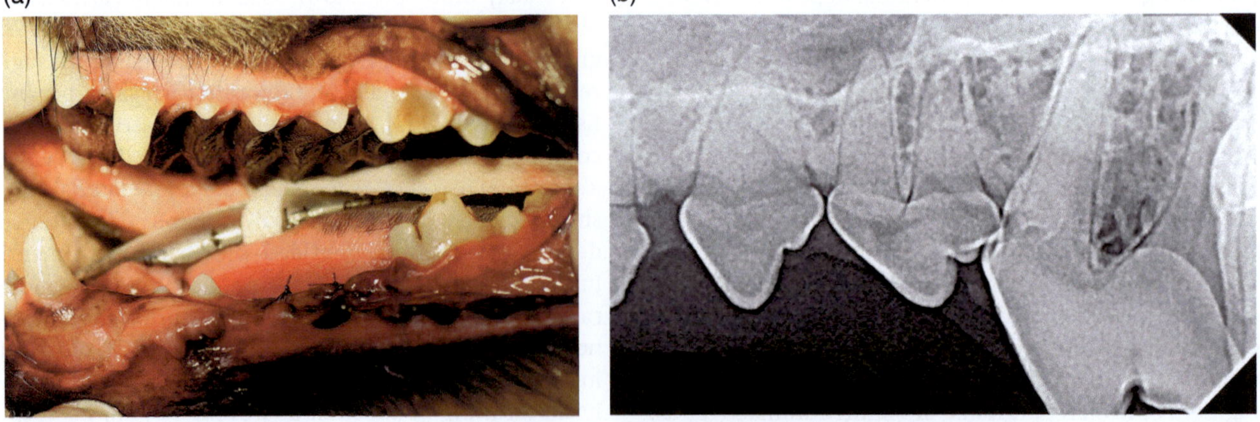

Figure 8.4 (a) bluish discoloration and translucency of teeth due to dentinogenesis imperfecta; (b) homogeneous appearance of internal material in teeth with diminished root canals.

intrapulpal hemorrhage can introduce iron sulfides into the tooth and discolor dentin as well. The longer a tooth has either had pulpal necrosis or intrapulpal hemorrhage, the more severe the discoloration [178] (see Chapter 15 – Basic Endodontic Therapy).

Teeth that are treated with root canal therapy, pulpotomies, or even amalgam fillings can change color. Depending on the sealer choice, if adequate removal of sealer and gutta percha is not achieved, the dentinal tubules can become discolored, changing the shade of the tooth. In pulpotomies, gray MTA (mineral trioxide aggregate) can also leach into dentinal tubules and cause tooth discoloration. A newer white MTA has become available and can be a more esthetic option to use.

8.13.5 Cementosis

Hypercementosis is an increase in the deposition of cementum customarily along the root surface of the tooth. It typically appears as a bulbous enlargement of the root tip, as compared to the normal tapering contour of the apex. Hypercementosis can occur due to the occlusal trauma and can be observed in the teeth of cats with inflammatory resorptive lesions. Hypercementosis can also occur due to chronic inflammation of pulpal tissues. These teeth will often require root canal therapy. Hypercementosis may be a complication seen in human patients suffering from Paget's disease (a bone disease). Cementomas (fibro-osteoma) are generally benign proliferations of the connective tissues in the jaws that produce cementum or cementum-like tissue.

References

1 Klokkevold, P.R. and Carranza, F.A. (2015). Acute gingival infections. In: *Carranza's Clinical Periodontology*, 12e (ed. M.G. Newman, H.H. Takei, P.R. Klokkevold and F.A. Carranza), 224–251. St. Louis, MO: Elsevier.

2 Maltha, J.C., Mikx, F.H.M., and Kuijpers, F.J. (1985). Necrotizing ulcerative gingivitis in beagle dogs. *J. Periodontal. Res.* 20: 522–531.

3 Sykes, J.E., Hartmann, K. et al. (2010, 2011). ACVIM small animal consensus statement on leptospirosis: diagnosis, epidemiology, treatment and prevention. *J. Vet. Intern. Med.* 25: 1–13.

4 Parpagalia, M.L., Vercelli, A. et al. (2007). Nodular lesions of the tongue in canine leishmaniosis. *J. Vet. Med.* 54 (8): 414–417.

5 Levy, E., Mylonakis, M.E. et al. (2006). Nasal and oral masses in a dog. *Vet. Clin. Pathol.* 35 (1): 115–118.

6 Koutinas, A.F. and Koutinas, C.K. (2014). Pathologic mechanisms underlying the clinical findings in canine leishmaniasis due to *Leishmania infantum/chagasi*. *Vet. Pathol.* 51 (2): 527–538.

7 Nardoni, S., Dini, M., Taccini, F., and Mancianti, F. (2007). Occurrence, distribution and population size of *Malassezia pachydermatis* on skin and mucosa of atopic dogs. *Vet. Microbiol.* 122 (1–2): 172–177.

8 Jadhav, V.J. and Pal, M. (2006). Canine mycotic stomatitis due to *Candida albicans*. *Rev. Iberoam. Micol.* 23 (4): 233–234.

9 Rees, T.D. (2015). Pathology and management of periodontal problems in patients with human immunodeficiency virus infection. In: *Carranza's Clinical Periodontology*, 12e (ed. M.G. Newman, H.H. Takei, P.R. Klokkevold and F.A. Carranza), 335–344. St. Louis, MO: Elsevier.

10 Giordano, C., Gianella, P. et al. (2010). Invasive mould infections of the naso-orbital region of cats: a case involving *Aspergillus fumigatus* and an aetiological review. *J. Feline Med. Surg.* 12 (9): 714–723.

11 Olson, G.A. and Wowk, B.J. (1981). Oral lesions of histoplasmosis in a dog. *Vet. Med.* 79 (10): 1449–1451.

12 Radford, A.D., Addie, D. et al. (2009). Feline calicivirus infection: ABCD guidelines on prevention and management. *J. Feline Med. Surg.* 11: 556–564.

13 Thiry, E. and Addie, D. (2009). Feline herpesvirus infection. ABCD guidelines on prevention and management. *J. Feline Med. Surg.* 11 (7): 547–555.

14 Martella, V., Pinto, P. et al. (2015). Detection and full-length genome characterization of novel canine vesiviruses. *Emerg. Infect. Dis.* 2 (8): 1433–1436.

15 Joffe, D.J. and Allen, A.L. (1995). Ulcerative eosinophilic stomatitis in three Cavalier King Charles Spaniels. *J. Am. Anim. Hosp. Assoc.* 31 (1): 34–37.

16 Helton, R.K. (2011). Pemphigus. In: *Blackwell's Five-Minute Veterinary Consult: Canine and Feline*, 5e (ed. L.P. Tilley and F.W.K. Smith), 968–969. Ames, IA: Wiley-Blackwell.

17 Fukushima, K. (1982). Pathogenesis of pemphigus vulgaris in dog and man – a review. *Can. Vet. J.* 23 (4): 135–137.

18 Heimann, M., Beco, L. et al. (2007). Canine hyperplastic intraepidermal pustular and suprabasal acantholytic dermatosis with features of human pemphigus vegetans. *Vet. Pathol.* 44 (4): 550–555.

19 Olivery, T., Dunston, S.M. et al. (2001). A spontaneous canine model of mucous membrane (cicatricial) pemphigoid, an autoimmune blistering disease affecting mucosae and mucocutaneous junctions. *J. Autoimmun.* 16 (4): 411–421.

20 Hill, P.B. and Boyer, P. (2008). Epidermolysis bullosa acquisita in a Great Dane. *J. Small. Anim. Pract.* 49 (2): 89–94.

21 Scott- Moncrief, J.C. and Thompson, M.F. (2011). Lupus erythematosus, systemic. In: *Blackwell's Five-Minute Veterinary Consult: Canine and Feline*, 5e (ed. L.P. Tilley and F.W.K. Smith), 764–765. Ames, IA: Wiley-Blackwell.

22 Nemec, A., Zavodovskaya, R., Afolter, V.K., and Verstraete, F.J. (2012). Erythema multiforme and epithliotropic T-cell lymphoma in the oral cavity of dogs: 1989 to 2009. *J. Small Anim. Pract.* 53 (8): 445–452.

23 Scully, C. and Bagan, J. (2008). Oral mucosal diseases: erythema multiforme. *Br. J. Oral Maxillofac. Surg.* 46 (2): 90–95.

24 Woldemeskel, M., Liggett, A. et al. (2011). Canine parvovirus-2b-associated erythema multiforme in a litter of English Setter dogs. *J. Vet. Diagn. Invest.* 23 (3): 576–580.

25 Mason, K.V. and Fadok, V.A. (1994). Cutaneous drug eruptions with epidermal necrosis: a discussion of pathophysiological and comparative aspects. *Clin. Dermatol.* 12 (4): 525–528.

26 Tepper, L.C., Spiegel, I.B., and Davis, D.J. (2011). Diagnosis of erythema multiforme associated with thymoma in a dog and treated with thymectomy. *J. Am. Anim. Hosp. Assoc.* 47 (2): e19–e25.

27 Noli, C., Koeman, J.P., and Willemse, T. (1995). A retrospective evaluation of adverse reactions to trimethoprim-sulphonamide combinations in dogs and cats. *Vet. Q.* 17 (4): 123–128.

28 Voie, K.L., Campbell, K.L., and Lavergne, S.N. (2012). Drug hypersensitivity reactions targeting the skin in dogs and cats. *J. Vet. Intern. Med.* 26 (4): 863–874.

29 Davis, E.M. (2015). Oral manifestations of chronic kidney disease and renal secondary hyperparathyroidism: a comparative review. *J. Vet. Dent.* 32 (2): 87–98.

30 Kelly, A., Pomarico, L., and de Souza, I.P. (2009). Cessation of dental development in a child with idiopathic hypoparathyroidism: a 5-year follow-up. *Oral Surg. Oral Med. Oral Pathol. Oral Radiol. Endod.* 107 (5): 673–677.

31 Dudhia, S.B. and Dudhia, B.B. (2014). Undetected hypothyroidism: a rare dental diagnosis. *J. Oral Maxillofac. Pathol.* 18 (2): 315–319.

32 Cheville, N.F., Cutlip, R.C., and Moon, H.W. (1970). Microscopic pathology of gray collie syndrome: cyclic neutropenia, amyloidosisi, enteritis and bone necrosis. *Pathol. Vet.* 7 (3): 225–245.

33 Gowda, T.M., Thomas, R. et al. (2013). Gingival enlargement as an early diagnostic indicator in therapy-related acute myeloid leukemia: a rare case report and review of the literature. *J. Indian Soc. Periodontol.* 17 (2): 248–252.

34 Manzon, L., Rossi, E., and Fratto, G. (2015). Management of osteoradionecrosis of the jaws induced by radiotherapy in oncological patients: preliminary results. *Eur. Rev. Med. Pharmacol. Sci.* 19 (2): 194–200.

35 Collen, E.B. and Mayer, M.N. (2008). Acute oropharyngeal effects of full-course radiation treatment of tumors of the head. *Can. Vet. J.* 49 (5): 509–512.

36 Serra, D.A. and White, S.D. (1989). Oral chrysotherapy with auranofin in dogs. *J. Am. Vet. Med. Assoc.* 194 (9): 1327–1330.

37 Cutright, D.E. and Bauer, H. (1967). Cell renewal in the oral mucosa and skin of the rat I. Turnover time. *Oral Surg. Oral Med. Oral Pathol.* 23 (2): 249–259.

38 Sheffy, B.E. and Williams, A.J. (1982). Nutrition and the immune response. *J. Am. Vet. Med. Assoc.* 180 (9): 1073–1076.

39 Lanska, D.J. (2012). The discovery of niacin, biotin, and pantothenic acid. *Ann. Nutr. Metab.* 61 (3): 246–253.

40 De-Fornel-Thibaud, P., Blanchard, G. et al. (2007). Unusual case of osteopenia association with nutritional calcium and vitamin D deficiency in an adult dog. *J. Am. Anim. Hosp. Assoc.* 43 (1): 52–60.

41 Hayes, K.C. (1982). Nutritional Problems in Cats: Taurine Deficiency and Vitamin A Excess. *Can. Vet. J.* 23: 2–5.

42 Cline, J.L., Czarnecki-Maulden, G.L. et al. (1997). Effect of increasing dietary vitamin A on bone density in adult dogs. *J. Anim. Sci.* 75 (11): 2980–2985.

43 Stocks, I.C. and Lindsey, D.E. (2008). Acute corrosion of the oral mucosa in a dog due to ingestion of Multicolored Asian lady beetles (*Harmonia axyridis: Coccinellidae*). *Toxicon* 52 (2): 389–391.

44 Billen, F., Day, M.J., and Clercx, C. (2006). Diagnosis of pharyngeal disorders in dogs: a retrospective study of 67 cases. *J. Small Anim. Pract.* 47 (3): 122–129.

45 Allen, H.S., Broussard, J., and Noone, K. (1999). Nasopharyngeal disease in cats: a retrospective study of 53 cases (1991-1998). *J. Am. Anim. Hosp. Assoc.* 35 (6): 457–461.

46 Deitz, K. (2011). Dysphagia. In: *Blackwell's Five-Minute Veterinary Consult: Canine and Feline*, 5e (ed. L.P. Tilley and F.W.K. Smith), 391–391. Ames, IA: Wiley-Blackwell.

47 Fasanella, F.J., Shively, J.M., Wardlaw, J.L., and Givaruangsawat, S. (2010). Brachycephalic airway obstructive syndrome in dogs: 90 cases (1991–2008). *J. Am. Vet. Med. Assoc.* 237: 1048–1051.

48 Grand, J.G. and Bureau, S. (2011). Structural characteristics of the soft palate and meatus nasopharyngeus in brachycephalic and non-brachycephalic dogs analysed by CT. *J. Small Anim. Pract.* 52 (5): 232–239.

49 Talavera Lopez, J., Fernandez del Palacio, J., Gil Cano, F., and Bayon del Rio, A. (2008). Nasopharyngeal stenosis secondary to soft palate dysgenesis in a cat. *Vet. J.* 200–204.

50 Griffon, D.J. and Tasker, S. (2000). Use of a mucosal advancement flap for the treatment of nasopharyngeal stenosis in a cat. *J. Small Anim. Pract.* 41: 71–73.

51 Corgozinho, K.B., Pereira, A.N. et al. (2012). Recurrent pulmonary edema secondary to elongated soft palate in a cat. *J. Feline Med. Surg.* 14 (6): 417–419.

52 Kirberger, R.M., Steenkamp, G. et al. (2006). Stenotic nasopharyngeal dysgenesis in the dachshund: seven cases (2002-2004). *J. Am. Anim. Hosp. Assoc.* 42 (2): 290–297.

53 Hayes, G.M., Friend, E.J., and Jeffery, N.D. (2010). Relationship between pharyngeal conformation and otitis media with effusion in Cavalier King Charles spaniels. *Vet. Rec.* 167 (2): 55–58.

54 Gregory, S.P. (2000). Middle ear disease associated with congenital palatal defects in seven dogs and one cat. *J. Small Anim. Pract.* 41 (9): 398–401.

55 White, R.N., Hawkins, H.L., Alemi, V.P., and Warner, C. (2009). Soft palate hypoplasia and concurrent middle ear pathology in six dogs. *J. Small Anim. Pract.* 50 (7): 364–372.

56 Woodbridge, N.T., Baines, E.A., and Baines, S.J. (2012). Otitis media in five cats associated with soft palate abnormalities. *Vet. Rec.* 171 (5): 124.

57 Peterson, N.W. and Buote, N.J. (2011). Soft palate cyst in a cat. *J. Feline Med. Surg.* 13 (8): 594–596.

58 Reed, N. and Gunn-Moore, D. (2012). Nasopharyngeal disease in cats: 2. Specific conditions and their management. *J. Feline Med. Surg.* 14 (5): 317–326.

59 Kudnig, S.T. (2002). Nasopharyngeal polyps in cats. *Clin. Tech. Small Anim. Pract.* 17 (4): 174–177.

60 Salinardi, B.J., Marretta, S.M. et al. (2003). Pharyngeal-laryngeal blastomycosis in a dog. *J. Vet. Dent.* 20 (3): 146–147.

61 Doran, I.P., Wright, C.A., and Moore, A.H. (2008). Acute oropharyngeal and esophageal stick injury in forty-one dogs. *Vet. Surg.* 37 (8): 781–785.

62 Bright, S.R., Mellanby, R.J., and Williams, J.M. (2002). Oropharyngeal stick injury in a Bengal cat. *J. Feline Med. Surg.* 4 (3): 153–155.

63 Kang, H.M., Lim, B.Y., and Park, H.M. (2011). Nasopharyngeal tooth foreign body in a dog. *J. Vet. Dent.* 28 (1): 26–29.

64 Haynes, K.J., Anderson, S.E., and Laszlo, M.P. (2010). Nasopharyngeal trichobezoar foreign body in a cat. *J. Feline Med. Surg.* 12 (11): 878–881.

65 Dobromylskvj, M.J., Dennis, R., Ladlow, J.F., and Adams, V.J. (2008). The use of magnetic resonance imaging in the management of pharyngeal penetration injuries in dogs. *J. Small Anim. Pract.* 49 (2): 74–79.

66 Miller, A.D., Alcaraz, A., and McDonough, S.P. (2008). Tonsillar lymphangiomatous polyp in an adult dog. *J. Comp. Pathol.* 138 (4): 215–217.

67 Montague, A.L., Markey, B.K. et al. (2002). A study of greyhounds with tonsillar enlargement and a history of poor racing performance. *Vet. J.* 164 (2): 106–115.

68 Dennis, M.M., Ehrhart, N. et al. (2006). Frequency and risk factors associated with lingual lesions in dogs: 1, 196 cases (1995-2004). *J. Am. Vet. Med. Assoc.* 228 (10): 1533–1537.

69 Evermann, J.F., McKeirnan, A.J. et al. (1985). Isolation and identification of caliciviruses from dogs with enteric infections. *Am. J. Vet. Res.* 46 (1): 218–220.

70 Buelow, M.E., Marretta, S.M., Barger, A., and Lichtensteiger, C. (2011). Lingual lesions in the dog and cat: recognition, diagnosis, and treatment. *J. Vet. Dent.* 28 (3): 151–162.

71 Yagci, B.B., Ural, K., Ocal, N., and Haydardedeoglu, A.E. (2008). Azithromycin therapy of papillomatosis in dogs: a prospective, randomized, double-blinded, placebo-controlled clinical trial. *Vet. Dermatol.* 19 (4): 194–198.

72 Fracassi, F., Gandini, G. et al. (2007). Acromegaly due to a somatroph adenoma in a dog. *Domest Anim Endocrinol.* 32 (1): 43–54.

73 Balme, E., Thuilliez, C. et al. (2009). Multiple atypical mucosal xanthomas in a dog similar to human verruciform xanthoma. *J. Vet. Diagn. Invest.* 21 (1): 124–128.

74 Collados, J., Rodriguez-Bertos, A. et al. (2002). Lingual calcinosis circumscripta in a dog. *J. Vet. Dent.* 19 (1): 19–21.

75 Tafti, A.K., Hanna, P., and Bourque, A.C. (2005). Calcinosis circumscripta in the dog: a retrospective pathological study. *J. Vet. Med. Physiol. Pathol. Clin. Med.* 52 (1): 13–17.

76 Marcos, R., Santo, M. et al. (2006). Cytochemical detection of calcium in a case of calcinosis circumscripta in a dog. *Vet. Clin. Pathol.* 35 (2): 239–242.

77 Jeong, W. and Noh, D. (2004). Calcinosis circumscripta on lingual muscles and dermis in a dog. *J. Vet. Med. Sci.* 66 (4): 433–435.

78 Cornegliani, L., Gracis, M. et al. (2011). Sublingual reactive histocytosis in a dog. *J. Vet. Dent.* 28 (3): 164–170.

79 Arnjberg, J. (1978). Pasteurella multocida from canine and feline teeth, with a case report of glossitis calcinosis in a dog. *Nordisk Vet.* 30 (7–8): 324–332.

80 Ito, D., Okada, M. et al. (2009). Symptomatic tongue atrophy due to atypical polymyositis in a Pembroke Welsh Corgi. *J. Vet. Med. Sci.* 71 (8): 1063–1067.

81 Toyoda, K., Uchida, K. et al. (2010). Inflammatory myopathy with severe tongue atrophy in Pembroke Welsh Corgi dogs. *J. Vet. Diagn. Invest.* 22 (6): 876–885.
82 Simison, W.G. (1997). Sialadentitis associated with periorbital disease in a dog. *J. Am. Vet. Med. Assoc.* 202 (12): 1983–1985.
83 Spangler, W.L. and Culberston, M.R. (1991). Salivary gland disease in dogs and cats: 245 cases: (1985-1988). *J. Am. Vet. Med. Assoc.* 198 (3): 465–469.
84 Mutsaers, A.J. (2011). Adenosarcoma, salivary gland. In: *Blackwell's Five-Minute Veterinary Consult: Canine and Feline*, 5e (ed. L.P. Tilley and F.W.K. Smith), 30. Ames, IA: Wiley-Blackwell.
85 Cannon, M.S., Paglia, D. et al. (2011). Clinical and diagnostic imaging findings in dogs with zygomatic sialadentitis: 11 cases (1990-2009). *J. Am. Vet. Med. Assoc.* 239 (9): 1211–1218.
86 McGill, S., Lester, N., McLachlan, A., and Mansfield, C. (2009). Concurrent sialocele and necrotizing sialadentitis in a dog. *J. Small. Anim. Pract.* 50 (3): 151–156.
87 Brown, P.J., Bradshaw, J.M., Sozmen, M., and Campbell, R.H. (2004). Feline necrotizing sialometaplasia: a report of two cases. *J. Feline Med. Surg.* 6 (4): 279–281.
88 Boydell, P. (2000). Presumptive sialadenosis in a cat. *J. Small Anim. Pract.* 41 (12): 573–574.
89 Gibbon, K.J., Trepanier, L.A., and Delaney, F.A. (2004). Phenobarbital-responsive ptyalism, dysphagia, and apparent esophageal spasm in a German Shepherd puppy. *J. Am. Anim. Hosp. Assoc.* 40 (3): 230–237.
90 Gilor, C., Gilor, S., and Graves, T.K. (2010). Phenobarbital-responsive sialadenosis associated with an esophageal foreign body in a dog. *J. Am. Anim. Hosp. Assoc.* 46 (2): 115–120.
91 Canapp, S.O. Jr., Cohn, L.A. et al. (2001). Xerostomia, xerophthalmia and plasmacytic infiltrates of the salivary glands (Sjogren's-like syndrome) in a cat. *J. Am. Vet. Med. Assoc.* 218 (1): 59–65.
92 Ritter, M.J., von Pfeil, D.J.F. et al. (2006). Mandibular and sublingual sialoceles in the dog: a retrospective evaluation of 41 cases, using the ventral approach for treatment. *N. Z. Vet. J.* 54 (6): 333–337.
93 Clarke, B.S. and L, Eplattenier, H.F. (2010). Zygomatic salivary mucocele as a postoperative complication following caudal hemimaxillectomy in a dog. *J. Small Anim. Pract.* 51 (9): 495–498.
94 Muir, P. and Rosin, E. (1995). Parotid duct obstruction after caudal maxillectomy in a dog. *Vet. Rec.* 136 (2): 46.
95 Guthrie, K.M. and Hardie, R.J. (2014). Surgical excision of the parotid salivary gland for treatment of a traumatic mucocele in a dog. *J. Am. Anim. Hosp. Assoc.* 50: 1–5.
96 Philp, H.S., Rhodes, M., Parry, A., and Baines, S.J. (2010). Canine zygomatic salivary mucocele following suspected oropharyngeal penetrating stick injury. *Vet. Rec.* 171 (6): 402.
97 Adams, P., Halfacree, Z.J. et al. (2011). Zygomatic salivary mucocoele in a Lhasa apso following maxillary tooth extraction. *Vet. Rec.* 168 (17): 458.
98 Guinan, J., Willis, A.M., Cullen, C., and Walshaw, R. (2007). Post-enucleation orbital sialocele in a dog associated with prior parotid duct transposition. *Vet. Ophthalmol.* 10 (6): 38–389.
99 Prassinos, N.N., Tontis, D.K. et al. (2005). Metaplastic ossification of a cervical sialocele in a dog. *Aust. Vet. J.* 83 (7): 421–423.
100 Lauer, S.K. (2011). Salivary mucocele. In: *Blackwell's Five-Minute Veterinary Consult: Canine and Feline*, 5e (ed. L.P. Tilley and F.W.K. Smith), 1124–1125. Ames, IA: Wiley-Blackwell.
101 Benjamino, K.P., Birchard, S.J., Niles, J.D., and Penrod, K.D. (2012). Pharyngeal mucoceles in dogs: 14 cases. *J. Am. Anim. Hosp. Assoc.* 48 (1): 31–35.
102 Tivers, M.S. and Moore, A.H. (2014). Surgical treatment of a parotid duct sialolith in a bulldog. *Vet. Rec.*
103 Torad, F.A. and Hassan, E.A. (2013). Clinical and ultrasonographic characteristics of salivary mucoceles in 13 dogs. *Vet. Radiol. Ultrasound* 54 (3): 293–298.
104 Atkins, R.M., Hecht, S., Westermeyer, H.D., and McLean, N.J. (2010). What is your diagnosis? A zygomatic salivary gland mucocele. *J. Am. Vet. Med. Assoc.* 237 (12): 1375.
105 Boland, L., Gomes, E. et al. (2013). Zygomatic salivary gland diseases in the dog: three cases diagnosed by MRI. *J. Am. Anim. Hosp. Assoc.* 49: 333–337.
106 Cannon, M.S., Paglia, D. et al. (2011). Clinical and diagnostic imaging findings in dogs with zygomatic sialadenitis: 11 cases (1990–2009). *J. Am. Vet. Med. Assoc.* 239 (9): 1211–1218.
107 Stuckey, J.A., Miller, W.W., and Almond, G.T. (2012). Use of a sclerosing agent (1% polidocanol) to treat an orbital mucocele in a dog. *Vet. Ophth.* 15 (3): 188–193.
108 Smith, M.M. (2010). Step-by-step surgery for cervical, sublingual and pharyngeal mucocele. *J. Vet. Dent.* 27 (4): 268–273.
109 Vallefuoco, R., Jardel, N. et al. (2011). Parotid salivary duct sialocele associated with glandular duct stenosis in a cat. *J. Feline. Med. Surg.* 13 (10): 781–783.
110 Harrison, J.D., Fouad, H.M., and Garrett, J.R. (2001). Variation in the response to ductal obstruction of feline submandibular and sublingual salivary glands and the importance of the innervation. *J. Oral. Pathol. Med.* 30 (1): 29–34.
111 Ryan, T., Welsh, E., McGorum, I., and Yool, D. (2008). Sublingual salivary gland sialolithiasis in a dog. *J. Small. Anim. Pract.* 49 (5): 354–356.

112 Boy, S.C., Van Heerden, W.F., and Steenkamp, G. (2005). Diagnosis and treatment of primary intraoral leimyosarcomas in four dogs. *Vet. Rec.* 156 (16): 510–513.

113 Schulttheiss, P.C. (2006). Histological features and clinical outcomes of melanomas of lip, haired skin and nail bed locations of dogs. *J. Vet. Diagn. Invest.* 18 (4): 422–425.

114 Jakab, C. and Balka, G. (2012). First report of a malignant collision skin tumor with malignant melanoma and anaplastic sarcoma components in a dog. *Acta Vet. Hung.* 60 (2): 245–255.

115 Esplin, D.G. (2008). Survival of dogs following surgical excision of histologically well-differentiated melanocytic neoplasms of the mucous membranes of the lips and oral cavity. *Vet. Pathol.* 45 (6): 889–896.

116 Hall, B.P. (2006). Full-thickness labial advancement flap following mast cell tumor excision. *J. Vet. Dent.* 23 (1): 27–31.

117 Koshino, A., Mauldin, G.E., Dickinson, R.M., and Mauldin, G.N. (2011). A clinical oncology case report. *Can. Vet. J.* 52 (8): 899–902.

118 Taney, K. and Smith, M.M. (2009). Resection of mast cell tumor of the lip in a dog. *J. Vet. Dent.* 26 (1): 28–34.

119 Gendler, A., Lewis, J.R., Reetz, J.A., and Schwartz, T. (2010). Computed tomographic features of oral squamous cell carcinoma in cats: 18 cases (2002-2008). *J. Am. Vet. Med. Assoc.* 236 (3): 319–325.

120 Sakuma, A., Nishiyama, S. et al. (2010). A case of canine cutaneous clear cell adnexal carcinoma with prominent expression of smooth muscle actin. *J. Toxicol. Pathol.* 23 (4): 265–269.

121 Shiomitsu, K. and Bauer, R.W. (2012). Cutaneous epitheliotropic lymphoma with dual CD3 and c-kit expression in a dog. *Vet. Clin. Pathol.* 41 (4): 592–598.

122 Snead, E., Kerr, M., and Macdonald, V. (2013). Cutaneous lymphoid hyperplasia mimicking cutaneous lymphoma in a hyperthyroid cat. *Can. Vet. J.* 54 (10): 974–978.

123 Mohebali, M., Malmasi, A. et al. (2011). Disseminated Leishmaniasis caused by Leishmania tropica in a puppy from Karaj, Central Iran. *Iran J. Parasitol.* 6 (2): 69–73.

124 Baneth, G., Zivotofsky, D. et al. (2014). Mucocutaneous Leishmania tropica infection in a dog from a human cutaneous leishmaniasisfocus. *Parasit Vectors.* 7: 118.

125 Evans, J., Levesque, D., and Shelton, G.D. (2004). Canine inflammatory myopathies: a clinicopathologic review of 200 cases. *J. Vet. Intern. Med.* 18 (5): 679–691.

126 Shelton, G.D. and Paciello, O. (2006). Evidence for MHC-1 restricted CD8+ T-cell-mediated immunopathy in canine masticatory muscle myositis and polymyositis. *Muscle Nerve* 34 (1): 122–123.

127 Pacielo, O., Shelton, G.D., and Papparella, S. (2007). Expression of major histocompatibility complex class I and class II antigens in canine masticatory muscle myositis. *Neuromuscul. Disord.* 17 (3): 313–320.

128 Bishop, T.M., Blass, E.N., DeLahunta, A., and Shelton, G.D. (2008). Imaging diagnosis – masticatory muscle myositis in a young dog. *Vet. Radiol. Ultrasound* 49 (3): 270–272.

129 Cauduro, A., Paolo, F. et al. (2013). Use of MRI for the early diagnosis of masticatory muscle myositis. *J. Am. Anim. Hosp. Assoc.* 49 (5): 347–352.

130 Reiter, A.M. and Schwarz, T. (2007). Computed tomographic appearance of masticatory muscle myositis in dogs: 7 cases (1999–2006). *J. Am. Vet. Med. Assoc.* 231 (6): 924–930.

131 Pitcher, G.D. and Hahn, C.N. (2007). Atypical masticatory muscle myositis in three Cavalier King Charles spaniel littermates. *J. Small Anim. Pract.* 48 (4): 226–228.

132 Clooten, J.K., Woods, J.P., and Smith-Maxie, L.L. (2003). Myasthenia gravis and masticatory muscle myositis in a dog. *Can. Vet. J.* 44 (6): 480–483.

133 Nanai, B., Phillips, L., Christiansen, J., and Shelton, G.D. (2009). Life threatening complication associated with anesthesia in a dog with masticatory muscle myositis. *Vet. Surg.* 38 (5): 645–649.

134 Vamvakidis, C.D., Koutinas, A.F. et al. (2000). Masticatory and skeletal muscle myositis in canine leishmaniasis. (Leishmania infantum). *Vet. Rec.* 146 (26): 698–703.

135 Illanes, O.G. (2002). Juvenile parameningeal rhabdomyosarcoma in a dog causing unilateral denervation atrophy of masticatory muscles. *J. Comp. Pathol.* 126 (4): 303–307.

136 Panciera, R.J., Richey, J.W., Baker, J.E., and DiGregorio, M. (2002). Trigeminal and polyradiculoneuritis in a dog presenting with masticatory muscle atrophy and Horner's syndrome. *Vet. Pathol.* 39 (1): 146–149.

137 Schultz, R.M., Tucker, R.L. et al. (2007). Magnetic resonance imaging of acquired trigeminal nerve disorders in six dogs. *Vet. Radiol. Ultrasound* 48 (2): 101–104.

138 Mayhew, P.D., Bush, W.W., and Glass, E.N. (2002). Trigeminal neuropathy in dogs: a retrospective study of 29 cases (1991–2000). *J. Am. Anim. Hosp. Assoc.* 38 (3): 262–270.

139 Pfafff, A.M., March, P.A., and Fishman, C. (2000). Acute bilateral trigeminal neuropathy associated with nervous system lymphosarcoma in a dog. *J. Am. Anim. Hosp. Assoc.* 36 (1): 57–61.

140 Strøm, P.C., Arzi, B., Cissell, D.D., and Verstraete, F.M.J. (2016). Ankylosis and pseudoankylosis of the temporomandibular joint in 10 dogs (1993–2015). *Vet. Comp. Orthop. Traumatol.* 29: 409–415.

141 Dickie, A.M. and Sullivan, M. (2001). The effect of obliquity on the radiographic appearance of the temporomandibular joint in dogs. *Vet. Radiol. Ultrasound* 42 (3): 205–217.

142 Hammond, G., King, A., and Lapaglia, J. (2012). Assessment of five oblique radiographic projections of the canine temporomandibular joint. *Vet. Radiol. Ultrasound* 53 (5): 501–506.

143 Arzi, B., Cissell, D.D. et al. (2013). Computed tomographic findings in dogs and cats with temporomandibular joint disorders: 58 cases (2006-2011). *J. Am. Vet. Med. Assoc.* 242 (1): 69–75.

144 Roza, M.R., Silva, L.A. et al. (2011). Cone beam computed tomography in the diagnosis of temporomandibular joint alterations in cats. *J. Feline Med. Surg.* 13 (6): 393–398.

145 Macready, D.M., Hecht, S., Craig, L.E., and Conklin, G.A. (2010). Magnetic resonance imaging features of the temporomandibular joint in normal dogs. *Vet. Radiol. Ultrasound.* 51 (4): 436–440.

146 Schwarz, T., Weller, R. et al. (2002). Imaging of the canine and feline temporomandibular joint: a review. *Vet. Radiol. Ultrasound.* 43 (2): 85–97.

147 Vollmerhaus, B. and Roos, H. (1996). The transverse movement of the temporomandibular joint (translation movement) of the dog, also with reference to dysplasia of this joint in the dachshund. *Anat. Histol. Embryol.* 25 (3): 145–149.

148 Gatineau, M., El-Warrak, A.O. et al. (2008). Locked jaw syndrome in dogs and cats: 37 cases (1998–2005). *J. Vet. Dent.* 25 (1): 16–22.

149 Klima, L.J. (2007). Temporomandibular joint luxation in the cat. *J. Vet. Dent.* 24 (3): 198–201.

150 Beam, R.C., Kunz, D.A. et al. (2007). Use of three-dimensional computed tomography for diagnosis and treatment planning for open-mouth jaw locking in a cat. *J. Am. Vet. Med. Assoc.* 230 (1): 59–63.

151 Eisner, E.R. (1995). Bilateral mandibular condylectomy in a cat. *J. Vet. Dent.* 12 (1): 23–26.

152 Lantz, G.C. and Cantwell, H.D. (1986). Intermittent open-mouth lower jaw locking in five dogs. *J. Am. Vet. Med. Assoc.* 188 (12): 1403–1405.

153 Lobprise, H.B. and Wiggs, R.B. (1992). Modified surgical treatment of intermittent open-mouth mandibular locking in a cat. *J. Vet. Dent.* 9 (1): 8–12.

154 Reiter, A.M. (2004). Symphysiotomy, symphysiectomy, and intermandibular arthrodesis in a cat with open-mouth locking: case report and literature review. *J. Vet. Dent.* 21 (3): 147–158.

155 Soukup, J.W., Snyder, C.J., and Gengler, W.R. (2009). Computed tomography and partial coronoidectomy for open-mouth jaw locking in two cats. *J. Vet. Dent.* 26 (4): 226–233.

156 Frazho, J.K., Tano, C.A., and Ferrell, E.A. (2008). Diagnosis and treatment of closed-mouth jaw locking in a dog. *J. Am. Vet. Med. Assoc.* 233 (5): 748–751.

157 Seiler, G., Rossi, F. et al. (2007). Computed tomographic features of skull osteomyelitis in our young dogs. *Vet. Radiol. Ultrasound* 48 (6): 544–549.

158 Ellenberger, S. and Snyder, C. (2013). Bilateral extracapsular soft-tissue ossification affecting range of TMJ motion in an Airedale terrier. *J. Am. Anim. Hosp. Assoc.* 49 (2): 115–121.

159 Hodik, V., Loeb, E., and Ranen, E. (2012). Chondroma of the vertical ramus of the feline mandible. *J. Feline Med. Surg.* 14 (12): 924–927.

160 Fricke, J., Linn, K., and Anthony, J.M. (2008). Treatment for traumatic craniofacial deformation with restriction of the temporomandibular joint in a dog. *J. Vet. Dent.* 25 (4): 246–248.

161 Van Ee, R.T. and Pechman, R.D. (1987). False ankyloses of the temporomandibular joint in a cat. *J. Am. Vet. Med. Assoc.* 191 (8): 979–980.

162 Greci, V., Travetti, O. et al. (2011). Middle ear cholesteatoma in 11 dogs. *Can. Vet. J.* 52 (6): 631–636.

163 Travetti, O., Guidice, C. et al. (2010). Computed tomography features of middle ear cholesteatoma in dogs. *Vet. Radiol. Ultrasound* 51 (4): 374–379.

164 Yoshikawa, H., Mayer, M.N. et al. (2008). A dog with squamous cell carcinoma in the middle ear. *Can. Vet. J.* 49 (9): 877–879.

165 Maas, C.P. and Theyse, L.F. (2007). Temporomandibular joint ankylosis in cats and dogs: a report of 10 cases. *Vet. Comp. Orthop. Traumatol.* 20 (3): 192–197.

166 Cetinkaya, M.A. (2012). Temporomandibular joint injuries and ankyloses in the cat. *Vet. Comp. Orthop. Traumatol.* 25 (5): 366–371.

167 Meomartino, L., Fatone, G. et al. (1999). Temporomandibular ankyloses in the cat: a review of seven cases. *J. Small Anim. Pract.* 40 (1): 7–10.

168 Lyon, K.F. and Bard, R.A. Mandibular osteomyelitis caused by *Coccidiodes immitis*. *J. Vet. Dent.* 5 (2): 5–6.

169 Johnston, K.A. (1994). Osteomyelitis in dogs and cats. *J. Am. Vet. Med. Assoc.* 204 (12): 1882–1887.

170 Thompson, D.J., Rogers, W., Owen, M.C., and Thompson, K.G. (2011). Idiopathic canine juvenile cranial hyperostosis in a Pit Bull terrier. *N. Z Vet. J.* 59 (4): 201–205.

171 Brachthauser, L., Pingen, C.H., Hecht, W., and Reinacher, M. (2013). Rubber jaw in a Weimeraner dog due to juvenile nephropathy. A case without

evidence for genetic involvement. *Tierarztl Prax Ausq Kleintiere Heimtiere.* 41 (3): 198–202.

172 Hale, F.A. (1998). Dental caries in the dog. *J. Vet. Dent.* 15 (2): 79–83.

173 Peralta, S., Verstraete, F.J., and Kass, P.H. (2010). Radiographic evidence of the classification of the extent of tooth resorption in dogs. *Am. J. Vet. Res.* 71 (7): 794.

174 Nemec, A., Arzi, B. et al. (2012). Prevalence and types of tooth resorption in dogs with oral tumors. *Am. J. Vet. Res.* 73 (7): 1057.

175 Eikenberg, S., Loheide, H., and Arens, F.C. (1998). Treatment of asymptomatic internal resorption of a maxillary premolar tooth in a military working dog. *J. Vet. Dent.* 15 (4): 175–178.

176 Hale, F.A. (2001). Localized intrinsic staining of teeth due to pulpitis and pulp necrosis in dogs. *J. Vet. Dent.* 18 (1): 14–20.

177 Charbonneau, D.L. and Snider, A.G. (1997). Reduced chlorhexidine stain coverage by sequential administration of monoperoxyphthalic acid in the beagle dog. *J. Dent. Res.* 76 (9): 1596–1601.

178 Nutting, E.B., Poe, G.S. (1967). Chemical bleaching of discolored endodontically treated teeth. *Dent. Clin. North Am.* 655–62.

9

Anesthesia and Pain Management

Lindsey C. Snyder[1], Christopher Snyder[1], and Donald Beebe[2]

[1] School of Veterinary Medicine, University of Wisconsin-Madison, Madison, WI, USA
[2] Apex Dog and Cat Dentistry, Englewood, CO, USA

9.1 Introduction

It has been well documented that periodontal disease is extremely prevalent in the canine and feline populations (see Chapter 5 – Periodontology). The high prevalence of disease equates to a large number of small animal veterinary patients being anesthetized yearly for dental cleanings, diagnostics, and treatments. Since most patients will have justifiable reason to undergo general anesthesia multiple times in their lives for the purpose of maintaining a healthy and pain-free oral cavity, considerations should be made to make general anesthesia as safe as possible. One study reported that the most common adverse events associated with general anesthesia (hypotension, cardiac dysrhythmias, blood loss, hypercapnea, or hypoxemia) occurred in as many as 12% of dogs and 10.5% of cats [1]. The use of pre-anesthetics medications and regional anesthetic techniques with local anesthetics both offer the advantage that polypharmacy has to offer – a multimodal approach to delivering anesthesia and decreasing perception of noxious stimulation. Use of hydromorphone or oxymorphone as premedications have shown a reduction in minimum alveolar concentration (MAC) (hydromorphone decreased by 48% and oxymorphone by 43%) to respond to a noxious stimulus [2]. The administration of a local anesthetic alone has demonstrated a 23% reduction in MAC in dogs [3].

9.2 Pathophysiology of Pain

Pain, by definition, is an unpleasant sensory and emotional experience associated with actual or potential tissue damage. In 1986, the International Association for the Study of Pain (IASP) defined pain as a sensory and emotional experience associated with real or potential injuries [4]. Pain begins at the site of tissue injury and is initiated by specialized nerve fibers called nociceptors. Nociceptors are free nerve ending receptors of sensory neurons responsible for sensing potentially damaging stimuli in response to tissue injury and are found throughout the tissues of the body. Nociceptors can be activated by mechanical, thermal, or chemical stimuli through the process of transduction.

High threshold nociceptors are stimulated at the site of injury. With a high degree of mechanical stimulation induced by surgical trauma, mechanical, polymodal, and mechanothermal nociceptors would all be stimulated. The stimulus would then be transduced into electrical impulses that would be *transmitted* to the dorsal horn of the spinal cord via fast, myelinated A-delta fibers and slower, unmyelinated C-fibers. The afferent nerve, either A-delta or C-fibers, enters the spinal cord via the dorsal nerve root and terminates on the cells in the dorsal horn of the gray matter. Nerves may then ascend or descend one or two segments in Lissauer's tract. The majority of A-delta fibers terminate in the most superficial layer of the spinal cord, lamina I, or the marginal zone. Most C-fibers also terminate in the superficial horn, lamina II, or the substantia gelatinosa. It is in the dorsal horn that modulation of nociceptive input occurs. The impulse is then projected to the cortex via the ascending spinal tracts. The spinothalamic tract is the most prominent nociceptive pathway. Originating in the dorsal horn, it crosses midline and courses cranially until it terminates in the thalamus. The spinoreticular tract also carries impulses to several midbrain sites. At supraspinal levels, nociceptive neurons have been identified in portions of the pons, midbrain, thalamus, hypothalamus, and cerebral cortex. The cortex modulates both the cognitive and aversive aspects of pain sensation and mediates complex behavior patterns through the perception of pain. Opioid, gamma aminobutyric acid (GABA), serotonin, and norepinephrine receptors are present in supraspinal centers.

Wiggs's Veterinary Dentistry: Principles and Practice, Second Edition. Edited by Heidi B. Lobprise and Johnathon R. (Bert) Dodd.

Descending pathways include motor pathways to alleviate pain as well as inhibitory pathways responsible for release of endogenous opioids affecting the dorsal horn.

Peripherally, tissue damage by injury, disease, or inflammation releases endogenous algogenic substances into the extracellular fluid surrounding nociceptors. The substances (H+, K+, serotonin, histamine, prostaglandins, bradykinin, substance P) are directly excitatory to the nociceptor membrane, as well as indirectly through their effects on microcirculation (peripheral sensitization).

In the dorsal horn of the spinal cord, glutamate, the major excitatory neurotransmitter in the nervous system found in almost every pain fiber [1], and aspartate act at excitatory *N*-methyl-D-aspartate (NMDA) receptors (central sensitization). Activation of the NMDA receptor for glutamate leads to wind-up pain, a state where a constant stimulus elicits responses that are 4–5 times increased despite the peripheral input remaining the same [5]. Substance P, a pain neuropeptide, is released in the spinal cord. Spinal neurons that become hyperexcitable have been shown to demonstrate reduced thresholds to stimulus, an increase in receptive field sizes, and ongoing activity despite the stimulus. These are the mechanisms that are likely to be the basis for allodynia, hyperalgesia, and spontaneous pain states [5]. Unlike inflammatory hyperalgesia that has a protective role, allodynia has no obvious biological utility to the organism [6].

Inhibitory receptors are also present in the dorsal horn, and include GABA, opioid, alpha-2, and adenosine receptors. Within the supraspinal centers, release of endogenous opioids is connected to the periaquaductal gray area. The periaquaductal gray area is a major source of descending pathways responsible for modulatory control of spinal nociceptors [7].

Pain can be separated into inflammatory pain, where pain is induced by direct stimulation of nociceptors by inflammatory mediators released by damaged tissue (surgical or otherwise) and neuropathic pain, where pain is caused by a direct disease or trauma to a sensory nerve. Inflammatory pain is induced by chemical mediators, whereas neuropathic pain is induced by altered electrical signaling secondary to changes in the ion channels that produce action potentials within the nerves [5]. Pain can be further divided into visceral and somatic in origin. With the different types of pain, their management is different as well. For example, neuropathic pain is notoriously more difficult to treat than inflammatory pain. Cancer pain in the bone, either a primary tumor or via metastasis, is a severe type of pain that will become chronic if not treated appropriately [5]. Even small areas of pain can have enhancing effects on overall pain sensitivity. The chronic pain from myofascial temporomandibular joint (TMJ) disease can profoundly increase pain sensitivity of remote areas [8]. Non-odontogenic sources of dental pain are reported in humans but have yet to be proven in veterinary patients [9].

Analgesics work at several sites along the pain pathway. Transmission can be inhibited by the use of local anesthetics at the site of injury as well as alpha-2 agonist drugs. Transduction may be inhibited by administration of non-steroidal anti-inflammatory drugs(NSAIDs), opioids, local anesthetics, and corticosteroids. The modulation of the spinal pathways can be altered by the use of local anesthetics (epidural, spinal), opioids (epidural, spinal, systemic), NSAIDs, NMDA antagonists (systemically, epidurally, spinally), tricyclic antidepressants, and anticonvulsants. Perception at supraspinal levels can be inhibited by the administration of anesthetics, opioids, alpha-2 agonists, benzodiazepines, and phenothiazines.

9.3 Management of Pain

Due to the complexity of the pain pathway, the management of pain is complex as well. As a painful impulse passes through the many parts of the brain, the pathways become increasingly complex. At each level, the impulse is subject to enhancement and modulation [5], making management challenging. The intensity of the pain experience is variable in individuals, adding another layer to the challenge of treating pain. Pain is a multifaceted sensation involving the entire nervous system [5], thus using drugs that affect the various levels of the pain pathway, in combination, can be more effective than using one analgesic alone. This multimodal approach to pain management is now widely used in veterinary medicine to decrease the dose of individual analgesic drugs, thereby decreasing the side effects of individual drugs.

The chronicity associated with many commonly presenting dental and oral conditions emphasize the need for multimodal techniques in the approach to pain management. A common method of pain management is to approach the pain pathway itself. By affecting the many steps in the pathway, pain can be minimized most effectively by utilizing multiple mechanisms. For example, using hydromorphone and dexmedetomidine as premedications for a younger dog, then inducing with propofol and maintaining anesthesia with isoflurane and supplementing with local anesthetic dental blocks, an NSAID and a fentanyl constant rate infusion, combined, would affect transduction, transmission, modulation, and perception. This would be an ideal plan, as all of the steps in the pain pathway are affected (Table 9.1).

Individual drug pharmacology dictates the dosing and dosing intervals. For drugs with short half-lives, a constant rate of infusion might be necessary for administration. Often, if using a longer acting drug, re-dosing may

Table 9.1 Various steps of the pain pathway with associated medications providing anesthetic and analgesic activities.

Transduction	The process in which afferent nerve endings take part *in translating noxious stimuli* (e.g., a needle stick) into a nociceptive impulse	Local anesthetics NSAIDs
Transmission	The process in which impulses are sent to the dorsal horn of the spinal cord	Local anesthetics
Modulation	The process of *decreasing or amplifying* the pain-related neural signals, primarily in the dorsal horn of the spinal cord, with input from ascending and descending pathways	Local anesthetics Opioids Alpha-2 agonists NSAIDs
Projection	The process of sending the pain impulse from the dorsal horn of the spinal cord to the higher levels of conscious perception	Local anesthetics
Perception	The subjective experience of pain that results from the interaction of transduction, transmission, modulation, and awareness of nociception	Opioids Alpha-2 agonists Centrally acting analgesics NSAIDs

be necessary mid-procedure for surgeries lasting longer than the half-life of the drug. Additionally, the chronicity of most dental conditions and wind-up associated with chronic pain, pain management should not end with the completion of the procedure. Instead, pain management may require days to weeks of treatment for success. The authors refer the reader to other texts for pharmacokinetic and pharmacodynamic information of various analgesics in veterinary species, as that is beyond the scope of this chapter.

9.4 Airway Management

Dental cleanings and oral treatment procedures both require access to the oral cavity while maintaining the patient under general anesthesia. Palatal surgeries involving the caudal oral cavity, caudal maxillectomy or mandibulectomy and maxillomandibular trauma reconstruction are all procedures in which the endotracheal tube may be a hindrance to surgical exposure or monitoring occlusion. Alternatives to conventional orotracheal intubation in various species include: pharyngostomy [10, 11], temporary tracheostomy [12], transmylohyoid intubation [13], and nasotracheal intubation [14, 15]. Alternatives to orotracheal intubation should be considered to improve visualization and surgical exposure, especially if a symphysiotomy approach is deemed necessary. Modifications to create a shortened endotracheal tube have been proposed as an alternative to repeatedly extubating the patient when verifying occlusion during fracture repair and placing orthodontic or prosthodontics devices [16].

9.5 Feline Oral Pain Syndrome (FOPS)

Feline oral pain syndrome (FOPS) refers on a disorder affecting cats, resulting in an exaggerated response to a painful or non-painful stimuli resulting in discomfort and mutilation [17]. The condition is believed to be a result of a nervous system dysfunction that either centrally or peripherally affects the ganglion of the trigeminal nerve. Burmese cats were overrepresented in one study (88%), which suggests a heritability component of the condition [17]. The condition may be analogous with other allodynic conditions and similarly responds to distracting the patient or use of anticonvulsants. Bimodal age distribution of cats (<12 months of age and 7 years of age) demonstrated that young and middle-aged cats are predisposed. No specific sex predilection has been reported. Some cats have been shown to demonstrate clinical signs during permanent tooth eruption and pain subsides following eruption of the canine teeth, while others commonly demonstrate signs following triggers such as eating, drinking or grooming. Most cats demonstrate unilateral discomfort affecting one side of the face. All patients should be closely evaluated for signs of oral lesions or pathology. While the specific trigger or etiology of the condition may not be specifically known, some cats show improvement of signs following dental treatments suggesting that other sources of oral pain may contribute to this behavioral disorder. Response to therapy seems individual and variable regarding which medications may be most helpful at managing the condition. Medications reported as being helpful have included: NSAIDs, corticosteroids, antibiotics, phenobarbital, diazepam, amitriptyline, and opioids. Reported successful treatment of FOPS cases treated with phenobarbital and diazepam support the belief that this is a manifestation of neuropathic pain.

9.6 Local and Regional Anesthesia for Dentistry and Oral Surgery Patients

9.6.1 Intraoral Regional Nerve Blocks

Local anesthetic agents should be considered as part of the overall analgesic management of the dental patient. These agents decrease transmission of nociception to the central nervous system (CNS) by selectively binding ion-selective Na^+ channels, thereby preventing nerve impulse transmission. This results in a preemptive analgesic effect. Removal of noxious stimulation should also result in a decreased need for general anesthetics, and potentially promote a faster smoother recovery from general anesthesia. Longer-acting local anesthetic medications may help attain a smoother transition from the peri-operative period to the post-operative period. Incorporation of local and regional anesthesia will decrease requirements for other analgesic agents, allowing for formulation of a more balanced multimodal approach to pain control.

Pain perception occurs via simulation of A-delta and C nerve fibers in the dental pulp. Acute pain is perceived by stimulation of A-delta fibers while C-fibers are associated with chronic, dull discomfort and chronic stimulation. Stimulation of nerve fibers occurs by transduction of stimuli into the nerve terminus and propagation of the signal through nerve fibers (transmission) and opening and closing of sodium channels. Pain is modulated at the level of the central nervous system after propagation of the signal through the pre-ganglionic trunk. Sensitization is the phenomenon by which the threshold of nerve stimulation is lowered. Sensitization can also occur centrally, resulting in an exaggerated perception of pain for stimuli that would normally be perceived as non-painful. Considering the prevalence of periodontal disease, conditions of hyperalgesia (increased response to a normally painful stimulus) and allodynia (perceived pain resulting from a non-painful stimulus) are likely to impact many veterinary patients.

Regional anesthetic alone has demonstrated a reduction in minimum alveolar concentration by 23% in one study [3]. Lidocaine is labeled for veterinary use, but benefits of longer acting local anesthetics are used off-label for the benefits of increased duration of action. While other local anesthetics are recognized to demonstrate prolonged effects, one study has questioned the efficacy of the local anesthetic in the porcine model evaluating a palatal nerve block [18]. Anatomic landmarks for the local anesthetics are listed below; however, it remains difficult to accurately assess the successful placement of the drug when performing either the caudal maxillary nerve block [19] as well as potential unreliable effects when performing the middle mental nerve block [20].

The proper placement of local and regional nerve blocks requires comprehensive knowledge of neuroanatomy and relevant anatomical landmarks. Sensory innervation to the oral cavity is primarily from two branches of the trigeminal nerve (cranial nerve V), the maxillary nerve, and the mandibular nerve and their branches. The maxillary nerve originates from the round foramen and courses rostrally along the dorsal margin of the medial pterygoid muscle to the pterygopalatine fossa. At this location the maxillary nerve branches, giving rise to the zygomatic and pterygopalatine nerves and continues as the infraorbital nerve as it passes through the maxillary foramen into the infraorbital canal. The pterygopalatine nerve branches into the major and minor palatine nerves, which innervate the soft and hard palate. Immediately before entering the infraorbital canal, the infraorbital nerve gives rise to the caudal superior alveolar nerve, which innervates the first and second molars. Within the infraorbital canal the middle and rostral superior alveolar nerves branch from the infraorbital nerve, supplying sensory innervation to the premolars via small foramina at the floor of the canal, and to the canines and incisors via the incisivomaxillary canal. The infraorbital nerve exits at the infraorbital foramen branching into the external nasal, internal nasal, and superior labial nerves. At the level of the infraorbital foramen, sensory innervation to the dentition and its associated bone and soft tissue structures has already disseminated. Desensitization of these tissues requires deposition of local anesthetic caudal to the infraorbital foramen, either within the canal or at the pterygopalatine fossa.

The mandibular nerve originates from the round foramen, courses rostrally along the medial side of the TMJ and gives rise to the buccal, the masseteric, and the auriculotemporal nerves. The buccal branch courses laterally and provides sensory innervation to vestibular mucosa and skin ventral to the zygomatic arch. The masseteric branch supplies motor innervation to the masseter muscle. The mandibular nerve continues rostrally to the medial surface of the caudal mandible. The mandibular nerve continues rostrally as the inferior alveolar nerve as it enters the mandibular canal via the mandibular foramen, where alveolar sensory branches are given off to the teeth. Just caudal to the mandibular canal entrance, two branches arise, the lingual and mylohyoid or inferior alveolar nerves. The lingual nerve provides sensory innervation to the rostral two-thirds of the tongue and, via the sublingual branch, to the sublingual mucosa. The mylohyoid innervates the mylohyoid muscle and rostral belly of the digastricus muscle; it also provides sensory innervation to the caudal two-thirds of the intermandibular mucosa. The inferior alveolar nerves course rostrally within the mandibular canal, providing sensory input to the mandibular teeth via foramina in the canal wall. The nerve branches rostrally into the caudal, middle, and rostral mental nerves, exiting at three corresponding mental foramina. The mental nerves provide sensory innervation to the lower lip and rostral one-third of the intermandibular area. At the level of the middle mental foramen, the inferior alveolar nerve has already passed on sensory innervation to the teeth; to desensitize dentition and associated structures requires infiltration of local anesthetic caudal to foramen.

9.6.2 Drugs and Materials

Local anesthetic medication can be easily administered using a one milliliter syringe and small gauge needle. Size 25- to 30-gauge needles are commonly used with needle lengths ranging from 5/8 to 1.5 inches. Regular needles for injection are frequently used for local block administration but short, atraumatic "b-bevel" needles are also available and in unconfined spaces may be more efficient at displacing rather than penetrating the nerve [21]. Large or giant breed dogs using certain intraoral approaches to the caudal maxillary nerve block may require additional needle length and an over-the-needle catheter or spinal needle may be necessary.

Glass cartridges preloaded with a local anesthetic agent may be used with a metal administration syringe. However, the availability of disposable syringes is commonplace in veterinary dentistry.

Multiple local anesthetic agents have been used in companion animal analgesia. Two of the most commonly used medications used for local anesthesia are lidocaine and bupivacaine. Other local anesthetics used occasionally are mepivacaine and carbocaine. In veterinary medicine, lidocaine is typically used as a 2% solution, with or without epinephrine. Lidocaine offers the advantage of rapid onset (two to five minutes), but the duration is limited (30 minutes to 2 hours) [22]. The maximum dose of lidocaine recommended for dogs and cats is 4 mg/kg [22] and efforts should be focused on dosing the patient based on volume and number of local block administration sites and less on calculating a mg/kg dose and feeling compelled to use the complete volume.

Bupivacaine requires more time to take effect (6–10 minutes), but results in a longer duration of action (four to eight hours dependent on location) [23]. One study suggests that in dogs, bupivacaine's activity as a local anesthetic may extend for one or more days [24]. Bupivacaine is available in 0.25%, 0.5%, and 0.75% solutions. Bupivacaine is particularly cardiotoxic due to lipophilicity of the drug and affinity for cardiac myosites [21] and care should be taken to be consistent in the concentration of drug used. The most common injectable local anesthetics used in veterinary medicine (lidocaine, bupivacaine, mepivacaine) are amide local anesthetics. Local inflammation at the site of injection may result in an acidic local tissue pH, in turn causing an increased amount of the unionized, inactive form of the drug. The dose of bupivacaine should not exceed 2 mg/kg in dogs or cats.

In some cases, a mixture of both lidocaine and bupivacaine has been advocated to achieve both the immediacy of action and the duration of effect. However, in most cases this may not be necessary; the addition of lidocaine provides little advantage if bupivacaine is the primary agent to be considered, since both lidocaine and bupivacaine will each have an onset of effect within about five minutes [22]. The addition of bupivacaine mixed with lidocaine compared with lidocaine alone demonstrated greater than a doubling of the duration of action (120 minutes compared with 277 minutes) when testing effects of the maxillary canine teeth after placing an infraorbital nerve block [25]. However, "the duration of the combination was at the lower end of the reported duration of action (4–8 hours) for bupivacaine alone [23] and was much shorter than the potential for bupivacaine's activity alone which has been suggested to last for days in some dogs" [24]. Preferential use of short-acting local anesthetics may be advantageous for perioperative pain management for palatal surgery and for maxillectomy or oronasal fistula repair patients. Prolonged activity may increase the risk that facial rubbing or scratching or tongue thrusting will excessively traumatize the surgery site. Aggressive post-operative injectable, constant rate infusion or oral pain medications should be instituted for these patients to address the central perception of pain.

The volume of the local anesthetic used should be calculated between the total dosage of drug used across multiple block locations. The amount of drug calculated for a four-quadrant block should be such that the patient does not risk receiving greater than the calculated maximum dose for the individual drug being used. Determination of the dosage of drug required should be based on lean, rather than actual, body mass. Also, the volume used is site-dependent. It would be expected that placement of a local anesthetic within a confined space such as a bony canal will result in a longer duration of effect compared to deposition at sites, primarily encased in soft tissue due to the local area's ability to clear the drug. Less anesthetic agent therefore may be necessary in the infraorbital or mandibular canals as local anesthetic absorption and clearance will be slower. Accuracy in local block placement also aids in reduction of the necessary amount of drug required to be effective. Due to the compact anatomy and accessibility for regional block placement in canines and felines, use of saline to dilute the local anesthetic or bicarbonate to buffer the acidic pH of local anesthetics and reduce injection site discomfort are ordinarily not necessary for local block success.

The addition of epinephrine to local anesthetics has been proposed to extend the duration of activity for local anesthetic drugs. Vasoconstriction may reduce the speed of tissue clearance of the drug while epinephrine has also been proposed to have a primarily nociceptive activity [26]. The addition of epinephrine has also been suggested to result in peripheral nerve ischemia also contributing to extended duration of activity [21].

In a study evaluating the duration of effect of buprenorphine mixed with bupivicane versus bupivacaine alone, the mixture demonstrated increased duration of activity despite being statistically insignificant. Bupivacaine alone was shown in some cases to last longer than 24 hours while bupivacaine + buprenorphine may last 48–96 hours [24]. Human patients have reported a threefold increase in the duration of action when buprenorphine was mixed with local anesthetic in patients receiving axillary brachial plexus blocks [27]. Human oral surgery patients have also demonstrated an increase in post-operative analgesia when opioids are mixed with local anesthetics [28]. Up-regulation of peripheral *mu* receptors appear to be the target for the mechanism of action for the opioids administered peripherally in patients with conditions of chronic pain or inflammation [27, 29]. Experimental investigation as to the effectiveness of opioid and local anesthetic mixtures in veterinary dentistry is a current area of active exploration. Experimental placement of low-dose morphine into the ligamental space of chronically inflamed teeth has shown to result in pain relief [30].

After withdrawal of anesthetic from the bottle, the needle should be changed prior to administration of the block [31]. When performing more than one block, a new needle should be used for each site. A gentle technique should be employed during insertion of the needle, with care to avoid unnecessary side-to-side movement. Ideally the needle is placed in close proximity to the targeted nerve without direct penetration through the nerve sheath. The needle bevel should be oriented parallel to the targeted nerve fibers to decrease the chance of cutting through nerve fibers [32]. Using a small-gauge needle with a gentle technique will help decrease intravascular penetration. Prior to administration of a local anesthetic, the syringe should be aspirated to ensure no vessel penetration. The needle should then be rotated and reaspirated to ensure extravascular positioning, in case the bevel was in contact with a vessel wall. Brief tachycardia may be noted during nerve block administration, due to paresthesia and transient local irritation of tissues; in some cases, the concentration of the gas anesthetic should be briefly increased. Hematomas may be avoided by immediate digital pressure following withdrawal of the needle. Applying pressure will also help facilitate diffusion of the medication.

9.6.3 Techniques

9.6.3.1 Middle Mental Nerve Block

The middle mental regional nerve block will desensitize ipsilateral teeth, bone, intraoral soft tissues, and some haired skin rostral to the mandibular second premolar on the infiltrated side. The middle mental foramen is typically the largest of the three mental foramina. The middle mental foramen is located ventral to the mesial root of the mandibular second premolar in the dog (recall cats do not have mandibular first or second premolar teeth) and just caudal to the mandibular labial frenulum. Needle placement through soft tissues immediately rostral to the labial frenulum will maximize anesthetic retention following needle withdrawal. The needle is inserted intraorally through the oral mucosa in a rostrocaudal direction. The needle should be advanced to a point just over, or just inside, the foramen and into the mandibular canal (Figures 9.1a,b and 9.2a,b). Consideration should be made for the needle gauge and anatomic opening size in small patients. If concern for lacerating the middle mental artery, vein, and nerve exists then administration of the local anesthetic over the mental foramen with digital pressure following injection should help maximize distribution of the block into the canal.

9.6.3.2 Inferior Alveolar Nerve Block

The inferior alveolar regional nerve block will desensitize ipsilateral teeth, bone, and intraoral soft tissues on the infiltrated side. The mandibular foramen is located on the medial (lingual) aspect of the ramus, approximately midway between an imaginary line drawn from the third molar to the angular process (Figure 9.3a). The foramen can usually be palpated intraorally by strumming a finger along the mucosa, following the palpable neurovascular bundle as it enters into the mandibular canal. The local anesthetic medication is deposited just superficial to the foramen via either an intraoral or extraoral approach. Of note, if the anesthetic drug is placed too far caudally, or in an excessively large volume, desensitization of the lingual nerve may occur, possibly risking self-trauma to the tongue by the patient.

9.6.3.2.1 Intraoral Approach

The index finger of the non-injecting, non-aspirating hand is placed on the angular process of the mandible as a visual guide (outside the mouth). An imaginary line is drawn from the distal aspect of the third mandibular molar tooth to the index finger at the angular process. The needle should be directed ventrocaudally toward the angular process. The needle is inserted into the alveolar mucosa just caudal to the third molar and advanced along the lingual (medial) surface of the ramus (Figure 9.3b). At the approximate midpoint between needle entry in the mucosa and the angular process, the needle should be positioned just superficial to the mandibular foramen.

9.6.3.2.2 Extraoral Approach

Alternatively, the needle may be advanced from an extraoral approach via the skin of the ventral aspect of the

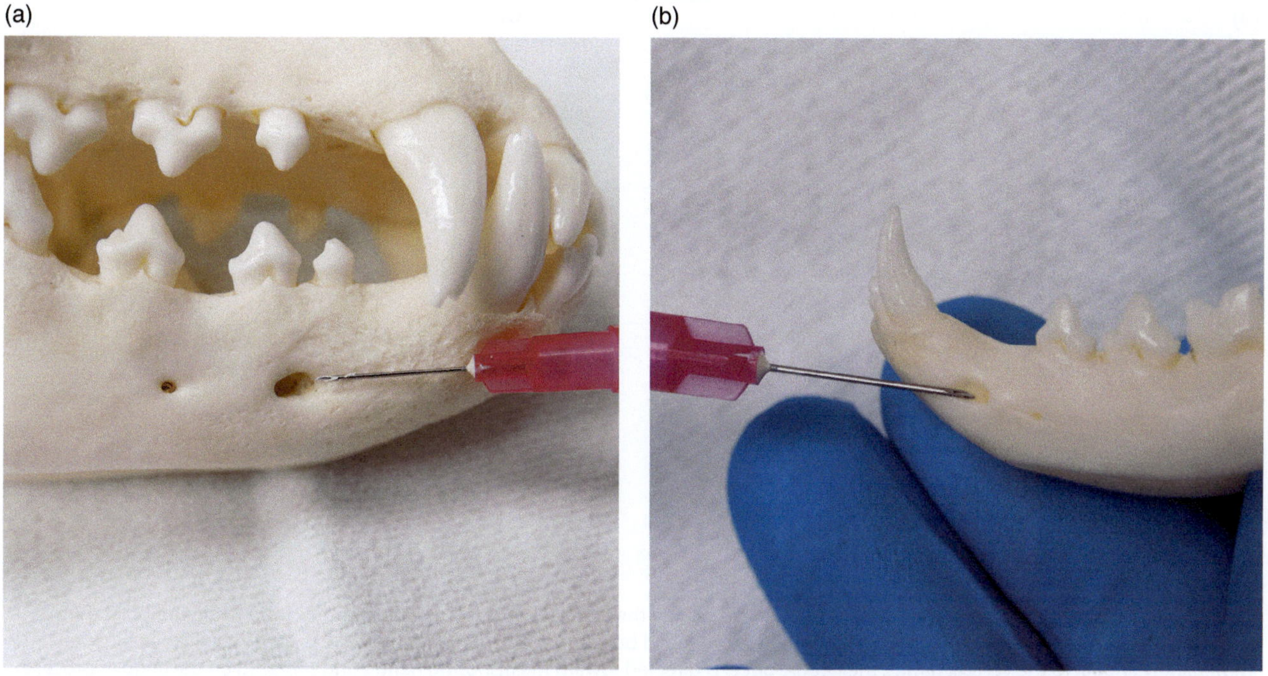

Figure 9.1 (a) The targeted placement of the needle bevel over the middle mental foramen in a dog; (b) similar placement in a feline. Efforts should be made for anesthetic placement rostral to, or right over, the foramen to avoid inadvertent threading of the needle into the foramen in small patients, which risks laceration or transection of the neurovascular bundle.

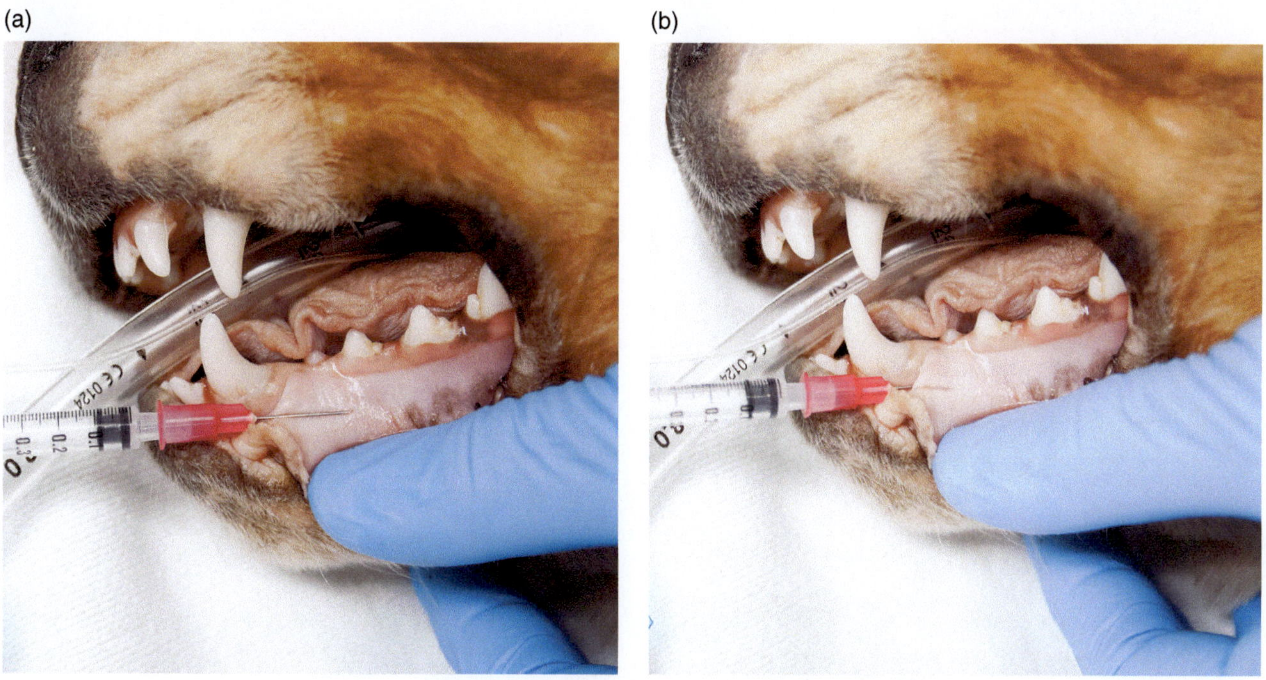

Figure 9.2 Demonstration of needle placement in a cadaver specimen. Approximation for the depth of needle placement can be assessed by overlying the needle (a) on top of soft tissue prior to needle placement (b).

mandible. Immediately rostral to the angular process is the prominent ventral notch of the mandible (Figure 9.4a). This anatomic location is less prominent and more difficult to palpate in cats. At the midpoint of the ventral notch, on the lingual surface of the ramus, the mandibular foramen will be located 0.5–1 cm dorsal to the ventral cortex at this location. The extraoral approach relies on palpation of the ventral notch, locating the midpoint and walking the

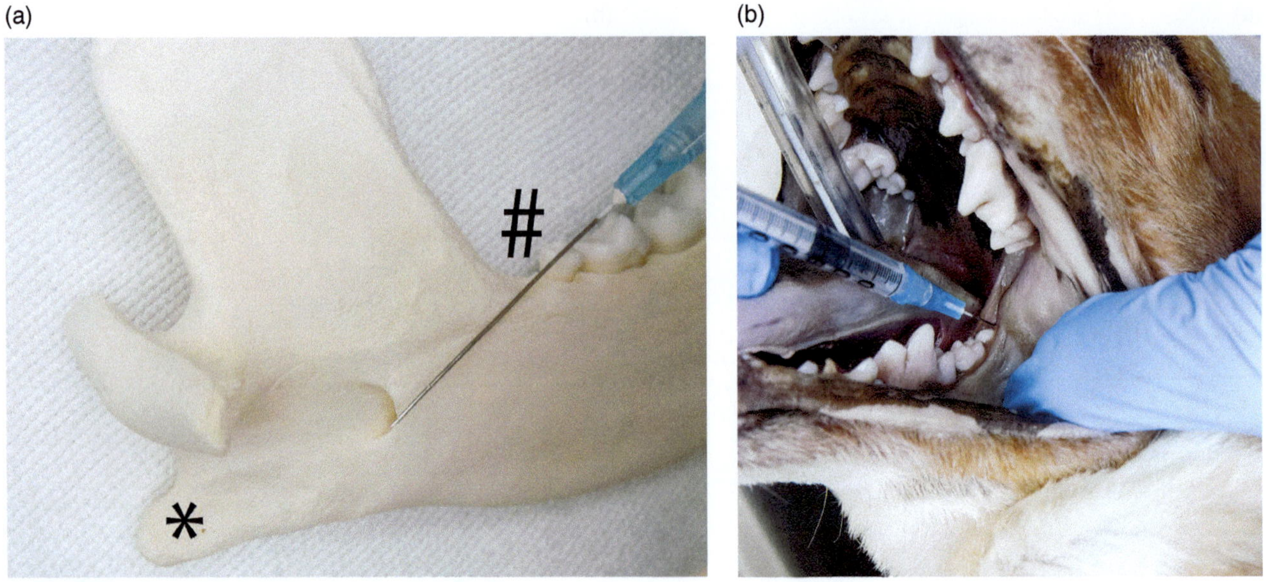

Figure 9.3 (a) Landmarks for needle placement in a canine include the angular process (*) of the mandible and the mandibular third molar (#). Half the distance between the two landmarks is the mandibular foramen. (b) With the needle placed into alveolar mucosa immediately lingual to the vertical ramus, the needle bevel is directed toward the opposing hand's finger placed on the angular process.

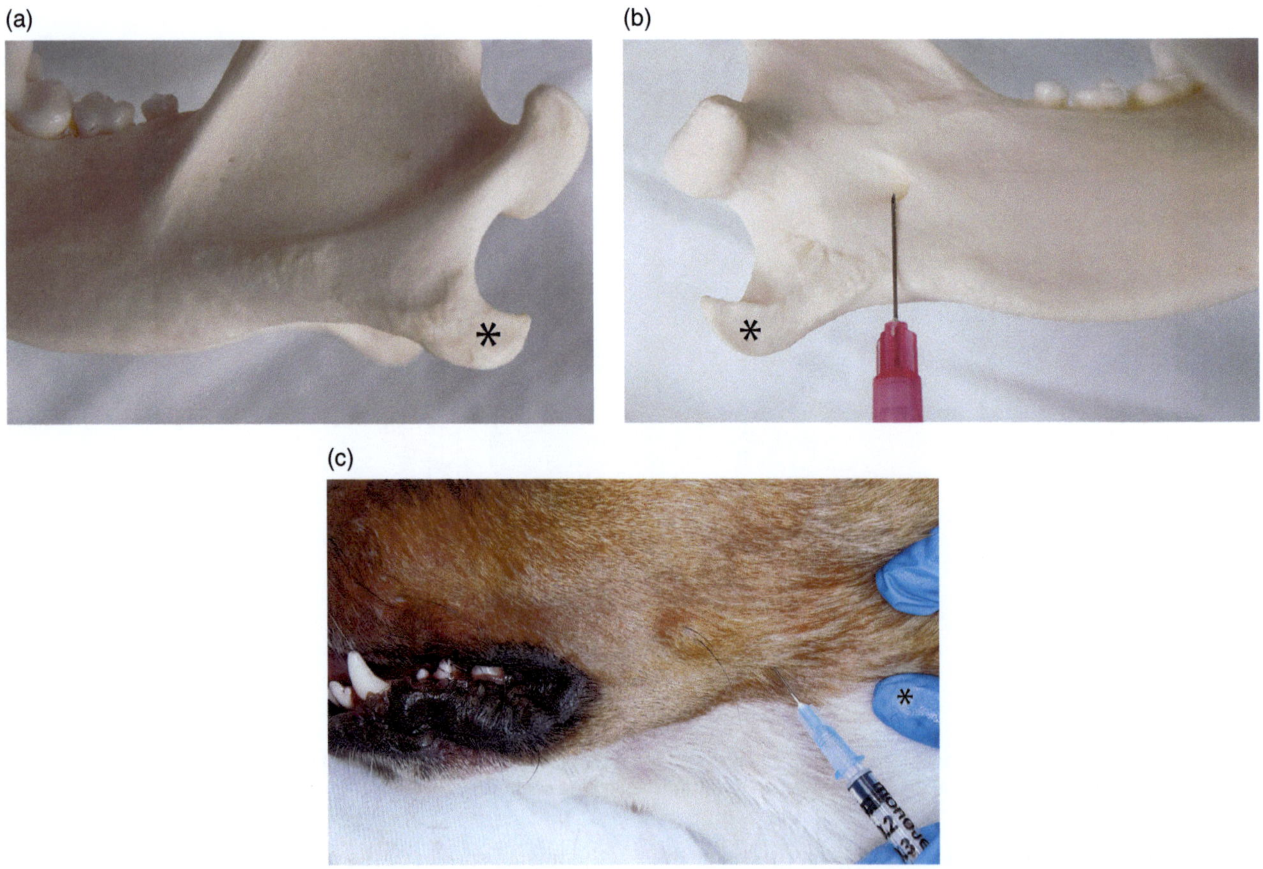

Figure 9.4 (a) The needle should be inserted along the lingual surface of the ramus, at the center of the mandibular notch, rostral to the angular process (*) and advanced 0.5–1 cm along the lingual border to the approximate location of the mandibular foramen. (b) On a clinical patient, the angular process should be identified and used for orientation to palpate the ventral notch of the mandible.

needle off the ventral cortex until the needle bevel courses along the periosteum to the depth of the foramen (Figure 9.4b). Following administration of the local anesthetic, digital pressure should be placed intraorally against the injection location to reduce hematoma formation and to encourage spreading of the local anesthetic.

Regional anesthetic techniques targeted at placement at the inferior alveolar nerve have been compared using the extraoral and intraoral techniques. The intraoral technique has been associated with increased accuracy in proximity to the inferior alveolar nerve [33].

9.6.3.3 Infraorbital Nerve Block

Intraoral and extraoral techniques have both been described for performing the infraorbital nerve block. The intraoral technique has been shown to demonstrate a significantly greater propensity for medication delivery, affecting the infraorbital and pterygopalatine nerves while showing no evidence in this study that intravascular or intraneural injections occurred [19].

The infraorbital regional nerve block will desensitize ipsilateral teeth, bone, and intraoral soft tissues on the infiltrated side. Depending on the level of the needle insertion, desensitized tissues extend caudally from the incisors and canine tooth to the fourth premolar ± ipsilateral molars. Because the caudal superior alveolar nerve branches off the infraorbital caudal to the maxillary foramen, desensitization of the maxillary molars requires deposition of medication at or caudal to the pterygopalatine fossa (Figure 9.5). In some patients, this may be obtained via caudal advancement of a long needle through the infraorbital canal using the infraorbital nerve block approach. Alternatively, a caudal approach to the maxillary nerve block can be considered.

9.6.3.3.1 Administration

The infraorbital foramen is palpated intraorally as an oval-shaped depression in the alveolar mucosa on the buccal aspect of the maxilla, dorsal to the distal root of the maxillary third premolar tooth. Sometimes it is helpful to palpate the submucosal neurovascular bundle above the maxillary premolars and trace it caudally to its exit at the infraorbital foramen. A needle is inserted through the alveolar mucosa just rostral to the foramen opening, directed in a rostrocaudal direction (Figure 9.6a). The needle should be advanced slowly and through mucosa and far enough for reasonable assurance that the needle bevel is placed within the infraorbital canal (Figure 9.6b). To reduce potential risk for globe perforation, the needle, and syringe should be maintained parallel to the dental arcade (Figure 9.6c). The infraorbital canal is noticeably shorter in felines and brachycephalic breeds of dogs (Figure 9.6d).

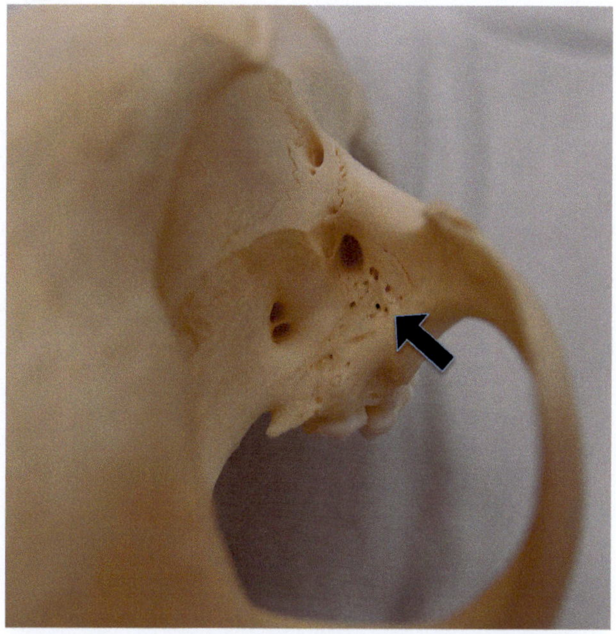

Figure 9.5 A view from within the orbital space demonstrates the multiple alveolar foramina (arrow) responsible for entry by the branches of the superior alveolar nerve. The prominent maxillary foramen is located immediately dorsal to the alveolar foramina.

9.6.3.4 Maxillary Nerve Block

The caudal maxillary nerve block will desensitize the entire maxillary quadrant, including teeth, alveolar bone, associated gingiva, alveolar mucosa, and mucosa of the hard palate. Extraoral soft tissues blocked include some of the nose, upper lip, and haired skin of the rostral muzzle. For this block, the local anesthetic agent is deposited in the pterygopalatine fossa and includes blockade of the major palatine branch of the maxillary nerve. Bilateral maxillary nerve block administration has also demonstrated local anesthesia to structures including the caudal nasal cavity [34]. Various approaches have been described for this nerve block including a dorsal approach with the needle through conjunctiva [22].

9.6.3.4.1 Administration

Two common intraoral options exist for the maxillary nerve block.

1) With the patient's mouth held open wide, the needle is inserted into the soft tissue space caudal to the last molar tooth, with the needle directed dorsally into the pterygoid fossa. The needle tip should not need to be advanced further than 1–3 mm into mucosa caudal to the second molar tooth [35] (Figure 9.7a and b).
2) Alternatively, the infraorbital approach offers the advantage of accurate needle placement through the use of the anatomic landmarks. Traumatic nerve sheath injury may be less likely since the needle is

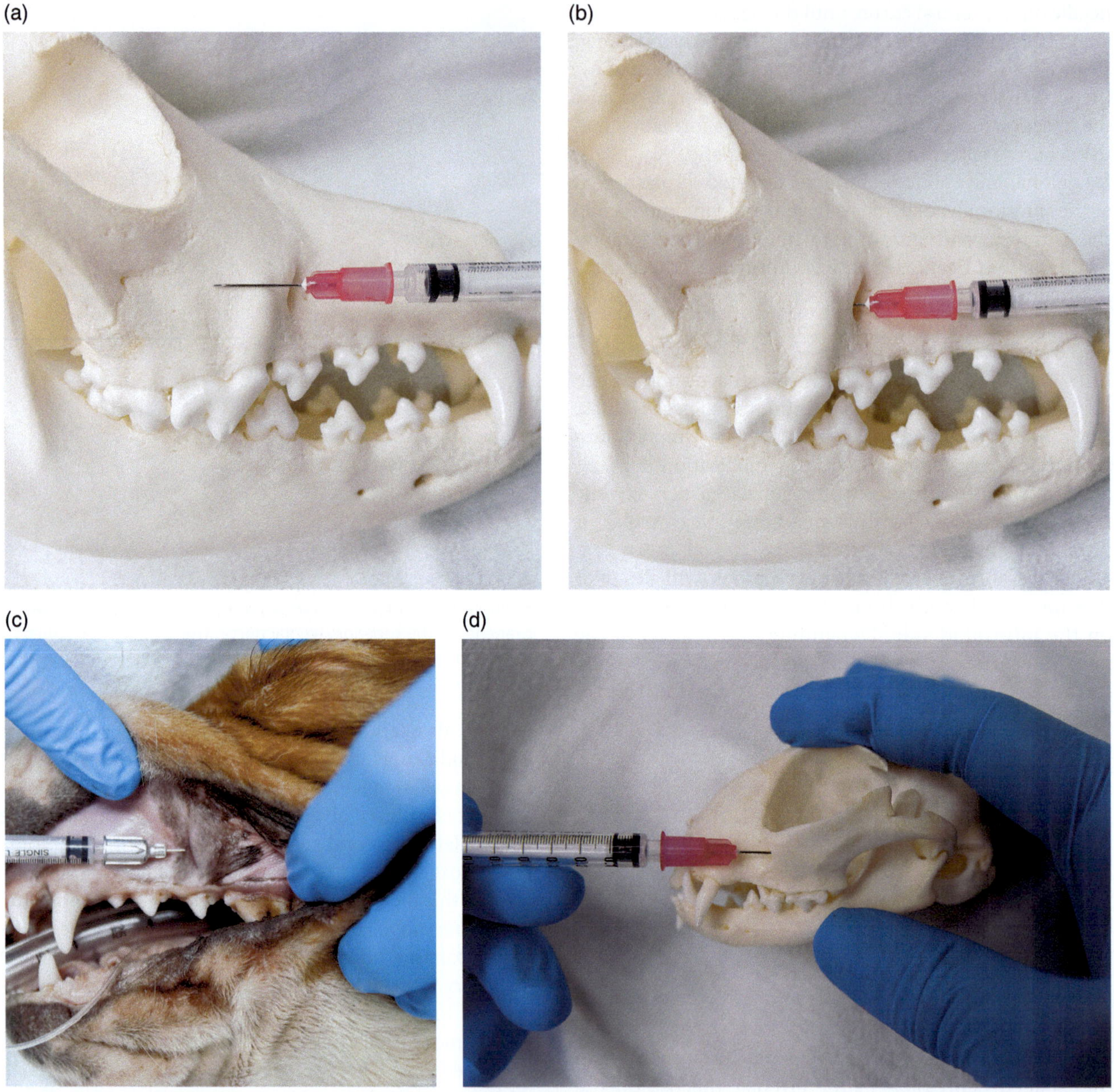

Figure 9.6 (a) The injection needle is overlying the buccal cortical plate superficial to the infraorbital canal to approximate the depth of needle placement into the canal. (b) Correct needle placement includes safely advancing the needle through the infraorbital canal without attempting to exit into the pterygopalatine fossa. (c) Needle placement demonstrated in a clinical patient. Note that the needle is advanced only to the point of assurance of placement into the infraorbital canal and that the syringe and needle are maintained parallel to the dental arcade. (d) A feline skull demonstrates the minimal distance necessary to place the needle into the infraorbital canal.

passed parallel to the nerve as opposed to perpendicular to it (as would be with the previous method described) to the pterygopalatine fossa. Both maxillary nerve block techniques would be preferred over the infraorbital technique to achieve blockade to the maxillary molars and mucosa of the hard palate. Flexibility in technique for local block placement may offer variation and flexibility depending on skull types or concurrent pathology (fracture, neoplasia, abscessation). Due to variability in needle placement and nerve location, larger volumes of local anesthetic may be necessary to see acceptable results.

An extraoral approach can be performed by inserting the needle at the rostroventral border of the zygomatic arch caudal to the lateral canthus of the eye, and directing the needle rostrally toward the nostril on the opposite side. This keeps the needle parallel to the plane of the palatal bone as it approaches the caudal opening of the infraorbital canal and the multiple alveolar foramina ventral to it (Figure 9.8a to d).

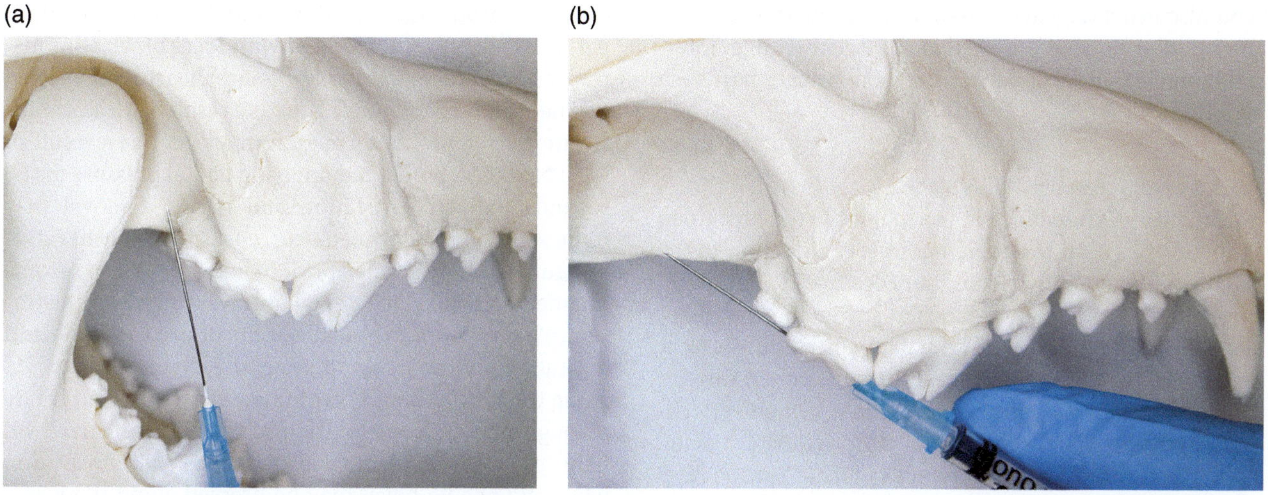

Figure 9.7 (a) With correct placement, the patient is placed into an open-mouth position, a needle is oriented dorsally, caudal to the maxillary second molar into the pterygopalatine fossa. Bending the needle to achieve orientation may be helpful, but the syringe should not be rotated through one revolution if the needle is no longer straight. (b) Incorrect needle placement results in the needle bevel top located too caudally and therefore inaccurately placing the block.

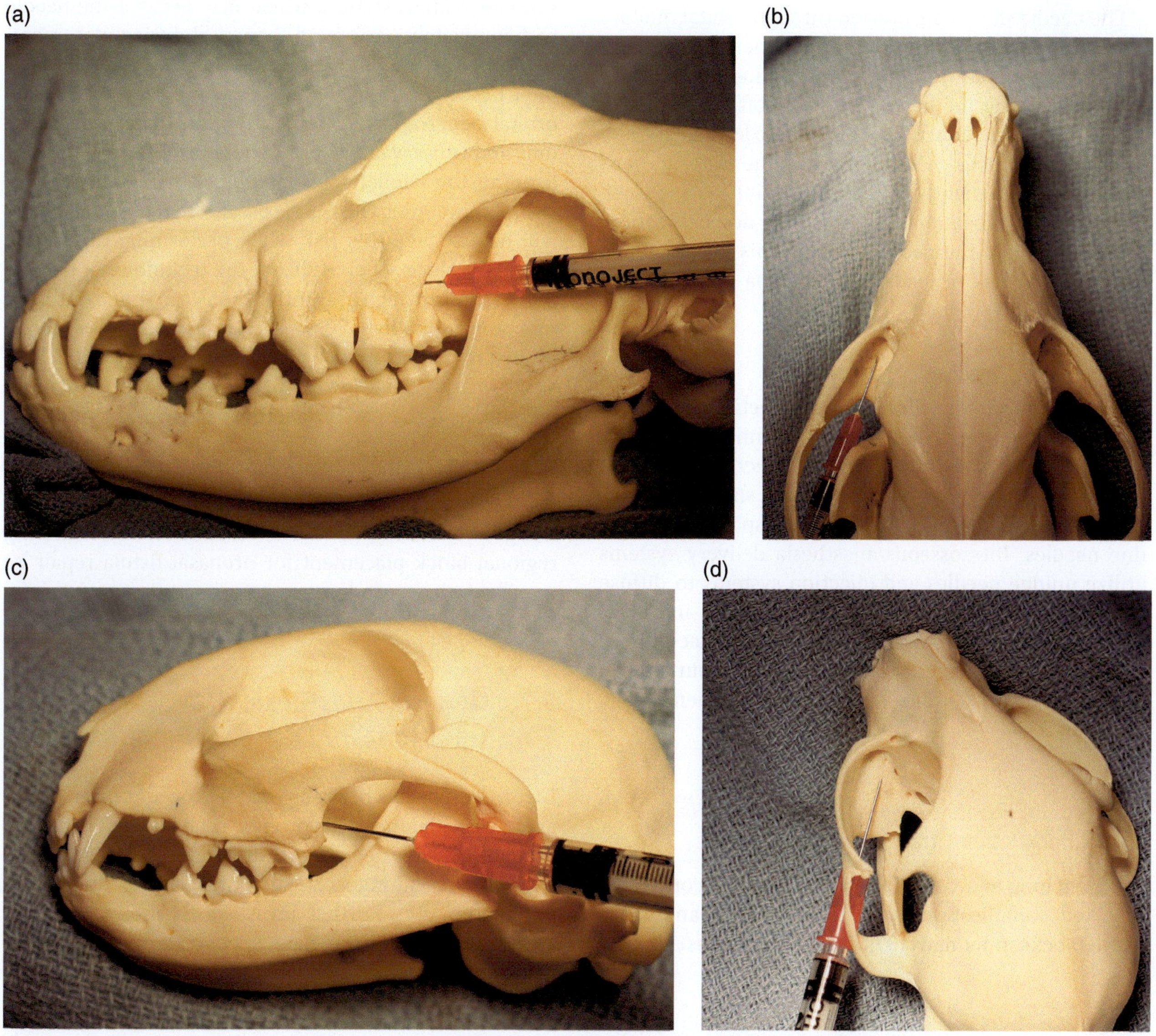

Figure 9.8 Caudal maxillary nerve block: (a) external caudal approach guides the needle rostrally under the zygomatic arch with the needle and syringe parallel to the palatal bone and (b) directed toward the opposite nostril in the dog; (c and d) in the cat.

This also avoids any inadvertent advancement of the needle into the globe of the eye that can occur with an internal approach in the dorsal direction, which has been reported [36].

9.6.3.5 Major Palatine Nerve Block

The major palatine block at the major palatine foramen is sometimes used to supplement desensitization of the palate. This block is usually unnecessary if the maxillary nerve is adequately blocked using the maxillary nerve block techniques. The palate epithelium is very thick, making digital palpation of this foramen unrealistic. The major palatine nerve lies in a trough superficial to the palatal bone and deep to the palatal epithelium. The foramen is typically located at the level of the mesial edge of the maxillary first molar, about halfway between the dental arch and palate midline (Figure 9.9a). Anatomical variations are common, with supplemental foramina located rostral to the major foramen reported [23].

The needle should be inserted through palatal mucosa several millimeters rostral to the foramen in a rostral-to-caudal direction and along the periosteum (Figure 9.9b). Threading the needle through soft tissue in this fashion will help reduce local anesthetic leakage following needle removal. Anecdotally, some veterinarians place this block slightly rostral to account for anatomic variation in location to ensure desensitization. Advancement of the needle through this narrow canal increases the risk of inadvertent trauma to the neurovascular bundle [22].

9.6.3.6 Alternative Techniques

Alternative techniques for local anesthetic administration have been described and are commonly used in humans when a focal anesthetic effect is desirable. Intraligamentary injections include small volumes injected into the periodontal ligament space using very fine needles. Intraosseous anesthesia delivery systems utilize unique needles and injection systems to diffuse local anesthetic into cancellous bone. Both intraligamentary [37] and intraosseous [38] injection techniques have been experimentally evaluated in dogs but clinical effects of the injections have yet to be scientifically objectified.

9.6.4 Complications Associated with Local/Regional Nerve Block Administration and Prevention

Fist clenching and vocalization are the most commonly reported complications with local/regional anesthetic nerve blocks in humans [39]. General anesthesia is necessary for orodental procedures and therefore will reduce patient discomfort associated with local block administration. Elevations in blood pressure, heart rate, or head and neck movement may occur as a result of local administration. Hematoma formation may occur as a result of local block placement but applying digital pressure for 60 seconds following injection and needle removal may reduce the likelihood of occurrence. Drawing negative pressure with the syringe prior to injection is also recommended to avoid accidental intravascular administration. Placement of the needle at the desired location and aspirating followed by rotating the syringe barrel 90° along the long axis and continuing to aspirate and rotate through one entire revolution of the syringe barrel will help prevent accidental intravascular administration when the needle bevel may be pressed along the vessel wall and therefore not result in flashback into the syringe. Despite not receiving flashback during aspiration, the local anesthetic should be administered in its entirety prior to needle withdrawal to prevent inadvertent intravascular administration, which may occur if the needle had completely perforated the vessel during placement. Inappropriate or careless needle control during infraorbital or caudal maxillary nerve block placement risks orbital penetration. Careful attention to regional anatomy and conservative placement of the needle while performing the caudal maxillary block will reduce these risks. Maintaining the needle parallel to the dental arcade will help reduce this risk when performing the caudal maxillary block when utilizing the technique of placing the needle through the infraorbital canal and into the pterygopalatine fossa. Care should be taken to avoid retropulsing the globe when performing the maxillary block as well as consideration for alternative pain management techniques if the patient demonstrates bupthalmos or if the needle placement will encroach upon a potential tumor and result in tumor seeding. Determination and consideration for the optimal duration of anesthesia and analgesia should be taken into account when considering regional block placement for oronasal fistula repair or maxillectomy procedures.

9.7 General Anesthesia Considerations for Dentistry Patients

Inconclusive links between dental procedures and post-anesthesia deafness have been reported in dogs and cats [40]. In cats, dental procedures have been associated with post-anesthetic cortical blindness following dental procedures [41]. Further investigation into the impact that mouth gags/props have on maxillary artery blood

(a) (b)

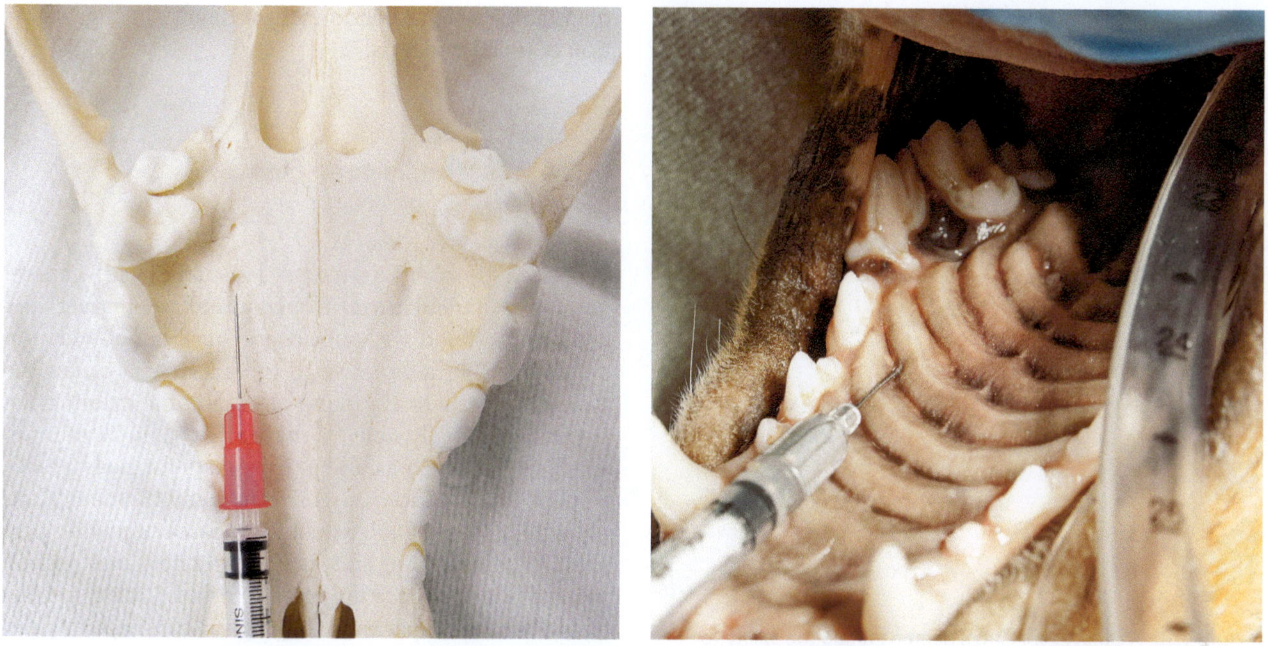

Figure 9.9 (a) The major palatine foramen is usually located halfway between midline of the hard palate and the distal surface of the fourth premolar tooth and along the mesial aspect of the first molar in a rostrocaudal direction. (b) Placement of the needle through mucosa and passing along the periosteum to the desired location helps reduce backflow of local anesthetic following needle removal.

flow demonstrated alteration in blood flow without the development of blindness or deafness [42]. In cats studied, an open-mouth position inconsistently creates compression of the maxillary arteries without consistently inducing collateral circulation [43]. Use of mouth props, and not spring-loaded mouth gags, appear to induce less alterations in blood flow and should be considered if a device is necessary to maintain an opened mouth position [44]. In addition to care and consideration for dental patients and the use of mouth gags, care should be taken to disconnect the endotracheal tube from the breathing circuit when repositioning the patient. Tethering the endotracheal tube to the breathing circuit when rotating or moving the patient risks the inflated endotracheal tube being associated with tracheal damage [45].

9.8 Special Consideration for Airway Management During General Anesthesia in Dental Patients

There are a variety of procedures performed in the oral cavity where the presence of the endotracheal tube creates challenges. Anesthetic delivery is necessity for the safe practice of orodental procedures and aside from maintaining the patient at an anesthetic plane while on inhalant anesthesia, an appropriately inflated endotracheal tube cuff aids in the prevention of aspiration. Alternatives to traditional orotracheal intubation may be beneficial when a more unobstructed access to the oral cavity is necessary. Procedures necessitating unobstructed access to the caudal oral cavity including caudal oronasal fistula repair, soft palate surgery, or pharyngeal surgery may have improved surgical exposure by using alternative methods of intubation. Pharyngostomy [10, 46, 47] intubation and temporary tracheostomy techniques both afford unobscured access to the oral cavity.

Success of certain procedures involving the oral cavity also may be impacted by the veterinarian's ability to check and maintain occlusion. Custom orthodontic devices fabricated chairside and oral fracture repair are two specific procedures where frequent evaluation of occlusion is critical to treatment success. Modifications to the endotracheal tube length have been described to permit disconnecting the patient from the anesthetic circuit [22]. Cutting short and splicing together the endotracheal tube within the patient's mouth allows for briefly disconnecting the patient and checking occlusion without completely extubating the patient. When planning to customize endotracheal tube length, consideration should be made to not sever the endotracheal tube pilot line. A transmylohyoid intubation technique has also been described permitting the passage of the

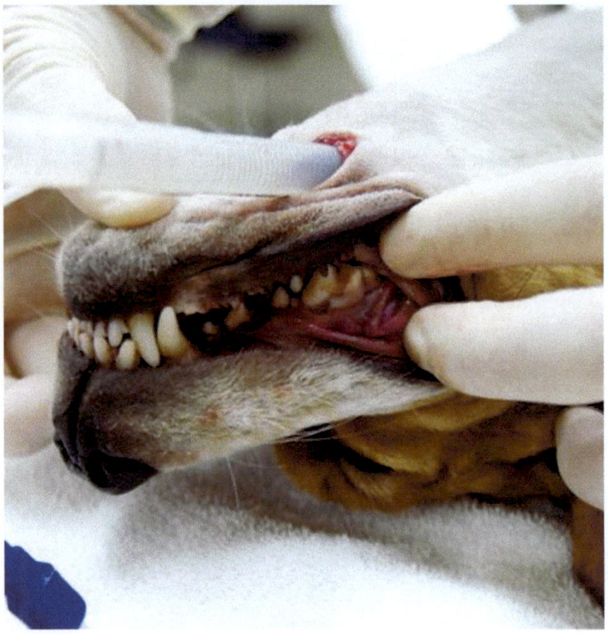

Figure 9.10 A cadaver specimen demonstrating the ability to maintain and check occlusion using the transmylohyoid intubation technique.

endotracheal tube through a stoma created through the skin of the ventral mandible, through the mylohyoideus muscle, and entering the oral cavity through mucosa lingual to the first molar tooth [13] (Figure 9.10). The use of custom created endotracheal tubes and the transmylohyoid intubation technique both offer the capacity for easy assessment of occlusion without the need for frequent extubation. By not extubating the patient the risk for tracheal irritation is decreased and the airway is maintained with the endotracheal tube reducing aspiration of fluids or debris.

9.9 Anesthesia-Free Dental Procedures

Propelled by client concerns associated with general anesthesia, a trend has developed whereby dental services are being offered without general anesthesia. Sedation dentistry as an alternative to full anesthesia places the patient under a heavy plane of sedation, rendering the patient minimally able to respond to painful stimuli. Use of drugs such as alpha-2 agonists for heavy sedation typically reduces the concerns about premedication drug-associated hypotension. Risks associated with performing dental scaling and polishing in a non-anesthetized patient include an unprotected airway from debris, limited ability to perform subgingival curettage or periodontal probing and risk to patient injury from intraoral use of sharp dental instruments. Considering the high prevalence of periodontal disease in the veterinary patient population, many patients are likely to need general anesthesia for treatment of dental and periodontal disease. Insufficient evidence exists at the time of this chapter's preparation as to the patient safety and clinical effectiveness of anesthesia-free dentistry (AFD). Current recommendations by the American Veterinary Dental College regarding AFD can be found at the organization's website (www.avdc.org).

References

1 Gaynor, J.S., Dunlop, C.I., Wagner, A.E. et al. (1999). Complications and mortality associated with anesthesia in dogs and cats. *J. Am. Anim. Hosp. Assoc.* 35 (1): 13–17.

2 Machado, C.E.G., Dyson, D.H., and Grant Maxie, M. (2006). Effects of oxymorphone and hydromorphone on the minimum alveolar concentration of isoflurane in dogs. *Vet. Anaesth. Anal.* 33 (1): 70–77.

3 Snyder, C.J. and Snyder, L.B. (2013). Effect of mepivacaine in an infraorbital nerve block on minimum alveolar concentration of isoflurane in clinically normal anesthetized dogs undergoing a modified form of dental dolorimetry. *J. Am. Vet. Med. Assoc.* 242 (2): 199–204.

4 Almeida, T.F., Roizenblatt, S., and Tufik, S. (2004). Afferent pain pathways: a neuroanatomical review. *Brain Res.* 1000 (1–2): 40–56.

5 Falk, S. and Dickenson, A.H. (2014). Pain and nociception: mechanisms of cancer-induced bone pain. *J. Clin. Oncol.* 32 (16): 1647–1654.

6 Lolignier, S., Eijkelkamp, N., and Wood, J.N. (2015). Mechanical allodynia. *Pflugers Arch.* 467 (1): 133–139.

7 Lei, J., Sun, T., Lumb, B.M., and You, H.J. (2014). Roles of the periaqueductal gray in descending facilitatory and inhibitory controls of intramuscular hypertonic saline induced muscle nociception. *Exp. Neurol.* 257: 88–94.

8 Staud, R. (2011). Peripheral pain mechanisms in chronic widespread pain. *Best Pract. Res. Clin. Rheumatol.* 25 (2): 155–154.

9 Mattscheck, D. and Law, A. (2006). The nonodontogenic toothache. In: *Pathways of the Pulp*, 9e (ed. S. Cohen and K.M. Hargreaves), 59–79. St. Louis, MO: Mosby.

10 Smith, M.M. (2004). Pharyngostomy endotracheal tube. *J. Vet. Dent.* 21: 191–194.

11 Hartsfield, S.M., Genfreau, C.L., Smith, C.W. et al. (1977). Endotracheal intubation by pharyngostomy. *J. Am. Anim. Hosp. Assoc.* 13: 71–74.

12 Nicholson, I. and Baines, S. (2012). Complications associated with temporary tracheostomy tubes in 42 dogs (1998–2007). *J. Small. Anim. Pract.* 53: 108–115.

13 Soukup, J.W. and Snyder, C.J. (2015). Transmylohyoid orotracheal intubation in surgical management of canine maxillofacial fractures; an alternative to pharyngostomy endotracheal intubation. *Vet. Surg.* 44 (4): 432–436.

14 Stephens Devalle, J.M. (2009). Successful management of rabbit anesthesia through the use of nasotracheal intubation. *J. Am. Assoc. Lab. Anim. Sci.* 48: 166–170.

15 Riebold, T.W., Engel, H.N., Brubb, T.L. et al. (2004). Orotracheal and nasotracheal intubation in llamas. *J. Am. Vet. Med. Assoc.* 1994: 779–784.

16 Holmstrom, S., Frost Fitch, P., and Eisner, E. (2004). Dental equipment and care. In: *Veterinary Dental Techniques for the Small Animal Practitioner*, 3e (ed. S. Holmstrom, P. Frost Fitch and E. Eisner), 129. Philadelphia, PA: Saunders.

17 Rusbridge, C., Heath, S., Gunn-Moore, D.A. et al. (2010). Feline orofacial pain syndrome (FOPS): a retrospective study of 113 cases. *J. Feline Med. Surg.* 12: 498–508.

18 Holman, S.D., Gierbolini-Norat, E.M., Lukasik, S.L. et al. (2014). Duration of action of bupivacaine hydrochloride used for palatal sensory nerve block in infant pigs. *J. Vet. Dent.* 31 (2): 92–95.

19 Viscasillas, J., Seymour, C.J., and Brodbelt, D.C. (2013). A cadaver study comparing two approaches for performing maxillary nerve blocks in dogs. *Vet. Anaesth. Analg.* 40: 212–219.

20 Krug, W. and Losey, J. (2011). Area of desensitization following mental nerve block in dogs. *J. Vet. Dent.* 28 (3): 146–150.

21 Greensmith, J.E. and Bosseau Murray, W. (2006). Complications of regional anesthesia. *Curr. Opin. Anaesthesiol.* 19: 531–537.

22 Pasco, P.J. (2012). Anesthesia and pain management. In: *Oral and Maxillofacial Surgery in Dogs and Cats* (ed. F.J.M. Verstraete, M.J. Lommer and A.J. Bezuidenhout), 23–42. London, UK: Saunders Elsevier.

23 Lantz, G.C. (2003). Regional anesthesia for dentistry and oral surgery. *J. Vet. Dent.* 20 (3): 181–186.

24 Snyder, L.B.C., Snyder, C.J., and Hetzel, S. (2016). Effects of buprenorphine added to bupivacaine infraorbital nerve blocks on isoflurane minimum alveolar concentration using a model for acute dental/oral surgical pain in dogs. *J. Vet. Dent.* 33 (2): 90–96.

25 Pascoe, P.J. (2016). The effects of lidocaine or a lidocaine-bupivacaine mixture administered into the infraorbital canal in dogs. *Am. J. Vet. Res.* 77 (7): 682–687.

26 Förster, J.G. and Rosenberg, P.H. (2003). Clinically useful adjuvants in regional anesthesia. *Curr. Opin. Anaesthesiol.* 16: 477–486.

27 Candido, K.D., Winnie, A.P., Ghaleb, A.H. et al. (2002). Buprenorphine added to the local anesthetic for axillary brachial plexus block prolongs postoperative analgesia. *Reg. Anesth. Pain Med.* 27 (2): 162–167.

28 Modi, M., Rastogi, S., and Jumar, A. (2009). Buprenorphine with bupivacaine for intraoral nerve blocks to provide postoperative analgesia in outpatients after minor oral surgery. *J. Oral Maxillofac. Surg.* 67 (12): 2571–2576.

29 Lamont, L.A. (2008). Multimodal pain management in veterinary medicine: the physiologic basis of pharmacologic therapies. *Vet. Clin. North Am. Small Anim. Pract.* 38 (6): 1173–1186.

30 Dionne, R.A., Lepinski, A.M., Gordon, S.M. et al. (2001). Analgesic effects of peripherally administered opioids in clinical models of acute and chronic inflammation. *Clin. Pharmacol. Therapeutics.* 70 (1): 66–73.

31 Rout, P.G., Saksena, A., and Fisher, S.E. (2003). An investigation of the effect on 27-gauge needle tips following a single local anaesthetic injection. *Dent. Update* 30 (7): 370–374.

32 Hirasawa, Y., Katsumi, Y., Kusswetter, W. et al. (1990). Experimentelle Untersuchungen zur peripheren Nervenverletzung durch Injektionsnadeln. *Reg. Anesth.* 13: 11–15.

33 Goudie-DeAngelis, E.M., Snyder, C.J., Raffe, M.R., and David, F.H. (2016). A pilot study comparing the accuracy of two approaches to the inferior alveolar nerve block in canine cadavers. *Intern. J. Appl. Res. Vet. Med.* 14 (1): 49–58.

34 Cremer, J., Sum, S.O., Braun, C. et al. (2013). Assessment of maxillary an infraorbital nerve blockade for rhinoscopy in sevoflurane anesthetized dogs. *Vet. Anaesth. Anal.* 40: 432–439.

35 Beckman, B.W. and Legendre, L. (2002). Regional nerve blocks for oral surgery in companion animals. *Comp. Cont. Ed. Prac. Vet.* 24 (6): 439–444.

36 Alessio, T.L. and Krieger, E.M. (2015). Transient unilateral vision loss in a dog following inadvertent intravitreal injection of bupivacaine during a dental procedure. *J. Am. Vet. Med. Assoc.* 246 (9): 990–993.

37 Cromley, L. and Adams, D.F. (1991). The effect of intraligamentary injections on diseased periodontiums in dogs. *Gen. Dent.* 389 (1): 33–37.

38 Smith, G.N. and Pashley, D.H. (1983). Periodontal ligament injection: evaluation of systemic effects. *Oral Surg. Oral Med. Oral Pathol.* 56 (6): 571–574.

39 Brand, H.S., Bekker, W., and Baart, J.A. (2009). Complications of local anesthesia. An observational study. *Int. J. Dent. Hyg.* 7 (4): 270–272.

40 Stevens-Sparks, C.K. and Strain, G.M. (2010). Post-anesthesia deafness in dogs and cats following dental and ear cleaning procedures. *Vet. Anaesth. Analg.* 37 (4): 347–351.

41 Stiles, J., Weil, A.B., Packer, R.A., and Lantz, G.C. (2012). Post-anesthetic cortical blindness in cats: twenty cases. *Vet. J.* 193 (2): 367–373.

42 Barton-Lamb, A.L., Martin-Flores, M., Scrivani, P.V. et al. (2013). Evaluation of maxillary arterial blood flow in anesthetized cats with the mouth closed and open. *Vet. J.* 196 (3): 325–331.

43 Scrivani, P.V., Martin-Flores, M., van Hatten, R. et al. (2014). Structural and functional changes relevant to maxillary arterial flow observed during computed tomography and nonselective digital subtraction angiography in cats with the mouth closed and opened. *Vet. Rad. Ultrasound* 55 (3): 263–271.

44 Martin-Flores, M., Scrivani, L.E. et al. (2014). Maximal and submaximal mouth opening with mouth gags in cats: implications for maxillary artery blood flow. *Vet. J.* 200 (1): 60–64.

45 Hardie, E.M., Spodnick, G.J., Gilson, S.D. et al. (1999). Tracheal rupture in cats: 16 cases (1983-1998). *J. Am. Vet. Med. Assoc.* 214 (4): 508–512.

46 Harvey, C.E. (1993). Oral cavity: the tongue, lips, cheeks, pharynx, and salivary glands. In: *Textbook of Small Animal Surgery*, 2e (ed. D. Slatter), 510–530. Philadelphia, PA: W.B. Saunders.

47 Lantz, G. (2012). Pharyngotomy and Pharyngostomy. In: *Oral and Maxillofacial Surgery in Dogs and Cats* (ed. V. FJM and M.J. Lommer), 543–546. London, UK: Saunders Elsevier.

10

Oral Surgery – Periodontal Surgery

Heidi B. Lobprise[1] *and Kevin Stepaniuk*[2]

[1] *Main Street Veterinary Dental Clinic, Flower Mound, TX, USA*
[2] *Veterinary Dentistry Education and Consulting Services, LLC, Ridgefield, WA, USA*

10.1 Introduction

In Chapter 5 – Periodontology – the basic concepts of periodontal disease and management were discussed, including the steps of complete dental assessment, dental cleaning and polishing, and home care. The roles of host modulation in combination with professional care and cleaning outlined the efforts to help manage the patient's inflammatory response to periodontal disease and how both aspects need to be addressed. Appropriate selection of antibiotics, including perioceutic therapy, was also discussed. This chapter continues periodontal treatment with the topics of periodontal surgery and other advanced therapies.

The goal of all periodontal therapy to arrest the progression of the disease is combined with efforts to minimize attachment loss, including efforts to eliminate periodontal pockets. Preservation of the periodontal tissues, with an emphasis on maintaining the attached gingiva (AG) and underlying tissues, is a primary objective of initial treatment, and efforts to restore or regenerate some of those lost tissues is possible in select cases.

10.1.1 Selection of Cases

The selection of cases, in fact, is a critical factor in determining which teeth should be treated and which teeth should be extracted. The opportunities to treat teeth with advanced lesions will be limitless, but several factors need to be considered, including the tooth/teeth, the patient and the client. Certainly, the extent and type of attachment loss on a tooth is evaluated closely, and the relative importance of the tooth can help determine if the effort is justified. Strategic teeth such as canines and carnassial teeth often deserve special consideration. Less strategic teeth, however, particularly those adjacent to the larger ones, may be selected for extraction to allow better access to the juxtaposed teeth for more effective treatment. Consideration of the quality of the tissues of attachment can influence prognosis as well. Toy breeds have been shown to have significantly thinner gingiva and alveolar bone than larger dogs and these dimensions may be predictors for the potential severity of the disease and can influence clinical outcome [1].

Advanced periodontal therapy will often result in longer and more frequent anesthetic episodes, so patients with increased anesthetic risks may be poor candidate choices. Extracting a potential source of chronic inflammation and infection may be preferable in those patients with ongoing systemic disease. Client education as to the importance of regular and effective home care and more frequent periodontal assessment may help identify those willing and able to commit to the extra work and financial investment to have satisfactory results.

Application of concepts and advanced treatments used in human dentistry has greatly enhanced the level of periodontal care we can provide our veterinary patients. Distinct differences in oral anatomy and function requires us to adjust definitions, classifications, and even anticipated prognoses for our patients. A shorter life span and the emphasis of function over aesthetics should make us question if a procedure that might be possible to perform would actually be best for the patient.

10.2 Goals of Periodontal Therapy

As stated in Chapter 5 – Periodontology – "The goal with periodontal disease is to stop the disease, minimize further attachment loss, and treat compromised teeth," as well as to "remove the plaque biofilm" and eliminate pockets. Modulating the host response to "address the inflammatory response to the plaque biofilm" is important as well.

Wiggs's Veterinary Dentistry: Principles and Practice, Second Edition. Edited by Heidi B. Lobprise and Johnathon R. (Bert) Dodd.

The efforts to minimize attachment loss are fundamental in attempting to keep optimal levels of the patient's attached gingiva, periodontal ligament, alveolar bone and healthy cementum on the root. In Chapter 1 – Oral Anatomy and Physiology – "The attached gingiva is arranged as mucoperiosteum with direct attachment .... The width of the attached gingiva is important in planning periodontal treatment." While a general guideline of needing a minimal width of attached gingiva for optimal health has been considered, in human patients with good, atraumatic oral hygiene, no minimum width of attached gingiva has been established as a necessary standard [2]. Such hygiene practices are unlikely to occur with veterinary patients, so the presence of keratinized gingiva (minimum of 2–3 mm of attached gingiva) can provide some level of protection.

Another specific consideration in periodontal therapy is to eliminate or minimize pockets, to facilitate healing and treatment. A variety of methods can minimize pocket depth, from reducing inflammation of soft tissue to excising excessive tissue or trying to build back tissues of attachment. Certainly, every effort at periodontal therapy includes the removal of any plaque biofilm or calculus, as well as necrotic or infected tissues in the area.

10.3 Evaluation/Classification of Disease

10.3.1 General Classification of Periodontal Disease

The basic definitions of the stages of periodontal disease are covered well in Chapter 5 – Periodontology – with specific references to the guidelines provided by the American Veterinary Dental College (AVDC). Typically, teeth in stage 3 to stage 4 periodontal disease have attachment loss significant enough to warrant advanced periodontal therapy, but some stage 2 teeth (up to 25% attachment loss) can be classified as stage 3 if stage 2 furcation involvement is present (F2) or as stage 4 with stage 3 furcation involvement (F3).

10.3.2 Attachment Loss Categorization

Determining both the extent and nature of attachment loss is critical in forming the appropriate treatment plan for the tooth or portion of the tooth. Measurement of all pockets/sulci, extent of gingival recession (GR) or marginal tissue recession (MTR), areas of root exposure and furcation involvement, tooth mobility, and evaluation of the remaining attached gingiva are critical parameters. Dental radiography and even advanced imaging will help determine the extent and type of periodontal bone loss (see Chapter 3 – Oral Radiology and Imaging).

Dividing the general groups of attachment loss or periodontal lesions into suprabony and intrabony (infrabony) highlights the special considerations when attachment loss extends apical to the alveolar bone height. In such lesions, there are both the challenges of access, as well as the opportunities for therapy. The descriptions of attachment loss in Chapter 5 include root exposure, suprabony pockets, intrabony(infrabony) pockets, and pseudopockets.

10.3.3 Suprabony Attachment Loss or Periodontal Lesion

10.3.3.1 Suprabony Periodontal Pocket

If there is horizontal bone loss without loss of the gingiva or at a rate greater compared to the loss of gingiva, the progression of attachment loss proceeds through the junctional epithelium (JE) and causes a soft tissue pocket with the base of the pocket coronal to the alveolar bone.

10.3.3.1.1 Pseudopocket

When there is gingival enlargement with no apical movement of the level of the JE or alveolar bone, the increased gingival height will give the appearance of periodontal pockets. Simple inflammation of the gingival margin can cause an increase in the "pocket" or sulcus depth, but with appropriate cleaning and therapy, the inflammation should subside and the sulcus depth can return to normal. True gingival enlargement (often termed gingival hyperplasia) will cause false pocket formation, which then requires treatment.

10.3.3.2 Gingival Recession – Marginal Tissue Recession

The term gingival recession is used more commonly than MTR, but if the loss of soft tissue extends beyond the mucogingival junction (MGJ), then mucosal tissue is also lost. Multiple classifications of soft tissue loss have been established, most notably Miller's Classification of MTR and Norland and Tarnow's classification of the loss of interdental papilla tissue [3, 4]. A newer classification by Kumar includes additional parameters that are not defined well in the Miller classification [5]. These measurements are not always applicable to veterinary cases, as interdental architecture can be quite variable, but basic concepts of how the extent and pattern of attachment loss can affect prognosis can be extrapolated.

10.3.3.3 Root Exposure and Furcation Involvement

If gingival tissue and alveolar bone height are both lost, there is exposure of the root apical to the neck of the tooth. This pattern is generally seen where there is horizontal bone loss around one tooth or several teeth, though focal clefts may occur. In dogs, a Stillman's cleft (mucogingival triangular-shaped defect on the buccal surface of a

Table 10.1 Furcation involvement/exposure index – FI [7].

Stage 1	F1, furcation involvement	Exists when a periodontal probe extends less than halfway under the crown in any direction of a multirooted tooth with attachment loss.
Stage 2	F2, furcation involvement	Exists when a periodontal probe extends greater than halfway under the crown of a multirooted tooth with attachment loss but not through and through.
Stage 3	F3, furcation involvement	Exists when a periodontal probe extends under the crown of a multirooted tooth, through and through from one side of the furcation out the other.

root can sometimes be found on the maxillary canine tooth [6]. If the attachment loss is pronounced at a multirooted tooth, then furcation involvement may be present (Table 10.1) [7]. Any level of furcation involvement can impact the prognosis for the tooth, as they can be more challenging to treat and to provide effective home care.

In some older cats, chronic osteitis and supereruption of the teeth can also result in root exposure of the canine teeth (particularly the maxillary canines), but is not due to gingival and alveolar recession. These teeth may also have additional pocket formation, so full assessment is needed.

10.3.4 Intrabony (Infrabony) Attachment Loss

When attachment loss of alveolar bone extends in a vertical or angular fashion down the root of a tooth, the intrabony defect has a base that is apical to the surrounding bone margin. This bone loss adjacent to a tooth root is further defined by the pattern of remaining "walls" of bone that surround the pocket. Each pattern – one-wall, two-wall, three-wall, and four-wall (cup or crater defect) – necessitates selection of appropriate treatment approaches for optimal results. From Chapter 5:

Three-wall infrabony pocket. The defect is formed by the root acting as one wall and three osseous surfaces as the other walls (Figure 10.1a).

Two-wall infrabony pocket. Extends interdentally to communicate with the root of an adjacent tooth; the two tooth surfaces make up two walls and the other two walls are formed by bone on the labial and lingual surfaces (Figure 10.1b). The two walls can also be formed if there is bony dehiscence of a buccal or lingual wall of a three-walled defect (Figure 10.1c).

One-wall infrabony pocket. The two-wall infrabony extends to include destruction of the labial or lingual osseous wall resulting in replacement by connective and inflammatory tissue and leaving only one bony surface (Figure 10.1d).

Cup defect or four-wall infrabony pocket. A defect surrounding the tooth like a moat (Figure 10.1e).

Combined osseous defect. Number of walls in the apical portion of the defect is often greater than in its occlusal portion [8].

Bone loss of the thin cortical bone can occur in a focal defect through the overlying periosteum and gingiva as a fenestration, and if this loss extends to the alveolar margin, then a dehiscence defect is present. Such defects may not be readily apparent radiographically and are found once the gingival flap is elevated.

10.4 Periodontal Healing and Treatment Planning

When the complete examination, including radiographs, has mapped out the picture of altered tissues, various factors have to be considered in the process of selecting the course of action.

10.4.1 Initial Prognostic Factors

Keratinized gingiva, as a band of attached gingiva, can be a factor in determining prognosis, particularly if oral hygiene will not be optimal. Teeth with a short root in comparison to crown size may also be a factor that put the tooth at risk for treatment failure, due to the decrease in reserve functional tissues of attachment [9]. Decreased attachment surface area and loss of tissue can lead to mobility, which is distinctly a prognostic risk, as the mobility is not likely to be corrected [9]. While mobile mandibular incisors have been treated successfully in dogs with a periodontal splint [10], the extent of care that is needed with subsequent periodontal therapy and continued home care is often unattainable, so extractions are usually done.

The biggest factor in determining prognosis in the veterinary dental field is likely to be the effectiveness of oral hygiene care that can be provided. Rarely does the patient–client combination exist that can guarantee meticulous control of plaque bacteria, so most procedures should be planned with the concept that a lower level of hygiene will be the reality of the situation compared to human periodontal patients.

10.4.2 Healing Goals/Rationale for Treatment

All efforts in periodontal therapy are aimed at restoring the function, if not the anatomy, of the periodontal structures [11]. Epithelial surfaces should be restored and connective tissue returned such that root cementum is predominantly attached to bone via the periodontal ligament.

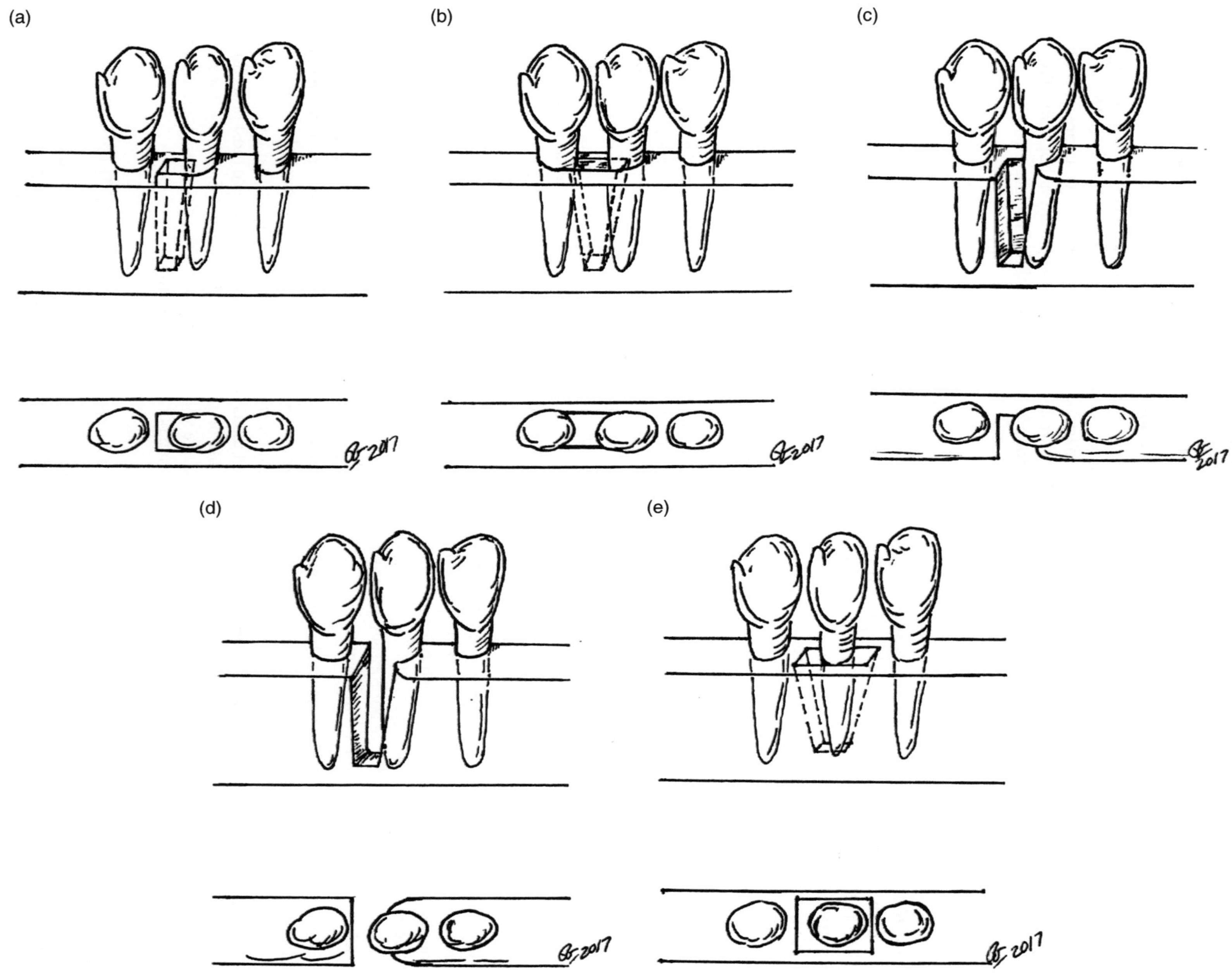

Figure 10.1 (a) Three-wall defect; (b) two-wall (crater) defect between two teeth; (c) two-wall defect – dehiscence of three-wall defect; (d) one-wall defect; (e) four-wall (circumferential) defect. *Source*: Illustration by Josephine Banyard, DVM, DAVDC, adapted from First Edition.

In addition, supporting bone height is preferred. The balance between formation and resorption of osseous tissues should be maintained. Depending on what tissues remain, and in what state, along with the availability of special materials and techniques, the goals for treatment will help maximize these tissue responses.

The American Association of Periodontists provide a glossary with some of the following terms [12]:

- *Repair.* Healing of a wound by tissue that does not fully restore the architecture or function of the part.
- *Regeneration.* The reproduction or reconstitution of a lost or injured tissue.
- *Periodontal regeneration.* The restoration of lost periodontium or supporting tissues, includes the formation of new alveolar bone, new cementum (NC) and new periodontal ligament (PDL).
- *New attachment.* The union of connective tissue or epithelium with a root surface that has been deprived of its original attachment apparatus. This new attachment may be epithelial adhesion or connective tissue adaptation or attachment and may include new cementum.
- *Reattachment.* Reunion of epithelial and connective tissue with a root surface (not exposed by disease, but by treatment) [11].
- *Guided tissue regeneration.* Describes procedures attempting to regenerate lost periodontal structures through differential tissue responses and typically refers to regeneration of periodontal attachment. Barrier techniques are used for excluding connective tissue and gingiva from the root in the belief that they interfere with regeneration.

In our efforts of periodontal therapy, we remove irritants (bacteria, granulation tissue, debris) that can interfere with natural regeneration and we can encourage selected tissues (PDL, bone, cementum) by excluding gingival connective tissue and epithelial cells into the region by use of barriers and membranes. Melcher's concept of "compartmentalization," dividing these tissues into groups, helps us anticipate the healing outcome based on the sequence of events [13]. If the more rapidly growing epithelial cells are allowed to repopulate the defect (they migrate approximately 10 times faster than other periodontal cell type [14], there will be a long junctional epithelium (LJE). With gingival connective tissue healing, the collagen fibers will be parallel to the tooth surface with remodeling of the bone but no attachment to the cementum, with potential exposure for resorption [15]. Repopulation with osteoblasts will at times result in ankylosis and root resorption, while in the presence of PDL cells there can be new formations of cementum and the PDL [11]. In studies of space-providing membranes, wound stability and space provision are critical to allow the repopulation of the defect with bone and periodontal ligament [16]. Studies have also shown that the "migration rate of periodontal ligament cells is at least as high as that of bone" [15], with possibly even a higher maturation or regeneration potential [16].

10.4.3 Host Modulation Therapy (HMT)

As the understanding of how a host's immunoinflammatory response determines the extent and severity of tissue destruction, part of any periodontal management should include considerations of modulating this host response [17]. The discussion of host modulation therapy (HMT) was briefly covered in Chapter 5 – Periodontology. The term "perioceutic" was once trademarked, but is now used to discuss the use of pharmacotherapeutic agents (antimicrobials and HMT) in periodontal management. The key is to help control excessive immune and inflammatory response without negating the beneficial effects in response to the bacterial presence.

10.4.3.1 Systemic HMT

Matrix metalloproteinases (MMPs) can degrade the extracellular matrix and modify cytokines and osteoclasts [18]. If unchecked by endogenous inhibitors, substantial tissue destruction can occur. The most common synthetic MMP inhibitor is a subantimicrobial dose of doxycycline (subantimicrobial dose doxycycline (SDD) – doxycycline hyclate 20 mg), used twice daily in humans for at least three months and up to a maximum of nine months [19]. Doxycycline is more effective in inhibiting collagenases than tetracycline or minocycline [20].

Non-steroidal anti-inflammatory drugs (NSAIDS) have been shown to inhibit prostaglandin synthesis and slow the rate of alveolar bone loss. This occurs with daily therapy over time, though, if stopped, not only can the improvement be stopped but a rebound effect with accelerated bone loss may occur [19]. Potential side effects of prolonged NSAID therapy should also be considered.

Endogenous lipoxins (LX) can reduce neutrophil infiltration, block cytokines and reactive oxygen species generation [17]. Lipid-inflammatory mediators (resolvins, protectins, maresins) can also inhibit neutrophil recruitment, helping to counter-regulate excessive acute inflammation and may help stimulate events that lead to resolution of inflammation [18]. Milk from hyperimmunized cows (HIMF) provides a substance that can decrease the impact of hyperactive neutrophils [21], decrease their recruitment [22], and have an impact in the dysbiotic oral community in periodontitis [23]. Cytokine antagonists bind against specific sites, with multiple anticytokine antibody products available in human medicine [17].

Targeting and disrupting cell-signaling pathways can help to inhibit the production of pro-inflammatory cytokines or stimulate anti-inflammatory cytokine production [17]. Pentoxifylline (PTX) can inhibit cytokine synthesis, particularly tumor necrosis factor (TNF) [24]. Endogenous osteoprotegrin can block the binding of RANKL to RANK (receptor activator of nuclear factor-kappa B ± ligand) to support a better equilibrium between bone formation and bone destruction [25]. RANKL inhibitors in humans have demonstrated increased bone mineral density and decreased bone resorption [25].

Bisphosphonate compounds disrupt osteoclasts and may interfere with lysosomes, which can lead to a decrease in bone turnover as bone resorption is inhibited [19]. Anticollagenase activity has also been described [26]. In other species, an increase in bone density and decrease in alveolar bone resorption has been demonstrated [27, 28]. Unfortunately, with intravenous products and long-term oral administration, a bisphosphonate-related osteonecrosis of the jaw (BRONJ) has been reported in humans [29]. Likewise, bisphosphonates can cause severe deleterious bone-related osteonecrosis of the jaw in dogs [30, 31]. There are discussions of cases in feline patients as well, but no peer-reviewed publications are available to date.

Selective estrogen receptor modulators (SERM) and hormone replacement therapy (HRT) are based on osteoporotic effects due to a lack of estrogens in postmenopausal women [17]. While estrogen may have bone-sparing effects, the potential side effects of HRT is likely to negate its universal use.

Low levels of nitric oxide maintain homeostasis but when endotoxins increase, inducible nitric oxide synthase enzyme (iNOS), producing NO and peroxynitrite, DNA damage, protein damage and cytokine release may occur. Selective inhibition of iNOS, such as with mercaptoethylguanidine (MEG) has been shown to prevent alveolar bone resorption [32].

10.4.3.2 Local HMT

Local treatments that are used in periodontal pocket, particularly during surgical treatment, will be discussed in a later section. Other local medicaments may include oral rinse or mouthwashes with compounds such as NSAIDS (ketoprofen) or chlorotaurine [17]. Topical cimetidine has been shown to inhibit neutrophil chemotaxis and superoxide production, down-regulating cytokines. It has even been shown to inhibit *Porphyromonas gingivalis*-elicited periodontal inflammation, modulating tissue destruction and influencing cell population in the infiltrate [33].

10.4.4 Periodontal Treatment Equipment [34]

In addition to some of the basic periodontal equipment discussed in Chapter 5 – Periodontology – probe/explorer, scaler, and curette, additional pieces will facilitate surgical periodontal efforts. Heavier curettes (Prichard curette) and sickle scalers (Ball scaler) can be used to surgically remove tough fibrous and granulation tissue. Gingivectomy knives such as the Kirkland knife provides an entire cutting edge along the periphery of the blade, either single-ended or double-ended. For interdental areas, an Orban knife or Merrifield knife has a cutting edge on each side of its spear-shaped blade (again, single- or double-ended).

The narrow 15C surgical blade can be used to follow scalloped contours, or in interdental spaces. The beak-shaped 12D blade can also be used interdentally with cutting edges on both sides of the blade. The 15C or 15-blade can be used to make the releasing and crevicular incisions for debridement or flap design. To elevate flaps after initial incisions are made, the thin edge of a periosteal elevator can be introduced to lift the flap, including the periosteum, from the bone surface. Woodson, Pritchard, or Molt periosteal elevators come in varying sizes. Once the flap is elevated, straight chisels such as the Wedelstadt or Ochsenbein can be used with a push motion to help debride exposed surfaces.

Care of the delicate periodontal tissues can be enhanced by using less traumatic instruments such as DeBakey forceps, appropriately sized and sharpened scissors such as Goldman-Fox no. 16, and needle-holders, either regular types or the Castroviejo needle-holder for precise techniques. The monofilament suture material, poligecaprone 25, is pliable, has low tissue drag, good knot security, ease of handling, and high initial tensile strength and strength-to-size ratio. For cutting through keratinized gingiva and mucosa, a reverse cutting needle is useful, while a taper-cut needle can be used for more delicate tissue [35].

If electrosurgery or radiosurgery is used, whether for electrosection (incising, reverse bevel) or electrocoagulation, the tip should always be moving. Soft tissue diode lasers have been used for treatment of periodontal pockets, to help resect small areas of gingival enlargement or provide hemostasis when larger amounts of tissue need to be removed [36].

10.4.5 Treatment Planning

For any procedure to be moderately successful, deliberate planning with diagnostics, treatment steps, and reassessment are necessary. More advanced lesions require more planning, which can be a challenge in some veterinary practices where clients expect a "one-stop shop" experience.

Adequate communication is essential to determine if the client wants optimal therapy, which may include staged procedures and meticulous home care.

10.4.5.1 Phase I

Before any advanced surgical periodontal therapy is selected, complete dental assessment and radiographs, scaling and root planning (SRP), and conservative management procedures should be done. A surgical attempt should only be performed if there is a lack of resolution in response to the SRP, as in human dentistry, after one to three months of oral hygiene. This first phase will identify those that have the potential of healing with conservative methods, but should also identify those clients that may be less willing to comply with the strict home care guidelines for optimal results. If a client is unwilling to return for regular care and provide home care, the tooth/teeth should be considered for possible extraction, if considered best for the patient's health.

10.4.5.1.1 Non-surgical Periodontal Therapy

Non-surgical periodontal therapy may be provided during the Phase I period for moderate cases or when return visits are unlikely. They may also be part of the Phase II procedures, particularly when inflamed areas improve after Phase I, but need additional treatment.

Considerations for non-surgical treatment typically rely on the pocket depth encountered. In human patients, based on outcomes data, the critical probing depth (PD) of 5.4 mm has been used to determine whether or not to proceed to surgical intervention [37]. It was also confirmed that in a pocket of 4–6 mm, SRP resulted in better attachment gain than a surgical procedure [37].

The local delivery of antimicrobial products can be added to the SRP protocol to provide additional antibacterial effects directly at the site, while eliminating the need for patient compliance [38]. Fibers containing tetracycline (no longer available), microspheres that release minocycline (2%) and a 10% doxycycline gel are available as human products, with a similar doxycycline gel (8.5%) labeled for veterinary use. Some, not all, studies show a moderate reduction in pocket depth and gingival bleeding as compared to SRT alone [39]. These are to be used as an adjunct to SRP, not as a standalone treatment, and combining SDD with local antibiotic delivery after a thorough SRP has been shown to be significantly effective [40]. While the complete benefit may be somewhat debatable, since meticulous home care is unlikely in most veterinary patients, the potential benefit may be considered.

10.4.5.2 Phase II

When the probing depth is greater than 5.4 or 6 mm, the decision for surgical intervention is likely to result in better clinical attachment than non-surgical efforts [41]. This 5 mm standard, as adopted from human dentistry, closely corresponds to the extent that a 5 mm pocket, with bone level situated 2 mm apical to that, adds up to 7 mm of attachment loss in an average tooth length of 13 mm. With only half of the bony support remaining for this compromised human tooth, surgical intervention is often deemed necessary.

In the veterinary field, a 6 mm pocket can signify greater than 50% attachment loss (incisor or small premolar), making extraction the treatment of choice. In a large dog with a pocket on a canine tooth, this could only be considered Stage 2 periodontal disease attachment loss, but a surgical approach would still be needed for adequate access to the site. The variations in the tooth and root size that veterinarians experience is a reason why it is good to rely on the wealth of knowledge from the human dental field, but also to be able to apply the concepts according to the patient's needs. This will also be addressed in concepts related to interdental tissue involvement.

This is why additional factors must be considered in surgical decisions beyond just the pocket depth [42, 43]. The full extent (amount and character) of bone loss and the root length will help determine the percentage of attachment loss or the tooth. Mobility of the tooth can play a significant role in deciding between treatment and extraction, as a lack of stability will decrease the chance of success. If the location of attachment loss is at a furcation, or between crowded teeth, the effectiveness of SRP may be questionable. Even the relative importance of the tooth and the probability of success ("restorability") will factor into treatment choices. Beyond the tooth, the patient's health status should be closely evaluated, due to the likely need for multiple anesthetic procedures. In addition, as stated previously, a dedicated owner will be essential for follow-up care.

10.4.5.2.1 Surgical Periodontal Therapy

The objectives of this surgical phase include eliminating pathological changes in the pocket wall to help maintain stable site(s) and to even regenerate periodontal tissues [43]. Surgical techniques first provide access to the area to be treated in order to reduce or eliminate pocket depth and to reshape tissues to help maintain periodontal health [43].

Reduction of pocket depth provides an area that is easier to keep clean and is less favorable to anaerobic bacterial proliferation. An active pocket with inflammation and bone loss can become inactive or quiescent with Phase I therapy, sometimes healing with a long junctional epithelial attachment [43]. While inactive pockets can be maintained with regular SRP and meticulous home care, creating a healthy sulcus (depth) surgically will provide better results.

Pocket depth is closely considered in treatment options: for example, SRP in pockets less than 2.9 mm (critical probing depth value) will induce loss of attachment, but result in a gain of attachment in deeper pockets [44]. The level of attachment in relation to the distance from the cementoenamel junction (CEJ) is even more important in considering the progression of the disease. Deeper pockets can be present in situations with gingival enlargement, with no attachment loss present.

Removal or resolution of the diseased pocket wall is the most common pocket therapy, whether SRP resolves the inflammation and shrinks the pocket depth or by employing surgical methods for removal or resection if needed. An apically repositioned flap with a resective technique will expose more root surface, but provides a pocket/sulcus depth that is easier to maintain. New attachment with regeneration of periodontal tissues is the ideal end result, though advanced techniques and materials are needed. In theory, extraction also treats the pocket by eliminating the tooth – or root.

Aesthetic considerations in human dentistry, particularly for the anterior dentition, are not as critical in veterinary patients, so greater detail can be given to maintaining function and comfort.

10.5 Treatment Considerations

10.5.1 Periodontal Surgical Principles

In order to provide the planned treatment, various principles should be followed, using appropriate techniques. Many techniques used in veterinary dentistry rely on experience in human dentistry, but specific differences must be kept in mind. For human patients, aesthetics in the rostral dentition is as important as function, so techniques such as papillary preservation may not be as critical in our patients. The distance in between teeth can also play a role in trying to extrapolate principles and techniques from the human field. Our goals should be to maximize the health and stability of functional teeth while maximizing our patients' systemic health.

When starting these procedures, we should keep in mind that we are trying to provide access for the procedure, to reduce pocket depth either with resective or regenerative (additive) techniques and to reshape tissues for a more harmonious topography [43]. The critical zones to evaluate include the soft tissue pocket wall, the tooth surface, the underlying bone, and the attached gingiva [43].

In providing access, tissue either needs to be removed (gingivectomy) or displaced (flaps). Once accessed, the area in question is debrided of all irritants (plaque, calculus, diseased cementum, and soft tissue), treatment performed, and then the flap is closed. No matter what treatment is chosen, it has been shown that a certain pocket depth will recur, unless regenerative steps are taken. Therefore, the minimal goal for resective techniques (pocket reduction) will be to maintain the site without further loss of attachment [45]. One last scenario that will reduce the pocket depth is extraction; with complete removal of the tooth/teeth and pocket(s), the end stage of periodontal disease is accomplished.

10.5.2 Access by Displacement – Incisions

Displacement of a portion of the surrounding soft tissue is a common method of providing access to the depth of the periodontal pocket encountered. Using the parameters of the extent and nature of the pocket, the flap can be designed with keeping the final result – flap closure and pocket reduction – in mind. While adequate access is necessary, a gingival flap should be elevated only as far as is necessary for the approach. There will be a loss of at least 0.5 mm in bone thickness anywhere the periosteum is elevated off the bone surface, so a larger flap is not necessarily better. Mandibular first molars with pockets at the mesial and distal aspects may benefit from two separate flaps (often associated with adjacent tooth extractions) while leaving the interradicular region (furcation area) intact. Starting the coronal portion of the flap at full thickness and then transitioning to partial thickness (sharp dissection) can help preserve the apical portion of exposed bone [46].

Selecting the correct placement and type of incisions will allow you to both access the site and begin removal of affected tissues. Horizontal incisions are performed across the width of the defect to start tissue removal and facilitate flap displacement, and vertical incisions are made mesially and distally to the defect to provide release for flap displacement. It is important to use a new, sharp blade for delicate periodontal surgery. Do not use the same blade that may have been used to create flaps for surgical extractions in the same patient.

10.5.2.1 Horizontal Incisions

Horizontal incisions following the tooth contour will be the internal (reverse) bevel and the crevicular (sulcular) incisions. The internal bevel, or first incision, is started a short distance from the gingival margin (depending on the character of the lesion) and is directed toward the alveolar crest (Figure 10.2). The scalpel blade is directed down toward the bone, following the scalloped contour of the teeth involved in the flap [48]. The second incision, the crevicular incision, is made from the base of the sulcus/pocket to the alveolar crest. These two incisions isolate a wedge-shaped segment of tissue that is removed once the flap is elevated and the interdental (third)

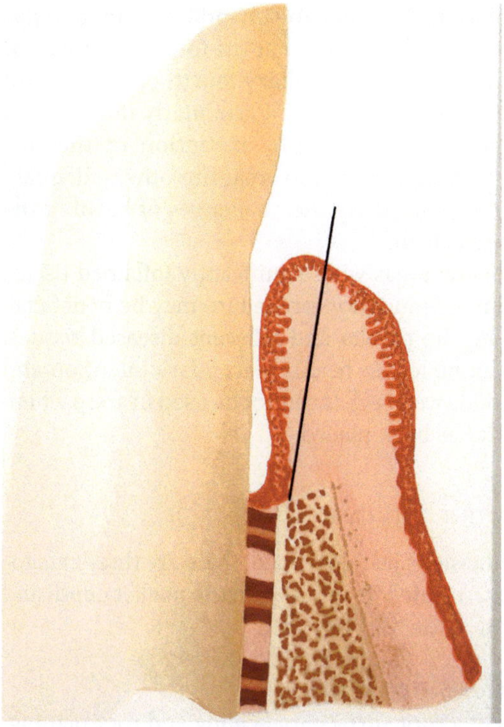

Figure 10.2 Reverse bevel incision. *Source:* Reprinted with permission from reference [47].

incision is made to separate the tissue from the bone in the interdental spaces, often with an Orban knife [46] (Figure 10.3).

A conservative approach for papilla management (interseptal or interdental incisions) includes incising the tissue between the contact point of the two adjacent teeth, with reflection of the buccal and lingual mucosa [44]. This approach is often done for flaps that will be displaced upon closure (apically, laterally repositioned).

Papillary preservation can be performed if there is sufficient interdental space and if the flap will be non-displaced (closed into its original location). With this, the base of the papilla remains with one of the flaps (buccal or lingual) and is replaced into the interdental space at closure. With interdental lesions, this method is preferred (especially in anterior teeth in humans), because it protects the interdental area more effectively [43]. This can extrapolated to the incisors in dogs, but may not be as crucial in the other regions while sacrificing juxtaposed teeth (e.g., for treatment of the mandibular first molar).

The papillary preservation technique (PPT) uses sulcular incisions with a semi-lunar incision that dips apically (at least 5 mm from the gingival margin) lingual/palatal to the papillary tissue with full thickness elevation. This keeps the papilla intact with the buccal flap, and is replaced and sutured after treatment is complete. The modified PPT (MPPT) moves the horizontal incision apical to the papilla at the buccal aspect, with an initial horizontal internal crossed mattress suture to relieve tension on tissue closure. A second incision (vertical internal mattress suture) is used for primary closure [49]. A simple papillary preservation technique (SPPT) is used for narrow interdental spaces and extends from the buccal line angle of the affected tooth to the midinterproximal portion of the papilla under the contact point [50].

In many veterinary cases (in the authors' experiences), this papillary tissue is well-defined only with healthy tissue where the teeth are closely positioned – at the incisor areas and at the fourth premolars through molar regions. Demonstrating this in cadaver specimens is possible, but once there is a need of periodontal surgery, this tissue is often so damaged that the PPT is of little value.

Figure 10.3 The three incisions necessary for flap surgery: (a) first (internal bevel) incision; (b) second (crevicular) incision; (c) third (interdental) incision. *Source:* Illustration by Josephine Banyard, DVM, DAVDC, adapted from reference [46].

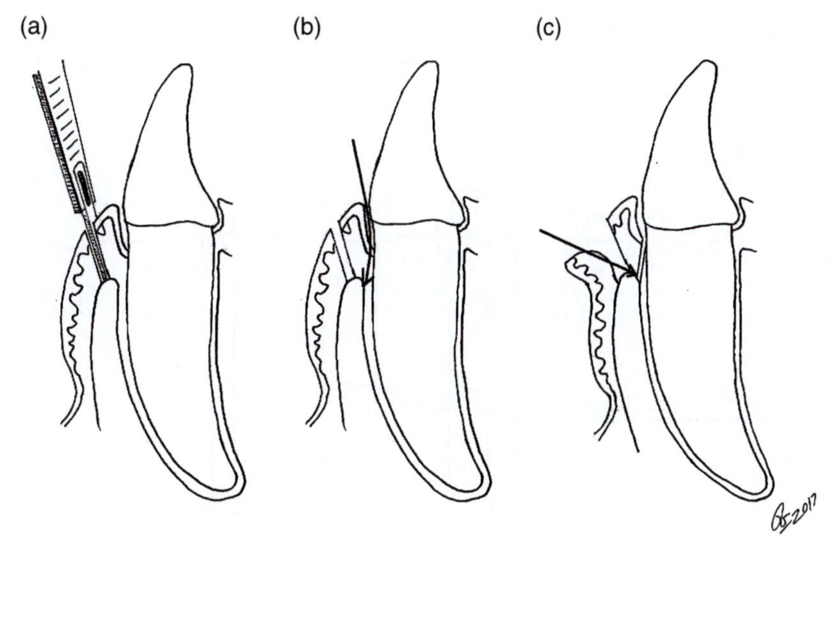

Incisions in the palatal mucosa are handled differently from buccal or lingual incisions. With keratinized tissue that is all attached, release and repositioning is typically not possible. The primary goal is to create a thin flap that will be replaced at the root–bone region. An internal bevel incision may be adequate or a horizontal incision followed by an internal bevel can be used for internal gingivectomy [51].

10.5.2.2 Vertical Incisions – Releasing Incisions

Vertical incisions are made to provide additional release of a flap, as far as is needed for conservative therapy, or past the mucogingival line for release of the flap and full displacement, particularly if the flap is to be repositioned. These vertical incisions should be made at a line angle on an adjacent tooth mesial or distal to the area being treated [52]. The term line angle is defined as dividing lines formed at the junction of two of the tooth's surfaces (e.g., mesiobuccal) (Figure 10.4). Determining the angle can be challenging at times, but the designation is meant to avoid making incisions in areas that would be detrimental to the treatment. By a process of elimination, a close interdental incision would not be chosen, as this would damage the papilla and result in closure in an area difficult to clean. Radicular incisions, at the midpoint of the root, would result in too much tension and difficulty in closure. Interradicular incisions can be made but the furcation area is generally avoided.

If there is sufficient space (diastema) between the tooth to be treated and the nearest tooth, then the incision can be made just beyond the treatment site, into healthy gingiva of the interdental area [52]. Frequently the site to be treated would benefit from extraction of an adjacent, less strategic tooth. The releasing incision can be made at the extent of the extracted tooth furthest from the treated tooth for optimal access. Common areas that benefit from these selective extractions are the mandibular third incisor extracted to treat mandibular canine; the mandibular first molar treated with extraction of either the fourth premolar or second molar; and the maxillary fourth premolar with the third premolar extracted. Particularly if the defect is interdental to these teeth, extraction of the one allows much better access to treat the other, adequate closure, and minimizing the challenges of keeping the crowded area clean.

In interdental areas with significantly inflamed tissue, an interdental denudation procedure may be beneficial. By removing the papilla and adjacent diseased tissues, this area can be left to heal by secondary intention and often responds well [46]. It cannot be used in areas where a bone graft has been placed.

10.5.3 Access by Displacement – Flaps

Using the incisions just described, there are three categories of flaps, selected depending on the pocket depth and the location of the MGJ.

10.5.3.1 Modified Widman Flap

For access of a root surface for scaling and root planing, and to eliminate the pocket lining, the modified Widman flap is used. Its primary goal is not for pocket reduction, though the pocket depth may decrease as the tissues heal [51]. The internal beveled incision will follow the scalloped outline of the gingiva, 1–2 mm from the margin and teeth, down to the alveolar crest. Vertical releasing incisions are generally not done and an attempt can be made to maintain the thickness of the interdental papilla [51]. The gingiva is reflected and the second (crevicular) incision is made to the apical extent of the pocket epithelium. The third incision horizontal is made in order to remove the supracrestal pocket tissue (not into any deeper pockets). This provides access and visualization for root debridement. Interdental or periodontal sling sutures are placed to keep the trimmed tissue close to the tooth surface [43, 53].

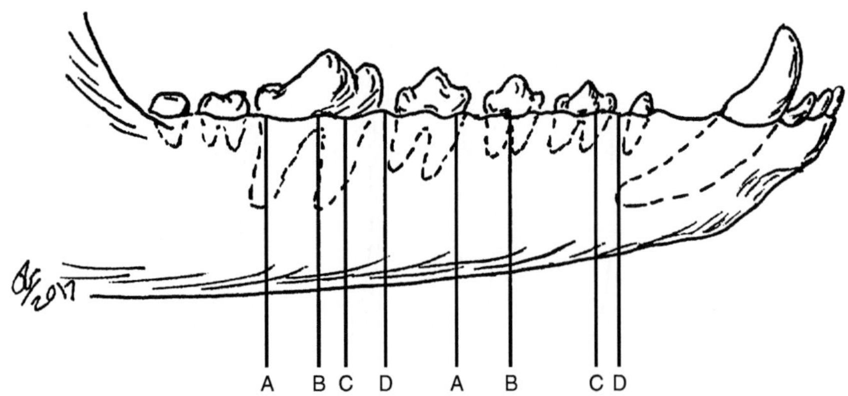

Figure 10.4 Line angles. Line angles incisions (a) and interradicular incisions (b) are considered appropriate for releasing incisions, while radicular midface incisions (c) and interproximal incisions (d) are not considered appropriate. *Source:* Illustration by Josephine Banyard, DVM, DAVDC, adapted from First Edition.

10.5.3.2 Undisplaced Flap

An undisplaced flap will provide access and help to remove the pocket wall, excising the diseased gingiva, and can be considered an internal bevel gingivectomy. Sufficient attached gingiva must be present once the pocket wall is removed. After marking the depth of the pockets, an internal bevel incision is made to a point apical to the alveolar crest, depending on the thickness of the tissue, if there is enough attached gingiva. If there is less attached gingiva, this internal bevel incision may need to be directed to the alveolar crest instead. This initial incision should attempt to remove as much of the excess thickness of the flap as possible, both buccally and palatally. Once the crevicular and interdental incisions are made, the excess tissue is removed and the pocket debrided (SRP). Vertical releasing incisions are typically not needed. The final flap edge should rest on the root–bone junction, if the incisions are properly planned. If not, the flap edge can be recontoured (if too long) or the bone contoured (if too short). A continuous sling suture (described later) holds the flap edges in place [51].

10.5.3.3 Apically Repositioned Flap

If there is limited attached gingiva, and a portion or all of the attached gingiva is overexposed root, not bone, then an apically repositioned flap will allow this band of gingiva to be placed over the tooth–bone junction. The initial internal bevel incision is made close to the gingival margin, directed to the crest of the bone [51]. After this is elevated, the crevicular incision is made, followed by interdental incisions and debridement. Vertical incisions are made past the MGJ and the full- or split-thickness flaps are elevated (Figure 10.5). Thorough SRP and osseous recontouring is done prior to closure of the flap in a more apical position (Figure 10.6). Movement of the attached gingiva to a position over the alveolar bone will expose the root(s), but will help reduce the periodontal pocket by transforming the previously unattached keratinized gingiva into attached tissue [51].

10.5.3.4 Coronally Advanced Flap

In areas of gingival recession, a displaced flap can be repositioned coronally to cover the exposed root. Issues in human dentistry with GR include aesthetics, root hypersensitivity, and challenges in plaque control [54]. The most predictable results in treating minor GR defect (Miller Class I and II) traditionally rely on a coronally advanced flap (CAF) with root conditioning, sometimes the use of a enamel matrix derivative (EMD – discussed later in the chapter), and often with the placement of a connective tissue graft (CTG) [55, 56]. In dog model studies of Class I GR defects, the addition of CTG or collagen membranes (CMs) did not have a significant advantage over CAF alone [57].

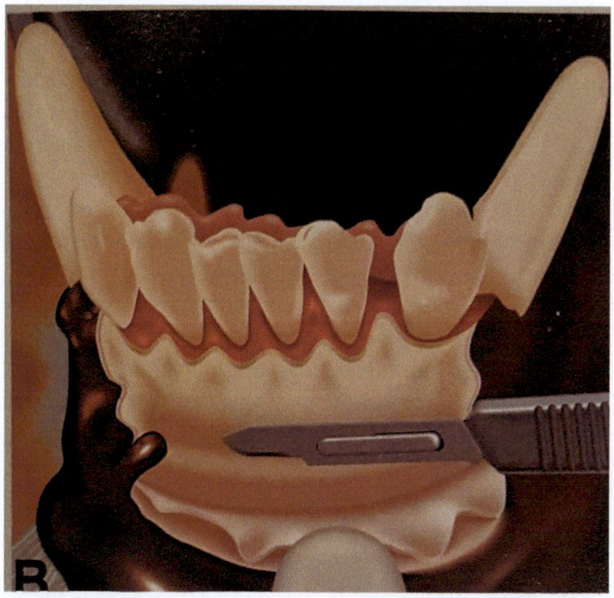

Figure 10.5 Diagram showing elevation of full-thickness mucogingival flap to expose several millimeters of bone. The flap is transitioned to a partial thickness flap apically. *Source:* Reprinted with permission from reference [47].

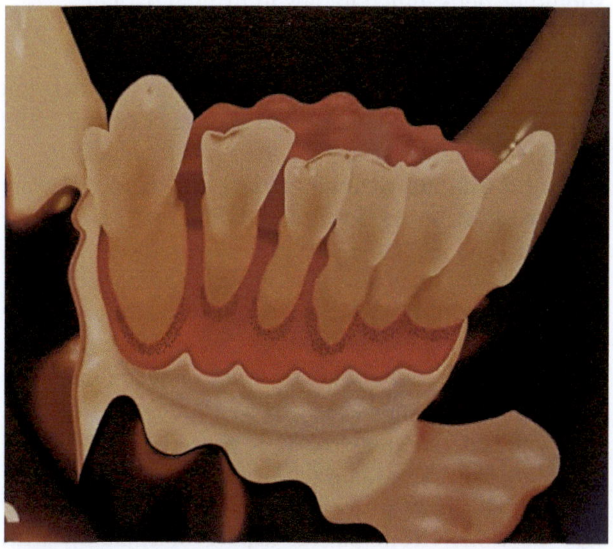

Figure 10.6 Diagram showing alveolar bone contouring and removal of sharp bone edges to remove all diseased tissues before flap is replaced apically. *Source:* Reprinted with permission from reference [47].

While a CAF may be effective in covering the defect, unless EMD products are used, fibroblasts may repopulate more quickly than PDL cells, so the healing will be only a new attachment, with a chance of resorption [55]. The CTG can be harvested from a distal wedge incision or a palatal donor site. Even if complete root coverage (CRC) is obtained, often the flap tissue remains fairly thin, a risk factor for future recession. A modified microsurgical tunnel technique has been described, using tunneling knives that undermine the buccal gingiva (split-thickness), creating a continuous tunnel. A CTG inserted into the tunnels appears to result in thicker gingiva (0.8 mm for critical flap thickness) and improved clinical outcomes [56]. These delicate flaps require meticulous home hygiene and avoidance of any trauma, including lingual trauma, to the healing graft, which is typically unrealistic in most canine veterinary patients. Determining the relative impact of a shallow gingival recession defect in a veterinary patient should be evaluated when contemplating advanced procedures and considering oral hygiene levels.

10.5.3.5 Lateral Pedicle Sliding Flap (LPSF)

Lateral pedicle sliding flaps (LPSFs) utilize grafting healthy periodontal tissue from a site adjacent to an area of gingival recession or fenestration. Details of the procedure will be covered later in the chapter. Any flap should have a wide base with sufficient harvested tissue to cover 1.5 times the width of the defect itself. Again, the risk to the clinical outcome-to-benefit ratio should be determined for any individual patient.

10.5.3.6 Free Gingival Graft

Free gingival grafts (FGG) have been used since the 1960s initially to provide gingival extension, replacing alveolar mucosa with an autogenous graft apical to the area of a thin attached gingival height. It can also be used to cover an exposed root surface and to increase the width and thickness of attached gingiva [58]. Though relatively easy to perform, with a high predictability in human patients, there are issues with acquiring a donor site of sufficient size and leaving the donor site open to heal by second intention [59]. A difference in the color of the donor tissue can impair aesthetics, as well as a mismatch in the gingival width and alignment of the MGJ [58]. Variations of the procedure include developing a gingival unit graft, including marginal and papillary portions (from palatal aspect of molars), with better vasculature potential [58]. In a partially epithelialized FGG, the apical portion of graft (that would lie apical to the MGJ) is de-epithelialized, to avoid the appearance of a mismatch of the MGJ between donor and recipient tissue. A graft can also be crafted to keep an epithelized "island" of the graft that corresponds to the defect, with the remaining de-epithelized portion of the graft placed on top of the surrounding connective tissue in a tunneling technique [58]. Once more, the risk-to-benefit ratio, including consideration for the level of oral hygiene, should be considered before performing advanced procedures on veterinary patients. Replacement material, such as an acellular dermal allograft (ADM – discussed later in chapter) may not provide quite as much coverage, but can be an alternative to free graft techniques [59].

10.5.3.7 Crescent Flap

Specific flaps can be developed to manage individual teeth, such as using a crescent shaped flap to access a deep pocket on the palatal aspect of maxillary canine teeth. The initial incision extends mesially from the mesial aspect of the canine tooth, then arcs into the palatal mucosa, to provide a flap that exposes the mesial and palatal aspect of the root once elevated. This flap can incorporate the palatal artery into its base, with ligation at the rostral aspect. Once the pocket is treated, slight debridement of the leading edge of the flap can bring the tissue into close approximation with the tooth, to keep the underlying regenerative material in place. A slight gap may be present at the crescent incision site at the palatal aspect, but this will heal by second intention. Alternatively, releasing incisions at the distal and mesial aspects of the tooth can be made.

10.5.3.8 Oblique Incision

An oblique incision can be made from the gingival margin of a mandibular canine to allow for collar expansion of the attached gingiva when sutured [60]. This is primarily performed for crown lengthening during prosthodontic treatment, but can also be used for apically repositioned flap techniques on the tooth.

10.5.4 Access by Removal – Gingivectomy/Gingivoplasty

If a pseudopocket is formed by gingival enlargement, simple reduction of the excess tissue (gingivectomy) removes the pocket wall and provides access for scaling and root planing [61]. Keratinized tissue will be removed from the external surface using a beveled incision, preserving at least 3 mm of attached gingiva. This can also be used to reduce suprabony pockets and areas of suprabony abscessation. If the pocket depth is apical to the MGJ, or if osseous recontouring is needed, then a flap technique should be employed.

Gingivoplasty refers to the reshaping of the gingiva in the absence of pockets. Small areas of gingival enlargement, clefts, and craters can be recontoured to restore the gingival margins to a healthier state. Scalpel blades, periodontal knives, diamond stones or 12-fluted burs can be used for this procedure.

Details of these procedures, including wedge resection and crevicular debridement, will be discussed later in this chapter.

10.5.5 Debridement of Irritants

A main objective in surgical periodontal therapy is to provide access to remove all irritants – plaque, calculus, diseased cementum, bone, and soft tissue – from the area to be treated. The basics of closed root planing and subgingival (gingival) curettage were described in Chapter 5 – Periodontology. Further definition separates gingival curettage (removal of the inflamed soft tissue lateral to the pocket wall and the JE) as compared to subgingival curettage that is performed apical to the JE (which is seldom indicated) [61]. The excisional new attachment procedure (ENAP) is definitive subgingival curettage performed with a knife, making an internal bevel incision from the free gingival margin to a point just apical to the bottom of the pocket (Takei CP 577). The excised tissue is removed with curettes and sutures placed if needed. In most human patients, it has been shown that with a thorough SRP, most of the bacteria is eliminated, and the granulation tissue present is slowly resorbed [61].

Removing the chronic granulation tissue and diseased or scarred epithelial lining is essential in flap surgery for better access to underlying surfaces. It is an important step when attempting to encourage new attachment or if aggressive surgical techniques cannot be used to help reduce inflammation. Ultrasonic curettage has been shown to be effective in debriding the epithelial lining of periodontal pockets. Chemical debridement (decontamination) has been proposed [62], but with concerns over a lack of controlled effect, additional tissue destruction may occur.

The concept of root conditioning – demineralizing the scaled root surface to expose collagen fibers to enhance the repopulation of periodontal cells – has been demonstrated *in vitro*. However, studies are lacking to show any benefit of root conditioning on periodontal surgery outcomes (discussed later in the chapter).

10.5.6 Flap Closure

When a flap is closely adapted to the alveolar process at the tooth/bone junction. there will be minimal inflammatory response, and the space in which the blood clot was formed (present within 24 hours after surgery) gets thinner within one to three days [46]. Gingiva and mucosa heal more rapidly than skin, so the minimal coaptation time is about five days [63].

Suturing techniques will vary according to the function of the closure (extraction versus membrane or flap placement). A simple interrupted pattern is used frequently, with the suture material placed at 2–3 mm from the gingival margin or papilla. In human dentistry, an interrupted pattern is used, with the suture passed from the epithelium to connective tissue on the buccal aspect, and again from the epithelium to connective tissue on the lingual/palatal tissue. This results in good apposition of the two portions of the flap, but the suture material will be in contact with the incision line itself, so should not be used if primary adaptation is needed. A horizontal mattress can be placed to distribute the tension of the suture, either in an external or internal pattern. The internal pattern will result in a smaller amount of external suture material buccally and labially/palatally, but some incision edge eversion may be possible. A further modification carries the needle back through the loop, bringing that portion externally by securing it during the knot placement [65]. The external pattern can have either crossed (cruciate) or parallel suture material resting on top of the interdental tissue [66]. A vertical internal mattress has the suture holes placed 2 and 3 mm from the papilla, with both inversion and eversion to keep the papilla more upright [66].

A sling suture is often used to position a flap in a position different from the opposite flap (buccal versus lingual). In humans, the contour of the teeth (neck) is used for coronal positioning of the flap, but few teeth provide this placement in veterinary dentistry. The sling suture can also be used to secure a membrane during regenerative procedures. After the suture is passed through the mesial aspect of the flap or membrane, it is directed through the interdental space (buccal to lingual), looped around the tooth, passed through the distal interdental space (lingual to buccal), with a bit to suture the distal aspect of the flap or membrane. The suture material is then doubled back on itself through the interdental spaces and tied at the mesial aspect. This pattern uses the tooth as anchorage for the flap. Two teeth can be incorporated into the sling suture pattern for a wider based flap [66]. (Authors' note: attempts to provide an adequate description or images for basic movements can be challenging, although a number of videos can be found on the Internet that demonstrate these techniques.)

As discussed previously, a flap may be designed to be undisplaced, so it will be sutured back into the area from which it was elevated. Repositioned flaps rely on a more extensive flap release with vertical incisions that will extend past the MGJ. For teeth with furcation involvement, the flap may be sutured further coronally than its original location, but sufficient underlying connective tissue and bone are needed to support attachment [67]. For teeth with periodontal pockets and limited attached gingiva, an apically repositioned flap can help align the band of attached gingiva over alveolar bone to encourage reattachment and diminish the pocket depth, though there will be additional root exposure. Laterally repositioned pedicle sliding flaps can be designed to harvest attached gingiva from an adjacent site to cover a gingival defect, such as a Stillman cleft on a maxillary canine. The descriptions of these specific therapies are discussed later in the chapter.

10.6 Periodontal Surgery – Flow Chart – Suprabony Attachment Loss

The wide range of possible periodontal treatments may seem daunting, but a step-wise approach can logically follow the goals of treatment: removal of irritants (debridement), minimizing attachment loss, and pocket depths. Complete evaluation, including visual, radiographical, and physical (periodontal) probing, will provide a reasonable picture of the level of remaining periodontal tissues and their relationship to each other. Advanced imaging (e.g., cone beam computed tomography) can provide an optimal assessment of bone loss patterns in particular. This treatment flow chart takes into consideration the extent and pattern of bone loss, the position and the depth of the sulcus or pocket, and the amount of attached gingiva.

10.6.1 Bone and Gingival Loss at Similar Levels

When alveolar bone and gingival tissues are lost at similar rates, often in a horizontal pattern, there may be root and furcation exposure but minimal pocket depth. The primary periodontal treatment goal is the removal of irritants, so cleaning of the exposed surfaces is performed. Gentle cleaning of the subgingival pocket can be done, but significant closed root planing in a pocket less than 2.9 mm in depth can result in additional attachment loss [43].

10.6.1.1 Furcation Exposure

If the bone and gingival loss has progressed enough around a multirooted tooth, the resulting tissue recession can exposure the furcation area. In addition to the three stages of furcation exposure defined on the AVDC. Nomenclature web page [7], Class (Grade) IV furcation exposure in human dentistry describes a lesion where the gingival recession exposes the furcation to view [8]. Due to the complex anatomy of exposed furcational areas, there are challenges with SRP and routine oral hygiene to maintain periodontal health. Proximity to other teeth and additional vertical or angular bone loss patterns can further complicate treatment efforts. Furcation-involved teeth with advanced periodontitis are given a less favorable diagnosis, and in the AVDC staging of periodontal disease, any tooth with stage 2 furcation involvement (F2) is then classified as stage 3 periodontal disease (PD3) and a stage 3 furcation involvement (F1) advances that tooth to PD4.

Conservative treatment is directed toward facilitating maintenance therapy and preventing further attachment loss. Thorough SRP therapy for F1 teeth with meticulous home care may be sufficient, but surgical treatment may be needed to make the area more accessible for continued care. In a stage 2 furcation involvement, a localized flap procedure with odontoplasty and osteoplasty to reduce the dome of the furcation can result in an area easier to maintain. In the past, surgical efforts were done to actually create a fully open, visible furcation area with better access for cleaning in humans. Now implants are more readily considered for resolution. Extraction of the tooth is a viable option in the face of poor oral hygiene, or with adjacent teeth impacted by the disease. In special cases of strategic teeth, regenerative methods may also be considered, as discussed later in the chapter.

Furcation involvement does not mean automatic extraction, in the authors' opinions, particularly in long-rooted teeth that have clearly visible stage 3 furcation exposure with no additional complications such as vertical bone loss or adjacent teeth at risk. Teeth with long roots, a short root trunk length (distance from the CEJ to the entrance of the furcation), and wide inter-radicular dimension (root separation) can be more readily treated [68]. Full access to the region allows for effective SRP, and if home care can be provided, the teeth can remain stable. It is important that all inflammatory tissue be removed from the furcation region. In some cases, advancing a flap of gingival tissue into the region will better protect the underlying bone and root surfaces (coronally advanced flap).

Teeth with additional vertical or angular bone defects of one or more roots can be more challenging to maintain without some surgical regenerative efforts, which will be discussed later in the chapter. Regenerative efforts in teeth with horizontal patterns of loss have shown variable results at best, and generally offer little benefit as compared to controls [68] from the use of barrier membranes to PDL fibroblast seeding and other methods [69]. Class II furcation defects have been treated in human dentistry with coronally advanced flaps (CAF) as a control, as well as with many combinations of membranes, graft placements, and biological modifiers [70–72].

In some patients, furcation involvement can be managed with the resection of a single root, to allow access to a previously inaccessible plaque-retentive area. If the remaining tooth structure has sufficient attachment to preserve its function, removing that section can eliminate the furcation exposure, as well as manage extension of periodontal disease on adjacent teeth [73]. Again, oral hygiene must be maintained, and in the absence of such, extraction remains a viable option.

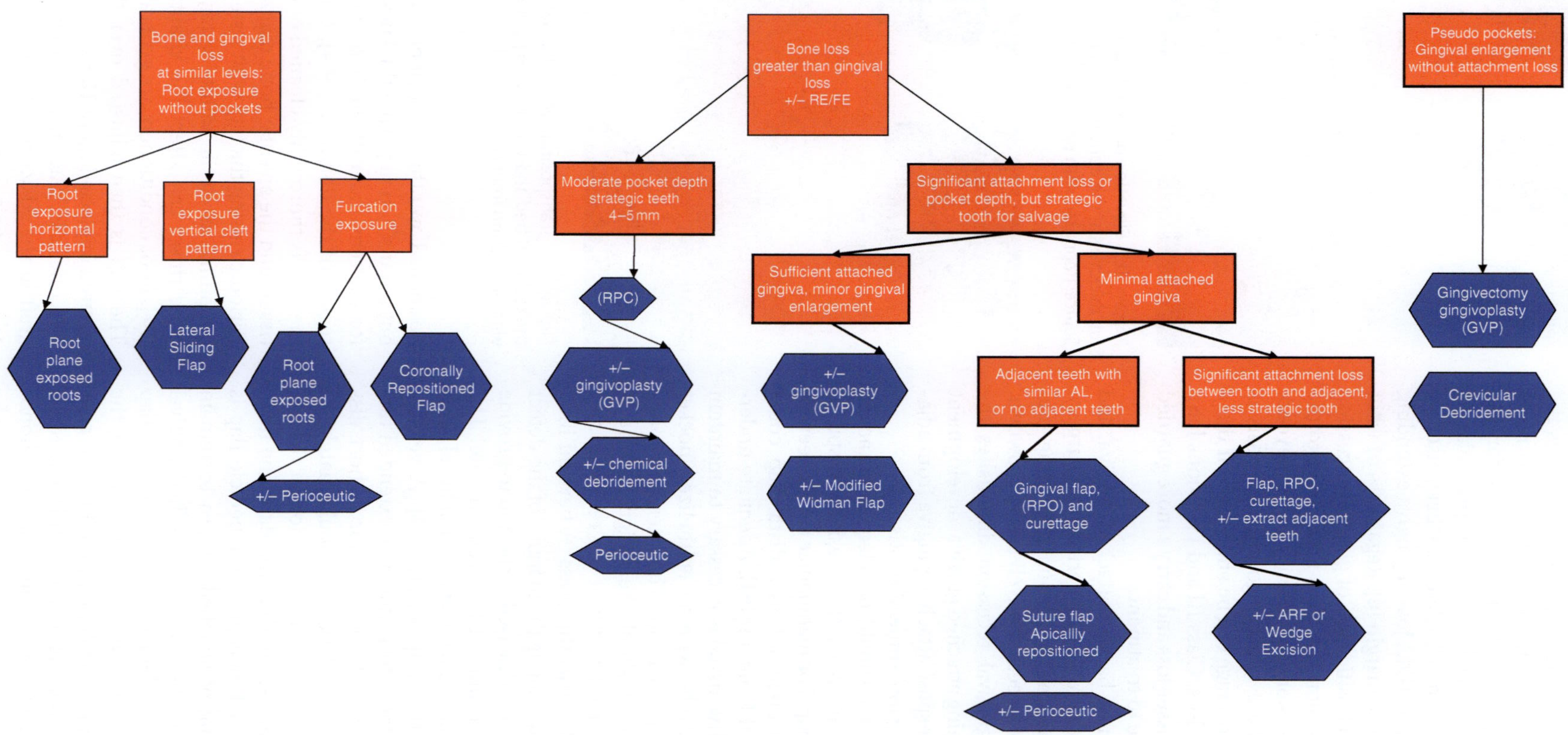

Bone and gingival loss at similar levels: Root exposure without pockets
Root exposure horizontal pattern
Root exposure vertical cleft pattern
Furcation exposure
Root plane exposed roots
Lateral Sliding Flap
Root plane exposed roots
Coronally Repositioned Flap
+/– Perioceutic
Bone loss greater than gingival loss +/– RE/FE
Moderate pocket depth strategic teeth 4–5 mm
(RPC)
+/– gingivoplasty (GVP)
+/– chemical debridement
Perioceutic
Significant attachment loss or pocket depth, but strategic tooth for salvage
Sufficient attached gingiva, minor gingival enlargement
+/– gingivoplasty (GVP)
+/– Modified Widman Flap
Minimal attached gingiva
Adjacent teeth with similar AL, or no adjacent teeth
Gingival flap, (RPO) and curettage
Suture flap Apicallly repositioned
+/– Perioceutic
Significant attachment loss between tooth and adjacent, less strategic tooth
Flap, RPO, curettage, +/– extract adjacent teeth
+/– ARF or Wedge Excision
Pseudo pockets: Gingival enlargement without attachment loss
Gingivectomy gingivoplasty (GVP)
Crevicular Debridement

10.6.1.2 Gingival Cleft

The buccal surface of the maxillary canine (dog) is the most common site for the development of a gingival cleft, though treatment has been described for the mandibular canine and maxillary fourth premolar as well [64]. The term "Stillman's Cleft" has been used to describe a triangular or slit-like loss of gingiva extending apically from the gingival margin [6]. Regardless of what term is used, Miller's classification of gingival recession defines Class I as recession that does not extend to the MGJ and Class II recession that extends to, or beyond, the MGJ [3]. With these two categories, prognosis is good and 100% root coverage can be anticipated if there is no interdental bone loss. Class III and IV lesions have interdental bone and tissue loss and carry a more guarded prognosis for response to treatment.

If there is still a slender band of attached gingiva, and the client does not want to pursue periodontal surgery, meticulous home care and professional cleaning and treatment can keep these teeth relatively stable. However, once the region of gingival recession diminishes the integrity of the remaining attached gingiva, development of a pedicle flap to transpose attached gingiva from adjacent tissue may help restore some of the tissue.

In case selection, there should be adequate attached gingiva from an adjacent area, either mesial or distal, in order to develop the flap. For mandibular canine teeth, a mesial flap would be preferred, as a distal flap could compromise the lateral frenulum [64]. Adequate underlying bone or connective tissue is necessary to maintain the repositioned AG; otherwise an epithelized pocket will form or recession will recur. The laterally repositioned sliding flap (LRSP) should be designed to be at least 1.5 times the greatest width of the recipient site, elevated to full or full/partial thickness. A beveled incision is made in a V-shape along the margins of the defect to remove at least 1 mm of diseased tissue and to provide access for thorough cleaning of the recipient site. The donor site should be incised with an external bevel, with an internal bevel on the recipient site [74]. A vertical incision at the "V" of the defect should be extended further apically into the alveolar mucosa for a short distance. The donor site vertical incision should match the entire length of the recipient vertical incision, at the site determined by the planned width of the flap. The horizontal, internally beveled incision of the pedicle flap is made to allow 2–3 mm of attached gingiva to remain near the donor site, with the remaining attached gingival band (at least 2–3 mm) to be incorporated into the flap [75]. If the flap is harvested from the incisor region, the horizontal incision can be scalloped to follow the contour of the AG in the area (Figure 10.7). Adjacent edentulous areas can potentially provide the best donor tissue, as more of the AG can be used. The portion to be positioned over the recipient bed should be full thickness, but a transition to partial thickness can be implemented for the remainder of the flap that will be covering the region of the donor site [64]. Once the flap is raised, the area is thoroughly cleaned of irritants and diseased tissue, and the alveolar bone margins are gently beveled. Periodic rinsing the flap with a sterile polyionic solution is optimal as sterile saline, water, and dilute chlorhexidine rinses can affect the vitality of periodontal cells [77]. Root conditioners are generally not recommended. The flap is then adjusted over the recipient bed and sutured in place (Figure 10.8).

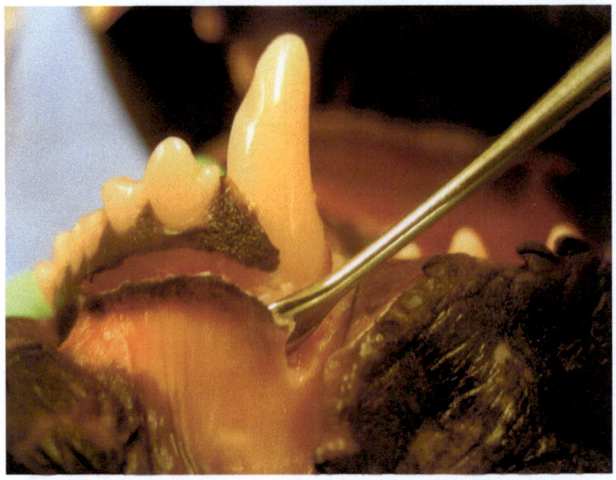

Figure 10.7 Elevation of the lateral sliding pedicle flap donor site, full thickness at the bony edge, and partial thickness mesially. *Source:* Reprinted with permission from reference [64].

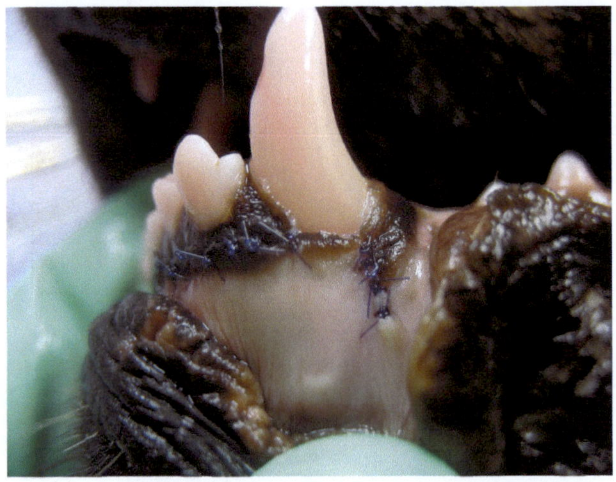

Figure 10.8 Transposition of the flap laterally (distally) to cover the recipient bed and sutured into position. *Source:* Reprinted with permission from reference [64].

In one case, placement of a synthetic particulate bone graft in the adjacent alveolus of the extracted 205 and adjacent original defect resulted in maintenance of the alveolar bone height [75]. In the absence of connective tissue and bone regeneration, a long epithelial junction may form or recession may occur. The extent of new attachment is unpredictable and any lack of oral hygiene or continuing therapy would put the prognosis at risk.

Other gingival grafts have been proposed to reestablish the presence of attached gingiva over areas of recession, including free gingival grafts, free CTGs and pouch-and-tunnel techniques [56]. While these carry a good prognosis in humans, the need for extended and repeated anesthetic events and meticulous home care make them less reasonable for most veterinary patients.

10.6.2 Bone Loss Greater than Gingival Loss

10.6.2.1 Suprabony Pocket – Moderate Depth

When soft tissue periodontal pockets (suprabony) are encountered in Phase I or Phase II therapy, the most important periodontal goal must be applied – remove the irritants. As discussed in Chapter 5 – Periodontology – scaling, closed root planing (SRP), and gingival curettage are an important part of the complete dental treatment. These pockets may be formed with alveolar bone recession alone (gingival height maintained) or can be found in conjunction with additional root exposure (some gingival recession, with more extensive alveolar bone recession). The extent of root exposure added to the depth of the pocket gives the true assessment of attachment loss: that distance from the CEJ to the apical aspect of the pocket.

Generally speaking, moderate pocket depths of 5 mm are amenable to closed root planing, either with sharpened hand curettes or with appropriate subgingival sonic, ultrasonic scalers, or Er/YAG lasers, with comparable microbiological results [78]. Ultrasonic instruments through high-speed action produce a cavitational activity and acoustic microstreaming that some believe may help enhance the disruption of the bacteria in subgingival biofilms [79]. Ultrasonic instrumentation of the root surface (root surface debridement – RSD) removes less cementum than with hand instruments [80, 81]. The thin tips can be used in furcations and tight spaces, and reach the depth of the pockets [74]. A combined ultrasonic debridement and use of a topical desiccant showed a significantly greater bacterial load reduction than ultrasonic debridement alone in one study of hospitalized patients with chronic periodontitis [62].

According to the American Academy of Periodontics, locally delivered agents can be used by the clinician when probing depths of more than 5 mm with inflammation which are still present after conventional therapy [82]. In human dentistry these agents include chlorhexidine chips, tetracycline fibers, doxycycline gel, minocycline microspheres, and metronidazole gel [83]. While there generally are moderate differences seen, these agents can reduce the clinical signs of inflammation, probing depths, and subgingival microflora [83]. However, if multiple sites are present, additional or alternate therapy should be considered. In one study, a combination of a locally applied doxycycline gel with SDD and SRP resulted in more than a 2 mm improvement in mean attachment gain and probing depth reductions compared to SRP alone [40].

10.6.2.2 Suprabony Pocket Greater than 5 mm – Strategic Tooth

10.6.2.2.1 Sufficient Attached Gingiva ± Minor Gingival Enlargement

With suprabony pockets deeper than 5 mm, surgical intervention is often considered, with a flap to open the site for better access. However, when evaluating the tissues of attachment at the defect, first determine the extent of attached gingiva. If there is sufficient width/depth of the attached gingiva, and even mild enlargement, it is reasonable to consider resecting a portion of that AG to immediately decrease the depth of the pocket. In Phase I therapy, this marginal gingiva may be enlarged due to inflammation alone that could respond to conventional therapy. Any true degree of gingival enlargement may not be appreciable, but as long as sufficient AG remains (3 mm or more), reduction of the pocket by lowering the soft tissue walls can be simply accomplished with a 12-fluted bur on a high-speed handpiece. Any remaining pocket depth (less than 5 mm now) can then be treated appropriately. During Phase II treatment, the edema and swelling should be reduced, allowing for a more accurate assessment of fibrous gingival enlargement that can be excised. This is not resection gingivectomy as is needed for advanced gingival enlargement with pseudopockets (described later), but a conservative removal of unsupported, excessive gingiva that can improve probing depths around teeth and in interdental spaces.

In evaluating sites with sufficient height of attached gingiva, but increased thickness due to inflammation and infection of the inner lining of the pocket, specific periodontal surgical incisions can then be made to both remove the diseased lining and decrease pocket depth. This crevicular debridement would be performed in a similar fashion to the modified Widman flap, with internal bevel incision and secondary vertical incisions to the base of the pocket with removal of the supracrestal pocket tissue.

10.6.2.2.2 Minimal Attached Gingiva – Adjacent Teeth with a Similar AL Pattern or No Adjacent Teeth

If deeper soft tissue pockets are encountered in the presence of minimal attached gingiva, then the techniques employed must preserve as much of the AG as possible, while still working to minimize the pocket depth and clean the area. If the AG is still associated with underlying alveolar bone, then access by displacement (discussed previously) can be started with a reverse bevel flap. Moderate pockets may just need an open flap with removal of fibrotic epithelium, without exposure of the crestal bone [74]. If osseous defects or minor intrabony pockets are present, the access may be extended further apically, just enough to expose the diseased region. Depending on the site, releasing vertical incisions may not be needed, but should be employed when indicated [74]. These flaps are then returned to their original position and interdental and vertical incision sutures placed.

At times, these pockets extend below the level of the MGJ, so that whatever AG is left is no longer positioned over alveolar bone. A horizontal incision (reverse bevel) is made 0.5–1 mm from the gingival margin [47], with vertical releasing incisions past the MGJ in order to release the gingival flap for access. Once the area is thoroughly cleaned, the flap will be positioned further apically, bringing the free gingival margin just coronal to the alveolar bone. Vertical mattress sutures apically will help retain the tissue in this position, though some redundant tissue may remain [74]. This will expose additional root and even furcations, but with the AG now over supporting bone, maintenance of healthier tissues of attachment will carry a better prognosis.

While the procedure of apically positioned flaps are frequently described using mandibular incisors, extensive surgery such as this for relatively non-strategic teeth should be carefully considered. In the authors' opinion, if this procedure is utilized on mandibular incisors, mobility of the incisors is often present. Therefore, periodontal splinting is needed in addition to the open root planing and apically repositioned flap. Additional sites to consider ARF would be with partially erupted teeth such as the mandibular canine or first molar. With enamel situated under the attached gingiva, apical to the free gingival margin, there is often a type of pseudopocket, as these tissues cannot attach directly to enamel. If there are no adjacent teeth, or if they need to be extracted (see the section below), the apically repositioned gingival margin can minimize the pocket encountered, even if done only on one aspect of the tooth (partial apically repositioned flap).

10.6.2.2.3 Minimal AG – AL Between Strategic and Less Strategic Teeth

If the decision has been made to provide periodontal surgery, it is probably because a strategic tooth is at risk. In evaluating adjacent teeth, many times extraction of a less strategic tooth will greatly enhance access at the site and facilitate later cleaning and oral hygiene in the area. In the dog, the most common teeth considered for tactical extraction are the mandibular fourth premolar and second molar adjacent to the first molar, the mandibular third incisor adjacent to the canine, the maxillary third premolar adjacent to the mesial furcation of the fourth premolar, the maxillary second molar, and any crowded teeth. Interceptive extractions of non-strategic teeth can help save strategic teeth.

(a) (b)

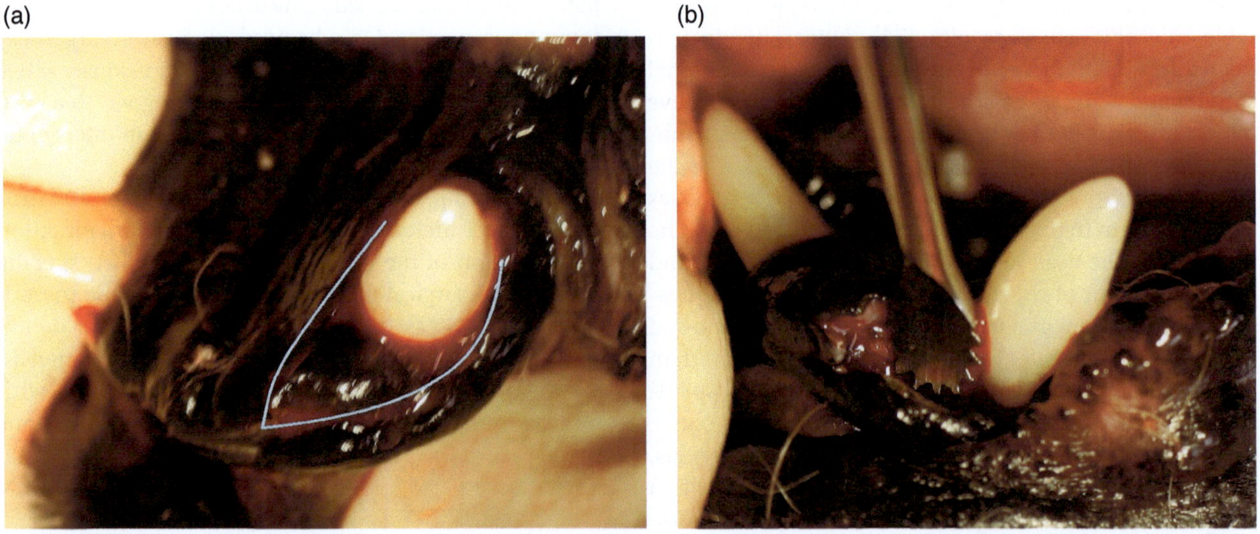

Figure 10.9 (a) Redundant tissue at the mesial aspect of the mandibular canine, creating pseudopockets and the planned reverse bevel incision to remove a wedge of affected tissue. (b) Debridement of the osseous defect and open root planing of the canine, after which bone graft material can be placed in an intrabony defect and the gingival edges are sutured, often in a more apical position.

Extraction of an adjacent tooth will allow placement of the vertical incision at a distance away from the periodontal defect to be treated. Using techniques previously described to access the area and remove diseased and fibrous pocket epithelium, complete debridement is much easier with good access. Whether or not regenerative techniques are then used, the gingiva is sutured to provide a complete collar of attached gingiva around the site treated. If is important to have the gingiva adapted back to the tooth surface without a gap. If alveolar bone has been lost in the area, some degree of apical repositioning may occur, exposing more dentin and root, and deliberate apical repositioning can also be employed.

At times, the remaining soft tissue adjacent to a strategic tooth remains thickened or fibrous, not encircling that portion of the tooth with healthy attached gingiva. Whether the previously adjacent tooth/teeth was/were extracted or lost, lack of curettage of unhealthy tissue or redundant tissue can result in a persistent pocket. Similar to wedge excisions described in human literature for the distal aspect of the maxillary or mandibular second molars, this has also been described for treatment of a pocket distal to the maxillary first molar in a dog [84]. Excision of the tissue allows access for regenerative techniques as well as to thin the remaining tissue for optimal approximation of the two edges when sutured. This procedure can also be performed as a wedge excision at the mesial aspect of the mandibular canine teeth when incisors have been extracted or lost (Figure 10.9a and b), in order to manage the redundant inflamed and poorly healing tissue with a potential defect or pocket at the canine tooth.

10.6.3 Pseudopockets

When periodontal probing is increased due to the coronal extension of the gingival margin and not due to loss of the tissues of attachment, a pseudopocket is formed. The level of attachment is typically still at the level of the CEJ. Whether the gingival enlargement is due to hyperplasia or hypertrophy, or whether the enlargement is a thin extension of the gingival margin coronally or involves extensive thickening of the tissue (think mandibular incisors of Boxers), the goal is the same: return the structure and function of the area to a healthy sulcus.

The term gingivectomy means "excision of the gingiva" [61], but is clinically not meant to remove all gingiva present. Elimination of fibrous suprabony pocket walls was previously discussed. The term gingivoplasty refers to the reshaping of gingiva in the absence of pockets to restore physiological contours, though in most cases this may reduce probing depth as well.

Treatment planning starts with mapping out the apical extent of the sulci, either using a probe and marking bleeding spots or using a pocket marker instrument. Cold steel instruments may include a Kirkland knife for incisions on the buccal and lingual surface or distal teeth, an Orban periodontal knife for interdental incisions, and scalpel blades. The incision should be started apical to the marked points and directed coronally to a point between the depth of the pocket (the points) and alveolar crest, without exposing the bone [61] (Figure 10.10). Alternate descriptions include marking the points 2 mm coronal to the depth of the sulcus and directing the incision to a point just coronal to the depth of the sulcus [76]. Beveled at a 45° angle, this incision is continued across the region of enlargement, following the scalloped pattern of normal gingiva [61]. Fully rectified electrosurgery electrodes, radiosurgery, or carbon dioxide lasers have also been used for gingivectomy, but care must be taken to avoid damaging teeth and bone in the area [48]. Crown-and-collar scissors can be effective to de-bulk

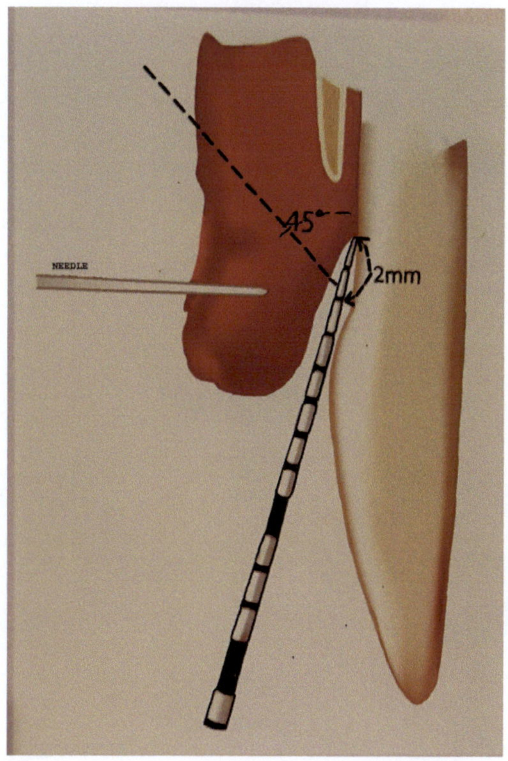

Figure 10.10 Illustration showing the approach (dotted line) to create a 45° bevel coronally oriented incision to the bleeding point line creating an approximation of the normal gingival margin. *Source:* Reprinted with permission from reference [76].

large sections of gingival enlargement, advancing one blade of the scissors in the gingival sulcus/pseudo-pocket while trimming away the excess tissue. Recontouring the edges with a 12-fluted bur or coarse tapered diamond bur [76] on a water-cooled high-speed handpiece is then needed to avoid a broad, flat fibrous plateau that will take longer to develop a physiological contour. The 12-fluted bur also helps provide some hemostasis. Of course, any abnormal-looking tissue should be submitted for histopathology.

Simple removal of the coronal aspect of highly thickened gingiva will not be able to restore these contours without significant removal of buccal and labial tissue. As best demonstrated at the mandibular incisors of a Boxer, the "original" keratinized gingival surface can often be distinguished from the enlarged tissue. By following this scalloped margin, an exaggerated internal (reverse) bevel can be made to lift a flap that will facilitate removing a wedge of labial-to-lingual tissue (crevicular debridement). After the tissue is removed, the site cleaned, and the flaps sufficiently thinned, they can be sutured interdentally, similar to an undisplaced flap closure. A similar case has been described in a dog with gingival enlargement due to cyclosporine therapy. The flaps were started with reverse bevel incisions and scissors and diamond burs were used to re-scallop the edges and thin the flap before they were repositioned apically [85].

10.7 Periodontal Surgery – Flow Chart – Infrabony/Intrabony Attachment Loss

As mentioned earlier in the chapter, case selection is critical in improving the chance of a successful procedure, and this is true when the vertical or angular bone defect extends apically along a root. While resection of minor defect walls with an apically repositioned flap can decrease the impact of the defect [86], with intrabony lesions, the pocket can also be minimized or eliminated with regenerative or repair techniques. The AAP terms reviewed earlier in the chapter makes distinctions between periodontal regeneration (restoration of lost periodontium, including formation of new bone (NB),

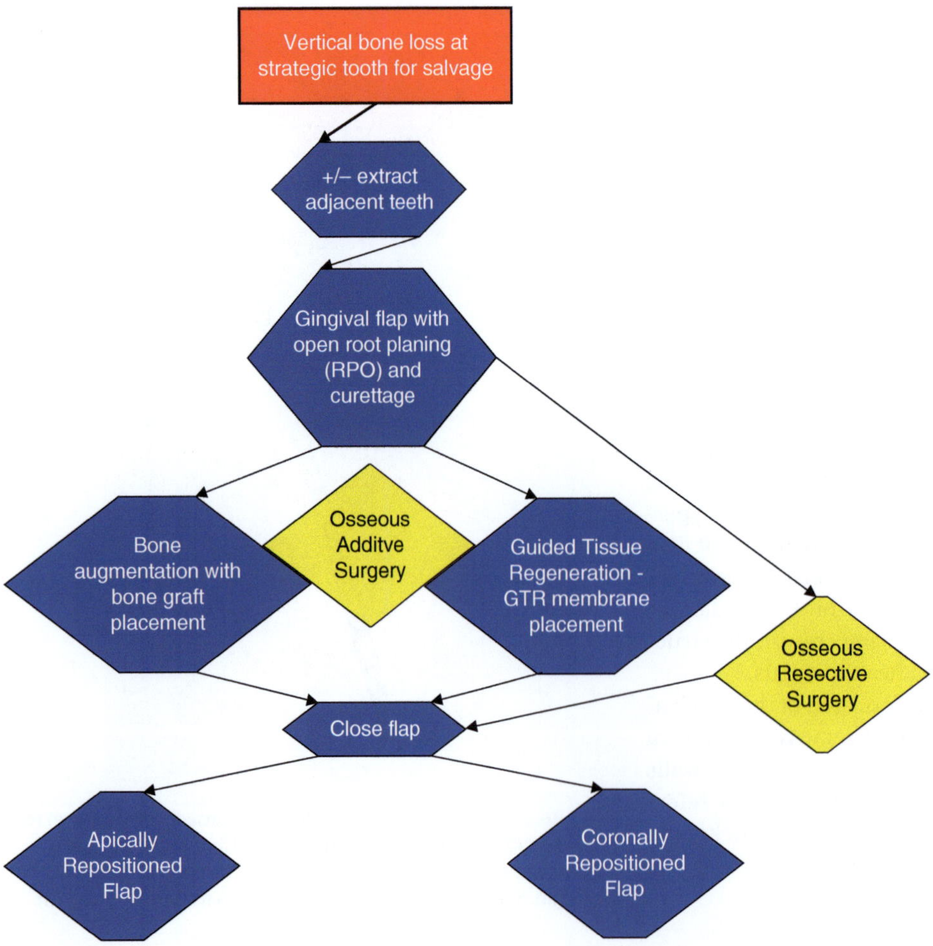

new cementum (NC), and new periodontal ligament) as compared to repair (healing of a wound that does not fully restore the architecture or function). This distinction can only be assessed histologically and a variety of healing endpoints can be identified. An LJE or connective tissue adhesion (CTAd), where the connective tissue contacts the root without cementum formation, will not restore the full architecture. Connective tissue attachment (CTA) will have new cementum with inserting collagen fibers, but they will not be in contact with new bone formation. Osseous repair (OR) will show new bone filling the defect, but without integration with the connective tissue. A further description of histological variations in bone fills will be covered when discussing bone graft materials later in the chapter. Full regeneration (REG) includes the presence of NC, NB, and new inserting fibers, restoring the full periodontal ligament and periodontal structures [86]. If a particular procedure has demonstrated histological regeneration potential during a study, then positive clinical outcomes can be correlated with regeneration [87]. A review of periodontal regeneration using various biomaterials and combinations in human histological studies showed that the amount of REG with NC and inserting fibers was similar among most treatments, with the exception of monotherapy alloplasts and biological factors [88].

Clinical assessment will include determining the clinical attachment level (CAL) and pocket or probing depth (PD), as well as bone fill/gain or OR [89]. Unfavorable outcomes may include continued infection, gingival growth into defect, connective tissue repair with root resorption, ankylosis, or an LJE, which may result in a persistent pocket [90]. Residual pockets (PPD > or = 6 mm) can have an influence on the risk factors for periodontal disease progression and tooth loss [91].

While the ultimate goal of complete tissue regeneration is optimal, in veterinary patients with shorter life spans than humans, the clinical relevancy of stable bone and reduced pocket depth may be considered as reasonable outcomes. This is where discerning the difference between statistical success, sometimes associated with small physical gains, needs to be compared to clinical success.

In veterinary dentistry, advanced procedures are typically reserved for strategic teeth, such as the mandibular first molars and canines, and the maxillary canine and fourth premolars. Lesions that extend into the apical region of a tooth will often necessitate extraction, but a root resection of the distal root of the mandibular first molar with endodontic therapy of the mesial root can combine both the root canal procedure and regenerative efforts. In most cases where palatal bone loss of the maxillary canines has already resulted in an oronasal fistula, extraction and appropriate closure is usually performed, but with smaller defects some regenerative procedure might be considered.

10.7.1 Wound Healing Principles [92]

Soft tissue healing has been previously discussed and those dynamics play an important part in intrabony lesions as well [93, 94]. Melcher's compartmentalization concept was also discussed, recognizing the different cell types that can populate the defect once all irritants are removed. Thorough scaling and root planing, closed or open, while improving the health of the defect, will generally result in an LJE or persistent pocket, with occasional, but inconsistent, new tissue formation. Due to the complexity and interaction of the periodontal tissues, only a portion of the lost tissue will be fully recovered, even with the best techniques and products [87].

The ultimate goal of periodontal regeneration will require a barrier that excludes epithelium and gingival tissues, selectively guiding the repopulation of the defect with appropriate tissues for establishing a healthy new attachment with new cementum, new bone, and new PDL. While it was once thought that only PDL cells were capable of regenerating attachment [15, 95], bone cells and possibly cementoblasts are now considered to have regenerative potential [14, 92], as well as the periosteum, which is rich in osteoprogenitor cells [96]. Paravascular cells from the endosteal region are thought to migrate into the periodontal ligament and progenitor cells have been found predominantly adjacent to blood vessels [97]. Other biological requirements for regeneration include the presence and stabilization of a blood clot and space maintenance to support the healing process [90, 96].

Once the defect is accessed appropriately, the area and tooth surface need to be treated to encourage proper tissue regrowth and attachment to the root, with reduction of the pocket depth. All irritants, inflammatory tissue, and diseased cementum should be thoroughly removed, though healthy cementum and root structure should not be damaged [90]. Aggressive root planing can unnecessarily remove cementum that could play an important role in the reattachment process. Traditional efforts to remove any endotoxin-containing layers (detoxification) [66] with aggressive root planing to achieve a smooth surface is likely to be detrimental [80]. RSD with ultrasonic instrumentation is probably sufficient to disrupt and remove the biofilm located superficially on the root surface, even on rough or uneven surfaces, with minimal damage to the tooth structure [81, 98]. Cortical perforations to create bleeding at the defect site to allow the entry of progenitor cells has also been suggested [92].

The process of root conditioning in theory uses a compound to demineralize the root surface, removing the smear layer and exposing fibrils that should enhance blood clot adhesion to the fibrils and root. *In vitro* studies have shown that citric acid treatment results in a dentinal surface with a thick network of fibrin directly attaching to the surface and trapping cellular elements [99]. This may even improve the mechanical interface bonding between the treated root surface and newly forming cementum, helping to prevent cementodentinal tears [87]. However, the actual clinical benefits of root demineralization are still debated [96, 100]. The use of citric acid has been shown to contribute to ankylosis, but the lower acidity of EDTA solutions may cause less damage to surrounding tissues [92].

An important aspect of the healing process is the presence and maintenance of the fibrin clot between the flap margin and the root surface. The stabilization of the coagulum and provisionary matrix of the fibrin clot may have a positive effect on wound healing, which is important in regeneration [101]. Mobility of the flap adjacent to the site can exceed the tensile strength of the fibrin clot and result in a tear [101]. A connective tissue matrix will gradually replace the clot and become attached to the root surface [101]. Both the formation of new cementum and a new CTA are critical for regenerative success [87].

10.7.2 Prognostic Factors

The characteristics of the intrabony pocket are considered prognostic factors: defects that are three-walled and are at least 4 mm or greater in depth carry the best prognosis [102] (Table 10.2). The healing of a defect can be greatly influenced by constituents from the surrounding PDL, bone, and gingiva, including vascular and cellular resources [88]. Defects with a non-supportive anatomy, such as a one-walled defect or the presence of thin gingiva are at higher risk for failure [103]. The angle of the defect, formed by two lines – the line of the lateral bony wall (CEJ to the base of the defect) should also be evaluated as well as the line from the base of the defect to the most coronal extension of the lateral bony wall [104]. A narrow defect angle would be 25° or less and a wide angle is considered to be 37° or more, with a higher probability of CAL gains in the narrow angle defects [105]. The greater surface area of a wide defect may encounter more exposure to the oral environment [106]. The quality of the gingiva is also critical: passive flap adaptation with adequate gingival thickness is optimal [88].

Table 10.2 Anatomical factors influencing GTR outcomes [102].

Positive effect	Negative effect
Deep (≥4 mm) intrabony defect	Shallow intrabony defect
Narrow defect angle (<45°)	Wide defect angle (>45°)
Vertical bone loss	Horizontal bone loss
Three-wall defects	One- or two-wall defects
Minimal furcation involvement	Deep furcation involvement
Adequate tissue thickness (>1.1 mm)	
Adequate keratinized gingiva (2 mm)	

The need to create and maintain space is a key objective of periodontal regenerative procedures [106]. Space provision has a significant effect on bone regeneration following GTR, which is a major function of barrier membranes and can be enhanced by filling materials. In a study model, when the alveolar ridge was narrow and contributed to a collapse of the membrane, the regenerative potential was diminished [107]. In the review of human histological studies, new CTA formation may not depend primarily on the physical exclusion of the epithelial downgrowth, with wound stability and space provision being of "paramount importance" [88].

The level of oral hygiene is a critical factor as well, so case selection, including evaluation of client commitment to their pet's after-care, is essential. For advanced periodontal procedures, the oral cavity should have thorough management (cleaning, polishing, extraction of compromised teeth) at an initial visit prior to the periodontal surgery itself. In humans, the clinical outcomes are considered to be more influenced by patient behavior (oral care, smoking) and the surgical approach than by the tooth and defect characteristics [108].

10.7.3 Regeneration Procedures and Materials

Effective regeneration of periodontal tissues requires additional concepts, materials, and techniques. In addition to the more general goals of periodontal therapy, such as debriding all irritants and eliminating pockets, efforts to promote blood clot stabilization, space maintenance, and preventing the apical growth of gingival epithelium and connective tissue, are also desired in these lesions. Without some type of barrier, chronic disease will continue with the presence of an LJE or persistent pocket. There may be repair and healing, but without full restoration of the structure or new attachment with nonfunctional scar tissue [109]. The ultimate periodontal regeneration will include the restoration and formation of new alveolar bone, new cementum, and new periodontal ligament. With guided tissue regeneration through differential tissue responses, structure and function of the periodontium can be returned. This process is very complex with interrelated factors, or, as Diaz-Sanchez describes it, "periodontal regeneration is an orchestrated process with the coordinated migration, proliferation and differentiation of cells" [110].

10.7.3.1 Barriers – Membranes

The ideal barrier membrane is biocompatible, favors selective cell line repopulation of the wound, protects the blood clot, and maintains space to allow the new tissues to form. It should be easy to use and handle, and should remain in place for around six weeks [111], with some studies evaluating them to be in place for eight weeks [16]. There is a critical period of at least three to four weeks in which the membrane should allow the complete repopulation by the selected progenitor cells [112]. For guided bone regeneration (GBR) around implants and for ridge augmentation, membranes are typically in place for six to nine months [112].

Membranes are grouped as synthetic non-resorbable, synthetic resorbable, and natural biodegradable. Most studies have not shown a significant difference between absorbable and non-absorbable membranes [92], and if the membrane is rigid enough, grafting material is not necessarily required, particularly in three-walled, Class II furcation or fenestration defects [90, 113]. There is some indication, however, that a bone graft with a membrane is better than either alone in non-contained periodontal defects (two-walled, supra-alveolar) with unfavorable architecture [113–115]. This is likely to be of higher importance when a less rigid absorbable membrane is used on an implant surface or over a large non-space making defects [115, 116].

The earliest membranes used, of methycellulose acetate, were fragile and could tear. Then ePTFE (extended polytetrafluoroethylene) membranes were developed with an inner cell-occlusive area and an outer cell-adherent region [117], with some titanium reinforced products. Complete tissue exclusion with occlusive membranes may provide optimal results, but substantial bone, cementum, and PDL regeneration occurs with macroporous and microporous membranes as well [16]. However, these membranes must be removed after four to six weeks and have been shown to experience early spontaneous exposure [118]. The degree of bacterial contamination at the time of removal can be an indicator of potential success or failure of the treatment [119]. These membranes may be utilized more for GBR around implants.

To avoid the need for a second surgical procedure, synthetic resorbable membranes were developed of collagen, synthetic aliphatic polymers (polylactic and polyglycolic acids), and calcium sulfate [120]. Features of collagen products (bovine and porcine type I) include a hemostatic function (platelet aggregation), which can support clot formation, and a fibroblast chemotactic function, to facilitate primary wound closure [96]. Modifications (cross-linkage with metal ions) are used to prolong collage retention, though after six weeks, greater periodontal regeneration is not found [121]. In one study, when healing was uneventful (two cross-linked collagen membranes (CCM) had early failures), the CCM sites had statistically greater bone fill than CM sites at 16 weeks [122]. More highly cross-linked, slow-resorbing collagen membranes typically resulted in membrane exposure in one study [121].

Aliphatic polymers typically use combinations of polyglycolic acid (PGA) and polylactic acid (PLA), and copolymers have been used safely and successfully for years in suture material and meshes. They are inert, non-antigenic, and are viscoelastic, becoming malleable at body temperature [118]. Degraded by hydrolysis, there is typically minimal inflammatory reaction [123] unless additional impurities are released during degradation or if the byproducts are slowly removed in a poorly vascularized area [116]. Resorption starts at four to six weeks with complete resorption at 6–12 months [112]. Degradable polymer membranes can be integrated into the overlying soft tissues, while still preventing epithelial downgrowth [124].

Calcium sulfate can provide a good adaptation to the margins of the periodontal defect, but is typically resorbed in 30 days [125]. It has also been used as a binder and barrier in combination with grating material.

Laminar bone sheets have been described in studies and for human implant sites [126, 127]. For dogs, an osseous bone membrane is available as thin, flexible sheets that are made of demineralized cortical bone and cancellous bone chips. It was evaluated in a small clinical study combined with the use of a dried bone allograft (DFDBA) and produced clinically significant periodontal attachment gains [90]. A liquid polymer gel (*N*-methyl-2-pyrrolidone) and poly (DL-lactide) combined with 8.5% doxycycline hyclate was formed into a membrane for use in another small clinical study of intrabony defects in dogs. A decrease in probing depth and increase in bony fill was seen at all four sites evaluated [128]. A membrane made of the same material also resulted in clinical improvement (increased radiographic bone fill and decreased probing depth in a dog) [129].

10.7.3.2 Bone Replacement Graft Materials

These biocompatible materials are primarily placed in osseous defects to fill the voids and to provide the structure or scaffold to support clot development, maturation, and remodeling of bone [130]. While most have properties limited to osteoconduction (scaffolding), others may contain substances that can be osteoinductive or even contain living cells for osteogenesis. Compared to open flap debridement alone in the treatment of intrabony defects, the use of bone grafts increases bone level and clinical attachment level, and reduces probing depth and loss of crestal bone [130].

10.7.3.2.1 Terminology

Autogenous bone graft is a tissue graft transferred from one part of a patient's body to another site.

Allogenic bone graft is a tissue graft from a donor of the same species as the recipient but is not genetically identical.

Xenogenic bone graft. A tissue graft from a donor of one species to an individual of another species.

Alloplastic graft. Inorganic material implanted into living tissue.

Osteoconductive. The quality of a graft material that allows it to serve as a scaffold (permit cellular attachment, proliferation, and migration) for deposition of an osteoid.

Osteointegrative. The quality of a graft material that allows a direct structural and functional connection with living bone.

Osteoinductive. The quality of a biologic adjunct, growth factor, or graft material that leads to differentiation of osteoprogenitor cells (mesenchymal stem cells) into osteoblasts.

Osteogenesis. Having tissues or cells capable of differentiation that become involved in the development, growth, or repair of bone.

Bone replacement grafts from the iliac crest and intraoral cancellous bone are means of providing an autogenous graft. A published case report utilizing a reusable cortical bone grafter harvesting an autograft from an extraction site provided material for placement in an intrabony defect in a dog with clinical results [129]. These are potentially osteogenic with the presence of osteoblasts, but root resorption has been seen with fresh graft placement [96]. Additional surgery for the patient and need for sufficient volume of graft can make this process challenging. A range of histologic evidence, from regeneration and new CTA to the presence of an LJE show variable results.

Bone allografts are available commercially, often as freeze-dried particulates that are mineralized or demineralized (demineralized freeze-dried bone allograft – DFDBA). The mineralized freeze-dried bone allograft (FDBA) mainly provides an osteoconductive function as a scaffold for bone formation. The demineralization process presumably exposes bone morphogenic proteins (BMP) that can potentially impart some osteoinductive properties to the product. There is a range of variability in manufacturing, so this property is not always consistent. Decalcification can cause this graft to resorb more quickly, providing less time for "scaffolding" [14].

Xenografts for periodontal surgery are inert, absorbable anorganic bone grafts with all cells and proteinaceous materials removed, in order to decrease antigenicity [14, 96]. While some periodontal regeneration has been reported with anorganic bovine bone mineral (ABM) and ABM with collagen membrane (CM) [131], xenografts are more suited for GBR around implants and for ridge augmentation with slower resorption rates [132–135]. Another ABM product combines the bone matrix with a synthetic peptide clone of type 1 collagen (ABM/P-15) that further promotes the binding of fibroblasts and osteoblasts [14, 72]. Grafts made of coral exoskeletons with calcium carbonate are also considered to be xenografts. Converted to hydroxyapatite (HA) by hydrothermal processes, with a variety of pore size and porosity, the graft provides a scaffold for osteoconduction and is resorbed as the forming bone remodels [136].

Alloplasts are inorganic synthetic bone grafts that are biocompatible, sometimes bioactive, generally osteoconductive, and classified as polymers or ceramics. As the graft supports new bone formation and its remodeling, the character of reaction or integration of the graft should involve a minimal fibrotic reaction [92]. The final tissue or substance in the defect should have strength and elasticity similar to cortical and cancellous bone [92]. In areas of limited osteoconduction, new bone may only be present in close proximity to existing bone [92]. These materials can also be used for periapical defects [14].

Ceramic-based materials include calcium phosphates (tricalcium phosphate (TCP) and hydroxyapatite (HA)), calcium sulfate, and bioactive glass, considered to be osteointegrative due to the bone formed between the graft material and bone [137]. Synthetic HA exhibits osteoconduction, with ossification of the porous structure of the graft. Beta-TCP has similar calcium and phosphorous ratios as cancellous bone [138], and often becomes fibroencapsulated, resulting in a primarily periodontal repair with an LJE. Bioglass with a surface layer of carbonated HA is thought to promote adsorption and concentrations of osteoblast-derived proteins for mineralization of the extracellular matrix [139]. It has also been shown to have the potential to reduce bacterial colonization *in vitro* [140]. While clinical benefits of increased CAL and bone fill have been shown, histologic evaluation shows a connective tissue encapsulation with minimal new cementum or CTA [141, 142]. Its osteoconduction properties have been shown in extraction sockets and in maxillary sinus grafts with a bone filling to minimize alveolar ridge resorption, even in the presence of a centripetal post-extraction bone healing response (optimal healing adjacent to host bone) [143, 144].

Natural polymers have limited use as bulk materials and most synthetic polymers are more frequently used as barrier membranes [130]. A composite material (HTR bone graft) of polymethylmethacrylate (PMMA), polyhydroxylethylmethacyrlate (PHEMA), and calcium hydroxide aids in stabilization of the clot through its hydrophilic and osteophilic properties [145]. A six-year study showed favorable results using the combination graft in Grade II furcation defects, similar to reports of other graft materials (but not directly compared) [145]. A comparison of the combination graft (HTR), with or without an ePTFE membrane, demonstrated similar clinical results to a defect treated with a membrane alone [146]. The same combination (PPCH) used with a polyanhydride (PA) in a chemically hardened graft material showed a better bone–implant contact interface for immediate bridging and stability in extraction sites prepared for implantation [147].

10.7.3.3 Biologic Modifiers – Tissue Engineering

The use of barrier membranes and defect fillers have demonstrated varying levels of regenerative potential and other factors have been evaluated in the biomimetic roles they play in the regenerative process. This class of biologic modifiers includes compounds and products, including growth factors and proteins that have been found in the development and healing of periodontal tissues.

10.7.3.3.1 Growth Factors

A variety of growth factors or cytokines has been evaluated for their role in periodontal regeneration. Normally stored in the extracellular matrix (ECM), these polypeptides are released by the ECM, cells, and platelets after an injury [148]. As key components of functional bone regeneration, these compounds modulate cellular activity, often with multiple cell types targeted in a highly complex process. The challenges of periodontal regeneration (as compared to appendicular bone treatment) include a variety of tissue types in a "mosaic structure" with compounds that work "singly, synergistically and synchronously" [149]. Osteoprogenitor migration is enhanced by BMPs, platelet-derived growth factors (PDGFs), fibroblast growth factors (FGFs), and vascular endothelial growth factors (VEGFs). PDGFs and FGFs stimulate the proliferation of periosteum-derived cells in the early stages, with differentiation of osteoprogenitor cells impacted by certain BMPs, transforming growth factor B (TGF-B) and insulin growth factors (IGFs) [148]. Since many of the products are developed using recombinant human technology, immunological reactions are possible, and the tumor-promotion effects of some factors (BMP2, VEGF) [150] remains unknown [148].

Bone Morphogenic Proteins (BMPs) Bone morphogenic proteins are a group of 30 non-collagen osteoinductive proteins obtained from non-mineralized bone matrix. They are considered osteoinductive with an anabolic effect as they stimulate the differentiation of pluripotent mesenchymal cells to osteoprogenitor cells [14, 110]. They are part of the superfamily of transforming growth factor-β (TGF-β), to which osteogenic proteins (OPs) also belong. Recombinant human OP-1 has been shown to preferentially initiate cementogenesis, with a highly cellular cementoid attaching to exposed dentin and inserted Sharpey's fibers [149]. RhOP-1 has also exhibited angiogenic properties [149].

BMP-2 and BMP-7 are known for their osteoinductive capabilities, and recombinant human products are available. Specific delivery systems, such as collagen sponges, platelet gels, or demineralized bone matrix, are combined with the proteins for application. As described earlier, the osteoinductive capabilities of DFDBM is attributed to the exposure of collagen fibrils and BMPs during the demineralization process. Often used for GBR in sinus lift augmentation or around implants, their use in periodontal regeneration is also advocated [110]. While there may be some concern with ankylosis when using BMP-2 [149–151], BMP-7 has been shown to promote periodontal regeneration and differentiation of cementoblasts in addition to potent bone-producing factors [108]. Combinations of BMPs with other factors have varying results, though enhancement was found in combination with biphasic calcium phosphate (BCP) ceramics, and they have also been used with adipose stem cells [152]. Even on the human side, however, the need for high doses at enormous costs to treat relatively small and non-threatening lesions (as opposed to orthopedic needs) [87] shows the limitations for practical and widespread clinical use in veterinary dentistry.

Platelet-Derived Growth Factors (PGDFs) In early studies using cell cultures, PDGF compounds exhibited potent mitogenic and chemotactic factors that can impact wound healing [109]. Recombinant human PGDF (rhPDGF-BB) has been developed and studied extensively, and has been shown to be comparable (when combined with β-TCP) to treatment standards of GTR with DFDMA in intrabony defects [153]. A 36-month follow-up to that study showed that bone fill and linear bone growth continued to improve over the three year period [154]. The rhPDGR/β-TCP product requires no membrane, is easy to use, and is consistent in concentration [108]. RhPDGF-BB in bone allograft has also been studied with histological evidence of new calcified tissue with inserting collagen fibers in treating Class II furcation defects [71]. A low-dose PDGF preparation with IGF did not improve results over the control in a study, but a higher dose level of PDGF resulted in a significant difference in bone regeneration [155].

10.7.3.3.2 Enamel Matrix Derivatives and Proteins

EMD, a semipurified protein prepared from developing porcine teeth, is a mixture of low molecular weight proteins (amelogenins) that enhance cementum formation [66]. Their presence in a thin layer between the dentin and cementum appears to be a precursor to acellular cementum in the process of cementogenesis in developing teeth [142]. Acellular cementum is integral for the insertion of collagen fibers, signaling PDL fiber development in regenerative processes. EMDs have been shown to promote fibroblast proliferation and growth as well as to inhibit epithelial cell proliferation and growth [142]. Studies (animal and human) have shown application of EMD to enhance periodontal wound healing with the formation of new root cementum, PDL, and alveolar bone as the proteins are absorbed into the hydroxyapatite and collagen fibers on the root surface [108]. Clinical parameters include a gain in clinical attachment and formation of new bone. Compared to GTR with membranes, the use of EMD shows similar results in stable defects, but no additional benefit to combining the therapies [156]. Some improvement has been shown when using EMD concurrently with DFDBA and in combination with autologous bone graft [156, 157]. Regenerative response can be unpredictable, as developing consistent batches is challenging [108].

10.7.3.3.3 Platelet Products

Platelet-rich plasma (PRP), prepared from autologous plasma, can deliver a number of polypeptide growth factors and fibrin that can help stabilize the blood clot and graft material [158]. Platelet pellets (PP) contain more platelets than PRP and have better adhesive properties [159]. While cheaper than bone graft materials, the harvesting process of these platelet products does take additional time, and clinical results from their use have varied [160, 161].

10.7.4 Techniques in Veterinary Dentistry

Case selection is critical when regenerative procedures are performed, to justify the additional anesthetic time (initial Phase I treatment, GTR procedure, and evaluation at six months) and materials used. Strategic teeth with periodontal defects are the most likely candidates, including intrabony defects at the mesial or distal aspect of mandibular first molars, palatal defects at maxillary canines, mesial defects at mandibular canines, and even Class II furcation lesions at the mesial aspect of maxillary fourth premolars in dogs. The defects at the distal aspect of mandibular first molars and the palatal aspects of maxillary canine teeth will often be three-walled in nature [162]. At the mesial aspect of the maxillary fourth premolar, a Class II furcation defect (with the third premolar extracted or missing) will create a defect that can often be classified as two-walled [90]. In several of these, loss or extraction of an adjacent, less strategic tooth may have contributed to the bone defect, but can also help provide access to the angular bone loss associated with the tooth to be treated [129]. The mandibular molar may also be treated with a root resection of the distal root to effectively treat the mesial root (with additional endodontic treatment) [73]. An owner dedicated to additional therapy and meticulous home care is vital, as is a patient healthy enough to withstand the multiple anesthetic procedures. Advanced periodontal therapy should be done once the benefits of the Phase I therapy is optimal, at a second procedure.

10.7.4.1 Access

For adequate access to the site being treated, a displacement flap is typically required. The flap should extend 3 mm beyond the defect edges [90]. This may be provided with a vertical incision at the extraction site of the adjacent tooth, with the release distant from the defect. Excessive gingival elevation should be somewhat limited, as alveolar bone exposure can lead to some bone loss and decrease in thickness. An internal bevel incision can be used to excise diseased tissue from the inside of the soft tissue of the pocket, if present. The flap should be full thickness through the extent of the attached gingival band and converted to partial thickness at the MGJ [151]. Access to the palatal aspect of the maxillary canine can be provided with an envelope flap that extends from the third incisor to the first premolar, again with an internal horizontal incision to start the debridement of the pocket lining.

10.7.4.2 Site Preparation

Adequate treatment of the site is critical to the eventual outcome. All debris and irritants must be completely removed, from plaque and calculus, to granulation tissue and disease bone and cementum [151]. Periodontal curettes and even fine diamond burs can be used to debride granulation tissue [90], with hand instruments to contour any root irregularities [151]. Aggressive debridement should be avoided, as every effort should be made to maintain whatever healthy cementum remains and to circumvent damaging the root surface unnecessarily. The benefits of using root conditioners has previously been discussed.

10.7.4.3 Placement of Bone Graft Material and Membranes

Once the defect is prepared, the materials for implantation are readied. The membrane is measured and trimmed so that the edge extends 2–3 mm past the defect in all directions [151]. Materials such as DFDBA need to be rehydrated according to the manufacturer's directions and then placed in the intrabony defect to the height of the remaining alveolar bone (not packed down) [90]. The membrane is then placed over the defect and secured with absorbable sutures (individual or sling sutures) or other methods [90]. The flap is then repositioned and secured with sutures. A modified horizontal mattress suture has

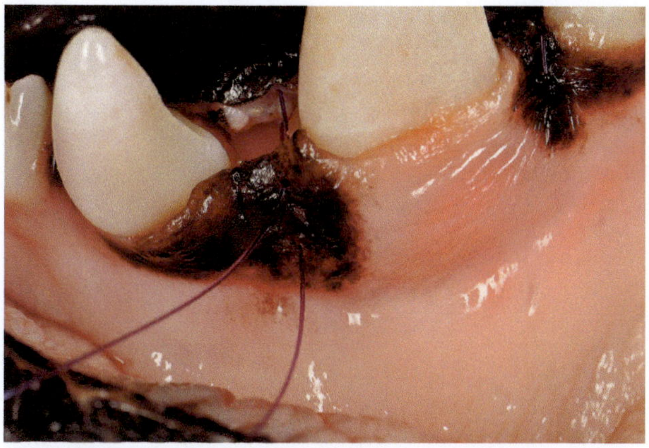

Figure 10.11 A modified horizontal mattress technique is used for interdental suturing. Following suture placement for a standard horizontal mattress, the needle is carried back through the loop of the mattress suture and then tied. This prevents placement of knots directly over the incision line and facilitates wound edge approximation rather than eversion. *Source:* Reprinted with permission from reference [65].

been described as well [65] (Figure 10.11). Membrane fixation has also been studied with the application of a resin [163]. Placement of a periodontal dressing is seldom done in veterinary medicine and is not used frequently in human dentistry. After-care includes chlorhexidine rinses, antibiotics, and pain management with a recheck at two weeks. Follow-up examination, radiographs, and complete dental cleaning is recommended at six months.

10.7.5 Other Techniques

10.7.5.1 Frenectomy and Frenotomy

If any of the frenula exert excessive pull upon the gingival margin or interdental papilla causing gingival recession, a frenectomy can be performed to release that tension [66]. Complete excision of the frenulum (frenectomy) removes the entire mucous membrane fold, along with the underlying musculature, and simple closure [164]. This is more commonly done with the maxillary frenulum in people. In dogs, a frenotomy or frenoplasty can be performed on either of the inferior labial mandibular frenula, with a horizontal incision across the tissue followed by a vertical or transverse closure to release the tension [165].

10.7.5.2 Minimally Invasive Techniques

Minimally invasive techniques can be used to reduce surgical trauma and increase flap stability, but surgical operating microscopes, magnification, and microsurgical instruments are required [166]. MIS, or minimally invasive surgery, described by Harrel, utilizes reflection of the papilla to expose a local defect, with vertical mattress suture closure [167]. The MIST (minimally invasive surgical technique) uses MPPT or SPPT with a modified internal mattress suture closure [166]. The modified minimally invasive surgery (MMIST) develops access through a tiny buccal incision window apical to the papilla, which is left undisturbed. These procedures are limited to isolated interproximal defects and there are issues with visibility of the defect field. Without microsurgical equipment, standard treatment with open flaps are needed.

10.7.5.3 LANAP – Laser Assisted New Attachment Procedure

The use of lasers has previously been described for soft tissue resection and moderate periodontal disease, but techniques have been studied using Nd:YAG lasers for minimally invasive regenerative procedures as well [168, 169]. With a first pass of the laser, the diseased pocket epithelium is removed, which also relaxes the tissues so they can be gently reflected for aggressive scaling and root planing [168]. A second laser pass is performed to stimulate the blood clot [168] and to "seal" the pocket [169]. Later en-bloc extraction of the treated teeth (initially selected for extraction prior to the studies) showed regeneration (cementum, PDL, and bone) in some (2 of 6 in the Yukna study, 5 of 10 in the Nevins study), new attachment (4 of 6 in the Yukna study, 1 of 10 in the Nevins study) and LJE (4 of 10 in the Nevins study) [168, 169]. Patient discomfort was minimal (some dentin sensitivity), with no significant side effects, other than occasional gingival recession. Therefore, the improved wound stability, as seen in MIST procedures, appears to be directly related to wound-healing results [168].

10.8 Summary

By the time this text has been written and published, the amount of new studies and techniques will continue to provide updated information on an ever-changing field. The science of periodontal therapy contains so many facets and variables that the one perfect procedure or process will never be fully defined, but a myriad of options can be considered. All of the information then needs to be assessed on a practical level, to determine what extent of treatment is appropriate for disease found in our veterinary patients, while balancing the risks and benefits, as well as costs.

10.9 AVDC Resource Abbreviations

See Table 10.3.

Table 10.3 AVDC abbreviation list for periodontal surgery (https://www.avdc.org/traineeinfo.html; accessed 3 March 2018).

	Definition
BG	Bone graft (includes placement of bone substitute or bone stimulant material)
CRL	Crown lengthening
F	Flap
F/AR	Apically repositioned periodontal flap
F/CR	Coronally repositioned periodontal flap
F/L	Lateral sliding periodontal flap
FGG	Free gingival graft
FRE	Frenoplasty (frenotomy, frenectomy)
GH	Gingival hyperplasia/hypertrophy
GR	Gingival recession
GTR	Guided tissue regeneration
GV	Gingivoplasty (gingivectomy)
IMP	Implant
ONF	Oronasal fistula
ONF/R	Oronasal fistula repair
PDI	Periodontal disease index
PD0	Normal periodontium
PD1	Gingivitis only
PD2	<25% attachment loss
PD3	25–50% attachment loss
PD4	>50% attachment loss
PRO	Periodontal prophylaxis (examination, scaling, polishing, irrigation)
RPC	Root planing – closed
RPO	Root planing – open
RRX	Root resection (crown left intact)
SC	Subgingival curettage
SPL	Splint

References

1 Kyllar, M., Doskarova, B., and Paral, V. (2013). Morphometric assessment of periodontal tissues in relation to periodontal disease in dogs. *J. Vet. Dent.* 30 (3): 146–149. http://www.ncbi.nlm.nih.gov/pubmed/24371921.

2 Takei, H.H., Scheyer, E.T., Azzi, R.R. et al. (2015). Periodontal plastic and Esthetic surgery. In: *Carranza's Clinical Periodontology*, 12e (ed. M.G. Newman, H.H. Takei, P.R. Klokkevold and F. Carranza), 628–631. St. Louis, MO: Elsevier Inc.

3 Miller, P. (1985). A classification of marginal tissue recession. *Int. J. Periodontics Restorative Dent.* 5 (2): 8–13. doi: 10.1016/0002-9416(82)90445-6.

4 Nordland, W.P. and Tarnow, D.P. (1998). A classification for loss of papillary height. *J. Periodontol.* 69 (10): 1124–1126.

5 Kumar, A., Gupta, G., Puri, K. et al. (2015). Comparison of the clinical applicability of Miller's classification system to Kumar and Masamatti's classification system of gingival recession. *J. Indian Soc. Periodontol.* 19 (5): 563–568. doi: 10.4103/0972-124X.167164.

6 Cassini, M.A., Cerroni, L., Ferlosio, A. et al. (2015). The gingival Stillman's clefts: histopathology and cellular characteristics. *Ann. Stomatol. (Roma)* 6 (3–4): 100–103. doi: 10.11138/ads/2015.6.3.100.

7 The American Veterinary Dental College. (2017). Furcation Involvement Index. AVDC Nomenclature. https://www.avdc.org/Nomenclature/Nomen-Perio.html#periofm. Published. accessed March 5, 2017.
8 Carranza, F.A., Camargo, P.M., and Takei, H.H. (2015). Bone loss and patterns of bone destruction. In: *Carranza's Clinical Periodontology*, 12e (ed. M.G. Newman, H.H. Takei, P.R. Klokkevold and F. Carranza), 290–299. St. Louis, MO: Elsevier Inc.
9 Novak, K.F., Takei, H.H., and DJ (2015). Determination of prognosis. In: *Carranza's Clinical Periodontology*, 12e (ed. M.G. Newman, H.H. Takei, P.R. Klokkevold and F. Carranza), 394–403. St. Louis, MO: Elsevier Inc.
10 DuPont, G. (1995). Tooth splinting for severely mobile mandibular incisor teeth in a dog. *J. Vet. Dent.* 12 (3): 93–95. http://www.ncbi.nlm.nih.gov/pubmed/9693632.
11 Carranza, F.A. and Takei, H.H. (2015). Rationale for periodontal treatment. In: *Carranza's Clinical Periodontology*, 12e (ed. M.G. Newman, H.H. Takei, P.R. Klokkevold and F. Carranza), 404–407. St. Louis, MO, Elsevier Inc.
12 American Academy of Periodontology Glossary of periodontal terms. *J. Periodontol.* doi: 10.1902/jop.1999.70.12.1575.
13 Melcher, A.H. (1985). Cells of periodontium: their role in the healing of wounds. *Ann. R Coll. Surg. Engl.* 67 (2): 130–131.
14 Bashutski, J.D. and Wang, H.L. (2009). Periodontal and endodontic regeneration. *J. Endod.* 35 (3): 321–328. doi: 10.1016/j.joen.2008.11.023.
15 Gottlow, J.A.N., Nyman, S., Karring, T., and Lindhe, J.A.N. (1984). New attachment formation as the result of controlled tissue regeneration. *J. Clin. Periodontol.* 11 (8): 494–503.
16 Wikesjö, U.M.E., Lim, W.H., Thomson, R.C., and Hardwick, W.R. (2003). Periodontal repair in dogs: gingival tissue occlusion, a critical requirement for GTR? *J. Clin. Periodontol.* 30 (7): 655–664.
17 Gulati, M., Anand, V., Govila, V., and Jain, N. (2014). Host modulation therapy: an indispensable part of perioceutics. *J. Indian Soc. Periodontol.* 18 (3): 282–288. doi: 10.4103/0972-124X.134559.
18 Preshaw, P.M. (2015). Periodontal pathogenesis. In: *Carranza's Clinical Periodontology*, 12e (ed. M.G. Newman, H.H. Takei, P.R. Klokkevold and F. Carranza), 76–100. St. Louis, MO: Elsevier Inc.
19 Ryan, M.E. and GY (2015). Host modulation. In: *Carranza's Clinical Periodontology*, 12e (ed. M.G. Newman, H.H. Takei, P.R. Klokkevold and F. Carranza), 525–534. St. Louis, MO: Elsevier Inc.
20 Burns, F.R., Stack, M.S., Gray, R.D., and Parerson, C.A. (1989). Inhibition of purified collagenase from alkali-burned rabbit corneas. *Invest. Ophthalmol. Vis. Sci.* 30 (7): 1569–1575.
21 Lamster, I.B. and Novak, M.J. (1992). Host mediators in gingival crevicular fluid: implications for the pathogenesis of periodontal disease. *Crit. Rev. Oral Biol. Med.* 3 (1–2): 31–60. doi: 10.1177/10454411920030010501.
22 Ormrod, D.J. and Miller, T.E. (1993). Milk from hyperimmunized dairy cows as a source of a novel biological response modifier. *Agents Actions* 38: SCpec No: C146-9.
23 Uriarte, S.M., Edmisson, J.S., and Jimenez-Flores, E. (2016). Human neutrophils and oral microbiota: a constant tug-of-war between a harmonious and a discordant coexistence. *Immunol. Rev.* 273 (1): 282–298. doi: 10.1111/imr.12451.
24 Lima, V., Vidal, F.D.P., Rocha, F.A.C. et al. (2004). Effects of tumor necrosis factor-alpha inhibitors pentoxifylline and thalidomide on alveolar bone loss in short-term experimental periodontal disease in rats. *J. Periodontol.* 75 (1): 162–168. doi: 10.1902/jop.2004.75.1.162.
25 Bartold, P.M., Cantley, M.D., and Haynes, D.R. (2010). Mechanisms and control of pathologic bone loss in periodontitis. *Periodontol 2000* 53 (1): 55–69. doi: 10.1111/j.1600-0757.2010.00347.x.
26 Shah, D.V., Dave, D., Deshpande, N. et al. (2013; April). Bisphosphonates in periodontal therapy. *Indian J. Res.* 293–295.
27 Shoji, K., Horiuchi, H., and Shinoda, H. (1995). Inhibitory effects of a bisphosphonate (risedronate) on experimental periodontitis in rats. *J. Periodontal. Res.* 30 (4): 277–284.
28 Weinreb, M., Quartuccio, H., Seedor, J. et al. (1994). Histomorphometrical analysis of the effects of bisphosphonate alendronate on bone loss caused by experimental periodontitis in monkeys. *J. Periodontol.* 29: 35–40.
29 Carter, G.D. and Goss, A.N. (2004). Bisphosphonates and avascular necrosis of the jaws. *Aust. Prescr.* 27 (2): 32–33.
30 Stepaniuk, K. (2011). Bisphosphonate related osteonecrosis of the jaws: a review. *J. Vet. Dent.* 28 (4): 277–281.
31 Lundberg, A.P., Roady, P.J., Somrak, A.J. et al. (2016). Zoledronate-associated osteonecrosis of the jaw in a dog with appendicular osteosarcoma. *J. Vet. Intern. Med.* 30 (4): 1235–1240. doi: 10.1111/jvim.13980 Epub 2016 Jun 14.
32 Leitão, R.F.C., Ribeiro, R.A., Chaves, H.V. et al. (2005). Nitric oxide synthase inhibition prevents alveolar bone resorption in experimental periodontitis in rats. *J. Periodontol.* 76 (6): 956–963. doi: 10.1902/jop.2005.76.6.956.
33 Hasturk, H., Kantarci, A., Ebrahimi, N. et al. (2006). Topical H2 antagonist prevents periodontitis in a rabbit

model. *Infect. Immun.* 74 (4): 2402–2414. doi: 10.1128/IAI.74.4.2402-2414.2006.

34 Klokkevold, P.R., Takei, H.H., and Carranza, F. (2015). General principles of periodontal surgery. In: *Carranza's Clinical Periodontology*, 12e (ed. M.G. Newman, H.H. Takei, P.R. Klokkevold and F. Carranza), 566–575. St. Louis, MO: Elsevier Inc.

35 Domnick, E. (2014). Suture materials and needle options in oral and periodontal surgery. *J. Vet. Dent.* 31 (3): 204–211.

36 Bellows, J. (2013). Laser and radiosurgery in veterinary dentistry. *Vet. Clin. North Am. Small Anim. Pract.* 43 (3): 651–668. doi: 10.1016/j.cvsm.2013.02.012.

37 Heitz-Mayfield, L.J., Trombelli, L., Heitz, F. et al. (2002). A systematic review of the effect of surgical debridement vs non-surgical debridement for the treatment of chronic periodontitis. *J. Clin. Periodontol.* 9 (Suppl 3): doi: 10.1034/j.1600-051X.29.s3.5.x 92-102-162.

38 Southard, G.L. and Godowski, K.C. (1998). Subgingival controlled release of antimicrobial agents in the treatment of periodontal disease. *Int. J. Antimicrob. Agents* 9 (4): 239–253.

39 Graca, M.A., Watts, T.L., Wilson, R.F., and Palmer, R.M. (1997). A randomized controlled trial of a 2% minocycline gel as an adjunct to non-surgical periodontal treatment, using a design with multiple matching criteria. *J. Clin. Periodontol.* 24 (4): 249–253.

40 Novak, M.J., Dawson, D.R. 3rd, Magnusson, I. et al. (2008). Combining host modulation and topical antimicrobial therapy in the management of moderate to severe periodontitis: a randomized multicenter trial. *J. Periodontol.* 79 (1): 33–41.

41 Perry, D.A. and TH (2015). Phase I Periodontal therapy. In: *Carranza's Clinical Periodontology*, 12e (ed. M.G. Newman, H.H. Takei, P.R. Klokkevold and F. Carranza), 484. St. Louis, MO: Elsevier Inc.

42 Carranza, F.A. and Takei, H.H. (2015). The treatment plan. In: *Carranza's Clinical Periodontology*, 12e (ed. M.G. Newman, H.H. Takei, P.R. Klokkevold and F. Carranza), 408–410. St. Louis, MO: Elsevier Inc.

43 Carranza, F.A. and Takei, H.H. (2015). Phase II periodontal therapy. In: *Carranza's Clinical Periodontology*, 12e (ed. M.G. Newman, H.H. Takei, P.R. Klokkevold and F. Carranza), 552–556. St. Louis, MO: Elsevier Inc.

44 Lindhe, J., Socransky, S.S., Nyman, S. et al. (1982). Critical probing depths in periodontal therapy. *J. Clin. Periodontol.* 9 (4): 323–336. doi: 10.1111/j.1600-051X.1982.tb02099.x.

45 Rosling, B., Nyman, S., Lindhe, J., and Jern, B. (1976). The healing potential of the periodontal tissues following different techniques of periodontal surgery in plaque-free dentitions: a 2-year clinical study. *J. Clin. Periodontol.* 3 (4): 233–250. doi: 10.1111/j.1600-051X.1976.tb00042.x.

46 Takei, H.H., Carranza, F.A., and Do, J.H. (2015). The periodontal flap. In: *Carranza's Clinical Periodontology*, 12e (ed. M.G. Newman, H.H. Takei, P.R. Klokkevold and F. Carranza), 582–586. St. Louis, MO: Elsevier Inc.

47 Beckman, B.W. (2004). Treatment of an infrabony pocket in an American Eskimo dog. *J. Vet. Dent.* 21 (3): 159–163. doi: 10.1177/089875640402100303.

48 Lewis, J. and Reiter, M. (2005). In a dog – Management of generalized gingival enlargement in a dog – Case report and literature review. *J. Vet. Dent.* 22 (3): 160–169.

49 Cortellini, P., Pini Prato, G., and Tonetti, M.S. (1996). The modified papilla preservation technique with bioresorbable barrier membranes in the treatment of intrabony defects. Case reports. *Int. J. Periodontics Restorative Dent.* 16 (6): 546–559. http://www.ncbi.nlm.nih.gov/pubmed/9242093.

50 Cortellini, P., Prato, G.P., and Tonetti, M.S. (1999). The simplified papilla preservation flap. A novel surgical approach for the management of soft tissues in regenerative procedures. *Int. J. Periodontics Restorative Dent.* 19 (6): 589–599.

51 Takei, H.H., Carranza, F.A., and SK (2015). The flap technique for pocket surgery. In: *Carranza's Clinical Periodontology*, 12e (ed. M.G. Newman, H.H. Takei, P.R. Klokkevold and F. Carranza), 593–603. St. Louis, MO: Elsevier Inc.

52 Smith, M.M. (2003). Line angle inisions. *J. Vet. Dent.* 20 (4): 241–244.

53 Shoukry, M., Ben, A.L., Abdel, M., and Soliman, M. (2007). Repair of plaque-induced experimental periodontal disease in dogs. *J. Vet. Dent.* 24 (3): 152–165.

54 Molnár, B., Aroca, S., Keglevich, T. et al. (2013). Treatment of multiple adjacent Miller Class I and II gingival recessions with collagen matrix and the modified coronally advanced tunnel technique. *Quintessence Int.* 44 (1): 17–24. doi: 10.3290/j.qi.a28739.

55 Cheng, Y.F., Chen, J.W., Lin, S.J., and Lu, H.K. (2007). Is coronally positioned flap procedure adjunct with enamel matrix derivative or root conditioning a relevant predictor for achieving root coverage? A systemic review. *J. Periodontal. Res.* 42 (5): 474–485. doi: 10.1111/j.1600-0765.2007.00971.x.

56 Rebele, S.F., Zuhr, O., Schneider, D. et al. (2014). Tunnel technique with connective tissue graft versus coronally advanced flap with enamel matrix derivative for root coverage: a RCT using 3D digital measuring methods. Part II. Volumetric studies on healing dynamics and gingival dimensions. *J. Clin. Periodontol.* 41 (6): 593–603. doi: 10.1111/jcpe.12254.

57 Sculean, A., Mihatovic, I., Shirakata, Y. et al. (2015). Healing of localized gingival recessions treated with coronally advanced flap alone or combined with either a resorbable collagen matrix or subepithelial connective tissue graft. A preclinical study. *Clin. Oral Investig.* 19 (4): 903–909. doi: 10.1007/s00784-014-1299-x.

58 Shah, R., Thomas, R., and Mehta, D.S. (2015). Recent modifications of free gingival graft: a case series. *Contemp. Clin. Dent.* 6 (3): 425–427. doi: 10.4103/0976-237X.161910.

59 Agarwal, C., Kumar, T., and Mehta, D. (2015). Comparative evaluation of free gingival graft and Alloderm(R) in enhancing the width of attached gingiva: a clinical study. *Contemp. Clin. Dent.* 6 (4): 483–488.

60 Reiter, A.M. and Lewis, J.R. (2008). Dental bulge restoration and gingival collar expansion after endodontic treatment of a complicated maxillary fourth premolar crown-root fracture in a dog. *J. Vet. Dent.* 25 (1): 34–45. http://www.ncbi.nlm.nih.gov/pubmed/18512624.

61 Takei, H.H., Carranza, F.A., and SK (2015). Gingival surgical techniques. In: *Carranza's Clinical Periodontology*, 12e (ed. M.G. Newman, H.H. Takei, P.R. Klokkevold and F. Carranza), 576–581. St. Louis, MO: Elsevier Inc.

62 Lombardo, G., Signoretto, C., Corrocher, G. et al. (2015). A topical desiccant agent in association with ultrasonic debridement in the initial treatment of chronic periodontitis: a clinical and microbiological study. *New Microbiol.* 38 (3): 393–407.

63 Silverstein, L.H., Kurtzman, G.M., and Shatz, P.C. (2009). Suturing for optimal soft-tissue management. *J. Oral Implantol.* 35 (2): 82–90. doi: 10.1563/1548-1336-35.2.82.

64 Startup, S. (2011). Lateral sliding pedicle flap for gingival cleft at the mandibular canine tooth. *J. Vet. Dent.* 29 (1): 60–66.

65 Gingerich, W. and Stepaniuk, K.S. (2011). Guided tissue regeneration for infrabony pocket treatment for dogs. *J. Vet. Dent.* 28 (4): 282–288.

66 Wolf, H.F., Rateitschak-Pluss, E.M., Rateitschak, K.H., and Hassell, T.M. (2005). Therapy. In: *Color Atlas of Dental Medicine*. 3e. New York: Theme, 201–458.

67 Luskin, I.R. (2000). Reconstruction of oral defects using mucogingival pedicle flaps. *Clin. Tech. Small Anim. Pract.* 15 (4): 251–259. doi: 10.1053/svms.2000.21044.

68 Sims, T.N. and Takei, H.H. (2015). Furcation involvement and treatment. In: *Carranza's Clinical Periodontology*, 12e (ed. M.G. Newman, H.H. Takei, P.R. Klokkevold and F.A. Carranza), 621–627. St. Louis, MO: Elsevier Inc.

69 Dogan, A., Ozdemir, A., Kubar, A., and Oygur, T. (2002). Assessment of periodontal healing by seeding of fibroblast-like cells derived from regenerated periodontal ligament in artificial furcation defects in a dog: a pilot study. *Tissue Eng.* 8 (2): 273–282. doi: 10.1089/107632702753725030.

70 Gantes, B., Martin, M., Garrett, S., and Egeiberg, J. (1988). Treatment of periodontal furcation defects. *Clin. Periodontol.* 9 (I): 69–89. http://onlinelibrary.wiley.com/doi/10.1111/j.1600-051X.1988.tb01576.x/abstract.

71 Camelo, M., Nevins, M.L., Schenk, R.K. et al. (2003). Periodontal regeneration in human Class II furcations using purified recombinant human platelet-derived growth factor-BB (rhPDGF-BB) with bone allograft. *Int. J. Periodontics Restorative Dent.* 23 (3): 213–225.

72 Khashu, H. and Vandana, K.L. (2012). Clinical and radiographic evaluation of human periodontal osseous defect (mandibular grade II furcation) treated with PepGen P-15 and a bioresorbable membrane (Atrisorb). *J. Indian Soc. Periodontol.* 16 (4): 569–576. doi: 10.4103/0972-124X.106917.

73 Reiter, A.M., Lewis, J.R., Rawlinson, J.E., and Gracis, M. (2005). Hemisection and partial retention of carnassial teeth in client-owned dogs. *J. Vet. Dent.* 22 (4): 216–226.

74 Holmstrom, S., Frost, P., and Eisner, E. (1998). Periodontal therapy and surgery. In: *Veterinary Dental Techniques*, 2e, 167–213. Philadelphia, PA: W.B. Saunders Company.

75 Rawlinson, J.E. and Reiter, A.M. (2005). Repair of a gingival cleft associated with a maxillary canine tooth in a dog. *J. Vet. Dent.* 22 (4): 234–242.

76 Force, J. and Niemiec, B. (2009). Gingivectomy and gingivoplasty for gingival enlargement. *J. Vet. Dent.* 26 (2): 132–137.

77 Buffa, E.A., Lubbe, A.M., Verstraete, F.J., and Swaim, S.F. (1997). The effects of wound lavage solutions on canine fibroblasts: an in vitro study. *Vet. Surg.* 26 (6): 460–466. http://doi.wiley.com/10.1111/j.1532-950X.1997.tb00517.x%5Cnpapers3://publication/doi/10.1111/j.1532-950X.1997.tb00517.x.

78 Derdilopoulou, F.V., Nonhoff, J., Neumann, K., and Kielbassa, A.M. (2007). Microbiological findings after periodontal therapy using curettes, Er:YAG laser, sonic, and ultrasonic scalers. *J. Clin. Periodontol.* 34 (7): 588–598. doi: 10.1111/j.1600-051X.2007.01093.x.

79 Jahn, C.A. (2015). Sonic and ultrasonic instrumentation. In: *Carranza's Clinical Periodontology*, 12e (ed. M.G. Newman, H.H. Takei, P.R. Klokkevold and F. Carranza), 507–514. St. Louis, MO: Elsevier Inc.

80 Ciantar, M. (2014). Time to shift: from scaling and root planing to root surface debridement. *Prim. Dent. J.* 3 (3): 38–42. doi: 10.1308/205016814812736592.
81 Apatzidou, D.A. and Kinane, D.F. (2010). Nonsurgical mechanical treatment strategies for periodontal disease. *Dent. Clin. North Am.* 54 (1): 1–12. 10.1016/j.cden.2009.08.006. S0011-8532(09)00071-8.
82 AAP (2006). American Academy of Periodontology Statement on Local delivery of sustained or controlled release antimicrobials as adjunctive therapy in the treatment of periodontitis. *J Periodontol.* 77 (8): 1458–1458. doi: 10.1902/jop.2006.068001.
83 Ciancio, S.G. and MA (2015). Anti-infective therapy. In: *Carranza's Clinical Periodontology*, 12e (ed. M.G. Newman, H.H. Takei, P.R. Klokkevold and F. Carranza), 515–524. St. Louis, MO: Elsevier Inc.
84 Klima, L.J. and Goldstein, G.S. (2010). Modified distal wedge excision for access and treatment of an infrabony pocket in a dog. *J. Vet. Dent.* 27 (1): 16–23. http://www.ncbi.nlm.nih.gov/pubmed/20469791.
85 Furman, R. (2014). Apically repositioned flap for gingival enlargment. *J. Vet. Dent.* 31 (3): 183–189.
86 Ivanovic, A., Nikou, G., Miron, R.J. et al. (2014). Which biomaterials may promote periodontal regeneration in intrabony periodontal defects? A systematic review of preclinical studies. *Quintessence Int.* 45 (5): 385–395. doi: 10.3290/j.qi.a31538.
87 Bosshardt, D.D. and Sculean, A. (2009). Does periodontal tissue regeneration really work? *Periodontol 2000* 51 (ii): 208–219. doi: 10.1111/j.1600-0757.2009.00317.x. PRD317.
88 Sculean, A., Nikolidakis, D., Nikou, G. et al. (2015). Biomaterials for promoting periodontal regeneration in human intrabony defects: a systematic review. *Periodontol 2000* 68 (1): 182–216. doi: 10.1111/prd.12086.
89 Kao, R.T., Murakami, S., and Beirne, O.R. (2009). The use of biologic mediators and tissue engineering in dentistry. *Periodontol 2000* 50 (1): 127–153. doi: 10.1111/j.1600-0757.2008.00287.x.
90 Stepaniuk, K.S. and Gingerich, W. (2015). Evaluation of an osseous allograft membrane for guided tissue regeneration in the dog. *J. Vet. Dent.* 32 (4): 226–232. doi: 10.1177/089875641503200403.
91 Matuliene, G., Pjetursson, B.E., Salvi, G.E. et al. (2008). Influence of residual pockets on progression of periodontitis and tooth loss: results after 11 years of maintenance. *J. Clin. Periodontol.* 35 (8): 685–695. doi: 10.1111/j.1600-051X.2008.01245.x.
92 Wang, H.-L. and Cooke, J. (2005). Periodontal regeneration techniques for treatment of periodontal diseases. *Dent. Clin. North Am.* 49: 637–659, vii. doi: 10.1016/j.cden.2005.03.004.
93 Hämmerle, C.H.F. and Giannobile, W.V. (2014). Biology of soft tissue wound healing and regeneration - Consensus Report of Group 1 of the 10th European Workshop on Periodontology. *J. Clin. Periodontol.* 41 (November 2013): S1–S5. doi: 10.1111/jcpe.12221.
94 Sculean, A., Gruber, R., and Bosshardt, D.D. (2014). Soft tissue wound healing around teeth and dental implants. *J. Clin. Periodontol.* 41: S6–S22. doi: 10.1111/jcpe.12206.
95 Nymann, S., Gottlow, J., and Karring, T. (1987). New attachment formation by guided tissue regeneration. *J. Periodontal Res.* 22 (3): 252–254.
96 American Academy of Periodontology (2005). Position Paper Periodontal Regeneration. *J. Periodontol.* 76 (September): 1601–1622. doi: 10.1902/jop.2006.069001.
97 McCulloch, C.A.G., Nemeth, E., Lowenberg, B., and Melcher, A.H. (1987). Paravascular cells in endosteal spaces of alveolar bone contribute to periodontal ligament cell populations. *Anat. Rec.* 219 (3): 233–242. doi: 10.1002/ar.1092190304.
98 Corbet, E.F., Vaughan, A.J., and Kieser, J.B. (1993). The periodontally involved root surface. *J. Clin. Periodontol.* 20 (6): 402–410. doi: 10.1111/j.1600-051X.1993.tb00380.x.
99 Baker, P.J., Rotch, H.A., Trombelli, L., and Wikesjö, U.M. (2000). An *in vitro* screening model to evaluate root conditioning protocols for periodontal regenerative procedures. *J. Periodontol.* 71 (7): 1139–1143. doi: 10.1902/jop.2000.71.7.1139.
100 Mariotti, A. (2002). Efficacy of chemical root surface modifiers in the treatment of periodontal disease. A systematic review. *Ann. Periodontal.* 8 (1): 205–226.
101 Polimeni, G., Xiropaidis, A.V., and Wikesjö, U.M.E. (2006). Biology and principles of periodontal wound healing/regeneration. *Periodontol 2000* 41 (1): 30–47. doi: 10.1111/j.1600-0757.2006.00157.x.
102 Lommer, M. and Wiggs, R.B. (2011). Guided tissue regeneration. In: *Oral and Maxillofacial Surgery in Dogs and Cats* (ed. F.J.M. Verstraete and M. Lommer), 1–8. Philadelphia, PA: Saunders.
103 Cosyn, J., Cleymaet, R., Hanselaer, L., and De Bruyn, H. (2012). Regenerative periodontal therapy of infrabony defects using minimally invasive surgery and a collagen-enriched bovine-derived xenograft: a 1-year prospective study on clinical and aesthetic outcome. *J. Clin. Periodontol.* 39 (10): 979–986. doi: 10.1111/j.1600-051X.2012.01924.x.
104 Kim, C.K., Choi, S.H., Kim, T.S. et al. (2006). The infrabony defect and its determinants. *J. Periodontal Res.* 41 (6): 498–502. doi: 10.1111/j.1600-0765.2006.00895.x.
105 Tsitoura, E., Tucker, R., Suvan, J. et al. (2004). Baseline radiographic defect angle of the intrabony defect as a prognostic indicator in regenerative periodontal

surgery with enamel matrix derivative. *J. Clin. Periodontol.* 31 (8): 643–647. doi: 10.1111/j.1600-051X.2004.00555.x.

106 Tonetti, M.S., Prato, G.P., and Cortellini, P. (1996). Factors affecting the healing response of intrabony defects following guided tissue regeneration and access flap surgery. *J. Clin. Periodontol.* 23 (6): 548–556. doi: 10.1111/j.1600-051X.1996.tb01823.x.

107 Polimeni, G., Albandar, J.M., and Wikesjö, U.M.E. (2005). Prognostic factors for alveolar regeneration: effect of space provision. *J. Clin. Periodontol.* 32 (9): 951–954. doi: 10.1111/j.1600-051X.2005.00763.x.

108 Kao, R.T. and Nares, S.R. (2015). Periodontal regeneration – Intrabony defects: a Consensus Report from the AAP Regeneration Workshop. *J. Periodontol.* 86 (2-s): S105–S107. doi: 10.1902/jop.2015.140378.

109 Kao, R.T., Takei, H.H., Cochran, D.L., and Nevins, M.L. (2015). Periodontal regeneration and reconstructive surgery. In: *Carranza's Clinical Periodontology*, 12e (ed. M.G. Newman, H.H. Takei, P.R. Klokkevold and F. Carranza), 611. St. Louis, MO: Elsevier Inc.

110 Diaz-Sanchez, R.M., Yanez-Vico, R.M., Fernandez-Olavarria, A. et al. (2004). Current approaches of bone morphogenetic proteins in dentistry. *J. Oral Implantol.* 41 (3): 337–342. doi: 10.1563/AAID-JOI-D-13-00012.

111 Gottlow, J., Laurell, L., Lundgren, D. et al. (1994). Periodontal tissue response to a new bioresorbable guided tissue regeneration device: a longitudinal study in monkeys. *Int. J. Periodontics Restorative Dent.* 14 (5): 436–449. http://www.ncbi.nlm.nih.gov/pubmed/7751110.

112 Simion, M., Trisi, P., and Piattelli, A. (1996). GBR with an e-PTFE membrane associated with DFDBA: histologic and histochemical analysis in a human implant retrieved after 4 years of loading. *Int. J. Periodontics Restorative Dent.* 16 (4): 338–347. http://www.ncbi.nlm.nih.gov/pubmed/9242101.

113 Sculean, A., Nikolidakis, D., and Schwarz, F. (2008). Regeneration of periodontal tissues: combinations of barrier membranes and grafting materials – Biological foundation and preclinical evidence: a systematic review. *J. Clin. Periodontol.* 35 (Suppl. 8): 106–116. doi: 10.1111/j.1600-051X.2008.01263.x.

114 Paolantonio, M. (2002). Combined periodontal regenerative technique in human intrabony defects by collagen membranes and anorganic bovine bone. A controlled clinical study. *J. Periodontol.* 73 (2): 158–166. doi: 10.1902/jop.2002.73.2.158.

115 Nociti, F., Machado, M., Stefani, C. et al. (2001). Absorbable versus nonabsorbable membranes and bone grafts in the treatment of ligature-induced peri-implantitis in dogs : a Histometric investigation. *Clin. Oral Impl. Res.* 12: 115–121.

116 Mellonig, J.T., Nevins, M., and Sanchez, R. (1998). Evaluation of a bioabsorbable physical barrier for guided bone regeneration. Part II. Material and a bone replacement graft. *Int. J. Periodontics Restorative Dent.* 18 (2): 139–149. https://www.scopus.com/inward/record.uri?eid=2-s2.0-0032041476&partnerID=40&md5=f9753d17081b833a52f1be0f668dcd63.

117 Jovanovic, S.A. and Nevins, M. (1995). Bone formation utilizing titanium-reinforced barrier membranes. *Int J Periodontics Restorative Dent.* 15 (1): 56–69. http://www.ncbi.nlm.nih.gov/pubmed/7591524.

118 Hutmacher, D., Hürzeler, M.B., and Schliephake, H. (1996). A review of material properties of biodegradable and bioresorbable polymers and devices for GTR and GBR applications. *Int. J. Oral Maxillofac Implants* 667–678.

119 Selvig, K., Kersten, B., Chamberlain, A. et al. (1992). Regenerative surgery of intrabony periodontal defects using ePTFE barrier membranes: scanning electron microscopic evaluation of retrieved membranes versus clinical healing. *J. Periodontol.* 63 (12): 974–978. doi: 10.1902/jop.1992.63.12.974.

120 Villar, C.C. and Cochran, D.L. (2010). Regeneration of periodontal tissues: guided tissue regeneration. *Dent. Clin. North Am.* 54 (1): 73–92. doi: 10.1016/j.cden.2009.08.011.

121 Crigger, M., Bogle, G.C., Garrett, S., and Gantes, B.G. (1996). Repair following treatment of circumferential periodontal defects in dogs with collagen and expanded polytetrafluoroethylene barrier membranes. *J. Periodontol.* 67 (4): 403–413. http://www.ncbi.nlm.nih.gov/pubmed/8708967.

122 Bornstein, M.M., Bosshardt, D., and Buser, D. (2007). Effect of two different bioabsorbable collagen membranes on guided bone regeneration: a comparative histomorphometric study in the dog mandible. *J. Periodontol.* 78 (10): 1943–1953. doi: 10.1902/jop.2007.070102.

123 Caffesse, R.G., Mota, L.F., Quiñones, C.R., and Morrison, E.C. (1997). Clinical comparison of resorbable and non-resorbable barriers for guided periodontal tissue regeneration. *J. Clin. Periodontol.* 24 (10): 747–752. doi: 10.1111/j.1600-051X.1997.tb00192.x.

124 Sallum, E.A., Sallum, A.W., Nociti, F.H. et al. (1998). New attachment achieved by guided tissue regeneration using a bioresorbable polylactic acid membrane in dogs. *Int. J. Periodontics Restorative Dent.* 18 (5): 502–510. http://www.ncbi.nlm.nih.gov/pubmed/10093526.

125 Bell, W.H. (1964). Resorption characteristics of bone and bone substitutes. *Oral Surg. Oral Med. Oral Pathol.* 17 (5): 650–657.

126 Majzoub, Z., Cordioli, G., Aramouni, P.K. et al. (1999). Guided bone regeneration using demineralized laminar bone sheets versus GTAM membranes in the treatment of implant-associated defects. A clinical and histological study. *Clin. Oral Implant Res.* 10 (5): 406–414. http://www.ncbi.nlm.nih.gov/pubmed/10551065.

127 Fugazzotto, P.A. (1996). The use of demineralized laminar bone sheets in guided bone regeneration procedures: report of three cases. *Int. J. Oral Maxillofac Implants* 11 (2): 239–244.

128 Alterman, J. and Huff, J. (2016). Guided tissue regeneration in four teeth using a liquid polymer membrane: a case series. *J. Vet. Dent.* 33 (3): 185–194.

129 Rice, C.A., Snyder, C.J., and Soukup, J.W. (2012). Use of an autogenous cortical graft in combination with guided tissue regeneration for treatment of an infrabony defect. *J. Vet. Dent.* 29 (3): 166–171. http://www.ncbi.nlm.nih.gov/pubmed/23193710.

130 Reynolds, M.A., Aichelmann-Reidy, M.E., and Branch-Mays, G.L. (2010). Regeneration of periodontal tissue: bone replacement grafts. *Dent. Clin. North Am.* 54 (1): 55–71. doi: 10.1016/j.cden.2009.09.003.

131 Nevins, M.L., Camelo, M., Lynch, S.E. et al. (2003). Evaluation of periodontal regeneration following grafting intrabony defects with Bio-Oss collagen: a human histologic report. *Int. J. Periodontics Restorative Dent.* 23 (1): 9–17.

132 Hallman, M., Lundgren, S., and Sennerby, L. (2001). Histologic analysis of clinical biopsies taken 6 months and 3 years after maxillary sinus floor augmentation with 80% bovine hydroxyapatite and 20% autogenous bone mixed with fibrin glue. *Clin. Implant Dent. Relat. Res.* 3 (2): 87–96. doi: 10.1111/j.1708-8208.2001.tb00236.x.

133 Yildirim, M., Spiekermann, H., Handt, S., and Edelhoff, D. (2001). Maxillary sinus augmentation with the xenograft Bio-Oss and autogenous intraoral bone for qualitative improvement of the implant site: a histologic and histomorphometric clinical study in humans. *Int. J. Oral Maxillofac Implants* 16 (1): 23–33.

134 Valentini, P., Abensur, D., Wenz, B. et al. (2000). Sinus grafting with porous bone mineral (Bio-Oss) for implant placement: a 5-year study on 15 patients. *Int. J. Periodontics Restorative Dent.* 20 (3): 245–253.

135 Maiorana, C., Santoro, D.D.S.F., Rabagliati, D.D.S.M., and Salina, S. (2001). Evaluation of the use of iliac cancellous bone and anorganic bovine bone in the reconstruction of the atrophic maxilla with titanium mesh : a clinical and histologic investigation. *Int. J. Oral Maxillofac Implants* 16: 427–432.

136 Guillemin, G., Meunier, A., Dallant, P. et al. (1989). Comparison of coral resorption and bone apposition with two natural corals of different porosities. *J. Biomed. Mater. Res.* 23 (7): 765–779. doi: 10.1002/jbm.820230708.

137 Boccaccini, A.R. and Blaker, J.J. (2005). Bioactive composite materials for tissue engineering scaffolds. *Expert Rev. Med. Devices* 2 (November): 303–317. doi: 10.1586/17434440.2.3.303.

138 Hashimoto-Uoshima, M., Ishikawa, I., Kinoshita, A. et al. (1995). Clinical and histologic observation of replacement of biphasic calcium phosphate by bone tissue in monkeys. *Int. J. Periodontics Restorative Dent.* 15 (2): 205–213. http://www.ncbi.nlm.nih.gov/pubmed/8593983.

139 Chopra, P.M., Johnson, M., Nagy, T.R., and Lemons, J.E. (2009). Clinical device-related article micro-computed tomographic analysis of bone healing subsequent to graft placement. *J. Biomed. Mater. Res. Part B Appl. Biomater.* 88 (2): 611–618. doi: 10.1002/jbm.b.31232.

140 Allan, I., Newman, H., and Wilson, M. (2002). Particulate Bioglass reduces the viability of bacterial biofilms formed on its surface in an *in vitro* model. *Clin. Oral Implants Res.* 13 (1): 53–58. doi: 10.1034/j.1600-0501.2002.130106.x.

141 Nevins, M., Marcelo, M., Nevins, V. et al. (2000). Human histologie evaluation of bioactive ceramic in the treatment of periodontai osseous defects. *Int. J. Periodontics Restorative Dent.* 459–467.

142 Sculean, A., Barbé, G., Chiantella, G.C. et al. (2002). Clinical evaluation of an enamel matrix protein derivative combined with a bioactive glass for the treatment of intrabony periodontal defects in humans. *J. Periodontol.* 73 (4): 401–408. doi: 10.1902/jop.2002.73.4.401.

143 Galindo-Moreno, P., Ávila, G., Fernández-Barbero, J.E. et al. (2008). Clinical and histologic comparison of two different composite grafts for sinus augmentation: a pilot clinical trial. *Clin. Oral Implants Res.* 19 (8): 755–759. doi: 10.1111/j.1600-0501.2008.01536.x.

144 Stvrtecky, R., Gorustovich, A., Perio, C., and Guglielmotti, M.B. (2003). A histologic study of bone response to bioactive glass particles used before implant placement: a clinical report. *J. Prosthet Dent.* 90 (5): 424–428. doi: 10.1016/S0022391303005857.

145 Yukna, R.A. and Yukna, C.N. (1997). Six-year clinical evaluation of HTR synthetic bone grafts in human Grade II molar furcations. *J. Periodontal Res.* 32 (8): 627–633. https://www.scopus.com/inward/record.uri?eid=2-s2.0-0031262085&partnerID=40&md5=9336ceff0425e18bd9c5c4a7c0b72f64.

146 Calongne, K., Aichelmann-Reidy, M., Yukna, R., and Mayer, E. (2001). Clinical comparison of microporous biocompatible composite of PMMA, PHEMA and

calcium hydroxide grafts and expanded polytetrafluoroethylene barrier membranes in human mandibular molar Class II furcations. A case series. *J. Periodontol.* 72 (10): 1451–1459. doi: 10.1902/jop.2001.72.10.1451.

147 Hasturk, H., Kantarci, A., Ghattas, M. et al. (2011). The use of light/chemically hardened polymethylmethacrylate, polyhydroxyethylmethacrylate, and calcium hydroxide graft material in combination with polyanhydride around implants in minipigs: part I: immediate stability and function. *J. Periodontol.* 82 (9): 1339–1352. doi: 10.1902/jop.2011.100617.

148 Devescovi, V., Leonardi, E., Ciapetti, G., and Cenni, E. (2008). Growth factors in bone repair. *Chir. Organi. Mov.* 92 (3): 161–168. doi: 10.1007/s12306-008-0064-1.

149 Ripamonti, U. and Renton, L. (2006). Bone morphogenetic proteins and the induction of periodontal tissue regeneration. *Periodontol. 2000* 41 (1): 73–87. doi: 10.1111/j.1600-0757.2006.00155.x.

150 Raida, M., Clement, J.H., Leek, R.D. et al. (2005). Bone morphogenetic protein 2 (BMP-2) and induction of tumor angiogenesis. *J. Cancer Res. Clin. Oncol.* 131 (11): 741–750. doi: 10.1007/s00432-005-0024-1.

151 Wang, H.-L., Greenwell, H., Fiorellini, J. et al. (2005). Periodontal regeneration. *J. Periodontol.* 76 (9): 1601–1622. doi: 10.1902/jop.2005.76.9.1601.

152 Bozic, D., Grgurevic, L., Erjavec, I. et al. (2012). The proteome and gene expression profile of cementoblastic cells treated by bone morphogenetic protein-7 *in vitro*. *J. Clin. Periodontol.* 39 (1): 80–90. doi: 10.1111/j.1600-051X.2011.01794.x.

153 Nevins, M., Camelo, M., Nevins, M.L. et al. (2003). Periodontal regeneration in humans using recombinant human platelet-derived growth factor-BB (rhPDGF-BB) and allogenic bone. *J. Periodontol.* 74 (9): 1282–1292. doi: 10.1902/jop.2003.74.9.1282.

154 Nevins, M., Kao, R.T., McGuire, M.K. et al. (2012). PDGF promotes periodontal regeneration in localized osseous defects: 36 month extension results from a randomized, controlled, double-masked clinical trial. *J. Periodontol.* 84 (4): 1–10. doi: 10.1902/jop.2012.120141.

155 Howell, T.H., Fiorellini, J.P., Paquette, D.W. et al. (1997). A phase I/II clinical trial to evaluate a combination of recombinant human platelet-derived growth factor-BB and recombinant human insulin-like growth factor-I in patients with periodontal disease. *J. Periodontol.* 68 (12): 1186–1193. doi: 10.1902/jop.1997.68.12.1186.

156 Sculean, A., Schwarz, F., Becker, J., and Brecx, M. (2007). The application of an enamel matrix protein derivative (Emdogain®) in regenerative periodontal therapy: a review. *Med. Princ. Pract.* 16 (3): 167–180. doi: 10.1159/000100386.

157 Cochran, D.L., Jones, A., Heijl, L. et al. (2003). Periodontal regeneration with a combination of enamel matrix proteins and autogenous bone grafting. *J. Periodontol.* 74 (9): 1269–1281. doi: 10.1902/jop.2003.74.9.1269.

158 Carvalho, M.D., Suaid, F.F., Santamaria, M.P. et al. (2011). Platelet-rich plasma plus bioactive glass in the treatment of intra-bony defects: a study in dogs. *J. Appl. Oral Sci.* 19 (1): 82–89. doi: 10.1590/S1678-77572011000100016.

159 Keles, G.C., Cetinkaya, B.O., Baris, S. et al. (2009). Comparison of platelet pellet with or without guided tissue regeneration in the treatment of class II furcation defects in dogs. *Clin. Oral Investig.* 13 (4): 393–400. doi: 10.1007/s00784-008-0245-1.

160 Gurgel, B.C.D.V., Gonçalves, P.F., Pimentel, S.P. et al. (2007). Platelet-rich plasma may not provide any additional effect when associated with guided bone regeneration around dental implants in dogs. *Clin. Oral Implants Res.* 18 (5): 649–654. doi: 10.1111/j.1600-0501.2007.01383.x.

161 Shayesteh, Y.S., Eshghyar, N., Moslemi, N. et al. (2012). The effect of platelet-rich plasma on healing of palatal donor site following connective tissue harvesting: a pilot study in dogs. *Clin. Implant Dent. Relat Res.* 14 (3): 428–433. doi: 10.1111/j.1708-8208.2009.00263.x.

162 Greenfield, B. (2010). Open root planing for a periodontal pocket of a naxillary canine tooth. *J. Vet. Dent.* 27 (1): 34–39.

163 Tomita, S., Yamamoto, S., Shibukawa, Y. et al. (2010). Application of 4-META/MMA-TBB resin for fixation of membrane to tooth in guided tissue regeneration in dog. *Dent. Mater. J.* 29 (6): 690–696. JST.JSTAGE/dmj/2010-021 [pii].

164 Devishree, Gujjari, S.K., and Shubhashini, P.V. (2012). Frenectomy: a review with the reports of surgical techniques. *J. Clin. Diagnostic Res.* 6 (9): 1587–1592. doi: 10.7860/JCDR/2012/4089.2572.

165 Holmstrom, S.E. (2011). Inferior labial frenoplasty and tight-lip syndrome. In: *Oral and Maxillofacial Surgery of the Dog and Cat* (ed. F.J.M. Verstraete and M. Lommer), 515–518. Philadelphia PA: Saunders.

166 Cortellini, P. (2012). Minimally invasive surgical techniques in periodontal regeneration. *J. Evid Based Dent. Pract.* 12 (3 Suppl): 89–100. doi: 10.1016/S1532-3382(12)70021-0.

167 Harrel, S.K. (1999). A minimally invasive surgical approach for periodontal regeneration: surgical technique and observations. *J. Periodontol.* 70 (1): 1547–1557. doi: 10.1902/jop.1999.70.12.1547.

168 Nevins, M.L., Camelo, M., Schupbach, P. et al. (2012). Human clinical and histologic evaluation of laser-assisted new attachment procedure. *Int. J. Periodontics Restorative Dent.* 32 (5): 497–507.

169 Yukna, R.A., Carr, R.L., and Evans, G.H. (2007). Histologic evaluation of an Nd:YAG laser-assisted new attachment procedure in humans. *Int. J. Periodontics Restorative Dent.* 27: 577–587.

11

Oral Surgery – Extractions

Cynthia Charlier

VDENT Veterinary Dental Education, Networking and Training, Elgin, IL, USA

The most commonly performed oral surgery is exodontia or extraction of teeth. While the primary goal of dentistry is to preserve tooth structure, situations may exist where removing the tooth results in a better outcome for the patient. The objective of oral surgery is to remove the entire tooth and root without damaging the surrounding soft tissue and bone.

A maxillofacial and intraoral examination should be completed as part of every physical examination. A tentative treatment plan can be formulated based on grossly visible pathology and should be reviewed with the client during the initial exam. The discussion with the client should include information about general anesthesia, pain management, the oral surgery procedure, potential complications, and postoperative care. Ultimately, the decision to extract a tooth or teeth is dependent on the patient's health status, physical examination, laboratory evaluation, intraoral examination under general anesthesia, and intraoral radiograph findings in combination with the wishes of the client. Whether tooth extraction is the best treatment option for a particular patient is also dependent upon the ability of the owner to provide home care for their pet. Client consent is required before any tooth extraction. An examination under general anesthesia, including dental charting and full mouth intraoral radiographs, allows the practitioner to identify all oral pathology and formulate a definitive treatment plan. A complete evaluation of the status of the tooth and periodontal tissues includes a visual exam, utilization of a probe and explorer, and radiographic evaluation of the tooth and surrounding structures.

The skill and knowledge of the veterinarian should always be considered. If you are not comfortable with a particular procedure based on your equipment, knowledge, skill, and/or the pathology that is present, it is best to refer the patient to a board certified veterinary dentist.

11.1 Indications

Periodontal disease is the most common reason for tooth extraction in veterinary practice. Other indications for tooth extraction include: malocclusions, crowded teeth, impacted or unerupted teeth, supernumerary teeth that predispose adjacent teeth to periodontal disease, teeth with advanced caries, tooth resorption, and inflammatory conditions (stomatitis). Additionally, all teeth affected by pulp necrosis or irreversible pulpitis that are not amenable to endodontic treatment or for which the owner does not wish to complete endodontic treatment should be extracted. Teeth that are potentially non-vital include: complicated or uncomplicated crown or crown root fractures; discolored teeth; teeth with severe periodontitis that results in endodontic disease; and teeth that have radiographic findings consistent with endodontic disease. Advanced periodontal surgery and endodontic treatment may be considered for diseased teeth and should be offered to clients as an alternative to extraction if indicated. Indications for exodontia in immature patients include: persistent deciduous teeth; fractured deciduous teeth; and interceptive orthodontics for treatment of deciduous malocclusions.

Contraindications for extraction may include: poor general health of the patient (general anesthesia is not possible or when the benefits of the procedure do not outweigh the risk to the patient), patients with coagulation disorders or those on medications that might affect coagulation, and teeth in an area previously treated with radiation therapy [1].

Wiggs's Veterinary Dentistry: Principles and Practice, Second Edition. Edited by Heidi B. Lobprise and Johnathon R. (Bert) Dodd.

11.2 Equipment and Instrumentation

Intraoral radiographs are essential to formulate a treatment plan and must be completed prior to extraction of any tooth. Radiographs allow the veterinarian to visualize the root structure and the condition of the surrounding alveolar bone. The typical number of tooth roots for a given tooth is known, but radiographs may reveal supernumerary roots, abnormally shaped roots, convergent roots, fused roots, dilacerated roots, fractured roots, or root resorption, all of which may change the surgical approach to extraction of that tooth. Radiographs are also important to evaluate the alveolar bone surrounding the tooth root for pathology. In the mandibles, periapical pathology and horizontal or vertical bone loss may cause weakening of the surrounding bone and make the area more prone to fracture during the extraction procedure. This information is critical to avoid potential complications when formulating a treatment plan.

Availability of proper equipment and the use of sharp hand instruments assist in the successful extraction of teeth. A water-cooled highspeed handpiece is required to facilitate the removal of buccal alveolar bone (alveolectomy) and to section multirooted teeth. Fiberoptics incorporated into the high-speed handpiece provide an additional light source at the surgical site. Adequate surgical lighting and magnification with a light source will facilitate exodontic procedures and are very helpful for retrieval of fractured root tips.

Gloves, eye protection, masks, and surgical caps should be worn by veterinarians performing oral surgery and by the technician assisting with the procedure. Although the oral cavity cannot be considered a sterile site for oral surgery, surgical instruments that are used to penetrate soft tissue or bone should always be sterilized after each use [2]. An autoclaved, sterile oral surgery pack should be available for each patient.

The following instruments are commonly utilized for tooth extractions and should be contained within the oral surgery/extraction pack (Figure 11.1):

- A highspeed handpiece should be held between the thumb and first two fingers at the working end of the handpiece in a modified pen grasp while resting a finger on the patient. This allows the operator to have more control and better tactile sense while using the highspeed drill.
- Carbide burs in a water-cooled highspeed handpiece are used to remove buccal bone (alveolectomy) and to section multirooted teeth into single roots prior to extraction. Commonly utilized burs include round burs (number 1/2, 1, 2, 4, 6), taper fissure crosscut burs (699L, 701, 701L, 702), and diamond burs.
- A number 15 or 15C scalpel blade with a standard scalpel blade handle or a round scalpel blade handle is utilized to incise gingival and mucosal tissues.

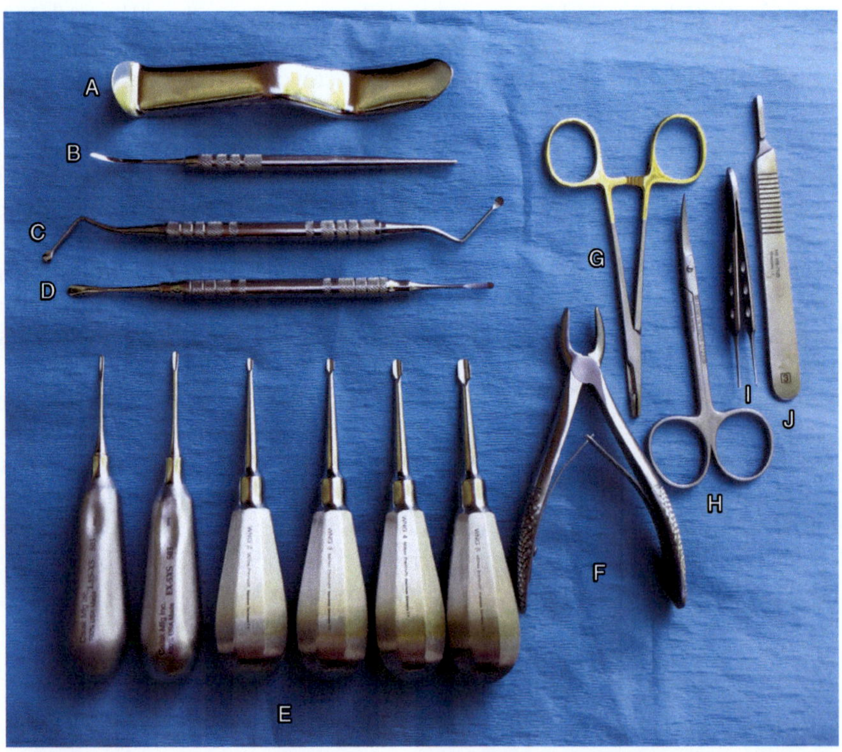

Figure 11.1 Oral surgery/extraction pack: (a) Minnesota lip retractor; (b) feline lip retractor; (c) Miller bone curette; (d) periosteal elevator; (e) straight and winged elevators; (f) small breed extraction forceps; (g) needle holders; (h) iris scissors; (i) thumb forceps; (j) scalpel blade handle.

- A periosteal elevator (Freer or Molt) is utilized to elevate the periosteum away from the underlying bone. It is placed in the palm of the operator's hand with the index finger placed close to the working end of the instrument. This short finger stop prevents inadvertent damage to surrounding soft tissue should the instrument slip. The periosteal elevator is used in a pushing or prying motion to elevate the attached gingival tissue and periosteum of the alveolar mucosal tissues from the underlying alveolar bone.
- Dental elevators vary in size and shape. The elevator is placed into the periodontal ligament space utilizing a short finger stop and is rotated to stretch and fatigue the periodontal ligament and facilitate extraction. The size of the elevator should conform to the size of the root being extracted. Wing-tipped elevators are very useful as they have curved sides that easily conform to the root. The size of the elevator corresponds with the width of the elevator in millimeters. The sizes most commonly used in veterinary dentistry are sizes 2 through 5 mm. A 2 mm elevator may be utilized to assist in the elevation of a cat premolar tooth and a 5 mm elevator may be utilized to assist in elevation of a canine tooth in a large dog.
- Dental luxators vary in size and shape. The luxator is placed in the periodontal ligament space and utilized as a wedge to cut and break down the periodontal ligament. The tip of the luxator is very thin, which allows it to be easily introduced into the periodontal ligament space in an apical direction. Luxators are not to be used with rotational pressure as rotational pressure will damage the luxator tip.
- Root tip picks come in various shapes and sizes and are utilized to assist in the removal of fractured root tips from within the alveolus.
- Extraction forceps are available in a variety of shapes and sizes. Small breed extraction forceps are most commonly used in veterinary dentistry. The size of the forceps should conform to the operator's hand and the tooth size. The forceps are utilized only after the tooth is mobile following successful elevation or luxation. They are placed on the tooth at the cementoenamel junction, and the tooth is then rotated along its long axis to displace it from the alveolus.
- Root tip extraction forceps have small tips and are utilized to remove root tips from within the alveolus.
- A Miller bone curette is used to debride granulation tissue, bone fragments, and debris from within the alveolus following tooth extraction.
- Thumb forceps are used to hold gingival tissue. Commonly utilized thumb forceps include Adson tissue forceps (with or without teeth) and Bishop Harmon (1 × 2) forceps. The tissue forceps should be used to gently hold the tissue while avoiding crushing the gingival tissue.
- Scissors are utilized to debride tissue and may be used to release the periosteum of the mucoperiosteal flap. Curved iris scissors work well for this purpose but some veterinary dentists prefer LaGrange scissors or Metzenbaum scissors.
- Small needle holders should be used for oral surgery. 4½–5 inch Mayo Hegar (without scissors) or Olsen Hegar (with scissors) needle holders may be utilized depending on the preference of the surgeon.
- Retractors are utilized by an assistant to retract the cheek, tongue, and/or mucoperiosteal flap to increase exposure for the operator. A Minnesota retractor or small feline retractor may be utilized for this purpose.
- Suture material for extraction sites is based on the size of the patient, condition of the tissue, and surgeon preference. A 4-0 and 5-0 absorbable suture with a reverse cutting or tapered needle is most commonly utilized.

11.3 Pain Management in Exodontia

Use of preemptive multimodal pain management provides oral surgery patients with a more comfortable intraoperative and postoperative period. Tooth extraction and the manipulation of oral tissues stimulate local pain receptors and initiate local inflammation. It is best to interrupt these afferent impulses before a painful stimulus occurs. Opioids, alpha-2 agonists, non-steroidal anti-inflammatory drugs, and intraoral regional nerve blocks may be utilized in pain management protocols for oral surgery cases (see Chapter 9 – Anesthesia and Pain Management).

11.4 Anatomy

Knowledge of basic anatomy of the maxilla and mandible is critical to avoid key structures during extraction (see Chapter 1 – Oral Anatomy and Physiology). Knowing the number of roots in each tooth and the location of the furcation facilitates multirooted tooth extractions, allowing the practitioner to section the teeth into single root segments. Although individual variations exist, three rooted teeth are located only in the maxilla. In the dog, they include the maxillary fourth premolars and first and second molars, and in the cat include only the maxillary fourth premolar tooth. Two rooted teeth in the dog include the maxillary second and third premolars and the mandibular second, third, and fourth premolars, and first and second molars. In the cat two rooted teeth include the maxillary third premolar and mandibular third and fourth premolars and molar. The maxillary second premolar and the maxillary molar in a cat have either two roots, fused roots, or a single root. All the remaining teeth in the dog and cat are single rooted [3]. Gingival connective tissue attaches directly to the root cementum between the base of the gingival sulcus and the alveolar crestal bone. A surgical blade or periosteal elevator can be used to sever this epithelial attachment circumferentially around the tooth as the first step in tooth extraction. The periodontal ligament has fibers that attach to the cementum of the tooth root and to the alveolus. Stretching and breaking down the periodontal ligament is the key to successful tooth extraction.

Neurovascular anatomy is an important consideration in oral surgery. In the dog, the infraorbital neurovascular bundle exits the infraorbital foramen apical to the distal root of the maxillary third premolar tooth. In the cat, the infraorbital neurovascular bundle exits the infraorbital foramen where the zygomatic arch meets the maxilla apical to the maxillary third premolar tooth. The caudal, middle, and rostral mental foramina are located in the rostral mandible in the dog and the cat. The middle mental foramen in the dog is in the ventral third of the mandible apical to the mesial root of the mandibular second premolar. In the cat, the middle mental foramen is in the ventral half of the mandible beneath the lip frenulum in the interdental space between the mandibular canine tooth and third premolar tooth. The mandibular canal, containing the inferior alveolar neurovascular bundle, is located in the ventral third of the mandible. The parotid and zygomatic salivary ducts are present in the mucosal ridge distal to the maxillary fourth premolar in dogs and should be identified prior to extraction of the caudal cheek teeth.

11.5 Simple versus Surgical Extraction

A simple tooth extraction is completed without elevation of a mucoperiosteal flap or removal of alveolar bone. Simple extractions are indicated for small single-rooted teeth or teeth that have attachment loss from severe periodontal disease. The gingival attachment to the tooth is severed with a number 15 or 15C scalpel blade. The dental elevator is inserted into the periodontal ligament space to elevate and extract the tooth. Non-surgical extractions of multirooted premolars or molars are indicated when they are very mobile secondary to severe periodontal disease or periapical pathology. The procedure for non-surgical extraction of multirooted teeth is the same as for simple extraction except that after the gingival attachment is severed, the tooth is sectioned into single-rooted segments and then extracted.

A surgical extraction involves creation of a mucoperiosteal flap to remove the tooth. Elevation of a mucoperiosteal flap improves visibility and expedites access to the extraction site [4].

For all but the simplest extractions, consider a surgical extraction. Surgical extractions involve raising a mucoperiosteal flap, removing buccal or lingual alveolar bone, sectioning multirooted teeth into single root segments, and apposition of the mucoperiosteal flap to the palatal or lingual gingival tissues following extraction of the tooth. Surgical extractions are often necessary in dogs due to the large root-to-crown ratio and diverging root structure. Indications for surgical extractions include large single-rooted teeth (canine teeth), multirooted teeth with minimal mobility or disease present, and multirooted teeth that have periodontal or endodontic disease affecting only one root.

The alveolus of all extraction sites, regardless of whether the extraction was simple or surgical, should be debrided to remove debris, the surgical site should be lavaged, and the gingival tissue should be sutured. Closure of oral surgery sites allows for primary intention healing, which occurs more rapidly with a lower risk of infection than if the wound is left to heal by secondary intention. The soft tissue edges are opposed and sutured in essentially the same anatomic position they were in before the extraction. This method of wound repair lessens the amount of re-epithelialization, collagen deposition, contraction, and remodeling needed for healing [5].

11.6 Biomechanical Principles for Oral Surgery to Extract Teeth

Elevators are used primarily as levers. Levers transmit a modest force (with the mechanical advantage of a long lever arm and short effector arm) into a small movement against great resistance [6]. Elevators, when they are placed in the periodontal space and rotated, utilize the surrounding alveolar bone as a fulcrum.

A wedge is used when a luxator or small straight elevator is wedged into the periodontal ligament space and pressure is directed apically in a longitudinal direction along the long axis of the tooth to displace the tooth. Luxators are made of softer metal and are unsuitable for use as a lever.

A wheel and axle movement is utilized when an elevator is placed between two roots or between the root and the alveolus and rotated. The handle serves as the axle and the elevator as the wheel when it engages and elevates the tooth from the socket [6]. Teeth that are to remain in the mouth should never be used as a fulcrum as they could be fractured during the process of extraction of adjacent teeth.

11.7 Steps to Surgical Extractions

As with any surgical procedure, it is important to follow the same steps for all patients to ensure consistency in care and outcome.

11.7.1 Chlorhexidine Rinse

When surgery in the oral cavity is performed the oral cavity should be rinsed with chlorhexidine gluconate (0.12%). This procedure reduces the amount of skin and oral mucosal contamination of the surgical site, decreases the microbial load of any aerosols created while using highspeed drills during the surgical procedure, and decreases the number of microorganisms entering the patient's bloodstream [7].

11.7.2 Supragingival and Subgingival Scaling and Polishing

Basic oral care should be completed prior to beginning the oral surgery procedure to minimize contamination of the surgical site with calculus and bacteria.

11.7.3 Radiographs of the Affected Tooth or Teeth

Imaging is necessary to evaluate the tooth and root structure and the alveolar bone, and determine if there is pathology present in the surrounding alveolar bone that may predispose to extraction complications.

11.7.4 Preoperative Analgesia

Preemptive multimodal pain management including intraoral regional nerve blocks is recommended prior to any extractions [8] (see Chapter 9 – Anesthesia and Pain Management).

11.7.5 Intrasulcular Incision

Make an intrasulcular incision in the gingiva circumferentially around the tooth or teeth to be extracted utilizing a number 15 or 15C scalpel blade. This is the first step in all surgical extractions.

11.7.6 Create a Flap

Several principles of flap design must be considered when planning the mucoperiosteal flap. The base (apical portion) of the flap must be broader than the free margin (coronal portion). The flap must be large enough to allow for adequate visualization of the area. Soft tissue heals across the incision not along the length of the incision and sharp incisions heal more rapidly than torn tissue.

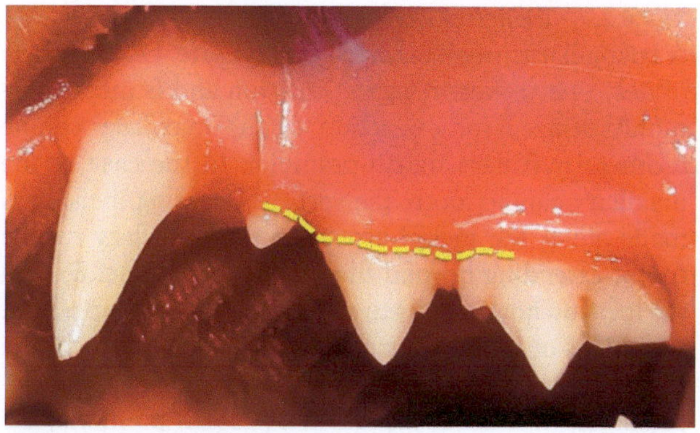

Figure 11.2 Envelope flap.

Therefore, a long straight incision heals more rapidly than a short, torn incision [9]. The flap should be designed to avoid injury to local vital structures, which include neurovascular bundles and salivary ducts. For oral surgery procedures in dogs and cats, an envelope flap, a triangular flap, or a broad-based pedicle flap may be utilized depending on the location of the tooth to be extracted, the patient, and surgeon preferences.

11.7.6.1 Envelope Flap

An envelope flap (Figure 11.2) is a full thickness flap created by a making a horizontal incision in the gingival sulcus at the crestal bone, followed by elevation of the attached gingival tissue with a periosteal elevator. The horizontal incision may extend to just the mesial and distal aspect of the tooth involved or it may be extended beyond the tooth to be extracted to incorporate adjacent teeth, which allows for greater flap reflection and exposure [10]. If the envelope flap is not elevated apical to the mucogingival line then it is considered a mucogingival flap not a mucoperiosteal flap.

11.7.6.2 Mucoperiosteal Flap

A mucoperiosteal flap is a full thickness flap, elevated beyond the mucogingival line to include the periosteum. A mucoperiosteal flap is utilized to improve visualization and facilitate exposure of the furcation and periodontal ligament space around the tooth roots. A triangular mucoperiosteal flap includes only one vertical releasing incision that extends apical to the mucogingival line. A pedicle or broad-based flap is a four-cornered flap created with two vertical releasing incisions. Triangular and broad-based flaps are often utilized when the removal of buccal alveolar bone (alveolectomy) is necessary. To prevent flap failure, adhere to the following principles: the apical portion of the flap should be wider than the coronal portion, the edges of the flap should be approximated over healthy bone, the flap should be gently handled, and the flap should be sutured without any tension [11].

11.7.6.2.1 Triangular Flap

A triangular (three-cornered) flap (Figure 11.3) consists of only one vertical releasing incision and is most commonly utilized for extraction of the maxillary canine tooth or maxillary fourth premolar. In the case of the maxillary canine tooth, the vertical releasing incision is made along the mesial aspect of the maxillary canine tooth, extending beyond the mucogingival line. Extend the incision horizontally to create an envelope flap within the sulcus of the teeth to the mid or distal aspect of the second premolar [12]. To create a triangular mucoperiosteal flap to extract the maxillary fourth premolar, the vertical incision is made starting 5 mm apical to the mucogingival line at the mesial aspect of the maxillary fourth premolar tooth along the mesial aspect of the alveolar juga of the mesiobuccal root. Continue the vertical releasing incision ventrally to the gingival attachment at the crown. The incision is then extended in a horizontal direction within the gingival sulcus, deep enough to reach the alveolar crestal bone, to the distal aspect of the maxillary fourth premolar. If more surgical exposure of the buccal bone over the distal root is needed, the incision can be extended to the distobuccal line angle of the maxillary first molar [13].

11.7.6.2.2 Pedicle Flap

To create a pedicle or broad-based (four-cornered) flap (Figure 11.4), make an intrasulcular incision around the tooth, then make two divergent vertical releasing incisions at the mesial and distal aspects of the tooth, which extend beyond the mucogingival line. The flap should be broad based to ensure adequate blood supply to the gingival margin. The vertical releasing incisions should be planned so the flap is wider than the area of the planned buccal bone removal. Properly placed incisions allow the wound margins to be sutured over intact, healthy bone that is a few millimeters away from the damaged bone, thereby providing support for the healing wound [11].

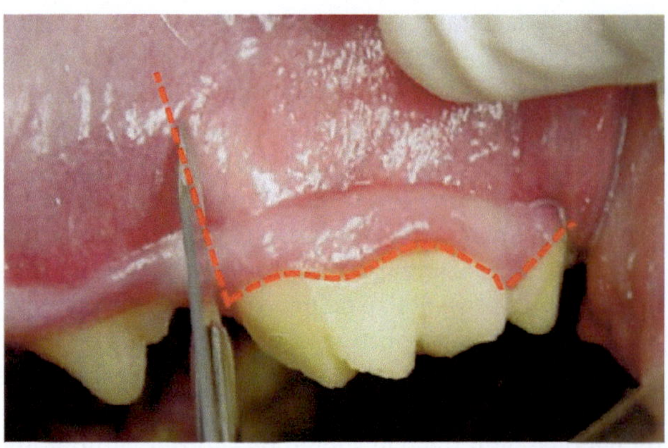

Figure 11.3 Triangular flap maxillary fourth premolar.

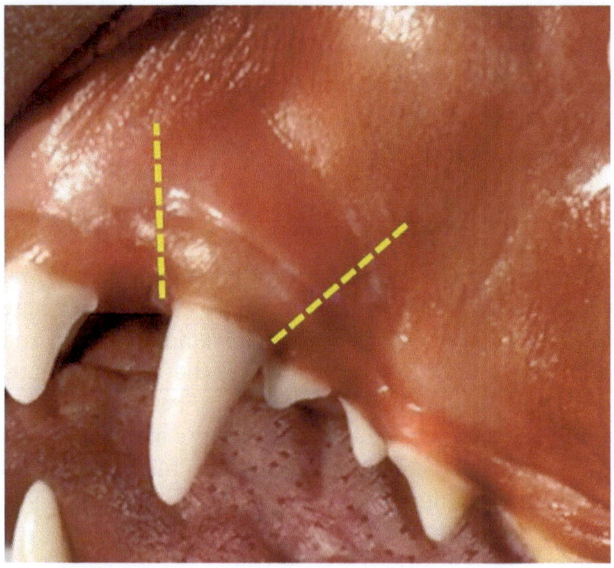

Figure 11.4 Broad-based pedicle flap canine tooth.

To make the vertical releasing incision, hold the alveolar mucosal tissue taught and use a number 15 or 15C scalpel blade with a firm, continuous stroke [11], pressing the scalpel blade down to the bone through the mucosa, submucosa, and periosteum. Care should be taken to avoid major vessels, nerves, and salivary ducts. After creating the vertical releasing incisions, carefully elevate the flap from the underlying alveolar bone using a freer or molt periosteal elevator. To reflect the attached gingival tissue, begin at the mesial or distal end of the free gingival margin. The attached gingiva is tightly adhered to the underlying alveolar bone and careful elevation in this area prevents tearing of the flap. Utilize the periosteal elevator in rotating lateral and pushing strokes to pry and elevate the attached gingival tissue from the underlying bone. Care must be taken to avoid perforation of the flap at the mucogingival line. Once apical to the mucogingival line, the elevator is then pushed apically and laterally to reflect the alveolar mucosa and periosteum from the underlying bone. When extraction of more than one tooth in a quadrant is indicated, a single mucoperiosteal flap is created to include all teeth that are being extracted.

11.7.7 Alveolectomy (Removal of Buccal Alveolar Bone)

Some buccal bone is removed from the root surface to facilitate tooth extraction. Use a small round bur in a highspeed handpiece with a light paintbrush or sweeping motion. The size of the round bur correlates with the size of the tooth being extracted. Some clinicians utilize a cross-cut fissure bur to remove alveolar bone by laying

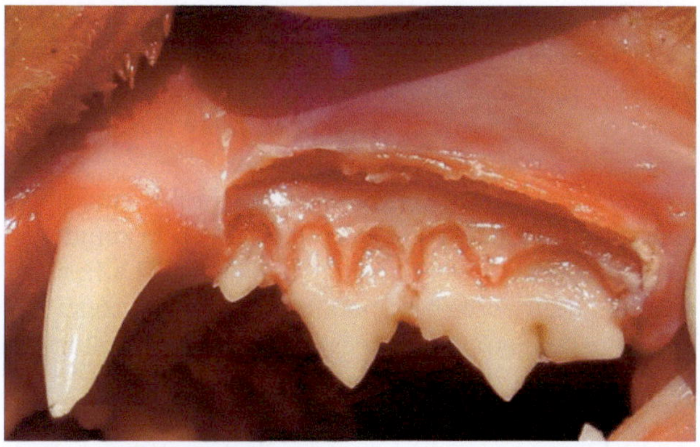

Figure 11.5 Buccal bone alveolectomy – maxilla cat.

the long axis of the bur against the alveolar bone. Start with the removal of the buccal bone from the coronal half of the root surface. The alveolar jugae (boney prominence over the root) is used to guide the removal of the buccal alveolar bone overlying the tooth root. Extend the bone removal mesially and distally to expose the periodontal ligament space on either side of the tooth root. The width of the buccal bone removal is the same width as the tooth root (Figure 11.5). Clear visualization of the periodontal ligament space allows the surgeon to properly place the dental elevator or luxator. The radiographic anatomy of the tooth root should be referenced during alveolectomy. A bulbous apical portion of the root may require additional bone removal to facilitate removal of the bulbous portion of the root through the smaller alveolus.

11.7.8 Section Multirooted Teeth

Section teeth into single root tooth segments to allow for easier extraction. Use either a crosscut taper fissure bur (701, 701L, 702) or a round bur in a highspeed handpiece with water irrigation, beginning at the furcation and working coronally. The tooth should be sectioned keeping in mind the anatomy of the tooth roots and the goal of placement of the dental elevator in the periodontal ligament space of each tooth root during elevation. Utilization of clear dental models allows the operator to visualize normal anatomy prior to sectioning. Remember that the tooth is being extracted, so removal of additional portions of the tooth crown is often helpful to facilitate proper placement of the elevators and luxators into the periodontal ligament space.

The tooth should be sectioned to allow "straight line" access to the periodontal ligament space with the dental elevator. If the tooth is sectioned perpendicular to the alveolar bone margin without taking into account the normal divergent anatomy of the tooth roots, it is difficult to properly place the dental elevator into the periodontal ligament space. When sectioning two rooted premolars in the dog and cat, begin at the furcation and create two separate cuts to remove a diamond-shaped piece of crown (Figure 11.6). Sectioning the teeth in this manner allows placement of the dental elevator into the periodontal ligament space in line with the tooth root as the diamond portion of the tooth crown is no longer present. To confirm that the tooth roots are appropriately sectioned, a dental elevator may be placed horizontally between the tooth roots at the level of the alveolar bone and gently turned. If properly sectioned each root should move independently of the other. If they move together, the sectioning is not complete.

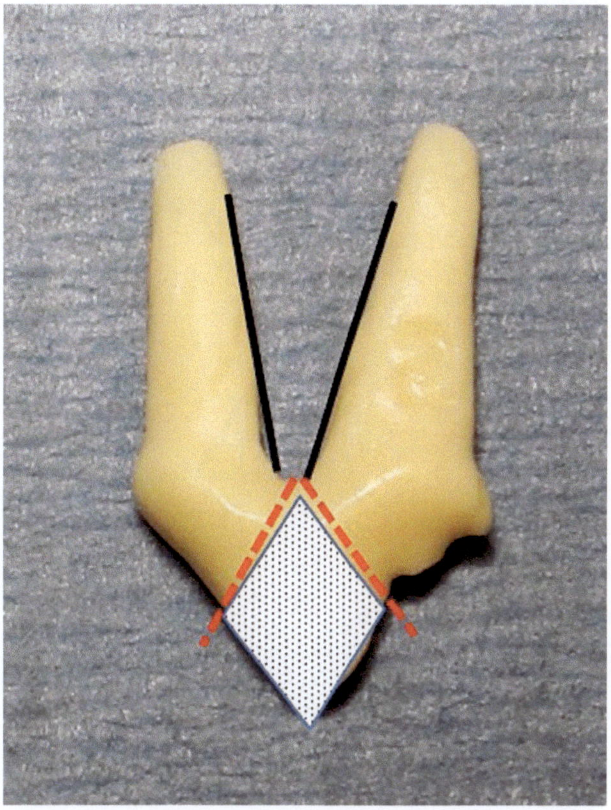

Figure 11.6 Sectioning premolar with diamond cuts.

When sectioning the mandibular first molar in the dog, two separate cuts allow for easier access to the periodontal ligament space of both roots (Figure 11.7). Extraction of the distal root first allows for easier access to the mesial root. If necessary the "bulge" of the distal and mesial crowns can be removed for easier access (yellow solid lines) [14].

When sectioning the mandibular first molar in a cat, begin at the furcation and proceed coronally in line with the mesial side of the distal root. Make an additional horizontal cut in the distal crown to remove a rectangular piece of the tooth crown (Figure 11.8). This additional cut decreases the incidence of breaking the distal root

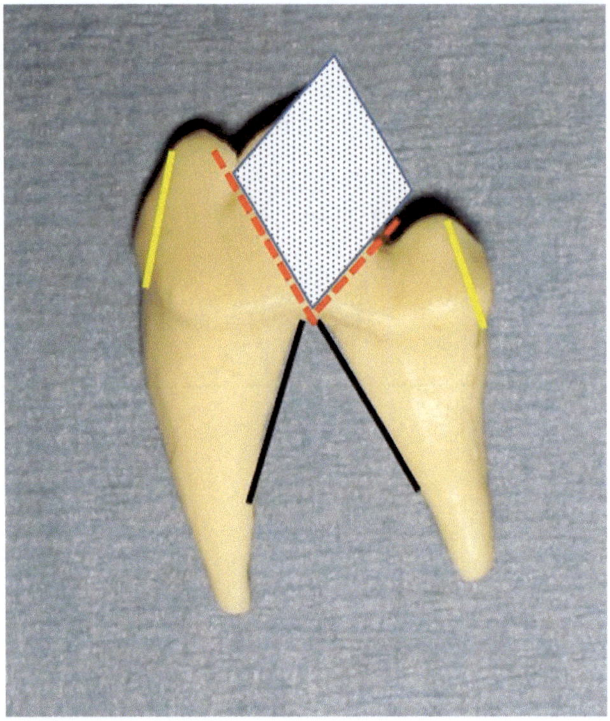

Figure 11.7 Sectioning the mandibular first molar in the dog.

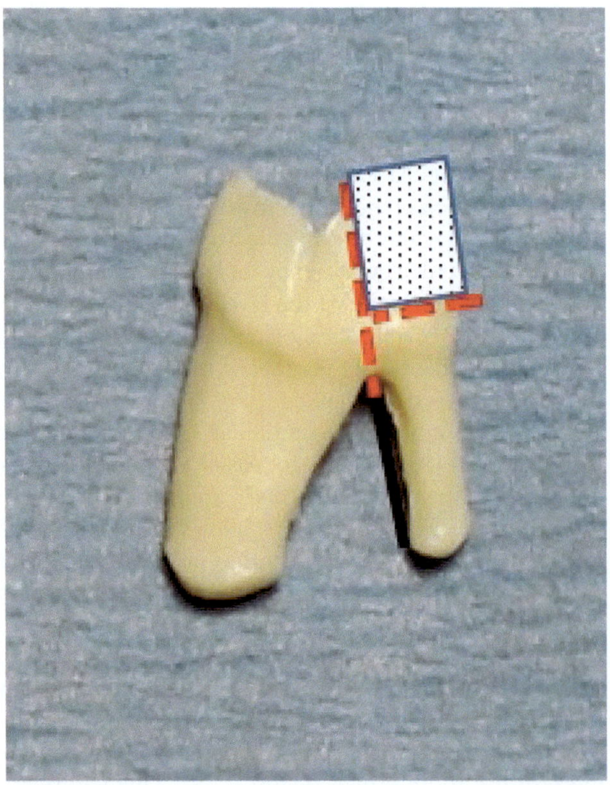

Figure 11.8 Sectioning the mandibular first molar in the cat.

during elevation and extraction as it eliminates the long "lever arm" of the distal crown and allows for easier access to the mesial portion of the distal root. Extract the distal root first. Once it is removed, there is clear access to the distal portion of the mesial root.

Sectioning the maxillary fourth premolar into single rooted segments involves two cuts. Keep in mind that the palatal root diverges slightly palatally. The first cut sections the two mesial roots from the distal root. The second cut separates the mesiobuccal and palatal roots. Do not begin elevation of tooth roots until all three roots are distinct and separate. The direction of the first cut is dependent upon which root will be elevated first. Sectioning as illustrated in Figure 11.9a allows easiest access to the mesial aspect of the distal root, and in this case the distal root should be elevated first. Alternatively, the operator may elect to make both cuts, removing the "diamond" portion of the tooth crown, as discussed previously for two-rooted premolar teeth (Figure 11.9b). If it is difficult to access the distal side of the distal root with the dental elevator, the distal "bulge" of the crown of the maxillary fourth premolar can be removed (yellow solid line). Care must be taken not to damage the maxillary first molar. The palatal root is sectioned by positioning the bur nearly parallel to the longitudinal axis of the tooth, perpendicular to the palate. Begin at the furcation between the two mesial roots and section mesial to distal (Figure 11.9c). It may be necessary to use a surgical length bur to section the mesiobuccal from the palatal root in large breed dogs. The palatal root of the maxillary fourth premolar should be elevated and extracted *after* the mesiobuccal and distal roots have been extracted. Removal of the interradicular alveolar bone on the buccal aspect of the palatal root provides better visualization of the palatal root and facilitates extraction.

The maxillary first molar in the dog is a three-rooted tooth, with a large palatal root and two smaller buccal roots. Sectioning of this tooth requires two cuts. The first cut begins at the furcation between the two buccal roots and extends to the buccal side of the palatal root. The second cut separates the palatal root from the two buccal roots (Figure 11.10). As with the fourth premolar tooth, do not begin elevation of the tooth roots until all three roots are distinct and separate [15].

11.7.9 Elevate Each Tooth Root Segment

When utilizing the dental elevator gently cradle the patient's head in your opposite hand to allow the delivery of controlled force and neutralize the pressure applied during tooth extraction. Always work with the apex of the tooth away from you so the periosteal elevator and dental elevator or luxator tip are directed away from you. Grasp the dental elevator or luxator with the handle in

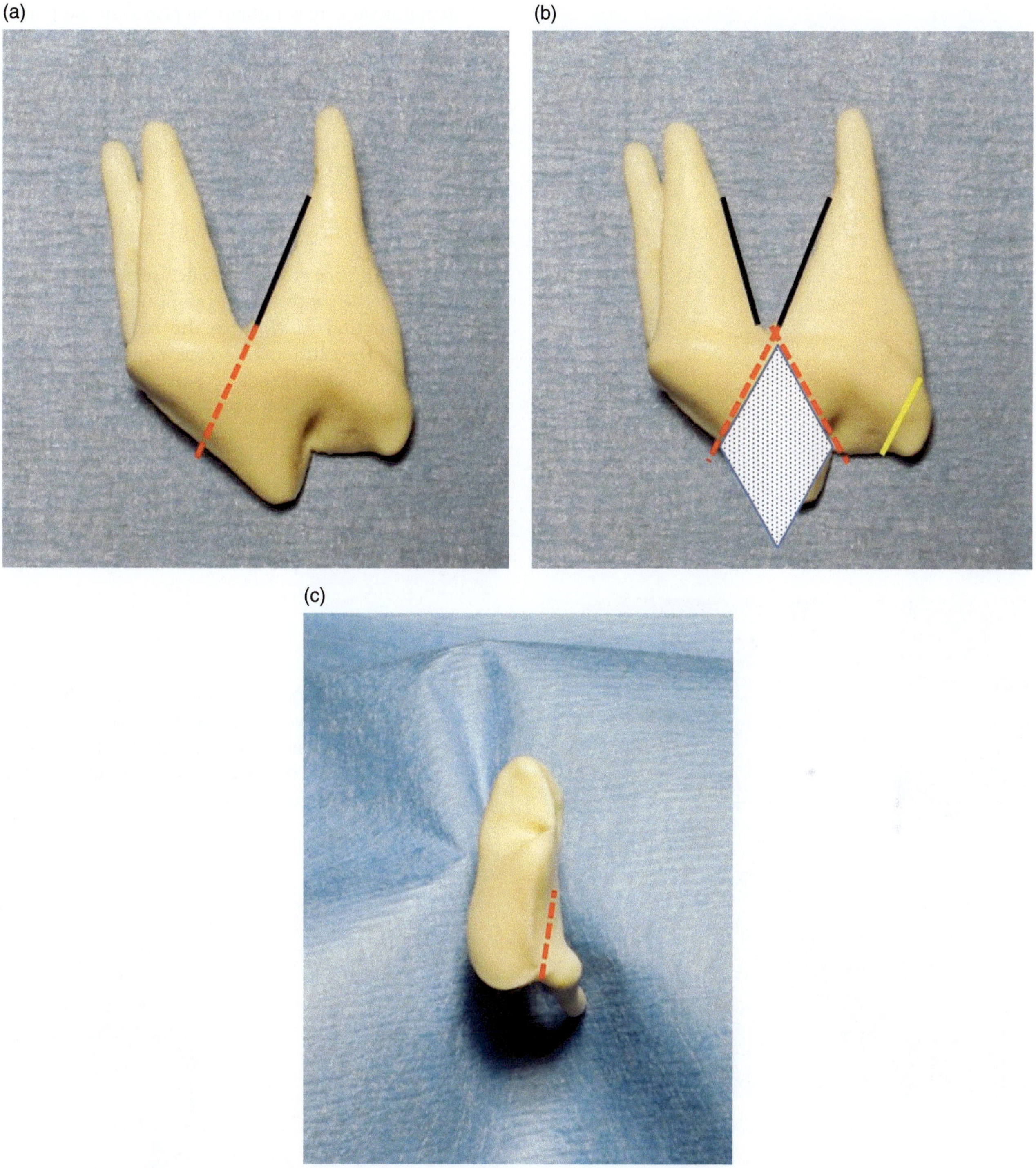

Figures 11.9 Sectioning the maxillary fourth premolar: (a) first cut; (b) diamond cut and distal bulge cut; (c) palatal root sectioning.

the palm of your hand and with your index finger extending down the shaft to within a few millimeters of the tip of the instrument (Figure 11.11). This short finger stop is very important as it prevents inadvertent penetration of the submandibular space, orbital region, or nasal cavity if the elevator slips.

Introduce a dental elevator into the space between the tooth and alveolar bone that is occupied by the periodontal ligament. Rotate the elevator and hold steady pressure for 15–30 seconds to facilitate stretching and tearing of the periodontal ligament fibers. Controlled force with prolonged steady pressure will assist in elevation

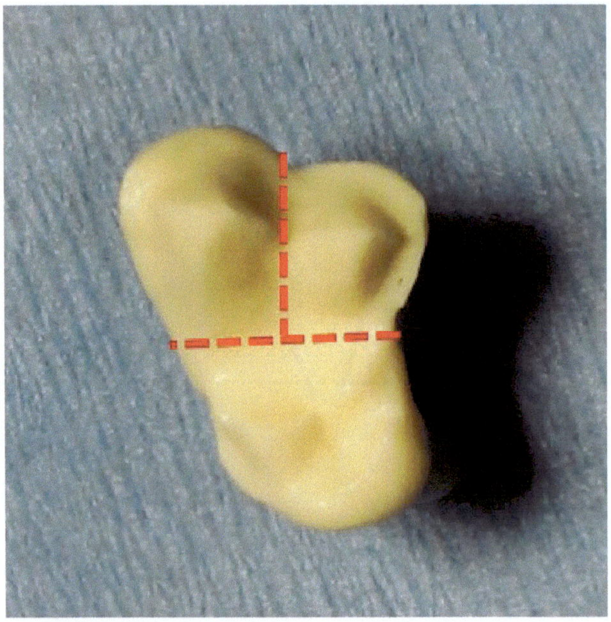

Figure 11.10 Sectioning the maxillary first molar.

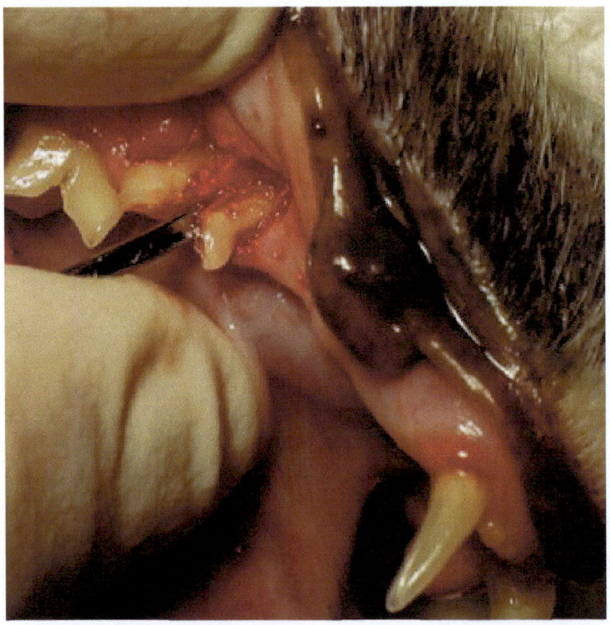

Figure 11.11 Short finger stop with elevator.

of the tooth and prevent inadvertent fracture of the root. As space allows, the elevator is then placed further apically into the periodontal ligament space and the process is repeated. Continue elevating circumferentially around the tooth until the tooth is loose. The dental elevator can also be used to create horizontal rotation by placing it perpendicular to the line of the tooth with a fulcrum point on the alveolar bone or on adjacent teeth if the tooth is also to be extracted [1].

A dental luxator may initially be placed in the periodontal ligament space and moved side to side to create a cutting action at the luxator tip. The luxator is pressed apically to sever the periodontal ligament creating a wedging force [1]. Luxators are made of softer metal and should not be rotated as the thin tip of the instrument will bend and break.

11.7.10 Extract Each Tooth Root Segment

After the tooth root is very mobile, use extraction forceps to grasp the tooth root segment near the cementoenamel junction as close to the root as possible. Gently rotate the extraction forceps along the long axis of the root and simultaneously pull the root segment coronally. Avoid applying excessive force as this may lead to tooth fracture. Carefully examine the extracted root. An intact root should have a smooth rounded apex. Obtain a postoperative radiograph to ensure that the entire tooth root segment has been removed and that no damage has occurred to the surrounding bone during the extraction process.

11.7.11 Alveoplasty (Alveoloplasty: Bone Recontouring)

Use a medium grit football or round diamond bur in a highspeed handpiece with water coolant to remove any diseased bone and to smooth rough alveolar bone edges (Figure 11.12). Palpate the extraction site to confirm that no sharp boney projections remain.

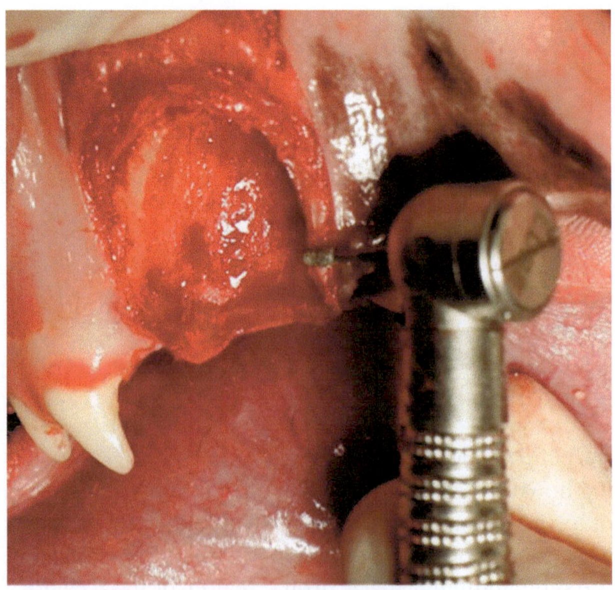

Figure 11.12 Alveoplasty (alveoloplasty).

11.7.12 Debride and Flush the Alveolus

Introduce a Miller bone curette or spoon curette into the alveolus to remove granulation tissue, debris, necrotic bone, and bone fragments from the alveolus. The empty alveolus is flushed with saline or 0.12% chlorhexidine to remove any persistent debris.

11.7.13 Release the Periosteum

Before the mucoperiosteal flap is closed, the periosteum must be incised along the entire width of the flap to eliminate tension on the flap. While holding the mucoperiosteal flap gently with thumb forceps, incise the periosteum on the alveolar bone side of the mucoperiosteal flap just apical to the mucogingival line to "release" the flap. This can be accomplished with a scalpel blade, the back side of the scalpel blade, or with iris scissors (Figure 11.13a and b). The periosteum is properly "released" when the mucoperiosteal flap easily covers the empty alveolus and allows tension-free closure of the flap. Elevate the lingual or palatal mucosa and 2–3 mm of the attached gingival tissue on the mesial and distal sides of the extraction site to allow for easier placement of the needle when suturing. Debride all tissue edges prior to flap closure.

11.7.14 Suture the Mucoperiosteal Flap

The suture line should be supported by intact healthy bone. When placing the sutures, place the needle though the mucosal tissue at a right angle to make the smallest possible hole in the mucosal flap [9]. With an envelope flap, sutures are placed in the interdental papilla only. When closing a mucoperiosteal flap the objective is to hold the flap in position and appose the wound edges. The purpose of the suture is to approximate the tissues; therefore, the sutures should not be tied too tightly. Knots should be placed so they do not fall directly on the incision line, but instead should be located to the side of the incision. Knots placed directly on the incision line cause additional pressure on the incision line [9].

The mucoperiosteal flap is apposed to the palatal or lingual mucosal tissue with simple interrupted 4-0 or 5-0 absorbable sutures utilizing a reverse cutting or tapered needle. Sutures should be placed 2–3 mm apart and 2–3 mm from the flap edges without tension [9]. Suture pattern and choice of suture material is at the discretion of the surgeon. Simple interrupted sutures are most commonly used in oral surgery as they can be placed quickly and if a knot becomes untied the remaining sutures are still present. Horizontal mattress sutures decrease the number of sutures needed, evert the wound edges, and compress the wound together slightly. A continuous suture pattern is quicker, with fewer knots to collect debris. The disadvantage of the continuous pattern is that if one suture pulls through the entire suture line loosens or if the knot becomes untied the entire suture line becomes untied [9].

(a)

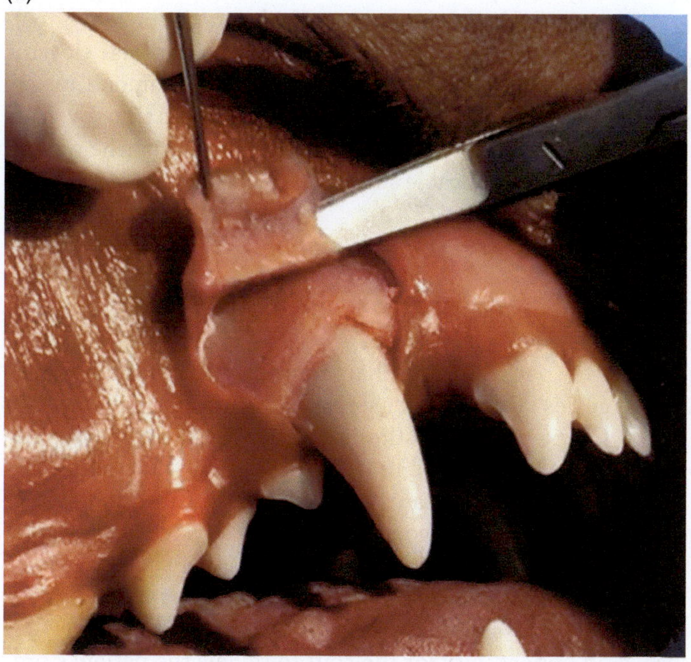

(b)

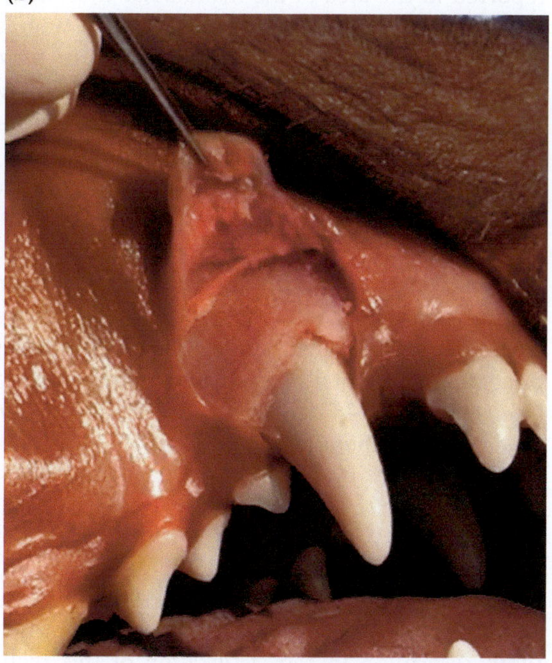

Figures 11.13 (a, b) Periosteal release maxillary canine tooth.

11.8 Specific Tooth Considerations

11.8.1 Extraction of Deciduous Teeth

Exodontia is indicated in immature patients with fractured deciduous teeth, persistent deciduous teeth, and maloccluded deciduous teeth. Awareness of the location of the developing permanent tooth bud is an important consideration during extraction of deciduous teeth as care must be taken not to damage the developing unerupted permanent tooth bud. All permanent teeth erupt lingual to their deciduous tooth counterpart except for the permanent maxillary canine tooth, which erupts mesial to the deciduous tooth. Closed extraction techniques are indicated when the deciduous tooth is mobile or there is a substantial amount of root resorption [16]. If little or no resorption has occurred, an open extraction technique may be preferred. The principles of mucoperiosteal flap creation and flap closure previously described apply to deciduous tooth extraction.

11.8.2 Canine Mandibular First Molar

In small breed dogs the apices of the mandibular first molar teeth are often in close proximity to the ventral cortex of the mandible. Severe periodontal or endodontic disease affecting the mandibular first molar tooth may result in significant bone loss and compromise the integrity of the mandible. Intraoral radiographs are necessary to evaluate the proximity of the apices of the tooth to the mandibular canal and the integrity of the surrounding alveolar bone. Pathologic fractures have been reported in the area of the mandibular first molar secondary to severe bone loss or as a result of trauma to a compromised mandible. Iatrogenic fracture may also occur during extraction of a severely diseased mandibular first molar in a small breed dog (see Chapter 13 – Oral Surgery – Fracture and Trauma Repair).

In cases where the distal root is severely affected by periodontal disease and the mesial root is unaffected, then hemisection of the tooth may be completed. The tooth is sectioned, the distal root is extracted, and the mesial root is treated endodontically. There are times where osseous regeneration techniques may be appropriate for periodontally diseased mandibular first molars (see Chapter 10 – Oral Surgery – Periodontal Surgery) for osseous regeneration techniques).

11.9 Coronectomy (Crown Amputation with Intentional Root Retention)

Coronectomy has been described as a treatment for tooth resorption in cats. Utilization of this technique requires preoperative dental radiographs to rule out concurrent endodontic or periodontal disease. Any tooth with concurrent endodontic or periodontal pathology must be treated by extraction. Any tooth associated with ulceroproliferative disease should be completely extracted. If a visible, normal periodontal ligament space is present on the radiographs (type 1 tooth resorption – TR), then proceed with surgical extraction as previously described [17, 18].

The practice of blindly pulverizing a fractured or resorbing root using a bur on a highspeed handpiece is contrary to the principles of oral surgery and is discouraged. Potential complications of root pulverization include air embolism, subcutaneous emphysema, inadvertent penetration of the nasal cavity, and displacement of the root apex into the nasal cavity or mandibular canal [1].

Radiographically, with type 2 tooth resorption (root replacement resorption) the periodontal ligament space is not visible, the root structure is not clearly defined, and is similar in density to the surrounding alveolar bone. In this instance, coronectomy may be performed. A small envelope flap is created with a periosteal elevator. The gingiva is minimally reflected to expose the tooth and marginal alveolar bone. If necessary, make two small interproximal gingival incisions located mesial and distal to the affected tooth. Retract the gingiva and use a number two round bur in a highspeed handpiece with water coolant to amputate the affected tooth at or slightly below the alveolar crest. It is important to remove all visible tooth structure. Cut almost all the way through the tooth but avoid cutting all the way through the tooth to avoid inadvertent damage to the lingual or palatal mucosal tissue. Use an extraction forceps to "break" the crown off. Elevate the lingual or palatal mucosa from the bone with a periosteal elevator (Figure 11.14). Utilize a medium grit diamond bur to remove the remaining tooth structure and smooth sharp boney projections (Figure 11.15) and suture the gingiva with an absorbable suture.

11.10 Oral Surgery Postoperative Care

The patient is discharged with postoperative analgesics that are customized to each patient (see Chapter 9 – Anesthesia and Pain Management). The client is instructed to feed the pet a soft diet (either softened kibble or canned food) for 7–14 days and the pet is not allowed access to treats or toys that may affect the sutures during the post-operative period. A two-week complimentary recheck examination allows the surgeon to recheck the oral surgery sites and provides an opportunity for the staff to review the patient's preventive oral health care program with the client.

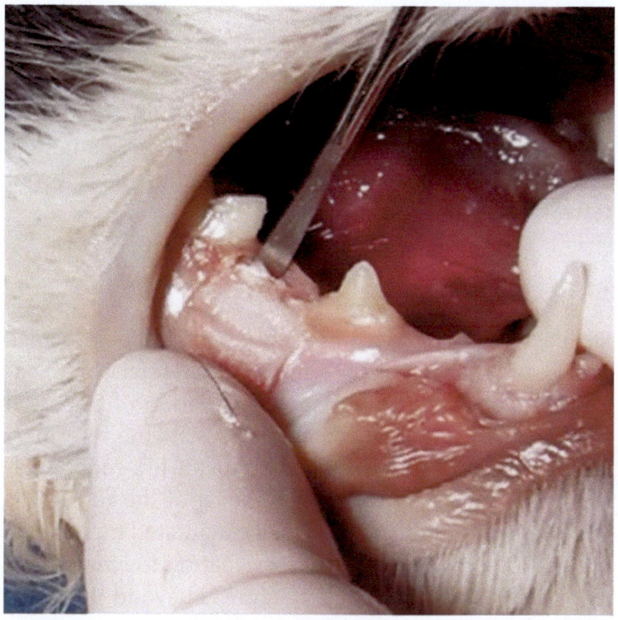

Figure 11.14 Elevate palatal or lingual mucosal tissue.

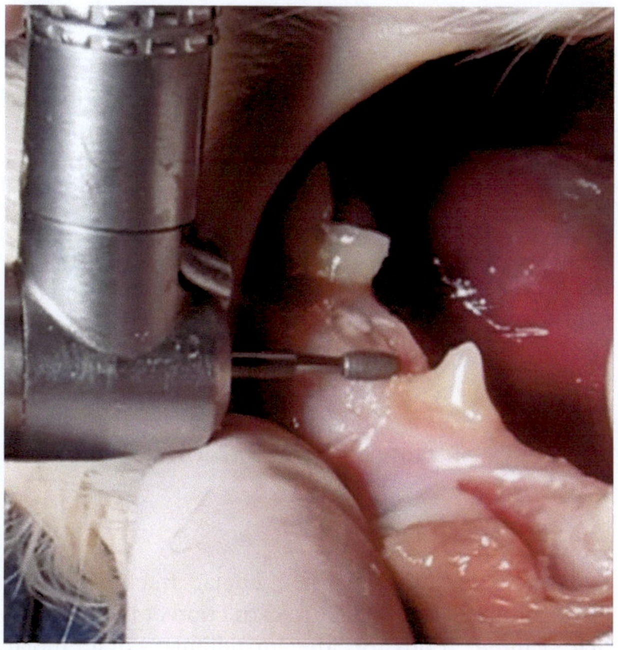

Figure 11.15 Alveoplasty with diamond bur.

11.11 Complications

The goal of all extractions is to extract the entire tooth without damage to surrounding structures. One of the most common complications during tooth extraction is fracture of the tooth root. Other potential extraction complications include: displacement of the root tip into the mandibular canal, nasal cavity or maxillary sinus, hemorrhage, trauma to adjacent structures, sublingual edema, salivary mucocele, emphysema, air embolism, mandibular and maxillary fractures, oronasal fistula, ophthalmic complications, and local or systemic infection [19, 20]. When the mandibular canine tooth is extracted in dogs, the tongue may occasionally hang out the mouth on the side of the extracted tooth. Lip entrapment by the mandibular canine tooth has been reported following extraction of a maxillary canine tooth [1].

The easiest way to avoid surgical complications is through adequate preparation. Preoperative radiographs should always be obtained prior to starting oral surgery to carefully evaluate the entire tooth, including the apex and the surrounding bone. Proper instrumentation, including a highspeed handpiece and sharp dental elevators, will assist in successful extraction. It is important that the operator use controlled forces and a proper technique when extracting teeth. In addition, the skill and knowledge of the veterinarian should always be considered. If you are not comfortable with a particular procedure based on your knowledge, skill, and/or the pathology that is present, it is best to refer the patient to a board certified veterinary dentist.

11.11.1 Fractured Tooth Roots

It is important to remove adequate alveolar bone and section all multirooted teeth prior to attempting elevation of the tooth roots. Anatomic variations in root structure, including hooked, curved, or bulbous roots can predispose the root to fracture during extraction [21]. In addition, many roots are not circular but often have longitudinal grooves along the apical–coronal axis [21]. The "bad sound" of a cracking root gives the surgeon a clue to the potential for an existing complication. Always inspect the extracted tooth root for a smooth round apex. If there is a rough or jagged edge to the root, there is probably still a root remnant remaining in the alveolus. Always take post-extraction radiographs to document complete extraction of the entire tooth and root without damage to the surrounding bone. Sometimes, despite our best attempts, tooth roots fracture during oral surgery to extract the tooth and additional surgery is needed to extract the root tip.

If the root was mobile prior to root fracture, it is sometimes possible to elevate and extract the remaining root tip without removal of additional bone using small elevators or root tip picks. In most instances it is advantageous to remove additional buccal bone to improve visualization and identification of the root tip. It may be quicker and less traumatic for the patient to complete an open exposure for retrieval of a fractured root tip [9]. Adequate lighting and magnification greatly assist in the retrieval of fractured root tips.

The end of the fractured root will usually be sharp and irregular. If the fracture is oblique, the direction of the fracture line provides valuable information about how the remaining tooth root is positioned within the alveolus. Intraoperative radiographs confirm the anatomy of the remaining root, the structures adjacent to the fractured root, and pathology associated with the surrounding bone. If the root tip is not mobile, removal of additional alveolar bone exposes the remaining root structure and assists in identification of the periodontal ligament space. Keep in mind the anatomy of the area, particularly the location of neurovascular bundles, the mandibular canal, and the nasal cavity. Place a small dental elevator into the periodontal ligament space of the root fragment and gently rotate. Do not use apical pressure as excessive apical pressure can displace the root tip into the nasal cavity, maxillary sinus, or mandibular canal. In the case of very small root tips, an 18- or 20-gauge needle can be utilized as an elevator. In addition, a small round bur (½ or 1) can be introduced into the alveolus to create a "moat" circumferentially around the root to allow introduction of an instrument (elevator, luxator, or root tip pick) into this expanded periodontal ligament space [21]. Root tip extraction forceps with fine tips may be utilized to assist in the removal of a mobile tooth root from the alveolus.

What if the attempt to remove the root tip is unsuccessful? When can root tips be left in place? Root tips can be left in place only if the risks of surgery to remove the root tip outweigh the benefits of removing the root tip. To leave a fractured root tip in place, the root tip must be small, deep within the alveolus, the tooth must not be infected, and there must be no periapical radiolucency visible radiographically. A root tip may *not* be left in place if there is any evidence of periodontal disease or potential for endodontic disease (complicated crown fracture, uncomplicated crown fracture, pulp hemorrhage, radiographic evidence of periapical pathology) associated with the root tip. The risks of proceeding with additional surgery that may outweigh the benefits of the root tip removal include: the patient is not stable under anesthesia; continued attempts at root retrieval may impact vital structures (nerves and vessels within the mandibular canal, the nasal cavity, or orbit); continued attempts may result in significant destruction of surrounding bone or soft tissues; or continued attempts may result in displacement of the root tip into the mandibular canal, nasal cavity, or retrobulbar space [9].

If the benefit of fractured root removal does not outweigh the risks, and the surgeon elects to leave the root tip in place, then an intraoral radiograph must be taken to document the remaining root structure. The clients must be informed of the decision, the reason for the decision, and the possible clinical sequelae that may result from the retained root tip. The medical record should document the decision to leave the root tip in place. Radiographs of the retained root should be obtained annually to determine if there is any pathology associated with the remaining root fragment and if root retrieval is indicated.

11.11.2 Displacement of Root Tips

Displacement of a tooth root into the mandibular canal, nasal cavity, or maxillary sinus is a potential complication of root tip retrieval. Careful elevation of fractured root tips with minimal apical force assists the veterinarian in preventing root tip displacement. If a root is displaced into a cavity or canal, removal of the root tip is recommended. Removal is usually facilitated by removal of additional bone and careful evaluation to identify the displaced root tip. If this procedure is beyond the capability of the veterinarian the case should be referred to a veterinary dentist.

11.11.3 Hemorrhage and Trauma to Soft Tissues

Excessive bleeding may originate from the extraction site or from trauma to vascular structures or soft tissue during the extraction. Hemorrhage usually results from the use of uncontrolled forces with the dental elevator and "slipping" into the sublingual area, buccal mucosal tissue, infraorbital vessels, or mandibular canal. Bleeding may occur after the tooth root is extracted if there is a large area of granulation tissue present at the tooth apex. Hemorrhage can usually be controlled with ligation of the lacerated vessel, direct pressure, use of an absorbable hemostatic gelatin sponge, or suturing of the gingiva over the alveolus to allow formation of a clot.

11.11.4 Mandibular and Maxillary Fractures

Pathologic or iatrogenic mandibular fractures occur most commonly secondary to extraction of the mandibular canine tooth or the mandibular first molar (Figure 11.16). The fracture may occur due to pre-existing periodontal or endodontic disease or excessive force used by the operator or a combination. Pre-extraction radiographs are always indicated to accurately evaluate the surrounding alveolar bone and to plan for a successful surgical extraction. Creation of a mucoperiosteal flap, removal of buccal bone, sectioning of the tooth into single root segments, followed by very careful elevation and extraction of the affected tooth with controlled forces will assist in prevention of mandibular fractures during tooth extraction.

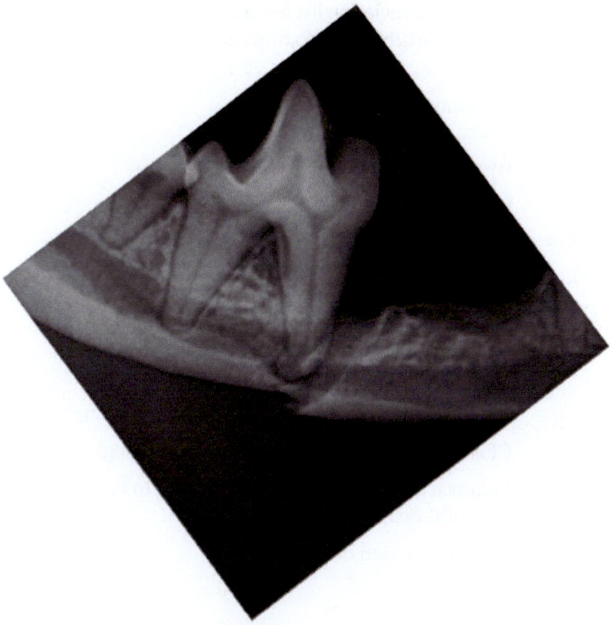

Figure 11.16 Radiograph of a pathologic fracture mesial to the mandibular first molar in a dog.

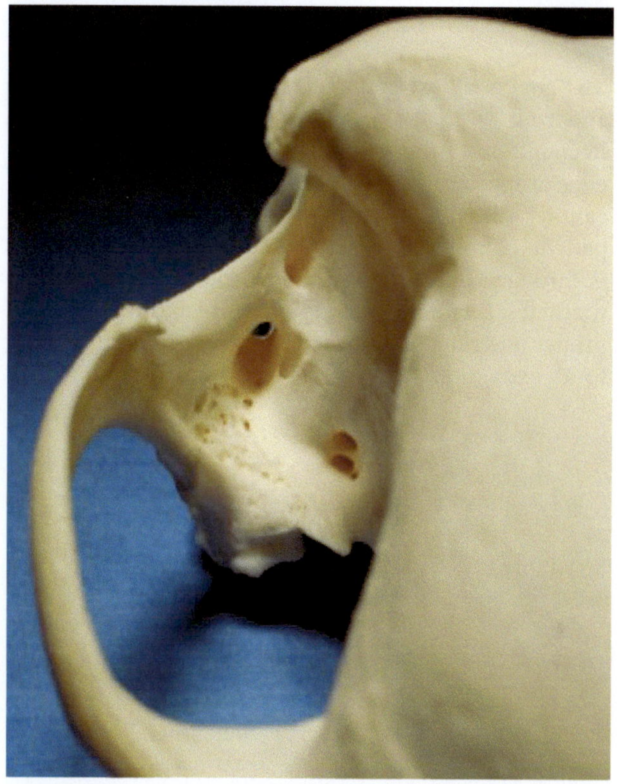

Figure 11.17 Caudal view of the orbit in a dog.

11.11.5 Oronasal Fistulas

Small breed dolichocephalic dogs are predisposed to the development of oronasal fistulas secondary to periodontal disease associated with the palatal aspect of the maxillary canine teeth. The shelf of bone separating the oral cavity from the nasal cavity is very thin on the palatal side of the maxillary canine tooth. Periodontal disease causing vertical bone loss in this area results in an oronasal fistula. An oronasal fistula may also occur if the maxillary first, second, and third premolars are affected by severe periodontal disease. If an oronasal fistula is visible at the time of extraction, debride the margins of the defect and create a mucoperiosteal flap to allow tension-free closure. Chronic oronasal fistulas can lead to rhinitis, resulting in mucopurulent or hemorrhagic nasal discharge and/or sneezing.

11.11.6 Ophthalmic Complications

Exodontic procedures performed in the caudal maxilla may be associated with orbital penetration, especially if there is concurrent periodontal disease [22]. The apices of the maxillary fourth premolar and first and second molars in the dog and the maxillary fourth premolar and first molar in the cat lie in close proximity to the ventral floor of the orbit and only a thin shelf of alveolar bone surrounds these tooth roots (Figure 11.17). The bony orbit of the dog and cat is incomplete. Soft tissues comprise the floor of the orbit and include the zygomatic salivary gland, orbital fat, and medial pterygoid muscle [23]. Inadvertent penetration of the orbital floor during caudal maxillary tooth extraction in dogs and cats is often multifactorial and related to regional anatomy, periodontal pathology, and improper or aggressive extraction techniques [22]. The orbit can easily be penetrated with a dental elevator if the tooth is affected by periodontitis and if a short finger stop is not utilized during extraction. Penetration of the globe may result in panophthalmitis and may ultimately result in enucleation of the affected eye. Use of controlled forces and a finger stop will assist the operator in prevention of this complication [20].

11.11.7 Neoplasia

Continued gingival inflammation in the area of previously extracted teeth or a non-healing oral surgery site may be due to the presence of underlying neoplasia. Pre-extraction radiographs identify abnormalities of the alveolar bone surrounding mobile teeth prior to extraction. Based on the radiographic findings, the operator may elect to biopsy the soft tissue and bone rather than extract mobile teeth. Mobile teeth always require intraoral radiographs prior to extraction.

11.12 Summary

The goal of all extractions is to extract the *entire* tooth and root without damage to surrounding structures. Recognition of the potential complications and knowledge of appropriate treatment methods for those complications will assist in minimizing pain and discomfort for patients. The easiest way to avoid surgical complications is through adequate preparation and evaluation of the tooth and surrounding bone structure and utilization of proper instrumentation with controlled forces during tooth extraction.

11.13 AVDC Resource – Abbreviations

See Table 11.1.

Table 11.1 AVDC abbreviation list for oral surgery – extractions (https://www.avdc.org/traineeinfo.html; accessed 3 March 2018).

	Definition
ALV	Alveolectomy/alveoloplasty
CR	Crown
CR/A	Crown amputation
DT	Deciduous tooth
DT/P	Persistent deciduous tooth
FX	Fracture (tooth or jaw; see T/FX for tooth fracture abbreviations)
X	Closed extraction of a tooth (without sectioning)
XS	Closed extraction of a tooth (with sectioning)
XS/ODY	Removal of interproximal crown tissue to facilitate transoral extraction of a tooth
XSS	Open extraction of a tooth

References

1 Holmstrom, S.E., Frost Fitch, P., and Eisner, E. (2004). *Veterinary Dental Techniques for the Small Animal Practitioner*, 3e, 291–338. Philadephia, PA: WB Saunders.

2 Anonymous. (2003). Recommendations and reports – guideline for infection control in dental health care settings. Atlanta: Centers for Disease Control – Morbidity and Mortality Weekly Report. 5 (2): (No. RR-17).

3 Verstaete, F.J.M. and Terpak, C.H. (1997). Anatomical variations in the dentition of the domestic cat. *J. Vet. Dent.* 14: 137–140.

4 Reiter, A.M. and Mendoza, K.A. (2002). Feline odontoclastic resorptive lesions. An unsolved enigma in veterinary dentistry. In: *Veterinary Clinic of a North American Small Animal Practice*, vol. 32(4) (ed. J. Harari), 791–837. Philadephia, PA: Saunders.

5 Hupp, J.R. (2014). Wound repair. In: *Contemporary Oral and Maxillofacial Surgery*, 6e (ed. J.R. Hupp, E. Ellis and M.R. Tucker), 43–53. St. Louis, MO: Elsevier Mosby.

6 Hupp, J.R. (2014). Principles of routine exodontia. In: *(eds) Contemporary Oral and Maxillofacial Surgery*, 6e (ed. J.R. Hupp, E. Ellis and M.R. Tucker), 88–118. St. Louis, MO: Elsevier Mosby.

7 Hupp, J.R. (2014). Infection control in surgical practice. In: *Contemporary Oral and Maxillofacial Surgery*, 6e (ed. J.R. Hupp, E. Ellis and M.R. Tucker), 54–64. St. Louis, MO: Elsevier Mosby.

8 Beckman, B. and Legendre, L. (2002). Regional nerve blocks for oral surgery in companion animals. *Compend. Cont. Ed. Pract. Vet.* 24: 439–444.

9 Hupp, J.R. (2014). Principles of more complex exodontia. In: *Contemporary Oral and Maxillofacial Surgery*, 6e (ed. J.R. Hupp, E. Ellis and M.R. Tucker), 119–142. St. Louis, MO: Elsevier Mosby.

10 De Bowes, L.J. (2005). Simple and surgical exodontia. In: *Veterinary Clinic of a North American Small Animimal Practice*, vol. 35(4) (ed. S.E. Holmstrom), 963–984. Philadephia. PA: Saunders.

11 Hupp, J.R. (2014). Principles of surgery. In: *Contemporary Oral and Maxillofacial Surgery*, 6e (ed. J.R. Hupp, E. Ellis and M.R. Tucker), 37–42. St. Louis, MO: Elsevier Mosby.

12 Beckman, B. (2012). Skills laboratory: how to extract a maxillary canine in dogs. *Vet. Med.* 107 (2): 68.

13 Peak, M. (2009; January). Surgical extraction maxillary fourth premolar tooth in a dog. *NAVC Clinician's Brief.* 59–62.

14 Manfra, M.S. (2005). Surgical extraction of the mandibular first molar in the dog. *J. Vet. Dent.* 19 (1): 46–50.

15 Vall, P. (2012). Maxillary molar tooth extraction in a dog. *J. Vet. Dent.* 29 (4): 276–284.

16 Hobson, P. (2005). Extraction of retained primary canine teeth in the dog. *J. Vet. Dent.* 22 (2): 132–135.

17 DuPont, G.A. (1995). Crown amputation with intentional root retention for advanced feline resorptive lesions – a clinical study. *J. Vet. Dent.* 12 (1): 9–13.

18 DuPont, G.A. (2002). Crown amputation with intentional root retention for dental resorptive lesions in cats. *J. Vet. Dent.* 19 (2): 107–110.

19 Reiter, A.M., Brady, C.A. et al. (2004). Local and systemic complications in a cat after poorly performed dental extractions. *J. Vet. Dent.* 21: 215–221.

20 Smith, M.M., Smith, E.M. et al. (2003). Orbital penetration associated with tooth extraction. *J. Vet. Dent.* 20: 8–17.

21 Woodward, T.M. (2006). Extraction of fractured tooth roots. *J. Vet. Dent.* 23 (2): 126–129.

22 Ramsey, D.T., Manfra M, S., Hamor, R.E. et al. (1996). Ophthalmic manifestations and complications of dental disease in dogs and cats. *J. Am. Anim. Hosp. Assoc.* 32: 215–226.

23 Murphy, C.J. and Pollock, R.V.S. (1993). The eye. In: *Miller's Anatomy of the Dog*, 3e (ed. H.E. Evans), 1030. Philadephia: WB Saunders.

12

Oral Surgery – General

Heidi B. Lobprise

Main Street Veterinary Dental Clinic, Flower Mound, TX, USA

12.1 Introduction

Tissues other than teeth, bone, and periodontal structures require surgical intervention at times. Basic surgical skills and rules for other body systems are often applicable, with some modifications. A good aseptic technique in the clean-contaminated environment of the oral cavity can be challenging, but should be followed when possible. Specific aspects from tissue healing to instrumentation and techniques are covered in greater detail in other texts that are good resources (see Suggested Reading).

12.1.1 Basic Surgical Principles

Tissues of the oral cavity tend to heal rapidly due to several factors, including more extensive monocytic phagocytic activity and epithelialization (compared to skin), warmer temperatures, high metabolic activity, higher mitotic rate, and an excellent blood supply [1]. The oral cavity's excellent blood supply can prove to be both a benefit and a hindrance to surgery: while hemostasis must be provided for proper visualization, preservation of major vessels is essential. The most significant vessels and nerves typically encountered are the maxillary and palatine structures of the maxilla, and the inferior alveolar neurovascular bundle of the mandible. Where possible, vascular structures should be preserved, even incorporated into retained tissue. If resection is necessary, then vessel identification, ligation, and hemorrhage control is vital.

Smaller scalpel blades are often an advantage in the restrictive spaces of the oral cavity. Tissue handling instruments (forceps, scissors) should be selected to provide delicate handling of the gingiva and mucosa, particularly when they are friable. Smaller, curved Metzenbaum scissors with serrated blades and delicate Adson 1X2 rat-tooth thumb forceps can be useful [2]. Right-angled forceps can be helpful to isolate vascular bundles for ligation and non-crushing forceps can secure tissues such as the tongue for temporary hemorrhage control during the procedure [1].

Preference for suture material may vary, but typically an absorbable product of 4-0 to –5-0 size with a swaged-on needle works best. The type and size of suture can be adjusted according to the size of the patient, condition, and thickness of the tissue and goal of the procedure. For extractions, synthetic absorbable material is recommended, and products that will stay intact longer (polyglacton 910 or polyglycolic acid) are preferred with oronasal fistula repair and other complicated procedures. In thin, friable tissue, a tapered needle may be preferred while a reverse cutting needle may be needed for thicker mucosa and gingiva.

A suture technique may also be adjusted according to need, often using a simple interrupted pattern and specialized patterns where indicated. Sutures should incorporate adequate bites of tissue and be secured snugly to resist loosening due to movement of the tongue and lips. A good rule of thumb to follow is the "3 × 3 × 3" rule, where the sutures are 3 mm apart, 3 mm from the incisional border, and the ends of the sutures are cut 3 mm long. For oral surgery, five to six throws should complete the knot due to the moist environment and tongue movement. Interdental sutures should allow for good approximation of tissues, and will keep the gingiva securely against the tooth. Position knots away from the incision line to prevent an accumulation of debris in the area. It is best not to have an incision line over a defect, but, most importantly, a suture line should never be placed under tension. Any suture line with tension should be expected to fail. It is also vital to provide a fresh edge or surface for adequate healing. Any chronic area or intact epithelial surface should be debrided to provide a fresh bleeding surface to promote rapid healing.

Hard tissues also require proper handling, as it is possible to injure or burn the bone surface with inappropriate use

Wiggs's Veterinary Dentistry: Principles and Practice, Second Edition. Edited by Heidi B. Lobprise and Johnathon R. (Bert) Dodd.

of burs on high-speed handpieces, lasers, or electro/radiosurgical units. All sharp and/or rough bony crests with spicules should be smoothed as in an alveoloplasty to avoid any further soft tissue damage, but excessive amounts of supportive bone should not be removed. Generally, no area of denuded bone should be left uncovered by soft tissue.

Pain management is an essential consideration with any form of surgery (see Chapter 9 – Anesthesia and Pain Management). Post-operative patient support with nutritive care and analgesia is critical in some cases.

12.1.2 Hemostasis During Oral Surgery

Digital pressure with a moist sponge for a short period of time will often be all that is needed for minor oral surgery. When more extensive oral surgery is anticipated, other means may be used to prevent blood loss, improve visualization, and decrease surgical time. Products to aid hemostasis include bone wax, oxidized regenerated cellulose, gelatin matrix (sponge or powder), microporous polysaccharide spheres (potato starch), microfibrillar (bovine) collagen and topical thrombins in gelatin matrix [2].

Electrosurgery or radiosurgery can provide either a cutting or hemostatic action, depending on the type of current used [3]. Fully rectified current provides easy cutting of most oral soft tissue, providing a good degree of hemostasis (50% cutting, 50% coagulation). It is useful for gingivectomy, gingivoplasty, palatal soft tissue surgery, frenectomy, and small soft tissue mass removal. A fully filtered current is the least traumatic of the four types and is used for delicate cutting, but little hemostasis is afforded (90% cutting, 10% coagulation). Any surgery close to cementum or bone benefits from this type of current, as well as biopsy specimens, gingival grafting, or even widening of the gingival sulcus for crowns. Partially rectified currents coagulate soft tissues for hemostasis where bleeding is a problem (90% coagulation, 10% cutting). The spark gap technique used at high power settings to produce the fulgurating current is the most destructive of the four and should be used cautiously. A variety of tip shapes and techniques (cutting action, point application) provide options for the practitioner.

12.1.3 Surgical Suction

Suction is an important part of maintaining good visualization and hemostasis during oral surgery. With the often times excellent blood supply, visualization to identify the source of bleeding can be difficult. Suction provides a dynamic means of visualizing bleeders and it is also very beneficial when searching for fractured roots. Bone generally bleeds when cut but a retained root does not, allowing for the surgeon to distinguish between bone and tooth root. "Look for the white pearl in the red sea."

12.1.4 Laser Surgery

Laser techniques in the oral cavity have been recommended with a variety of surgical applications including correction of elongated soft palates [4], tonsillectomy, and gingivectomy or gingivoplasty. Proliferative tissue can be removed in an alternating ablate and wipe technique, often as one part of multimodal therapy, and repeated as necessary. CO_2 lasers interact with water molecules in soft tissue, resulting in shallow thermal necrosis zones, while diode lasers penetrate deeper. Lower level laser therapy can be used as adjunctive therapy for analgesia and wound healing [3].

12.2 Palatal Defects

12.2.1 Repair Techniques for the Palate

When palatal defects disrupt the separation of the oral and nasal cavities, proper surgical techniques are essential for reconstruction. Surgical sites can be under constant stress due to the relative inelasticity of palatal mucosa and constant movement from both respiratory efforts and constant movement of the tongue. Two goals in flap design include tension-free flaps and the incorporation of an adequate blood supply. All tissue edges and any intact epithelial surface in the surgical field should be freshly debrided. Any flap design should be at least 1.5–2 times the size or width of the defect to be covered to allow for contracture of tissue, and sutures should not lie directly over the defect.

12.2.2 Congenital Defects

Primary and secondary palatal cleft (with accompanying lesions) are some of the more common defects seen in newborn puppies. Some advocate surgical repair by six to eight weeks of age, with any delay contraindicated as the defect is likely to get larger [5]. Other guidelines recommend supporting the patient with alternate feeding (orogastric tubes) until they reach 8–12 weeks of age [6]. Surgery can interfere with the growth of the palatal and maxillary tissues if performed any time prior to 16 weeks of age [7]. Custom-made nursing teats have proven successful in research-based puppies, with removable, flexible prosthetic plugs placed at the time of weaning [8]. In one case, the patient was maintained on dry kibble and a suspended water bottle and surgery was performed finally at 14 months of age, at which time the defect had partially closed spontaneously [6]. Additional craniomaxillofacial abnormalities are often seen in these patients, and the extent of the osseous lesion is often greater than the soft tissue defect and is hidden [9].

A number of defects can also be seen in the soft palate, with or without hard palate involvement [10]. These could include an extension of a secondary cleft to an asymmetric unilateral defect, or bilateral soft palate hypoplasia [11]. With unilateral hypoplasia, two- or three-layer appositional repair with ipsilateral tonsillectomy may be adequate if there is minimal tension at closure. In bilateral hypoplasia, where the small caudal portion on the midline looks like a uvula, repair of one side can be followed with repair of the other side four to six weeks later. However, if there is considerable tension, then a nasopharyngeal mucosal flap may be needed [11]. Sager describes using two buccal mucosal flaps, each based on a palatoglossal arch (harvested rostrally – finger shaped), with the first positioned and sutured so its mucosa faces the nasal cavity and the second rotated for its mucosa to face the oral cavity [12]. In a feline case, one flap from the hard palatal mucosa and two lateral pharyngeal flaps were required [13]. A similar case in a dog with bilateral hypoplasia and no pseudouvula utilized an initial split thickness hinged soft palate flap. When released, the flap expanded the length of the palate caudally. Bilateral U-shaped rotational flaps from the adjacent buccal mucosa were placed over the opened palatal flap, with less tension than a pharyngeal flap would have caused [14]. If full function cannot be returned, treatment for palatal hypoplasia may be reconsidered [15].

Nasopharyngeal stenosis due to dysplasia of the palatopharyngeal muscles in the Dachshund is not amenable to surgery in most cases [16, 17]. In one case of nasopharyngeal stenosis due to soft palate dysplasia, the caudal portion adhered dorsally to the pharyngeal mucosa, and anti-inflammatory medication decreased the edema sufficiently to relieve the dyspnea [18]. In a separate feline case, a mucosal flap for correction and release of the laryngeal webbing avoided the complication of recurrence that has been seen in other cases [19].

By far the most common soft palate defect is an extension of a secondary cleft into the hard palate. If the defect is small to moderate in size, and the two edges can be gently apposed without extensive tension, then a simple two- or three-layer closure may be sufficient [10, 20]. Once the edges are excised, the nasal mucosa should be sutured from a caudal to rostral direction in a simple interrupted pattern with the knots facing the nasal cavity. While some elect not to close the muscle layer to minimize suture material, a continuous pattern can provide additional closure. The final oral mucosa layer is then closed, with knots facing the oral cavity. Tension-releasing incisions may be made laterally and the tissues can be separated from the pterygoid hamulus.

The more complicated bilateral overlapping mucosal single-pedicle flaps may be performed if simple closure would result in excessive tension [21]. On one side of the defect, a mucosal flap is harvested with an initial incision 5 mm away from the defect edge, for the length of the defect (Figure 12.1a). Two incisions are made to the midline at the caudal and rostral edges of the initial incision. The oral mucosa is undermined to harvest a flap that will be "flipped" on the hinge formed by the edge of the defect on that side. This flap is positioned dorsal to the soft palate on the other side of the defect, with the mucosa facing the nasal cavity (Figure 12.1b). The mucosal flap on the other side is harvested in a similar manner from the nasal aspect of the tissue, and when undermined and opened and flipped, will be placed on the ventral aspect of the two flaps, with the mucosa facing the oral cavity (Figure 12.1c). The initial flap can be sutured to the lateral-most aspect of the second flap harvest site to secure the mucosa facing the nasal cavity. The second flap is also sutured to secure its edge facing the oral cavity (Figure 12.1d). This technique was successful in a number of cases with suture lines placed away from the defect and tissue closure over the harvest sites [21].

Elongated soft palates are a common finding in brachycephalic breeds, along with a combination of lesions including stenotic nares, everted tonsils, and laryngeal ventricles, known as Brachycephalic Airway Obstruction Syndrome (BAOS) [22–25]. Correction of an elongated soft palate may be accomplished with cold steel (scissors), electrocautery, low-temperature, high-frequency radiotherapy [26], carbon dioxide laser, a bipolar sealing device, or harmonic scalpel. In one study, a CO_2 laser and electrocautery had favorable outcomes, with the laser having a shorter surgical time and less bleeding, while diode laser therapy had more complications [27]. The bipolar sealing device provides firm compression and electrothermal energy that is feedback controlled, without the safety precautions necessary for laser devices [28]. The ultrasonic motion of the blades of the harmonic scalpel are purported to cause less post-operative pain and swelling, and a decrease in bleeding [29].

No matter what method is used, the basic approach is similar: using lateral stay sutures caudal to the level of the tonsils, retracting the tissue carefully, and resecting enough so the new edge will be positioned just caudal to the epiglottis. With scissors, a cut is made a third of the way across at a time, closing the nasopharyngeal and oropharyngeal mucosal layers for each section, but not incorporating the muscle layer [14]. Crushing the tissues may cause excessive edema and improper use of electrocautery can be damaging.

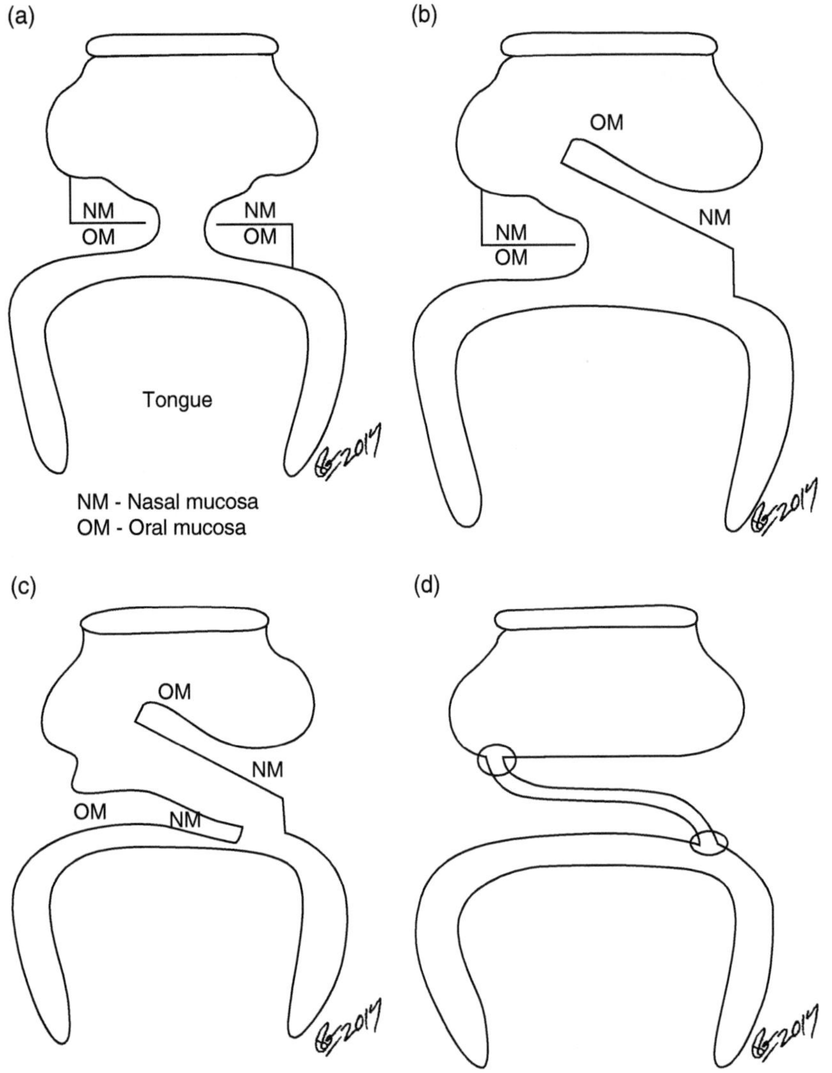

Figure 12.1 Secondary cleft extending into soft palate closed with two layers – bilateral overlapping mucosal single-pedicle flaps which are cut and rotated 180° and closed. *Source:* Courtesy of Josephine Banyard. Adapted from reference [15].

12.2.3 Midline Defect Repair – Acquired

12.2.3.1 Narrow Defect, Acute – Primary Appositional Closure

With minor midline defects (<1 mm), whether due to congenital cleft or trauma (high-rise syndrome in cats) [30], primary closure of the narrow space is often simple [10]. After debriding the soft tissue to freshen the edges, and using digital pressure to realign any displaced osseous structures, the mucosal edges can often be closely reduced and repositioned for simple interrupted suture closure.

12.2.3.2 Narrow to Medium Defect – von Langenbeck Technique

This technique has also been called the medially repositioned double flap or sliding bipedical flap technique [31, 32]. In some moderate midline lesions, a releasing flap at the lateral aspect by each dental arch can provide enough flexibility to bring the two medial edges together at the midline. The lateral releasing incisions often must be fairly long, should incorporate the palatine arteries, with the medial edges freshened before suturing. Full thickness releasing incisions may allow the most flexibility, but partial thickness flaps have been shown to minimize the scar tissue that could potentially affect maxillary growth in the young patient [33]. This is best used if there is minimal tension, though the sutures are placed over a defect (Figure 12.2a to c).

12.2.3.3 Wide Defect (Linear) – Overlapping Flap ± Releasing Incision

After making an incision palatal to the maxillary teeth on one side, releasing incisions are made at the rostral and caudal extents, toward the cleft defect, perpendicular to

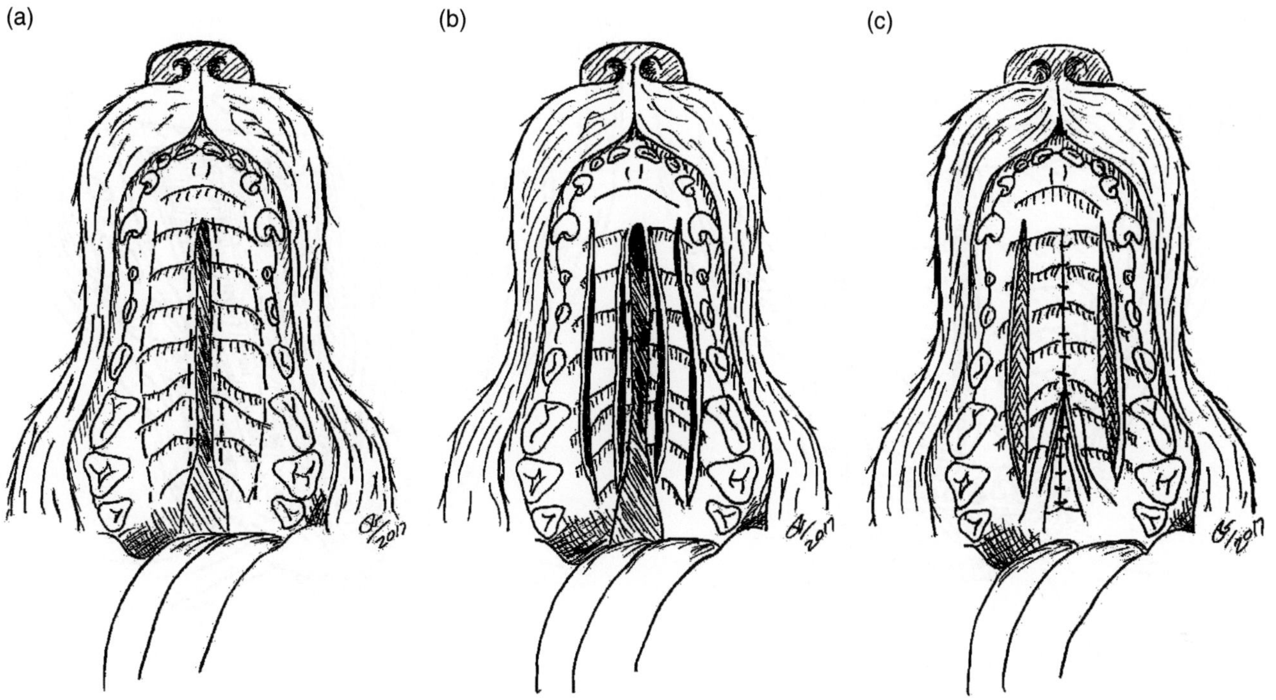

Figure 12.2 Medially repositioned double flap or sliding bipedicle flap technique (von Langenbeck Technique). *Source:* Courtesy of Josephine Banyard. Adapted from reference [31].

the first incision and incorporating the palatal artery into the flap [10]. The defect margin on the opposite side is incised to elevate the mucoperiosteum off the underlying palatal bone, preserving the artery on that side as well. Once the original flap is raised, it is flipped on the hinge of tissue at the edge of the defect and is secured with vest-over-pants sutures under the mucoperiosteum on the other side (Figure 12.3a to c). This is best used with wider defects, as the suture line has underlying bone for support. This can be paired with a two- or three-layer closure of the soft palate if the defect extends distally.

12.2.3.4 Wide Defect – Midline Caudal Hard Palate – Advancement Flap

Once the site around the defect is prepared (edges freshened), incisions are made caudally at each side of the defect [20]. The advancement flap is elevated, starting with full thickness over the hard palate and transitioning to partial thickness over the soft palate. Once sufficient tissue is released to provide closure without tension, the flap is advanced rostrally and sutured to the prepared margins. This allows the suture line to be supported by underlying bone.

12.2.4 Asymmetrical Defect Repair – Acquired

The size and position of the defect, as well as the available vascularized tissue for repair, will help determine the type of surgical technique for a variety of palatal defects.

12.2.4.1 Small, Circular Defects – Transposition (Rotation) Flap

Smaller defects rostral to the level of the maxillary fourth premolars can be covered with a U-shaped flap, incorporating the palatal artery, from the opposite side. Design the rostral edge of the flap to align with the rostral extent of the defect. Once released, the flap is positioned into the prepared area of the defect. Incisions extended back into the soft palate should be adjusted from a full thickness flap to partial thickness in this region to provide a mobile caudal base for rotation. The flap is secured by sutures over the prepared defect site, with some sutures preplaced in small holes drilled into the palatal bone on the donor side. The harvest site is allowed to heal by second intention. This flap allows large coverage with sutures supported by underlying bone.

12.2.4.2 Central Defect at Level of Maxillary Fourth Premolars – Split Palatal U-Flap

Here a large full-thickness U-shaped flap is created rostral to the defect, extending to the level of the first premolars [34]. The flap is divided at the midline and the rostral extent of the palatine artery is ligated, with preservation of the rest of the artery for vascularization of the flap. The first half of the flap is rotated 90° so the medial border is sutured to the caudal aspect of the defect. The second flap is then rotated to suture the now rostral extent of the first flap (Figure 12.4a and b). This is

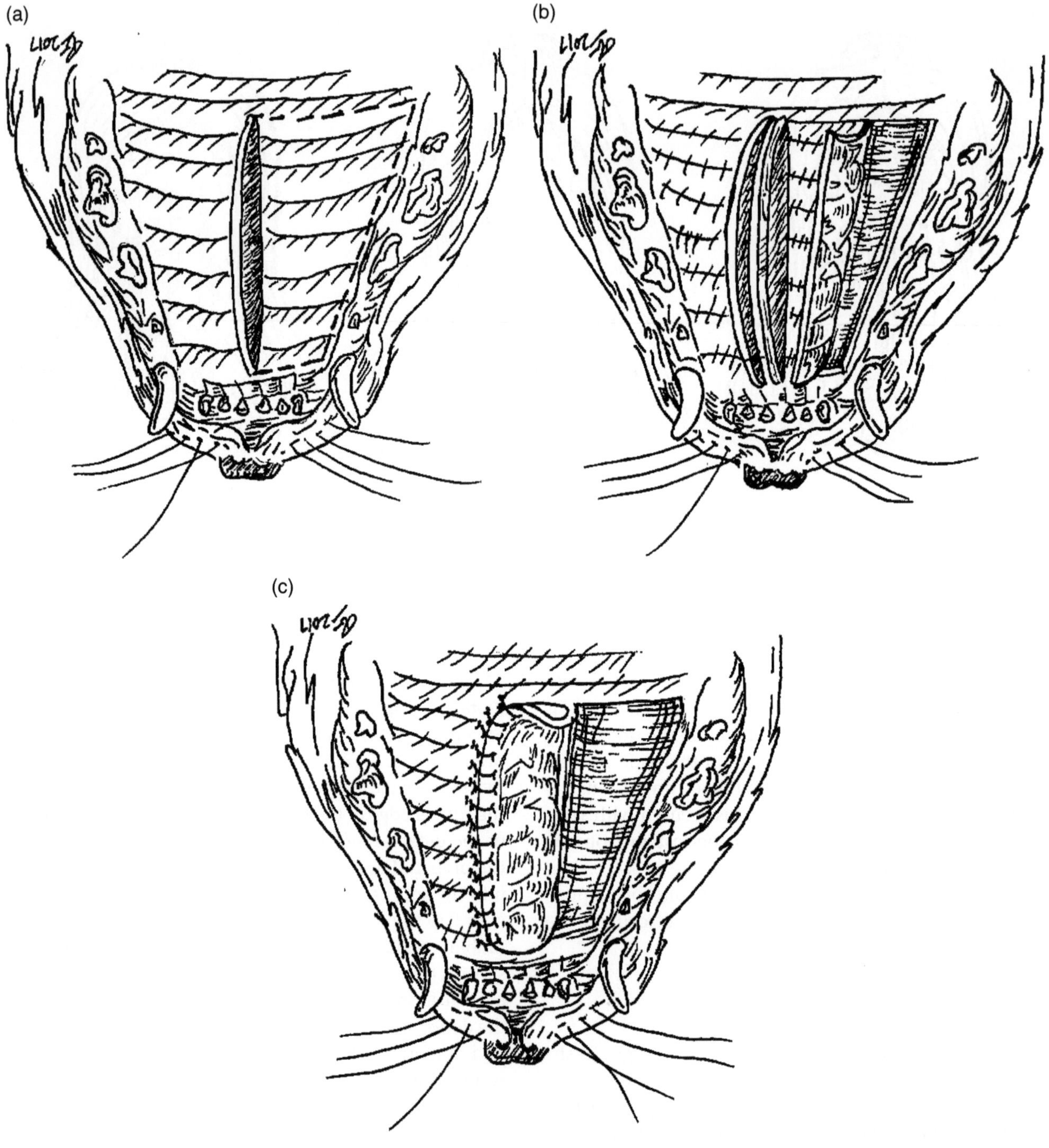

Figure 12.3 Overlapping flap – "vest over pants" technique to close a midline palatal defect. *Source:* Courtesy of Josephine Banyard.

best used when there is minimal tension or wound contraction in the harvested tissue.

12.2.4.3 Large Caudal Defects – Island Axial Pattern Flap

In areas where there is less viable tissue on one side to harvest for a flap, a variation of the split palatal U-flap can utilize healthier tissue on the other side, incorporating the palatal artery [35]. The caudal extent of the flap will extend to the level of the second maxillary molar, with full thickness release of the mucoperiosteum from the underlying palatal bone. This preserves the major palatine neurovascular bundle as the pedicle of the flap. This flap can be rotated up to 180° to be positioned at the prepared defect site.

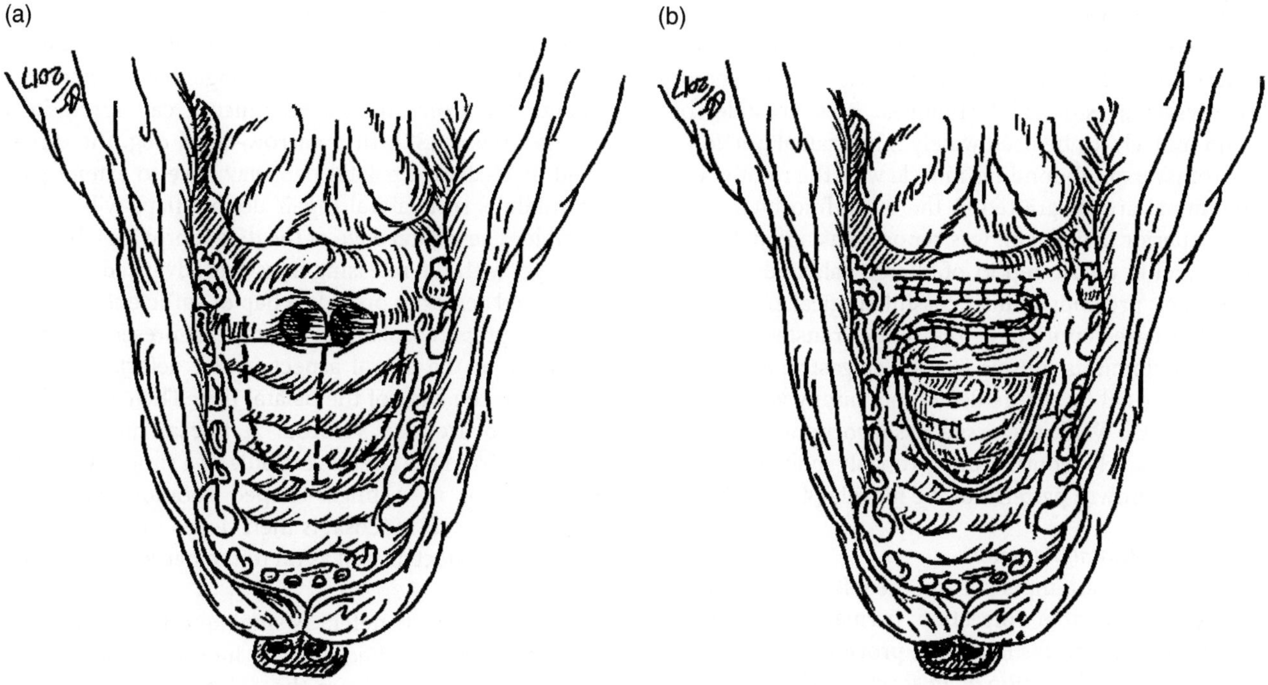

Figure 12.4 Split palatal U flap to correct a central caudal palatal defect. *Source:* Courtesy of Josephine Banyard.

12.2.4.4 Large Rostral Defects

For extensive palatal defects with limited tissue from which to harvest a flap, the dorsum of the tongue can be incorporated to cover the defect. The tongue surface is incised and undermined to use the cut surfaces as flaps, sutured to the palatal defect edges once rotated 180°. After four weeks of assisted feeding, the tongue is separated from the palate, with enough tissue left to close the defect permanently. This procedure is not tolerated well and should be used if other techniques have proven unsuccessful.

12.2.4.5 Large Defects – Complicated – Previous Surgical Attempts

12.2.4.5.1 Unilateral or Bilateral Vestibular Mucosal (Overlapping) Flap(s)

If there is a lack of healthy, tension-free tissue for flap development, premolars and molars are first extracted unilaterally or bilaterally [10, 36]. This can provide a wide section of tissue that can be released up into the vestibular buccal mucosa once the extraction sites have healed sufficiently. With a lateral defect, just one arch may be needed for harvesting a flap, but with an extensive defect, both sides can be developed to create a bilateral overlapping flap [10].

12.2.4.5.2 Angularis Oris Axial Pattern Buccal Flap (APBF)

An axial flap can be harvested from the caudal buccal mucosa on the affected side, incorporating the angularis oris branch of the facial neurovascular branch [37, 38]. After skin preparation, the vessel is located by palpating the buccal mucosa of the cheek, finding the pulse of the artery, or by transillumination. A skin incision is made, extending caudally from the commissure of the lips, reflecting the skin ventrally and dorsally. A full thickness (except for the skin) rectangular flap is harvested, ligating the vessels at the rostral aspect, and continuing the flap caudally to the extent at which the artery travels deep to the masseter muscle. This base is maintained for rotation of the flap to allow its positioning over the defect, with the buccal mucosa facing the oral cavity and secured with sutures. Depending on the patient's size, this flap could reach rostrally to the extent of the maxillary canines. The submucosa and mucosa are closed with two layers, and the skin is closed externally. Reports of complications of distal tip necrosis could be attributed to trauma from the upper molars if they are not extracted [38]. Early intervention with repositioning of the flap if the rostral extent fails has been shown to result in eventual flap success.

12.2.4.5.3 Superficial Cervical Axial Pattern Skin Flap Variation

While previously used for extensive head and neck reconstruction procedures, the axial skin flap harvested with the superficial cervical artery (prescapular branch – SCA) has been proposed as a possible palatal defect flap [39]. However, since this procedure requires the use of a pneumatic dermatome and would need an extended (bilateral) flap to reach the oral cavity, it is unlikely to be used widely.

12.2.4.5.4 Myoperitoneal Free Flap [40, 41]

Harvesting a portion of a muscle with associated vasculature for grafting into the oral cavity would require microvascular surgical techniques. It is possible, but again unlikely, to be used widely. The cranial portion of the transversus abdominus muscle with the right cranial abdominal artery, grafted to the left infraorbital artery and superior labial vein, was reported as an anatomical study and in a case report of a large palatal defect that had many previously unsuccessful surgical treatments. Another case report of a free tissue transfer from the rectus abdominus muscle (caudal epigastric artery and vein) was used in a large defect in a puppy with a traumatic defect. While the tissue was incorporated into the patient, muscle contracture probably contributed to abnormal growth patterns of the maxilla [41].

12.2.4.5.5 Palatal Obturators

When surgical attempts fail and there is insufficient viable tissue for further correction, permanent or removal obturators can be fashioned to provide closure of the region. Direct fabrication of an acrylic device carries the risk of tissue damage (thermal reaction of some acrylics), while obturators made off-site will require two anesthetic episodes. A titanium plate was designed for a patient with a severe defect, secured with screws with a glass ionomer repair for additional coverage [42]. Several reports describe using a small, flexible silastic nasal septal button with thin flanges that can be trimmed to the defect's size (up to 30 mm) [43–45]. The central post is typically round and 7 mm in diameter. Other versions are available with elliptical central posts that can be sized to the perforation to minimize slippage. There can be challenges with prosthodontic devices, including difficulties attaching to certain tooth structures, contributing to periodontal disease formation and requiring regular care by the owner [43].

12.3 Oronasal Fistula Repair

12.3.1 Vestibular Flaps

12.3.1.1 Single Mucoperiosteal Flap

If sufficient healthy tissue is present at the time of oronasal fistula detection or extraction of the corresponding tooth, simple closure with the full thickness mucoperiosteal flap developed for the extraction may be sufficient, if no tension is present. Making releasing incisions away from the defect edge will produce a broader based flap and provide underlying osseous support for the suture line. Due to the constant strain on the sutures due to inspiration and expiration, however, the client should always be cautioned that a persistent opening may occur, and additional surgery may be necessary.

12.3.1.2 Double-Layer Flap Technique

If the defect is large or chronic, or insufficient tissue is present to provide a tension-free single flap, providing a second flap from the palatal mucosa can result in a stronger repair [32]. In a narrow-faced dog, the three-sided or U-shaped palatal flap may have to extend past the midline, so bilateral repair double flaps will not be possible. The palatal edge of the defect provides the base or hinge, with the releasing incisions advanced palatally and joined across to provide a flap of sufficient size. The defect is prepared, with an attempt to preserve part of the tissue at the dorsal aspect of the defect to be the anchor for the edge of the palatal flap. The edges of the palatal flap are also secured. A buccal mucosa flap, extending from the lateral vestibule as a simple advancement flap or as a finger-shaped rotation flap from the rostral buccal mucosa, is then closed over the site of the original defect as well as on to the harvest site on the palate.

Alternately, if the defect is small and the perifistular tissue is relatively healthy, an incision made at an appropriate distance from the defect margin can provide a shelf of tissue that can be elevated and hinged toward the nasal cavity, suturing the edges together while trimming the mesial and distal sections. A buccal mucosal flap can then be used to cover the perifistular closure.

12.3.2 Free Auricular Cartilage Autograft [46]

For persistent, chronic oronasal fistulation, a section of auricular cartilage can be harvested from the patient. It is sized to fit within the compartment made by undermining the mucoperiosteum at least 3–4 mm around the defect to accept the graft (with edges debrided). With the external surface of the ear prepped, a U-shaped incision (base positioned toward the base of the ear) is made and elevated with blunt dissection. The scapha cartilage graft is carefully cut to fit the dimensions of the defect compartment (no shrinkage will occur), elevated from the inner dermis of the pinna, and placed on a moistened gauze sponge. The graft is placed in between the mucosal edges of the graft and the underlying bone and sutured in a vest-over-pants pattern. If sufficient tissue is present, closure over the graft may be attempted. At two months after a reported case, the graft was epithelialized and the donor site (sutured at the time of surgery) had healed [46].

Any attempts at palatal surgery should be accompanied by regular re-checks, as persistent fistulation or communication into the nasal cavity is always possible. If minor defects persist, additional surgical techniques are usually sufficient to provide adequate correction. If persistent defects occur, additional surgery may be successful. However, multiple procedures often have to rely on tissues that already have some fibrotic areas, so options can be limited.

12.4 Tongue

With resective surgery of the tongue, the amount of healthy tissue remaining tends to be more critical for cats than for dogs. Canine patients can often learn to adjust to extensive loss of the tongue, while cats typically do not. Their inability to groom themselves properly often leads to severe secondary problems with infections, not to mention challenges with eating [47].

12.4.1 Congenital

While some congenital conditions of the tongue such as microglossia obviously have no surgical remedy, other conditions can benefit from procedures. Dogs with ankyloglossia (tongue-tie) show some benefit to the individual when the sublingual frenulum was excised [48–50]. Individuals with extremely long tongues may benefit from resection of the rostral portion.

12.4.2 Acquired

Other than lingual tumors, most of the problems associated with the tongue are due to some type of trauma – physical (foreign body, laceration), electric or chemical. Lacerations should be sutured where possible, without causing excessive deviation of the tongue once healing is complete. Necrotic tissue as a result of electrical cord or chemical burns should be debrided conservatively, trying to preserve as much normal tissue as possible. If necessary, additional tissue can be removed at a later date. Abscesses, often sublingual, should be drained and marsupialized or a drain placed, with any foreign objects removed [51, 52].

The ventral surface and sublingual areas should be closely examined for injury, string foreign body, masses, and even sublingual proliferative tissue ("gum-chewer's"). If the gum-chewer's lesion is interfering with mastication, it can be carefully resected, avoiding major vessels and salivary ducts, and submitted for histopathology [53].

Simple excision of lesions such as calcinosis circumscripta may be needed if the masses are causing discomfort [53]. One large eosinophilic granuloma complex (EGC) lesion on the distal aspect of a cat's tongue was successfully removed with the successful use of a diode laser [54]. Excision of a tongue with lateral protrusion in a dog with a neurological deficit can provide sufficient correction.

12.4.2.1 Glossectomy

When the lesion is extensive (damage caused by paper shredders) or significant amounts of tissue should be removed due to the presence of a tumor, then a glossectomy procedure is required. A classification scheme for the extent of tongue removal (transverse) has been established [55]. With appropriate support (feeding tubes) post-operatively and adjusting feeding habits, most dogs do very well with extensive tongue loss.

Marginal (partial thickness) and wedge (full thickness) excision of smaller benign lesions in the rostral free tongue is not likely to involve the lingual vessels or salivary ducts, so simple closure is sufficient. A longitudinal excision can help preserve one lingual artery when resecting a unilateral mass, though the remaining rostral tongue will be very narrow [10].

For malignant tumors that often need 2 cm margins, a non-crushing clamp can be placed at the base of the tongue to provide some hemorrhage control for the transverse glossectomy procedure [1]. Care must be taken to identify and ligate the paired lingual arteries and sublingual salivary ducts. A wedge incision should leave sufficient mucosa for closure with a combination of through-and-through mattress sutures for the bulk of the tissue and apposition of the epithelial edges [1]. Incise step by step through the dorsal mucosa, and then the ventral lingual mucosa and frenulum. This is followed by excising portions of the musculature with subsequent closure of the mucosa, eventually making it across the width of the tongue [56]. Preserving sufficient mucosa on the floor of the mouth when the frenulum is excised can help with final closure. A straight or U-shaped incision can be closed transversely, while a V-shaped incision (with the tip of the V facing caudally in order to provide better margins for a central mass) can be closed longitudinally [57].

12.5 Tonsils

Surgical resection of a tonsil or tonsils is warranted in cases of refractory infection, where hyperplasia interferes with swallowing, for mass removal or debulking prior to ancillary therapy, to aid in soft palate surgery, and to address the everted tonsils found in BAOS (brachycephalic airway obstruction syndrome). Some advocate the use of pre-operative dexamethasone to decrease post-operative edema [58], and the use of epinephrine in the base to help with hemorrhage is debated [59].

Long-handled instruments can be used to first retract the edge of the tonsillar crypt caudodorsally, allowing the base of the tonsil to be grasped with Allis tissue forceps [58]. Cross-clamping the base prior to transaction is one method. Another is transaction of the hilar mucosa followed by ligation or cautery. The fossa can be closed, depending on personal preference. Efforts should be made to select procedures that will minimize postoperative swelling.

12.6 Salivary Glands

12.6.1 Salivary Ducts

Focal trauma to a salivary duct may be repaired with microsurgery and stent placement [60], but complications due to the damage may result in the development of a sialocele [61]. In some cases, particularly with the parotid gland, duct disruption or blockage can lead to glandular atrophy. Duct ligation can be used as treatment for feline parotid duct sialocele, though formation of sialocele may also occur with duct ligation. If a sialolith is present, surgically opening the duct to remove the obstruction may initiate a full healing process if there is just partial blockage [62, 63]. With severely affected ducts [64] or if problems continue, the gland should be removed.

12.6.2 Sialocele

A majority of sialoceles are due to the disruption of the sublingual duct, with cervical, sublingual, and pharyngeal sites forming (in order of occurrence). Drainage or marsupialization of the defect is often unsuccessful, so surgical removal of both the sublingual gland and mandibular glands with their common capsule is required. While removal of the parotid duct has been described and performed [65], there is evidence to indicate that ductal ligation may be sufficient to result in eventual glandular atrophy [64]. In a patient with chronic exophthalmos due to a zygomatic sialocele, surgical intervention was declined [66]. Placement of polidocanol (sclerotherapy) successfully resolved the case.

12.6.3 Sialadenectomy

12.6.3.1 Mandibular – Sublingual Salivary Gland Chains

Since the mandibular and sublingual (monostomatic portion) salivary glands are closely associated within a common capsule, their removal is performed together. Description of sialadenectomy of this grouping may include incision of the capsule and removal of the glands from the capsule for treatment of sialocele, but extracapsular excision is performed for removal of suspected neoplasia [67] (Figure 12.5a and b).

12.6.3.1.1 Lateral Approach [68]

A lateral approach to these glands is most commonly used, unless the sialocele or defect is rostral to the region of the lingual nerve. In that case, a ventral approach would provide the best access. With large sialoceles, place the patient in dorsal recumbency, noting the dependent displacement of the accumulated saliva to identify the affected side [69]. With the patient in lateral recumbency and a bolster placed under the neck, make an incision using the bifurcation of the jugular nerve near the angular process of the mandible as the starting point, and extend the incision to the caudal aspect of the mandible, over the gland [68]. Once the platysma and parotidoauricularis muscles are incised and reflected, the mandibular gland is isolated at the caudal aspect and dissected to reveal the

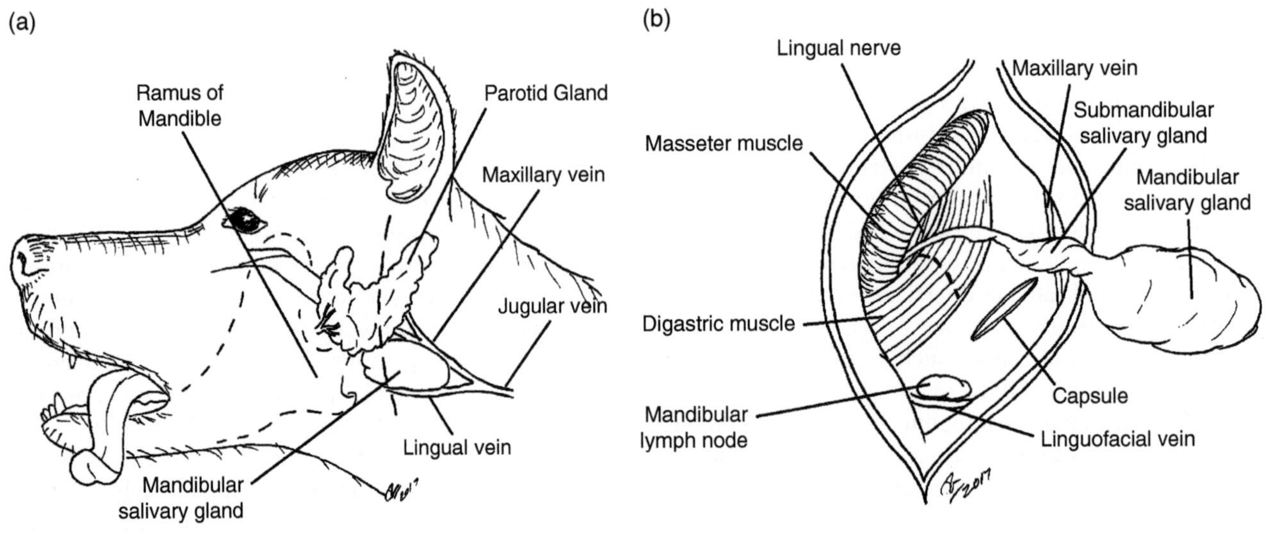

Figure 12.5 Approach for removal of mandibular and sublingual salivary glands. *Source:* Courtesy of Josephine Banyard. Adapted from reference [67].

vascular supply at its rostromedial aspect. Dissection continues forward to incorporate the monostomatic portion of the sublingual gland and then the polystomatic portion until the level of the defect is visualized [66]. The duct is ligated at its most rostral aspect, often near the level of the lingual nerve, in uncomplicated surgeries. Continuous drainage of the secretions should be performed during surgery, but no attempt should be made to remove the sialocele due to its infiltration into tissues. A passive draining system (Penrose drain) can be used for three to five days post-operatively.

Options for following the duct dissection as it travels under the digastricus muscle (tunneling) can help improve exposure of the gland/duct complex further rostrally. Increased caudal retraction on the sublingual gland/duct complex or rostral retraction of the muscle may be needed [66]. This will increase the total length of duct incision and allow removal of increased amounts of the polystomatic sublingual salivary gland [70]. A combined lateral and oral approach allows better access, though is more invasive and some surgeons prefer a ventral approach [71].

If a pharyngeal sialocele is present, additional correction may be needed to relieve the pressure of the defect in the pharyngeal region. After a standard lateral procedure, an oral approach may then be needed to drain, partially excise, or marsupialize the pharyngeal portion [72].

12.6.3.1.2 Ventral Approach [73]

Though technically more difficult and invasive, a ventral approach has the benefits of providing better access for more rostral defects, and options for bilateral surgery [73, 74]. In dorsal recumbency, with the neck distended, an incision medial to the ramus of the mandible is extended longitudinally beyond the angular process to the region of the mandibular salivary gland. In the presence of a cervical sialocele, the approach may have to go through the defect itself. Access to the salivary glands/ducts complex is similar to the lateral approach, dissecting the portions free, ligating appropriate vasculature and extending the exposure rostrally.

The rostral portion of the salivary duct is dissected from between the tongue and mandible, splitting the mylohyoid and styloglossal muscles longitudinally [73]. The sublingual chain can then be bluntly freed up as it passes under the digastricus muscle and then ligated at its most rostral aspect.

12.6.3.2 Parotid Salivary Gland

If ligation of the parotid gland duct has not been successful, the gland itself can be removed, though complete dissection can be challenging [66]. The incision is made from the ventral aspect of the ear canal to the caudal extent of the ramus of the mandible. The platysma and parotidoauricularis muscles are incised and reflected and the gland is dissected free from surrounding muscles. Avoid injury to the superficial temporal artery and facial nerve branches. Trace the duct to the sialocele and ligate and then provide drainage of the sialocele with placement of a Penrose drain.

12.6.3.3 Zygomatic Salivary Gland

There are several approaches to the zygomatic salivary gland as it lies in the floor of the orbit, protected below the zygomatic arch. The ventral approach includes an incision on the zygomatic arch, dissecting between the aponeurosis of the masseter muscle and the periosteum, then removing the ventral portion of the arch. Orbital fat can be cleared and then the gland dissected with gentle traction [73]. A modified lateral orbitotomy can provide better exposure, reflecting a portion of the zygomatic arch released with rostral and caudal osseous cuts. Predrilled holes are made to facilitate the replacement of the arch at closure. The aponeurosis of the temporalis and masseter muscles are reflected dorsally and ventrally, and the orbital ligament does not need removal [75, 76].

12.7 Lip and Cheek Defects

12.7.1 Cleft Repair – Lip

While some mild abnormalities can be seen, at times more serious changes are present. Any form of cleft lip (in combination with a secondary cleft palate) or signs of a failure of tissues to fuse should always alert the practitioner to look for any other abnormalities. Complete reconstruction of the facial contours can be quite challenging at times, and more advanced procedures beyond two-layer closure of simple defects may be necessary. Utilizing a fascia lata implant or auricular cartilage graft may help provide additional support to the soft tissue to aid in repair (Figure 12.6a to d). It is important to try to preserve the line of the mucocutaneous junction of the lips and patency of the nasal passage, if affected.

12.7.2 Tight Lip Repair

In more severe cases, a surgical procedure must be performed to release the tension and to provide for a healing period without additional scar formation. Most surgery is based upon attempts to reestablish a proper vestibular depth, with the dog positioned in sternal recumbency and the maxilla gently suspended from above. An incision is made at the mucocutaneous junction of the lip, extending from the inferior labial frenulum on one side to the frenulum on the other side [77–79]. This flap is dissected free from underlying tissues to be used as a graft to enlarge the vestibule. A second incision is made to elevate a periosteal

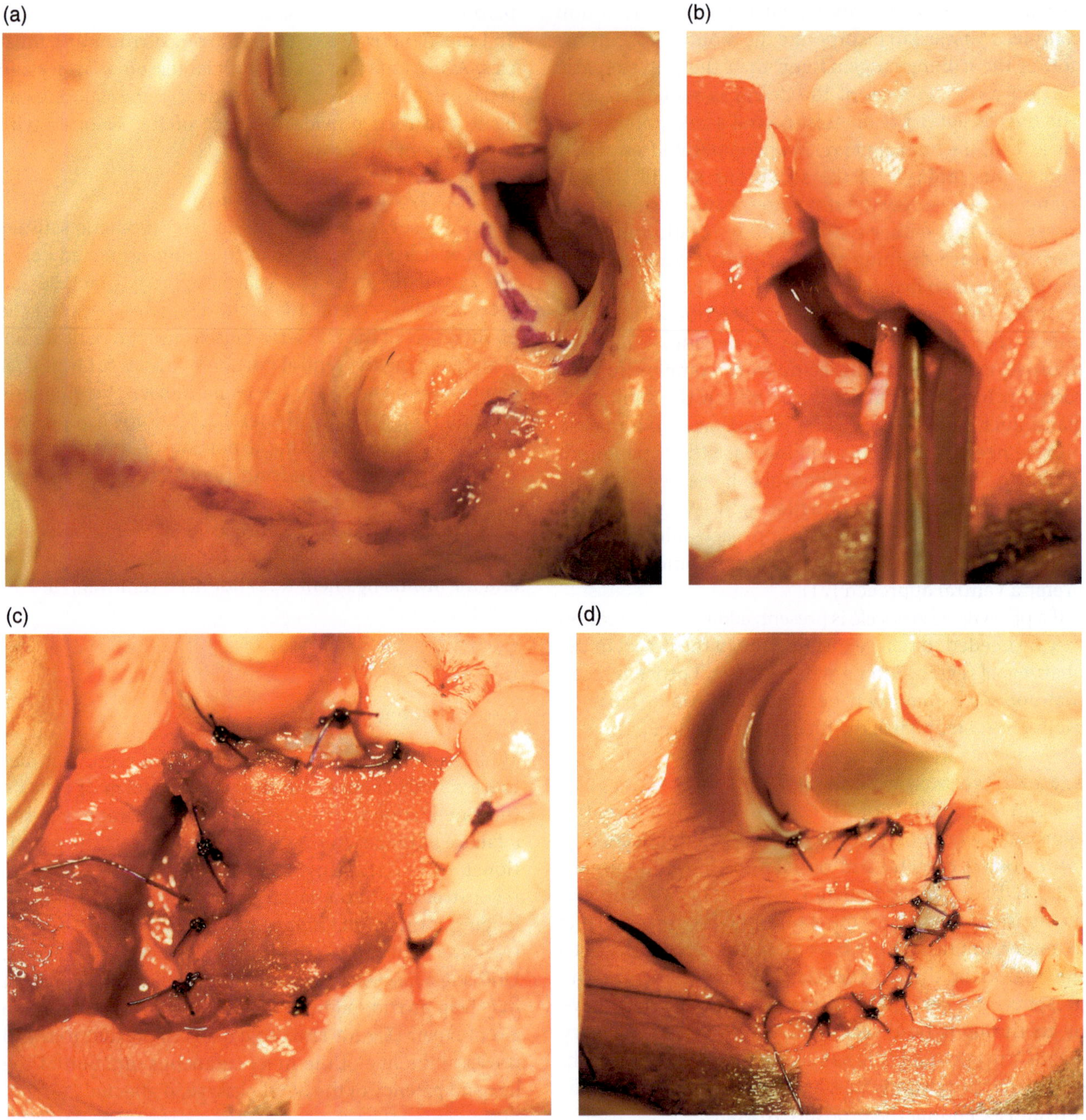

Figure 12.6 Repair of cleft lip defect using fascia lata implant to support soft tissue closure: (a) surgical marker for incising defect edge and forming a buccal sliding flap from tissue distal/caudal to defect; (b) splitting the defect edges to receive the fascia lata implant; (c) securing the fascia lata sandwiched in between nasal and mucosal layers with mattress sutures; (d) initial closure of the mesial portion of the sliding flap released to cover fascia lata.

flap at the level of the mucogingival line that has been exposed with the primary flap, providing a recipient site for the first flap [78]. This flap is secured with pre-placed sutures with the edge of the flap placed deep into the newly formed vestibule. The periosteal flap can then be sutured to the inner portion of the lip at the mucocutaneous margin. Digital manipulation of the site has been described to prevent adherence [78], or graft material cut from a Penrose drain or harvested from buccal mucosa may be placed [77]. Concurrent bilateral mandibular frenectomy may also be performed to release further tension. After the incised edges of the defect have sufficiently epithelialized, the Penrose drain may be removed. Ideally, enough tension is relieved on the initial surgery because subsequent attempts may not be as successful.

A ventral approach can be made with a craniocaudal incision over the mandibular symphysis [77]. After undermining the skin from muscle layers, a suture is placed dorsally toward the lip to pull the lip ventrally, tacking it down to the periosteum on the caudal symphysis. In older patients, a fusiform incision in the skin, parallel to the incisors, can be made to remove a ventral portion of the redundant lip [80].

12.7.3 Inferior Labial Frenoplasty

In an area such as that distal to a mandibular canine, a tight frenulum can contribute to periodontal disease. Release of the tension is achieved by excising the frenulum parallel to the dental arcade (sagittal cut) [77]. The mesial and distal cut points are then brought together and sutured side to side, perpendicular to the dental arcade (transverse direction).

12.7.4 Cheiloplasty

Excessive or redundant lip tissue, normal in some breeds, can be a focal point for saliva and food collection with resulting cheilitis and dermatitis. Cheiloplasty can be performed to remove some of the excess tissue, including any pendulous folds that have become infected.

A simple resection of the deep lateral furrow will not slow down the salivation, but it can help in the natural cleansing effect. A fusiform incision is made parallel to the body of the mandible to include the affected area [81].

Alternately, a more involved commissuroplasty (commissurorhaphy) may be performed to reduce the actual oral opening, allowing the saliva to remain more in the oral cavity. Resection of the tissue should be planned in advance to determine the proper extent of the oral opening and the new position of the commissures. The mucosal margins should be closely approximated to avoid any defects intraorally, with a subcutaneous layer, and the dermal layers should match as well. This procedure can also be used after a mandibulectomy or in cases of non-union to help provide additional stability to the area and to help keep the tongue in the mouth [82]. It should be recognized that any future attempts to clean or treat structures in the caudal portion of the oral cavity will be compromised. Conversely, with fibrotic scarring of the lips due to previous injury, commissuroplasty can be performed to open the stoma further.

The lower lip can also be adjusted into a more dorsal position using an elective antidrool chelioplasty to reduce the loss of saliva and food [81]. The mucocutaneous margin of the lower lip is grasped approximately 20–30 mm rostral to the commissure and lifted dorsally until taut with the mouth opened. The placement of incision on the upper lip/cheek will be made at the level where the lower lip was lifted, typically at the level of the maxillary fourth premolar. A 25–30 mm horizontal incision in the upper cheek is made with the caudal aspect on a line from the commissure and medial canthus of the eye. Dissect through to the buccal mucosa, avoiding the superior labial vein. The lower lip is prepared by excising a 25 mm long mucocutaneous border and splitting the edges of the lower lip to create separate mucosal and cutaneous flaps to a depth of 7.5–10 mm, which are then everted. The everted edges are brought into contact with the upper lip incision, using pre-placed horizontal mattress sutures to appose the incised edges of the lip and cheek.

12.8 Repair of Trauma

Most of the acquired lesions of the cheeks and lips, other than tumors, are due to trauma of some type. Vehicular injuries can contribute to the nearly complete avulsion of the mandibular soft tissue from the bone, and can be quite extensive. Barring any additional injuries to the mandible or other oral structures, repair is typically rewarding if sufficient tissue is present. The area should be thoroughly cleaned and any debris irrigated away. With adequate tissue, the lip can be held into position with sutures from the soft tissue incorporating the canines or incisors, or using sutures through pre-drilled holes in the mandible if teeth are missing [83].

Lacerations or cuts of the lips should be sutured back into a normal anatomical position whenever possible, freshening wound edges and realigning mucocutaneous margins with a two-layer closure. Injury to the tissues due to chemical, thermal, or electrical trauma must be evaluated as to the extent of the injury [84]. If no bone is exposed, debridement of the necrotic areas should be performed with an attempt to preserve as much healthy tissue as possible.

With extensive lesions due to trauma, or even tumor removal, reconstruction of defects can often be accomplished through a variety of flap techniques. A single pedicle advancement flap can be used for both the dorsal and ventral regions [84]. Full thickness labial advancement flaps have been used for maxillary lip reconstructions both unilaterally and bilaterally [85, 86]. Techniques of nasal skin fold transposition flap [87] and even palatal mucoperiosteal flaps (after incisal bone removal) [88] have been described for maxillary reconstruction. Axillary flaps such as an angularis oris cutaneous flap have been helpful in repair of extensive ventral chin and rostral lip defects due to tumor removal [89].

More extensive facial reconstruction procedures can be found in other oral surgical texts and in individual case reports. In such patients, a creative outlook to incorporate remaining vascularized tissues can provide unique solutions.

12.9 AVDC Resource – Abbreviations

See Table 12.1.

Table 12.1 AVDC abbreviation list for oral surgery – general (https://www.avdc.org/traineeinfo.html; accessed 3 March 2018).

	Definition		Definition
CFL	Cleft lip	LIP/X	Lip/cheek resection
CFL/R	Cleft lip repair	N	Nose/nasal/nasopharyngeal
CFP	Cleft palate	N/EN	Rhinoscopy
CFP/R	Cleft palate repair	N/LAV	Nasal lavage
CFS	Cleft soft palate	N/NS	Naris stenosis
CFS/R	Cleft soft palate repair	N/NS/R	Naroplasty
CFSH	Soft palate hypoplasia	N/NPS	Nasopharyngeal stenosis
CFSH/R	Soft palate hypoplasia repair	N/NPS/R	Nasopharyngeal stenosis repair
CFSU	Unilateral cleft soft palate	N/POL	Nasopharyngeal polyp
CFSU/R	Unilateral cleft soft palate repair	OFF	Orofacial fistula
CFT	Traumatic cleft palate	OFF/R	Orofacial fistula repair
CFT/R	Traumatic cleft palate repair	ONF	Oronasal fistula
COM	Commissurotomy	ONF/R	Oronasal fistula repair
CPL	Cheiloplasty/commissuroplasty	OP	Operculectomy
ESP	Elongated soft palate	PDE	Acquired palate defect
ESP/R	Elongated soft palate reduction	PDE/R	Acquired palate defect repair
FB	Foreign body	PHA	Pharynx
FB/R	Foreign body removal	POB	Palatal obturator
FRE	Frenuloplasty (frenulotomy, frenulectomy)	SG	Salivary gland
		SG/ADC	Salivary gland adenocarcinoma (check abbreviations under OM for other tumors)
IOF	Intraoral fistula		
IOF/R	Intraoral fistula repair	SG/ADS	Sialadenosis
LAC	Laceration	SG/IN	Sialadenitis
LAC/B	Laceration (cheek skin/buccal mucosa)	SG/MAR	Marsupialization
LAC/G	Laceration (gingiva/alveolar mucosa)	SG/MUC/S	Sublingual sialocele
LAC/L	Laceration (lip skin/labial mucosa)	SG/MUC/P	Pharyngeal sialocele
LAC/O	Laceration (palatine tonsil/oropharyngeal mucosa)	SG/MUC/C	Cervical sialocele
		SG/NEC	Necrotizing sialometaplasia
LAC/P	Laceration (palatal mucosa)	SG/RC	Mucous retention cyst
LAC/R	Laceration repair	SG/SI	Sialolith
LAC/T	Laceration (lingual/sublingual mucosa)	SG/X	Salivary gland resection
LIN	Tongue	TON	Palatine tonsil
LIN/X	Tongue resection	TON/IN	Tonsillitis
LIP	Lip/cheek	TON/X	Tonsillectomy

Suggested Reading

Fossum, T.W. and Hedlund, C.S. (2007). *Small Animal Surgery*. St. Louis, MO: Mosby Elsevier.

Verstraete, F. and Lommer, M. (2012). *Oral and Maxillofacial Surgery in Dogs and Cats*. Philadelphia, PA: Saunders Elsevier.

References

1 Hedlund, C.S. and Fossum, T.W. (2007). Surgery of the digestive system: surgery of the oral cavity and Oropharynx. In: *Small Animal Surgery*, 3e (ed. T.W. Fossum, C.S. Hedlund, et al.), 348. St. Louis, MO: Mosby Elsevier.

2 Reiter, A.M. (2013). Equipment for oral surgery in small animals. *Vet. Clin. North Am. Small Anim. Pract.* 587–608.

3 Bellows, J. (2013). Laser and radiosurgery in veterinary dentistry. *Vet. Clin. North Am. Small Anim. Pract.* 651–658.

4 Peavy, G.M. (2012). Wilder-Smith. Laser surgery. In: *Oral and Maxillofacial Surgery in Dogs and Cats* (ed. F. Verstraete and M. Lommer), 79–88. Philadelphia, PA: Saunders Elsevier.

5 Hale, F.A. (2005). Juvenile veterinary dentistry. *Vet. Clin. North Am. Small Anim. Pract.* 35 (4): 789–817.

6 Davidson, A.P., Gregory, C., and Dedrick, P. (2014). Successful management permitting delayed operative revision of cleft palate in a Labrador retriever. *Vet. Clin. North Am. Small Anim. Pract.* 325–329.

7 Hedlund, C.S. and Fossum, T.W. (2007). Surgery of the digestive system: surgery of the oral cavity and oropharynx. In: *Small Animal Surgery*, 3e (ed. T.W. Fossum, C.S. Hedlund, et al.), 351. St. Louis, MO: Mosby Elsevier.

8 Martinez-Sanz, E., Casado-Gomez, K. et al. (2011). A new technique for feeding dogs with a congenital cleft palate for surgical research. *Lab Anim.* 45 (2): 70–80.

9 Nemec, A., Danaiux, L. et al. (2014). Craniomaxillofacial abnormalities in dogs with congenital palatal defects: computed tomographic findings. *Vet. Surg.*

10 Zacher, A.M. and Marretta, S.M. (2013). Oral and maxillofacial surgery in dogs and cats. *Vet. Clin. North Am. Small Anim. Pract.* 609–649.

11 White, R.N., Hawkins, H.L., Alemi, V.P., and Warner, C. (2009). Soft palate hypoplasia and concurrent middle ear pathology in six dogs. *J. Small Anim. Pract.* 50: 364–372.

12 Sager, M. and Nefen, S. (1998). Use of buccal mucosal flaps for the correction of congenital soft palate defects in three dogs. *Vet. Surg.* 27: 358–363.

13 Headrick, J.F. and McAnulty, J.F. (2004). Reconstruction of a bilateral hypoplastic soft palate in a cat. *J. Am. Anim. Hosp. Assoc.* 40: 86–90.

14 Mulins, R.A. (2016). Use of a split-thickness soft palate hinged flap and bilateral buccal mucosal rotation flaps for one-stage repair of a bilateral hypoplastic soft palate in a dog. *J. Am. Vet. Assoc.* 248 (1): 91–95.

15 Manfra, M.S. (2012). Cleft palate repair techniques. In: *Oral and Maxillofacial Surgery in Dogs and Cats* (ed. F. Verstraete and M. Lommer), 351–361. Philadephia, PA: Saunders Elsevier.

16 Kirberger, R.M., Steenkamp, G. et al. (2006). Stenotic nasopharyngeal dysgenesis in the dachshund: seven cases (2002–2004). *J. Am. Anim. Hosp. Assoc.* 42: 290–297.

17 Dvir, E., Spotswood, T.C., Lambrechts, N.E., and Lobetti, R.G. (2003). Congenital narrowing of the intrapharyngeal opening in a dog with concurrent oesophageal hiatal hernia. *J. Small Anim. Pract.* 44: 359–362.

18 Talavera Lopez, J., Fernandez del Palacio, J., Gil Cano, F., and Bayon del Rio, A. (2008). Nasopharyngeal stenosis secondary to soft palate dysgenesis in a cat. *Vet. J* 200–204.

19 Griffon, D.J. and Tasker, S. (2000). Use of a mucosal advancement flap for the treatment of nasopharyngeal stenosis in a cat. *J. Small Anim. Pract.* 41: 71–73.

20 Sivarolundhu, R.K. (2007). Use of local and axial flaps for reconstruction of the hard and soft palate. *Clin. Tech. Small Anim. Pract.* 22: 61–69.

21 Griffiths, L.G. and Sullivan, M. (2001). Bilateral overlapping mucosal single-pedicle laps for correction of soft palate defects. *J. Am. Anim. Hosp. Assoc.* 37: 183–186.

22 Fasanella, F.J., Shively, J.M., Wardlaw, J.L., and Givaruangsawat, S. (2010). Brachycephalic airway obstructive syndrome in dogs: 90 cases (1991–2008). *J. Am. Vet. Med. Assoc.* 237: 1048–1051.

23 Flanders, J.A. and Thompson, M.S. (2009). Dyspnea caused by epiglottic retroversion in two dogs. *J. Am. Vet. Med. Assoc.* 235: 1330–1335.

24 Lodato, D.L. and Hedlund, C.S. (2012). Brachycephalic airway syndrome: pathophysiology and diagnosis. *Comp. Contin. Ed.* E1–E5.

25 Riecks, T.W., Birchard, S.J., and Stephens, J.A. (2007). Surgical correction of brachycephalic syndrome in dogs: 62 cases (1991–2004). *J. Am. Vet. Med. Assoc.* 230: 1324–1328.

26 Brdecka, D., Rawlings, C.R. et al. (2007). A histopathological comparison of two techniques for soft palate resection in normal dogs. *J. Am. Anim. Hosp. Assoc.* 43: 39–44.

27 Dunie-Merigot, A. and Poncet, B.B. (2010). C. Comparative use of CO_2 laser, diode laser and monopolar electrocautery or resection of the soft palate in dogs with brachycephalic airway obstructive syndrome. *Vet. Rec.* 167: 700–704.

28 Brdecka, D.J., Rawlings, C.A., Perry, A.C., and Anderson, J.R. (2008). Use of an electrothermal, feedback-controlled, bipolar sealing device for resection of the elongated portion of the soft palate in dogs with obstructive upper airway disease. *J. Am. Vet. Med. Assoc.* 233: 1265–1269.

29 Michelsen, J. (2011). Use of the harmonic scalpel for soft palate resection in dogs: a series of three cases. *Aust. Vet. J.* 89: 511–514.

30 Bonner, S.E., Reiter, A.M., and Lewis, J.R. (2012). Orofacial manifestation of high-rise syndrome in cats: a retrospective study of 84 cases. *J. Vet. Dent.* 29 (1): 10–18.

31 Hedlund, C.S. and Fossum, T.W. (2007). Surgery of the digestive system: surgery of the oral cavity and oropharynx. In: *Small Animal Surgery*, 3e (ed. T.W. Fossum, Hedlund, et al.), 353. St. Louis, MO: Mosby Elsevier.

32 Manfra, M.S. (2012). Repair of acquired palatal defects. In: *Oral and Maxillofacial Surgery in Dogs and Cats*

(ed. F. Verstraete and M. Lommer), 363–372. Philadelphia, PA: Saunders Elsevier.

33 Leenstra, T.S., Kuijpers-Jagtman, A.M., and Maltha, J.C. (1999). The healing process of palatal tissues after operations with and without denudation of bone: an experimental study in dogs. *Scand. J. Plast. Reconstr. Hand Surg.* 33: 169–176.

34 Manfra Marretta, S., Grove, T.K., and Grillo, J.F. (1991). Split palatal U-flap: a new technique for repair of caudal hard palate defects. *J. Vet. Dent.* 8 (10): 5–8.

35 Smith, M.M. (2001). Island palatal mucoperiosteal flap for repair of oronasal fistula in a dog. *J. Vet. Dent.* 18 (3): 127–129.

36 Peralta, S., Nemec, A., Fiani, N., and Verstraete, F.J.M. (2014). Staged double-layer closure of palatal defects in 6 dogs. *Vet. Surg.* 1–9.

37 Bryant, K.J., Moore, K., and McAnulty, J.F. (2013). Angularis Oris axial pattern buccal flap for reconstruction of recurrent fistulae of the palate. *Vet. Surg.* 42: 113–119.

38 Cook, D.A. and Thomson, M.J. (2013). Complications of the angularis oris axial pattern buccal flap for reconstruction of palatine defects in two dogs. *Aust. Vet. J.* 92: 156–160.

39 Dundas, J.M., Fowler, J.D., Shmon, C.L., and Clapson, J.B. (2005). Modification of the superficial cervical axial pattern skin flap for oral reconstruction. *Vet. Surg.* 34: 206–213.

40 Degner, D.A., Lanz, O.I., and Walshaw, R. (1996). Myoperiotoneal microvascular free flaps in dogs: an anatomical study and a clinical case report. *Vet. Surg.* 25: 463–470.

41 Lanz, O.I. (2001). Free tissue transfer of the rectus abdominus myoperitoneal flap for oral reconstruction in a dog. *J. Vet. Dent.* 18 (4): 187–192.

42 Kuipers, R.G., Worth, A.J. et al. (1012). Rapid prototype modeling and customized titanium plate fabrication for correction of a persistent hard palate defect in a dog. *J. Am. Vet. Med. Assoc.* 240: 1316–1322.

43 Smith, M.M. and Rockhill, A.D. (1996). Prosthodontic appliance for repair of an oronasal fistula in a cat. *J. Am. Vet. Med. Assoc.* 208 (9): 1410–1412.

44 Hale, F.A., Sylvestre, A.M., and Miller, C. (1997). The use of a prosthetic appliance to manage a large palatal defect in a dog. *J. Vet. Dent.* 14 (2): 61–64.

45 DeSouza, H.J., Amorim, F.V., Corgozinho, K.B., and Tavares, R.R. (2005). Management of the traumatic oronasal fistula in the cat with a conical silastic prosthetic device. *J. Feline Med. Surg.* 7: 129–133.

46 Soukup, J.W., Snyder, C.J., and Gengler, W.R. (2009). Free auricular cartilage autograft for repair of an oronasal fistula in a dog. *J. Vet. Dent.* 26 (2): 86–95.

47 Stauffer, V.D. (1973). Loss of the tongue in a cat and the resulting skin problem. *Vet. Med. – Small Anim. Clin.* 68 (11): 1266–1267.

48 Grundmann, S. (2006). Ankyloglossia in an Anatolian Shepherd dog. *Schweizer Arch. Tier* 148 (8): 417–420.

49 Karahan, S. and Cinar Kul, B. (2009). Ankyloglossia in dogs: a morphological and immunohistochemical study. *Anat. Histol. Embryol.* 38: 118–121.

50 Temizsoylu, M.D. and Avki, S. (2003). Complete ventral ankyloglossia in three related dogs. *J. Am. Vet. Med. Assoc.* 223 (10): 1443–1445.

51 Kelmer, E., Kelmer, G., and Kerl, M.E. (2007). Diagnosis and successful treatment of a caudal lingual abscess in a geriatric dog. *Can Vet. J.* 48 (8): 852–854.

52 Von Doernberg, M.C., Peeters, M.E., ter Haar, G., and Kirpensteun, J. (2008). Lingual abscesses in three dogs. *J. Small Anim. Pract.* 49: 413–416.

53 Buelow, M.E., Marretta, S.M., Barger, A., and Lichtensteiger, C. (2011). Lingual lesions in the dog and cat: recognition, diagnosis, and treatment. *J. Vet. Dent.* 28 (3): 151–162.

54 Kovacs, K., Jakab, C., and Szasz, A.M. (2009). Laser-assisted removal of a feline eosinophilic granuloma from the back of the tongue. *Acta Vet. Hungarica.* 57 (3): 417–426.

55 Dvorak, L.D., Beaver, D.P. et al. (2004). Major glossectomy in dogs: a case series and proposed classification system. *J. Am. Anim. Hosp. Assoc.* 40: 331–337.

56 Buelow, M.E. and Manfra Marretta, S. (2011). Step-by-step – major glossectomy in the dog. *J. Vet. Dent.* 28 (3): 210–213.

57 Sequin, B. (2012). Surgical treatment of tongue, lip and cheek tumors. In: *Oral and Maxillofacial Surgery in Dogs and Cats* (ed. F. Verstraete and M. Lommer), 431–449. Philadelphia, PA: Saunders Elsevier.

58 Hedlund, C.S. and Fossum, T.W. (2007). Surgery of the digestive system: surgery of the oral cavity and oropharynx. In: *Small Animal Surgery*, 3e (ed. T.W. Fossum, Hedlund, et al.), 347. St. Louis, MO: Mosby Elsevier.

59 Matthews, K.G. (2012). Tonsillectomy. In: *Oral and Maxillofacial Surgery in Dogs and Cats* (ed. F. Verstraete and M. Lommer), 553–556. Philadelphia, PA: Saunders Elsevier.

60 Dumpis, J. and Feldmane, L. (2001). Experimental microsurgery of salivary ducts in dogs. *J. Maxillofac Surg.* 29 (1): 56–62.

61 Peeters, M.E. (2012). Principles of salivary gland surgery. In: *Oral and Maxillofacial Surgery in Dogs and Cats* (ed. F. Verstraete and M. Lommer), 495–500. Philadelphia, PA: Saunders Elsevier.

62 Tivers, M.S. and Moore, A.H. (2014). Surgical treatment of a parotid duct sialolith in a bulldog. *Vet. Rec.*

63 Jeffreys, D.A., Stasiw, A., and Dennis, R. (1996). Parotid sialolithiasis in a dog. *J. Small Anim. Pract.* 37 (6): 296–297.
64 Trumpatori, B.J., Geissler, K., and Matthews, K.G. (2007). Parotid duct sialolithiasis in a dog. *J. Am. Anim. Hosp. Assoc.* 43: 45–51.
65 Guthrie, K.M. and Hardie, R.J. (2014). Surgical excision of the parotid salivary gland for treatment of a traumatic mucocele in a dog. *J. Am. Anim. Hosp. Assoc.* 50: 1–5.
66 Stuckey, J.A., Miller, W.W., and Almond, G.T. (2012). Use of a sclerosing agent (1% polidocanol) to treat an orbital mucocele in a dog. *Vet. Ophth.* 15 (3): 188–193.
67 Hedlund, C.S. and Fossum, T.W. (2007). Surgery of the digestive system: surgery of the oral cavity and oropharynx. In: *Small Animal Surgery*, 3e (ed. T.W. Fossum, Hedlund, et al.), 371. St. Louis, MO: Mosby Elsevier.
68 Smith, M.M. (2010). Step-by-step – surgery for cervical, sublingual and pharyngeal mucocele. *J. Vet. Dent.* 27 (4): 268–273.
69 Waldron, D.R. and Smith, M.M. (1991). Salivary mucoceles. *Prob. Vet. Med.* 3 (2): 270–276.
70 Marsh, A. and Adin, C. (2013). Tunneling under the digastricus muscle increases salivary duct exposure and completeness of excision in mandibular and sublingual sialoadenectomy in dogs. *Vet. Surg.* 42: 238–242.
71 Ritter, M.J., von Pfeil, D.J.F. et al. (2006). Mandibular and sublingual sialoceles in the dog: a retrospective evaluation of 41 cases, using the ventral approach for treatment. *NZ Vet. J.* 54 (6): 333–337.
72 Benjamino, K.P., Birchard, S.J., Niles, J.D., and Penrod, K.D. (2012). Pharyngeal mucoceles in dogs: 14 cases. *J. Am. Anim. Hosp. Assoc.* 48 (1): 31–35.
73 Lane, J.G. (2012). Surgical treatment of sialoceles. In: *Oral and Maxillofacial Surgery in Dogs and Cats* (ed. F. Verstraete and M. Lommer), 501–510. Philadelphia, PA: Saunders Elsevier.
74 Papazoplou, L.G., Tzimtzimis, E., Rampidi, S., and Tzimitris, N. (2015). Ventral approach for surgical management of feline sublingual sialocele. *J. Vet. Dent.* 32 (3): 201–203.
75 Bartoe, J.T., Brightman, A.H., and Davidson, H.J. (2007). Modified lateral orbitotomy for vision-sparing excision of a zygomatic mucocele in a dog. *Vet. Ophth.* 10 (2): 127–131.
76 Boland, L., Gomes, E. et al. (2013). Zygomatic salivary gland diseases in the dog: three cases diagnosed by MRI. *J. Am. Anim. Hosp. Assoc.* 49: 333–337.
77 Holmstrom, S.E. (2012). Inferior labial frenoplasty and tight-lip syndrome. In: *Oral and Maxillofacial Surgery in Dogs and Cats* (ed. F. Verstraete and M. Lommer), 515–518. Philadelphia, PA: Saunders Elsevier.
78 Eisner, E.R. (2008). Vestibule deepening procedure for tight lip syndrome in the Chinese Shar-Pei dog. *J. Vet. Dent.* 25 (4): 284–289.
79 Lobprise, H.B. and Wiggs, R.B. (2000). Oral surgery. In: *The Veterinarian's Companion for Common Dental Procedures*, 89–92. Lakewood: CO. AAHA Press.
80 McCoy, D.E. (1997). Surgical management of the tight lip syndrome in the Shar-Pei dog. *J. Vet. Dent.* 14 (3): 95–96.
81 Smeak, D.D. (2012). Cheiloplasty. In: *Oral and Maxillofacial Surgery in Dogs and Cats* (ed. F. Verstraete and M. Lommer), 511–514. Philadelphia, PA: Saunders Elsevier.
82 Durand, C. (2017). Commissurorraphy in the dog (step-by-step). *J. Vet. Dent.* 34 (1): 36–40.
83 Vicari, E. and Stepaniuk, K. (2014). Mandibular lip avulsion repair in the dog and cat. (step-by-step). *J. Vet. Dent.* 31 (3): 212–2217.
84 Swaim, S.F. (2012). Facial soft tissue injuries. In: *Oral and Maxillofacial Surgery in Dogs and Cats* (ed. F. Verstraete and M. Lommer), 243–257. Philadelphia, PA: Saunders Elsevier.
85 Hall, B.P. (2006). Full-thickness labial advancement flap following mast cell tumor excision. *J. Vet. Dent.* 23 (1): 27–31.
86 Taney, K. and Smith, M.M. (2009). Resection of mast cell tumor of the lip in a dog. *J. Vet. Dent.* 26 (1): 28–34.
87 Benlloch-Gonzales, M., Lafarge, S., Bouvy, B., and Poncet, C. (2013). Nasal-skin-fold transposition flap for upper lip reconstruction in a French bulldog. *Can. Vet. J.* 54: 983–986.
88 Kurach, L., Plesman, R. et al. (2013). Use of a hard palate mucoperiosteal flap for rostral muzzle reconstruction in a dog after a traumatic premaxillary degloving injury. *Vet. Surg.* 42: 192–197.
89 Bradford, M., Degner, D.A., and Ghandal, J. (2011). Use of the angularis oris cutaneous flap for repair of a rostral mandibular skin defect in a cat. *V Comp. Orthop. Traum.* 303–306.

13

Oral Surgery – Fracture and Trauma Repair

Kendall Taney[1] and Christopher Smithson[2]

[1] *Center for Veterinary Dentistry and Oral Surgery, Gaithersburg, MD, USA*
[2] *The Pet Dentist at Tampa Bay, Wesley Chapel, FL, USA*

13.1 Introduction

The main goal in repair of maxillofacial trauma is a rapid return to normal function for the patient. This can be most reliably achieved by utilizing repair techniques that simultaneously reduce fractures where possible and restore or maintain proper occlusion. Occlusion must constantly be evaluated as fractures are reduced. In some cases anatomic reduction may not be possible due to severe comminution of fracture fragments. Even with a non-anatomic repair technique patients are able to aliment on their own shortly after surgery in most cases. Nutritional support with feeding tubes is recommended in the immediate postoperative period as an insurance policy in case the patient is still unwilling to eat on its own. Examination of the patient at regular short intervals allows assessment of the occlusion as the fracture is healing. Without evaluation at regular intervals failure of the repair can lead to non-union as well as lifelong morbidity of the patient due to malocclusion. Many different repair styles and techniques exist for management of this common traumatic injury. Some are similar to techniques used in the appendicular skeleton, but special considerations exist for repairs of the oral cavity. Difficult exposure, the presence of many overlapping vital structures, and lack of sterility are some of the challenges that can be faced during repair. In addition to these challenges the presence of concurrent periodontal, metabolic disease, or other traumatic injuries can further complicate the treatment of the patient.

13.2 Osseous Healing

In summary, fractures of bones heal fastest with anatomic reduction and rigid or semi-rigid fixation. Anatomic reduction will allow for direct healing or osteonal reconstruction of the bones. This requires rigid stability at the fracture site to occur. Direct healing is further divided into gap and contact healing. Contact healing can only occur where the defect between fragments is less than 0.01 mm and interfragmentary strain must be less than 2%. Interfragmentary strain is defined as the deformation occurring at the fracture site relative to the size of the gap and it influences the type of tissue that will form in the fracture gap [1, 2]. Primary osteonal reconstruction results in direct healing of lamellar bone oriented in the normal axial direction. Gap healing occurs in gaps less than 800 μm to 1 mm and interfragmentary strain must also be less than 2%. Direct healing in the maxilla and mandible can be more difficult to achieve due to limitations of performing rigid internal fixation techniques.

Without anatomic reconstruction and rigid fixation, maxillofacial and mandibular fractures will undergo indirect healing. Minimally invasive fracture repair techniques can be very successful and may be preferable depending on the fracture type and location. These types of repairs are less likely to achieve anatomic reduction that allow for direct healing. Fortunately the bones of the maxilla and mandible do not bear large portions of the body weight, and mostly need to be able to withstand muscular forces. Multiple mechanisms are set in motion by the body to attempt to stabilize fractures. Initially the muscles contract and blood supply to the area of injury is increased. This inflammatory phase is characterized by hematoma formation and increased extraosseous blood supply. Resorption of the ends of the bone fragments occurs, which reduces interfragmentary strain. The repair phase follows and is initially characterized by callus formation. Orderly repair of the tissues can then occur, depending on the stability of the fracture environment. Each stage of fracture healing is characterized

Wiggs's Veterinary Dentistry: Principles and Practice, Second Edition. Edited by Heidi B. Lobprise and Johnathon R. (Bert) Dodd.

by development of specific tissues that have a certain level of tolerance for interfragmentary motion. As callus formation progresses from soft callus to hard callus the interfragmentary motion/strain is reduced and new bone formation can occur. At the end of the repair phase the bone should be strong enough to withstand normal forces. The final phase is the remodeling phase and can last for years [3].

13.3 Diagnostics

Definitive assessment of maxillofacial injuries should be performed once the patient has been stabilized from the initial trauma. High-impact forces such as automobile trauma or a fall from heights commonly result in maxillofacial fracture or luxation of the temporomandibular joint (TMJ) and often have sequelae such as pulmonary contusions, hemorrhage, myocardial damage, and neurologic effects. Primary repair of maxillofacial trauma should be delayed if abnormalities of the respiratory, circulatory, or neurologic systems are present. Serial neurologic examinations should be performed to assess final neurologic status. A gentle, awake examination can be performed as an initial assessment. Obvious abnormalities of the occlusion such as open-mouth appearance (not associated with respiratory distress), lateral deviation of the mandible, or inability to close the mouth can be indicative of a maxillofacial, mandibular fracture or TMJ luxation or fracture. Changes in the appearance of the normal facial structure can indicate a depressed or displaced maxillofacial fracture, and similarly changes in the position of the globe can indicate an orbital or zygomatic fracture.

Once the patient has been stabilized, more comprehensive diagnostic modalities can be initiated. General anesthesia should be safely administered to allow for full evaluation of the oral cavity and skull without causing excessive pain or resistance from the patient. Digital palpation may reveal crepitus, instability, or physical inability to completely close the mouth. Visualization of bony structures is common since the trauma often causes damage to the thin layer of soft tissues overlaying the bones. Sharp fracture fragments can also penetrate the soft tissues and result in an open fracture. Following gross examination of the skull and oral cavity, dental and survey radiographs can be made and evaluated. Computed tomography (CT) with three-dimensional reconstruction provides excellent detail of injuries present, especially in complex cases with fractures of multiple bones of the skull and the mandible [4, 5]. Results of the diagnostics will help shape the final treatment plan.

13.4 Surgical Principles

Surgical approaches for treatment of maxillofacial and mandibular injuries will vary by the particular injury and can be intraoral, extraoral, or both. Patients should be anesthetized safely, carefully monitored, and positioned to allow for the best approach to the fracture repair. The naturally contaminated environment of the oral cavity provides an additional challenge not always present in appendicular skeletal fracture repair. The presence of advanced periodontal disease also further complicates treatment and healing by perpetuating a contaminated environment if left untreated. Infection and persistent periodontal disease can lead to osteomyelitis and non-union of fracture fragments. Extractions, judicious debridement of tissues, and systemic antimicrobial therapy may be indicated under these conditions. The use of antimicrobials is controversial as to time of administration and duration of use. Some advocate only peri-operative use of intravenous antibiotics based on human and canine studies showing minimal benefit for post-operative usage [6–8]. Other studies indicate that post-operative antimicrobial usage is justified in cases of open fractures that communicate with the oral cavity or the paranasal sinuses in humans [8, 9]. The main concern for generalized usage of antimicrobials is resistance. Amoxicillin-clavulanic acid, clindamycin, doxycycline, and metronidazole are common choices for treatment of the anaerobic types of bacteria often present in periodontitis in humans [8, 10, 11]. Clipping of the hair and preparation of skin for sterile surgery is advised for an extraoral approach. Decontamination of the oral cavity with antiseptic agents can reduce the bacterial load present in the mouth to foster a clean-contaminated environment [8, 12].

When utilizing normal occlusion as a way to gauge successful fracture reduction, steps must be taken to allow for evaluation of the occlusion at any time throughout the surgery. Removing as many obstructions from the oral cavity will greatly increase exposure and reduce the difficulty of repair. Esophageal monitoring equipment or temperature probes should be replaced by external electrocardiogram monitoring, auscultation by stethoscope, and rectal temperature probes. The endotracheal tube will also reduce access and visibility in the oral cavity. Extubation–reintubation practices are not a great option as the chance of malocclusion occurring is increased and maintaining reduction of fracture fragments is much more difficult. A better alternative would be to place the endotracheal tube via pharyngotomy or through a transmylohyoidal approach [13–16]. The patient is initially intubated through an oral approach and attached to the anesthesia delivery system.

Reintubation or repositioning of the endotracheal tube through one of the aforementioned approaches is performed. For the pharyngotomy approach, the caudal mandible and lateral cervical area is clipped and prepped for aseptic surgery. A long-handled angled forcep is placed into the mouth and directed just caudal to the angle of the mandible. This approach avoids several vital structures in this area such as the hypoglossal nerve, external carotid artery, external jugular vein, the lingual artery, and the linguofacial vein [15, 17]. A skin incision is made over the tip of the angled forcep. The tip of the forcep is protruded through the sphincter colli muscle and through the skin incision. The tissues are stretched by repeated opening of the forceps to allow for passage of a second appropriately sized endotracheal tube [13–15]. The tip of the second endotracheal tube is grasped and advanced through the pharyngotomy and into the oral cavity. The per os endotracheal tube is removed and the pharyngotomy endotracheal tube is placed into the trachea. The tube is secured with a finger trap suture to prevent dislodgement [14]. Once surgery is completed the pharyngotomy tube is removed and the per os endotracheal tube is replaced for recovery of the patient. For the transmylohyoid approach, the patient is placed in dorsal recumbency and the ventral aspect of the mandible is clipped and prepared aseptically for surgery. A skin incision is made medial to the ventral border of the mandible at the level of the mandibular first molar tooth. Blunt dissection of the subcutaneous tissues and the mylohyoideus muscle along the lingual cortex of the mandible is performed to allow for passage of the endotracheal tube that has been previously placed per os. A hemostat is placed into the incision directed toward the oral cavity and an intraoral mucosal incision is made over the tip of the instrument. The tissue is again stretched to allow for passage of the endotracheal tube. The anesthesia circuit is disconnected, the connector of the endotracheal tube is removed, and the hemostat placed into the incision is used to grasp the end of the endotracheal tube passing it through the incision into an extraoral position (Figure 13.1). The tube is secured with a finger trap suture or gauze tie as preferred [16]. The connector is replaced and the anesthesia circuit is reconnected. With this approach it is possible to direct a single endotracheal tube into an oral or extraoral position through the same incision, thus avoiding the extra step of reintubation. After a final check of the occlusion post-fracture repair, the patient's per os endotracheal tube is removed and the patient is again intubated through an oral approach for recovery from anesthesia. The incision made for pharyngotomy or the transmylohyoid approach should not be closed and is left to heal by second intention [13–16].

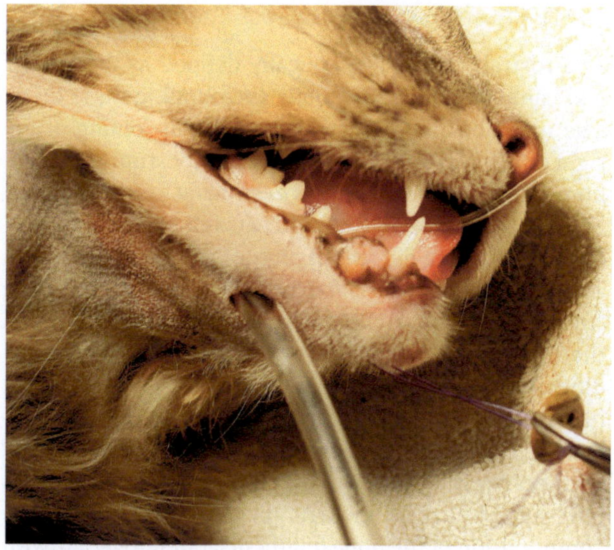

Figure 13.1 Placement of endotracheal tube through a transmylohyoid approach.

Fracture repair principles apply to treatment of maxillofacial trauma in the same manner as for appendicular fractures. Determining the best method of repair depends on knowledge of not only the anatomy but also of the forces that are applied to the bones during physiologic movement. Appliances or implants used to repair fractures must be placed appropriately to counteract these forces. Excessive strain placed on the implant will lead to failure of the device, and improper stabilization and alignment of a fracture may lead to non-union. The tension band principle states that all fixation devices are strongest in tension. As long as all stresses are acting parallel to the long axis of the implant it should be able to neutralize the normal physiologic forces after fixation [18, 19]. In the mandible the tension band surface is the alveolar border, and, as such, implants or appliances should be placed in this location whenever possible. The maxilla also has lines of stress and areas of buttressed support that should be considered during repair. Anatomic reduction and compression of fracture fragments along with maintenance of occlusion are the cornerstones of successful maxillofacial fracture repair.

13.5 Treatment Planning

In this section, the different types of fractures that may be encountered will be addressed, with brief discussions of recommended treatments. The specific treatments themselves will be covered later in the chapter. Each location has specific anatomic features that will influence fracture repair type.

13.5.1 Rostral Mandibular Fractures

The rostral mandible is typically defined as the incisor and canine teeth and the bone surrounding these teeth. The mandibular symphysis is the fibrous joining of the right and left mandibles in this rostral location. Unlike in humans where the mandibles eventually fuse at the midline, the symphysis in dogs and cats is a fibrous joint and can have varying degrees of physiologic movement [20]. Therefore mandibular symphyseal fracture is not a true "fracture" but a disruption of this fibrous union between the mandibles. This is one of the most common mandibular injuries in the cat [21, 22]. The degree of trauma in this region will determine the extent of treatment necessary [21]. In type I injuries, there will be a separation with no break in the soft tissues, while type II injuries have soft tissue disruption. A type III lesion will also have comminution of the bone fragments, often together with broken teeth [21]. Stabilization of a straightforward symphyseal separation is relatively simple to achieve with circumferential osseous wiring around the rostral mandibles just distal to the canine teeth. Care must be taken to ensure the incisor teeth remain in alignment, as step defects can be easy to create. Interdental wiring can also be used in these types of injuries and may allow for more precise maintenance of tooth alignment. Parasymphyseal fractures are a common iatrogenic injury during extraction of the mandibular canine tooth. Osseous circumferential wiring may still be successful in this type of fracture or, if the canines and incisors are missing, intraosseous wiring or use of a heavy grade suture can provide appropriate stabilization, especially in smaller patients.

13.5.2 Mandibular Body Fractures

Fractures of the body of the mandible are the most frequent oral fractures seen in the dog [23, 24]. A unilateral fracture may cause the jaw to be deviated toward the side of the injury, the same as with a caudoventral luxation of the TMJ, while rostroventral luxation of the TMJ will deviate away from the injured side [25, 26]. With minimal displacement, particularly with a unilateral defect and intact symphysis, a conservative approach with a gauze or tape muzzle may be sufficient. One way to determine the feasibility of a muzzle would be to see if the mouth closes easily while maintaining proper occlusion [24]. With the mandible, however, there are a few factors that determine what treatment is best, particularly the considerations of the biomechanical effects the muscles of mastication have on the mandible and any fracture segments. The bulk of the muscles, the masseter, temporal and pterygoid, work to swing the mandible dorsally as in closing the mouth, with their insertion on the caudal end of the body of the mandible [24, 27]. This movement can lift the caudal mandible in a rostrodorsal direction [28]. The digastricus muscle works in opposition to these muscles, tending to pull the rostral portion of the mandible caudoventrally, as in opening the mouth.

Fracture biomechanics indicate that the tension side of the mandible is the dorsal or alveolar border of the mandible where the teeth are [18]. Stabilization on this border will provide for a natural compressive force on the ventral surface. This can be provided with methods such as interdental wires and splints. Plate placement at the tension side of the mandible is much more difficult due to presence of the teeth and roots. Use of miniplates or larger plates in buttress fashion on the ventral border of the mandible is possible and can be used in combination with interdental or interfragmentary wire to counteract distractive and bending forces [19].

13.5.2.1 Favorable/Unfavorable Fractures

Biomechanical muscular forces have a particular influence on the type of stabilization needed for fractures in the region. If the fracture line is perpendicular to the long axis of the mandible, some dorsal distraction may occur [29]. With a fracture line that runs caudodorsally, the forces tend to keep the segments compressed together, classifying it as a favorable fracture (Figure 13.2). While some of these can be adequately treated with conservative methods such as a tape muzzle, often a single interosseous wire placed perpendicular to the fracture line will provide sufficient reduction and resistance to displacement forces. This is often true when the fracture is unilateral, there is no symphyseal mobility, and the intact opposite mandible provides both a good basis for reduction as well as stability [24].

When the fracture line runs in a caudoventral direction, however, the larger muscles of mastication exert force upward on the distal segment and the digastricus tends to pull the rostral segment down and caudally, with subsequent displacement and classification as an unfavorable fracture (Figure 13.3). Two intraosseous wires can be placed, one dorsally and one ventrally, or just one ventrally with acrylic splint stabilization to compensate for any dorsal gap should be sufficient [24]. Alternatively, two wires may be placed with a common placement site in the rostral segment and two sites in the distal segment to approximate a perpendicular relationship of the two wires. This triangular method helps to provide additional stabilization against the muscular forces. A good indication for use of miniplates in the mandible would be the presence of an unfavorable fracture. This more rigid type of fixation can adequately counteract the muscular forces pulling the fracture fragments apart [19].

Acrylic splints may be used, alone or in combination with wire placement. The combination of interdental wire and acrylic together is significantly stronger than

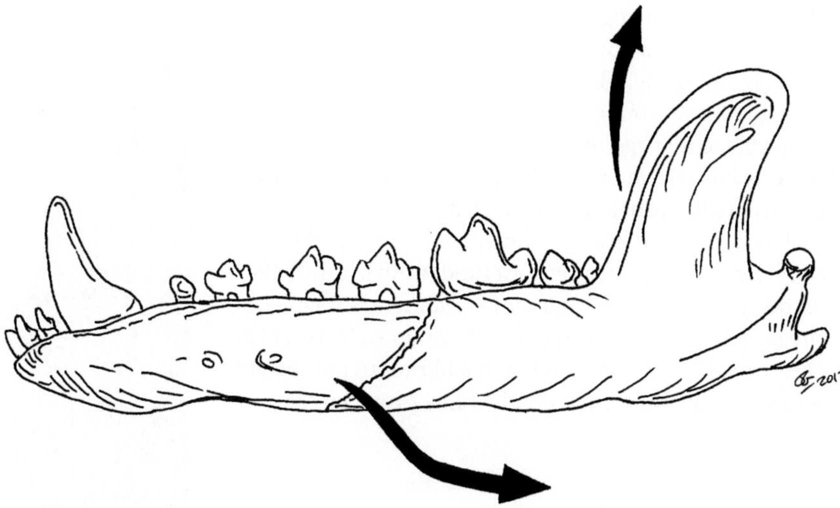

Figure 13.2 Favorable mandibular fracture. Courtesy of Josephine Banyard.

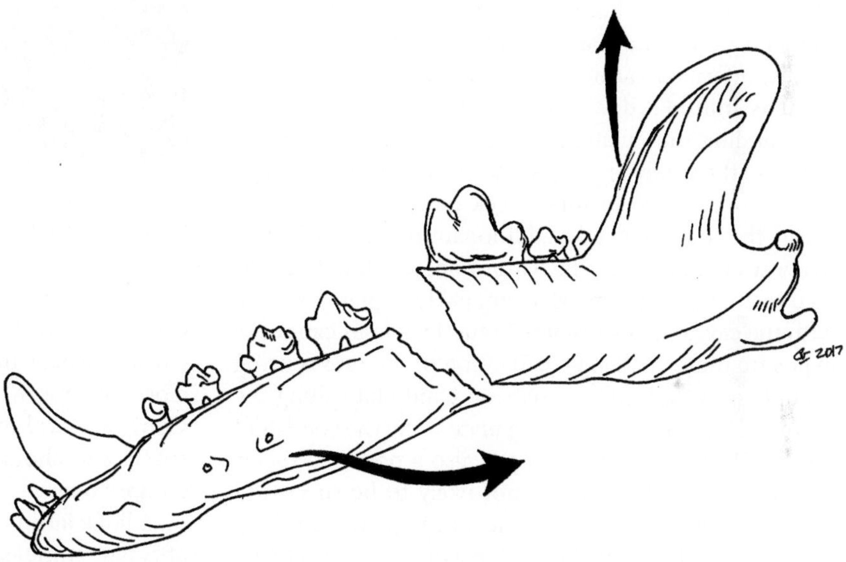

Figure 13.3 Unfavorable mandibular fracture. Courtesy of Josephine Banyard.

either material alone [30]. Incorporating wires into acrylic in edentulous areas can be one means of fixation of pathologic fractures due to periodontal disease at the lower first molars. Similarly, a direct acrylic splint can be secured to the mandible with cerclage wires when interdental wiring is not an option [31]. Maxillo-mandibular fixation (MMF), immobilizing the mouth in partial occlusion, prevents excessive movement while still allowing some ability to drink and eat is another less invasive method of fracture repair [32].

Severely comminuted fractures that have gaps or non-viable tissues often require more complicated means of fixation. While some appendicular skeletal fixation means do not translate as well to the oral cavity, such as intramedullary pinning, plating and screws, some forms of external fixation have been successfully employed [28, 33]. The combination of using Kirschner wires or Steinmann pins on either side of the fracture site, even bilaterally, with an acrylic-filled tube to engage the pin ends can provide immediate stabilization. Areas of substantial bone loss, either due to fragmentation or necrosis, can be held in position with this method to allow the defect to eventually fill in, though this can be a long-term solution (several months if more than 4–6 cm). Alternately, grafts of cancellous bone chips or even ribs can be used to facilitate bone regrowth [24]. If the area is grossly contaminated, delaying implantation until the epithelial surfaces have healed, then placing the material through a sterile, ventral approach may be the optimum method [34]. More recently other treatment options have been attempted such as the use of bone morphogenic proteins to regenerate bone in a large defect. Recombinant human bone morphogenic protein 2 (rhBMP-2) is infused into a compression-resistant matrix and placed into a large mandibular defect, followed by placement of a large plate or plates in buttress fashion [35–39].

Fractures of this region that become a non-union may be manageable as a fibrous union if unilateral with a stable opposite mandible. Bilateral lesions, particularly ones instigated by severe periodontal disease are often nearly impossible to manage, and while long-term mouth closure methods (muzzle, interarcade fixation, commissuroplasty) may eventually provide a functional "bite," the management and possible complications are often challenging [28]. Continuing research into methods utilizing rhBMP-2 has the potential to provide new treatments in cases of non-union, malunion, repair of large defects from osteomyelitis, or severe trauma in addition to immediate reconstruction after a mandibulectomy procedure.

13.5.3 Fractures of the Mandibular Ramus

Mandibular ramus fractures are less common than ones of the mandibular body or symphysis [23]. In the far caudal region of the mandibular body and even up in the ramus, internal fixation may not be needed if displacement is minimal due to the supportive effect of the surrounding musculature [25, 28]. Unilateral fractures dorsal to the condylar process may respond well to a tape muzzle over a two to three week period, but fractures below that level may take additional time, up to four to five weeks. If unstable, the flatter bones, without associated teeth, make it somewhat amenable to plate fixation, with the caveat that substantial muscle masses can make exposure more challenging. Fixation of the ramus using miniplates would utilize a tension band plate along the coronoid crest and a stabilizing plate along the condyloid crest [19]. Intraosseous wiring is also a potential repair method. External fixation is not likely to be successful given the thin nature of the bone for pin placement [25]. If there is significant malocclusion associated with a suspected ramus fracture, the TMJs should be closely examined for any signs of concurrent fracture or luxation [24]. Future problems may occur with larger callus formation during conservative management if there is any interference with normal oral movements. Zygomaticomandibular ankylosis occurs when there is fusion of the coronoid process to the zygomatic arch, which can also restrict movement of the TMJ [26]. If restricted TMJ movement and morbidity exists after treatment for a caudal mandibular fracture then excision arthroplasty can be considered to alleviate discomfort. Mandibular condylectomy can be performed to prevent contact of the mandible with the temporal bone. Fibrous tissue formation will occur to create a false joint [25].

13.5.4 Fractures of the Temporomandibular Joint

As with other portions of the vertical ramus, fractures in this region are uncommon and usually the result of trauma [22, 23, 26, 40] (Figure 13.4). The most common clinical finding with TMJ fracture or luxation is a malocclusion, which may present as the inability to open or close the mouth, or lateral shifting of the mandible [26]. Complete oral examination is performed under anesthesia and should also include diagnostic imaging for comprehensive evaluation of the TMJ and concurrent maxillofacial injuries. If any structures of the TMJ are affected, complete evaluation with radiographs and/or CT is indicated for diagnosis and treatment planning [41]. In a recent study utilizing a CT scan for evaluation of TMJ disorders, TMJ fractures were the most common TMJ disorder identified in cats and the second most common TMJ disorder identified in dogs. Cats in this study were all noted to have fractured the condylar process of the mandible. Dogs were found to have fractures of either the condylar process or the temporal bone. It was suggested that differences in skull anatomy between dogs and cats resulted in the variance of fracture types [41].

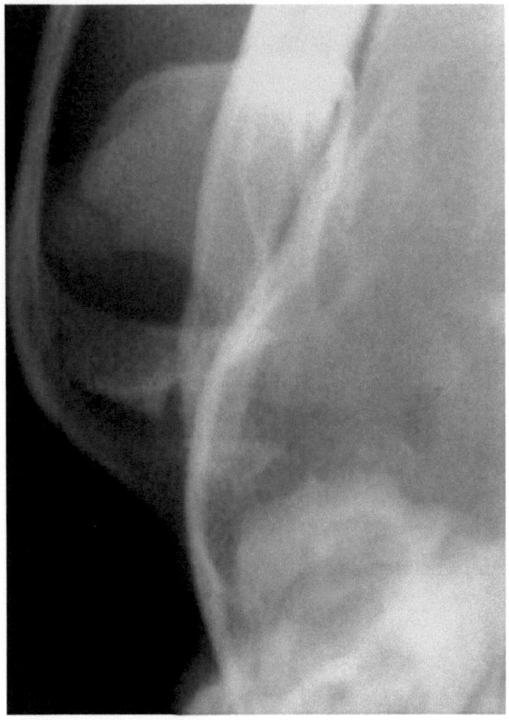

Figure 13.4 Fracture of the condyloid process of the temporomandibular joint.

Subluxation of the TMJ may not result in significant clinical signs and usually is managed conservatively by feeding a soft diet and pain medications [26]. Joint luxations most commonly occur in a rostrodorsal direction. Caudoventral luxations occur less frequently and are usually accompanied by fracture of the retroarticular process. Unilateral rostrodorsal luxations usually result in shifting of the mandible toward the contralateral side. Unilateral caudoventral luxations tend to shift the mandible toward the ipsilateral (affected) side [26]. Fractures of the TMJ may result in crepitus when the mandible is manipulated, but usually the mandible can be easily placed into occlusion, whereas the mandible may be resistant to reduction in the case of a luxation injury. Fractures of the caudal mandible and condyle may cause displacement of the mandible caudally, resulting in a shifting of the mandible toward the affected side. Luxation injuries can be seen radiographically with ventrodorsal, dorsoventral, or laterodorsal oblique projections. Radiographs may also reveal fractures of the retroarticular process, condylar neck, or condyle [42, 43]. Computed tomography is particularly useful for visualization of fractures with multiple fragments or condylar fractures that may not be appreciated on radiographs, given its ability to isolate the regional anatomy without superimposition of other structures and to provide three-dimensional reconstruction [41, 44].

13.5.5 Fractures of the Maxilla

Discussion of maxillary trauma for the purpose of this section will include fractures of the incisive, palatine, zygomatic, lacrimal, frontal, nasal bones, and the maxillary bone proper [45, 46]. Maxillary fractures are less common than mandibular lesions and may be more difficult to detect and evaluate fully with skull and dental radiographs due to overlapping structures. Epistaxis, swelling, discomfort, and malocclusion may be indications of damage, but displacement at times can be minimal. If such is the case, and the occlusion is still correct, little may need to be done. Occasionally the simple act of suturing any soft tissue defects after digital realignment will provide sufficient stabilization [24, 34], though some cases benefit from other methods such as tape muzzles or acrylic splints, with or without interdental wiring. For more complex fractures and obvious facial deformity, computed tomography is indicated to fully evaluate the injuries present. Three-dimensional reconstruction provides added information [46]. Miniplates have been utilized for comminuted and depressed fractures of the maxillofacial bones. Depression fractures of the bones that make up the borders of the nasal cavity can cause significant impairment of airflow and can result in long-term morbidity with chronic nasal obstruction [47]. Most of the maxillary bones are relatively thin and surround larger areas of space such as the nasal cavity and paranasal sinuses [48]. The bones of the maxilla can be thought of as a frame surrounding these voids. This strong and lightweight frame connects the base of the skull to the occlusal surfaces [46, 49]. The human skull was found to have buttresses of projecting support and similar buttresses are noted in the dog and cat skulls [49, 50]. Damage to these buttressed areas of support will cause the frame to collapse. Understanding the anatomy and support of the maxillofacial frame will facilitate proper management of fractures to this area. Three primary buttresses exist: medial, lateral, and caudal. Generally, repair of two of the three main buttresses will restore the position of the maxilla in relation to the skull and mandible [46, 50, 51].

13.6 Treatment Modalities

Repair techniques of maxillofacial injuries can be generally described as non/less-invasive or invasive. Non-invasive techniques may include tape muzzle, MMF/immobilization, interdental wiring, acrylic splinting, or combination of interdental wiring and acrylic splinting. External fixation is another minimally invasive technique for fracture stabilization. In general non-invasive techniques allow for preservation of vital structures such as the teeth and neurovascular anatomy. Minimal disruption of the periosteum is also beneficial for encouraging bony healing [52]. The location of the injury often dictates which type of repair is likely to be most successful. Some areas such as the ramus of the mandible and certain areas of the maxilla can be repaired with an invasive technique such as plating with fewer concerns of interfering with structures such as teeth or neurovascular anatomy. The mandible provides a challenge for use of traditional plating techniques due to the volume occupied by tooth roots and the structures within the mandibular canal.

13.6.1 Tape Muzzle

The conservative use of a tape muzzle has many applications when dealing with oral fractures [23]. It is helpful as a first aid treatment with any oral fracture that results in significant displacement to help protect the segments and avoid any further damage [23]. In unilateral mandibular fractures or maxillary fractures with minimal displacement, it may be the only modality needed to provide sufficient stabilization [53]. The oral cavity, with its rich blood supply and lack of heavy weight bearing, does not need complete rigid fixation for adequate healing [33], though the callus formation will be larger in areas that are not totally immobilized. Due to the muscular support afforded in fractures of the mandibular ramus, a tape muzzle may provide additional support for sufficient healing [53], as well as in minimally displaced condylar process fractures. Muzzles may also be used as an adjunctive treatment after primary fracture repair [53].

In addition to fractures with minimal displacement, a tape muzzle may also be used when other methods of fixation are not possible, such as the bilateral pathological fracture of the mandibles due to severe periodontal disease or cases where owner's finances do not allow definitive treatment. Often complete union is not likely, even with attempted osseous regeneration, but if sufficient stability can be afforded initially, a fibrous union may result.

Tape muzzles can be made readily with non-porous tape. They are cheap and disposable once they become soiled. Several can be made for the owner to have at home and change out as needed. Alternatively, a cloth muzzle can be used for support. It is beneficial to have more than one muzzle available so that soiled ones can be washed. The tape muzzle should be placed with the canines in correct occlusion, allowing a 0.5 to 1.0 cm (up to 1.5 cm) gap in the incisors to allow for lapping of water and soft food. The first layer of tape is placed around the muzzle with the adhesive side out, and a second layer around it, with the two adhesive sides touching each other. The head strap is fashioned in a similar fashion, extending from the tape around the nose back behind the ears and to the other side to keep the muzzle held comfortably in place. Some contraindications for a muzzle include a brachycephalic head and any problems with vomition, where the material can be retained in the mouth and aspirated. A patient with respiratory distress would not be a good candidate for a muzzle, and nor does it allow for panting if the animal gets overheated. Long-term use of a tape muzzle can also cause a significant dermatitis problem [54].

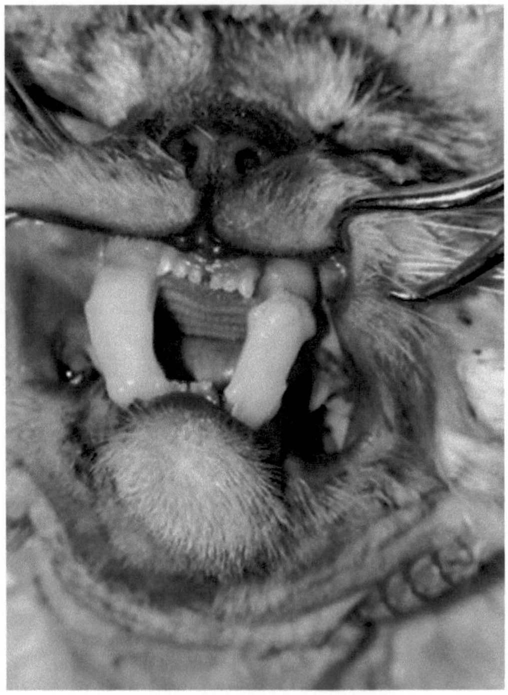

Figure 13.5 MMF (maxillomandibular fixation) of a cat with composite spanning ipsilateral canine teeth.

13.6.2 Maxillomandibular Fixation

There are other means of limiting oral movements while maintaining occlusion, such as MMF [21, 29, 33]. Many methods of immobilizing the movement of the mandible exist and the goal of treatment is similar to a tape muzzle – immobilize the movement of the jaws to allow healing of the fracture. However, the success rate with MMF would be expected to be higher because complete immobilization can be achieved. Invasive methods of immobilizing the mandible can include placing circumferential wires around both the maxilla and mandible or with transosseous placement of wires or screws with stabilization between the two arcades [29, 55]. Less invasive methods are also quite successful and with less potential side effects. The patient should be properly anesthetized and positioned for oral surgery. Placement of an endotracheal tube via pharyngotomy or a transmylohyoid approach is performed to facilitate application of the chosen technique and allow for simple extubation on recovery. With the mouth held in proper occlusion and a slight space between the incisors, the canines can be joined together with a composite bridge (Figure 13.5). Various techniques and materials for joining the canines have been reported. The canine teeth are scaled, polished with flour pumice, and acid etched in preparation for placement of an acrylic dental composite material. The canine teeth are placed in occlusion and a normal caudal dentition relationship should be confirmed. The maxillary and mandibular canines should overlap about one-third of the crown height, enough to allow for the patient to drink water and lap up gruel-consistency food. Self-curing acrylic or composite is applied on the canine teeth to create two pillars of material. Syringe cases can also be placed on the canines to act as a mold for the composite and are left in place until the appliance is removed [54, 56]. A feeding tube should be placed to ensure nutritional needs can be met if the patient will not aliment voluntarily while the appliance is in place. The same factors of concern with respiratory distress or vomiting apply as with the tape muzzle.

13.6.3 Wiring Techniques

Wire provides advantages of being a simple, inexpensive, and versatile tool for repair of osseous fractures of the oral cavity. Wire is useful not only in the reduction of fractures but also, when used properly, can provide an excellent realignment of the dentition. Wiring is used in four basic techniques: osseous, interdental, adjunct, and interarcade.

13.6.3.1 Osseous Wiring

Osseous wiring places wire in direct contact with bone to provide direct reduction and support to portions of a bony fracture. It can be performed either by open or closed surgical approaches, but the visualization attained by open techniques allows for a more accurate assessment and realignment of the fractured segments. This also allows for the possible visualization of potential complications from hidden foreign bodies and loose bone fragments. Osseous wiring's primary function is to reduce fractures and prevent their displacement by the passive function of the muscles of mastication. However, by itself, osseous wiring cannot be relied upon for stable fixation if the jaw is to be functional and non-immobilized during the initial healing period. If this is to be the case, the osseous wiring should be augmented by interdental wiring or some additional form of acrylic or dental composite splinting. The first rule of osseous wiring is to do no harm, or attempt to avoid injury to other structures within the jaws, such as the mandibular canal, roots of teeth, and the periodontal ligament. The second rule is to always endeavor to reestablish normal functional occlusion. In the osseous category there are three fundamental forms of wiring: circumferential/cerclage, intraosseous, and transcircumferential.

13.6.3.1.1 Circumferential/Cerclage

In circumferential or cerclage wiring the wire is typically placed by using a suitable shaped and size of suture needle or large gauge injection needle to guide its placement. When using a large bore needle, it is initially placed from the vestibule behind the canine on one side down into the intermandibular space through a small ventral incision. The wire is placed into the needle bore hole and the combination is retracted back through the soft tissue. The wire is then passed distal to the two canines and exits back out of the incision. The wire is then tightened to oppose the two mandibles (Figure 13.6). Alternatively, the wire can be tightened on the oral side and the twist covered with a small bead of composite to prevent tongue trauma. The wire is placed in a similar fashion utilizing a ventral skin incision. Removal of wire placed in this manner does not involve recreating a skin incision to locate the wire twist [57, 58]. Care must be taken to avoid excessive force while tightening the cerclage wire, which can deviate the mandibular canines medially, contributing to a malocclusion when the mouth is closed. The same concern applies in cases where there is more extensive osseous damage or missing fragments of bone. Circumferential wires can also be used in edentulous areas in combination with an acrylic splint. The wire itself can be incorporated in the acrylic. Further discussion on the use of acrylic splints with cerclage wires is found later in this chapter.

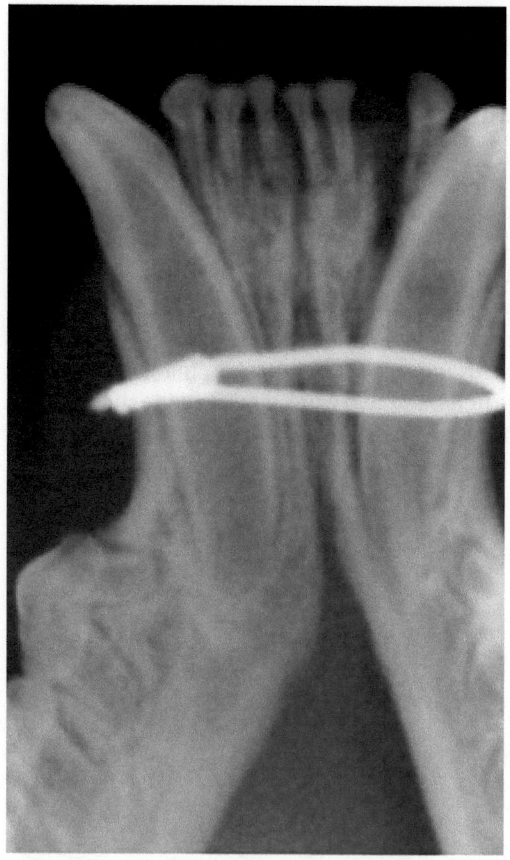

Figure 13.6 Circumferential wiring to stabilize symphyseal separation.

13.6.3.1.2 Intraosseous

In intraosseous wiring, 20 to 28 gauge stainless steel wire, typically 24 gauge, is used. A large gauge heavy-duty injection needle, 14 to 20 gauge, and a #4 to #6 surgical length round bur can be used for anchorage hole placement. Every effort should be made to avoid injury to the roots and periodontal ligament of the teeth and the mandibular canal during placement of the anchorage holes through the bone. When done, open soft tissue is seldom a problem, but in closed placement a small cut with a #11 blade will reduce soft tissue tangling with the bur. In some cases the large-bore needle can actually be passed through the bone with some twisting manipulations, but the surgical bur is typically faster. However, even the surgical length burs will not always pass entirely though some mandibles. This is circumvented by placing the guide hole with the bur and then finishing the hole either with the large-bore injection needle or an intramedullary pin of a similar size. Intraosseous wiring is most successful when all fragments can be reduced by the intraosseous wires, thus allowing the fragments and wire to share load-bearing [18].

For fractures of the body of the mandible, placement and number of anchorage holes is primarily dependent upon the adjacent structures and the type of fracture. Most body fractures are vertical obliques resulting in either a favorable or unfavorable type of fracture line. On favorable fractures that reduce well, a single horizontal intraosseous wire may provide the needed fixation (Figure 13.7). However, when dealing with an unfavorable fracture line, additional anchorage is customarily required if intraosseous wiring is to be used (Figure 13.8). A combination of a horizontal and vertical intraosseous wire in a triangular configuration, made with three anchorage holes and two wires, may provide the required stabilization. Two of the holes are placed vertically or at an oblique to one another in the caudal segment, with one in the rostral segment. Both wires will make use of the single anchorage hole in the rostral segment. The first wire is placed horizontally and the second placed obliquely. The wires should be tightened to realign the segment, while providing the needed retraction to close the fracture line. In some cases, unfavorable fractures will be stabilized with the combination of a horizontal intraosseous wire and interdental wiring.

13.6.3.1.3 *Transcircumferential*

Transcircumferential wiring is a single-wire technique that has both a transosseous anchorage and goes circumferentially around the bone (Figure 13.9). It is used most

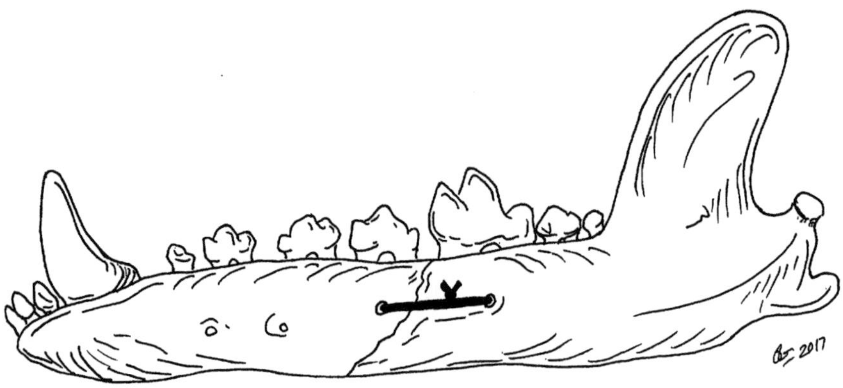

Figure 13.7 Single horizontal transosseous wire to stabilize favorable fracture. Courtesy of Josephine Banyard.

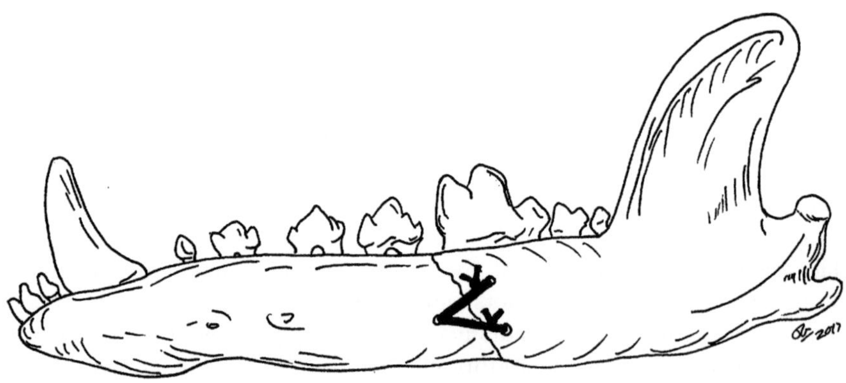

Figure 13.8 Additional anchor with double transosseous wire in a triangular configuration to stabilize unfavorable fracture. Courtesy of Josephine Banyard.

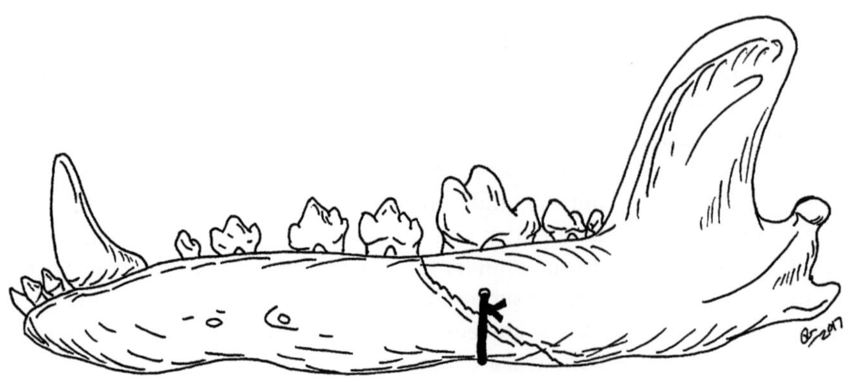

Figure 13.9 Transcircumferential wire technique with both a transosseous anchorage and going circumferentially around the mandible.

commonly for unfavorable body fractures. The transosseous anchorage hole is placed 3 to 4 mm from the alveolar crest over the fracture site, possibly even between two roots of a tooth. The wire is passed through the anchorage hole and then run circumferentially under the mandible with the aid of needles. The lead ends are twisted together and tightened. Interdental wiring performed in combination with transcircumferential wiring provides greater stability for these fractures.

13.6.3.2 Interdental Wiring

Interdental wiring is the placement of wires around adjacent teeth to provide reduction and support to a bony fracture that extends between the teeth. Interdental wiring is one of the techniques that can be used for closed fracture repair [33, 54]. However, it is used in both closed and open techniques, and adjunct procedures where a combination of acrylics, composites or other devices may be used in association with the wire to provide the needed support once reduction is accomplished. The size of wire used, 22 to 30 gauge, is dictated by the size of the oral cavity and the teeth involved. Most wire comes dead soft in rolls. The natural curling of such wire should be corrected by stretching the segment of wire to be used between with two forceps. Many types of wire handling and twisting instruments are available for use with wire, but needle holders can be used in most cases.

Wires can usually be placed below the cervical bulge of the tooth either with instrument pressure or with the aid of 18 to 20 gauge needles. A W-3 or cord packing instrument can many times assist in holding the wire below the bulge during the tightening phase. Alternatively, a needle can be placed through the gingiva below the bulge to expedite passage of the wire at the proper depth. In most healthy animals this will cause a transitory inflammation that resolves when the wire is removed. On occasion, notching a tooth with a vertical groove may be required to maintain the wire in either the correct position, or at a preferred height above the gingiva. Wire placed at this level will commonly cause gingival irritation. Prevention of infection can generally be accomplished by the routine use of oral hygiene solutions until the wires are removed, at which time healing is typically rapid and complete. However, if pre-existing periodontal disease is present, wire at the gingival level must be inspected routinely and oral hygiene of the highest caliber must be done. If meticulous care cannot be provided, then other forms of support should be considered. A simple alternative is the placement of the wires higher on the tooth by the assistance of composite bonding, notching of the tooth, or both.

There are four basic types of interdental wiring most commonly used: Ivy loop, Stout multiple loop, Essig, and Risdon. The Ivy and Stout multiple loops incorporate a single-wire technique, while the Essig and Risdon require two wires. Placement of these patterns does take some practice, but once the techniques are mastered, they become invaluable in fracture reduction. If the twisted wire ends or any of the loops are irritating to the soft tissues, they can be padded by covering them with a small amount of acrylic or dental composite.

13.6.3.2.1 Ivy Loop

The Ivy loop wiring technique is used most commonly for reduction of simple fractures between two teeth, securing acrylic appliances, or as an anchorage for other attachments. It is the fastening of two teeth together by a single ligating wire (Figure 13.10). The wire is folded in half and an instrument placed between the two ends at the fold. The wire is then twisted around the instrument to form a loop. The two loose ends are passed through the interdental space between the two teeth to be ligated together to the lingual surface. One end goes around each tooth and back around to the facial side. The distal lead is then passed through the loop and twisted together with the other lead, approximately at the mesiofacial line angle of the mesial tooth. The loop is then lightly tightened over the lead wire that passed through it. The leads and loop are each delicately tightened until the desired tension develops. A slight apical tension on the leads will

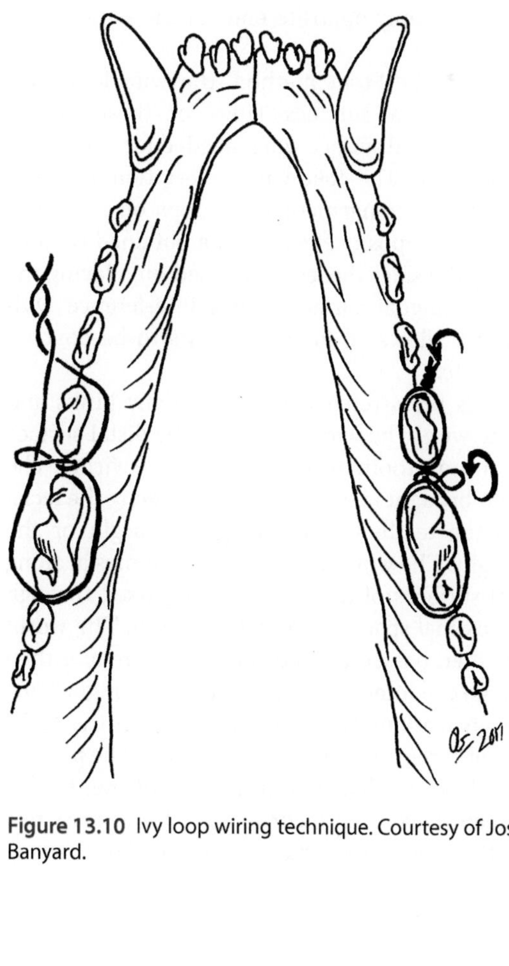

Figure 13.10 Ivy loop wiring technique. Courtesy of Josephine Banyard.

help to keep the wire in place below the cervical bulge. Care must be taken not to over tighten the wire or it will fatigue and break, and the process will have to be repeated. If the Ivy loop is to act as an anchorage for an acrylic appliance on the lingual surface, loops may need to be created with the leads before they are passed back around to the facial surface. When tightening the leads or loops, they should be grasped as near the tooth or bone as is reasonable to obtain the required reduction of the fracture. The loop and twisted ends can be tucked interdentally if small enough or, if needed, pressed tightly against the tooth and covered with composite where appropriate.

13.6.3.2.2 Stout Multiple Loop

The Stout multiple loop wiring technique is another single-wire method, but incorporates more than just two adjacent teeth. It is in fact a simple continuation of an Ivy loop technique. It is used in the same applications as the Ivy loop, but provides greater stability and strength.

The lead ends in the Stout technique are known as the static wire and the working wire. The working wire is the lead end that is passed back and forth through the interproximal spaces and forms the tightening loops. The static wire is the lead that lies against the tooth and is fixed in place by the loops of the working wire lead. It should be kept in mind that the working lead and static lead are simply opposite ends of the same single piece of wire.

Classically in the Stout method, the wire loops are placed on the facial surfaces. However, these can be placed on the lingual surface when needed for anchorage or other support. The following description is based upon the classic arrangement with loops on the facial surface, but the opposite effect can be obtained by simply reversing the sides the leads are used on. Placing the loops on the lingual surface avoids interference with occlusion and allows all loops or twists to be covered with composite.

The wire is pre-stretched to remove any kinks and laxity in the wire. The wire is taken to the distal surface of the distal-most tooth to be included in the wiring. The static lead is brought mesially or rostrally along the facial surface of the teeth near the gingival margin or the desired height. The working lead is brought mesial along the lingual surfaces of the teeth and is passed through the interproximal space between each tooth. The working lead is then passed around the static wire and then back through the interproximal space to the lingual surface. Enough working wire should be left on the facial surface to form the needed tightening loops. The process is continued up the dental arch until all of the desired adjacent teeth have been incorporated, for at least two teeth on either side of the fracture if possible. The working and static lead ends of the wire are then twisted together. The tightening loops should now each be lightly and evenly tightened. Once all have been evenly snugged, the loops and twisted ends can be tightened to the desired reduction point (Figure 13.11). Care should be taken not to overtighten the wire or it may fatigue and break.

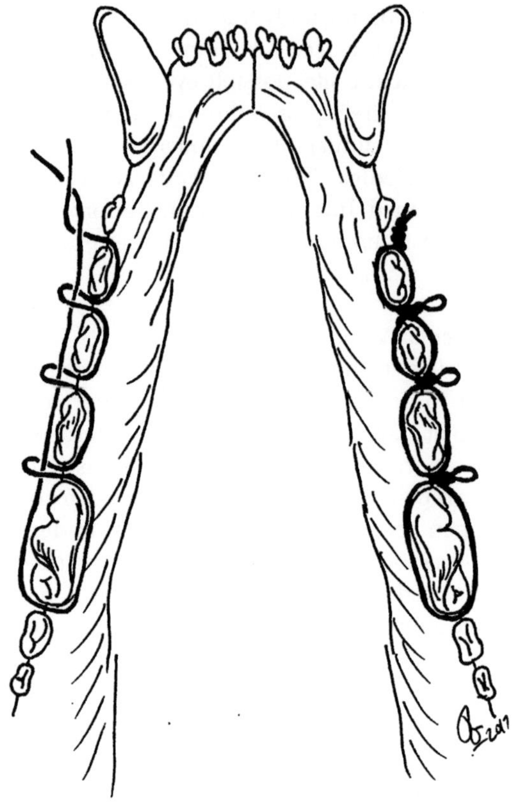

Figure 13.11 Stout multiple loop wiring technique. Courtesy of Josephine Banyard.

13.6.3.2.3 Essig

The Essig wiring method is most commonly used in stabilizing incisor teeth loosened from trauma, or for fracture reduction. It is formed by a primary wire and multiple secondary wires. The primary wire is the master wire that is passed around all of the teeth to be incorporated in the support, usually the incisors, but sometimes the canines as well, and the ends lightly twisted together. The secondary wires are short segments passed interdentally through the interproximal spaces, between each adjacent tooth in the wiring pattern, from the facial surface to the lingual surface and back facially, circling both the lingual and facial strands of the primary wire. Each secondary wire is lightly tightened to hold it in place until all of the secondary wires are placed. The wires are then tightened evenly to the desired tension (Figure 13.12).

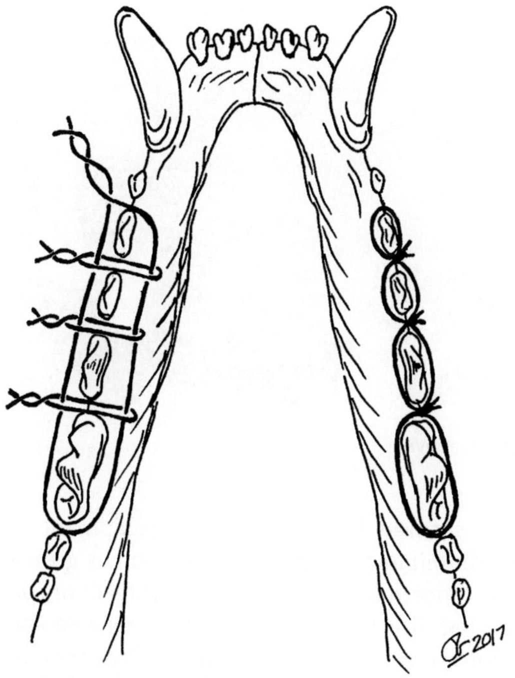

Figure 13.12 Essig wiring technique. Courtesy of Josephine Banyard.

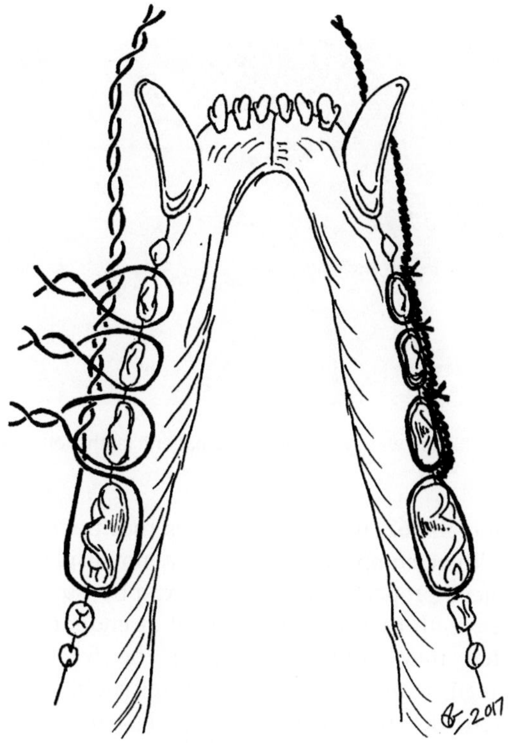

Figure 13.13 Risdon wiring technique. Courtesy of Josephine Banyard.

13.6.3.2.4 Risdon

The Risdon wiring technique is used when greater strength of reduction is required, such as in some rostral and symphyseal fractures of the mandible. In this technique, there are two sets of primary wires, a left and a right. In addition, there will be numerous secondary wires. The primary wire is passed distally around the anchorage tooth bilaterally, which is typically the mandibular carnassial tooth if healthy. The anchorage tooth should be healthy, have a substantial root surface, and be supported in an adequate degree of solid bone. The primary wire is looped around the tooth below the cervical bulge with the ends meeting at the mesial buccal line angle, leaving two long leads of approximately equal lengths. The two leads are then twisted together in a long braid that reaches past the midpoint of the mandibular symphysis. The secondary wires are looped around the teeth mesial to the anchor tooth, with one end looped over and one under the primary wire, either lingually or buccally. The ends of the secondary wires should then be twisted together over the primary braided wire. This is repeated on as many teeth as needed for support and stability of the primary braided wire, and to align the incisors properly (Figure 13.13). This technique can be used in fractures that require additional support such as bilateral mandibular fractures. The primary braided wire from each mandible can be twisted together mesially (Figure 13.14a and b).

13.6.3.3 Teeth in the Fracture Line

If teeth are present in the fracture line or have been traumatized, immediate extraction may be contraindicated. Extraction of teeth within the fracture line can further destabilize the fracture fragments and make proper reduction more difficult. These teeth may also be needed for placement of an intraoral appliance for the fracture repair. A recent study compared the strength of various non-invasive repair techniques based on the presence or absence of the crown (roots were not removed) of the mandibular first molar (M1). Maintenance of the M1 significantly increased stiffness in the interdental wire and acrylic appliances, although ultimately strength of the appliance was not reliant on the presence of the M1 crown. Further research is needed to determine the benefits of retaining teeth in the fracture line, but it would be expected that fixation devices with greater ultimate strength and stiffness should reduce micromotion in the fracture environment. Conditions resulting from a more rigid construct should facilitate primary bone healing. Presence of the crown of the M1 would be expected to contribute to the overall stability and rigidity of the fracture repair appliance [59]. Human maxillofacial trauma management has gravitated toward maintenance of teeth in the fracture line [60, 61]. Based on these principles it may be prudent to leave these teeth until the fracture has healed and subsequently reevaluated at

(a) (b)

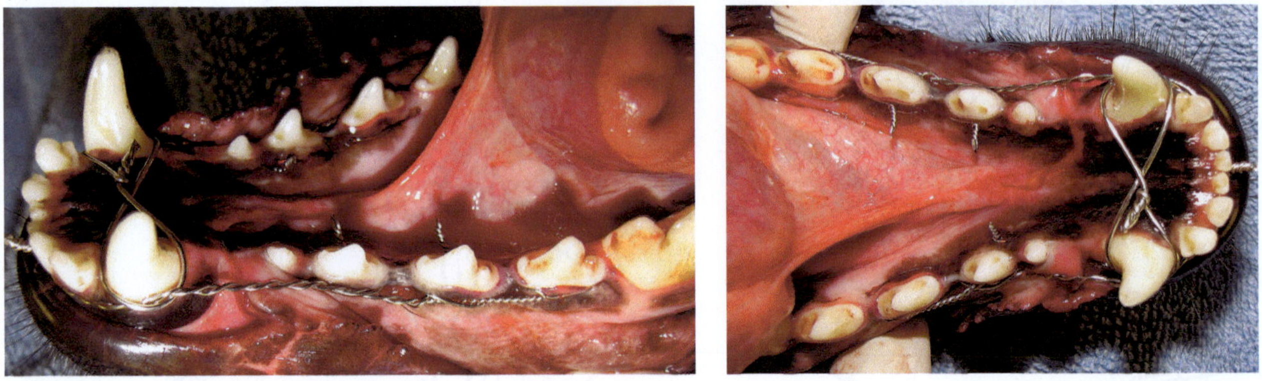

Figures 13.14 Risdon wiring technique in a patient: (a) the left side; (b) both sides, from above.

certain intervals [62, 63]. In some cases root fractures may heal with no complications if they are not displaced or are reduced properly. The obvious exception to this practice are teeth that have periodontal or endodontic disease that may inhibit healing of the fracture. Diseased teeth within pathologic fractures should also be extracted. If a particular tooth has just one root extensively affected by periodontal disease, tooth or root resection can be performed to salvage the healthy portion of the tooth (See Chapter 16 – Advanced Endodontic Therapy).

13.6.3.4 Adjunct Wiring

Adjunct wiring is when a wiring technique is used as an adjunct to some other form of stabilization or device, such as cerclage wiring to secure acrylic or composite splints [31, 54], or some form of orthodontic appliance.

13.6.3.5 Interarcade Wiring

The process of interarcade wiring or fixation was briefly discussed under tape muzzle, because the final effect is similar. Interarcade wiring has largely been replaced with less-invasive procedures such as dental composite bonding of the canine teeth, placement of orthodontic brackets with elastic power chains, or camouflage procedures that extend the crown of the maxillary canine to prevent shifting of the mandible.

13.6.4 Acrylic and Composite Splints

Acrylics and composites are widely used in the oral cavity due to their non-invasive nature, ease of use, versatility, and low cost [33]. The acrylic or composite splint can either be formed directly in the oral cavity or on a model in an indirect fashion, and then attached in an appropriate manner. Indirect splint formation requires taking impressions in order to create a stone model on which to form the splint. The cured splint is then placed on to the patient and secured by wires. The development of materials with minimal exothermic reaction has greatly lessened the concern for heat damage to the teeth or soft tissues, making direct application more amenable and also the more time-efficient technique. Wires may be used within the acrylic to provide additional strength or can be incorporated around other structures such as teeth to enhance retention of the appliance. Self-curing bis-acryl composite material for temporary crown and bridge placement is an excellent material with a minimal exothermic reaction that can be used for splinting.

Some inherent problems with acrylic or composite include the possibility of rough edges irritating the soft tissue or enhancing the retention of food particles and debris, contributing to stomatitis. In order to minimize problems, the acrylic edges should be smoothed and well-formed to the contours of the oral cavity, the owner should rinse the splint regularly, and the patient should be reevaluated at regular, short intervals (weekly or biweekly) until the appliance is removed to monitor for shifting or failure. Once the splint is removed, any inflammation usually subsides within a short period of time.

It is a fact that an acrylic splint generally incorporates the teeth associated with a fracture; thus it is applied to the tension band side, which is optimum. Keeping the occlusal forces also in mind, forming the bulk of a mandibular splint on the lingual surface and a maxillary splint on the buccal surface will minimize any occlusal interference by the opposing dentition [33, 54].

With the availability of self-curing or light-cured acrylics and composites it is not generally necessary to use materials that have an excessive exothermic reaction. Previous generations of acrylic materials produced a large amount of heat during polymerization and required cooling techniques to prevent soft tissue or pulpal damage [64]. The oral tissues should be prepared prior to splint placement by first minimizing any open wound areas.

(a) (b)

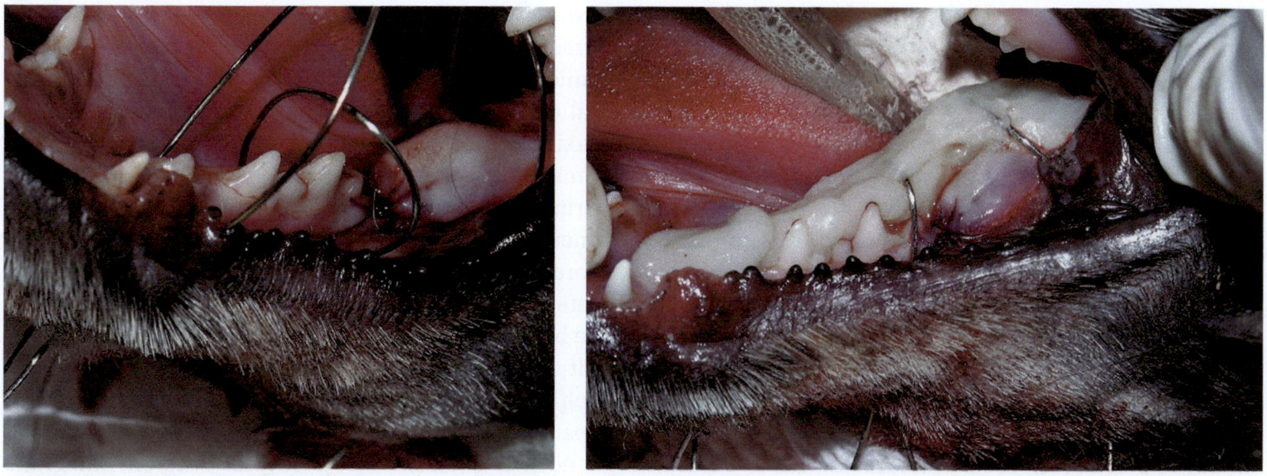

Figures 13.15 (a) Cerclage wires pre-placed for splint; (b) composite or acrylic incorporated with cerclage wires for splinting across partially edentulous areas.

The teeth to be incorporated into the splint should be cleaned, polished with flour pumice, and acid-etched. As the fracture is held in a reduced position, acrylic or composite is placed directly on to the teeth and mandible [54]. The thickness of the acrylic should be around 7–10 mm in diameter [54]. A wire may be placed after the initial layer of acrylic is set, by conforming the piece of wire to the arcade to be stabilized or by placing a U-shaped pieced of wire around teeth incorporated in the splint with the free ends embedded in the acrylic. Any edges of the splint should be rounded and smoothed to avoid excessive soft tissue trauma. The splint can be trimmed with acrylic or diamond burs to provide a more accurate fit, paying particular attention to the occlusion. Regular examination and client monitoring is essential to flush any debris from the edges. Studies show that acrylic and composite in combination with techniques such as interdental wiring are significantly stronger than wire or acrylic alone [65, 66]. Acrylic and composite splints are also useful in edentulous areas. Acrylic is applied directly after reduction of the fracture and secured to the mandible with the appropriate number of cerclage wires, ideally two wires on either side of the fracture but with a minimum of one wire per fracture fragment. Wires are placed in a similar manner to cerclage wiring for symphyseal separation. Small ventral skin incisions are made for placement of each wire and an 18 or 20 gauge needle is passed through the incision in a dorsal direction along the buccal or lingual surface of the mandible. The needle is directed to the opposite surface of the man;dible and the wire is passed back through the incision via the needle. After reduction of the fracture an acrylic or composite splint is placed and allowed to undergo initial stages of curing until moderately firm. The wires are tightened ventrally to secure the splint to the mandible. An additional layer of acrylic is applied over the wires and any rough edges of the splint are contoured [31, 54] (Figures 13.15a and b).

13.6.5 Internal Fixation

The use of internal fixators in the oral cavity has many challenges due to the presence of the teeth and neurovascular structures [67]. Although it has been attempted, the mandibular canal is not a good site for intramedullary pin placement, due to its curvature and function in protecting the mandibular artery, mandibular vein, and the inferior alveolar nerve. Placement of a pin down the canal can lead to disruption of the reduction, occlusal misalignment, and the loss of important nerves and vessels within it. An IM pin by itself provides no rotational stability to the fracture site [68, 69]. For these reasons other internal fixation techniques are preferable.

Plating of maxillofacial fractures requires care to avoid damage to the structures noted above. The roots of the teeth occupy up to two-thirds of the volume of the mandible. Additionally the bones of the maxillofacial region are typically thin, making screw placement more challenging. Without careful planning, including radiographs and/or computed tomography, it is very possible to cause substantial damage to the roots if placed incorrectly. While it is optimal to place a plate on the tension side of the mandible, since this is the alveolar ridge, optimal placement is very difficult [67]. To counteract the forces of mastication an implant should be placed on the tension band side or if placed on the compression side it must be strong enough to neutralize these forces without failure. Screw placement of larger plates such as dynamic compression, locking compression, or reconstruction plates on the alveolar border is difficult without damaging tooth roots. Skipping multiple screw holes or using the plate in a buttress fashion may avoid this but places more stress on the implant. Ventral placement of these types of plates may be feasible but places the plate on the compression side. Combining ventral plating with some form of fixation on the tension side, such as interdental or intraosseous wiring, would be preferred. Miniplates developed for human maxillofacial fractures are applicable to similar injuries in the dog and cat (Figure 13.16). Miniplates are available in a low profile and allow for three-dimensional contouring. Non-locking plates allow the direction of the screw to be manipulated more easily than a locking plate. This is beneficial in an area such as the mouth to avoid tooth roots or neurovascular structures or in the thin bones of the maxilla. The tension band principle applies for placement of miniplates in the mandible; however, they can also function in a buttress fashion to span defects or severely comminuted fragments of the maxilla or mandible [19]. Ideally the miniplate would be placed along the alveolar border to counteract the bending forces on the mandible, and placement of a second miniplate in a more ventral location counteracts rotational forces and enhances stability of the repair. Alternatively, a larger dynamic compression or reconstruction plate can be placed ventrally on the mandible, with care being taken to avoid drilling into tooth roots or the mandibular canal [28, 70].

Internal fixation of maxillary fractures is not as common as many are treated conservatively. In cases of minimal bony displacement, simple suturing of the soft tissues is all that may be needed [71, 72]. An example of a fracture that could be treated in this manner would be a midline maxillary symphyseal separation where normal occlusion remains. If the structural support of the maxilla has been compromised or in the case of highly comminuted or depressed fractures, use of intraosseous wiring and/or miniplate fixation can restore form and function. Use of larger standard plates in the maxilla is more challenging due to the difficulty in contouring the plates in three dimensions to shape it to the contours of the bones. The larger screw threads can also have difficulty making purchase in the thinner bones [70, 71]. For multiple maxillofacial fractures the mandible should be repaired first to allow for more accurate determination of normal occlusion [70]. Several different miniplate systems exist but in general they are available in a low profile, about 1 mm in thickness, and come in a variety of shapes and lengths. Miniplates in the maxilla should be placed across fracture lines and along areas of thicker boney support wherever possible [50, 70].

13.6.6 External Fixation

Various means of external or percutaneous skeletal fixation can be adapted for use in the oral cavity, to provide immobilization of fractures with pins or screws placed through the fragments, and then connected externally with a metal or acrylic device [73]. With a good technique that avoids root structures and places the implant on either side of the defect, particularly in comminuted

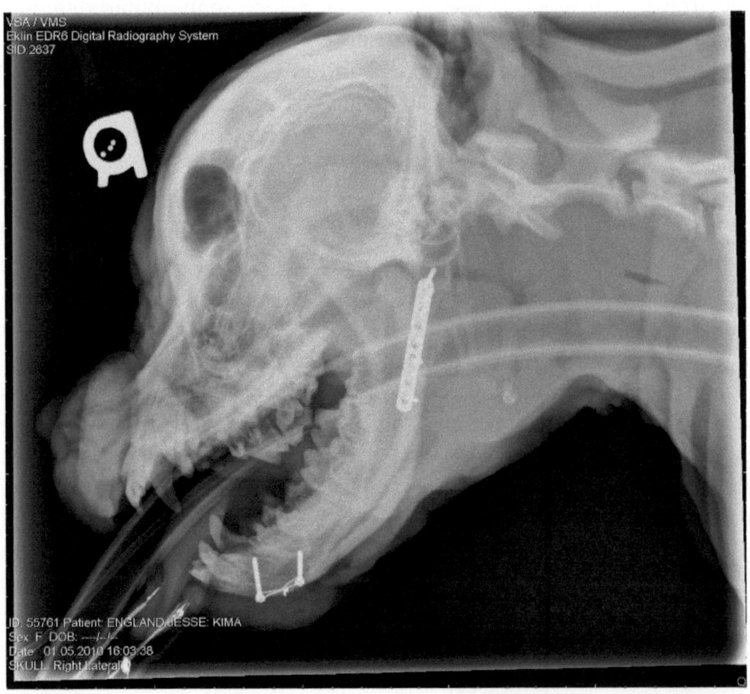

Figure 13.16 Pins, wires, and plating of mandibular fractures.

fractures, minimal trauma to the soft tissue is produced [73, 74]. The size of a typical Kirschner-Ehmer apparatus is typically too bulky to use in the oral cavity and the linear nature of the clamps can limit pin placement choices [75]. Transmandibular fixation, even if for a lesion that is unilateral and rostral to the first molar, can still cause excess damage to the sublingual tissues and is generally not recommended [28]. Pins should engage a minimum of six cortices per major fracture fragment where possible. Positive profile threaded pins are less likely to pull out or loosen when compared to smooth pins. Negative profile pins may be prone to breakage. Pre-drilling with a smaller pin can reduce thermal damage to the bone that may lead to pin tract osteomyelitis [76, 77]. An alternative method of pin placement in the rostral mandible has been described. A medium full-length centrally threaded pin is secured to the distal aspect of the mandibular teeth with a figure-of-eight 18 gauge orthopedic wire. Acrylic or composite is placed over the wire and pin construct for further stability. This allows pin placement rostrally without damaging the mandibular canine tooth roots [78]. Once pins are placed, the fracture site is reduced and an acrylic bridge can be formed to incorporate the exposed ends of the pins to stabilize them (Figure 13.17). A piece of tubing can be connected to each of the pin ends and acrylic injected into the tubing, which is then allowed to cure [74, 76]. Epoxy resin can also be formed around the pin ends as a connecting material [74]. After healing (four to six weeks), the pins are cut close to the acrylic and removed from the bone.

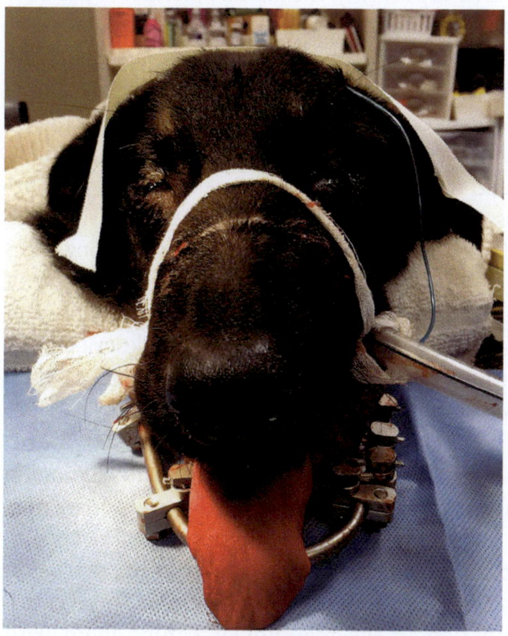

Figure 13.17 Dog with external fixation for mandibular fractures.

13.7 Temporomandibular Joint Surgery

Conservative management of TMJ disease may be appropriate for cases of subluxation or minimally displaced condylar fractures [26]. Minimally displaced TMJ fractures may be managed with a tape or nylon muzzle for a period of four to six weeks or until radiographic evidence of healing is seen. Fractures of the joint surfaces that are treated conservatively may develop TMJ ankylosis, which presents clinically as a progressive inability to open the mouth [79]. Acute luxation of the TMJ can be treated by closed reduction. A rostrodorsal luxation is treated by the use of a wooden or plastic dowel fulcrum in the caudal mouth (molar region, caudal to the primary cusp of the mandibular first molars) [26, 40, 80]. The mouth is closed on the fulcrum, causing ventral displacement of the condyle while the mandible is moved caudally to position the condyle into the articular fossa. Caudoventral luxations can be reduced with rostral pressure on the mandible. Radiographs should confirm reduction of the luxation (Figures 13.18a and b). If the luxation reduces easily and does not recur upon intraoperative manipulation of the mandible, then no other treatment is recommended other than feeding a soft diet and avoiding hard chew toys for four to six weeks. If the luxation recurs intraoperatively with manipulation of the mandible, then a tape muzzle, labial buttons, or MMF should be used to prevent recurrence of the luxation [81, 82] (Figure 13.19). Cases of chronic or recurring TMJ luxation may develop fibrosis of the joint space, reducing the effectiveness of a closed technique. Open reduction of TMJ luxations have been described [26]. Condylectomy is indicated for cases of chronic or recurring TMJ luxation, non-reducible luxations, TMJ fractures with multiple displaced fragments of the joint surface, or TMJ ankylosis [83].

Other problems can exist in the region of the TMJ, particularly with dysplastic or degenerative processes. The syndrome of dysplastic TMJs, with lateral deviation of the coronoid process getting locked past the zygomatic arch, has previously been discussed [84–86]. Clinically, dogs and cats with this problem present with the mouth locked in a wide open position and usually the patients are experiencing pain. Reduction of the displacement may require sedation, but can be performed manually by maximally opening the mouth to free the dorsal aspect of the coronoid from the lateral aspect of the zygoma. Zygomectomy and/or coronoidectomy has been described for recurrent entrapment of the coronoid process lateral to the zygoma [84, 87–89]. Severe cases of dysplasia or degeneration, including ankylosis, can be treated with reasonable success by excision of the ankylosed area, which may include portions of the caudal mandible, mandibular condyle, zygomatic arch, or articular process

(a) (b)

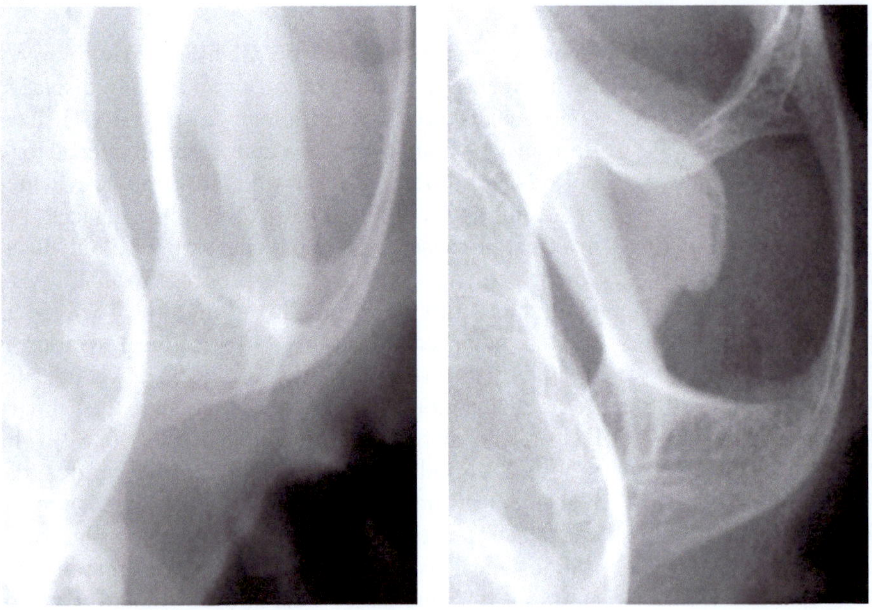

Figures 13.18 Radiographs of (a) TMJ luxation and (b) reduction.

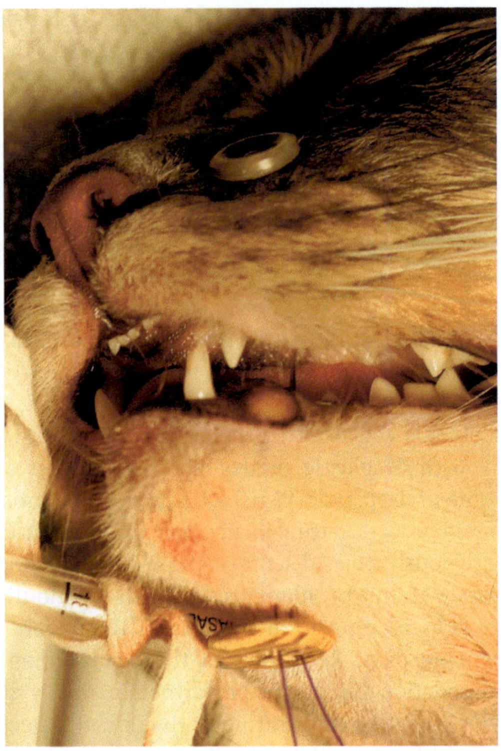

Figure 13.19 Labial buttons placed with suture material to limit oral opening for modified maxillary–mandibular fixation.

of the temporal bone [90]. True ankylosis is due to a bony union across the joint surface, which is an intracapsular process [26]. True ankylosis may occur secondary to trauma but it has also been reported in young animals without a history of trauma [91]. These cases will often present with the inability to open the mouth, but this can also be seen in cases of false ankylosis where extracapsular pathology can limit the movement, such as one case of squamous cell carcinoma of the ear canal that extended to the TMJ area [92].

Surgical approach to the TMJ for open reduction or condylectomy is achieved with access through the masseter muscle at the caudoventral aspect of the zygomatic arch [26, 93]. For condylectomy, the lateral ligament of the TMJ is identified and opened. Care should be taken to avoid transecting the facial nerve and parotid salivary duct. The articular condyle is then resected and removed with rongeurs or a bone cutting bur on a high-speed handpiece. Removal of the articular disk may increase the likelihood of ankylosis and is therefore not recommended [94]. The surgical site is closed routinely. In most cases, condylectomy will allow for a normal range of motion and good long-term function [90, 92]. A malocclusion with lateral drifting of the mandible can be seen. A technique for placement of an elastic chain anchored to the teeth has been described.

Orthodontic buttons are placed on the side of the mouth from where the mandible drifts away and are anchored to the buccal aspect of the maxillary fourth premolar and the buccal aspect of the mandibular canine tooth. An elastic chain is then placed between the buttons with enough tension to maintain normal occlusion [26]. Bilateral condylectomy can result in malocclusion due to caudal movement of the mandible. In these cases, crown reduction of the mandibular canine teeth with vital pulp therapy or a root canal may be needed [90].

13.8 Complications

Two of the more common complications in attempted fracture repair are osteomyelitis and delayed union or non-union [33]. Delayed union precedes non-union, where non-union is defined as a cessation of the progression of fracture healing, where motion is present at the fracture site, and healing is unable to occur without intervention. Instability of the fracture has been stated as the most common cause [95, 96]. Many factors can contribute to delayed or non-union including loss of blood supply, infection, missing bone fragments, instability at the fracture site, and improper reduction of fracture fragments [95, 96]. When persistent signs of infection are present, culture and sensitivity with appropriate antibiotic usage and curettage of the affected area may be sufficient to allow the oral cavity to continue the healing process. Implant materials in areas of persistent infection should be removed. With unresponsive cases, extensive curettage or removal of sequestra may cause a defect or gap in the bone structure. The same may also be true with a non-union or in cases of pathological fracture. If such is the case, applying fixation to stabilize both ends stops any movement in the area and the defect can eventually fill itself in, though the time period may be extensive, up to several months [24]. Implantation of osteoconductive or even osteoinductive materials, including cancellous bone chips may be used in gaps over 4–6 cm. A rib autogenous graft has been described, but post-operative care can be difficult and some degree of failure can be anticipated [24]. As mentioned previously, success has been achieved in healing of large defects with the use of rhBMP-2 in a compression-resistant matrix, secured to the bone ends with a buttress plate or plates. In severe cases of infection or non-union, sometimes excision of the affected area with a maxillectomy or mandibulectomy can resolve continuing problems [97]. At times, delaying the grafting procedure until all infection is under control and then approaching the lesion aseptically from a ventral skin incision may be preferable [34]. Some patients can eventually adjust to areas of non-union, and a commissuroplasty may give the area more support [98]. Commissuroplasty is the alteration of the commissure location of the lips. By the removal of the edges of the lips in the commissure area and suturing the opposing edges together, the commissure level can be moved rostrally, providing additional support to the mandible in holding it closer to the maxilla. During the healing stage (two weeks) a tape muzzle is required to prevent the commissuroplasty from being separated. It should be kept in mind that this procedure reduces access to the oral cavity, which may cause difficulties in future dental procedures and intubation.

A malunion fracture is one that has healed in a non-anatomical position [99]. Non-functional malunions result in significant morbidity to the patient and should be alleviated with surgical intervention. In the case of a maxillofacial malunion fracture that has resulted in malocclusion, selective extraction of teeth or crown reduction followed by direct pulp capping can alleviate discomfort. In severe cases where TMJ movement is severely restricted, osteotomy and/or primary repair may be required.

It has already been emphasized several times that to maintain correct occlusion when reducing a fracture, major complications are certain to arise when malocclusions result from surgical attempts at fracture repair. This is even more significant when dealing with younger animals that have not completed their growth. Not only can the initial injury itself impair the natural growth of the affected jaw, but rigid fixation may also cause complication problems in growth patterns, interference with dental eruptions, injuries to tooth buds, perforations of roots, and damage to the periodontium. When dealing with immature animals, less invasive fracture repair techniques are preferred. Younger animals have a higher frequency of greenstick fractures that can be managed with closed reduction and stabilization with a muzzle [47]. Often, with minimal assistance, the tremendous healing capability of young animals may overcome extensive injuries in the oral cavity [100].

Other complications that can be encountered in maxillofacial trauma repair include oronasal fistula formation, damage to teeth, and restriction or immobilization of the TMJ. Oronasal communication can result from tissue destruction due to trauma and requires surgical treatment to repair the defect. Multiple techniques utilizing palatal flaps, buccal mucosal flaps, ear cartilage or other tissue grafts, and palatal obturators have been described [101–110]. The type of technique utilized will depend on the size and location of the defect [47]. The sequelae of traumatized teeth and subsequent treatment is described in detail in the dentoalveolar trauma chapter (Chapter 6 – Traumatic Dentoalveolar Injuries). Trauma in the region of the TMJ can lead to fibrosis, muscular contracture, and exuberant callus formation, all of which can result in restriction of the movement of the joint. Excision arthroplasty of the joint can restore more normal function but fibrosis and muscular contracture can be difficult to counteract. Physiotherapy after trauma or after revision procedures may reduce the incidence of fibrosis. MMF appliances should be removed as early as possible to prevent permanent restriction of the movement of the TMJ. Knowledge of appropriate repair techniques as they relate to the specific maxillofacial injury will give the clinician the best advantage in successful treatment and healing of maxillofacial trauma.

13.9 AVDC Resource – Abbreviations

See Table 13.1.

Table 13.1 – AVDC nomenclature – abbreviations. https://www.avdc.org/traineeinfo.html; accessed 3 March 2018.

COM		Commissurotomy
CON		Condylar process of the mandible
	CON/X	Condylectomy
FX		Fracture (tooth or jaw; see T/FX for tooth fracture abbreviations)
	FX/R	Repair of jaw fracture
	FX/R/EXF	External skeletal fixation
	FX/R/IAS	Interarch splinting (between upper and lower dental arches)
	FX/R/IDS	Interdental splinting (between teeth within a dental arch)
	FX/R/IQS	Interquadrant splinting (between left and right upper or lower jaw quadrants)
	FX/R/MMF	Maxillomandibular fixation (other than muzzling and interarch splinting)
	FX/R/MZ	Muzzling
	FX/R/PL	Bone plating
	FX/R/WIR/C	Wire cerclage
	FX/R/WIR/OS	Intraosseous wiring
OMJL		Open-mouth jaw locking
	OMJL/R	Open-mouth jaw locking reduction
SYM		Mandibular symphysis
	SYM/R	Mandibular symphysis repair
	SYM/S	Mandibular symphysis separation
TMA		Trauma
	TMA/B	Ballistic trauma
	TMA/E	Electric trauma
	TMA/BRN	Burn trauma
	TMA/R	Trauma repair
TMJ		Temporomandibular joint
	TMJ/A	Temporomandibular joint ankylosis (true or false)
	TMJ/A/R	Temporomandibular joint ankylosis repair
	TMJ/D	TMJ dysplasia
	TMJ/FX	Temporomandibular joint fracture
	TMJ/FX/R	Temporomandibular joint fracture repair
	TMJ/LUX	TMJ luxation
	TMJ/LUX/R	Temporomandibular joint luxation reduction
ZYG		Zygoma (zygomatic arch)
	ZYG/X	Zygomectomy

References

1 Cheal, E.J., Mansmann, K.A., DiGioia, A.M. III et al. (1991). Role of interfragmentary strain in fracture healing: ovine model of a healing osteotomy. *J. Ortho. Res.* 9: 131–142.
2 Perren, S.M. and Rahn, B.A. (1980). Biomechanics of fracture healing. *Can. J. Surg.* 23: 228–232.
3 Perren, S.M. and Claes, L. (2000). Biology and biomechanics in fracture management. In: *AO Principles of Fracture Management* (ed. T.P. Ruedi and W.M. Murphy), 7–31. Stuttgart: Thieme.
4 Snyder, C.J., Soukup, J.W., Drees, R. et al. (2016). Caudal mandibular bone height and buccal cortical bone thickness measured by computed tomography in healthy dogs. *Vet. Surg.* 45: 21–29.
5 Arzi, B. and Verstraete, F.J.M. (2015). Internal fixation of severe maxillofacial fractures in dogs. *Vet. Surg.* 44: 437–442.
6 Davidson, J.R. and Bauer, M.S. (1992). Fractures of the mandible and maxilla. *Vet. Clin. North Am. Small Anim. Pract.* 22: 109–119.
7 Lovato, C. and Wagner, J.D. (2009). Infection rates following perioperative prophylactic antibiotics versus postoperative extended regimen prophylactic antibiotics in surgical management of mandibular fractures. *J. Oral Maxillofac. Surg.* 67: 827–832.
8 Miles, B.A., Potter, J.K., and Ellis, E. III (2006). The efficacy of postoperative antibiotic regimens in the open treatment of mandibular fractures: a prospective randomized trial. *J. Oral Maxillofac. Surg.* 64: 576–582.
9 Sarkiala-Kessel, E.M. (2012). Use of antibiotics and antiseptics. In: *Oral and Maxillofacial Surgery in Dogs and Cats* (ed. F.J.M. Verstraete and M.J. Lommer), 15–21. Edinburgh, UK: Saunders Elsevier.
10 Radice, M., Martino, P.A., and Reiter, A.M. (2006). Evaluation of subgingival bacteria in the dog and susceptibility to commonly used antibiotics. *J. Vet. Dent.* 23: 219–224.
11 Kuriyama, T., Williams, D.W., Yanagisawa, M. et al. (2007). Antimicrobial susceptibility of 800 anaerobic isolates from patients with dentoalveolar infection to 13 oral antibiotics. *Oral Microbiol. Immunol.* 22: 285–288.
12 Seymour, R.A. and Hogg, S.D. (2008). Antibiotics and chemoprophylaxis. *Periodontology* 2000 (46): 80–108.
13 Hartsfield, S.M., Gendreau, C.L., Smith, C.W. et al. (1977). Endotracheal intubation by phayrngotomy. *J. Am. Anim. Hosp. Assoc.* 13: 71.
14 Smith, M.M. (2004). Pharyngostomy endotracheal tube. *J. Vet. Dent.* 21: 191–194.
15 Lantz, G.C. (2012). Pharyngotomy and pharyngostomy. In: *Oral and Maxillofacial Surgery in Dogs and Cats* (ed. F.J.M. Verstraete and M.J. Lommer), 543–546. Edinburgh, UK: Saunders Elsevier.
16 Soukup, J.W. and Snyder, C.J. (2015). Transmylohyoid orotracheal intubation in surgical management of canine maxillofacial fractures: an alternative to pharyngotomy endotracheal intubation. *Vet. Surg.* 44: 432–436.
17 Smith, M.M. and Waldron, D.R. (1993). Head and neck surgery. In: *Atlas of Approaches for General Surgery in the Dog and Cat* (ed. M.M. Smith and D.R. Waldron), 82–85. Philadelphia, PA: WB Saunders.
18 Rudy, R.L. and Boudrieau, R.J. (1992). Maxillofacial and mandibular fractures. *Semin. Vet. Med. Surg. (Small Anim.)* 7: 3–20.
19 Boudrieau, R.J. and Kudisch, M. (1996). Miniplate fixation for repair of maxillary and mandibular fractures in 15 dogs and 3 cats. *Vet. Surg.* 25: 277–291.
20 Evans, H.E. and Christensen, G.C. (2013). Ligaments and joints of the skull: intermandibular joint. In: *Miller's Anatomy of the Dog*, 4e (ed. H.E. Evans and A. Delahunta), 161. St. Louis, MO: Elsevier Saunders.
21 Weigel, J.P. (1985). Trauma to oral structures. In: *Veterinary Dentistry* (ed. C.E. Harvey), 140. Philadelphia, PA: WB Saunders.
22 Umphlet, R.C. and Johnson, A.L. (1988). Mandibular fractures in the cat: a retrospective study. *Vet. Surg.* 17: 333–337.
23 Umphlet, R.C. and Johnson, A.L. (1990). Mandibular fractures in the dog: a retrospective study of 157 cases. *Vet. Surg.* 19: 272–275.
24 Harvey, C.E. and Emily, P.P. (1993). *Small Animal Dentistry*, 312. St. Louis, MO: Mosby, Year Book.
25 Piermattei, D.L., Flo, G.L., and DeCamp, C.E. (2006). Fractures and luxations of the mandible and maxilla. In: *Brinker, Piermattei, and Flo's Handbook of Small Animal Orthopedics and Fracture Repair*, 4e (ed. D.L. Piermattei, G.L. Flo and C.E. DeCamp), 716–736. Philadelphia, PA: Elsevier Saunders.
26 Lantz, G.C. and Verstraete, F.J.M. (2012). Fractures and luxations involving the temporomandibular joint. In: *Oral and Maxillofacial Surgery in Dogs and Cats* (ed. F.J.M. Verstraete and M.J. Lommer), 321–332. Edinburgh, UK: Saunders Elsevier.
27 Evans, H.E. and Christensen, G.C. (2013). Muscles: muscles of the head: muscles of mastication. In: *Miller's Anatomy of the Dog*, 4e (ed. H.E. Evans and A. Delahunta), 197–200. St. Louis, MO: Elsevier Saunders.
28 Verstraete, F.J.M. (1995). Advanced oral surgery in small carnivores. In: *Manual of Small Animal Dentistry* (ed. D.A. Crossley and S. Penman), 193. Gloucester, UK: British Small Animal Association.
29 Nibley, W. (1981). Treatment of caudal mandibular fractures: a preliminary report. *J. Am. Anim. Hosp. Assoc.* 17–27.

30 Kern, D.A., Smith, M.M., Grant, J.W. et al. (1993). Evaluation of bending strength of five interdental fixation apparatuses applied to canine mandibles. *Am. J. Vet. Res.* 54: 1177–1182.
31 Legendre, L. (2003). Intraoral acrylic splints for maxillofacial fracture repair. *J. Vet. Dent.* 20: 70–77.
32 Bennet, J.W., Kapatkin, A.S., and Manfra Marretta, S. (1994). Dental composite for the fixation of mandibular fractures and luxations in 11 cats and 6 dogs. *Vet. Surg.* 23: 190–194.
33 Manfra Marretta, S., Schrader, S.C., and Matthiesen, D.T. (1990). Problems associated with the management and treatment of jaw fractures. *Probl. Vet. Med. Surg. Dent.* 2: 220.
34 Schrader, S.C. (1990). Dental orthopedics. In: *Small Animal Oral Medicine and Surgery* (ed. M.J. Bojrab and M. Tholen), 241. Philadelphia, PA: Lea & Febiger.
35 Boudrieau, R.J., Mitchell, S.L., and Seeherman, H. (2004). Mandibular reconstruction of a partial hemimandibulectomy in a dog with severe malocclusion. *Vet. Surg.* 33: 119–130.
36 Lewis, J.R., Boudrieau, R.J., Reiter, A.M. et al. (2008). Mandibular reconstruction after gunshot trauma in a dog by use of recombinant human bone morphogenic protein-2. *J. Am. Vet. Med. Assoc.* 233: 1598–1604.
37 Arzi, B., Verstraete, F.J., Huey, D.J. et al. (2015). Regenerating mandibular bone using rhBMP-2: part 1- immediate reconstruction of segmental mandibulectomies. *Vet. Surg.* 44: 403–409.
38 Verstraete, F.J., Arzi, B., Huey, D.J. et al. (2015). Regenerating mandibular bone using rhBMP-2: part 2 – treatment of chronic, defect non-union fractures. *Vet. Surg.* 44: 410–416.
39 Arzi, B., Cissell, D.D., Pollard, R.E. et al. (2015). Regenerative approach to bilateral rostral mandibular reconstruction in a case series of dogs. *Front. Vet. Sci.* 2: 4.
40 Fossum, T.W. (2007). Diseases on the joints. In: *Small Animal Surgery*, 3e, 1143–1315. St. Louis, MO: Elsevier Mosby.
41 Arzi, B., Bissell, D.D., Verstraete, F.J. et al. (2013). Computed tomographic findings in dogs and cats with temporomandibular joint disorders: 58 cases (2006–2011). *J. Am. Vet. Med. Assoc.* 242: 69–75.
42 DuPont, G.A. and Technique, D.B.L.J. (2009). *Atlas of Dental Radiography in Dogs and Cats*, 229–254. St. Louis, MO: Elsevier Saunders.
43 Schwartz, T., Weller, R., Dickie, A.M. et al. (2002). Imaging of the canine and feline temporomandibular joint: a review. *Vet. Radiol. Ultrasound.* 43: 85–97.
44 Eubanks, D.L. (2013). Advanced imaging of the TMJ and other oral structures. *J. Vet. Dent.* 30: 180–182.
45 Evans, H.E. and Christensen, G.C. (2013). The skeleton: skull: bones of the face and palate. In: *Miller's Anatomy of the Dog*, 4e (ed. H.E. Evans and A. Delahunta), 99–105. St. Louis, MO: Elsevier Saunders.
46 Boudrieau, R.J. and Verstraete, F.J.M. (2012). Principles of maxillofacial trauma repair. In: *Oral and Maxillofacial Surgery in Dogs and Cats*, 1e (ed. F.J.M. Verstraete and M.J. Lommer), 233–242. Edinburgh, UK: Saunders Elsevier.
47 Manfra Marretta, S. (2012). Maxillofacial fracture complications. In: *Oral and Maxillofacial Surgery in Dogs and Cats*, 1e (ed. F.J.M. Verstraete and M.J. Lommer), 333–341. Edinburgh, UK: Saunders Elsevier.
48 Evans, H.E. and Christensen, G.C. (2013). The skeleton: skull: the skull as a whole. In: *Miller's Anatomy of the Dog*, 4e (ed. H.E. Evans and A. Delahunta), 106–110. St. Louis, MO: Elsevier Saunders.
49 Sorni, M., Guarinos, J., and Penarrocha, M. (2005). Implants in anatomical buttresses of the upper jaw. *Med. Oral. Patol. Oral. Cir. Bucal.* 10: 163–168.
50 Boudrieau, R.J. (2004). Miniplate reconstruction of severely comminuted maxillary fractures in two dogs. *Vet. Surg.* 33: 154–163.
51 Gruss, J.S. and Mackinnon, S.E. (1986). Complex maxillary fractures: role of buttress reconstruction and immediate bone grafts. *Plast. Reconstr. Surg.* 78: 9–22.
52 Wilson, J.W. (1991). Vascular supply to normal bone and healing fractures. *Semin. Vet. Med. Surg. (Small Anim.)* 6: 26–38.
53 Withrow, S.J. (1981). Taping of the mandible in treatment of mandibular fractures. *J. Am. Anim. Hosp. Assoc.* 17: 27.
54 Smith, M.M. and Legendre, L.F.J. (2012). Maxillofacial repair using noninvasive techniques. In: *Oral and Maxillofacial Surgery in Dogs and Cats*, 1e (ed. F.J.M. Verstraete and M.J. Lommer), 275–284. Edinburgh, UK: Saunders Elsevier.
55 Lantz, G.C. (1981). Interarcade wiring as a method of fixation for selected mandibular injuries. *J. Am. Anim. Hosp. Assoc.* 17: 27.
56 Beckman, B. and Smith, M.M. (2009). Interarcade bonding for non-invasive mandibular fracture repair. *J. Vet. Dent.* 26: 62–66.
57 Mulherin, B.L., Snyder, C.J., and Soukup, J.W. (2012). An alternative symphyseal wiring technique. *J. Vet. Dent.* 29: 176–184.
58 Matis, U. and Kostlin, R. (2012). Symphyseal separation and fractures involving the incisive region. In: *Oral and Maxillofacial Surgery in Dogs and Cats*, 1e (ed. F.J.M. Verstraete and M.J. Lommer), 265–274. Edinburgh, UK: Saunders Elsevier.
59 Lothamer, C., Snyder, C.J., Duenwald-Kuehl, S. et al. (2015). Crown preservation of the mandibular first molar tooth impacts the strength and stiffness of three non-invasive jaw fracture repair constructs in dogs. *Front. Vet. Sci.* 2: 18.

60 Flores, M.T., Andersson, L., Andreasen, J.O. et al. (2007). Guidelines for the management of traumatic dental injuries. I. Fractures and luxations of permanent teeth. *Dent. Traumatol.* 23: 66–71.

61 Flores, M.T., Andersson, L., Andreasen, J.O. et al. (2007). Guidelines for the management of traumatic dental injuries. II. Avulsion of permanent teeth. *Dent. Traumatol.* 23: 130–136.

62 Soukup, J.W., Hetzel, S., and Paul, A. (2015). Classification and epidemiology of traumatic dentoalveolar injuries in dogs and cats: 959 injuries in 660 patient visits (2004–2012). *J. Vet. Dent.* 32: 6–14.

63 Soukup, J.W. and Snyder, C.J. (2014). Traumatic dentoalveolar and maxillofacial injuries in cats: overview of diagnosis and management. *J. Feline. Med. Surg.* 16: 915–927.

64 Rice, C.A., Riehl, J., Broman, K. et al. (2012). Comparing the degree of exothermic polymerization in commonly used acrylic and provisional composite resins for intraoral appliances. *J. Vet. Dent.* 29: 78–83.

65 Kern, D.A., Smith, M.M., Grant, J.W. et al. (1993). Evaluation of bonding strength of five interdental fixation apparatuses applied to canine mandibles. *Am. J. Vet. Res.* 54: 1177–1182.

66 Kern, D.A., Smith, M.M., Stevenson, S. et al. (1995). Evaluation of three fixation techniques for repair of mandibular fractures in dogs. *J. Am. Vet. Assoc.* 206: 1883–1890.

67 Verstraete, F.J.M. and Ligthelm, A.J. (1992). Dental trauma caused by screws in internal fixation of mandibular osteotomies in the dog. *VCOT* 5: 104.

68 Cechner, P.E. (1980). Malocclusion in the dog caused by intramedullary pin fixation of mandibular fractures. *J. Am. Anim. Hosp. Assoc.* 16: 79.

69 Rough, J.K. and Wilson, J.W. (1989). Healing of mandibular body osteotomies after plate and intramedullary pin fixation. *Vet. Surg.* 18: 190.

70 Boudrieau, R.J. (2012). Maxillofacial fracture repair using miniplates and screws. In: *Oral and Maxillofacial Surgery in Dogs and Cats*, 11e (ed. F.J.M. Verstraete and M.J. Lommer), 293–308. Edinburgh, UK: Saunders Elsevier.

71 Verstraete, F.J.M. (2003). Maxillofacial fractures. In: *Textbook of Small Animal Surgery*, 3e (ed. D.H. Slatter), 2190–2207. Philadelphia, PA: WB Saunders.

72 Tsugawa, A.J. and Verstraete, F.J.M. (2012). Maxillofacial fracture repair using miniplates and screws. In: *Oral and Maxillofacial Surgery in Dogs and Cats*, 1e (ed. F.J.M. Verstraete and M.J. Lommer), 309–319. Edinburgh, UK: Saunders Elsevier.

73 Owen, M.R., Langley-Hobbs, S.J., Moores, A.P. et al. (2004). Mandibular fracture repair in dogs and cats using epoxy resin and acrylic external fixation. *Vet. Comp. Orthop. Traumatol.* 17: 189–197.

74 Moores, A.P. (2011). Maxillomandibular external skeletal fixation in five cats with caudal jaw trauma. *J. Small. Anim. Pract.* 52: 38–41.

75 Salisbury, S.K. and Cantwell, H.D. (1989). Conservative management of fractures of the mandibular condyloid process in three cats and one dog. *JAVMA* 194: 85.

76 Smith, M.M. and Kern, D.A. (1995). Skull trauma and mandibular fractures. *Vet. Clin. North. Am. Small. Anim. Pract.* 25: 1127–1148.

77 Sequin, B., Harari, J., Wood, R.D. et al. (1997). Bone fracture and sequestration as complications of external skeletal fixation. *J. Small. Anim. Pract.* 38: 81–84.

78 Cook, W.T., Smith, M.M., Markel, M.D. et al. (2001). Influence of an interdental full pin on stability of an acrylic external fixator for rostral mandibular fractures in dogs. *Am. J. Vet. Res.* 62: 576–580.

79 Gatineau, M., El-Warrak, A.O., Marietta, S.M. et al. (2008). Locked jaw syndrome in dogs and cats: 37 cases (1998–2005). *J. Vet. Dent.* 25: 16–22.

80 Klima, L.J. (2007). Temporomandibular joint luxation in the cat. *J. Vet. Dent.* 24: 198–201.

81 Somrak, A.J. and Marietta, S.M. (2015). Management of temporomandibular joint luxation in a cat using a custom-made tape muzzle. *J. Vet. Dent.* 32: 239–246.

82 Hoffer, M., Marretta, S.M. et al. (2011). Evaluation of composite resin materials for maxillomandibular fixation in cats for treatment of jaw fractures and temporomandibular joint laxations. *Vet. Surg.* 40: 357–368.

83 Cetinkaya, M.A. (2012). Temporomandibular joint injuries and ankylosis in the cat. *Vet. Comp. Orthop. Traumatol.* 25: 366–374.

84 Robins, G. and Grandage, J. (1977). Temporomandibular joint dysplasia and open-mouth locking in the dog. *J. Am. Vet. Med. Assoc.* 171 (10): 1072.

85 Lantz, G.C. and Cantwell, H.D. (1986). Intermittent open-mouth lower jaw locking in five dogs. *J. Am. Vet. Med. Assoc.* 188: 1403–1405.

86 Soukup, J.W., Snyder, C.J., and Gengler, W.R. (2009). Computed tomography and partial coronoidectomy for open-mouth jaw locking in two cats. *J. Vet. Dent.* 26: 226–233.

87 Lobprise, H.B. and Wiggs, R.B. (1992). Modified surgical treatment of intermittent open-mouth mandibular locking in a cat. *J. Vet. Dent.* 9: 8–12.

88 Lantz, G.C. (2012). Temporomandibular joint dysplasia. In: *Oral and Maxillofacial Surgery in Dogs and Cats* (ed. V. FJM and M.J. (e.) Lommer), 321–332. Philadelphia, PA: Elsevier Saunders.

89 Lantz, G.C. (1987). Intermittent open-mouth locking of the temporomandibular joint in a cat. *J. Am. Vet. Med. Assoc.* 190: 1574.

90 Eisner, E.R. (1995). Bilateral mandibular condylectomy in a cat. *J. Vet. Dent.* 12: 23–26.

91 Ellenberger, S. and Snyder, C. (2013). Bilateral extracapsular soft-tissue ossification affecting range of TMJ motion in an Airedale terrier. *J. Am. Anim. Hosp. Assoc.* 49: 115–121.

92 Anderson, M.A., Orsini, P.G., and Harvey, C.E. (1996). Temporomandibular ankylosis: treatment by unilateral condylectomy in two dogs and two cats. *J. Vet. Dent.* 13: 23–25.

93 Piermattei, D.L. (1993). The head, approach to the temporomandibular joint. In: *An Atlas of Surgical Approaches to the Bones and Joints of the Dog and Cat*, 3e (ed. D.L. Piermattei), 38–39. Philadelphia, PA: WB Saunders.

94 Minamoto, H., Kurita, K., Ogi, N. et al. (1999). The role of the disk in sheep temporomandibular joint ankylosis. *Oral. Surg. Oral. Med. Oral. Pathol. Oral. Radiol. Endod.* 88: 151–158.

95 Millis, D.L. and Jackson, A.M. (2003). Delayed unions, nonunions, and malunions. In: *Textbook of Small Animal Surgery*, 3e (ed. D.H. Slatter), 1849–1861. Philadelphia, PA: WB Saunders.

96 DeCamp, C.E., Johnston, S.A., Dejardin, L.M., and Schaefer, S.L. (2016). Delayed union and malunion. In: *Brinker, Piermattei, and Flo's Handbook of Small Animal Orthopedics and Fracture Repair*, 5e, 163–174. St. Louis MO: Elsevier.

97 Lantz, G.C. and Salisbury, S.K. (1987). Partial mandibulectomy for treatment of mandibular fractures in dogs: eight cases (1981–1984). *J. Am. Vet. Med. Assoc.* 191: 243.

98 Manfra, M.S. (1995). A salvage procedure for bilateral pathologic mandibular fractures in the dog. *World. Vet. Dent. Cong Proc.* 128.

99 Anson, L.W. (1991). Malunions. *Vet. Clin. North. Am. Small. Anim. Pract.* 7 (61): 21.

100 Schmitz, J.P. and Hollinger, J.O. (1985). The critical size defect as an experimental model for craniomandibular non-unions. *Clin Orthop.* 205: 299.

101 Manfra, M.S., Grove, T.K., and Grillo, J.F. (1991). Split palatal u-flap: a new technique for repair of caudal palatal defects. *J. Vet. Dent.* 8: 5–8.

102 Smith, M.M. (2001). Island palatal mucoperiosteal flap for repair of oronasal fistula in a dog. *J. Vet. Dent* 18: 127–129.

103 Smith, M.M. (2000). Oronasal fistula repair. *Clin. Tech. Small. Anim Pract.* 15: 243–250.

104 Beckman, B.W. (2006). Split palatal u-flap for repair of caudal palatal defects. *J. Vet. Dent.* 23: 267–269.

105 Lanz, O.I. (2001). Free tissue transfer of the rectus abdominus myoperitoneal flap for oral reconstruction in a dog. *J. Vet. Dent.* 18: 187–192.

106 Cox, C.L., Hunt, G.B., and Cadier, M.M. (2007). Repair of oronasal fistulae using auricular cartilage grafts in five cats. *Vet. Surg.* 36: 164–169.

107 Soukup, J.W., Snyder, C.J., and Gengler, W.R. (2009). Free auricular cartilage autograft for repair of an oronasal fistula in a dog. *J. Vet. Dent.* 26: 86–95.

108 Lorain, R.P. and Legendre, L.F. (2012). Oronasal fistula repair using auricular cartilage. *J. Vet. Dent.* 29: 172–175.

109 Hale, F.A., Sylvestre, A.M., and Miller, C. (1997). The use of a prosthetic appliance to manage a large palatal defect in a dog. *J. Vet. Dent.* 14: 61–64.

110 Edstrom, E.J. and Smith, M.M. (2014). Prosthetic appliance for oronasal communication obturation in a dog. *J. Vet. Dent.* 31: 108–112.

14

Oral Surgery – Oral and Maxillofacial Tumors

Heidi B. Lobprise[1] and Jason Soukup[2]

[1] Main Street Veterinary Dental Clinic, Flower Mound, TX, USA
[2] School of Veterinary Medicine, University of Wisconsin-Madison, Madison, WI, USA

14.1 Introduction

This chapter correlates closely with Chapter 7 – Oral and Maxillofacial Tumors, Cysts, and Tumor-Like Lesions. Important topics, such as "Principles of Staging," "Principles of Imaging," and "Principles of Biopsy Acquisition" are covered thoroughly in Chapter 7, as well as descriptions of lesions and, in most cases, the extent to which surgical techniques should be applied. This chapter will cover the basic tenets of surgical considerations in management of lesions, with frequent reference to a text devoted entirely to the discipline – *Oral and Maxillofacial Surgery of Dogs and Cats* by Verstraete and Lommer, currently the premier text on the topic in the field of veterinary dentistry and oral surgery [1]. Additional resources include relevant articles from the *Journal of Veterinary Dentistry*, including "Step By Step" and "Veterinary Dentist at Work" features, with detailed descriptions of particular procedures.

14.2 Treatment Considerations

This chapter starts with the premise that the lesion has been classified by histopathological assessment and the patient has been staged as to the extent (or lack) of systemic impact of the mass. A better understanding of the tumor type, and extent, stabilization and preparation of the patient (including basic hygiene care during biopsy), and a customized treatment plan for excision and closure will maximize the surgical efforts.

The reader should bear in mind that every patient and every surgical lesion is unique. Thus, the following pages on surgical technique and approaches should be read as general guidelines and principles. Modifications to the described approaches are nearly a 100% necessity as the uniqueness of the patient and lesion, the expectations of the client, and the preferences or comfort level of the surgeon will typically dictate some deviations, sometimes significant, from a textbook approach.

With a few decades of experiencing the benefits of improved outcomes, as well as improvements in imaging techniques, wide and radical excisions are often considered the standard of care for many oral tumors [2]. While the clinician may take for granted that aggressive surgery is needed and will likely work well, it is important to have complete communication with the client to educate them about expectations – from realistic survival times (STs) and possible post-surgical complications and challenges. Owners may often be concerned about issues such as facial disfigurement, the ability to eat, drink, and groom, and overall quality of life. A study looking at these points revealed that nearly 85% of clients were satisfied with their decision to proceed with the surgery for their dogs, with post-operative quality of life being equal to or exceeding pre-operative quality [3]. Once the hair grew back, even facial appearance did not appear to be a major concern. Up to 83% of cat owners were satisfied with mandibulectomy procedures and would do it again for their pet, even with 98% of the patients having immediate issues and nearly 75% having long-term issues post-operatively [4].

Meticulous attention must also be paid to the management of pain throughout and after the procedure time. Chapter 9 (Anesthesia and Pain Management) has excellent information on anesthetic protocols, pre-, peri-, and post-operative analgesic options, and chronic pain management. Return to full function through pain management and nutritional support is a key goal for surgical patients.

Wiggs's Veterinary Dentistry: Principles and Practice, Second Edition. Edited by Heidi B. Lobprise and Johnathon R. (Bert) Dodd.

14.2.1 Patient and Client Preparation

The ideal situation going into a major procedure for tumor removal includes gathering as much information as possible about the patient, the lesion (type, extent), and impact of disease on the patient. Standard preoperative diagnositics and anesthetic assessment should precede the initial biopsy (incisional), and a thorough oral assessment and basic dental cleaning will help identify any other oral issues and provide a healthier oral cavity prior to the planned surgery [5]. The incisional biopsy site should be selected in order to get a representive sample of the lesion, without compromising the eventual complete resection of the mass [6]. Lymph node (LN) assessment and thoracic radiographs are recommended, particularly if the incisional biopsy is indicative of a neoplastic mass. While only a small number of cases typically show evidence of thoracic metastasis at the time of initial diagnosis, the presence of metastasis would warrant a more guarded prognosis. Monitoring thoracic radiographs can also be used to track a response to any therapy or lack of a response, or even progression of signs. Full skull and intraoral radiographs are used to evaluate any osseous changes, which can be indicative of infiltrative lesions. Lack of obvious osseous involvement does not rule out microscopic extensions, particularly in fixed masses that would still be candidates for aggressive resection [6]. Advanced imaging can provide more precise information on the extent of many tumors, as radiographic signs of osteolysis do not occur until a substantial portion of the cortical bone is involved. Additionally, the three-dimensional capabilities of advanced imaging may enhance the surgical planning process. Advanced imaging such as scintigraphy can also be used to assess the presence of metastatic disease and its progression in response to therapy [7].

Staging of the lesion using the accepted tumor–node–metastasis (TNM) guidelines was discussed in Chapter 7 – Oral and Maxillofacial Tumors, Cysts, and Tumor-Like Lesions. In a review of lymph node staging of oral neoplasia in 31 dogs and cats, only 54.5% of cases with metastatic disease to regional lymph nodes had mandibular node involvement [8]. Therefore, while evaluation of the parotid and retropharyngeal lymphcentrums would reveal a higher percentage of metastatic cases, those areas are challenging to access with fine needle aspiration [8]. Full evaluation would require removal of the appropriate lymph nodes (Figure 14.1a and b).

Appropriate support for the patient, including complete analgesia management throughout the peri-operative period, monitoring, fluids (including transfusions if needed), and stringent recovery monitoring, is essential. Antibiotics may be used during the intraoperative period, up to four hours afterward. If there is any evidence of concurrent osteomyelitis at the site or elsewhere in the oral cavity, additional antibiotic therapy may be warranted [6]. Nutritional support intervention (feeding tube, feeding assistance) will vary with each case, but should be provided until the patient has full return to function.

Additional therapy such as radiation therapy (RT) (curative intent for microscopic remnant or palliative) and chemotherapy may be considered. For the most part, however, primary treatment for oral neoplasia involves surgical removal, as there are few studies for strong recommendations for multimodal approaches provided by evidence-based medicine [9]. Keep in mind that review

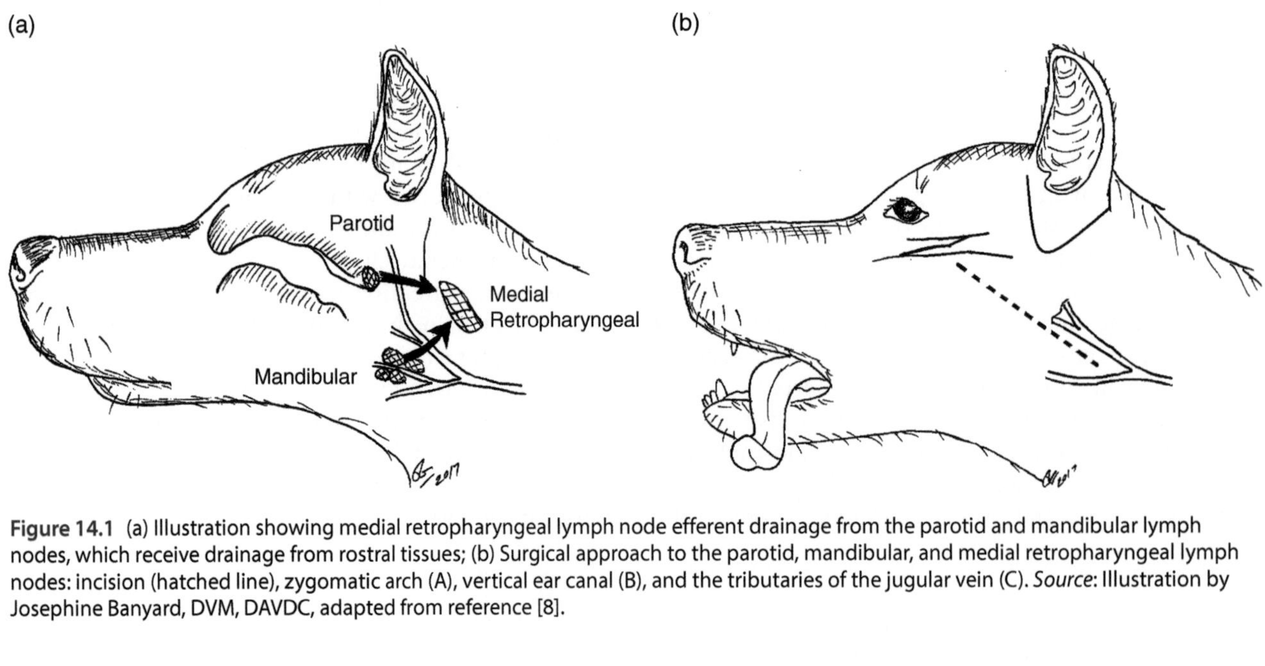

Figure 14.1 (a) Illustration showing medial retropharyngeal lymph node efferent drainage from the parotid and mandibular lymph nodes, which receive drainage from rostral tissues; (b) Surgical approach to the parotid, mandibular, and medial retropharyngeal lymph nodes: incision (hatched line), zygomatic arch (A), vertical ear canal (B), and the tributaries of the jugular vein (C). *Source*: Illustration by Josephine Banyard, DVM, DAVDC, adapted from reference [8].

of current studies is far more updated than what can be shared in a text.

14.2.2 Therapy Considerations – Biological Behavior and Adjunctive Therapy Options

14.2.2.1 Melanoma

Melanocytic tumors have always been a challenge for canine patients, being one of the most common oral malignancies found, with a highly variable metastatic rate depending on the biological behavior (see Chapter 7 – Oral Maxillofacial Tumors, Cysts, and Tumor-Like Lesions). Lymph node enlargement can be found, so full metastatic evaluation is recommended, as 70% of cases in one study had metastasis with lymphadenopathy, but 40% of metastatic patients had no lymph node enlargement [10]. Abdominal ultrasonography is recommended for patients [11]. Tumor size is an important prognostic factor, though relative size of tumor to patient size has not been standardized [11]. Incomplete margins have reported to be associated with a decreased prognostic outlook, but other studies have shown no significant decrease in ST and progression free intervals (PFIs) [12]. Patient age tends to have a negative impact on prognosis [13], but location, aside from contributing to tumor resection challenges, is not a prognostic factor [12].

Consideration of systemic treatment would be a likely choice for a metastatic disease, but melanomas in humans have been extremely chemoresistant [11]. The use of carboplatin has shown no significant difference in recurrence or survival time as compared to surgery alone [14, 15], and, in general, the inefficiency of chemotherapy is recognized [16]. Anecdotal results have been reported with complementary medicine efforts including hyperthermia and dendritic cell therapy [17]. Recent studies on canine melanoma cell lines that show apoptosis with high doses of celecoxib in Cox-2 expressing cells continue to explore options [18].

Previous studies with external beam radiation therapy had shown some promise in local disease control, though earlier reports had not determined the optional fraction selection [16]. Studies include use of hypofraction protocols, including one in cats (without a durable response) [19] and one in dogs evaluating hypofraction with cisplatin in dogs, the majority with incompletely excised Stage 1 disease (but local control similar to other methods) [20]. The use of megavoltage versus orthovoltage to palliatively treat local disease unamenable to surgery (similar results, but some severe complications) has also been studied [21].

In 2007, a conditional license was granted for a DNA vaccine (xenogenic human tyrosinase) based on a Phase 1 clinical trial or proof of concept trial. A safety and efficacy study demonstrated a significantly improved survival time in treated patients, when achieving sufficient local control to allow the activation of a host response, in the absence of disseminated disease [22]. Two later retrospective studies did not show the benefits of the vaccine on survival time or PFIs [23, 24].

Therefore the concept that resection with wide margins and complete excision to improve survival time remains the optimal goal for managing melanocytic tumors [12, 13]. Any time a melanocytic mass, pigmented or not, is diagnosed, surgical attempts should be aggressive with full metastatic evaluation. The one exception, a benign variant called a melanocytoma, typically less than 1 cm and well circumscribed, can often be managed with wide excision [25].

14.2.2.2 Squamous Cell Carcinoma

As the second most common oral malignancy in dogs and by far the most common in cats, squamous cell carcinoma (SCC), is often seen characterized by aggressive local infiltration, especially in cats. As stated in Chapter 7, the metastatic rate in dogs is low for rostral tumors and high for lingual and tonsillar tumors. Recent studies show a higher metastatic rate (to the mandibular lymph node, often the only one checked) of near or greater than 30% [26, 27], which is higher than previously thought. Though location is not a definitive prognostic factor, a tumor that is inoperable, either due to its size or location (non-maxillary), carries a poor to grave prognosis [27]. Truly resectable tumors followed by definitive radiation therapy carried the best prognosis in a small number of cats [28] and may also be true in dogs [9].

Few reports have shown significant improvement in therapy parameters when using chemotherapy for feline oral squamous cell carcinoma (FOSCC): cisplatin was shown to be ineffective [29] and carboplatin had one partial response of short duration [30]. However, an aggressive protocol using carboplatin and radiation therapy in cases of tonsillar FOSCC showed some long-term survival rates [31]. Other therapies look at adjunctive therapy to slow the pathological bone changes and tumor growth with the use of bisphosphonates [32] and toceranib, especially when combined with non-steroidal anti-inflammatory drugs (NSAIDs) [33]. In particular, the Cox-2 activity of some NSAIDs has been investigated, looking at the Cox-2 expression of oral SCC cells and the impact of medication [34]. The co-treatment of cells with masitinib and piroxicam significantly inhibited cell proliferation as compared to either drug alone [35]. Polyamine inhibitors that target a substance needed for cell proliferation have shown inhibited cell growth in mice [36], as well as tumor regression in 2 cats and stable disease in 6 cats out of 13 in one study [37].

While survival times may not change, such medications can provide clinical benefit and palliative treatment.

Additional medications include analgesics (tramadol, gabapentin, amitryptillyine) to decrease inflammation and pain and oral prednisolone instead of NSAIDs to maintain appetite in the patient [28].

Radiation therapy has been considered as adjunctive therapy in FOSCC to reduce the tumor size prior to surgery [38] and as palliative therapy for non-resectable tumors with varying responses [39, 40]. The previously noted responses for tonsillar SCC to radiation therapy and carboplatin [31], as well as an accelerated hypofraction protocol with 29% of cats lasting more than one year [41], show some promise, though tumor size is of a prognostic factor and most responses were of short duration [41].

As with melanocytic tumors, the standard of care remains early aggressive surgical removal of the entire mass, if possible, with adjunctive therapy in specific cases. Supportive care, particularly in cats, may include palliative medication and nutrition support.

14.2.2.3 Fibrosarcoma (FSA)

The third most common oral malignancy in dogs (and second in cats) is fibrosarcoma (FSA). FSA is known to be infiltrative and determining its full extent can be challenging (see Chapter 7 – Oral Maxillofacial Tumors, Cysts, and Tumor-Like Lesions). While generally thought to have a low metastatic potential (12% pulmonary, 20% regional LN) [42], a higher metastatic rate can be seen in patients with longer survival times, probably due to the extended time to metastasize [43]. Another challenge with FSA is the discrepancy that can be seen with apparently low-grade histological evaluation in a tumor with biologically high-grade activity ("high–low FSA") [42]. In this study of 25 dogs, 72% had bone lysis with aggressive infiltration of local tissues and local recurrence was the typical reason for euthanasia.

While surgical margin intent may be limited due to anatomical planes and anticipated post-operative function, the widest margins should be the goal [43]. Even if 2 cm margins cannot be reached, surgery should still be considered, as even a narrow excision (<15 mm) can potentially provide dogs with a good long-term outcome [43].

Adjunct treatment with radiation therapy has been proposed, with the optimal approach being aggressive surgery and definitive, rather than palliative, radiation therapy [41, 44]. Palliative RT alone in cases of non-resectable tumors can help to reduce tumor size and improve the patient's quality of life [41].

14.2.2.4 Osteosarcoma

Osteosarcoma (OSA) in the oral cavity tends to cause surrounding bone lysis rather than hard tissue proliferation (see Chapter 7), and low-grade tumors, as well as benign osteomas, need to be differentiated from fibro-osseous lesions by their clinical appearance, not just by histopathology [45]. While debulking an osteoma often results in minimal progression [46], OSA requires wide surgical margins of at least 1 cm, as incomplete resection will result in 100% recurrence [2].

While the roles of adjuvant therapy (radiation or chemo) have not been fully determined [2], with a reported 58% metastatic disease prevalence [47], further management needs to be addressed. Palliative radiation therapy for non-resectable tumors may be considered. A recent study also investigated the effects of a selective inhibitor of nuclear export (SINE), where apoptosis of appendicular OSA cell lines was demonstrated [48]. Aggressive surgery remains the standard of care.

14.2.3 Pre-operative Considerations

14.2.3.1 Surgical or Intraoperative Intent

With information gathered about the patient, the lesion, and the client's goals for therapy, decisions can be made as to the extent of the surgical procedure to be performed. The ideal situation is detecting a small lesion early in the course of the disease with adequate excision and clean margins for curative surgical intent. Complete local disease control and no indication of metastasis provides the best scenario. If the intent is curative surgery, or eradication of the pathological condition [49], it is important to make every effort to completely excise the tumor the first time. If additional surgery is needed, the region now has a distorted anatomical structure and even more radical surgery would be required [5]. Unfortunately, many oral tumors are discovered later in their progression, with extensive local invasion and even indications of early metastasis. With these more advanced lesions, a balanced decision looking at the size of the lesion and the attainment of reasonable margins will be considered, taking into account the size of the patient and surrounding anatomical structures. This intraoperative intent – the gross margins the surgeon is attempting to obtain via excision – can be restricted by anatomical planes, the ability to reconstruct the defect, and maintenance of post-operative functionality [43, 50]. If reconstruction is to be considered, a surgical plan for that reconstruction should occur prior to excision of the tumor [49].

On one extreme, removal of a cyst or cyst-like lesion can be as simple as enucleation, the shelling-out of the entire cystic lesion without rupture, including the entire epithelial lining. Often enucleation attempts are followed by curettage to remove 1–2 mm of bone around the entire periphery of the cyst to remove any remaining epithelial cells that could cause recurrence of the cyst [49]. Most tumors, however, require some degree of resection by incising through the uninvolved tissues around the tumor and delivering the tumor without direct contact during instrumentation (an en bloc resection) [49].

This determination of "involved" and "uninvolved" tissues can be described in the context of the zones around the tumor. The pseudocapsule is described as a grossly visible membrane consisting of normal and neoplastic cells, surrounded by a reactive zone of inflammatory cells [5]. An intracapsular excision (from within its pseudocapsule) would be a debulking of the tumor. This could be used for palliative therapy or for benign, well-differentiated tumors such as odontomas [5, 51] (Figure 14.2a to d). In relation to the described zones, a marginal resection would be outside the pseudocapsule but still within the reactive zone, and may be appropriate for some well-differentiated benign tumors. Another definition of marginal incision involves resection of a tumor without disruption of the continuity of the bone [49]. A wide excision would involve an en bloc resection of the tumor, pseudocapsule, reactive zone, and a wide margin of normal tissue [5]. The term "partial resection" parallels this description, with removal of a full-thickness portion of the mandible or maxilla [49]. Relatively small to medium sized malignant tumors are likely to be treated with such procedures. Radical excision

(a) (b) (c) (d)

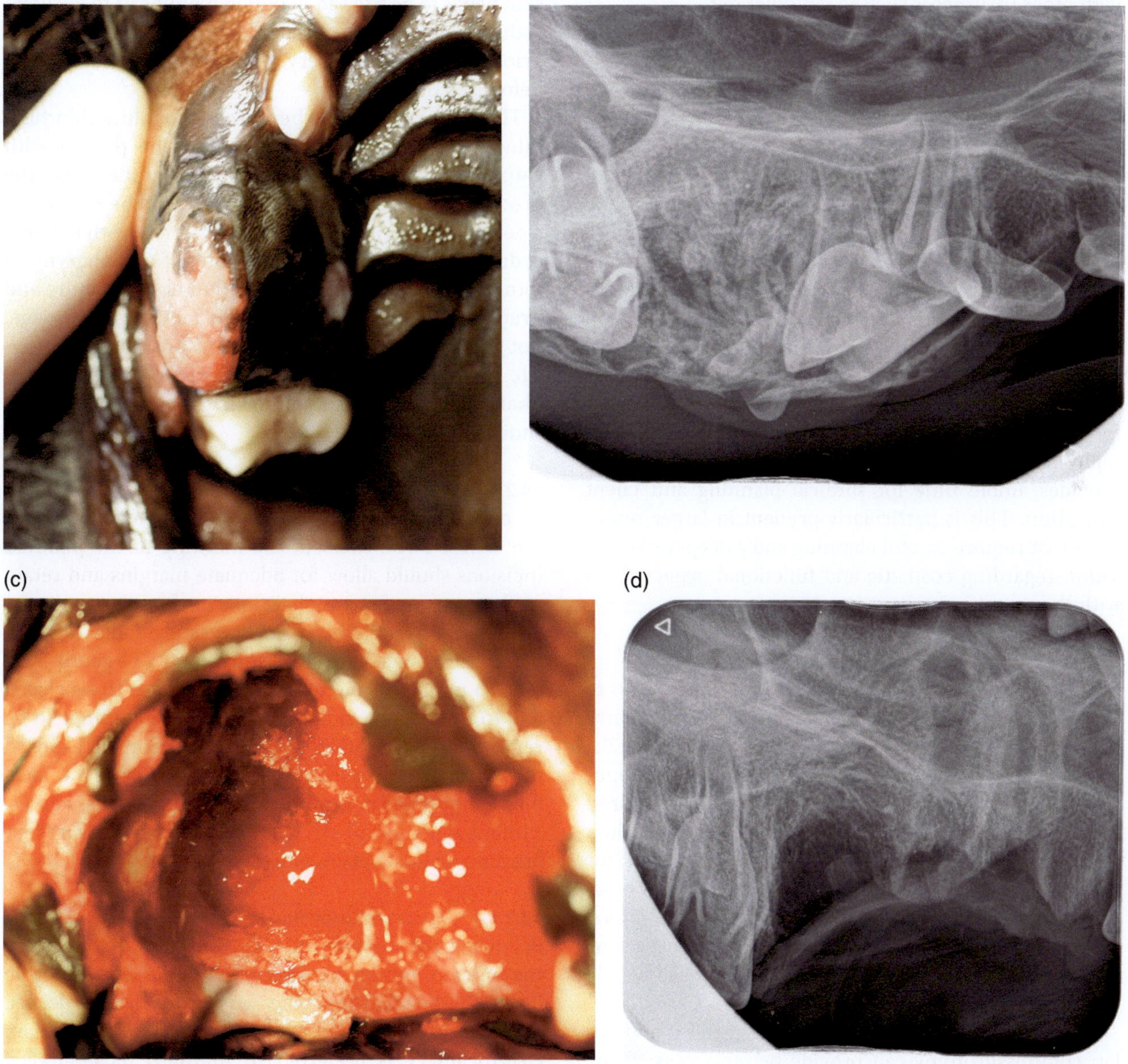

Figure 14.2 Conservative resection of an odontoma: (a) pre-operative appearance of mass at right maxilla; (b) radiograph of right maxilla; (c) intraoperative evaluation of site after tissue removal and curettage; (d) post-operative radiograph.

would involve removal of the entire involved bone or supporting tissue compartment (mandibulectomy). Ablative composite resection would extend the excision to include the bone, adjacent soft tissues, and contiguous lymph channels for malignant tumors [49].

For whatever reasons the client may have, sometimes providing palliative relief will be the limits of clinical efforts. Goals of such therapy would be to relieve clinical signs, restore or improve function, and to improve the quality of life of the patient, though not necessarily the life span [52]. Debulking or cytoreduction of the tumor is seldom recommended (see Chapter 7 – Oral Maxillofacial Tumors, Cysts, and Tumor-Like Lesions), as recurrence would be likely, though may be utilized in conjunction with other treatments such as radiotherapy.

14.2.4 General Surgical Principles

There are many excellent texts and articles covering oral and maxillofacial tumor surgery and many of the general concepts following are found in most of these resources. Specific acknowledgement (reference) will be made when a particular point is made. Having all materials organized ahead of time, including skulls for orientation, a camera for intraoperative photographs and all histopathology supplies ready (including marking inks), can facilitate the procedure and decrease anesthetic time. Additionally, in one of the author's experiences, it is often more appropriate to separate the anesthetic event for acquiring advanced imaging (i.e., computed tomography (CT)) from the actual surgical procedure, as this provides ample time for surgical planning and client education. This is particularly prudent in larger resections that require careful planning and a deeper conversation regarding cosmetic and functional expectations with the owner.

14.2.4.1 Access to Surgical Site

Positioning of the patient is critical for optimal access to the surgical site: for rostral procedures, dorsal recumbency has been described for working on the maxilla, and sternal recumbency for the mandible, with the opposite jaw suspended from a framework above. Dorsal recumbency or a "lazy lateral" position (mostly on their back but leaning to one side or the other) can work for most procedures, reserving ventral recumbency for nasal procedures. For central and caudal procedures, lateral recumbency affords good visualization of the buccal surfaces, though adjustment of the patient's head would facilitate palatal and lingual access.

For caudal procedures, both maxillary and mandibular, commissurotomy can provide better access to the lesion and surrounding tissues. Some variations for maxillectomy will be discussed in that section. Closure of the lips further rostrally (to the first or second premolar), a commissuroplasty, can help post-mandibulectomy to help prevent excessive drooling or tongue protrusion. This three-layer closure will, however, minimize access to the caudal maxillary teeth, making home care, professional care, or any future extractions quite challenging.

14.2.4.2 Surgical Preparation

In determining the intraoperative intent, evaluation of the tissues external to the oral cavity should also be evaluated. If any portion of the lips should be incorporated into the resection, a broad area around that region should receive complete surgical preparation, with isolation of the area with surgical draping. Likewise, if a section of skin needs to be excised to obtain margins or to facilitate esthetic closure, the area should be prepped and marked prior to the start of surgery, keeping final closure in mind before starting [53].

The oral cavity should be rinsed with dilute chlorhexidine solution and the pharynx can be packed with gauze sponges, which will be removed at the end of the procedure. The endotracheal tube should be secured in a position that will not allow it to interfere with the procedure (see options for transmylohyoid and pharyngeal intubation in Chapter 13 – Oral Surgery – Fracture and Trauma Repair). Appropriate soft mouth gags (wedge, not spring-loaded) can be placed to position the opposite jaw if other suspension devices are not used. Pharyngeal packs or suctioning in the back of the mouth should be provided.

14.2.4.3 Intraoperative Intent

In conjunction with the pre-operative evaluation of the tumor to be excised, the marking of the planned incisions should allow for adequate margins and retain sufficient tissue for complete, tension-free closure, hopefully with the possibility of harvesting large mucosal flaps to minimize tension. Tissues should be gently handled to minimize any trauma to the tissue to be closed and to minimize handling of tissues of the tumor to be removed. Visualization and identification of exposed neurovascular bundles will help to preserve the local blood supply and minimize damage to associated nerves. Minimize the use of electrocautery, using pressure and ligation of blood vessels where possible.

14.2.4.4 Mucosal and/or Skin Incision

Following the marked intended incisions, lightly score the mucosa, producing a bleeding line that will not be distorted when the time comes to make the incision deeper. When incising the mucosa, sharp dissection rather than electrocautery is preferred to minimize post-surgical dehiscence [54]. Carefully dissect through the soft tissue down to the bone, preserving neurovascular bundles as they are encountered, or ligating when necessary [51]. A periosteal elevator can be used to elevate the soft tissues with the periosteum of the bone to either side of the planned ostectomy line. Stay sutures may be used to retract these soft tissue layers with care. Protective gauze may be used over the tumor segment itself to minimize handling or potential dissemination of cells [51].

14.2.4.5 Osteotomy – Ostectomy

While an osteotome and mallet can be used, following pinpoint holes initially drilled into the line of the ostectomy, more precise cutting can be made with burs and power equipment. Ideally, a surgical handpiece with no air-insufflation and built-in sterile irrigation can be used for a precision ostectomy. A standard high-speed handpiece with cutting burs and irrigation certainly can also be used, adding the risk of compressed air being introduced into the surgical site. Carbide burs are commonly used for cutting teeth and bone, but will produce a rougher cut edge. Diamond burs with medium grit can be used for a smoother cut or for osteoplasty to smooth the sharp bone edges.

The potential risk of thermal injury using any rotating cutting instruments should be minimized with careful use and appropriate irrigation. This thermal injury can be avoided if ultrasonic piezoelectric units are utilized, with better protection of adjacent soft tissue and a lack of coagulative necrosis [55]. Surgical time can be increased with these piezoelectric units as they are less effective than mechanical saws, and it is said they have a learning curve, but the benefits should be considered [55]. In most resections, a 90° sharp-angled cut should be avoided, as a curvilinear ostectomy has been shown to have higher resistance to occlusal forces [56].

14.2.4.5.1 Teeth in Region of Intended Ostectomy

Once the margins of surgical intent have been marked, attention should be paid to any teeth in the region of excision. Teeth involved in the lesion, pseudocapsule, or reactive zones of the tumor should be removed with their entire alveolar structures, to avoid the potential presence of cells in the periodontal ligament (PDL) space, thus completely removing that tissue compartment. This is likely to be the reasoning behind performing a bilateral rostral mandibulectomy at the level between the second and third premolars, where the most caudal extent of the mandibular canines can be found (as well as the position of the middle mental foramina).

In many cases, the caudal-most aspect of the incision will involve one or more premolars (or a canine tooth). If the surgical intent incision is positioned in an interdental space and there will be sufficient osseous covering of the mesial root of the premolar in the retained section, the excision can be made, but this is not common. Typically there is minimal space in between teeth; planning to transect the next most caudal tooth (at the furcation) is preferred to leaving an unprotected or damaged mesial root and extracting the remaining root once the section is removed [51]. This also allows a segment of tissue that can be easily contoured before closure.

14.2.4.6 Closure Concepts

Once the mass is removed, general principles of closure are followed, including lavage of the area with dilute (0.12%) chlorhexidine or sterile saline. With certain tumors, changing gloves, instruments, and drapes may be warranted [5]. Further preparation of the remaining tissues may involve examination of the exposed bone margins and alveoloplasty with a fine to medium grit diamond bur. The soft tissues are also inspected and blunt dissection begun between the submucosa and deeper tissues to develop mucosal/submucosal flaps to reconstruct the vestibular area and close the surgical site. When possible, place suture lines over an osseous ridge, not over a defect. When possible, a two-layer closure is preferred, with absolutely no tension on the incision line [54]. For closure of a maxillectomy, elevation and excision of an additional 1–3 mm of the palatal mucoperiosteum will provide for suture placement over bone [57]. Plan pre-operatively to restore the vestibular space at closure by resecting a portion of the adjacent skin or lip. Align and suture the lip margins first and then close the mucosal and skin layers separately.

14.3 Procedures

The American Veterinary Dental College (AVDC) website is a good resource for oral surgery terminology (Table 14.1) and abbreviations (Table 14.2).

14.3.1 Mandibulectomy

14.3.1.1 Anatomical Considerations

An anatomical description of the mandible and maxilla can be found in Chapter 1 – Oral Anatomy and Physiology – but a brief description of relevant anatomical landmarks are mentioned here. Knowing the location of neurovascular bundles that supply the tissues to be managed is important to both preserve the viability of the remaining structures and to be able to handle these vessels and nerves in the operative field. The mandibular artery enters the mandibular canal at its distal opening and the inferior alveolar arteries supply the teeth and periodontium, as does the neural component. The mandibular branch of the trigeminal nerve also provides sensory innervation to the caudal two-thirds of the tongue, a fact to keep in mind when administering caudal mandibular

Table 14.1 AVDC nomenclature – surgical treatment procedures for oral tumors (https://www.avdc.org/Nomenclature/Nomen-Surgery.html; accessed July 4, 2017).

Term	Abbr	Definition
Surgery	S	Branch of medicine that treats diseases, injuries, and deformities by manual or operative methods
Buccotomy	BUC	Incision through the cheek (for example to gain access to an intraoral procedure)
Cheiloplasty/ Commissuroplasty	CPL	Reconstructive surgery of the lip/lip commissure
Commissurotomy	COM	Incision through the lip commissure (for example to gain access to an intraoral procedure)
Partial mandibulectomy	S/M	Surgical removal (en block) of part of the mandible and surrounding soft tissues
Dorsal marginal mandibulectomy	S/MD	A form of partial mandibulectomy in which the ventral border of the mandible is maintained; also called marginal mandibulectomy or mandibular rim excision
Segmental mandibulectomy	S/MS	A form of partial mandibulectomy in which a full dorsoventral segment of the mandible is removed
Bilateral partial mandibulectomy	S/MB	Surgical removal of parts of the left and right mandibles and surrounding soft tissues
Total mandibulectomy	S/MT	Surgical removal of one mandible and surrounding soft tissues
Partial maxillectomy	S/X	Surgical removal (en block) of part of the maxilla and/or other facial bones and surrounding soft tissues
Bilateral partial maxillectomy	S/XB	Surgical removal of parts of the left and right maxillae and/or other facial bones and surrounding soft tissues
Partial palatectomy	S/P	Partial resection of the palate

Table 14.2 AVDC abbreviation list for oral surgery – maxillofacial tumors (https://www.avdc.org/abbreviations.pdf; accessed July 4, 2017).

		Definition
B		Biopsy
	B/B	Bite biopsy
	B/CN	Core needle biopsy
	B/E	Excisional biopsy
	B/I	Incisional biopsy
	B/NA	Needle aspiration
	B/NB	Needle biopsy
	B/P	Punch biopsy
	B/S	Surface biopsy
COM		Commissurotomy
CPL		Cheiloplasty/commissuroplasty
LN		Lymph node (regional, i.e., facial, mandibular, parotid, lateral, and medial retropharyngeal)
	LN/E	Lymph node enlargement
	LN/X	Lymph node resection
MET		Metastasis
	MET/D	Distant metastasis
	MET/R	Regional metastasis
OM		Oral/maxillofacial mass
	OM/AA	Acanthomatous ameloblastoma
	OM/AD	Adenoma
	OM/ADC	Adenocarcinoma

Table 14.2 (Continued)

		Definition
	OM/APN	Anaplastic neoplasm
	OM/APO	Amyloid-producing odontogenic tumor
	OM/CE	Cementoma
	OM/FIO	Feline inductive odontogenic tumor
	OM/FS	Fibrosarcoma
	OM/GCG	Giant cell granuloma
	OM/GCT	Granular cell tumor
	OM/HS	Hemangiosarcoma
	OM/LI	Lipoma
	OM/LS	Lymphosarcoma
	OM/MCT	Mast cell tumor
	OM/MM	Malignant melanoma
	OM/OO	Osteoma
	OM/OS	Osteosarcoma
	OM/MTB	Multilobular tumor of bone
	OM/PAP	Papilloma
	OM/PCT	Plasma cell tumor
	OM/PNT	Peripheral nerve sheath tumor
	OM/POF	Peripheral odontogenic fibroma
	OM/RBM	Rhabdomyosarcoma
	OM/SCC	Squamous cell carcinoma
	OM/UDN	Undifferentiated neoplasm
S		Surgery
	S/M	Partial mandibulectomy
	S/MB	Bilateral partial mandibulectomy (removal of parts of the left and right mandibles)
	S/MD	Dorsal marginal mandibulectomy (marginal mandibulectomy, mandibular rim excision)
	S/MS	Segmental mandibulectomy (removal of a full dorsoventral segment of a mandible)
	S/MT	Total mandibulectomy (removal of one entire mandible)
	S/P	Partial palatectomy
	S/X	Partial maxillectomy
	S/XB	Bilateral partial maxillectomy (removal of parts of the left and right maxillae and/or other facial bones)
SG		Salivary gland
	SG/ADC	Salivary gland adenocarcinoma (check abbreviations under OM for other tumors)

(inferior alveolar) local anesthetic blocks. Disruption of these during a caudal or central mandibulectomy can impact structures rostral to the ostectomy, though some extraosseous arterioles that span the symphysis may be important to a rostral mandibular segment [53]. The sublingual artery, a branch from the facial artery, may be encountered on the medial aspect of the mandible. As the maxillary artery passes medial to the angular process of the mandible, it can be damaged during mandibulectomy if not protected. In cats, overextension of the mandibles with spring mouth gags can potentially compress these arteries that have been linked to sight and hearing loss [58].

Muscle attachments require handling during mandibulectomy, particularly in caudal procedures. The masseter muscle inserts in the masseteric fossa of the ramus, while the lateral and medial pterygoid muscles insert on the medial aspect of the condylar process and ventromedial aspect of the angular process, respectively. The fibrous raphe between the pterygoid and masseter muscles can be used as a surgical landmark for an approach to the caudal mandible. The ventral border of the mandible is the site for insertion of the digastricus muscle.

During rostral procedures, the sublingual caruncles should be identified, isolated, and preserved if possible. These small elevations on either side of the base of the lingual frenulum of the tongue lie on the floor of the mouth and can be cannulated for further delineation [59]. The ducts of the sublingual and mandibular salivary glands run in the sublingual folds on either side of the tongue.

14.3.2 Unilateral Rostral Mandibulectomy

For patients with small, non-invasive tumors that involve the mandibular incisors, canine or first premolar on one side, with surgical intent margins not crossing the midline, a unilateral rostral procedure may be indicated. This typically applies to larger dogs with small, non-infiltrative lesions, as a larger tumor on a smaller dog may necessitate resection of the complete symphyseal joint [60] or a bilateral procedure to get clean margins [61].

The surgical intent caudal margin will typically be in the interproximal area between the second and third premolars. The buccal mucosa is incised, transecting the lower labial frenulum, at which time the middle mental neurovascular bundle can be identified, ligated, and retracted. The sublingual caruncle should be avoided if possible on the lingual aspect of the incision. Once the soft tissues are elevated and retracted, the symphysis can be split with a thin osteotome and mallet [62]. If an asymmetrical osteotomy is planned in the contralateral rostral mandible, the cut will be made in between the incisors, or the third incisor and canine, leaving adequate medial cortex at that canine [61]. The caudal osteotomy placement will avoid transecting the canine root and should be just rostral to the middle mental foramen. Once the ostectomy is complete and the segment is removed, the labial vestibular flap is prepared with submucosal and mucosal closure. Resection of the lip is typically not needed [62].

14.3.3 Bilateral Rostral Mandibulectomy

In many cases surgical resection cases involving the rostral mandible, a bilateral procedure is indicated, particularly when the surgical intention approaches or crosses the symphyseal midline. Dorsal recumbency positioning offers the greatest exposure for dissection [60], with the neck extended and the end of the table lowered [62]. Some practitioners prefer sternal recumbency with the maxilla supported above, which gives the greatest exposure of the oral cavity for more difficult closures [60]. The procedure is the same as a unilateral rostral mandibulectomy, with the added option of being able to extend the ostectomy as far caudal as the interproximal space between the fourth premolar and first molar [62]. While some patients may have challenges with prehension and lingual function with any removal beyond the third premolar [61], some have shown a good return to function and adequate cosmesis with the extended resection [60]. If the osteotomy will involve the mandibular canal, care will be taken to identify and ligate the neurovascular bundle when exposed. Stabilization of the two mandibles is generally not necessary, and in fact may cause additional problems with medial drift and temporomandibular joint (TMJ) dysfunction [61].

Once the caudal osteotomy is complete, the soft tissue is elevated for 4–5 mm and the alveolar margin is tapered to approximately 30° to 60° caudodorsally to reduce the tension on the soft tissues at closure. This is facilitated if the ostectomy was performed at the furcation of a tooth, with the distal root elevated. If the mandibular canal has been breached, soft tissue closure should provide adequate protection. The redundant rostral lip tissue can be managed with a resection of a single rostral V-shaped wedge or two wedges placed at the level of the lower labial frenula [50, 61]. When recreating the vestibule, the lip margin should be higher than the alveolar margin and mucosa between the two mandibles, to minimize drooling [62]. For further support of the mucosal closure, a large interrupted suture can be placed circumferentially around each mandibular body for 7 to 10 days [11].

14.3.4 Symphyseal Sparing Rostral Mandibulectomy

For small, benign, or less-invasive tumors or cysts at or near the incisors or canines in larger dogs, a more rostrally placed ostectomy can preserve the caudal aspect of the symphysis. Careful planning of margin intent (1 or 2 cm) will remove a substantial portion of the rostral mandible, but can spare some of the symphysis to help prevent non-physiologic mandibular mobility and help maintain normal occlusion [63] (Figure 14.3a to d).

Determining the extent of the caudal aspect of the mandibular symphysis in relation to the mandibular first premolars and middle mental foramen will provide landmarks to guide the decision for ostectomy. Resection is likely to be made at or immediately rostral to the middle mental foramen, with identification and ligation of the neurovascular bundle in the region [63]. A bilateral rostral ostectomy will probably be made through the canine roots, so concerns of tumor extension into the PDL space would preclude this procedure in some cases. If performed at this level, the remaining root segments would be elevated. Appropriate resection for cosmetic and functional vestibular closure is similar to that of a standard bilateral rostral mandibulectomy.

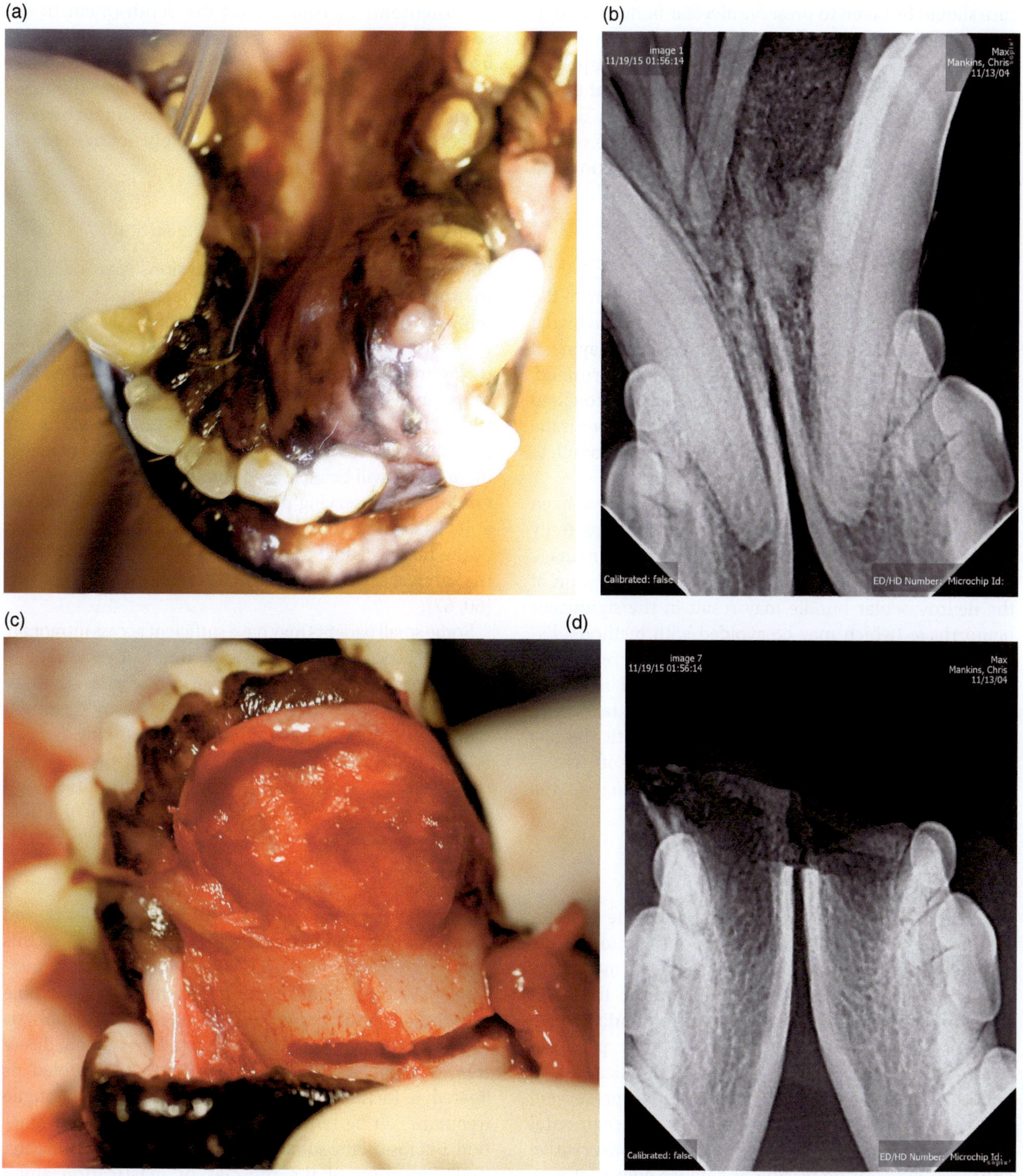

Figure 14.3 Symphysis sparing rostral mandibulectomy of a benign mass: (a) pre-operative appearance of mass at left mandible; (b) radiograph of rostral mandible; (c) osteotomy incision to remove mass yet preserve caudal aspect of symphysis; (d) post-operative radiograph.

A unilateral resection may be considered for a mass involving the buccal surface of one of the canine teeth, with ostectomy that may include the ipsilateral first and second premolars and incisors. This procedure can be considered if the planned margin is rostral to the caudal extent of the symphysis as the cut crosses the midline, and can include some of the contralateral incisors. Typically, the contralateral canine will be retained and care should be taken to preserve alveolar bone around it. Closure does not generally include a lip resection [63].

Occasionally a mass will be small enough in a large dog at the very rostral aspect of the mandible (buccal to the central incisors) to allow preservation of both canine teeth. An en bloc excision of the incisors and rostral mandibular bone can be closed without lip resection and proper stability of the symphysis maintained [63].

14.3.5 Segmental (Central) Mandibulectomy

For tumors involving the body of the mandible from the second premolar to the third molar, and not involving the ramus, an entire segment of the mandible may need resection. As the initial surgical margins are determined, if any malignant or aggressive tumor has approached the mandibular canal, the removal of the entire tissue compartment (mandibular canal), or even complete mandibulectomy, may be necessary.

Once the gingiva and soft tissue incisions have been made, the full thickness ostectomy is performed rostrally and caudally, taking extreme care to identify and manage the contents of the mandibular canal. Any disruption of the neurovascular bundle may result in the significant hemorrhage (which may be avoided with methods discussed above) or devitalization of teeth in the remaining rostral segment. Multiyear medical surveillance with oral examination and radiography of these teeth is a necessity as they may require future endodontic therapy or, alternatively, extraction [62]. Elevation of soft tissues at the cut margins and osteoplasty (rounding) of the bony corners can facilitate closure.

14.3.6 Marginal (Rim) Mandibulectomy

For benign or small malignant tumors on the alveolar margin of the body of the mandible, a variation of the segmental mandibulectomy can be performed [64]. If the size of the mandible allows for the intended incisions to be made dorsal to the mandibular canal, preservation of an intact ventral border provides several advantages (Figure 14.4a to e). Complications of malocclusion can be avoided, function can be preserved, and the cosmetic effect is better than full segmental procedures [64]. However, this more conservative approach may not be feasible is smaller dogs that may lack sufficient mandibular height to obtain clean margins. If the tumor invades the mandibular canal, this procedure may not be prudent.

The rostral and caudal extents of the ostectomy should be planned in a curvilinear manner, as right-angle cuts will introduce stress concentration points within the mandibular body, possibly making the mandible more susceptible to subsequent fracture [56]. When making the osteotomy incisions, limit the depth of cut to the cortical bone just dorsal to the mandibular canal and use the blunt end of a broad periosteal elevator to rotate the segment out [64]. Two-layer closure over the mandibular canal is typically sufficient. The resultant osseous defect will fill in with bone, but possibly not to the same pre-operative cortical height [65].

14.3.7 Unilateral (Total) Mandibulectomy

For large invasive or malignant lesions, particularly if the tumor extends into the mandibular canal, complete removal of the mandible may be necessary [53, 59]. In smaller patients, the surgical margin intent may include the entire mandible, even with less invasive tumors. Due to extensive soft tissue dissection, disarticulation at the TMJ and separation of the mandibular symphysis rostrally, post-operative pain, inflammation, and management issues will be increased with these procedures [66]. Options of preserving portions of the coronoid process at its base, the temporomanidublar joint, or any portion of the ramus caudal to the mandibular canal can reduce the surgical extent if the original lesion is rostrally located [60, 67].

Some small patients may have sufficient access intraorally in sternal recumbency [62], though dorsal recumbency may be preferred and lateral positioning with commissurotomy is often described [50, 60]. A modification with cutting from the commissure in an oblique incision following the direction of the coronoid process may provide better visualization of the operating field and possibly improved post-operative masticatory function, in that author's opinion [68]. It is these authors' experience that a commissurotomy is typically required for disarticulartion of the TMJ in larger dogs.

Identification and management of musculature and neurovascular bundles in the region are critical in this procedure. Once the buccal and lingual mucosal incisions have been made along the extent of the mandible (depending on soft tissue margins needed), the symphysis can be split and the dissection started in a caudal direction. Sublingual salivary ducts should be avoided or ligated if included in the resection [62]. The tongue frenulum can be removed with minimal effect on function, but loss of the sublingual muscle can impair function [53]. Elevation of the muscles of mastication along with the periosteum is preferred to incising them away from the bone at their insertion points [62]. The mental vessels are ligated on the rostral buccal surface and the inferior alveolar neurovascular is carefully isolated and ligated distally on the lingual aspect before it enters the mandibular canal.

The TMJ is carefully dissected, avoiding the branches of the maxillary artery on the caudal and medial aspect of

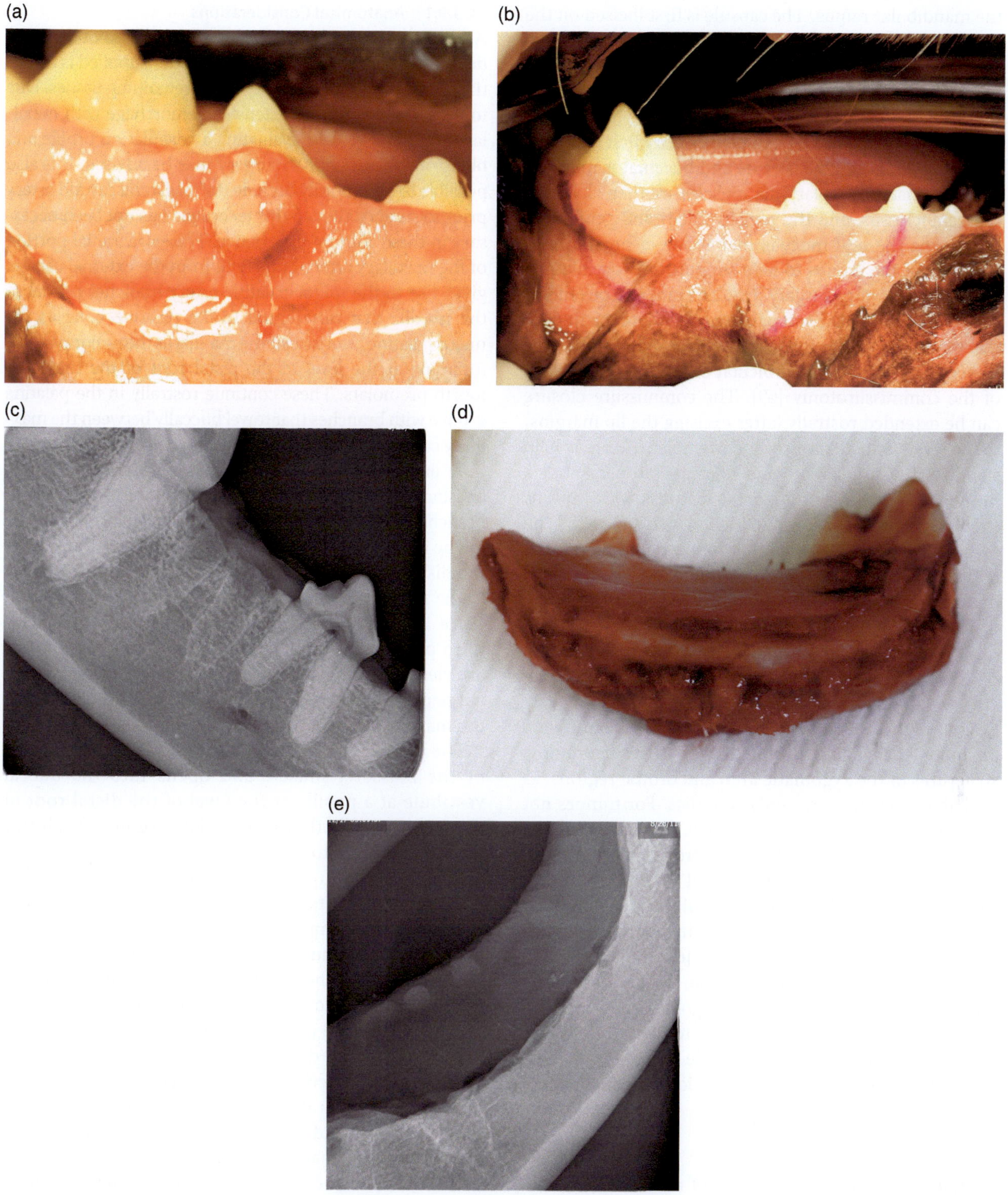

Figure 14.4 Marginal (rim) mandibulectomy: (a) preoperative appearance of mass prior to incisional biopsy (intermediate grade spindle cell carcinoma (fibrosarcoma) – clean margins); (b) pre-operative appearance of mandible with planned incision marked; (c) pre-operative radiograph; (d) dorsal segment of mandible post-operatively; (e) post-operative radiograph.

the mandibular ramus. The capsule is first incised on the medial aspect, surrounding soft tissue gently removed, and the incision is extended to the lateral capsule [53]. Once disarticulated, the temporal muscle is elevated from the coronoid process to release the mandible [62].

The associated muscles can be closed by first apposing the masseter to the digastricus and buccinator muscles. The buccinator and platysma muscles are then closed to the genioglossus, and the mylohyoideus and geniohyoideus bring the oral mucous membrane in proximity to the floor of the mouth to help support the contralateral hemimandible after surgery [69]. The oral mucous membrane is sutured to the soft palate caudally and the floor of the mouth rostrally, followed by a three-layer closure (mucosa, buccinator and orbicular oris muscles, and skin) of the commissurotomy [69]. The commissure closure can be extended rostrally (after excising the lip margins) to the level of the first or second premolar. This may help stabilize the surgical site and decrease drooling, but a muzzle or temporary horizontal mattress with buttons should be placed to prevent dehiscence [50, 62]. The owner should be cautioned that future home care of the maxillary teeth will be more challenging with the commissuroplasty procedure. Complications of drifting of the ipsilateral mandible will be covered later in the chapter.

14.3.8 Caudal Mandibulectomy

Lesions of the caudal body of the mandible or ramus can be more challenging to access with the surrounding structures of the zygomatic arch and orbital regions, as well as various neurovascular bundles. For tumors not associated with the mandibular canal, the ramus with the coronoid process, condyle and retroarticular process, with or without part of the caudal mandibular body, can be resected [62]. For more rostrally invasive tumors, the caudal resection can be combined with a central segment or a total mandibulectomy [61].

Removal of the ramus alone can be accessed with incision over, and removal of, the zygomatic arch [60]. An intraoral or lateral approach, similar to that for unilateral mandibulectomy, can also be made for central-caudal procedures. Commissurotomy with closure is also similar.

14.3.9 Maxillectomy

With few exceptions, the portion of maxillary structure that remains after a portion is removed is typically sufficient to maintain stability and function. Limits on the extent of a resection may include the location (especially caudal) if the surgical margins cross the midline or if extensive lip involvement is encountered. Often the limiting factor is the surgeon's ability and comfort level with reconstructive techniques, which are beyond the scope of this text.

14.3.9.1 Anatomical Considerations

As in the mandibulectomy section, knowledge of the location of neurovascular bundles and tissues supplied is essential for preserving the viability of the remaining tissues. Due to potential issues with extensive hemorrhage with maxillary and nasal vessels, evaluating a coagulation profile and blood-matching prior to surgery may be advised. It is also possible to temporarily occlude the ipsilateral carotid artery prior to surgery, though this technique has not been necessary in these authors' experience. The extracranial portion of the maxillary artery branching from the external carotid gives rise to the minor palatine artery branches caudal to the maxilla that run ventral to the palatine bone as the major palatine arteries exit the maxilla at the major palatine foramina at the level of the distal root of the maxillary fourth premolars. These continue rostrally in the palatine groove with branches that travel buccally between the maxillary canines and third incisors. The remainder of the palatine arteries passes through the palatine fissures to anastamose with the sphenopalatine arteries (the nasal branches of the maxillary arteries).

The infraorbital arteries enter the maxillary foramen at the distal aspect of the infraorbital canal, with branches to the zygomatic gland and alveoli of the maxillary teeth. Once it exits the canal, near the level of the maxillary third premolar, it branches into dorsal and lateral nasal arteries. The infraorbital nerve, a branch of the trigeminal nerve, follows with the vascular branches, supplying the maxilla and maxillary teeth.

The parotid salivary duct crosses the lateral surface of the masseter muscle and opens into the buccal vestibule at a papilla at the level of the distal root of the maxillary fourth premolar. The zygomatic salivary gland empties into the caudal buccal vestibule, just caudal to the last upper molar at the zygomatic papilla. Avoiding the ducts or ligating them can help avoid post-operative complications.

Masses of the caudal maxilla may require excision of tissues including the zygomatic arch and orbital bones, so additional neurovascular structures may be encountered. Identify and protect the nasolacrimal ducts, salivary papillae, and ducts that may be near the surgical site, or manage remaining portions if they are to be resected. Any rostral or central procedure that exposes the nasal cavity and turbinates will also need to address maintaining adequate air passage and complete closure. These issues will be addressed during the description of the applicable surgeries.

14.3.10 Terminology

Some basic terminology can be found on the AVDC website (Table 14.1). While this listing primarily covers partial maxillectomy and bilateral partial maxillectomy for purposes of reporting cases, the term total (unilateral)

(a) (b) (c)

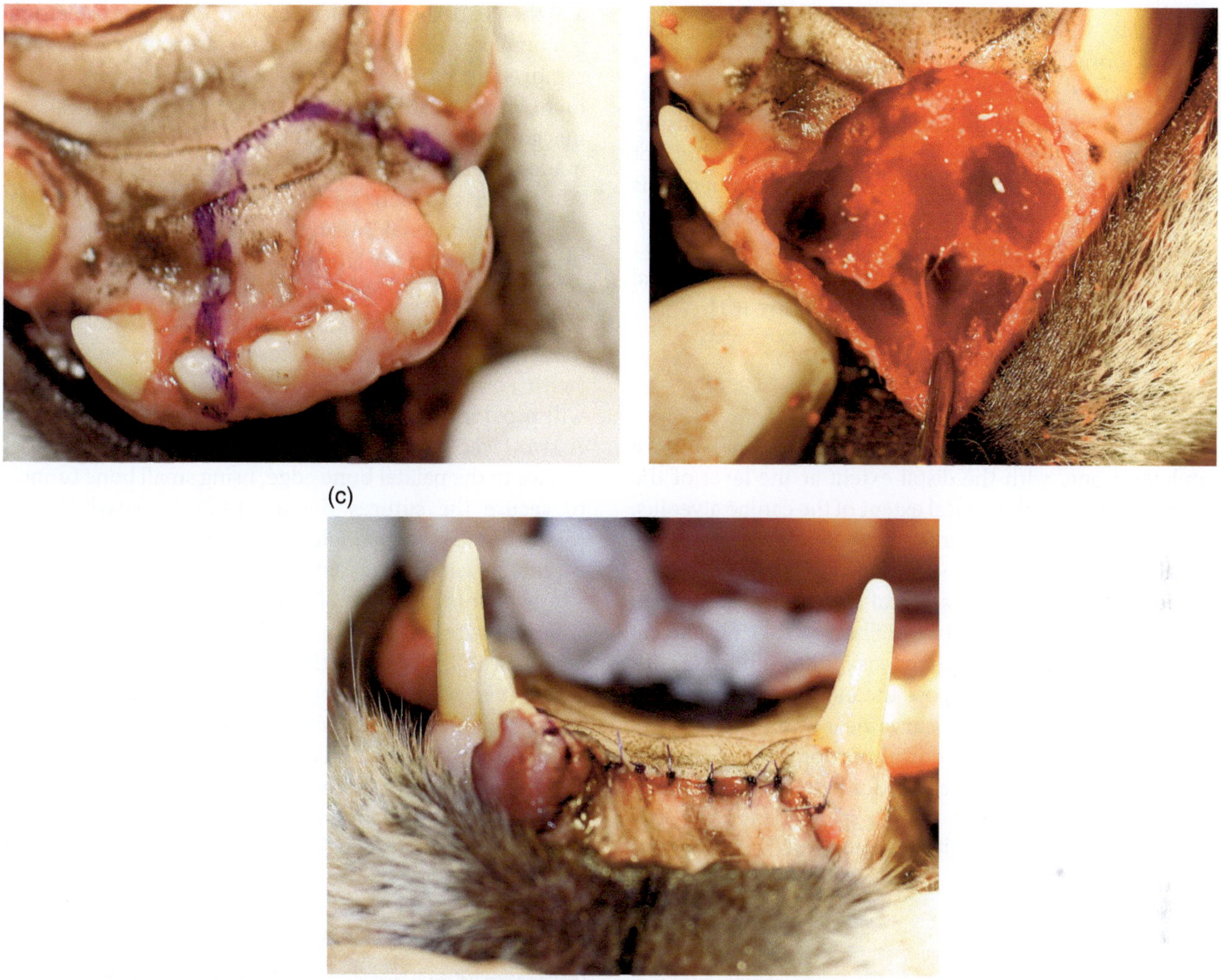

Figure 14.5 Rostral maxillary incisivectomy of a benign mass: (a) pre-operative appearance of mass at right maxilla; (b) resection into maxilla; (c) closure.

maxillectomy is used to describe the removal of one maxillary bone with all or parts of the incisive and palatine bones [69]. Incisivectomy has replaced that term premaxillectomy (anatomically more correct), though removal of just the incisive bone(s) is seldom indicated. Rostral maxillectomy will include removal of incisive bone(s) and the most rostral part of the maxilla(e) – either unilateral or bilateral. These rostral procedures may include a nasal planectomy if the surgical intent includes the soft tissues and cartilage that comprise the facial portions of the nose [69]. Other partial (typically unilateral) procedures include the central maxillectomy (midportion removal) or caudal maxillectomy (from the fourth premolar distally). With more invasive tumors, portions of the ventral orbital region, including the zygomatic arch and even the coronoid process of the mandible, may need to be included in the resection.

14.3.11 Incisivectomy

As stated earlier, seldom will a true incisivectomy be indicated, as most margins with rostral lesions will at least extend into the maxilla or palate. With a very small benign mass on a large dog, the ostectomy should be confined to the region of the distal line angles of the third incisor to avoid trauma to the canine teeth [62] (Figure 14.5a to c). Branches of the major palatine arteries should be avoided as they pass between the third incisors and canines. While the ventrolateral nasal cartilages may be exposed, the nasal cavity typically is not exposed [62]. A bilateral procedure may result in nasal droop and a unilateral surgery can have lateral deviation post-operatively (the correction technique is detailed later in the chapter) [69]. Simple vestibular flap closure is often sufficient, though releasing incisions may be necessary.

14.3.12 Unilateral Rostral Maxillectomy

If a small lesion is located on the buccal surface of the canine tooth and extensive margins are not needed, a unilateral rostral maxillectomy may be adequate. An incision line would be planned rostral to the second premolar, can extend to the incisive bone midline, but should not involve the nasal planum [6]. Dorsal recumbency is described [61], with the mandible secured out of the way. Additional details of excision are covered in the next section (bilateral rostral maxillectomy). A single intraoral mucosal flap is typically sufficient for closure [61].

14.3.13 Bilateral Rostral Maxillectomy

This procedure is more commonly performed than a unilateral one, with the distal extent at the level of the second premolar, the typical extent of the canine alveolus. The mucosal incision across the palate can follow the rugal pattern (if bilaterally symmetrical), with a deliberate identification and ligation of the palatal arteries on each side [62] (Figure 14.6). The rostral and buccal incisions are made through mucosa and submucosa with periosteal elevation to expose the incisive and maxillary bones of the planned curvilinear osteotomy [57]. Preserving the nasal and dorsal portions of the incisive bone will help support the nose for better cosmesis.

Initial osteotomy with a high-speed handpiece and burs of the incisive, maxillary, and palatal bones may be accompanied by careful use of an osteotome and mallet, and the use of the piezoelectric unit. When the ostectomy is complete, the nasal turbinates are cut sharply and removed en bloc with the surgical segment [57]. Placement of the osteotomy in relation to the soft tissue margins may be made at the same level [6] or may be made wider to provide sufficient soft tissue for closure. Alternatively, a soft palatal mucosal incision may be made an additional 2–3 mm caudal to the osteotomy in order to leave a bony ledge for suture line support [57].

Closure can be facilitated with strategically placed releasing incisions [57], though they are not always necessary [62]. Releasing the mucosa and submucosa (with some subcutaneous tissue) from the vestibule will provide sufficient tissue for a T-shaped closure [6]. A two-layer closure is started by securing submucosal tissues to the palatal bone edge, using small bone tunnels to secure the sutures (Figure 14.7). Mucosal closure (buccal to palatal) should be started from the caudal extent on each side, joining at the midline with final sutures joining right and left buccal mucosal flaps.

If the entire incisive bone and ventrolateral nasal cartilage area is included in the removal, pronounced nasal droop may occur. To correct this complication, a short incision over the dorsal midline is made at the junction of the nasal cartilages and nasal/incisive bones [69]. The dorsal lateral aspect of the incisive bone is exposed by shifting the incision laterally and a small hole is drilled through the bone. A suture is placed through the dorsolateral nasal

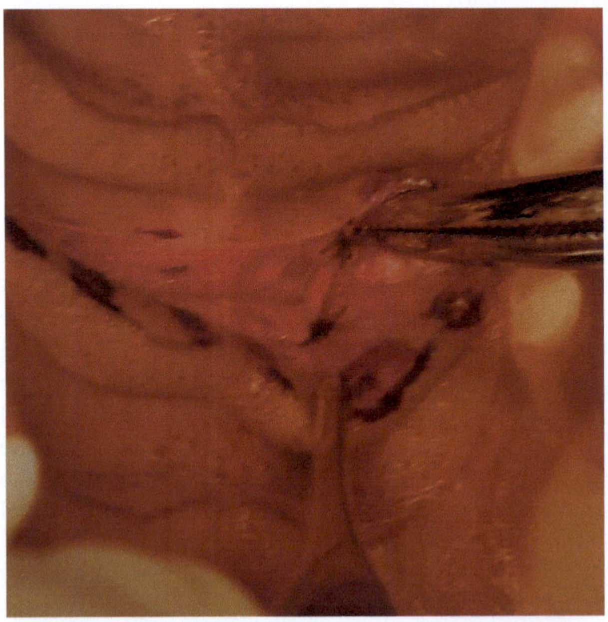

Figure 14.6 Demonstration of ligation of palatal arteries during a bilateral rostral maxillectomy. *Source:* Reprinted with permission from reference [57].

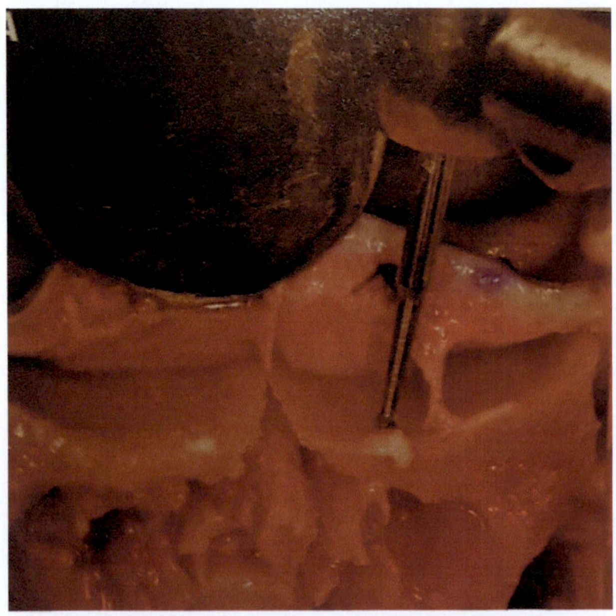

Figure 14.7 Demonstration of pre-placing holes in the maxilla (bone tunnels) for suture placement upon closure of bilateral rostral maxillectomy. *Source:* Reprinted with permission from reference [57].

cartilage, then through the hole, and tied to provide tension to correct the deviation [69]. This is repeated on the other side if a bilateral procedure has been done. For large maxillofacial tumors involving the maxilla and nares, the bilateral rostral maxillectomy can be combined with a nasal planectomy, with closure of the skin at the nasal bone rim, leaving the apertures open [70]. Alternatively, a more cosmetic, and in these authors' experience, more functional and complication-free, reconstruction of the nasal planum may be performed utilizing the lip mucocutaneous junction, as described by Gallegos et al., the details of which are beyond the scope of this text [71].

14.3.14 Central Maxillectomy

For lesions in the central or caudal regions of the maxilla, lateral or dorsal recumbency may be used. Surgical planning is likely to involve management of the nasal or sinus cavities, palatal arteries, and infraorbital canal with contents. Curvilinear excisions are preferred over rectangular incisions, which may be more likely to dehisce [50]. Due to the out-turn of the caudal maxillary arch, if an excision extends to the third premolar, removal of the remaining premolar and molars may help alleviate tension at closure [50].

Once initial mucosal incisions have been made with soft tissue elevated and retracted, initial osteotomy should be performed carefully to cut just through the bony structure of the maxilla and palate, avoiding the soft tissues. Alveolar incisions are made to connect the dorsal and ventral cuts, with management of any remaining tooth roots. As the tissue block is released, remaining soft tissue attachments are severed, and the nasal turbinates are cut sharply and removed with the block [6].

Closure with a released vestibular buccal mucosal/submucosal flap typically will be sufficient in resections that do not cross the palatal midline. In cases where the resection is more extensive, or if vestibular and lip tissue were included in the resection, additional steps may be taken. A palatal incision on the contralateral side, 2–3 mm from the alveolar ridge and teeth, can be made the approximate length of the initial surgical site. This edge of the palatal mucosa is then elevated full thickness from the palatal bone, keeping the palatal artery intact with the section of tissue. The elevation is completed to the palatal mucosal extent of the resection, to relieve tension on the final closure. The incision on the contralateral side is not sutured.

14.3.15 Caudal Maxillectomy

Surgical planning for a tumor of the caudal maxilla can be more challenging due to access and surrounding structures such as the orbit, salivary ducts, and vessels. Cheilotomy with the patient in lazy lateral or lateral recumbency may be adequate for less invasive tumors of the mandible, but more aggressive tumors that encroach upon the ventral orbital area and zygoma may need further exposure.

For removal of the caudal maxilla, the mucosal incision at the mucogingival junction is made from the rostral aspect of the intended margins back to the level of the second molar or as dictated by the extensiveness of the tumor [6]. It is optimal to preserve the salivary papillae if possible. Otherwise, ligate the ducts if they are included in the resection [69]. The palatal incision is made, managing the palatal artery if incorporated into the resection. Osteotomies are made in the rostral sections first, including at the rostral base of the zygomatic arch, with the caudal cut saved for last. Prior to the caudal cut, identify, ligate, and cut the maxillary artery. If it is difficult to completely isolate the complex of vessels (maxillary artery and branches) at the caudal aspect, remove the caudal segment quickly once the caudal osteotomy incision is complete, and immediately identify and ligate these vessels. If a dorsal resection involves the nasolacrimal duct, typically post-operative epiphora does occur due to healing of the proximal end with a new osteium formed. Any exposed turbinates are trimmed and hemorrhage controlled. Closure with a buccal mucosa flap separated from the vestibule is performed in a one- or two-layer pattern.

For more invasive tumors, such as those involving the zygoma and ventral orbital margin, an orbitectomy can be combined with the caudal maxillectomy. For better exposure, a combined dorsolateral skin and intraoral approach has been described [70]. In this method, an incision is begun in the dorsolateral skin near the dorsal midline and then the incision is advanced caudally below the orbit, following the zygomatic arch. The globe, with an intact conjunctival sac, is separated from the zygoma and the masseter muscle is separated from the ventral aspect of the zygomatic arch [70]. Intraorally, the buccal mucosal incision is made, undermining the bone, and is connected dorsally with the dorsolateral incision, which creates an isthmus of skin (bipedicle flap) between the dorsal and intraoral incisions. The facial vein and other vessels are ligated at the dorsocaudal aspect. This bipedicle flap can be reflected dorsally or ventrally as needed to access the surgical site.

Removal of the inferior orbit can be performed by carefully using an osteotome through the medial aspect of the orbit, angled to the second molar. The surgical segment can also be laterally displaced to separate the bone at the rostromedial aspect of the pterygopalatine fossa. The zygomatic arch is resected according to intended surgical margins if needed. The dorsal incision is closed in two layers and the masseter muscle is sutured to the fibrous tissue ventral to the globe if an orbitectomy is performed. A two-layer closure of the buccal mucosa may include sutures passing through holes made in the palate. The area between the skin and oral incisions is not closed [70].

14.4 Complications

Several complications associated with specific procedures have already been addressed, from incisions involving the orbit and nasolacrimal duct to management of salivary structures and correcting nasal droop. Intraoperative complications with hemorrhage can be substantial, particularly with maxillectomy procedures, so careful attention to vascular management and preparation with available blood products for transfusion may be needed. Post-operative dehiscence is a common event, particularly if closure was compromised by any tension on the suture lines. Careful monitoring of the patient post-operatively is critical to avoid serious complications. Teeth apposing a surgical site can cause trauma, but minor odontoplasty of sharp crowns may help alleviate some of this. Odontoplasty typically exposes some dentinal tubules and, thus, a bonding agent should be placed on the exposed surface. Of course, the pulp chamber canal of the tooth being shortened should be avoided if possible. If exposure of the root canal is unavoidable, proper endodontic therapy (see Chapter 15 – Basic Endodontic Therapy) or, alternatively, extraction is required.

With mandibulectomy procedures that remove an entire segment or an entire mandible, post-operative malocclusion is likely to occur and must be handled accordingly. Once that portion of the mandible is gone, the contralateral side may drift in that direction. The remaining mandibular canine(s) can cause trauma to the palate and changes to the TMJs can occur [61]. Orthodontic brackets or buttons can be cemented on to the lingual surface of the mandibular canine and the buccal surface of the maxillary fourth premolar. When an orthodontic elastic chain is placed between the two, the tension helps to correct the drift and maintain the occlusion [72]. In a study, half of the dogs reviewed in follow-up maintained TMJ stability after the appliance was removed. Good client compliance includes replacing the elastics, maintaining good oral hygiene, and follow-up visits.

References

1 Verstraete, F.J.M., V. and Lommer, M.J. (eds.) (2012). *Oral and Maxillofacial Surgery in Dogs and Cats*. Edinburgh, UK: Elsevier.

2 Farcas, N., Arzi, B., and Verstraete, F.J.M. (2014). Oral and maxillofacial osteosarcoma in dogs: a review. *Vet. Comp. Oncol.* 12 (3): 169–180. doi: 10.1111/j.1476-5829.2012.00352.x.

3 Fox, L., Geoghegan, S., Davis, L. et al. (1997). Owner satisfaction with partial mandibulectomy or maxillectomy for treatment of oral tumors in 27 dogs. *J. Am. Anim. Hosp. Assoc.* 33 (1): 25–31.

4 Northrup, N.C., Selting, K.A., Rassnick, K.M. et al. (2006). Outcomes of cats with oral tumors treated with mandibulectomy: 42 cases. *J. Am. Anim. Hosp. Assoc.* 42: 350–360. doi: 42/5/350 [pii].

5 Soderstrom, M. and Gilson, S. (1995). Principles of surgical oncology. *Vet. Clin. North Am. Small Anim. Pract.* 25 (1): 97–110.

6 Dernell, W.S., Schwartz, P.D., and Withrow, S.J. (1998). Maxillectomy and premaxillectomy. In: *Current Techniques in Small Animal Surgery*, 4e (ed. M.J. Bojrab, G.W. Ellison and B. Slocum), 124–131. Baltimore, MD: Williams & Wilkins.

7 Liuti, T., De Vos, J., Bosman, T. et al. (2009). 67 Gallium citrate scintigraphy to assess metastatic spread in a dog with an oral melanoma. *J. Small Anim. Pract.* 50 (1): 31–34. doi: 10.1111/j.1748-5827.2008.00652.x.

8 Herring, E., Smith, M.M., and Robertson, J. (2002). Lymph node staging of oral and maxillofacial neoplasms in 31 dogs and cats. *J. Vet. Dent.* 19 (3): 122–126.

9 Klein, M.K. (2003). Multimodality therapy for head and neck cancer. *Vet. Clin. Small Anim.* 33: 615–628.

10 Williams, L.E. and Packer, R.A. (2003). Association between lymph node size and metastasis in dogs with oral malignant melanoma: 100 cases (1987–2001). *J. Am. Vet. Med. Assoc.* 222 (9): 1234–1236.

11 Berg, J. (1998). Principles of oncologic orofacial surgery. *Clin. Tech. Small Anim. Pract.* 13 (1): 38–41. doi: 10.1016/S1096-2867(98)80025-X.

12 Tuohy, J.L., Selmic, L.E., Bv, M. et al. (2014). Outcome following curative-intent surgery for oral melanoma in dogs: 70 cases (1998–2011). *J. Am. Vet. Med. Asoc.* 245 (11): 1266–1273. doi: 10.2460/javma.245.11.1266.

13 Boston, S.E., Lu, X., Culp, W.T.N. et al. (2014). Efficacy of systemic adjuvant therapies administered to dogs after excision of oral malignant melanomas: 151 cases (2001–2012). *J. Am. Vet. Med. Assoc.* 245 (4): 401–407. doi: 10.2460/javma.245.4.401.

14 Dank, G., Rassnick, K.M., Sokolovsky, Y. et al. (2014). Use of adjuvant carboplatin for treatment of dogs with

oral malignant melanoma following surgical excision. *Vet. Comp. Oncol.* 12 (1): 78–84. doi: 10.1111/j.1476-5829.2012.00338.x.

15 Brockley, L., Cooper, M., and Bennett, P. (2013). Malignant melanoma in 63 dogs (2001–2011): the effect of carboplatin chemotherapy on survival. *N.Z. Vet. J.* 61 (1): 25–31. doi: 10.1080/00480169.2012.699433.

16 Proulx, R., Ruslander, M., and Hauck, L. (2003). Treated with external beam radiation. *Vet. Radiol. Ultra.* 44 (3): 352–359.

17 Itoh, H., Mukaiyama, T., Goto, T. et al. (2014). Non-surgical treatment of canine oral malignant melanoma: a case study of the application of complementary alternative medicine. *Oncol. Lett.* 7 (6): 1829–1830. doi: 10.3892/ol.2014.2041.

18 Seo, K.w., Coh, Y.r., Rebhun, R.B. et al. (2014). Antitumor effects of celecoxib in COX-2 expressing and non-expressing canine melanoma cell lines. *Res. Vet. Sci.* 96 (3): 482–486. doi: 10.1016/j.rvsc.2014.03.003.

19 Farrelly, J., Denman, D.L., Hohenhaus, A.E. et al. (2004). Hypofractionated radiation therapy of oral melanoma in five cats. *Vet. Radiol. Ultrasound.* 45 (1): 91–93. doi: 10.1111/j.1740-8261.2004.04015.x.

20 Freeman, K.P., Hahn, K.A., Harris, F.D., and King, G.K. (2003). Treatment of dogs with oral melanoma by hypofractionated radiation therapy and platinum-based chemotherapy (1987–1997). *J. Vet. Intern. Med.* 17 (1): 96–101. doi: 10.1892/0891-6640(2003)017<0096:TODWOM>2.3.CO;2.

21 Kawabe, M., Mori, T., Ito, Y. et al. (2015). Outcomes of dogs undergoing radiotherapy for treatment of oral malignant melanoma: 111 cases (2006–2012). *J. Am. Vet. Med. Assoc.* 247 (10): 1146–1153. doi: 10.2460/javma.247.10.1146.

22 Grosenbaugh, D.A., Leard, T.A., Bergman, P.J. et al. (2011). Safety and efficacy of a xenogeneic {DNA} vaccine encoding for human tyrosinase as adjunctive treatment for oral malignant melanoma in dogs following surgical excision of the primary tumor. *Am. J. Vet. Res.* 72 (12): 6–8. doi: 10.2460/ajvr.72.12.1631.

23 Ottnod, J.M., Smedley, R.C., Walshaw, R. et al. (2013). A retrospective analysis of the efficacy of oncept vaccine for the adjunct treatment of canine oral malignant melanoma. *Vet. Comp. Oncol.* 11 (3): 219–229. doi: 10.1111/vco.12057.

24 Treggiari, E., Grant, J., and SM N. (2016). A retrospective study of outcome and survival following surgery and adjuvant xenogenic DNA vaccination in 32 dogs with oral malignant melanoma. *J. Vet. Med. Sci.* 78 (5): 845–850.

25 Esplin, D.G. (2008). Survival of dogs following surgical excision of histologically well-differentiated melanocytic neoplasms of the mucous membranes of the lips and oral cavity. *Vet. Pathol.* 45 (6): 889–896. doi: 10.1354/vp.45-6-889.

26 Gendler, A., Lewis, J.R., Reetz, J.A., and Schwarz, T. (2010). Computed tomographic features of oral squamous cell carcinoma in cats: 18 cases (2002–2008). *J. Am. Vet. Med. Assoc.* 236 (3): 319–325. doi: 10.2460/javma.236.3.319.

27 Soltero-Rivera, M.M., Krick, E.L., Reiter, A.M. et al. (2014). Prevalence of regional and distant metastasis in cats with advanced oral squamous cell carcinoma: 49 cases (2005–2011). *J. Feline Med. Surg.* 16 (2): 164–169. doi: 10.1177/1098612X13502975.

28 Bilgic, O., Duda, L., Sánchez, M.D., and Lewis, J.R. (2015). Feline oral squamous cell carcinoma: clinical manifestations and literature review. *J. Vet. Dent.* 32 (1): 30–40.

29 Fox, L.E., Rosenthal, R.C., King, R.R. et al. (2000). Use of cis-bis-neodecanoato-trans-R, R-1, 2,-diaminocyclohexane platinum (II), a liposomal cisplatin analogue, in cats with oral squamous cell carcinoma. *Am. J. Vet. Res.* 61 (7): 791–795.

30 Kisseberth, W.C., Vail, D.M., Yaissle, J. et al. (2008). Phase I clinical evaluation of carboplatin in tumor-bearing cats: a veterinary cooperative oncology group study. *J. Vet. Intern. Med.* 22 (1): 83–88. doi: 10.1111/j.1939-1676.2007.0017.x.

31 Fidel, J., Lyons, J., Tripp, C. et al. (2011). Treatment of oral squamous cell carcinoma with accelerated radiation therapy and concomitant carboplatin in cats. *J. Vet. Intern. Med.* 25 (3): 504–510. doi: 10.1111/j.1939-1676.2011.0721.x.

32 Wypij, J.M., Fan, T.M., Fredrickson, R.L. et al. (2008). *In vivo* and *in vitro* efficacy of zoledronate for treating oral squamous cell carcinoma in cats. *J. Vet. Intern. Med.* 22 (1): 158–163. doi: 10.1111/j.1939-1676.2007.0010.x.

33 Wiles, V., Hohenhaus, A., Lamb, K. et al. (2017). Retrospective evaluation of toceranib phosphate (palladia) in cats with oral squamous cell carcinoma. *J. Feline Med. Surg.* 19 (2): 185–193. doi: 10.1177/1098612X15622237.

34 DiBernardi, L., Doré, M., Davis, J.A. et al. (2007). Study of feline oral squamous cell carcinoma: potential target for cyclooxygenase inhibitor treatment. *Prostaglandins Leukot. Essent. Fat Acids* 76 (4): 245–250. doi: 10.1016/j.plefa.2007.01.006.

35 Rathore, K., Alexander, M., and Cekanova, M. (2014). Piroxicam inhibits Masitinib-induced cyclooxygenase 2 expression in oral squamous cell carcinoma cells in vitro. *Transl. Res.* 164 (2): 158–168. doi: 10.1016/j.trsl.2014.02.002.

36 Lewis, J.R., O, Brien, T.G., Skorupski, K.A. et al. (2013). Polyamine inhibitors for treatment of feline oral

squamous cell carcinoma: a proof-of-concept study. *J. Vet. Dent.* 30 (3): 140–145.
37 Skorupski, K., O, Brien, T., Guerrero, T. et al. (2011). Phase I/II clinical trial of 2-difluoromethylornithine (DFMO) and a novel polyamine transport inhibitor (MQT 1426) for feline oral squamous cell carcinoma. *Vet. Comp. Oncol.* 9 (4): 275–282. doi: 10.1021/nl061786n.Core-Shell.
38 Mestrinho, L., Bernardo, E., Niza, M. et al. (2012). Neoadjuvant chemoradiotherapy and surgery as treatment for oral maxillary squamous cell carcinoma in a dog. *Aust. Vet. J.* 90 (7): 264–268. doi: 10.1111/j.1751-0813.2012.00928.x.
39 Sabhlok, A. and Ayl, R. (2014). Palliative radiation therapy outcomes for cats with oral squamous cell carcinoma (1999–2005). *Vet. Radiol. Ultrasound.* 55 (5): 565–570. doi: 10.1111/vru.12157.
40 Bregazzi, V.S., LaRue, S.M., Powers, B.E. et al. (2001). Response of feline oral squamous cell carcinoma to palliative radiation therapy. *Vet. Radiol. Ultrasound.* 42 (1): 77–79. doi: 10.1111/j.1740-8261.2001.tb00907.x.
41 Poirier, V.J., Bley, C.R., Roos, M., and Kaser-Hotz, B. (2006). Efficacy of radiation therapy for the treatment of macroscopic canine oral soft tissue sarcoma. *In Vivo (Brooklyn)* 20 (3): 415–420.
42 Ciekot, P.A., Powers, B.E., Withrow, S.J. et al. (1994). Histologically low-grade, yet biologically high-grade, fibrosarcomas of the mandible and maxilla in dogs: 25 cases (1982–1991). *J. Am. Vet. Med. Assoc.* 204 (4): 610–615.
43 Frazier, S.A., Johns, S.M., Ortega, J. et al. (2012). Outcome in dogs with surgically resected oral fibrosarcoma (1997–2008). *Vet. Comp. Oncol.* 10 (1): 33–43. doi: 10.1111/j.1476-5829.2011.00272.x.
44 Gardner, H., Fidel, J., Haldorson, G. et al. (2015). Canine oral fibrosarcomas: a retrospective analysis of 65 cases (1998–2010). *Vet. Comp. Oncol.* 13 (1): 40–47. doi: 10.1111/vco.12017.
45 Soltero-Rivera, M., Engiles, J.B., Reiter, A.M. et al. (2015). Benign and malignant proliferative fibro-osseous and osseous lesions of the oral cavity of dogs. *Vet. Pathol.* 52 (5): 894–902. doi: 10.1177/0300985815583096.
46 Volker, M. and Luskin, I. (2014). Oral osteoma in 6 dogs. *J. Vet. Dent.* 32 (2): 88–91.
47 Coyle, V.J., Rassnick, K.M., Borst, L.B. et al. (2015). Biological behaviour of canine mandibular osteosarcoma. A retrospective study of 50 cases (1999–2007). *Vet. Comp. Oncol.* 13 (2): 89–97. doi: 10.1111/vco.12020.
48 London, C.A., Bernabe, L.F., Barnard, S. et al. (2014). Preclinical evaluation of the novel, orally bioavailable selective inhibitor of nuclear export (SINE) KPT-335 in spontaneous canine cancer: results of a phase i study. *PLoS One* 9 (2): doi: 10.1371/journal.pone.0087585.
49 Ellis, E. (2007). Surgical management of oral pathological lesions. In: *Contemporary Oral and Maxillofacial Surgery*, 5e (ed. J.R. Hupp, E. Ellis and M.R. Tucker), 449–470. St. Louis, MO: Mosby Elsevier.
50 Hedlund, C.S. and Fossum, T.W. (2007). Surgery of the digestive system: surgery of the oral cavity and oropharynx. In: *Small Animal Surgery*, 3e (ed. T.W. Fossum, C.S. Hedlund, A.L. Johnson, et al.), 361–366. St. Louis, MO: Mosby Elsevier.
51 Lommer, M. and Verstraete, F.J.M. (2012). Principles of oral oncologic surgery. In: *Oral and Maxillofacial Surgery in Dogs and Cats* (ed. F.J.M. Verstraete and M.J. Lommer), 423–430. Edinburgh, UK: Elsevier.
52 Salisbury, S.K. (2002). Principles of oncologic surgery. In: *Cancer in Dogs and Cats: Medical and Surgical Management*, 2e (ed. W.B. Morrison), 217–248. Jackson, WY: Teton NewMedia.
53 Lantz, G.C. (2012). Mandibulectomy techniques. In: *Oral and Maxillofacial Surgery in Dogs and Cats* (ed. F.J.M. Verstraete and M.J. Lommer), 467–480. Edinburgh, UK: Elsevier.
54 Marretta, S.M. (1998 September). Maxillofacial surgery. *Vet. Clin. North Am. Small Anim. Pract.* 28 (5): 1285–1296, viii. Review.
55 Gleizal, A., Bera, J.C., Lavandier, B., and Beziat, J.L. (2007). Piezoelectric osteotomy: a new technique for bone surgery – advantages in craniofacial surgery. *Child's Nerv. Syst.* 23 (5): 509–513. doi: 10.1007/s00381-006-0250-0.
56 Melugin, M.B., Oyen, O.J., and Indresano, A.T. (2001). The effect of rim mandibulectomy configuration and residual segment size on postoperative fracture risk: an *in vitro* study. *J. Oral Maxillofac. Surg.* 59 (4): 409–413. doi: 10.1053/joms.2001.21879.
57 Gingerich, W. and Stepaniuk, K.S. (2013). Bilateral rostral maxillectomy in the dog. *J. Vet. Dent.* 30 (2): 125–130.
58 Martin-Flores, M., Scrivani, P.V., Loew, E. et al. (2014). Maximal and submaximal mouth opening with mouth gags in cats: implications for maxillary artery blood flow. *Vet. J.* 200 (1): 60–64. doi: 10.1016/j.tvjl.2014.02.001. Epub 2014 Feb 12.
59 Harvey, C.E. (1986). Oral surgery: radical resection of maxillary and mandibular lesions. *Vet. Clin. North Am. Small Anim. Pract.* 16 (5): 983–993. doi: 10.1016/S0195-5616(86)50312-0.
60 Dernell, W.S., Schwartz, P.D., and Withrow, S.J. (1998). Mandibulectomy. In: *Current Techniques in Small Animal Surgery*, 4e (ed. M.J. Bojrab, G.W. Ellison and B. Slocum), 132–142. Baltimore, MD: Williams & Wilkins.
61 Matthiesen, D.T. and Manfra Marretta, S. (1990). Results and complications associated with partial

mandibulectomy and maxillectomy techniques. *Probl. Vet. Med.* 2 (1): 248–275.

62 Verstraete, F.J.M. (2005). Mandibulectomy and maxillectomy. *Vet. Clin. North Am. Small Anim. Pract.* 35 (4): 1009–1039, viii.

63 Smithson, C.W. and Taney, K. (2009). Symphyseal sparing rostral mandibulectomy. *J. Vet. Dent.* 26 (4): 264–269.

64 Walker, K.S., Reiter, A.M., and Lewis, J.R. (2009). Marginal mandibulectomy in the dog. *J. Vet. Dent.* 26 (3): 194–198.

65 Arzi, B. and Verstraete, F.J.M. (2010). Mandibular rim excision in seven dogs. *Vet. Surg.* 39 (2): 226–231. doi: 10.1111/j.1532-950X.2009.00630.x.

66 Kosovsky, J., Matthiesen, D., Marretta, S., and Patnaik, A. (1991). Results of partial mandibulectomy for the treatment of oral tumors in 142 dogs. *Vet. Surg.* 20 (6): 397–401. doi: 10.1111/j.1532-950X.1991.tb00346.x.

67 Birchard, S. and Carothers, M. (1990). Aggressive surgery in the management of oral neoplasia. *Vet. Clin. North Am. Small Anim. Pract.* 20 (4): 1117–1140. http://www.ncbi.nlm.nih.gov/pubmed/2196733.

68 Felizzola, C., Martins, M., A S, D.A.N., and DeSousa, S. (2003). Compound odontoma in three dogs. *J. Vet. Dent.* 20 (2): 79–83.

69 Lantz, G.C. (2012). Maxillectomy techniques. In: *Oral and Maxillofacial Surgery in Dogs and Cats* (ed. F.J.M. Verstraete and M.J. Lommer), 451–466. Edinburgh, UK: Elsevier.

70 Lascelles, B.D.X., Thomson, M.J., Dernell, W.S. et al. (2003). Combined dorsolateral and intraoral approach for the resection of tumors of the maxilla in the dog. *J. Am. Anim. Hosp. Assoc.* 39 (3): 294–305. doi: 10.5326/0390294.

71 Gallegos, J., Schmiedt, C.W., and McAnulty, J.F. (2007). Cosmetic rostral nasal reconstruction after nasal planum and premaxilla resection: technique and results in two dogs. *Vet. Surg.* 36 (7): 669–674. PubMed PMID: 17894593.

72 Bar-Am, Y. and Verstraete, F.J.M. (2010). Elastic training for the prevention of mandibular drift following mandibulectomy in dogs: 18 cases (2005–2008). *Vet. Surg.* 39 (5): 574–580. doi: 10.1111/j.1532-950X.2010.00703.x.

15

Basic Endodontic Therapy

Robert C. Boyd

Montgomery, TX, USA

15.1 Introduction

Endodontics is that branch of dentistry that deals with the diagnosis and treatment of diseases of the pulp and their sequelae in the apical, periapical, radicular, and periradicular tissues. When pulpal tissue is compromised and its vitality threatened or destroyed, some form of endodontic treatment is necessary to preserve teeth that might be otherwise exfoliated or extracted.

Therapy may also serve to resolve dental and peridental infections that can result not only in local but possibly systemic complications [1]. To be able to diagnose endodontic disease and develop a treatment plan a thorough understanding of dental and endodontic morphology, anatomy, pathology, microbiology, immunology, and physiology is required. Because there is such a wide array of endodontic armamentarium and techniques it is imperative for the veterinary dentist to have a detailed working knowledge of the armamentarium and experience with various techniques employed in endodontic treatment.

When the pulp is injured and vitality is compromised the potential for complications, especially painful conditions, infections, and abscesses, is substantial. An indifferent attitude of ignoring the problem, particularly if it does not seem to bother the patient, can only lead to further dental problems, pain, infection, and eventual tooth loss. The option of extracting the affected tooth is preferable to ignoring the problem, but the endodontically aware clinician can offer the client the option of retaining a tooth for both function and esthetics. Most animals can function well with the loss one or more teeth, but many owners are committed to optimum care and even have true esthetic concerns about their pets. For these owners, endodontics may be an unexpected, but appreciated, alternative. Animals trained for special duties (military, police, tracking, patrol, retrieving, human assistance, and protection) usually require a sound, functional, complete, or near-complete dentition. For these animals, avoidance of tooth loss can be crucial.

15.2 Endodontic Anatomy and Morphology

A thorough working knowledge of the morphology of the normal dental endodontic system is essential in order to assess abnormalities and to make a logical decision concerning endodontic procedures [2]. Details of the anatomy and physiology of the structures pertinent to endodontic therapy are covered in previous chapters. The most clinically relevant aspects are reviewed here.

The external shape or morphology of the tooth is divided into three areas. The crown is that portion of the tooth visible above the gingival margin and the root is that portion of the tooth apical to the crown, lying under the gingiva and enclosed in the bony socket. The third area is the neck or cervical area, the junctional point between the crown and the root. The external tooth shape gives the practitioner an approximate localization of the internal structure (see Chapter 1 – Oral Anatomy and Physiology). The interior tooth vault that the pulp occupies is known as the root canal system. The portion in the crown is referred to as the pulp chamber, with its most coronal aspect identified as the pulp horns and the potion located in the root referred to as the root canal. Humans typically have an apical foramen in which the pulp communicates with the periapical periodontal tissues via a single opening, while dogs and cats have multiple microscopic foramina known as an apical delta [3–5]. There are typically between 5 and 20 of these small delta openings that penetrate the root within several millimeters of the root apex [3]. While it is impossible to clean and fill all the minute openings of this delta, sealing the canal in the apical one-third generally produces an effective treatment [6]. The internal root canal

Wiggs's Veterinary Dentistry: Principles and Practice, Second Edition. Edited by Heidi B. Lobprise and Johnathon R. (Bert) Dodd.

apex or apical terminus is located 1–3 mm from the actual external root apex. The apex of the tooth is the tip of the root and it may be considered to be open or closed. Human teeth are considered to have an open apex due to a large foramen opening but mature dogs and cats are considered to have a closed apex because the multiple foraminal openings are microscopic openings that are not detected on radiographs. Immature, developing teeth of dogs and cats have a large open apex that closes as the tooth matures. As the tooth develops, dentin and cementum are produced at the apex of the root and the root closes. Although the tooth physically appears to have a solid root apex microscopic foramina provide a pathway to connect the pulp to the periodontal tissue. This is customarily called a *closed apex*. Standard veterinary endodontics typically deals with mature permanent teeth with adequate root apex closure. Immature teeth require alternative procedures to deal with their extremely wide canals (blunderbuss) and possibly open apices that may require additional development prior to endodontic therapy [6].

Lateral or accessory canals may provide passage between the pulp cavity and periodontal tissues in locations other than at the apex. While these are fairly common in human teeth they are less common in dog and cat teeth [7].

The pulp emerges from the tooth and connects with the periodontal ligament at the apical foramen or delta foramina. It is composed of soft connective, vascular, lymphatic, and nervous tissue. It contains odontoblasts, fibroblasts, fibrocytes, collagen fibers, elastic fibers, blood vessels, lymph tissue, and nerves [8]. Dentin, a pale yellow, ivory-like substance comprised of collagen fibers and hydroxyapatite crystals, surrounds the pulp. The pulpal odontoblasts produce dentin. The odontoblasts function to produce dentin throughout the vital life of the tooth, resulting in thicker dentinal walls and narrower pulp cavities as the teeth mature. This maturing process is sometimes referred to as canal calcification [8]. Dentinal tubules perforate the dentin at right angles to the pulp and contain fluid, nerve fibers and cytoplasmic extensions or processes from the odontoblasts, called Tome's fibers. In addition to normal aging, attrition, bruxism, pulpal irritation, and some injuries may cause increased dentin production [3, 9]. This increased dentin and calcified canals can result in narrowed canals or constrictions that can be a problem during cleaning and shaping with endodontic instruments [10, 11].

It must be emphasized that there are a formidable number of variations in dental anatomy, not only between species but within as well. Even within the same individual, great variations occur in the degree of calcification, dilaceration, and apical status. One of the most reliable guides for the veterinary dentist on most individuals is multiple radiographic views [2, 12].

15.3 Etiology of Pulpal and Periapical Pathology

The fact that the tooth is a vital structure makes it important to understand the changes that may occur in response to various stimuli. Inflammation, infective or sterile, of the pulp is termed pulpitis, and can be reversible or irreversible. Reversible pulpitis is generally a symptom of pulpal inflammation caused by some form of short-term irritation such as caries, dental treatment, or trauma [8, 13]. If the cause can be removed or treated the pulp can return to a normal state, but if not and the irritation progresses or is long term then it can lead to irreversible pulpitis [8, 13]. Treatment for reversible pulpitis is generally of a restorative nature. Irreversible pulpitis and chronic inflammation is a pronouncement of impending pulpal death, termed pulpal necrosis, requiring root canal therapy or extraction. Chronic pulpal irritation and trauma-related pulpitis can result in pulp necrosis, but in the absence of bacterial contamination this necrosis does not cause periapical periodontitis [14]. In contrast, there is a large body of evidence indicating bacterial infection as the cause of pulpal necrosis as well as periapical pathology [8, 14, 15]. Tooth fracture with pulp exposure, severe blunt trauma, advanced caries, tooth resorption (TR) and exposed root dentin that communicates with the pulp can result in irreversible pulpitis. Pupal injury causing pulpitis or even periapical periodontitis could possibly expose these tissues to the anachoretic effect. Anachoresis is thought to occur when bacteria are attracted to an area of inflammation and cause a local infectious process [16]. Bacteria may be carried to the periodontal periradicular tissues by the bloodstream during transient bacteremia or by way of regional gingival lymphatics that extend from the sulcus and periodontal lesions. Although some doubt the validity of this effect, it may explain the sudden onset of acute or chronic periapical involvement of teeth that appear to be apparently sound [16]. Only those conditions that allow bacterial access to pulp tissue result in irreversible pulpitis, necrosis, and periapical periodontitis.

A tooth can be damaged and the pulp injured by blunt or concussive trauma, resulting in inflammation or rupture of pulp vasculature with intrapulpal hemorrhage. Intrapupal hemorrhage may cause the collapse of venules, stopping blood flow and strangling the pulp (pulp strangulation theory) [14]. Because the pulp is in a low compliance environment, enclosed in dentin, pulp inflammation causing vascular permeability and vasodilation increases pulpal interstitial fluid pressure. This pressure increase may compress blood vessels and prevent beneficial blood circulation [9]. Although trauma-induced pulpitis can potentially lead to pulpal necrosis, pulp is a resilient connective tissue and the inflammatory response usually resolves without necrosis [8, 14]. Some dental traumatic injuries may first present as a pink or blue tinged tooth due to rupture and vascular bleeding inside the pulp cavity. Once the blood or its breakdown components penetrate to near the dentinoenamel junction (DEJ) it becomes visible. If the pulpitis is reversible, the color may eventually diminish and the appearance of the tooth return to normal. If irreversible destruction has occurred, the color changes to a purple or gray as the pulp dies and the blood cell components are degenerated. Initial pain and discomfort during the period when the pulp is acutely inflamed tends to dissipate as the innervation undergoes necrosis. The necrotic pulp breaks down into noxious tissue substances that may escape the apical foramina and cause inflammation of the periodontal ligament and periradicular tissues [14].

Tooth avulsion or luxation interrupts the apical pulpal blood supply with a resultant inflammatory pulp response. With complete severance of the pulpal periapical blood supply an irreversible pulpitis will result in pulpal necrosis. However, with luxation the apical vascular supply may only undergo partial interruption, causing reversible pulpitis and then pulpal repair. Pulp hemorrhage and tooth discoloration may result from tooth luxation or avulsion [14].

Dental treatment has the potential to cause pulpitis due to frictional heat and vibration from motorized instruments, ultrasonic shock waves from ultrasonic instruments, chemicals, and medicaments used to treat exposed pulp and dentinal desiccation from using forced air to dry the tissue [13, 17]. Prevention of pulpitis during dental treatment is directed at using water-cooled rotary instruments and limiting the use of water-cooled ultrasonic dental scalers for no more than 30 continuous seconds per tooth [18]. Teeth with exposed dentin should not be completely air dried but remain moist during preparation and treatment. Some chemicals and medicaments used to treat pulp tissue can cause pulpitis but they usually are associated with reversible pulpitis [17]. Iatrogenic electrical shock from pets chewing an electrical cord can result in pulpitis and may be reversible or irreversible.

Another condition occasionally seen with an exposed pulp chamber or canal is hyperplastic pulpitis [19] (Figure 15.1). This condition exhibits itself in one of two forms, hyperplastic granulation and hyperplastic swelling pulpitis. Granulation tissue is usually a reddish rough overgrowth that partially or completely occludes the exposure opening. This results from the pulp attempting to construct a barrier between it and the source of inflammation. In primates, it is seen most commonly in carious lesions of the young. With carnivores, it is more commonly associated with pulp exposures due to fractures.

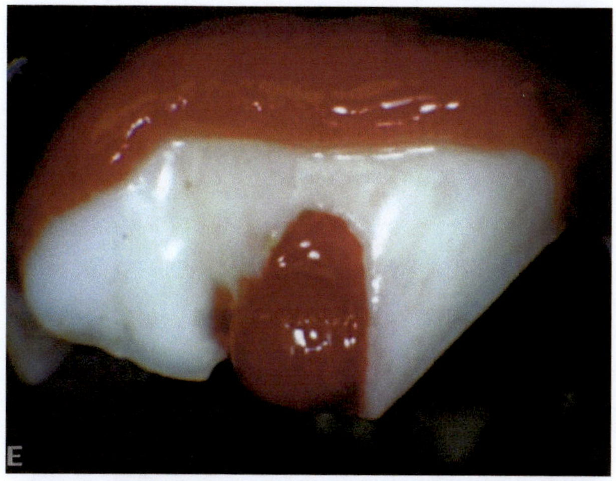

Figure 15.1 Pulp exposure caused by crown fracture of 108 has resulted in hyperplastic pulpitis.

This hyperplastic activity is an indication of the local immune system's effort to maintain pulp vitality. With simple pulpal swelling the tissue will appear either reddish to blue and have a smooth tight surface. Pulp tissue demonstrating this condition is usually in a terminal change of vital to non-vital and standard root canal treatment is indicated.

15.3.1 Periapical Pathology

In veterinary dentistry, periapical pathology is diagnosed from dental radiographs and appears as widening of the apical periodontal ligament space or periapical lucency and periradicular bone loss. Radiographic periapical lucencies do not all represent the same and their appearance can vary from tooth to tooth within a patient and among patients. Some will appear as diffuse and faint radiopacities in periapical tissue while others may be obvious circumscribed radiolucent halos surrounding the root apex (Figure 15.2). It should be noted that a definitive diagnosis of periapical pathology can only be made from histopathological evaluation of periapical lesions. Further determination of radicular or periapical cysts can only be made after complete sectioning and histopathological evaluation of all of the affected periradicular tissue [15]. Epithelial tissue reported on histopathology is not sufficient to diagnose apical cysts because it is found in apical granulomas as well as apical cysts, the difference being that cysts are sack-like structures with a complete epithelial lining whereas granulomas only contain a mixed cell population including epithelial tissue. Therefore, cyst diagnosis can only be made after complete evaluation of a periapical soft tissue lesion. Cysts have only been reported a few times in veterinary patients and are considered rare. Infected pulp tissue

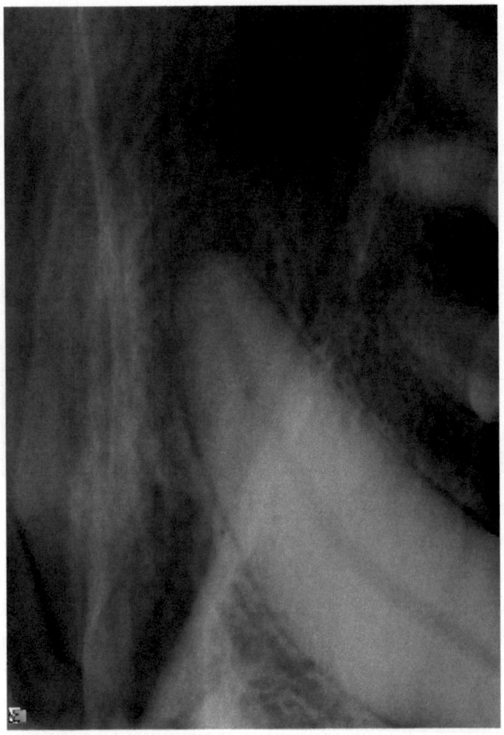

Figure 15.2 Radiograph showing a periapical lucency or "halo" lesion of a previously fractured tooth with pulp exposure.

is the primary cause of apical periodontitis. After the pulpal tissue becomes infected, bacterial toxins and metabolic byproducts escape from the root canal system through apical foramina to cause an immunoinflammatory response in the periradicular periodontal tissues. Over instrumentation, endodontic materials, medicaments, chemical irrigants, and trauma can cause periapical periodontitis. It is unlikely that sterile necrotic pulp can stimulate periapical periodontitis [14]. Periapical tissues have good collateral circulation, which allows for the building of a defensive barrier in an attempt to confine the pathogens and their toxins within the root canal system. Whether an acute or chronic process develops is dependent upon virulence of the organism, degree of organism challenge, and host immunoinflammatory response. Since bacterial infection in the pulp is the inciting factor, status of the pulp has to be considered together with periapical disease.

In human dentistry, several systems of categorization of apical periodontitis have been proposed that include clinical and histological findings in periapical pathology. These systems have included patient evaluation of pain perception and normal tissue parameters [14]. The World Health Organization (WHO) categorizes human apical periodontitis into five groups: acute apical periodontitis of pulpal origin, chronic apical periodontitis, periapical abscess with sinus, periapical abscess without sinus, and radicular cysts [14, 20]. The WHO categories will be used to define periapical pathology in this text as they are more suited to a discussion of veterinary periapical pathology [15].

Acute apical periodontitis of pulpal origin is the first line of defense initiated by the innate immune system in response to an extension of apical pulpitis into the apical periodontal tissues [3]. Acute apical periodontitis results in few periapical signs other than tenderness or pain on palpation or percussion, and this can be difficult to assess in the veterinary patient. Radiographs generally appear normal, although slight widening of the periapical periodontal ligament space may be seen. It may be associated with either vital or non-vital teeth. If left untreated, acute apical periodontitis may progress into one of the following: chronic apical periodontitis, periapical abscess, with or without sinus, or radicular cyst.

Chronic apical periodontitis is a long-term immunoinflammatory reaction involving the innate and adaptive immune systems in response to pulpitis [21]. With the advancing pulpal infection and inflammation, the inflammatory mediators stimulate osteoclast differentiation with resultant dissolution or resorption of periapical bone [14, 15]. This resulting disease produces the classical periapical lucency seen on radiographs [12, 15]. Although the immune systems are unable to eliminate the irritants they maintain an active defense response and there appears to be a balance between the pupal infection and the host immune response. Chronic apical periodontitis may establish itself as a chronic periapical granuloma. Granulomas have the same radiographic appearing lucencies as periapical cysts and they can only be differentiated histologically [14, 15]. Even though cysts and granulomas cannot be differentiated radiographically, they are caused by bacterial pulp infection and endodontic treatment is indicated.

Periapical abscess implies a painful collection of purulent exudate of sudden onset at the apex [14]. Technically, a periapical abscess cannot be diagnosed without histologic confirmation [14]. In man, signs are slight to severe swelling and pain, with some patients being febrile. The stoic nature of animals makes recognition of these signs difficult unless there is gross or obvious tissue swelling. Radiographically, as with acute apical periodontitis, no signs may be apparent, due to a lack of duration to cause dissolution or resorption of the periapical lamina dura. When radiographic changes are present, it may indicate the abscess is a flare-up of a previous asymptomatic chronic lesion, sometimes called a phoenix abscess. In some cases, development of a sinus tract allows for the escape of toxins and the suppression of symptoms, which is identified as a periapical abscess with sinus. These sinus tracts may be seen facially or suborbital, ventral-mandibular, or within the oral mucosa, either gingival or at the mucogingival line (Figures 15.3 and 15.4).

Radicular cysts may form as a result of stimulation of the epithelial cell rests of Malassez by inflammatory mediators [14, 15]. If the epithelial lined cyst communicates with the apical foramen or foramina it is a pocket cyst. If epithelium completely surrounds the cyst without communication with the pulp it is known as a true cyst. Radiographically cysts appear as periapical lucencies associated with the root apex. Periapical cysts have been rarely reported in veterinary literature [15, 22, 23]. While radicular cysts are recognized in humans, they are seldom diagnosed in dogs.

Condensing osteitis is a radiographic sign associated with chronic periapical periodontitis, causing reactive bone formation and increased radiodensity of periradicular alveolar bone. In this condition, pulpal inflammation may stimulate osteoblastic activity, causing reactive bone formation with resultant focal periapical radiodensity [12, 15]. It is the osseous response observed in teeth with previous endodontic treatment or low-grade pulpal infection with corresponding strong immune defense and local tissue resistance. Idiopathic or focal osteosclerosis is a similarly described radiodensity of the periapical alveolar bone seen on dental radiographs. Osteosclerosis is ascribed to teeth having no endodontic disease and it is most commonly seen as a benign condition in dogs with excessive chewing habits. This is relatively asymptomatic in most cases. Low-grade chronic pulpal inflammation of vital teeth, such as seen in occlusal stress (bruxing, excessive chewing, etc.) can induce this excessive periapical mineralization [15, 21]. Condensing osteitis and osteosclerosis are relatively asymptomatic and may be associated with some radiographic widening of the periapical periodontal ligament space [24].

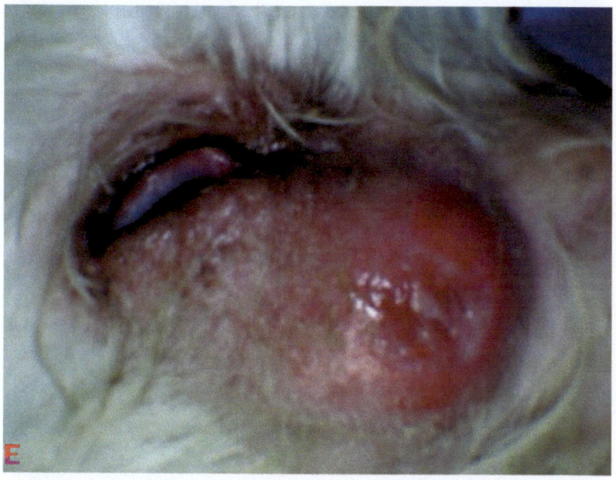

Figure 15.3 Facial swelling and draining sinus tract caused by an abscessed tooth 108.

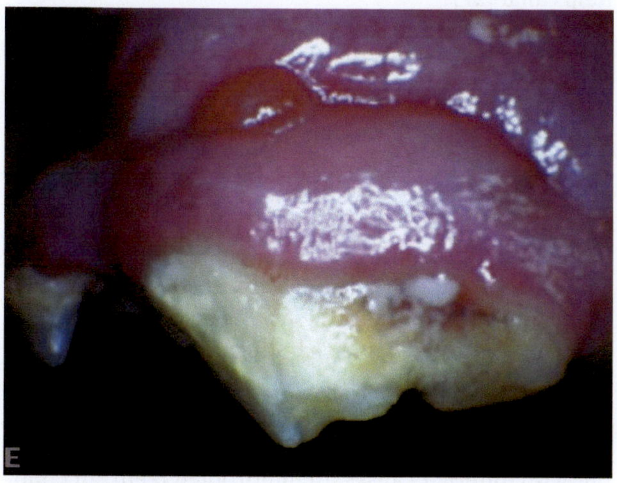

Figure 15.4 Gingival sinus tract from an abscessed tooth 208.

Radicular ankylosis and external root resorption can eventually occur in some chronically infected endodontic cases [24]. Radiographically this presents as the loss of the periodontal ligament space and root tissue, giving the appearance of tooth root merging with adjacent bone and resulting in the loss of a distinctive root image.

Periradicular osteomyelitis radiographically appears as an osteopenia and expansion effects of the alveolus seen in some cases of chronic pulpal inflammation [24]. This appears most commonly around the cuspids of the cat involved with tooth resorptive activity. It is not uncommon in these cases for a degree of osteosclerosis to be present.

The osseous radiographic conditions most commonly reported are condensing osteitis or chronic focal sclerosing osteomyelitis [24]. Condensing osteitis and periapical osteosclerosis are indistinguishable radiographic signs seen as increased bone density involving periapical and periradicular alveolar bone.

If endodontic disease remains undiagnosed and intraradicular infection persists, the periapical tissues can be in flux between the different types of apical periodontitis. Additionally, the patient may experience asymptomatic periods as well as intense pain dependent on the type and severity of apical periodontitis present. In order for the veterinarians to fulfill their advocacy role for animals, they must be able to perform and interpret dental radiographs and then couple those findings with presenting history and physical findings to properly assess endodontic dental disease. Inadequate training and facilities for dental diagnosis and treatment should not be an excuse because trained veterinary dentists are available to help with diagnosis and treatment.

If endodontic infection is certain and endodontic treatment is not an option then extraction is required.

15.3.2 Root Fractures

Fractures of the root structure are seen in domestic animals [3, 25]. Flexible, malleable, or padded objects are more common causes of root fractures, while sparing the crown of injury. The level at which the root is fractured principally determines the degree of mobility in the coronal segment and the need for immobilization. Fractures nearer the cervical area are generally more mobile and have an increased chance of bacterial contamination from the sulcus.

Clinically, root fractures are usually detected only if the coronal segment is displaced or serious mobility is observed. Radiographically, fractures are not always obvious or detectable. Horizontal fractures, in acute cases, are often obscured by trabecular bone patterns and have no marked radicular change, unless displacement has occurred. Fractures of this type can sometimes be delineated from bone patterns by close observation of whether the pattern extends beyond the bounds of the root structure image. Vertical fractures are seldom detectable on radiographs, except in advanced stages of separation.

Most root fractures, if reasonably stable and uncontaminated, heal unaided with the pulp remaining vital [3]. The alveolus acts as a natural splint, stabilizing and maintaining the segments in close proximity. New cementum or osseous material is laid down on the external root surface, while reparative dentin forms internally to heal the fracture. If mobility is a problem, a temporary acrylic or composite splint is advisable.

Periodontal disease and excessive mobility are problems that can lead to complications in treatment to salvage the tooth [3]. Displacement of the coronal segment may result in pulpal strangulation and necrosis. For this reason, displaced segments should be radiographed and suitably aligned as quickly as possible following the injury. If pulpal necrosis does occur, at times only the coronal segment is initially involved, allowing for pulpotomy and direct pulp capping in some cases. Should the entire pulp be involved, a standard root canal procedure will be required. Complications of advanced periodontal disease or that of fractures transgressing the sulcus can easily influence tooth vitality due to bacterial intrusion and/or mobility from loss of alveolar support. Loss of vitality can be addressed with root canal therapy, but mobility requires realignment and stabilization, which can be a challenge in many animals. Splinting with acrylics can provide a degree of stabilization, but the periodontal disease must also be addressed. When periodontal disease is progressive or extensive exodontia is most likely to be the treatment of choice.

15.4 The Endodontic/Periodontic Relationship

The stable function of a tooth is determined by its structural integrity, periodontal attachment, and support component. Endodontic and periodontic soft tissues are intimately related through accessory or lateral canals, furcation canals, apical foramen or delta, periodontal ligament, and exposed root dentinal tubules [26]. Therefore, it would seem logical that infection in either the endodontic system or the periodontal apparatus may cross-contaminate or infect the other system. This is generally true; however, there is lack of a large body of evidence and research to implicate periodontal infection as a frequent cause of endodontic infection [27]. Although it seems likely that periodontal disease can spread to the endodontic system through exposed dentinal tubules, lateral or accessory canals, and the apical foramen or delta, some research in animals indicates that it may not happen unless dentinal tubules are exposed [27]. Cementum protects the root dentin and prevents bacterial entrance from the periodontium to the dentinal tubules while a rich pupal blood supply protects the pulp from periodontal inflammatory mediators and bacterial toxins. When open dentinal tubules of the root surface are exposed to periodontal infection (bacteria) ensuing pulpitis may be either reversible or irreversible. With either reversible or irreversible pulpitis, sclerotic dentin can be produced on the adjacent pulp canal wall and effectively seal the dentinal tubules from further bacterial irritation. Chronic periodontal disease can also cause mineralization of the pulp canal, resulting in a narrowed pulp canal [27].

Because pulpal disease can be primarily endodontic in origin, or even possibly secondary to periodontal disease, classification of the lesions as to the primary and secondary elements can provide a speculative prognostic guide for treatment [26, 27]. The relationship can be classified as primary endodontic disease, primarily endodontic with secondary periodontal involvement, primary periodontal disease, primarily periodontal lesions with secondary endodontic involvement, true combined lesions, or concomitant lesions. True combined lesions are found in teeth that have both endodontic and periodontal disease in the same tooth. Another classification is concomitant endodontic and periodontal lesions where there are two separate lesions in the same tooth but with different causes. In multirooted teeth, an endodontic lesion may be found in one root and a separate periodontal lesion found in another root. True combined or concomitant lesions may be hard to differentiate once they coalesce.

In veterinary dentistry, classification of endodontic and periodontal lesions and their relationship to each other is largely dependent upon physical and radiographic findings. Physical findings are typically those related to external facial signs, oral cavity examination, dental evaluation, and periodontal probing [3]. Pulp testing, used in evaluating human teeth, is of little or limited value in veterinary dentistry because it requires cooperation and a positive or negative response from the patient [28].

Teeth showing primary endodontic disease usually have crown fractures with or without pulp exposure and typical radiographic periapical lucency or a "halo" at the root apex. They do not have any radiographic periodontal signs. Physical signs can include facial or mucosal swelling over the root, and sometimes a draining sinus or fistula can be found in the mucosa around the tooth or externally on the face or ventral to the jaws.

Teeth with primary endodontic and secondary periodontal disease have a radiographic periapical lucency or halo that continues into a wide periodontal ligament space that follows the root architecture to the gingival margin. These lesions are known as "J" lesions. A periodontal pocket may be found when probing these teeth.

Primary periodontal lesions have a "wedge"-shaped widened periodontal ligament space where the wide part of the wedge is coronal and the point of the wedge is apical. There can also be furcation bone loss noted on radiographs. Periodontal probing will reveal a periodontal pocket.

Primary periodontal lesions with secondary endodontic involvement have deep periodontal pockets and furcation bone loss from long-standing periodontal disease that exposes the endodontic tissues to infection through exposed dentinal tubules, accessory canals, or the apical delta. There may not be any clear radiographic signs that distinguish this condition from primary endodontic with secondary periodontal disease.

In the early stages of true combined or concomitant endodontic and periodontal lesions the radiographic and physical signs may be distinguishable as separate lesions in the same tooth; however, once the two lesions coalesce, they become indistinguishable from primary endodontic and secondary periodontal lesions. If endodontic and periodontal lesions occur in different roots of the same tooth they are readily distinguishable.

Because each classification carries a different prognosis it is important for the practitioner to be able to adequately evaluate the endodontic and periodontic disease relationship for proper treatment planning [26]. With regards to endodontics, when the crown still has good integrity and the roots have not been fractured, a tooth with a primary endodontic lesion has a very good to excellent prognosis while a tooth with primary endodontic lesion and secondary periodontal lesion has a good prognosis. Teeth with combined or concomitant lesions have a more questionable prognosis and treatment outcome depends upon the correct identification of pathology and tissue destruction. In veterinary dentistry these teeth have a fair to poor prognosis; however, a combination of endodontic and periodontic treatment can be successful. An alternate treatment for teeth with concomitant lesions would be endodontics and hemi-section or root resection to salvage part of a tooth and preserve some function [29] (Figures 15.5 and 15.6).

Generally, a tooth needs the periodontium to be in good health with its independent vasculature and nerve supply to maintain a healthy attachment. Therefore, extensive periodontal disease can give a tooth a poor prognosis, so the endodontic procedure may be unwise.

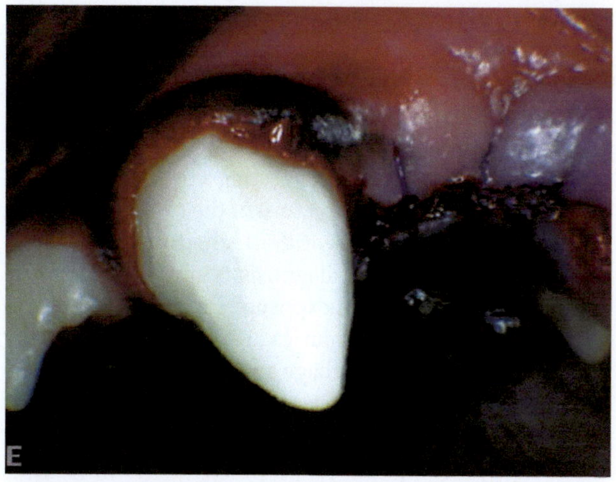

Figure 15.5 Photograph of the treated and restored mesial half of tooth 208 seen in Figure 15.4.

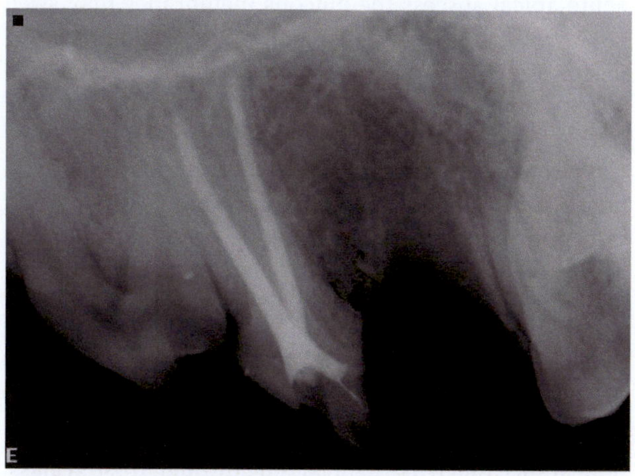

Figure 15.6 Radiograph of tooth 208 that has been hemi-sectioned. The distal root has been extracted and root canal therapy performed on the mesial roots.

15.5 Examination

The goal of the endodontic examination is to take subjective information and objective data to locate the origin of the problem and obtain an appropriate diagnosis for treatment planning. Subjective information indicating obscure pain, discomfort, lethargy, loss of appetite, and reluctance to play with toys are of limited help while information concerning pain at a specific area is beneficial.

Objective information from the owner can be helpful in arriving at an appropriate diagnosis [3]. These are typically traumatic injuries that cause immediate pain, discomfort, facial swelling, draining fistula, or oral bleeding that the owner readily recognizes. However, many endodontically compromised teeth are not presented with such obvious signs and require an objective examination for specific information. The objective oral examination entails visual examination, tactile exploration, palpation, percussion, thermal sensitivity testing, transillumination, and dental radiography.

The visual examination is the simplest, yet can be the most informative in many cases for the initial diagnosis. The most obvious finding suggesting a tooth is endodontically compromised is a fracture of the crown, including cracks and slab fractures still attached by the gingiva. If the canal is open the diagnosis is simple, but partial crown loss without canal exposure can also lead to irreversible pulpitis. When injuries are recent, the pulp may have conspicuous hemorrhage and be painful. With time the inflamed pulp becomes necrotic, the tooth generally becomes asymptomatic as far as pain is concerned, and the red or pink exposed pulp site turns brown, gray, or black. Tooth discoloration due to reversible or irreversible pulpitis may display a range of color shades progressing from pink to purple to gray or beige. In the later stages of acute apical abscess the mucous membranes may swell or discolor and facial swelling or even fistulation may be discovered.

Palpation, percussion, transillumination, and tactile assessment are diagnostic tests that are extensions of the visual examination. Digital palpation of the mucosa above teeth suspected of being compromised may elicit indications of discomfort or reveal a swelling. Palpation and percussion of the appropriate tooth may induce a suppurative flow from a fistulous tract or disclose tooth mobility or sensitivity. Transillumination, also known as diascopy, is the passage of a strong light through body tissues for the purpose of examination [30]. Crowns of vital teeth exposed to a light source have a translucent appearance much like light passing through frosted glass. Light penetrating through the tooth may also aid in the identification of coronal cracks or other defects. With time, non-vital teeth become more opaque due to hemoglobin breakdown in the pulp chamber and light does not readily pass through the crowns [31].

The tactile assessment can occasionally be performed on an alert animal, but a proper assessment is best performed under sedation or general anesthesia. This evaluation is performed using endodontic explorers to probe for an opening into the endodontic system or pulp cavity [32]. Fine line fractures can often be spread to identify and discriminate severity using gentle pressure with explorers, probes, or rubber-tipped instruments. Dyes, such as methylene blue, may be placed on teeth to aid in the delineation of fracture lines.

A pulpal response can be evoked by thermal and electric stimuli, but pain is the sensation that can be elicited from the patient. In man both tests are an objective diagnostic tool as the person verbally responds to the acute onset of sensitivity to stimulus. However, in veterinary dentistry it becomes more of a subjective test because the clinician must interpret the animal's response. Cold testing utilizes a small ice source that is applied to the crown to determine if the associated nerves are normal. In humans, a hyper-responsive reaction indicates acute pulpitis, no response indicates a non-vital pulp, while temporary pain relief indicates irreversible pulpitis. Heat testing is a more complex assessment, as all teeth respond to heat, but those with pulpitis have a more prolonged effect, and those with acute pulpitis respond severely and can be calmed quickly with cold [31]. Electrical and thermal pulp testing are too subjective or difficult to perform on alert animals to be of serious value.

15.5.1 Radiology

Radiology is the most important diagnostic, prognostic, and treatment evaluation tool used in veterinary endodontics [3, 21]. Digital radiography is employed by many veterinary dentists because it not only saves time but it greatly reduces the radiation exposure to the patient. Diagnostically, radiographs can confirm pulp canal exposure, pulp canal morphology, radicular and crown fractures, internal or external resorption, canal calcification or blockages (including endoliths), alveolar fractures, root abnormalities, dilacerations, periapical, and periodontal disease. Prognostically, radiographs determine the extent of the structural damage due to root fractures, as well as the degree of supportive structure loss due to periodontal and periapical periodontal disease.

With the exception of obvious visual or radiographic findings no one single method of diagnosis should totally be depended upon. Two or more of the diagnostic tools or methods should be used to aid in confirming the final diagnosis. The subjective and objective examinations provide information for the basis of the prognosis, as well as indicating treatment that can then be offered.

15.6 Endodontic Instruments and Materials

Endodontic instruments and materials are those used to treat the pulp of vital teeth or the pulp cavity of non-vital teeth. Understanding the endodontic armamentarium is essential to perform successful endodontic treatment. Variations found among species and individual teeth within species presents the dental operator with challenges that can be overcome with a broad knowledge of the endodontic armamentarium and its use. The appropriate use of individual instruments and materials as well as their limitations should be thoroughly understood by the veterinary endodontic practitioner.

15.6.1 History

Early instruments used for endodontics were developed by individual dental practitioners. Small flat blades, broaches, hickory pegs, and annealed piano wire were used [33]. Broaches, rasps, probes, and applicators are historically some of the oldest forms of endodontic instruments, dating back prior to the nineteenth century [34].

Ingle was primarily involved with recommending and working for standardization of endodontic instrumentation as early as 1955 [35, 36]. At the annual session of the American Association of Endodontists, in 1962, the association's research committee instituted meetings with manufacturers and suppliers of endodontic instruments and began dialogues for standardization. From these conferences, a working committee was formed under the endorsement of the North American Section of the International Association of Dental Research. The American Dental Association (ADA), the National Institute of Dental Research, and the National Bureau of Standards consolidated efforts with the North American Section group in 1964. Later, the American National Standards Institute (ANSI) and its committee Z-156 (Dentistry) were given the worldwide responsibility for standards development. The ANSI Committee Z-156 was later designated Committee MD-156 (Medical Devices). The Council on Dental Materials, Instrumentation, and Equipment of the ADA acts as secretariat for the United States [36].

Under the Federation Dentaire Internationale (FDI) and International Standards Organization's (ISO) joint guidance, the development of worldwide standards for endodontic instruments is governed by Technical Committee 106, Joint Working Group 1 (TC-106, JWG-1). It continues to advance the development of international standards for endodontic instruments in the areas of terminology, dimensions and measuring systems, physical properties, and quality control [37].

In 1976, the American National Standard (specification no. 28) was adopted. In this standard endodontic instrument terminology, shape, dimensions, and a color-code identification system is covered [38, 39].

15.6.2 Instruments

Originally endodontists used smooth broaches or probes to locate and negotiate root canals. Currently most operators use other instruments such as endodontic explorers, pathfinder files, or K-type files for this purpose [11, 40].

Most endodontic instruments and files were initially manufactured from carbon steel which provided an excellent edge on the file flutes for a superior cutting effect. Now most instruments are made from stainless steel or nickel titanium alloy (NiTi) that does not readily corrode. Both metals are a great deal more resistant to fracture and separation, although stainless steel will tend to straighten out when used in curved canals even though it can be pre-curved or pre-bent to try to conform to natural canal curvature [41]. Ledging, gouging, zipping, stripping, and translation are all caused by straight–stiff files working in curved canals and trying to regain their straight shape. Their tendency to straighten out in curved canals causes instrument binding coronal and apical to the outer curvature and at the inner curvature in mid canal. Instrumentation techniques such as balanced force and anticurvature filing can help reduce some of the problems encountered in using stainless steel hand files [41, 42].

NiTi is a superelastic metal that, when stressed, does not show the usual proportional strain found in stainless steel and its memory property allows it to return to its original shape after instrumenting curved canals [31]. The memory property of NiTi allows it to traverse curved root canals with little to no transportation or ledging [41–43]. Various manufacturing techniques have been employed when making stainless steel and NiTi instruments to prevent some of the problems encountered during instrumentation. Non-cutting tips, radial lands, and negative rake angles are some of the techniques used to help keep endodontic instruments centered in the canal.

15.6.2.1 Barbed Broach

The barbed broach primarily used to remove soft pulp tissue from the pulp canal can also be used to remove medicaments, treatment materials, and debris. It is slowly inserted into the canal until light contact is made with the pulp or material to be removed. It is then rotated 180° to entangle the tissue in its extended barbs and is then drawn back to extract the entangled pulp. Barbed broaches are produced by making small angular incisions into the metal shaft of a smooth broach. These incisions are forced open to form barbs that result in areas of weakness in the instrument. If the broach is forced into the canal the barbs can be compressed and when attempting to remove the instrument the barbs can spread, digging into the dentinal wall and locking it in place. Any twisting action at this point and the delicate instrument will usually fracture at one of the incision points. Forcing, twisting, and bending the broach may lead to instrument fracture and separation within the canal. A keen tactile sense is required when using the barbed broach, always keeping in mind the weakness of the instrument. When selecting the proper sized broach to use within the canal, the size selected should be slightly smaller than the canal so that little or no contact is made between the barbed tips and the dentinal walls of the canal. This determination of size is extrapolated from critical examination of the scout or diagnostic radiographs of the dentition. In small or finely curved canals, a file or rotary endodontic instrument will effectively remove pulp material in most cases, without the inherent danger of using a barbed broach [10, 44]. In a young animal with a very large canal, a pair of broaches twisted together and used simultaneously may be necessary to remove the pulpal tissue cleanly. Most files and endodontic instruments used to clean and shape the pulp canal will remove pulp tissue during instrumentation.

15.6.2.2 Kerr Files and Reamers

Kerr files (K-type or k-file) are endodontic instruments that are manufactured from stainless steel wires, cut into straight rods and machined into three- or four-sided tapered pyramidal blanks. In cross-section, the three-sided blank is an equilateral triangle and the four-sided blank is either a square or rhomboid. The tapered terminal end of the blank is then twisted to produce the series of spirals that are the operating head of the instrument. The number of twists introduced to the instrument determines whether the blank becomes a file or reamer. Blanks with one-tenth to less than one-quarter spirals per millimeter of length produce an instrument with 0.28–0.80 cutting flutes per millimeter of operating head, and are designated reamers. Blanks with one-quarter to over one-half spiral per millimeter of length produce instruments with 0.88–1.97 cutting flutes per millimeter of operating head, and are designated files. Reamers have a smaller helical angle of the edge of the flute as compared to files. This results in the reamers having a little better cutting efficiency but a poorer carrying ability than a file. Most operators believe they have a better tactile sense inside the canal with files as compared with reamers, because of the greater number of spirals producing more dentinal wall contact surfaces with the instrument. Reamers are used in a clockwise turning fashion. Files are used with a push–pull filing action or a quarter turn and pull mode [31].

Of clinical importance is the shape of the shaft. One-third rotation of a triangular instrument completes a cutting circle of the root canal. With a square shaft, only a quarter turn is necessary to complete a cutting circle, while a rhomboid shaft requires a half turn. Triangular blanks are more flexible than the square, but are not as strong. K-files are more flexible than K-reamers, but again are not as strong. K-reamers and files are stiffer and stronger than most comparable instrument types, size for size [31]. Many manufacturers alter steel, the number of twists, or the shape of the instrument blank in an effort to deliver an endodontic instrument that is more flexible while providing good cutting qualities. Many change their files and reamers from a square to a triangular blank in the larger sizes to improve flexibility. With the change in shape, a subsequent loss of strength occurs. The operator that is not aware of this is likely to experience an increase in instrument breakage at the point of the substitution [45].

During endodontic treatment instruments may break or become separated due to instrument failure or incorrect use. When instruments separate in the canal, the separated fragment may block the canal and be difficult, if not impossible, to remove. Magnification is essential when trying to locate and extract a separated instrument. There are many methods and extractor instruments used for removing separated instruments [46]. Some separated instruments can be removed with sterile saline (SS) irrigation, files, and barbed broaches loaded with small amounts of cotton and are used to entangle separated pieces, forceps, ultrasonic vibration, burs, and extractors. Extractors are instruments designed for retrieving separated fragments and are manufactured with many designs from tubes to snares. Some even utilize the use of adhesives to attach instrument pieces to an extractor. No method is totally reliable and when extraction efforts fail two options remain: bypass the separated piece and treat around it or perform surgical endodontic treatment. Prognosis varies with the location of the separated instrument and stage of treatment when the separation occurred [46].

15.6.2.3 Hedstrom Files

Hedstrom files (H-type or H-file) are machine cut from a round metal blank or wire that is shaped to produce a spiral groove on a tapered, pointed instrument. The spiral groove is machined to manufacture a continuous spiral flute that has a large diameter cutting blade with a positive rake angle. While this design feature produces an aggressive cutting instrument, it also results in a delicate instrument because the manufacturing process creates a large diameter blade with a small diameter core having multiple stress points where the blades have been cut from the core. Any bends in the long axis create greater stress points than bends in a K-file. This type of file can be deceptive in its strength because endodontic instruments are only as strong as their central core. The large helical angle (90° or less) contributes to its effectiveness when used in a push–pull filing action, but it will tend to thread into dentin if used in a turn and pull technique. If the operator threads and locks the H-file into the dentin, efforts to remove it may create a twist in the metal, making it more prone to fracture. Its flutes provide a good carrying effect for the removal of debris from the canal [31].

15.6.2.4 Standard File Sizes

Since endodontic instrument standards were established K-files and H-files are manufactured in standard lengths, diameters, and tapers. Standard human dental file lengths are 21, 25, and 31 mm. ISO series files or instruments of various types are color coded to match so that a 21 mm 0.02 taper ISO size 15 K-file matches an ISO 15 size H-file and both are color coded white. A 25 mm length ISO size 15 K-file having a taper of 0.02 means that the instrument is 0.15 mm diameter 1 mm from the tip and tapers 0.02 mm in diameter for each 1 mm in length up to 16 mm from the tip. File locations are designated by the letter "D" with D0 being the location at the tip and D16 being 16 mm from the tip where the cutting flutes stop. Therefore, an ISO 15 file is 0.15 mm in diameter at the tip and 0.47 mm in diameter where the cutting flutes end. The percentage change in file diameter is not the same when different ISO file sizes are examined. For example, when an ISO 10 file is compared to an ISO 15 file there is a 50% increase in diameter, but when an ISO 15 file is compared to an ISO 20 file there is only a 33.3% increase. To normalize the percentage increase in file size to a constant percentage increase the Series 29 file was manufactured with a 29% increase in diameter between each successive file size. As file diameters increase the Series 29 files actually have a greater percentage increase in diameter than the ISO series. Other manufacturers have changed the taper from 0.02 to 0.04, 0.06, and 0.08. These larger tapers are mostly found in motorized files. Standard human endodontic files are usually not long enough to reach the canal apex in a canine tooth.

Veterinary endodontic files are available in extended shaft lengths up to 60 mm for K-files and up to 120 mm for H-files (Shipp's lab). Additional length is necessary when treating long canine or cuspid teeth of various species because of their long root structure. Longer veterinary length files can have an operative head up to 30 mm from the tip. With the continued widening of the diameter to support this longer operative head the 60 mm instrument has a shaft almost twice the diameter of the shorter instruments. Therefore, these longer H-files are not interchangeable during a procedure. The extended length of the operative head has a superior effect in the long-wide dog canine tooth pulp canal of some young individuals. In older animals with narrow canals, this additional instrument width can sometimes be a problem. The extended operative head of the 60 mm H-file improves carrying capacity, provides a tapered preparation, and has had fewer reports of instrument separation or fracture. These variations from the standard are helpful for certain veterinary endodontic cases.

15.6.2.5 Engine-Operated Rotary Instruments

Newer generation engine-operated instruments are manufactured from NiTi alloys to make use of their strength and superelastic properties. Like hand files, most engine-driven instruments are tapered with the largest diameter at the handle and the smallest diameter at the tip so that pulp canals are prepared with a taper or cone shape to facilitate various obturation techniques. They are machined from an NiTi wire blank so that flutes and cutting edges can have positive rake angles that cut dentin or negative rake angles that scrape dentin to clean and shape pulp canal walls. Most have blunt or non-cutting tips and radial lands to keep them centered in the canal and prevent stripping, gouging, ledging, and transportation. Most engine-driven NiTi instruments are manufactured for human patients and are not long enough to be used in large canine teeth.

The most commonly used engine-operated NiTi instrument in veterinary dentistry is the LSX (Sybron Endodontics), designed with a small shaft and a neutral angle spade blade located at the tip of the instrument. It is manufactured in 50 mm veterinary length instruments. Unlike most NiTi endodontic instruments that have cutting blades along the shaft of the instrument, the cutting portion or spade blade located at the tip of the shaft cuts less than 0.5 mm of canal wall dentin as it rotates in the canal. As the operator pushes the rotating LSX down the root canal, the instrument engages and cuts dentin along its path. Because of its design characteristics, the operator knows exactly when and where the canal wall is being prepared through tactile and aural feedback. Other engine-driven instruments, having conical cutting blades along the tapered shaft, may be cutting dentin anywhere along the canal from the crown to the apex without the operator's knowledge.

15.6.3 K-File and H-File Instrument Use

Within the canal a smooth clean surface is produced with rotational or reaming motion when using K-type files.

In comparison, the H-type files produce a clean preparation when used in a rasping or translational motion, but they do not result in as smooth a preparation. H-type files are effective when cleaning oval or ribbon canals. Rotary motion used with K-type files produces a fairly rounded-conical apical preparation, where push–pull rasping actions are less likely to produce the rounded-conical preparation [31]. For this reason, K-type files are usually best used for the cylindrical apical retention preparation and the H-type files for the coronal flare [31, 41]. When using files in a push–pull action it is normally best to gently pre-bend them for use in noticeably curved canals. Acute bends or angles should be avoided as these stress and fatigue the metal and predispose instruments to premature failure.

15.6.4 Condensers and Spreaders

Condensers, also known as pluggers, are flat-ended metal instruments with smooth, round, and very-slightly tapered sides. They are used to compact or press filling materials vertically or apically into the root canal. Spreaders are round, smooth, tapered metal instruments with a point. They are used for laterally compacting filling material by spreading or pushing it against the walls of the canal. Hand-held spreaders and condensers of the endodontic group have handles that rest in the entire hand. Finger spreaders and condensers are short instruments having handles similar to files and they are held in the fingers. Hand-held veterinary length condensers and spreaders are available.

Heated pluggers are attached to electronic heating units and are used to soften gutta-percha for warm lateral and vertical compaction. Temperature can be controlled and some instruments heat from the tip to the shank for a continuous wave technique.

15.6.5 Spiral or Paste Filler

Lentulo spiral paste fillers are engine-driven instruments operated with slow-speed handpieces. They are made of an operative latch-type head and reverse spiral shaft that will move sealer and paste apically in root canals when operated in a clockwise rotation. If they are operated in reverse or counterclockwise they will thread or screw into the canal wall and break. They are delicate instruments that require a knowledgeable operator for safe use.

15.6.6 Engine-Driven Drills and Burs

Gates Glidden burs (G-type reamer) and Peeso reamers are latch-type engine-driven drills or burs that are primarily used for the enlargement of the coronal access and the straight part or coronal third of the canal. On occasion, the G-type reamer is used to aid in the removal of gutta-percha from the coronal part of the canal for restorative procedures. The delicate shaft size of these instruments lends itself to swift fracture and failure should the tip become bound when mechanically engaged. Those made from stainless steel should not be operated in curved canals.

15.6.7 Absorbent Paper Points

Absorbent points are cones of porous paper. These are used to dry the canal after instrumentation. Paper points may also be used to apply medicaments and sealer cements in the canal by dipping them in the medicine or sealer and then placing it within the canal. Spinning the point between the fingers will help disperse paste-type medicines and sealers on the canal walls. In some cases, the medicated points may be sealed within the canal temporarily. Soaking paper points in sterile saline and placing them on hemorrhaging pulp will control bleeding during partial pulpectomy. If needed, they can also be used in the same manner to control hemorrhaging at the apex during root canal treatment.

15.6.8 Gutta-Percha Cones and Points

Gutta-percha is a natural, rigid latex produced from the sap of Palaquim trees (*Palaquim gutta*). Gutta-percha, the *trans*-isomer of polyisoprene, is bio-compatible, inert and malleable [47]. Gutta-percha exists in two crystalline forms known as the beta and alpha forms. Gutta-percha cones, also known as points, are manufactured as crystalline beta form because they are more rigid than the alpha form. When heated, the beta form changes to the alpha phase and then an amorphous phase that is plastic and can be molded. The alpha phase is sticky, pliable, and flowable with application of pressure. The alpha phase remains as the alpha phase if cooled very, very slowly; however, with normal cooling and compaction it changes to the beta form. Compacting the softened amorphous alpha form of gutta-percha material will cause it to flow and fill canal irregularities. Compacting the alpha gutta-percha while it cools collapses internal voids and prevents shrinkage [47].

Gutta-percha was reported as being used as a root canal filling material as early as 1847 by Hill [48] and in 1887 gutta-percha points were manufactured for root canal obturation by the S.S. White Company.

Gutta-percha cones or points made for endodontic obturation are composed of about 18–22% gutta-percha and 59–76% zinc oxide, with the remainder being a combination of radiodense materials and plasticizers [47, 48]. These cones are regulated by ADA Specifications and are available in two basic types of cones, standard, and conventional (non-standard). Standard points correspond to the sizes of standard endodontic instruments, can be ISO color coded, and are used as primary or master points. Conventional points are manufactured to have a similar taper to endodontic spreaders and are used as accessory points in lateral compaction.

15.6.9 Irrigants and Irrigation Materials

Irrigants are liquid agents used to aid the instrumentation process in debridement and disinfection of the root canal. Irrigant solutions lubricate the root canal, dissolve organic pulp and necrotic debris, soften dentin, destroy bacteria, flush debris from the canal and remove the smear layer. The smear layer is formed during instrumentation and is caused by mechanical instruments or files cutting infected dentin and literally wiping fine inorganic particles, organic debris, and bacteria on the canal wall and forcing it into open dentinal tubules. The pulp cavity is an intricate and complicated system, which cannot be cleaned in all areas by instruments; therefore chemical solutions have been used to aid in debridement of the canal for many years [49]. It is further theorized that it is a chemomechanical action that allows these solutions to be effective. This is the chemical cleansing and disinfecting effect combined with instrumentation and the actual mechanical fluid flushing action that loosens and removes materials from the canal.

Irrigants should ideally possess the following properties: dissolve inorganic material, dissolve organic tissue, biocompatible, antibacterial, non-toxic, penetrate dentinal tubules, and easy to use. Commonly used irrigants that fit the aforementioned criteria are bleach or sodium hypochlorite (NaOCl), ethylenediaminetetraacetic acid (EDTA), chlorhexidine, hydrogen peroxide, sterile saline, and alcohol. Other solutions have been developed that combine acids, detergents, and antibiotics to broaden their effectiveness in disinfection and debris removal. However, NaOCl continues to be the most widely used irrigant because it satisfies most of the criteria for an ideal irrigant [43, 49–51]. NaOCl can be used at half (3%) or full strength (6%); however, full strength has been shown to provide better tissue hydrolyzation and antimicrobial properties while disrupting biofilms [52].

17% EDTA, a chelating agent, is used to decalcify dentin and to remove the inorganic tissue of the smear layer. The decalcifying effect of EDTA on dentin is self-limiting and when it is used as an irrigant during instrumentation it acts as a lubricant. Irrigation with EDTA for one minute followed by irrigation with 6% NaOCl for one minute is recommended as a final irrigation cycle for smear layer removal; 6% NaOCl has the added benefit of disrupting biofilms [52].

Chlorhexidine is a very safe and effective antimicrobial and has substantive properties when used at 2%. Chlorhexidine is not effective in removing the biofilm or dissolving necrotic organic tissue. Hydrogen peroxide is an effective antibacterial irrigant and removes debris by effervescing and fluid movement, but it has no effect on necrotic organic tissue and can be toxic to supporting tissues. Alcohol is an effective antimicrobial agent and it is safe, but it will not dissolve organic tissue or remove the smear layer. Sterile saline, when used as an irrigant, can safely and effectively reduce bacteria, but it is not an antimicrobial agent and it does not remove the smear layer, biofilm, or dissolve organic tissue [50].

15.6.10 Irrigation Equipment/Methods

For endodontic irrigation to be effective and accomplish the goals of cleaning and disinfecting canals, sufficient volumes of fresh irrigation solution needs to be supplied, replenished, and evacuated from the canal. To accomplish cleaning and disinfection, two basic methods of irrigation used during instrumentation are positive pressure irrigation and negative pressure irrigation.

With the positive pressure method, irrigants loaded into syringes are released in pulp canals, under pressure through endodontic needles 1–2 mm from the apical constriction in human teeth. In animal teeth, with a closed apex, irrigants are released to the canal apex (apical terminus). Endodontic needles are manufactured with either closed tips and side ports or open tips with side relief to allow irrigant fluids to escape around the needle and out the coronal access site if the needle becomes wedged in the apical constriction or terminus. Their use does not guarantee absolute safety; therefore cautious application is always recommended when using positive pressure irrigation. These built-in safety features are designed to help prevent the serious complications associated with accidently forcing toxic irrigant fluids into the periapical tissues. This is particularly important when using full or half-strength NaOCl as an irrigant, because apical extrusion of this solution can cause severe tissue damage and pain [50, 53, 54]. If irrigant is forced beyond the apex, the irrigation needle should be immediately replaced into the canal with an empty syringe attached and the canal aspirated to remove any remaining irrigant. After removing the remaining irrigant, the canal should be thoroughly irrigated with sterile saline. Irrigation needles are sometimes used to aid in drying the canal following irrigation. They should be used to aspirate fluids and never to blow them from the canal.

Negative pressure irrigation uses a system of tubes, syringes, and needles connected to dental vacuum systems to draw irrigation solutions from the access opening to the apical portion of the canal before evacuation through

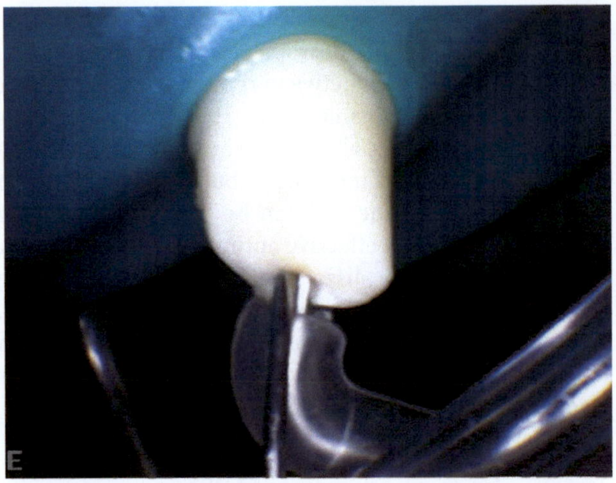

Figure 15.7 Canine tooth isolated with a rubber dam. Note that the rubber dam is secured with a composite place around the circumference of the tooth.

an endodontic needle. Negative pressure reverses the flow of irrigation solutions by drawing them from the coronal access, down along canal walls by apical negative pressure to an endodontic needle placed on the apical canal terminus. With negative pressure irrigation, there is no risk of fluids under pressure being forced through the apical delta openings. Negative pressure irrigant-dispensing syringes are also equipped with suction that covers the dispensing needle to prevent accidental spills from overfilling the coronal access with irrigant solutions (Figure 15.7).

Endodontic needles are manufactured in standard 31 mm lengths and their use in veterinary endodontics is limited to short canals because irrigant solutions need to reach the canal apex. Longer endodontic needles are required to carry irrigants to the canal apical terminus of medium to large dog canine teeth. Veterinary length needles have been manufactured and are available from some veterinary suppliers. Tom cat or long intravenous catheters can be adapted for irrigation in longer pulp canals.

15.6.11 Sonics and Ultrasonics

When used with irrigation solutions they greatly enhance canal cleaning, but have demonstrated a poor canal shaping efficiency [42]. Enhanced cleaning is due to the resonant vibration effect known as *acoustic streaming* and heat produced at the tip of the instrument [42, 49, 55]. As the tip vibrates it produces heat that can be transferred to NaOCl irrigation solution to enhance its activity [42]. Vapor lock or apical air bubbles formed through hydrolysis of organic tissues by NaOCl create an environment that could prevent acoustical streaming [56]. Previously considered cavitation effects are probably not produced due to the low power of dental ultrasonic equipment and the small confined space in the apical canal [31].

15.6.12 Measuring Pulp Canal Length

Accurate measurement of the root canal for instrumentation has always been a problem in human endodontics because two-dimensional radiographs may not accurately identify the location of the foramen. Human teeth have a large foramen that can be located several mm from the root apex. The ability to accurately locate and measure the length of the root canal provides the dental operator with a working length (WL) measurement. Knowing the WL is essential so the operator can keep root canal instruments working within the confines and limits of the canal. Electronic devices, known as apex locators, accurately measure WL in human patients and when used with radiographs they provide the most complete assessment of the pulp canal and WL. Apex locators are not utilized in veterinary dentistry because animal patients lack an apical foramen with associated soft tissue that is necessary for electronic measuring devices [57].

Veterinary dentists rely on measurements taken from endodontic instruments that have endodontic stops moved on the instrument shaft to the access opening after the instrument tip is placed to the canal apex. Radiographs are used to verify the instrument tip is contacting the canal apex and that the WL has been reached [6]. The instrument is withdrawn from the canal without moving the stop and the distance is measured from the instrument tip to the stop and recorded in millimeters.

15.7 Endodontic (Root Canal) Treatment

The objectives of endodontic therapy are to treat infection, alleviate discomfort, and preserve dental structure and function. Successful root canal treatment is accomplished by removing the affected canal contents, disinfecting the canal/s, providing an adequate canal obliteration, and sealing the endodontic complex.

15.7.1 Rubber Dams

Rubber dams are mandatory and are the standard of care for human endodontic treatment in the United States [58]. Rubber dams are used to isolate teeth, control infection, protect the patient from aspirating fluids or endodontic instruments, protect dental operators, and enhance the field of vision [59]. Because endodontic infections are caused by bacteria, isolation with a dental dam keeps infected material within the confines of the tooth. After instrumentation and disinfection are accomplished, the dam serves to protect sterile obturation materials from oral contamination. Even though dental dams are not the standard of care for veterinary endodontic procedures, they should be used to protect veterinary patients and veterinary dental operators.

15.7.2 Access

Access deals with the fundamental choice of the site of coronal entry and approach to the pulp chamber and pulp cavity. Straight line access provides a straight line to the first root canal curvature or to the apex in straight canals [40, 60]. Its purpose in endodontic therapy is to establish an unrestricted passageway from the crown and through the pulpal cavity to the apical terminus. When accessing intact teeth, the dental operator must know dental morphology and be able to visualize pulp canal access from radiographic and physical anatomical landmarks. Access sites have been identified and published for a dog's teeth [60]. Some intact, single-rooted teeth can be accessed through the crown tip if the access will accommodate the instruments chosen for root canal treatment. This approach is especially useful in mature teeth having a small mature pulp canal. Access can be made with a small round bur or the crown tip can be removed to expose the pulp chamber. Once the pulp chamber is exposed access preparation can begin. Removing the crown tip or performing access at the crown tip also facilitates cleaning the coronal pulp canal. Complicated crown fractures in single-rooted teeth present the veterinary dental operator with additional choices. Instead of creating a standard mesial-buccal access site on canine teeth that may further weaken the tooth structure, access can begin at the fracture site [10]. This access technique satisfies "straight line" principles that recommend establishing a straight line to the first curvature or the apex. These principles were established for the purpose of having unrestricted instrument access to the apical portion of the canal for complete cleaning, shaping, and disinfection. When using this technique for complicated crown fractures of cat canine teeth straight line access can be made from the exposed pulp chamber to the apex because the roots of these teeth are usually straight. Coronal access at fracture sites in single-rooted teeth of dogs can accommodate rigid files, but it is especially suited for long flexible NiTi instruments [10] (Figure 15.8).

Because there is variation among species and individuals within species, the dental operator has to use known access points and pre-operative survey radiographs of the dentition to adequately evaluate each tooth before access openings are made [60]. Pre-operative radiographs will aid in identifying pulp canals and provide a rough estimate of the canal diameter [10]. Dental radiographs, although only two dimensional, are essential to properly assess the anatomical relationship between the crown and root, angle of the root within the arch, and the general condition and position of the pulp cavity [40]. It is imperative that the dental operator have a thorough appreciation and understanding of the morphology of the whole tooth and its supporting structures in order to analyze radiographic details and correctly implement access [60]. Use of two-dimensional radiographs in a three-dimensional tooth can occasionally be misleading; therefore, several views should be taken to reduce the chance of deceptive information. With abnormalities of the crown or root configuration or rotation of teeth, radiographs commonly must be angled from mesial or distal aspects to provide the anatomical information required [40, 60]. Failure to establish proper access to the pulp chamber and root canals is one of the most common complicating factors in root canal therapy for veterinary practitioners [60]. The pulp chamber is generally situated in the central portion of the crown, with the root canals prone to be near the center of the root. However, each pulp cavity is individualistic in its confines, and is dynamic in that it changes during life. The pulp cavity in vital teeth diminishes in size with age, due to secondary dentinal development. Additionally, irritation to the pulp from caries and restorative procedures can lead to dimensional changes at the point of the disturbance due to sclerotic or reparative dentin deposition internally.

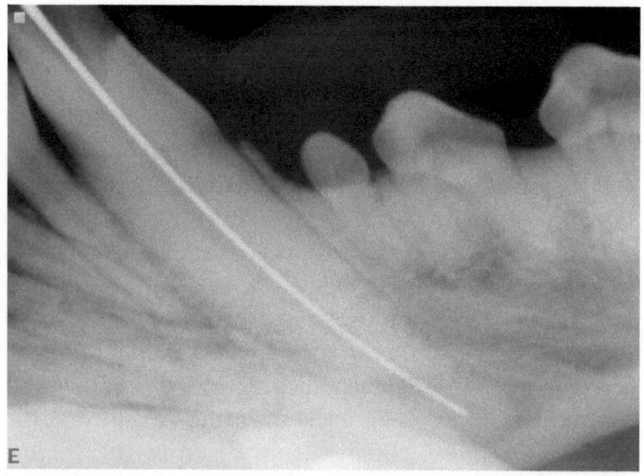

Figure 15.8 LSX in a long curved pulp canal. Note the coronal fracture access site provides straight line access for the LSX rotary instrument.

Even though each tooth must be evaluated as a distinctive individual, certain generalities may be drawn as to the characteristic position of approach to the access of dog teeth. One rule of thumb is to avoid making access openings directly over or through incisal edges, cusp tips, and other developmental ridges or margins, as these may predispose to vertical fractures. Typically, the entrance to the incisors is made on the central lingual facet of the crown 1–2 mm above the free gingival margin. However, a labial approach similarly positioned can be used, but due to esthetic considerations this is not commonly used. The cuspid or canine teeth can be accessed 1–3 mm from the free gingival margin on the mesial crown, which provides for a more direct line of access to the apex. Individual canals of premolars with two roots may have the access openings made on the buccal or facial surface over the center of each root near the cusp margin. Confirmation can be attained by palpation of the alveolar juga and dental radiographs. The mandibular first molars access is basically the same, except that the approach is most commonly made from the lingual aspect. These two rooted molars have access achieved on the occlusal surface directly over the roots to be entered, while avoiding cusp tips. The maxillary fourth premolar provides a slight challenge in the access to the mesial roots, especially the palatal. Whereas the distal root access is fundamentally the same as other premolars, a transcoronal approach is the easiest for the mesial roots [61] (Figure 15.9a and b). Access to these roots is determined through a mental extrapolation after palpation of the mesiobuccal root juga and a visual comparison of the actual location of the mesiopalatal root cusp tip. The actual opening is generally made between these two determined points and approximately 2–4 mm above the gingival margin on the buccal aspect of the tooth [61]. The maxillary molars are three-rooted and may be accessed with a Y- or V-shaped opening on the occlusal surface that exposes each individual canal system [62]. The first access point is usually made directly over the lingual or palatal root, with extension of the access using a high-speed bur and following the chamber to expose the two buccal root canals. Straight-line access of the buccal roots must be done cautiously as periodically perforation of the floor of the chamber occurs due to root angulation.

15.7.2.1 Access Preparation

Access preparation with straight-line access is one way to achieve an unrestricted access to the apex [60]. During access preparation, coronal enamel and dentin that impede or prevent rigid or semi-rigid endodontic instruments and materials from reaching the pulp canal are removed. One of the cornerstones of dentistry has always been the conservation of tooth structure; nevertheless, this should not overly influence access preparation. Rotary diamond and fissure burs, files, motorized rotary drills, and orifice shaping instruments are used to enlarge and pre-flare the coronal access and coronal portion of the pulp canal. Pre-flaring produces a tapering funnel design from the coronal access to the coronal portion of the pulp canal to facilitate instrumentation of the middle and apical pulp canal. Each step in the sequence from coronal access to pulp chamber and canal, when properly accomplished, facilitates the pathway to the apical canal or terminus. The goal of access design is to gain full unimpeded access to WL for instrumentation, disinfection, and obturation.

A tooth or restorative structure that is in the line of access should be removed prior to initiating endodontic treatment. Additionally, all compromised tooth structures and faulty restorative material should be removed prior to accessing the pulp chamber or pulp canals. This pre-emptive action assists in maintaining asepsis while improving visibility and providing a more complete evaluation of restorative requirements needed after canal therapy [59]. Failure to remove diseased tooth or restorative material prior to opening the access can lead

(a) (b)

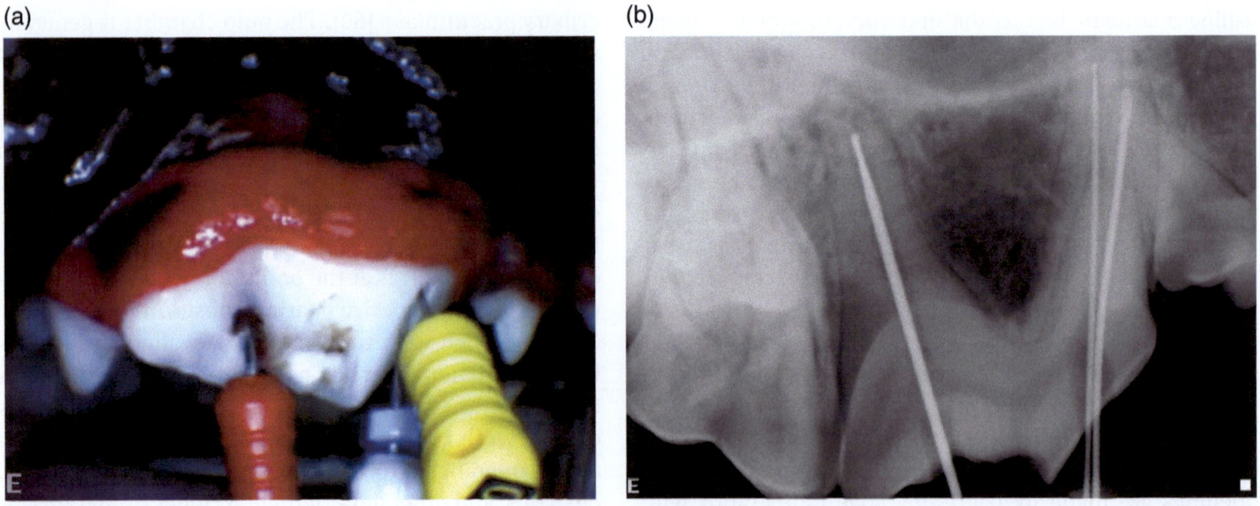

Figure 15.9 (a) 108 transcoronal access with K-files; (b) radiograph of tooth 108 transcoronal access with final apical size LSX rotary files.

to debris or contaminates falling or being carried into the canal. If restorations are incompletely removed, materials can unintentionally be transported into the root canal. Attempting the use of standard instrumentation to remove the material typically leads to the material being pushed further into the canal or being packed into the apical terminus, which if not removed may prevent achieving a proper apical seal.

Regardless of the type of root canal instrumentation and obturation chosen, access and access preparation remains the same. Many technical complications confronted in endodontic treatment can be diminished or prevented with appropriate access preparation. It can be an invitation to unnecessary complications when these basic concepts are not understood and employed.

15.7.3 Standard Root Canal Treatment Using Hand Instruments

In the standardized root canal technique, ISO size K-files are used in sequence from small to large to clean and shape the canal to WL. This technique produces a cleaned canal that matches the shape of the master file, which is the final file used to shape the canal [63]. A matching ISO size gutta-percha cone is then used to obturate the canal. Once access is attained, the pulp chamber is irrigated using an endodontic needle and syringe filled with 3–6% NaOCl or SS to remove debris. An endodontic explorer, pathfinder, or file can be used to determine the exact canal orifice location and the general shape or size of the canal. If pulp tissue is present an appropriate sized barbed broach is inserted until slight resistance is felt; it is then rotated 180° to entangle the pulp tissue before being gently pulled from the canal with the pulp tissue. When the pulp material separates and fails to be removed intact, the procedure may be repeated. Using barbed broaches to remove pulp tissue is optional because pulp tissue can be removed during instrumentation with files and rotary instruments. After removing pulp tissue, irrigation is again performed. Occasionally identifiable pulp tissue will be absent due to necrolysis. A small lubricated file with an endodontic stop is positioned in the canal and moved apically with watch winding motion to contact the apical terminus. At this juncture, the stop is slid down the instrument to make contact with the incisal or occlusal tooth margin. A radiograph is taken to confirm the instrument is reaching the canal apex or apical terminus, and after removing the file, the WL is measured from the endodontic stop to the instrument tip using an endodontic ruler [6]. The WL is recorded in mm and endodontic stops are affixed at the WL on each successively larger instrument used in the cleaning and shaping process. Files are coated with a lubricating or chelating agent and used in a watch winding motion or quarter-turn and pull motion to instrument the canal until the final file or master apical file (MAF) is determined. Determination of the MAF is based on file binding in the apical terminus and then enlarging the apical preparation to 2–3 file sizes larger than the first file to bind at the apical terminus. Irrigation is performed between every other file size change using 3–6% NaOCl. Recapitulation *or* re-instrumentation is performed between increasing file sizes using the previous smaller file to insure patency is maintained to the WL [41, 42]. After using the MAF, a final irrigation is performed using NaOCl and 17% EDTA. The canal is dried with paper points and a gutta-percha cone matching the size of the MAF is selected for obturation. The guta-percha cone is sterilized and trial fitted in the dry, treated canal while checking for slight resistance to removal or tug back [42]. This cone is the master cone and fit is confirmed with dental radiography. A spreader or finger spreader is selected to fit within 1–2 mm of WL; then a sealer is applied to the canal and the master cone is placed in the canal. Lateral compaction is applied to the master cone as the spreader is moved apically in the canal alongside the cone to 2 mm short of WL. The spreader is removed and additional or accessory cones matching the size of the spreader are placed until the apical two-thirds of the canal is completely obturated. Excess gutta-percha is removed with a heated instrument and the remaining gutta-percha is compacted with a plugger. The access site is cleaned and prepared for restoration.

15.7.4 Step-Back Technique

Like the standard instrumentation technique, the step-back procedure utilizes serially larger hand files to work from the apical terminus to the coronal portion of the canal [41, 42]. Pulp tissue removal can be accomplished using barbed broaches or files and irrigation performed routinely with NaOCl between file size changes. The MAF is determined when clean dentinal material is collecting on the tip of the largest file to instrument the apical terminus and it is shaped to the desired size. The next sequentially larger files are used to step back in 0.5–1.0 mm increments short of WL or short of the previous file, and this creates a 0.05 or 0.10 taper. Irrigation and recapitulation should be performed between each larger change in file size [42]. The MAF is used during recapitulation. The step-back procedure produces a tapered canal to the coronal portion of the canal where Gates-Glidden burs or motorized instruments can be used to flare or taper the coronal portion of the canal. After coronal shaping is performed recapitulation and irrigation are repeated to clear debris from the apical preparation. Some operators modify the step-back procedure and perform the coronal flaring prior to apical preparation.

After final irrigation, the canal is dried and a sterile master cone is selected to match the MAF and trial fit. Obturation followed by restoration is then completed in a manner similar to the standard technique.

15.7.5 Step-Down and Crown-Down Techniques

Step-down and crown-down instrumentation procedures are similar in that the coronal taper or pre-flaring is accomplished before cleaning and shaping the apical portion of the canal [41, 42]. However, in the step-down technique WL is determined prior to instrumentation or pre-flaring and in the crown-down technique WL is determined after coronal flaring. Gates-Glidden burs, orifice shapers, and NiTi files are typically used in motorized handpieces to save time while pre-flaring the coronal canal. Copious irrigation should be performed during coronal flaring to prevent canal blockage. If WL is determined prior to pre-flaring, a small file can be used to confirm canal patency and prevent canal blockage during pre-flaring. After pre-flaring the coronal portion of the canal, WL is determined using a small file or instrument. Endodontic stops are placed to WL on the instruments chosen to clean and shape the apical and middle portion of the canal. Starting with the smallest file or instrument it is worked to WL followed by successively larger instruments until the apical portion of the canal is properly cleaned and shaped. Pre-flaring accommodates endodontic instruments, irrigation instruments, and materials as well as obturation instruments and materials. Irrigation is performed during instrumentation to remove debris and final irrigation and restoration are completed similar to the other techniques.

Variations of the crown-down technique include a combination or double flare technique where instruments are used in a step-back technique after the apical crown-down preparation is completed [42]. Ascending size files are used to step-back and flare the apical and mid-portion of the canal. This technique is used to accommodate thorough irrigation and complete obturation, and is employed by veterinary dentists using rotary NiTi instruments and obturation with matching gutta-percha plugs as well as heated gutta-percha obturation [64].

15.7.6 Balanced Force Technique

Because of differing properties and uses, most endodontic instruments are suited to specific instrumentation techniques. Stainless steel K-files, Flex-R files, and GT hand files can be used for the balanced force technique where the files are used in a rotational clockwise and counterclockwise movement. Instruments are passively placed in the canal and rotated 90° clockwise to engage canal wall dentin and then rotated counterclockwise as axial force is applied to the instrument. The counterclockwise rotation breaks the engaged dentin and it can be removed for cleaning or the procedure can be repeated with the instrument remaining in the canal. When using the balanced force technique with K-files they will remain centered with fewer canal complications [42].

15.7.7 Engine-Driven Instrument Technique

The crown-down technique is recommended when using most NiTi rotary endodontic instruments. Because LSX instruments have been manufactured for use in veterinary patients they are the most commonly used engine-driven NiTi instrument. The technique requires coronal pre-flaring and copious irrigation followed by WL determination using either small hand files or small LSX instruments. Small endodontic files up to ISO 15 are used to WL to establish a glide path for the small LSX instruments before they are used in a motorized handpiece. Frequent irrigation is recommended between instrument size changes using 3–6% NaOCl while EDTA is used to soften and lubricate dentin during instrumentation [64]. LSX instrumentation requires the pulp canal to be flooded with EDTA solution before the instruments are rotating and working in the canal. LSX instruments are used in ascending order from the smallest instrument cutting dentin to the final apical size (FAS) instrument that completes the apical preparation. The FAS is determined when the last cutting instrument requires a firm push to complete the final 5–10 mm of apical preparation in short canals and 10–15 mm in long canals. Step-back preparation is completed with at least four successively larger instruments than the FAS. The first four step-back files are used at 4 mm short of WL followed by step-backs 6, 8, and 10 mm short of WL. Additional instruments are used for the midcanal as needed [64]. Recapitulation using the FAS should be performed after the step-back flaring is accomplished. Final disinfection with 3–6% NaOCl irrigation is done after the canal preparation is complete and 17% EDTA is used for one minute of irrigation to remove the smear layer. A final rinse with NaOCl and SS completes irrigation. The canal is dried with paper points and obturation is performed using sealer and a GP Plug®. A GP Plug matching the FAS ISO size instrument is placed in 6% NaOCl for one minute for disinfection and then rinsed in SS and dried. Sealer is placed in the dried canal using a lentulo spiral filler, paper point, or syringe and needle. Next the GP Plug is seated in the apical canal and a dental radiograph is taken to verify complete apical fill. The canal is then filled with sealer and a GP cone matching the ISO size GP Plug is selected, sterilized in 6% NaOCl, and dried before placing it in the canal. This cone should contact the GP Plug and displace the sealer as it is seated in the canal.

The excess cone is removed 4–5 mm deep in the canal and then compacted vertically using an endodontic plugger. The access is cleaned, prepared, and filled with a restorative material of the operator's choosing.

15.7.8 Canal Disinfection and Preparation for Obturation

Disinfecting the canal is accomplished during canal preparation through instrumentation and irrigation. Endodontic instruments or files cut and remove a portion of the dentinal walls and aid in transporting some of the debris and bacteria from the canal. Irrigation solutions such as alcohol, 2% hydrogen peroxide, 3–6% NaOCl, and 2% chlorhexidine can be used for root canal disinfection; however, 3–6% NaOCl and 2% chlorhexidine are more commonly used for final disinfection [50].

When hand or motorized instruments are working in the canal and cutting or instrumenting canal walls a matrix known as the smear layer is created. Some of this matrix, composed of inorganic and organic debris, is forced into dentinal tubules and may even occlude them. 17% EDTA is used in the final irrigation cycle to remove the smear layer and open the occluded dentinal tubules prior to a final irrigation of 3–6% NaOCl or 2% chlorhexidine. While both agents perform well as broad-spectrum antimicrobials, they have other different yet desirable properties: 3–6% NaOCl has the ability to disrupt biofilms and 2% chlorhexidine has substantive properties that provide a long-lasting effect. Therefore, either NaOCl or chlorhexidine are usually used as a final disinfecting irrigant.

15.7.9 Obturation

Obturation is the three-dimensional filling of all the root canal complexities with a biocompatible material to seal the root canal from the apex to the coronal access. This seal should prevent the entry of microbes and fluids from entering the root canal system. All the efforts of canal preparation and disinfection are useless without providing a complete seal during obturation [41, 65]. Although once considered the ultimate predictor of successful endodontics, obturation is no more important than diagnosis, morphology, access, cleaning, shaping, disinfection, and restoration [2].

15.7.9.1 Obturation Techniques

There are numerous ways to obturate the canal. Among these are lateral compaction, vertical compaction, SimpliFill™, thermomechanical obturation, thermoplastic obturation, chemoplastic obturation, and the paste method. No one method is reliable and recommended for all cases; instead the clinician should be versatile and proficient in several. No matter how the core material is placed, the primary objective is to completely obturate the canal, especially the apical one-third [6, 66].

15.7.9.1.1 Lateral Compaction

After canal instrumentation using standard ISO size files, a standard gutta-percha cone matching the MAF is selected and sterilized in NaOCl before trial fitting in the canal [67]. The master cone is inserted in the canal and checked for tug-back [48]. Tug-back is the slight back pull or resistance to dislodgement felt by the operator when removing the cone from the canal. This tug-back, if coming from the apical third would be an indication of a good fit; however, irregularities in the upper portions of the system may give a false tug-back sign. For this reason, it is still best to confirm proper fit radiographically. A spreader is also pre-fit in the canal to reach 1–2 mm short of WL. Sealer is then applied to the canal and the master cone is seated in the canal and the spreader is placed alongside the cone to laterally compact it in the canal. The spreader actually applies lateral and vertical forces to the cone. Note: care must be exercised to not split the root when performing lateral compaction. The spreader is rotated to remove it without pulling the gutta-percha cone from the canal. An accessory gutta-percha cone matching the spreader is selected and placed in the void caused by the spreader. The process is repeated and additional cones are placed until the apical two thirds of the canal are obturated.

Some large canals cannot be instrumented to provide a proper fit for a standard size prefabricated cone and a fabricated or customized single master gutta-percha cone is made. Three or more sterile gutta-percha points are heated and twisted together then rolled between two glass slabs held at a slight angle. Trial fit of the cone while still warm with a light apical pressure can increase the conformation of the fit. If additional cone adaptation is required, the tip can be heat softened or dipped in eucalyptol or chloroform for three to five seconds, and the cone replaced lightly pumping it down into the canal. The procedure is repeated until WL and adaptation is suitable. This procedure can also be used to adapt a standard master gutta-percha cone. When the cone properly fits the canal, it can be marked at its coronal access at a specific location of the tooth. This will allow the cone to be properly placed both directionally and in depth after the sealer cement is placed. Radiographic confirmation of the fit is recommended before seating the cone with sealer and performing lateral compaction as describes above.

Standard gutta-percha cones, accessory or custom gutta-percha cones are sterilized in 6% NaOCl, for one minute, rinsed in SS and dried before use. Custom cone fabrication is normally used in very large, immature canals.

Using lateral compaction does not produce a solid mass of gutta-percha, however, is does not shrink and sealer fills the spaces between cones.

15.7.9.1.2 *Warm Vertical Compaction*

Vertical compaction is used most commonly with various heated gutta-percha techniques, although it can be used on cold gutta-percha [6, 48]. A master gutta-percha cone with sealer is placed in the canal and an automated electronic heating instrument is used to remove excess material. The heated instrument is then used to heat the gutta-percha core and a plugger is used to vertically compact the material. If the instrument is not red hot, or it is allowed to remain in contact with the gutta-percha more than a brief second, the material will cling to the instrument and possibly be removed or dislodged as it is withdrawn. A non-heated plugger is used to vertically compact the gutta-percha while it is still warm. The plugger can be dipped in zinc oxide powder to reduce its adhesion to the heated mass. Additional segments of gutta-percha can be added, heated, and compacted until the canal is filled.

A variation of this technique, known as continuous wave compaction, utilizes a variable electric heat source with attached pluggers to heat and compact gutta-percha cones [48]. After premeasuring an appropriate size plugger to fit 5–7 mm short of WL, a master cone is seated with sealer in the prepared canal and excess material is removed with the heated plugger. Next, the plugger is placed vertically on the remaining cone material and the plugger is heated as it is moved 2–3 mm from the premeasured binding point. The plugger is allowed to cool as vertical force is maintained. After cooling, heat is again applied to the plugger tip and it is removed leaving the compacted, single gutta-percha cone to fill the apical canal. The remainder of the canal can be filled with sealer and heated gutta-percha.

15.7.9.1.3 *SimpliFill™*

SimpliFill™ is another type of vertical fill that is recommended to use with LSX instruments and the crown-down technique is an associated product. It is a 5 mm tapered ISO gutta-percha cone mounted by threads on a disposable carrier (GP plug) and used with a sealer to fill the apical preparation [66]. The plug can be trial-fitted prior to applying a sealer by placing it in a coronal to apical direction in the canal until slight resistance is felt. During a trial fit the plug should fit within 2–3 mm of WL. Using a lentulo spiral filler mounted in a slow-speed handpiece, the sealer is applied to the apical portion of the canal. Excess sealer is removed with a paper point that is placed to WL and then digitally rotated. The apical plug is sterilized in 6% NaOCl for one minute, rinsed, and dried and then digitally placed to WL with vertical pressure. Radiographic evaluation is used to verify a proper fit and seal with the apical plug. The middle and coronal portion of the canal is then filled with the sealer and a sterile gutta-percha cone matching the plug is seated in the canal until it contacts the plug. The excess cone is removed with heat and the cone is compacted vertically using a plugger. This GP plug and sealer provide a consistent and efficient apical seal when used in conjunction with LSX instruments [68, 69].

15.7.9.1.4 *Flowable Obturation Materials*

Guttaflow® is a polydimethylsiloxane containing small particles of gutta-percha that is supplied in mixing syringes or ampules requiring mixing in a titurator before placement [48, 70]. Sealers are not used with this product and canals are filled by injection or Lentulo spirals. Guttaflow can be used in any size of canal that will accommodate mixing syringe tips or Lentulo spiral fillers. After filling the canal, some operators place a single master gutta-percha cone to the WL and they may even add accessory cones when obturating large, wide, and long pulp canals.

15.7.9.1.5 *Thermoplastic Method*

With the thermoplastic method, gutta-percha is heated to soften it for improved fill in tapered root canal preparations. Sealer is placed prior to the heated gutta-percha using a small file, carrier, or paper point. Gutta-percha can be softened inside the pulp canal with electronically heated pluggers and lateral or vertical compaction can be employed to fill the apical canal and any irregularities or accessory canals. Other methods utilize electronic heating units to heat gutta-percha outside the canal before transport and placement in the canal. Depending upon the system used, the heated gutta-percha is placed in the canal with needles, cannulas, carriers, or obturators. Most of these methods, due to cooling, will have shrinkage or a volume loss similar to that of gutta-percha heated for lateral compaction. Heating will have caused slight expansion of gutta-percha, which will shrink as it cools [71]. Compacting heat-softened gutta-percha as it cools will compensate for shrinkage [47]. If carriers or obturators are used they are cut off at the level of the pulp chamber.

15.7.9.1.6 *Thermomechanical Compaction*

A compactor instrument mounted on a conventional slow speed hand-piece with a contra-angle running at 10 000–12 000 rpm is placed into a prepared canal that has had sealer and a master cone placed near WL [72]. When the compactor is inserted beside the master cone frictional heat from the dentinal walls is generated that melts the gutta-percha. The blades of the instrument force the softened gutta-percha apically and laterally.

Additional points can be fed into the canal as the instrument is being gradually withdrawn, until the canal is filled. These compactors are not typically used in veterinary endodontics.

15.7.9.1.7 Chemoplastic Method

Chemical solvents are utilized to soften gutta-percha or dissolve it prior to placement in the canal. The chemoplastic method is no longer in use due to shrinkage and lack of chemical solvent biocompatibility.

15.7.9.2 Obturation Complication Terms

Four terms are commonly used with problems of the fill or obturation of the root canal. These are underextension, overextension, underfilling, and overfilling. The differences are subtle, but distinct. Underextension and overextension refer solely to the vertical fill dimension, while underfilling and overfilling refer to obturation in any dimension [73, 74]. Gutta-percha points can be overextended into the periodontal ligament, while the canal still has voids around it having an underfill. Therefore, the obturation was overextended, but underfilled. A canal that is fully obturated and has material extruded beyond the apex into the periodontal ligament is overextended, but more appropriately termed overfilled. A canal that has the apex obturated correctly, but has voids is termed underfilled. One that is well obturated except at the apex is termed underextended. A canal with voids around a master cone that also has a void at the apex is both underextended and underfilled.

15.7.10 Coronal Restoration

Sealing and filling the pulp cavity openings at the fracture site and instrument access are essential to completing endodontic root canal treatment. Leaking restorative materials has often been overlooked as one of the common causes of root canal failure [2, 48, 69]. Cavity preparation is dictated by the type of fill or restorative material used to seal the access opening and the cavity or fracture site. Removal of excess gutta-percha and sealer cement and acid-etching the enamel and preparing the dentin is followed by the placement and finishing of an appropriate restorative. Because some sealer cements containing eugenol can inhibit the setting or curing of restorative composites, an intermediate restorative is used to sandwich a layer of non-eugenol restorative between the two materials. Glass ionomers are the more commonly used intermediate restoratives to separate eugenol sealers and composites.

15.7.11 Antibiotic Therapy

Antibiotic treatment in dental patients is controversial and antibiotics should be used judiciously and at the discretion of the practitioner. The American Heart Association guidelines indicate that antibiotics should be used in high-risk human patients receiving dental treatment or dental surgery. High-risk patients are those having a history of endocarditis, valve disease, prosthetic heart valves, or a lack of immunocompetancy [21, 75]. Dental surgery, periodontal treatment, endodontic treatment, tooth brushing, flossing, and dental manipulation during examination may cause transient bacteremias [16, 75, 76]. Transient bacteremias last from 10 to 60 minutes and according to research transient bacteremia lasting from 10 to 30 minutes can occur after dental extraction, periodontal treatment, and periapical manipulation [16]. Although transient bacteremia can be caused by endodontic treatment of teeth with associated periapical periodontitis, a healthy patient's immune defense system should be adequate to prevent disease.

Certain conditions or diseases other than periapical infection or abscess may also dictate antibiotic use in a particular patient. Antibiotics may also be indicated in patients with orthopedic implants. Consult with the orthopedic surgeon for their input and recommendations [21, 76].

References

1 DeBowes, L.J., Mosier, D., Logan, E. et al. (1996). Association of periodontal disease and histologic lesions in multiple organs from 45 dogs. *J. Vet. Dent.* 13 (2): 57–60.

2 Gutmann, J.L., Dumsha, T.C., and Lovdahl, P.E. (2006). Problem solving in the assessment of treatment outcomes. In: *Problem Solving in Endodontics*, 4e, 1–30. St. Louis, MO: Mosby.

3 Harvey, C.E. and Emily, P.P. (1993). Endodontics. In: *Small Animal Dentistry*, 156–212. St. Louis, MO: Mosby.

4 Hennet, P. and Harvey, C.E. (1996). Apical root canal anatomy of canine teeth in cats. *Am. J. Vet. Res.* 57: 1545–1547.

5 Orsini, P. and Hennet, P. (1992). Anatomy of the mouth and teeth of the cat. *Vet. Clin. N. Am. Small Anim. Pract.* 22 (6): 1265–1277.

6 Holmstron, S.E., Frost-Fitch, P., and Eisner, E.R. (2004). Endodontics. In: *Veterinary Dental Techniques for the Small Animal Practitioner*, 3e, 339–414. Pennsylvania, PA: Saunders.

7 Gioso, M.A., Knobl, T., Venturini, M.A.F.A. et al. (1997). Non-apical root canal ramifications in the teeth of dogs. *J. Vet. Dent.* 14 (3): 89–90.
8 (2008). Tencate's oral histology. In: *Development, Structure and Function*, 7e, 227–237. St. Louis, MO: Mosby.
9 Hargraves, K.M. and Cohen, S. (2011). Structure and function of the dentin-pulp complex. In: *Cohen's Pathways of the Pulp*, 10e, 452–503. St. Louis, MO: Mosby.
10 Boyd, R.C., Ross, D.L. (2010). LightSpeed and SimpliFil tips and tricks. Proceedings of the 24th Annual Veterinary Dental Forum.
11 Gutmann, J.L., Dumsha, T.C., and Lovdahl, P.E. (2006). Problem solving in locating and negotiating fine and calcified canals. In: *Problem Solving in Endodontics*, 4e, 115–142. St. Louis, MO: Mosby.
12 DuPont, G.A. and DeBowes, L.J. (2009). Endodontic disease. In: *Atlas of Dental Radiography in Dogs and Cats*. St. Louis, MO: Saunders.
13 Hargraves, K.M. and Cohen, S. (2011). Pulpal reactions to caries and dental procedures. In: *Cohen's Pathways of the Pulp*, 10e, 504–528. St. Louis, MO: Mosby.
14 Abbott, P.V. (2004). Classification, diagnosis and clinical manifestations of apical periodontitis. *Endod. Topics* 8: 36–54.
15 Menzies, R.A., Reiter, A.M., and Lewis, J.R. (2014). Assessment of apical periodontitis in dogs and humans: a review. *J. Vet. Dent.* 31 (1): 8–21.
16 Dezan, E., Holland, R., Consolaro, A. et al. (2012). Experimentally induced anachoresis in the periapical region after root canal filling. *Int. J. Odontostomatol.* 5-10: 5–10.
17 Schwartz, R.S., Summitt, J.B., and Robbins, J.W. (1996). Caries management and pulpal considerations. In: *Fundamentals of Operative Dentistry: A Contemporary Approach*, 51–66. Hanover Park, IL: Quintessence Publishing Co. Inc.
18 Verez-Fraguela, J., Valles, M.A.V., and Calvo, L.J.E. (2000). Effects of dental scaling on pulp vitality in dogs: an experimental study. *J. Vet. Dent.* 17 (2): 75–79.
19 Holmstrom, S. (1992). Feline dentistry. *Vet. Clin. N. Am. Small Anim. Pract.* 1433–1451.
20 World Health Organization. (2010). Diseases of the digestive system. In: *International Statistical Classification of Diseases and Related Health Problems*, 10th Revision; ICD-10.
21 Hargraves, K.M. and Cohen, S. (2011). Pathology of the periapex. In: *Cohen's Pathways of the Pulp*, 10e, 529–558. St. Louis, MO: Mosby.
22 French, S.L. and Anthony, J.M.G. (1996). Surgical removal of a radicular odontogenic cyst in a four-year-old Dalmatian dog. *J. Vet. Dent.* 13 (4): 149–151.
23 Beckman, B.W. (2003). Radicular cyst of the premaxilla in a dog. *J. Vet. Dent.* 20 (4): 213–217.
24 DuPont, G.A. and DeBowes, L.J. (2009). Miscellaneous conditions. In: *Atlas of Dental Radiography in Dogs and Cats*, 221–228. St. Louis, MO: Saunders.
25 DuPont, G.A. and DeBowes, L.J. (2009). Trauma. In: *Atlas of Dental Radiography in Dogs and Cats*, 208–220. St. Louis, MO: Saunders.
26 Manfra-Marretta, S., Schloss, A.J., and Klippert, L.S. (1992). Classification and prognostic factors of endodontic–periodontic lesions in the dog. *J. Vet. Dent.* 9 (2): 27–30.
27 Hargraves, K.M. and Cohen, S. (2011). Endodontic and periodontal interrelationships. In: *Cohen's Pathways of the Pulp*, 10e, 655–670. St. Louis, MO: Mosby.
28 Remeeus, P. and Verbeek, M. (1997). Use of dental pulp testers in veterinary dentistry. *J. Vet. Dent.* 14 (1): 23–28.
29 Swan, R.H., Rapley, J.W., and Schindler, W.G. (1991). Hemisection of a molar tooth in a dog: an alternative to total extraction. *J. Vet. Dent.* 8 (3): 12–14.
30 Tharaldsen (1927). *Diagnosis by Transillumination*, 18. Chicago, IL: Cameron's Publishing Co.
31 Hargraves, K.M. and Cohen, S. (2011). Instruments, materials and devices. In: *Cohen's Pathways of the Pulp*, 10e, 223–282. St. Louis, MO: Mosby.
32 Wiggs, R.B.. (1992). Endodontic anatomy, pathology and examination. *The North American Veterinary Conference Proceedings*. 106.
33 Sampeck, A.J. (1967). Instruments of endodontics. *Dent. Clin. N. Am.* 579.
34 D.D.R.(1983). *Materials, Instruments, and Equipment*, 2e, 311. Chicago, IL: ADA.
35 Ingle, J.I. (1955). The need for endodontic instrument standardization. *Oral Surg. Oral Med. Oral Path.* 8: 1211.
36 Ingle, J.I. and Levine, M. (1958). The need for uniformity of endodontic instruments, equipment, and filling materials. In: *Transactions of the Second International Conference on Endodontics* (ed. L.I. Grossman), 123. Philadelphia, PA: University of Pennsylvania.
37 (1979). American National Standards Institute, American Dental Association. Document No.41. *JADA* 99: 697.
38 American Dental Association, Council on Dental Materials and Devices (1976). New ADA Specification No.28 for endodontic files and reamers. *JADA* 93: 813.
39 American National Standards Institute, American Dental Association. Meeting of ISO Committee MD-156, Chicago, IL; 1982.
40 Hargraves, K.M. and Cohen, S. (2011). Tooth Morphology and access cavity preparation. In: *Cohen's Pathways of the Pulp*, 10e, 136–222. St. Louis, MO: Mosby.

41 Gutmann, J.L., Dumsha, T.C., and Lovdahl, P.E. (2006). Problem solving in canal cleaning and shaping: traditional and contemporary techniques. In: *Problem Solving in Endodontics*, 4e, 155–198. St. Louis, MO: Mosby.

42 Hargraves, K.M. and Cohen, S. (2011). Cleaning and shaping the root canal system. In: *Cohen's Pathways of the Pulp*, 10e, 283–348. St. Louis, MO: Mosby.

43 Boyd, R.C., and Ross, D.L. (2007). Rotary endodontics: How to improve the quality and speed of your root canal treatments LightSpeed rotary instruments and EndoVac Apical Negative Pressure Irrigation System. In: Proceedings of the 21st Annual Veterinary Dental Forum.

44 Gutmann, J.L., Dumsha, T.C., and Lovdahl, P.E. (2006). Problem solving the management of painful tooth emergencies. In: *Problem Solving in Endodontics*, 4e, 281–309. St. Louis, MO: Mosby.

45 Lilly, J.D. and Smith, D.C. (1966). An investigation of the fracture of root canal reamers. *Br. Dent. J.* 120: 364.

46 Hargraves, K.M. and Cohen, S. (2011). Non-surgical retreatment. In: *Cohen's Pathways of the Pulp*, 10e, 890–952. St. Louis, MO: Mosby.

47 Ingle, J.I., Bakland, L.K., and Baumgartner, J.C. (2008). Root canal filling material. In: *Ingle's Endodontics*, 6e, 1019–1053. Hamilton, Ontario: BC Decker Inc.

48 Hargraves, K.M. and Cohen, S. (2011). Obturation of the cleaned and shaped root canal system. In: *Cohen's Pathways of the Pulp*, 10e, 349–388. St. Louis, MO: Mosby.

49 Gutmann, J.L., Dumsha, T.C., and Lovdahl, P.E. (2006). Problem solving in the use of irrigants, chelating agents and disinfectants: their role in tissue removal and microbial control. In: *Problem Solving in Endodontics*, 4e, 143–154. St. Louis, MO: Mosby.

50 Glassman, G. (2011). Safety and efficacy considerations in endodontic irrigation. In: *Academy of Dental Therapeutics and Stomatology*, 1–12. PennWell Dental CE Digest.

51 Torabinejad, M. (2011). Root canal irrigants and disinfectants. *American Association of Endondontists Colleagues for Excellence Newsletter*. 1–7.

52 Clegg, M.S., Vertucci, F.J., Walker, C. et al. (2006). The effect of exposure to irrigant solutions on apical dentin biofilms *in vitro*. *J. Endod.* 32: 434–437.

53 Wiggs, R.B. (1991). Endodontic instrumentation. *J. Vet. Dent.* 8 (4): 4.

54 Hargraves, K.M. and Cohen, S. (2011). Endodontic records and legal responsibilities. In: *Cohen's Pathways of the Pulp*, 10e, 389–450. St. Louis, MO: Mosby.

55 Ahmad, M., Pitt Ford, T.R., and Crum, L.A. (1987). Ultrasonic debridement of canals: acoustic streaming and its possible role. *J. Endod.* 13 (10): 490.

56 Ross, D.L., and Boyd, R.C. (2009). Rotary endodontics: Using LightSpeed, EndoVac and SimpliFill. In: *23rd Annual Veterinary Dental Forum Proceedings*. 35–39.

57 Gioso, M.A., Teixeira, L.L., Souza, J.I.L. et al. (1995). Evaluation of electronic method in determining the root canal length in teeth of dogs. *J. Vet. Dent.* 12 (4): 141–142.

58 Cohen, S. and Schwartz, S. (1987). Endodontic complications and the law. *J. Endod.* 13: 191–197.

59 Gutmann, J.L., Dumsha, T.C., and Lovdahl, P.E. (2006). Problem solving in access openings orifice locations and initial preparation. In: *Problem Solving in Endodontics*, 4e, 85–114. St. Louis, MO: Mosby.

60 Manfra-Marretta, S., Golab, G., Anthony, J.M.G. et al. (1992). Development of a teaching model for coronal access to the canine dentition. *J. Vet. Dent.* 9 (4): 11–17.

61 Eisner, E.R. (1990). Transcoronal approach for endodontic access to the fourth maxillary premolar in dogs. *J. Vet. Dent.* 7 (4): 22–23.

62 Wiggs, R.B. (1993). Problem solving in veterinary endodontics. *J. Semin. Vet. Med. Surg. (Small Anim.)* 8 (3): 165.

63 Walton, R.E. and Torabinejad, M. (2002). Cleaning and shaping. In: *Principles and Practice of Endodontics*, 3e, 212–232. Philadelphia, PA: Saunders.

64 LSX and SimpliFill Veterinary Technique Guide. (2010). Sybron Endodontics, California.

65 Mendoza, K.A., Manfra-Marretta, S., Siegel, A.M. et al. (2000). Comparison of two heated gutta-percha and sealer obturation techniques in canine teeth of dogs. *J. Vet. Dent.* 17 (2): 69–74.

66 McCoy, T.E. (2012). SimpliFill obturation. In: Proceedings of the 26th Annual Veterinary Dental Forum.

67 Senia, S.E. et al. (1975). Rapid disinfection of gutta percha cones with 5.25% sodium hypochlorite. *J. Endod.* 1: 136.

68 Stein, K.E., Manfra-Maretta, S., Siegel, A.M. et al. (2004). Comparison of hand-instrumented, heated gutta-percha and engine driven, cold gutta-percha endodontic techniques. *J. Vet. Dent.* 21 (3): 136–145.

69 Krug, W., Manfra-Marretta, S., Thomas, M.W. et al. (2008). Comparison of cold GP/sealer and resin bonded obturation techniques in canine teeth in dogs. *J. Vet. Dent.* 25 (1): 10–14.

70 Goldstein, G.S. (2010). Guttaflow: use and various techniques in delivery methods. *Vet. Dent. Forum*.

71 Schilder, H., Goodman, A., and Aldrich, W. (1985). The thermomechanical properties of gutta-percha. Part V. Volume changes in bulk gutta-percha as a function of temperature and its relationship to molecular phase transformation. *Oral Surg. Oral Med. Oral Path.* 59: 285.

72 Wiggs, R.B. (1988). Use of the McSpadden compactor for root canal obturation in dogs and macaques. *J. Vet. Dent.* 5 (3): 9.

73 Schilder, H. (1987). Filling root canals in three-dimension. In: *Dental Clinics of North America*, 723. Philadelphia, PA: WB Saunders Co.

74 Chapter 8Gutmann, J.L., Dumsha, T.C., and Lovdahl, P.E. (2006). Problem solving in root canal obturation: traditional and contemporary techniques. In: *Problem Solving in Endodontics*, 4e, 197–238. St. Louis, MO: Mosby.

75 American Heart Association. (2014). Prevention of Infective Endocarditis: Circulation Journal of the American Heart Association. http://circ.ahajournals.org/content (accessed July 2014).

76 Gingrich, W. (2013). Evidence based recommendations for antibiotic prophylaxis prior to oral and dental procedures in dogs and cats. In: Proceedings of the 27th Annual Veterinary Dental Forum.

16

Advanced Endodontic Therapy

Michael Peak[1] and Heidi B. Lobprise[2]

[1] *Tampa Bay Veterinary Specialists, Largo, FL, USA*
[2] *Main Street Veterinary Dental Clinic, Flower Mound, TX, USA*

16.1 Principles

Standard therapeutic endodontics has rapidly progressed from an emerging science to an established part of veterinary dentistry. The excellent results from standard endodontic treatments, founded on scientifically established techniques, have resulted in the profession and the public accepting and expecting more ambitious treatments to more advanced problems [1]. Anticipation of every possible problem is not feasible; however, the more commonplace can be satisfactorily managed in a proficient manner when correctly identified. In complicated cases, however, advanced endodontic techniques may be employed to salvage teeth and circumvent procedural difficulties that might limit the success of standard techniques.

Many diverse areas of difficulty can be confronted in endodontic treatment [2, 3]. Some of the more common are access to the pulp cavity, attaining and maintaining working length, resolution of periapical pathology, complete obturation, and addressing iatrogenic injury. Perforations of the pulp cavity may result when access is complicated, tissues are diseased, or instrumentation is inappropriate for the situation. Canal abnormalities and blockages may present obstacles for adequate access, instrumentation to full working length, canal filing, canal shaping, and ultimately canal obturation. In addition, there are pedodontic endodontic considerations such as treatment of deciduous teeth and permanent teeth with immature or poorly developed root structure.

16.2 Endodontic Access

The fundamental purpose in the site of tooth access in standard endodontics is to establish an unrestricted passageway from the crown and through the pulpal cavity to the apical terminus of the endodontic canal [2]. An unimpeded pathway must be customized to expedite acceptable canal instrumentation and obturation according to specific tooth type and the individuality of the tooth's pulp system. The goal of access design is to gain full working length to the apical terminus of the canal while providing for obturation of the apical third of the canal, yet conserving as much tooth structure as possible.

Numerous technical difficulties can be diminished or eliminated with proper access preparation [2]. A cornerstone of good dentistry has always been the conservation of tooth structure; nevertheless this should not be allowed to influence the valid selection of site, design, or execution of the actual access opening [2]. This does not suggest that an excess of coronal structure should be removed indiscriminately. It does imply the need for a competent awareness of the pulp cavity and external root anatomy and the ability to properly assess radiographic details in order to appropriately implement access and prepare the coronal approach [2]. Until imaging modalities such as cone beam computed tomography (CBCT) are commonplace, the clinician must be thoroughly knowledgeable of pulpal and root anatomy as it is interpreted with proper two-dimensional radiographic assessment of a three-dimensional endodontic canal [2]. Failure to follow these basic steps may unnecessarily invite complications.

Tooth or restorative structure that is unsound or unsupported in the access pathway is better removed prior to initiation of endodontic treatment. Such action assists in maintenance of asepsis, provides for a better evaluation of restorative needs prior to root canal therapy, while enhancing visibility [2]. When all diseased structure is not removed prior to cleaning and shaping of the endodontic canal, contamination by debris falling or being carried into the canal may result. There are several techniques to remove material trapped in the root canal system, which are discussed in detail later in this chapter.

Wiggs's Veterinary Dentistry: Principles and Practice, Second Edition. Edited by Heidi B. Lobprise and Johnathon R. (Bert) Dodd.

Failure to establish proper access to the pulp chamber and root canals is one of the most common complicating factors in root canal therapy for veterinary practitioners [3]. The pulp chamber space is typically located in the center of the crown and the root canal in the center of the root. However, the pulp cavity is a dynamic, changing, cavernous space. With age, the cavity diminishes in size. In addition, pulpal irritation from caries, abrasion/attrition, tooth resorption, and restorative procedures can result in dimensional changes in the area of the irritation due to deposition of reparative or tertiary dentin internally. Diagnostic dental radiographs, while only two dimensional, are necessary to properly assess the anatomical relationship between the crown, the root, the angle of the root within the arch, and the general condition of the pulp cavity. When dealing with abnormal crown or root configurations or rotated teeth, radiographs often must be angled from mesial and distal aspects to provide the necessary information. Using two-dimensional radiographs as a guide for an access opening in a three-dimensional tooth can sometimes be misleading. CBCT has been shown to be superior to dental radiographs in the detection of small areas of bone loss in endodontically involved teeth and for mapping root canal morphology and finding extra roots/canals (see Chapter 3 – Oral Radiology and Imaging).

In some cases, access can be made through the pulp exposure at the fracture surface. If the access through the pulp exposure is not ideal, or if there is no pulp exposure, the pulp canal must be accessed independently. Although each tooth must be assessed individually, certain generalities can be made on the typical location of approach to the more commonly accessed teeth in the dog [4]. The typical entrance to the incisors may be found on the central lingual aspect of the crown 1–2 mm above the free gingival margin. Additionally, a similar labial approach may be used, though commonly not the choice in human dentistry due to esthetics. Cuspids or canine teeth are accessed 1–2 mm coronal to the free gingival margin on the mesial aspect of the crown to allow a straighter line access to the apex. The individual canals of two-rooted premolars should have the access openings made on the buccal aspect over the center of each root near the cusp's margin, as determined by physical palpation of the juga and radiographs. The approach to the lower first molars is similar except that access is most commonly made on the lingual surface for the mesial root and within the occlusal surface for the distal root. The other two rooted molars have access achieved on the occlusal surface directly over the roots to be entered. The maxillary fourth premolar presents a moderate challenge in the access to the mesial roots, especially the mesiopalatal root. While the distal root access is similar to other premolars, a transcoronal access has been described, using distinct angles [5]. This described technique is most useful to the novice clinician in gaining an understanding of the basic approach. In most fractured teeth, however, normal anatomy has been destroyed and determining an adequate exposure by mental extrapolation is required. Palpation of the mesiobuccal root juga and comparison to the actual location of the mesiopalatal root's cusp typically affords sufficient visualization to attain suitable lines of access determination. The actual opening is generally made between these two determined points and approximately 2–4 mm above the gingival margin on the buccal aspect of the tooth. One potential complication in access of the mesial roots is accidental perforation into the furcation between the mesial roots. To avoid this, once the pulp chamber has been identified and one of the pulp canals is found, the operator can insert a small (number 1/2 or number 1 size) round ball bur or small pear-shaped bur (*without* engaging power so the bur is not spinning) into the access until the bur encounters the pulp floor. Once the depth of the floor has been established, the power is engaged to the high-speed handpiece, causing the bur to spin. As the bur is spinning, it is removed from the canal in a sweeping motion to remove the ceiling of the pulp canal in the direction of the yet to be identified pulp canal. In many instances, this will remove only the dentin overhang that is blocking insertion of a small endodontic file into the desired canal. Use of this technique can help identify either the mesiobuccal or mesiopalatal canal yet helps reduce the chance of iatrogenic perforation. Three-rooted molars may be accessed with a Y- or V-shaped opening on the occlusal surface that exposes each individual canal system. The first access is typically made over the lingual or palatal root, with extension of the access with a high-speed bur and following the chamber to expose the two buccal root canals. Attempted straight-line access of the buccal roots initially will periodically lead to chamber perforation due to the angulation of the roots. Additionally, the V- or Y-shaped access aids in the detection of ribbon canals associated with fused distal and palatal roots, which are not uncommon in the upper first and second molars.

With calcified or difficult to find canals, magnification and transillumination can help with their location. In human endodontic therapy, complete preparation of the pulp chamber to visualize the chamber floor can be combined with placement of a dye or sodium hypochlorite, which will form bubbles over the canal [6]. When these basic parameters are not properly followed, problems such as failure to locate all canals, excessive gouging, and even perforations of the chamber walls and floor may occur [6].

16.3 Abnormal Canals

In veterinary endodontics, it is uncommon to encounter pulp canals that are of abnormal configuration, dystrophic, or have excessive linear calcification [7]. However, idiosyncrasies such as supernumerary roots and anomalous configured root systems like ribbon canals must be detected either by visualization or radiographs. Failure to recognize these quickly can lead to unnecessary delays and problems. Dystrophic canals may be confronted when standard root canal treatment is attempted on teeth that have previously had direct or indirect pulp capping performed with certain agents. Calcium hydroxide-type products can stimulate an increased layering of tertiary dentin within the pulp cavity, causing dystrophic areas for instrumentation [8].

Most cases exhibiting radiographically fine or unidentifiable canals or other calcification endodontic canal blockages are treatable with non-surgical root canal therapy. Successful identification of calcified orifices requires the use of a knowledge of normal dental anatomy, quality two-dimensional radiographs, and a good three-dimensional imagination. With these, access exploration is initiated using a small size ball bur directed toward the logical location of the endodontic cavity. Accurate pre-operative as well as frequent operative radiographs are an absolute necessity for assessment of bur orientation and depth penetration. The search for the canal can be aided with a smooth broach or Pathfinder® (Kerr Co., Romulus, MI) to assist the clinician in identification of the orifice.

Once located, the obstructed canal must be negotiated. At this juncture, the pathfinder can continue to be used or substitution with a No. 8 K-file is acceptable. The No. 6 K-file is usually too weak to allow appropriate pressure and the No. 10 may be too large. Instrumentation should be performed with a file that is long enough to reach the apex but not excessive in length as the longer the instrument the more tactile sense is lost [9]. If the canal is curved, a slight curve can be placed 1 mm from the apical tip of the instrument to aid in its correct direction of orientation. Endodontic stops should always be used, and if the instrument is curved, a directional stop is mandatory. The directional stop's pointer should be aligned to indicate the direction of the instrument's curvature.

Chelating agents such as ethylene-diamine-tetra-acetic acid (EDTA) can be used to aid in the dissolution of inorganic calcification within the canal. Products such as RC Prep® (Premier Corp., Plymouth Meeting, PA), a white paste-like substance, combine EDTA, urea peroxidase, and lubricant for use directly on instruments introduced into the canal. Frequent copious irrigation with EDTA solution, sterile saline, dilute chlorhexidine, or full or half-strength sodium hypochlorite (3–6% NaOCl) is important to remove debris as the instrument is advanced. Sodium hypochlorite should be used with care in suspect perforation or open apex cases as it can result in serious complications should it enter the periodontal or periapical tissues. Care should be taken to use true windowed or slotted endodontic irrigation needles in irrigating within fine canals as injection needles may easily occlude a canal, preventing irrigant from flushing around the needle, thereby forcing irrigant and debris through the apex.

When obstruction is met, the file (K-file or reamer) should have gentle force applied and be worked in a very delicate clockwise–counterclockwise rotation. This is sometimes called "stem winding" or balanced force instrumentation. This action is slowly continued, along with alternating larger files, removing dentinal shavings from the file flutes and flushing the canal frequently until the canal terminus is encountered. Once appropriate working length is verified radiographically, a filing or up and down action should be used until the instrument is functioning in a clean, free movement. Normal standard hand instruments can commonly be followed from this point as long as regular recapitulation of the canal with smaller files is employed to loosen any debris or dentin and maintain full length with each enlarging file. The use of ultrasonic activated endodontic instruments has been advocated for passive penetration of calcified or blocked canals [6].

16.4 Procedural Errors

16.4.1 Instrumentation Errors

Gouging is the penetration of the pulp chamber floor but not completely through the root/crown wall, typically with burs or files during exploration for root canals. Canals can also be gouged, but this is more appropriately termed ledging or hedging. If gouging results in compete extension into the periradicular tissues or outside the crown, this is called a perforation.

A ledge is a gouge or false canal created during instrumentation with excessive apical pressure primarily associated with curved canals (Figure 16.1). Ledging also causes loss of working length, but usually can be corrected with use of a proper treatment protocol. Prevention comes from avoidance of excessive apical instrument pressures until the file is working freely in the canal, use of lubricants on the files, use of flexible materials/files such as nickel titanium (NiTi files), and use of pre-bent files with properly placed directional stops when working in curved canals. Early recognition of the error is important and the dilemma is usually obvious if routine radiographs are being taken. Unfortunately, if missed, these errors may lead to perforation and a poorer

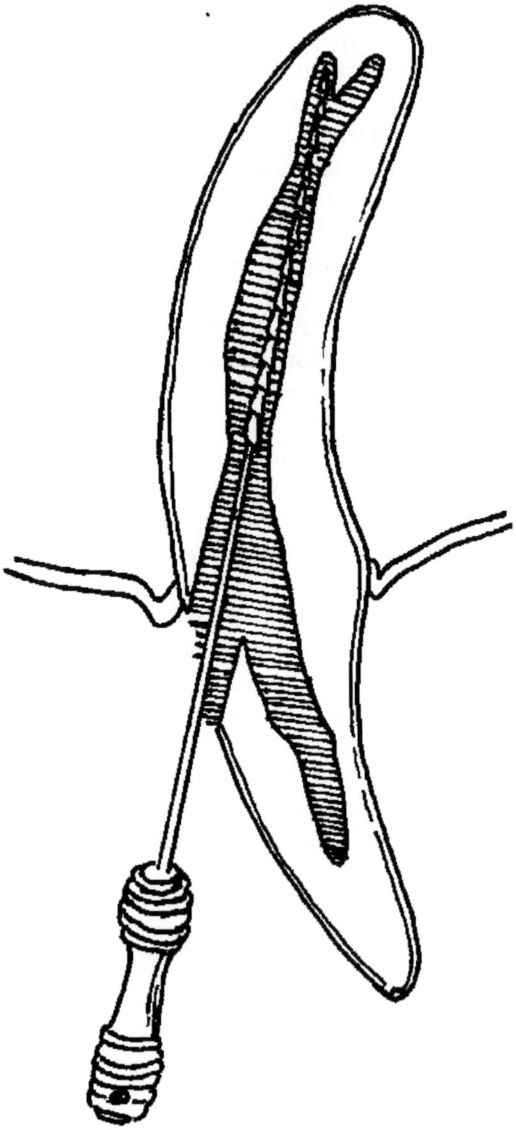

Figure 16.1 Ledging or transportation. *Source:* Courtesy of Josephine Banyard.

prognosis of the endodontic procedure. Even when caught early, the novice will find that attempts at reestablishment of the original canal pathway can be frustrating. This is overcome in most cases by placing a 45° acute bend 3 mm from the tip of a pathfinder or size 8–15 K-file. A directional endodontic stop should be placed so that it points to the direction of the angle of the instrument point. The instrument should be well lubricated. The tip of the instrument should be directed away from the ledge. The spring action of the bend of the instrument will normally force the tip to bypass the ledge and compel it to enter the true root canal passageway, thus allowing the correct working length to be achieved. Once the actual canal is patent, the subsequent files may be treated similarly until the filing is complete.

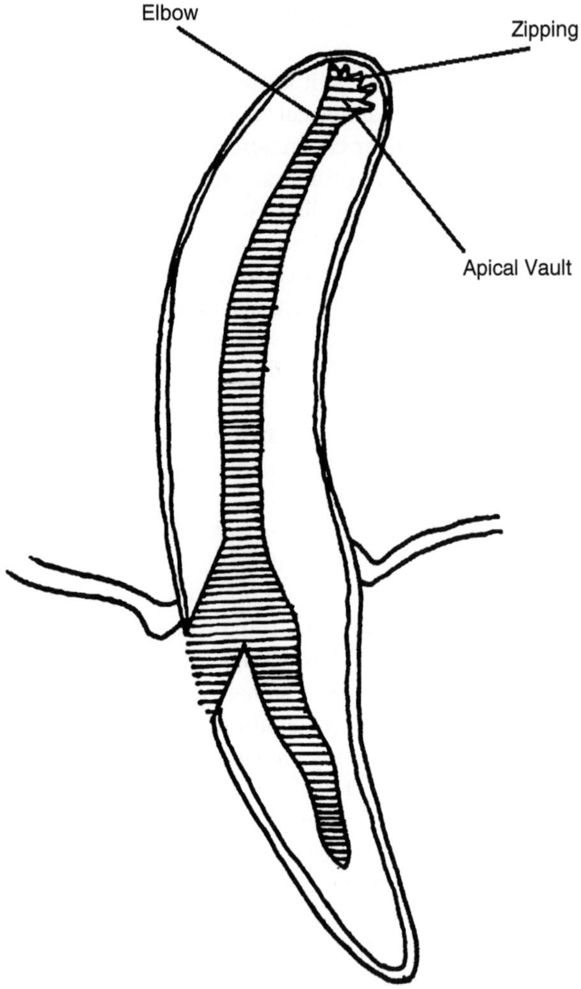

Figure 16.2 Elbowing within the apical portion of the root canal contributed to the apical vault and zipping or elliptication. *Source:* Courtesy of Josephine Banyard.

Another procedural error encountered that results in a change of working length is zipping or elliptication (Figure 16.2). These terms refer to when an overextended file transports the outer wall of the apical foramen [6]. The primary indicted cause of zipping is failure to prebend files, excessive rotation of instruments, and use of instruments in curved canal systems that are too stiff. Two complications are common with this phenomenon, elbow stricture and apical perforation. In elbow stricture, the root canal has decreased the diameter just before the actual terminus of the canal, creating a larger space just before the apical delta. When obturating the canal, this leaves a potential unfilled apical void or vault in which fluids can accumulate and result in the eventual failure of the endodontic procedure. The best approach to treat this problem is further enlargement of the canal to remove the stricture and frequent irrigation to remove any dentinal debris.

Stripping is an endodontic complication that results in lateral wall perforation (Figure 16.3). This refers to the thinning of a lateral root canal wall, usually in the direction of the root tip curvature. Overzealous instrumentation in the midroot areas is the primary suspected cause, with perforation eventually occurring if not caught early. Use of judicial filing pressure away from the curvature of the root tip and/or toward the bulkier portion of the tooth root (anticurvature filing) is normally sufficient to prevent stripping. Stripping, when detected early, can be handled by appropriate instrumentation, as previously described. Proper radiographs normally provide the differential diagnosis between lateral wall perforation of stripping and apical perforations. Treatment of lateral wall perforation is best dealt with in a two-stage non-surgical endodontic procedure. Non-affected roots can have standard endodontic treatment completed. The perforated root should be filled with mineral trioxide aggregate (MTA) (see the discussion regarding perforations that follows).

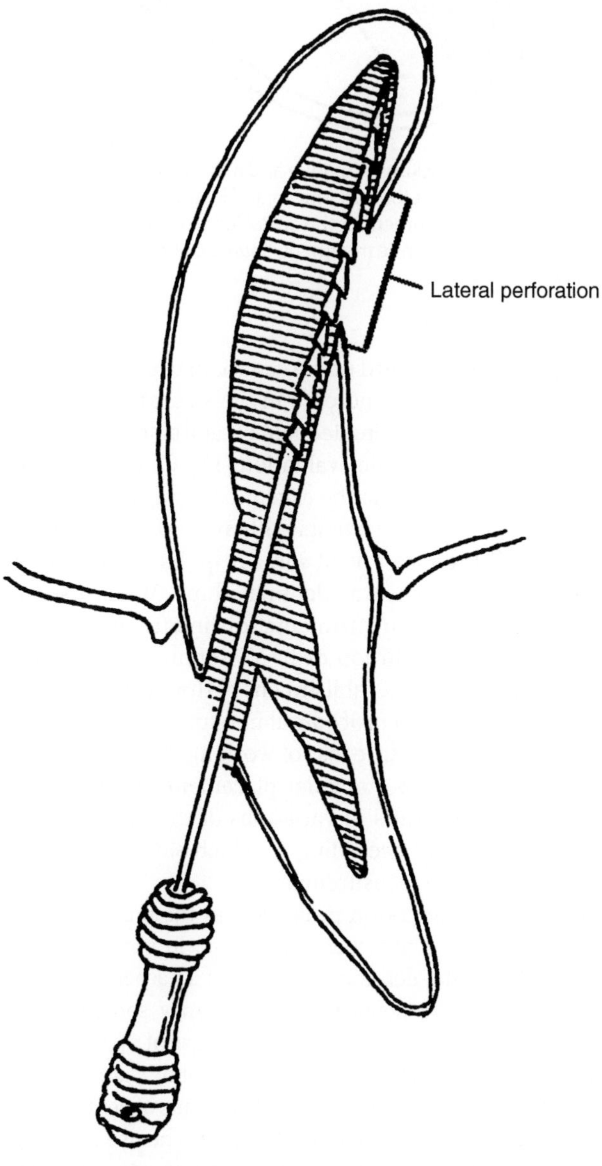

Figure 16.3 Stripping of the canal wall can result in lateral perforation. *Source:* Courtesy of Josephine Banyard.

16.4.1.1 Perforations

Perforation is an accidental mechanical extension through the pulp chamber into the oral cavity or the periodontal tissues [2]. Should this occur, recognition of the problem as soon as possible can reduce damage to the periradicular tissues. Canal hemorrhage, one of the most common clinical indications of perforation is continued bleeding into the chamber from the exposed periradicular tissues. When dealing with perforations into the gingival sulcus or coronal to the free gingival margin, bleeding may or may not be encountered. If this type of perforation is noted, the following treatment protocol can, in many instances, be employed. First, control any hemorrhage. This may be accomplished with a dry cotton pellet or the large blunt end of a paper point. If the patient is healthy, the use of epinephrine (1:50 000) or another hemostatic agent on the pellet can be considered [2]. Epinephrine-containing agents should be used cautiously in animals with endocrine imbalances or heart disease. This is followed by placement of a gutta-percha point or paper point into the yet to be filled root canals to prevent restoratives from entering and sealing them off. Next place a temporary filling material into the perforation, such as Cavit-G® (3M, St. Paul, MN) or Intermediate Restorative Material (IRM®) (Dentsply/Caulk Co., Milford, DE). The root canal procedure should now be completed. Once the root canal procedure is completed, permanent restoration should be placed to seal off the perforation. If the perforation is in the sulcus or furcation, there is a probability that a persistent periodontal lesion with migration of the gingival margin may occur [10]. Additional periodontal treatments, such as gingivectomies or apical repositioning, may prove necessary.

The prognosis for perforation repair is improved with more apical lesions, but these may be more difficult to access for the repair procedure [11]. The perforation should be attended to and sealed as soon as possible. Hemorrhage must be controlled to obtain a seal in most cases [2]. Control can be facilitated with placement of saline moistened followed by dry paper points. While waiting for any bleeding to stop, any additional canals may be treated with standard root canal therapy. If hemorrhage cannot be adequately controlled, then calcium hydroxide paste may be placed along with a temporary filling and allowed two to three weeks before final treatment is attempted. Once the bleeding has been controlled, filling of the endodontic canal with MTA coronal to the level of the perforation in the affected root may be completed [11]. Once the perforation has been sealed with MTA, final restoration may be placed. These endodontically treated teeth should be carefully followed with radiographs. No references for exact follow-up times are found for dogs, but the author usually recommends dental radiographs at 6, 12, and 18 months post-operatively, followed by annual radiographic examinations thereafter.

Apical perforation is the condition of an instrument extending beyond the apical delta. It is typically associated with one of two scenarios. Loss of the apical constriction (apical stop) commonly occurs due to root resorption from disease or excessive instrumentation. Either of these situations may lead to instrumentation damage of the periodontal ligament and alveolar bone, along with possible inoculation of the area with debris and bacteria. Additionally, in an open apex, overfilling and a poor apical seal, as well as potential patient discomfort, may occur. Continued hemorrhage into the canal is another common sign. Although continued hemorrhage can be an indication of over-instrumentation, it is more commonly an indication of under-instrumentation with pulp tissue remnants. Differential diagnosis is often evident with good-quality intraoral radiographs. Prevention comes from appropriate use of instrument stops, quality operative radiographs with periodic verification, and attention to detail during instrumentation. Once apical perforation and loss of apical stop occurs, control of hemorrhage is the first step. A new apical stop must then be established within the confines of the root canal system without excessive loss of structural integrity. This is accomplished by establishing a position with the endodontic file tip approximately 1–2 mm from the apex radiographically. With stops in place at this newly established working length, instrumentation should continue to two or three file sizes larger than the first file that shows binding at the tip. This is commonly known as the "Backup Technique" (Figure 16.4). Once the apical stop has been established, MTA can be placed at the apex of the root and the endodontic obturation completed thereafter. If the perforation is large enough to allow gross overextension of root canal obturation materials, a surgical approach to the root apex with apicoectomy and retrograde filling or extraction is advised.

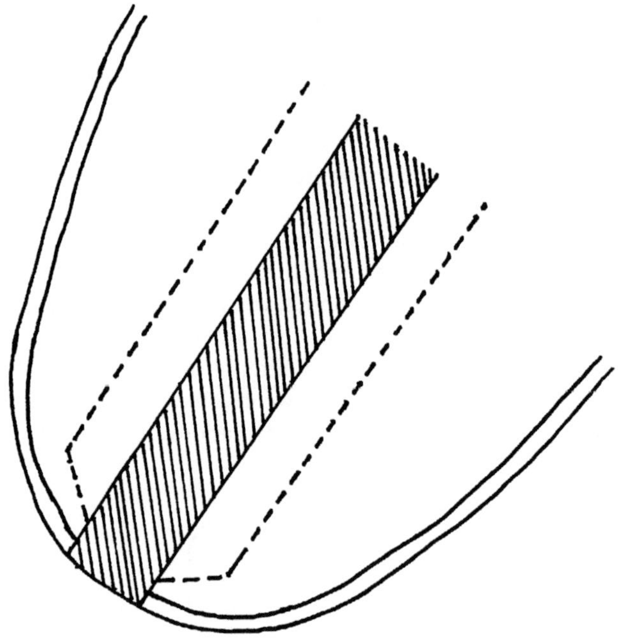

Figure 16.4 The backup technique and a tooth without an apical stop. The dotted lines indicate the area of instrumentation that allows the reestablishment of the apical ledge or stop for standardized endodontic treatment. *Source:* Courtesy of Josephine Banyard.

16.4.2 Procedural Blockage

Endodontic canal blockage is the obstruction of a once-patent canal preventing full instrument access to the canal terminus. Most blockages result from the packing of dentinal chips, cotton pellets, paper points, or a piece of fractured instrument within the canal [11]. Loss of working length due to dentinal chip accumulation (dentinal mud) at the apical third of the canal can usually be attributed to too rapid an increase in file size, an insufficient irrigation technique, inadequate recapitulation, and lack of routine radiographic evaluation [11]. Once the condition has occurred it can be exceptionally difficult to correct. Use of chelating agents with an EDTA component such as RC-Prep® can be of some help. Its action softens inorganic debris such as dentinal chips. When used in cooperation with reinstrumentation and frequent irrigation with EDTA solution or 3–6% sodium hypochlorite may facilitate the reestablishment of the working length. In other cases, it is a procedural measurement or recording error, and not a true loss of working length. This may occur from improper angular placement of the stop on the file, which results in variations of the measurement to working length according to which side of the file is used to make the measurement.

Paper points or cotton pellets lost in the pulp canal can pose a significant challenge. These can, in most cases, be removed with the delicate assistance of a barbed broach or file. Broken instruments in the canal may sometimes be removed by access enlargement and the use of a pair of mosquito forceps to grasp the instrument end. Care must be maintained not to remove excessive amounts of dental tissue, thus producing unsound tooth structure. The use of a magnetized file, spreader, or plugger can be of assistance with loose instrument pieces. Many spreaders and pluggers with a high ferrous content can be magnetized in the same fashion as screwdrivers with a strong magnet or magnetizer.

Ultrasonic instruments have been demonstrated to be one of the best ways to manage obstruction retrievals in the root canal [12]. Ultrasonic instruments and techniques involving them are commonly used to disengage cements and loosen solid objects and material from the frictional hold of the root canal. In some cases, by orienting the coronal canal access opening in a downward position and then placing an ultrasonic scaler in contact with the tooth, the fragment may vibrate out of the opening. With those that are more tenacious and in the coronal part of the canal, a different approach can be taken. The access can be slightly enlarged and the scaler placed against the exposed portion of the fragment to loosen it with activation of the ultrasonic tip. With deeper instrument fragments, a spreader or plugger may be placed in direct contact with the end of the instrument and the ultrasonic scaler touched to the spreader and activated to vibrate the fragment indirectly with the ultrasonic energy. In other cases when the instrument fragment cannot be loosened, a Gates Glidden drill can be used to widen the area immediately above coronal to the fragment. Canal obturation, in some cases, can then be attempted by leaving the fragment and bypassing it with instrumentation to complete the root canal procedure. Occasionally the bypass instrument, when in lateral contact with the instrument fragment, can be energized with an ultrasonic scaler tip and utilized to loosen the fragment. If the instrument fragment is bound firmly at the apex with no canal distal to the fragment, a sealer may be introduced around it, forming an apical seal, and the procedure can be completed. In these cases, the owner should be advised of the situation and routine rechecks performed for signs or symptoms of failure. The alternative to this would be surgical access of the apex of the root, apicoectomy, and retrograde filling (Figure 16.5a to c). If the fragment is not at the apex and cannot be bypassed, a surgical procedure with a retrograde filling would be advisable.

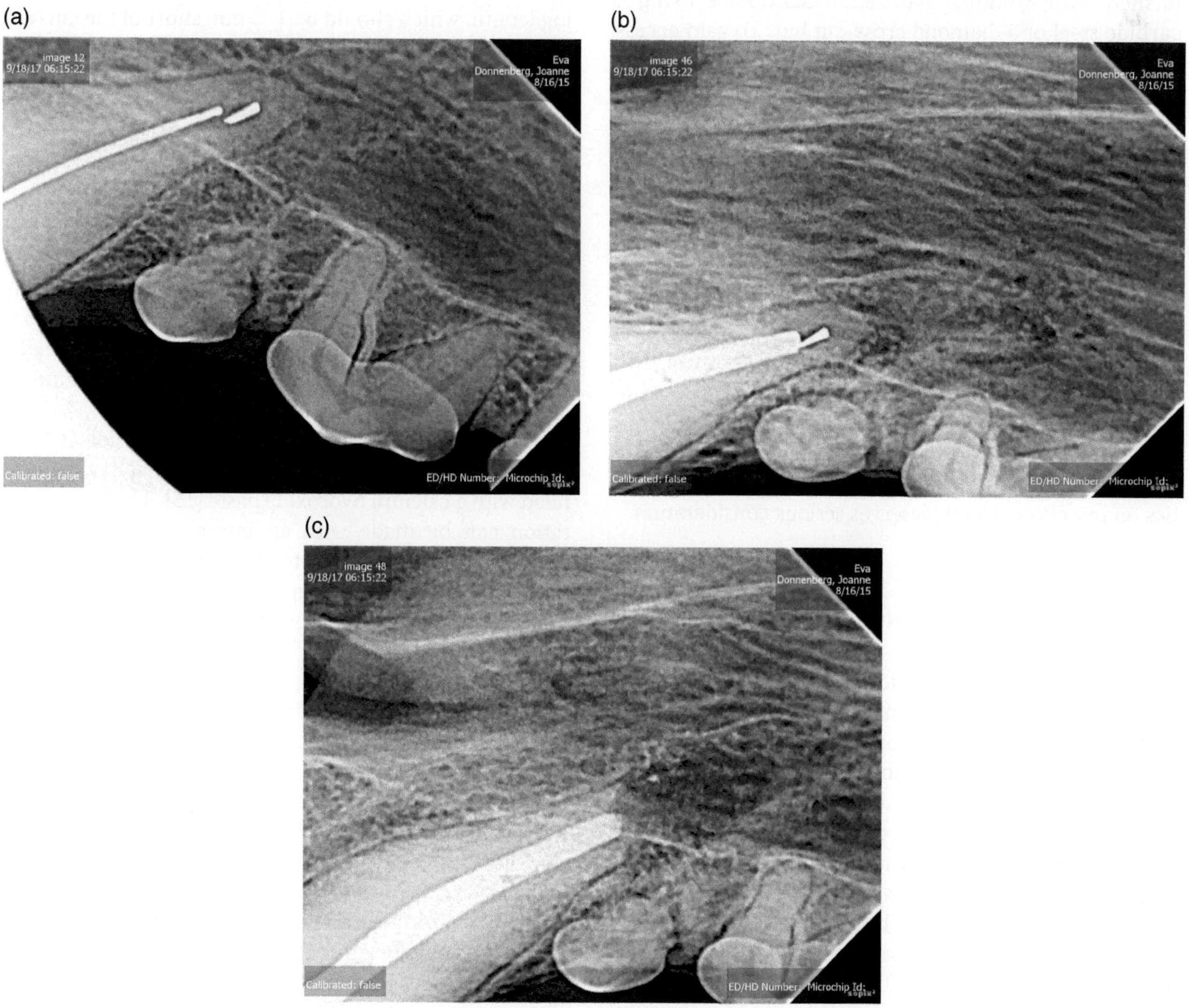

Figure 16.5 Radiographs of file tip separation and management: (a) tip of the file lodged in the apical region, unretrievable; (b) orthograde obturation of the canal to the level of the file tip; (c) completed apicoectomy and apical fill.

16.5 Tooth Resection, Root Resection and Hemisection

The term sectioning comes from the Latin word *sectus* meaning to cut, where resection comes from the Latin word *resectus* meaning to cut off. Root resection (root amputation) involves removing just the root portion, while retaining the entire crown [13]. Hemisection indicates a two-rooted tooth being cut through the furcational area into two pieces, and trisection is cutting a three-rooted tooth into three root–crown segments [13]. If any portion of the tooth is removed, there is partial tooth resection.

Resection is performed for many reasons such as root fracture, root perforation, root resorption, an endodontically inoperable tooth or root, periodontal disease, tumors of the jaws, or fractures of the jaws. Root resection involves a horizontal or angular cut to remove the root from the cervix of the tooth. This is usually accomplished with a high-speed dental handpiece using a carbide steel or a diamond cross-cut bur. To gain access to the furcation area, a gingival flap and possible slight alveolar bone reduction may be necessary in some cases, although in periodontal disease sufficient exposure may already be present. Root resection allows for the functional crown structure to remain intact, as compared to tooth resectioning. Currently in veterinary dentistry both are performed, but tooth resectioning is the more traditional because of the greater ease and speed of procedure. The mandibular first molar is a frequently resectioned tooth in the dog because of periodontal disease involving the distal root, or in cases of jaw fracture [13]. Vital resectioning should be approached with appropriate deliberation because of the risk of loss of pulpal vitality as in any pulp amputation and direct pulp capping (DPC) procedure. For this reason, complete standard endodontics on resectioned teeth deserves serious consideration.

16.6 Immature Deciduous Teeth

Disease and fractures of deciduous teeth occur in young animals. Treatment is determined by the extent of structural damage of the crown and root, degree of physiological or pathological resorption of the root, pulp vitality or lack of it, and the strategic value of the tooth.

As a rule, due to the short functionality (two to five months in most dogs and cats) of the deciduous teeth, extraction is usually the best treatment. On occasion, retention of the tooth may be considered advisable in order to maintain the occlusal spacing and/or interlock. The mandibular canine (#704/804) and the maxillary third incisors (#503/603) can be of strategic importance in maintaining the occlusal pattern in occlusions that are tight with an inclination toward a Class III malocclusion. Maintaining these teeth may aid in holding the occlusion in a more normal and functional pattern for the individual. Other teeth may also be of importance in maintaining proper spacing in certain situations. When it is desired to maintain a tooth that still shows indications of pulp vitality, a pulpotomy with DPC and a permanent restoration of composite or glass ionomer is advised. If the tooth shows indications of irreversible pulpitis, by continued pulpal hemorrhage following pulpotomy or other signs, the pulp should be extirpated and the tooth treated as non-vital.

In non-vital teeth, the treatment protocol is greatly influenced by the state of the root structure based upon pathological and/or physiological resorption. Instrumentation of the canal must be performed carefully so as not to injure the permanent tooth bud by apical perforation of instruments, irrigants, or debris and bacterial inoculation. Radiographs should be taken to establish the working length, which should be 1–3 mm short of the current apex, so preparation takes place inside of the root canal [14]. Endodontic stops should be placed at the working length on all instruments to insure safety of the permanent tooth bud. Irrigation should be made with liberal amounts of sterile normal saline and instruments coated with an EDTA chelating disinfectant. If the apex is intact the canal can be filled with a thick paste of zinc oxide and eugenol (ZOE) [15]. The material can be placed by syringe or spiral filler, and a cotton pledget used to gently compact the material. Should air be trapped at the apex a needle and syringe can be used to remove it. The needle is advanced to the site of the air bubble and a vacuum is created with the syringe to evacuate it.

If the apex has already begun normal physiological or abnormal pathological resorption, the canal may be best filled with a calcium hydroxide paste [15]. The final restoration can be made with an intermediate restorative, glass ionomer or a composite. With ZOE fills, a composite restoration will require an intermediate separating layer of a glass ionomer or the composite may fail to properly cure.

16.7 Immature Permanent Teeth

The permanent dentition of the dog has approximately only 50% of its expected root length present at the time of eruption [16]. This also means that the apex and apical stop has not formed and the root end is open. Teeth with undeveloped root apices are not good candidates for standard root canal therapy as a complete seal of the apex is extremely difficult to successfully attain [15]. Prior to the development of procedures to induce apical closure, treatment was typically a surgical approach with retrograde filling. Although this was successful in many cases, mechanical problems were commonly encountered. The thin, fragile dentinal walls proved challenging to attain an apical seal in the less-developed apices [15], and removal of a weak structure to a more substantial level would at times produce a poor crown-to-root ratio. For these reasons, two therapies have developed to treat these teeth to stimulate the eventual closure of the apex. In teeth with the presence of viable pulp, vital pulp therapy (VPT) is performed to protect and support the remaining healthy pulp to support its maturation and closure of the apex, or apexogenesis [15]. In non-vital teeth, treatment is provided to stimulate a hard-tissue closure at the apical region, or apexification [15].

16.7.1 Vital Pulp Therapy (VPT)

In VPT, the first step is to remove the infected coronal portion of the pulp (partial coronal pulpectomy). The underlying pulp is then treated by placing an appropriate medication (DPC – direct pulp capping) to maintain its vitality for continued maturation of the tooth. Pulp capping is mainly indicated for reversible pulp tissue injury of developing or mature teeth. A primary goal is to be able to induce the dentinogenic potential of pulpal undifferentiated mesenchymal cells for repair [17]. If the pulp is covered with an inert material (no stimulus), the pulp cells do not differentiate for odontoblastic activity [18]. Pulp capping with a material that stimulates the differentiation, with endogenous signaling molecules, results in initial fibrodentin formation with a non-polar arrangement of fibers. Experimentally, it has been shown that with the addition of a mechanical support (demineralized dentin matrix), the cells differentiate and migrate on the substrate, resulting in a more organized polarized reparative dentin [18].

The goals of the procedure are to stimulate continued root growth, root end closure, and thickening of the dentinal walls of the root. These are accomplished by maintaining the vitality of Hertwig's epithelial root sheath, to encourage continued root growth and closure, and to preserve pulp vitality and its associated odontoblast's function in laying down additional layers of dentin in order to thicken the root and bridge the access site. If the pulp eventually becomes non-vital, the continued maturation of the tooth may be sufficient for possible standard root canal therapy at a later date [19, 20].

It is important that the normal tissue architecture at the amputated dentin–pulp interface is restored in order to protect the pulp from secondary infection from bacterial leakage at the margins of the restoration [18]. This protection of the reparative dentin is necessary, but not at the expense of the underlying pulp. If the pulp is damaged, uncontrolled hard tissue formation can result in the obliteration of the pulp chamber [18]. Deep penetration of capping material into the pulp that can damage the tissue has also been associated with treatment failure [21].

16.7.1.1 Vital Pulp Materials

DPC entails using a suitable dental material over an exposed pulp to protect it from further damage and to initiate the formation of irritation dentin, permitting the preservation of the remaining pulp. Ideal characteristics of a pulp capping material include biocompatibility, minimal inflammatory response, good handling, reasonable setting times, and an appropriate reparative response.

Calcium hydroxide (CaOH or CH) has been used in the past, with its important antibacterial effect, as well as its ability to help promote the formation of a reparative dentinal bridge in order to help maintain pulp vitality. However, tunnel defects in the dentinal bridge and poor sealing properties are some disadvantages, with unpredictable results [22]. MTA, introduced in 1993 by Torabinejad, stimulates pulp healing with dentinal bridge formation and minimal inflammatory reactions [23]. It stimulates increased hard tissue formation as compared to CH and results in the intimate connection of cell processes and extracellular fluids with the crystals of the compound. Progressive mineralization of the dentinal bridge from the periphery to the central area is also seen when MTA is used in VPT [24]. It provides good sealing, has little cytotoxicity, exerts an antibacterial effect, is biocompatible, and is not affected by fluid or blood contamination [23]. However, it has poor handling characteristics and typically has a prolonged setting time, though fast setting products have been developed.

Calcium enriched mixtures (CEM) contain combinations of tricalcium phosphate (TCP), calcium sulfate, CaOH, calcium oxide, and other materials. These mixtures have the biocompatibility of MTA but have faster setting times and better handling characteristics. Water-soluble calcium and phosphate in the product help to immediately form hydroxyapatite crystals during and after the setting time. It forms an effective seal against microorganisms, has an antibacterial effect, and is resistant to washout. In a scanning electron microscopy (SEM) study, complete dentinal bridge formation has been found to an extent similar to MTA and is better than CH [25].

16.7.1.2 Vital Pulp Procedure

The degree of inflammation as determined by the intensity of traumatic insult, amount of debris and bacterial contamination, and duration of time from exposure until treatment all play a key role in the likelihood of success in preserving pulp vitality. It can be difficult to determine the true extent of pulpal inflammation. While numerous studies have indicated the depth of inflamed pulp typically does not exceed 2–3 mm from the exposed surface for up to 168 hours or seven days following traumatic exposures, bacterial ingress can put the pulp at risk if treated beyond this time period [26, 27]. Direct bacterial invasion via pulp tissue does not normally occur, even when left open to saliva, until food and debris contaminated with bacteria is compacted into direct contact with the pulp [26].

Once diagnosed and treatment is chosen, isolation, and aseptic conditions should be maintained to prevent further introduction of debris or bacteria. Only exposed pulp deemed inflamed should ordinarily be removed. The instrument of choice is a high-speed dental handpiece with a diamond bur and adequate water flow to remove inflamed tissue, as it has been shown to create the least damage to the underlying pulpal tissues [28]. The first few millimeters of inflamed or proliferative tissue should be removed until healthy pulp is encountered [29]. In some cases, it may be necessary to remove pulp tissue to a greater depth to reach non-inflamed tissue or to provide a suitable depth for restorative requirements, often up to 5–7 mm. All filaments of the pulp tissue coronal to the selected amputation level should be removed, otherwise hemorrhage will be difficult to control. Once severed, the stump should be thoroughly cleansed with a gentle flow of normal saline or sterile water. Excess moisture can be removed by a light syringe vacuum and sterile dry paper points. Blown air should not be used for this purpose as it can cause desiccation and additional tissue damage. Most hemorrhage can be controlled with sterile paper points dipped in saline and placed against the pulp. Dry cotton pellets or dry paper points should not be used for this purpose as they will be incorporated into the clot and when removed will dislodge the clot, stimulating additional hemorrhage. Dry paper points or cotton pellets may be placed on top of the wet in order to apply gentle pressure to aid in hemorrhage control. Should the hemorrhage persist, first check for filaments of pulp coronal to the amputation level and, if found, they should be removed with an endodontic spoon. Bleeding can usually be controlled with saline-soaked cotton pellets or a lavage with NaOCl. This solution may be left in contact with the pulp for 10–15 minutes (refreshing every few minutes) and has no adverse effect on pulpal healing [15]. Continued bleeding for longer than five or six minutes may indicate that not all inflamed hyperplastic tissue has been removed and pulpectomy should be extended more apically. Once amputation enters several millimeters into the root canal and hemorrhage is still insistent, a compromise treatment must be considered. The hemorrhage is then controlled using a hemostatic agent, such as aluminum chloride or ferric sulfate, applied with a cotton pellet or the blunt end of a paper point, even knowing the risk [15]. Once hemorrhage has been controlled, a small layer (1–2 mm) of calcium hydroxide (CaOH) or MTA is placed against the pulp. An amalgam carrier and blunt end of a paper point is customarily sufficient to accomplish this treatment. The material should not be forced into the pulp as this can result in pressure necrosis or stimulate excessive calcification within the canal [21]. While MTA is a viable alternative, if the tooth needs to be re-entered due to procedure failure, it is more difficult to bypass this material in comparison to CaOH [15]. A glass ionomer cement is placed (sandwich method), cured, and the access closed accordingly (Figure 16.6).

The patient should be recalled for radiographic evaluations at six- to nine-month intervals for up to two years to determine success. Once the apex has closed, the clinician must decide whether to leave the tooth as it is or to follow with a complete standard endodontic root canal procedure. Retrospective reports of success rates for VPT range from 85% to 100%, with optimal results seen for the immediate pulp capping of teeth after crown amputation under more sterile conditions [20, 21]. Success was increased with the use of MTA (92%) compared to CaOH (58%) and treatment failure increased with prolonged exposure after traumatic fracture and pulp exposure [20] or if the dressing extended into the pulp chamber [21].

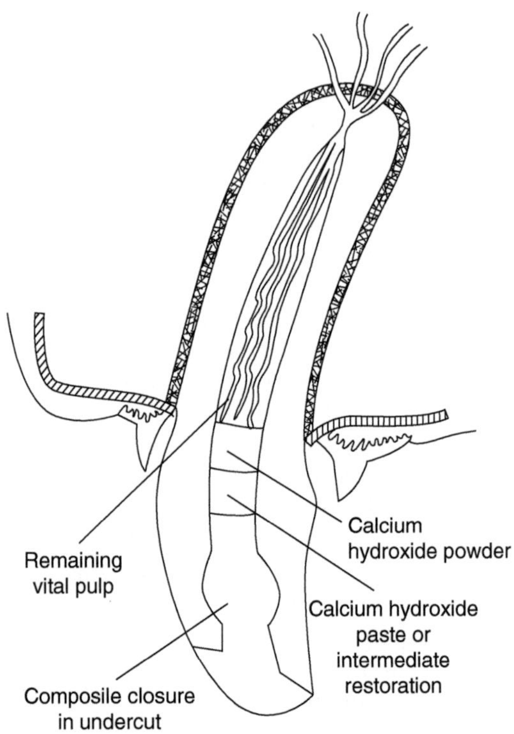

Figure 16.6 Illustration showing the layers of medicaments for vital pulp therapy. Source: Courtesy of Josephine Banyard.

16.7.2 Apexification

Apexification is a method of inducing a calcified barrier at the apex of a non-vital tooth with incomplete root formation. The goal is to stimulate root end closure (or a hard tissue barrier to serve as a closed root end), so that eventually a standard endodontic procedure may be carried out. This is accomplished by the removal of all infected or decaying pulp and debris from the canal, and then filling the root canal space with a material to stimulate formation of a calcified apical closure. Historical reports of numerous materials that successfully promote apexification have been found, with calcium hydroxide commonly used in the most recent past. Disadvantages of CaOH include the variability of treatment time, the number of appointments needed, and the possibility of increased tooth fracture after its extended use [30]. The use and placement of MTA into the prepared endodontic canal has developed into the most commonly accepted protocol for apexification [31].

Histological studies of the calcification that occurs at the apical foramen in apexification cases tends to be osteoid (bone-like) or cementoid (cementum-like) [15]. These have also indicated an absence of odontoblasts or Hertwig's epithelial root sheath, showing that these are not necessary for the process, though remnants may be present (Rests of Malassez). Cementoblasts present in the apical region and fibroblasts of the dental follicle and periodontal ligament can undergo differentiation and produce hard tissue [32]. However, to be successful, the apex must be completely within the confines of the cortical plate [15]. Additionally, this means if there is any degree of radiolucency periapically, apexification may be delayed or not occur. Therefore, radicular curettage and drainage to simulate bony healing may be required in these cases to improve the prospect of obtaining apexification.

The apexification technique is not complex, but the basic guidelines must be strictly followed for consistent results. The removal of all infected pulp and debris is the first step. In many cases the pulp will have decayed to a point of fragmentary debris or be totally dissolved, leaving a pulpless tooth. With the use of a file with the endodontic stop applied, it is advanced until light resistance is met. Radiographs then confirm the location of the tip to the tooth apex or suggests appropriate movement of the file. This is done in order to establish true working length for subsequent instrumentation to minimize periapical instrument trauma, which can affect the eventual outcome of the procedure. The canal should then be instrumented clean using sterile saline as the irrigant of choice. Although sodium hypochlorite greatly improves disinfection and removal of debris, it must be used with extreme caution as it can easily be forced into the periapical tissues with the large open apex, often with dire results. Once all debris has been removed, the canal is dried by syringe aspiration of excess fluid and the employment of sterile dry paper points. The endodontic canal fill material of choice is MTA. An initial plug of calcium sulfate can be pushed through the apex to provide a resorbable barrier against which to pack the MTA [15]. The cement can be placed into the canal with an amalgam carrier, disposable syringe, endodontic pressure syringe, spiral filler, or a McSpadden-type compactor. Care must be taken to avoid overextending the material into the periapical space. The blunt end of sterile paper points or large size pluggers with pre-measured endodontic stops can be helpful in packing the material to the apex [33]. A level or even apical fill or slight underfill is best, thereby avoiding introduction of material into periapical tissue, yet obtaining a complete fill [33]. Use of some dry powder mix on top of the paste is sometimes helpful in compacting the paste. The moisture from the open apex may be sufficient to offset the delayed setting time of the MTA [15]. Periodic radiographs are necessary to verify appropriate and adequate fill. Composite resin or glass ionomer filling material can be used for access closure [33].

Apexification normally requires six to twenty-four months [15]. The patient should be recalled at three- to six-month intervals for physical and radiographic evaluation and for symptoms or signs of infection or pathology. If these are found, the tooth should be considered for extraction or surgical exposure of the apex of the root, apical resection, and retrograde filling if the tooth is to be preserved. While replacement of the CaOH dressing is not necessary for apexification to occur, it can reduce the intensity of the inflammatory process [34].

16.8 Regenerative Endodontics

16.8.1 Introduction

An alternative to apexification with either MTA or CaOH is the concept of pulp regeneration. While apexification may have a relatively high success rate, there are potential disadvantages. For CaOH apexification, there may be multiple visits needed for removal and replacement of the CaOH before a hard tissue barrier is formed to allow for standard endodontic therapy. In addition, neither MTA or CaOH apexification procedures allow for continued root development, which, in some cases, may result in a shorter than normal root with less than desirable root-to-crown ratio. Pulp regeneration, the intentional revascularization and regeneration of pulp (or "pulp-like") tissue, has recently become a reality where non-vital, immature teeth may be treated such that pulp tissue is regained, allowing continued root end development in both width, length, increased thickness of dentinal walls, and apical end closure [35–39]. The potential future ramifications may also include eventual treatment of mature non-vital teeth such that it could change the concepts of obturation to allow for regeneration of pulp tissue and regaining vital teeth.

16.8.2 Principles

Pulp revascularization was first described in the 1960s by Professor Nygaard-Ostby and showed some slight promise in getting vascularization to repopulate vital and non-vital immature pulp canals [40]. Since those studies were only slightly successful, the thought of regenerating live pulp tissue into necrotic pulp space lost interest until recently. Recent advances in guided tissue regeneration, stem cell regeneration, newer pulp dressings (MTA), and canal sealing have created a renewed interest in attempts at reestablishing vital pulp tissue within the confines of the pulp canal.

It is important to note the difference in pulp revascularization and pulp regeneration. Pulp revascularization is the intentional regrowth of vascularity (blood vessels) into the pulp canal space in the hope that the other critical components of true pulp tissue also regenerate (neuronal tissue, collagen matrix, and odontoblasts). Pulp regeneration is aimed at intentional and focused regrowth of the entire pulp–dentin complex (blood vessels, nerves, collagen matrix, and odontoblasts [41]. Most clinical procedures use some method of revascularization coupled with advances in canal disinfection/debridement, indirect release of growth factors, and prevention of microleakage. To date, none of the published studies fully engage the concepts of tissue engineering. Instead, these studies are best described as revascularization procedures that attempt to regenerate biologic tissues within the root canal space, without necessarily replicating the pulp–dentin complex [41].

True pulp regeneration focuses on rebuilding all the lost tissues within the pulp canal. This healing has been suggested to be similar to the granulation phase of wound healing where growth factors stimulate the angiogenesis across a fibrin matrix [41]. Certain growth factors such as vascular endothelial growth factor (VEGF) and platelet-derived growth factor (PDGF) enhance this angiogenesis and may be helpful in stimulating revascularization of pulp tissues [42]. Demineralized dentin may release some of these growth factors found in dentin, helping not only to stimulate angiogenesis but also to regulate or enhance odontoblastic activity [41]. This may explain why EDTA has been helpful as an irrigant in pulp regeneration/revascularization. Attempts are also made at sterilizing the pulp canal or ridding the canal of as much bacteria and bacterial byproducts as possible to enhance the healing capabilities. Antibiotic pastes and honey bee resins have been advocated [43, 44]. Other drugs may also enhance odontoblastic activity, such as dexamethasone, insulin, and statin drugs [41]. In addition to growth factors, stem cells may play an important role in pulp regeneration. At least five different mesenchymal cells have been shown to differentiate into odontoblast-like cells: dental pulp stem cells (DPSC), stem cells of human exfoliated deciduous teeth (SHED), stem cells of the apical papilla (SCAP), dental follicle progenitor cells (DFPC), and bone marrow-derived mesenchymal cells (BMMSC). In most clinical cases, the SCAP are utilized to hopefully provide cells that eventually mature into odontoblasts or odontoblast-like cells [41, 43]. The third component of pulp regeneration is scaffolding. Appropriate scaffolding is necessary to provide a spatially correct cell location and regulation of differentiation, proliferation, and metabolism of pulp cells. An ideal scaffolding might bind and localize cells, contain growth factors, and undergo biodegradation over time. Platelet-rich plasma (PRP) has these properties and has been advocated to help with pulp revascularization. At least one study in dogs, however, did not show an enhancement of vascularization pulp tissue [44]. For these reasons, we see these products and materials being tested and incorporated into regenerative endodontic procedures.

16.8.3 Practice

The American Association of Endodontists (AAE) has proposed guidelines to help with protocol for pulp regeneration in human patients (http://www.aae.org/regeneration). These clinical considerations include case selection, informed consent, and protocol suggestions for the two visits and follow-up care. After local anesthesia, tooth isolation, and the access approach, the canal is copiously flushed with dilute NaOCl and then saline or EDTA using an apical negative pressure irrigation with the needle positioned 1 mm from the apical end. Once the canal is dried with paper points, CaOH or a low concentration antibiotic paste is placed. The access is sealed with a temporary restorative material. The second appointment is scheduled one to four weeks later to assess the response to initial treatment and determine if there is persistent infection, at which point additional irrigation and antibiotic placement is recommended. After copious irrigation with 17% EDTA, the canal is dried and then bleeding is stimulated by overinstrumenting with an endo file or explorer 2 mm past the apical opening. If a blood clot (to the level of the cementoenamel junction) cannot be created, PRP, platelet-rich fibrin (PRF), or an autologous fibrin matrix (AFM) can be placed. With the remaining coronal 3–4 mm, a resorbable matrix of a collagen product can be placed over the blood clot, with

MTA as a capping material (some discoloration may occur with MTA). A layer of glass ionomer is then placed over the MTA. Success is measured with the primary goal of the elimination of symptoms and evidence of bone healing. Additional goals include evidence of increased wall thickness and/or increased root length, and ultimately a positive response to vitality testing (more applicable in human dentistry).

16.8.4 Future Possibilities

As mentioned previously, to this point, these procedures have primarily been directed at immature non-vital teeth. In the future, it may be possible to regenerate lost pulp tissue in mature teeth, provided there is an apical foramen or opening to allow integration of surrounding vasculature, either by placing stem cells in the pulp canal or utilization of stem cells from remnants of the apical papilla to develop vital pulp tissue [45]. This may create special challenges in the dog since there is not naturally an apical foramen. It may be possible to instrument through the apical delta or, as was done in one study in dogs, apicoectomy, such that it allows for revascularization and regeneration techniques.

16.9 Surgical Endodontics

16.9.1 Introduction

Complicating factors in or around the apical third of a tooth may prevent its effective conservative standard endodontic treatment. Surgical endodontic procedures such as periradicular drainage, apical and periapical curettage, apical resection (apicoectomy), and retrograde obturation or filling in many cases are the sole alternatives to extraction. Surgical endodontics, although an advanced procedure, should not be considered radical, but another alternative to extraction in select cases. Surgical endodontics in dogs has been described for dogs and the success rate is excellent [46, 47].

16.9.2 Criteria for Selection

The most common indications for surgical treatment is when standard endodontic therapy is not possible or has been ineffective in resolving periapical problems [48]. In these cases, surgical procedures may offer resolution. Factors implicated for such problems are numerous, but typically can be placed in one of two categories, those that have an internal root apex inaccessibility and those with external root end complications.

Inaccessible apices can be present due to a number of reasons. Acute curvature of the canal can occasionally inhibit standard instrumentation, although with newer, highly flexible files, this is not as much of a problem as it once was. Reduced canal dimensions due to secondary or tertiary reparative dentin deposition from age or irritation may result in barrier problems in reaching the apex. Decisions of inaccessibility should not be based on radiographs alone. Many canals can be located with pathfinders and instrumented sufficiently for obturation with fine instruments, lubricants, and chelating agents. Broken instruments lodged in the canal may also prevent instrumentation to the apex. Pulp stones (endoliths), if unremovable or not bypassable, may preclude access to the apical canal. Malformations of the teeth may provide the same hindrances.

External root end complications can also be an indication for surgical endodontic procedures. Among these are failure of radiographic evidence of resolution of periapical destruction within a reasonable period of time (9–12 months). Failure of a periapical lesion to show indications of healing may indicate a periapical cyst formation. Cyst formation typically occurs when the rest of Malassez, an epithelial structure caught in a periapical granuloma, rapidly proliferates due to chronic irritation [49]. Surgical intervention is generally required to address the cystic pathology.

Incomplete root development may be a cause for surgical endodontics, but apexigenesis and apexification should be attempted first. Root fractures in the apical third may prevent complete instrumentation and in these cases surgery to remove the fractured root tips may be required. Perforation of the apex by instruments may necessitate surgical proceedings, but a backup technique to reestablish the apical stop can many times alleviate the condition (Figure 16.7a to c). A periapical ablation technique has been described in human dentistry with deliberate passage of instrumentation to debride and "mince" infected periapical tissues during conventional endodontic therapy. Such a technique is thought to enhance the healing of the area by removing inflammatory tissue, but would only be possible with an apical foramen present [50]. Extrusion of endodontic sealer and filling material will seldom require surgical intervention, unless it is associated with a poor apical seal and a non-healing lesion [46].

16.9.3 Contraindications

There are distinct contraindications for surgical endodontics. These are complex deviations of patient, root, crown, and periodontal health, as well as anatomical location. The patient must be systemically healthy enough to allow for required sedation and anesthesia for the procedure and for reasonable healing of the tissues following surgery [48]. Excessively weak or

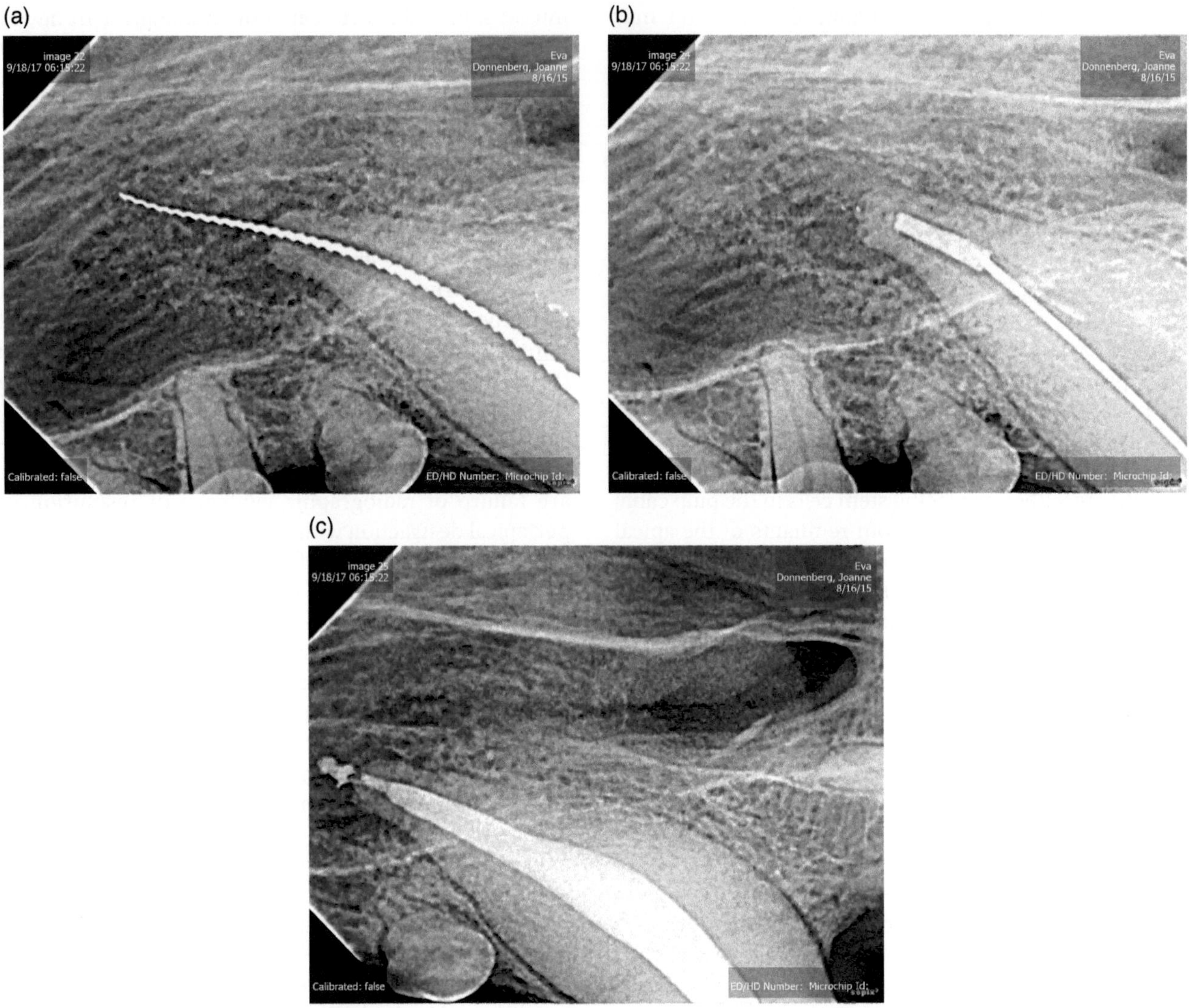

Figure 16.7 (a) Perforation of the apex during standard endodontic therapy; (b) backup technique used to establish an apical stop with placement of a gutta-percha plug and sealer; (c) completed fill with minor extrusion of the gutta-percha material.

damaged roots that require extensive root resection may leave an unfavorable crown-to-root ratio, allowing for easy exfoliation due to trauma or inflammatory disease. If the crown has been damaged beyond reasonable restoration and the root, if saved, serves no useful function, extraction may be best. In cases of advanced periodontal disease, the patient's general health may be best served also by exodontia. Anatomical conditions of the tooth include its location, value of bony support that must be removed for access, and the proximity of neural, vascular, sinus, and other important structures [48]. Location considerations have to do with the ability to attain access and visualize structures. In the anterior portion of the mouth this is not of major concern, but in the posterior region, especially in most herbivores, this can present a problem unless an external access to the mouth is utilized.

The value of the bony support tissue to be removed is also important. In the mandible, the posterior buccal cortical plate thickens. Removal of an excessive support structure to gain access to root apices can lead to a weakened mandible that may be more prone to fracture in the short term until complete healing has taken place. If periodontal or other disease has already compromised the mandibular strength, additional bone removal may not be judicious.

The proximity to various structures and organs must also be considered [48]. Vessels and nerves exiting from the infraorbital canal of the maxilla just above the mesiobuccal root of the maxillary fourth premolar should be located and isolated if needed to prevent their injury. The same is true in the mandible of those vessels and nerves exiting the mental foramina. The roots of the mandibular premolars and molars generally lie just above the mandibular canal except for the first molar's roots, which commonly lie just lateral to the canal. Injury to the structures within the canal can lead to nerve loss and other complications. Additionally, when perforation of a maxillary sinus or mandibular canal occurs, caution must be exercised not to allow debris, root tips, infected bone, or filling materials to be pushed into these openings. Reasonable attempts to remove such material should be made if this happens.

16.9.4 Prognosis

Most studies of prognostic factors associated with surgical endodontics are published for human dentistry, so factors such as age (less than 45 years of age) and the consistent use of microsurgical techniques may not be as applicable to veterinary patients [51, 52]. Other factors can be more relevant, such as the position of the tooth involved (in humans – better outcome with upper anterior or premolar teeth), as apical access is an important aspect, as is the strategic importance of the tooth. Non-cystic lesions that are less than 10 mm in size also tend to have a better outcome, indications that less severe, less chronic lesions (not yet transformed into a cystic lesion) may respond better to treatment [51]. Other factors associated with a better outcome may include the absence of pre-operative signs, teeth with an adequate root-filling length, MTA as root-end filling material, apical resection <3 mm, and teeth not associated with an oroantral fistula [51]. The presence of concurrent periodontal involvement or combined endodontic–periodontic lesions can greatly impact the potential success of surgical endodontic therapy [52, 53]. An apicomarginal defect or communication, particularly with the loss of the buccal bone plate, will typically not respond to endodontic treatment alone. Guided tissue regeneration to control the downgrowth of epithelial proliferation may be needed to manage the periodontal aspect of the lesion (see Chapter 10 – Oral Surgery – Periodontal Surgery).

16.9.5 Apical and Periapical Surgical Endodontic Procedures

Four categories of apical surgical intervention are periradicular drainage, periapical curettage, apical resection or apicoectomy, and retrograde obturation or filling. Each serves a distinct function and are not necessarily linked to one another in every case.

16.9.5.1 Periradicular Drainage

When exudate begins to accumulate due to acute, periapical inflammation, the adjacent alveolar bone can be destroyed [54]. Although not commonly done in the dog and cat, in cases of clinical discomfort when clients would like to preserve a tooth, establishment of periapical drainage to help relieve the pain, swelling, and discomfort may be of benefit. Maintenance of drainage can allow periapical healing and the successful use of standard endodontics in many cases. In an emergency situation, antibiotics, anti-inflammatories, and analgesics may give temporary relief. Drainage can be established by opening the tooth and extirpating the pulp to allow drainage through the tooth. This is primarily done in humans, because in the dog with an apical delta, this is an unreliable technique for complete relief.

Trephination through the bone at the site of periapical swelling can be performed in people to provide relief from pain. In veterinary dentistry, trephination is a primary step in the surgical endodontic procedure, once the site is accessed with an appropriate incision. Incisional site selection should take into consideration local anatomical structures such as vessels, nerves, and foramina. A mucosal/gingival flap should be designed to maintain a good blood supply and provide adequate exposure. Injection with a local anesthetic with epinephrine in a healthy patient can aid in hemorrhage control and post-operative discomfort. A regional block may also be utilized. In most teeth other than the mandibular canine (in dogs and cats), the access incision is made in the alveolar mucosa near the level of the tooth's apex [55] and ends curving apically. For the maxillary canine tooth, a curvilinear incision can be made perpendicular to the root of the maxillary second premolar, in the region of the apical juga [56]. In humans, the coronal-most aspect typically extends into the attached gingiva. This will provide a firm attachment point that prevents the flap from gathering in an irregular mucosal pattern when sutured, which would result in a post-surgical lump. A full thickness mucoperiosteal flap is elevated using a No. 2, 4, or 9 Molt periosteal elevator. Triangular and trapezoidal flaps will provide better exposure, but take longer to implement [46]. For the mandibular canine teeth, aseptic surgical preparation is followed by an incision made in the skin of the ventral mandible parallel to the tooth and centered over the apex [57] (Figure 16.8). The two buccal roots of a maxillary fourth premolar can be accessed in a similar manner, though the palatal root may need to be resected (Figure 16.9a and b).

16.9.5.2 Apical Access

Radiographs should be used to pinpoint the access site, which is generally 1–2 mm coronal to the root apex. The alveolar juga can be used to aid in apical locating, as well as needles or gutta-percha points pre-placed at intervals for radiographs (Figure 16.10). Care should be exerted during access, as an improper approach can result in problems, including drilling above the root tip into other tissues or organs, too lateral an approach resulting in

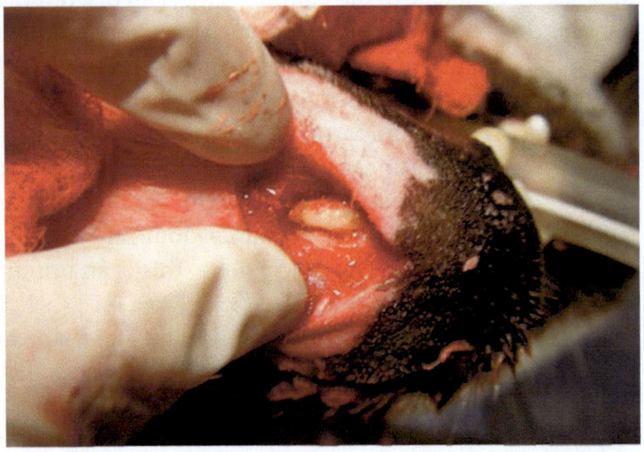

Figure 16.8 Ventral access to the apex of the mandibular canal for surgical endodontic therapy.

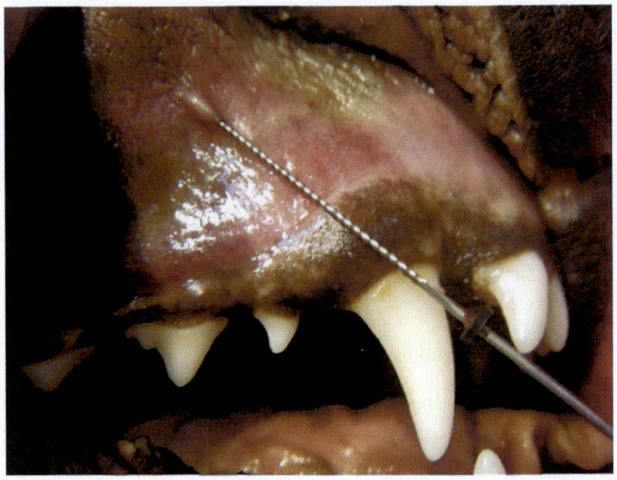

Figure 16.10 Periodontal probe used to help locate the maxillary canine apex.

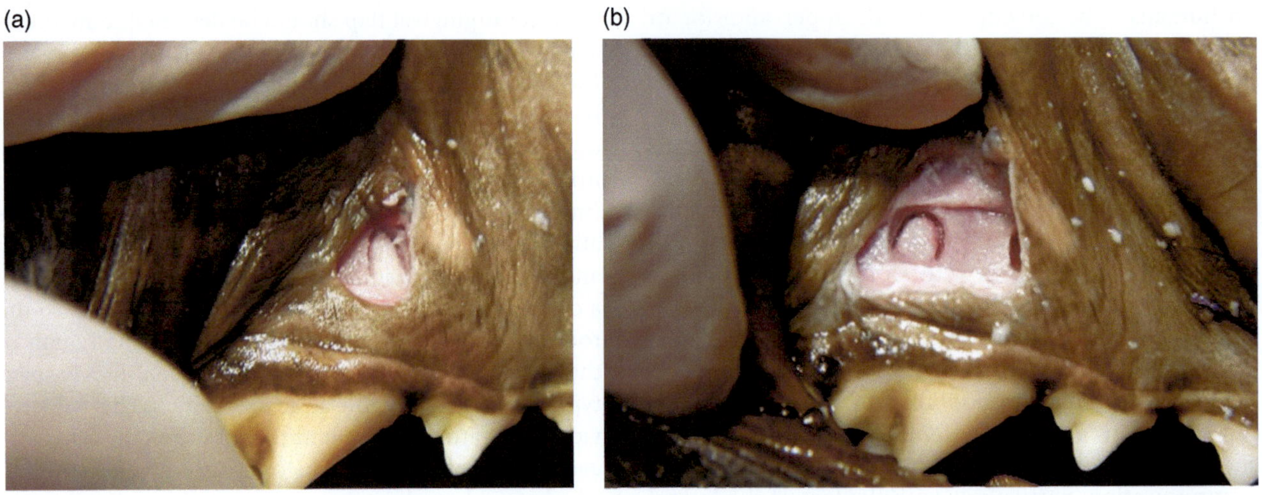

Figure 16.9 Access for surgical endodontic therapy of a maxillary fourth premolar to the apices of: (a) mesiobuccal root; (b) distal root.

damage to adjacent vital teeth, or one taken below the desired point requiring extension of the access. With the bone exposed, a No. 4 or 6 round ball bur on high-speed handpiece, with adequate water flow to prevent thermal injury to the bone, is used to bore a hole through the alveolus and into the diseased periapical space (Figure 16.11). Once the periapical space is encountered, remove the bone for 1–2 mm around the defect and avoid perforating the medial (palatal or lingual) aspect [46] (Figure 16.12).

Providing adequate hemostasis in the surgical field is important for adequate visualization and access. Caustic and styptic agents should be avoided as they can inhibit healing. Collagen-based agents stimulate platelet adhesion and aggregation, aid in the release of coagulation factors, and act mechanically at the wound interface. These materials produce minimal foreign body reactions and interfere minimally with wound healing [48]. As a physical hemostatic agent, regenerated alpha cellulose products serve as an artificial coagulum, but with their slow resorption, healing can be retarded. Gelatin-based sponges can stimulate the clotting pathway, but there is an increase in inflammation and decrease in the rate of healing. The use of bone wax is not recommended, due to poor healing, chronic inflammation, and potential infection. Ferric sulfate can be used, but as a necrotizing agent it must be thoroughly removed at the end of the procedure. Calcium sulfate can be placed in the crypt and allowed to set, carving away a portion to allow access for the procedure. As an alternate bone graft material, the residual material can be removed or left in the site [48]. Epinephrine-soaked cotton pellets can be used directly on the bone (all granulation tissue moved away) with minimal systemic effects [58], but all fibers must be removed. Using epinephrine on collagen pellets avoids the possibility of leaving behind fiber foreign bodies.

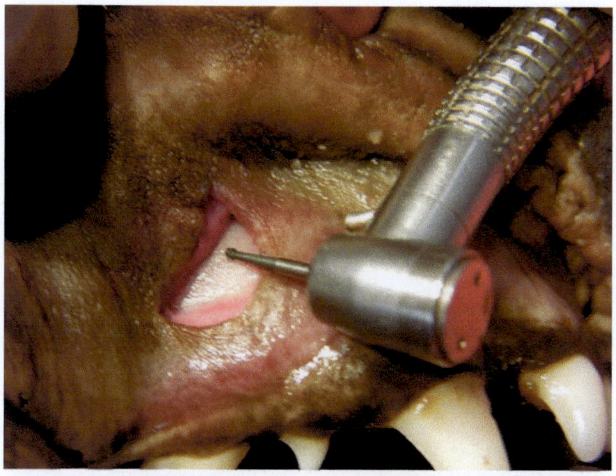

Figure 16.11 After making a semilunar incision to expose the buccal bone, a round bur is used to remove the bone over the apical area.

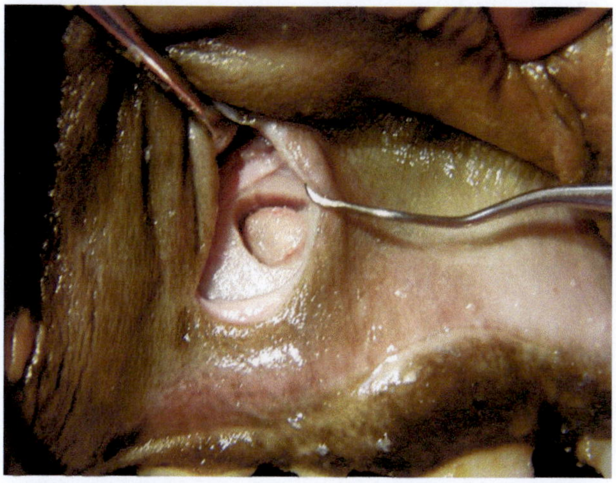

Figure 16.12 The round bur is used to isolate the apex from the surrounding tissue.

16.9.5.3 Periapical Curettage

While it is important to remove the diseased tissue, if the causative irritant is identified and removed, the elimination of all inflamed tissue may not be as critical. In fact, overly aggressive debridement should be avoided if neurovascular structures would be damaged in the process. Using sharp bone and periodontal curettes, the soft tissue should be first peeled away from the lateral extents of the osseous crypt. The remainder of the tissue can be gently debrided out of the lesion and submitted for histopathological assessment.

16.9.5.4 Apical Resection

Apical resection or apicoectomy is performed fundamentally for two reasons, removal of a diseased apex and for retrograde filling access. Resection for the removal of a necrotic or diseased apex is done in order to stimulate healing, in combination with a standard coronal access obturation. Retrograde filling is recommended in conditions where standard access obturation cannot be accomplished due to blockage, or where standard endodontic therapy has repeatedly failed. In either case, one of the most important considerations is the removal or extraction of the apical tip once resectioned. If left in place it will act as a nidus of continued infection, even if an excellent obturation and seal is accomplished.

Once the root tip is isolated it is then resected. This can be accomplished by burs on a standard high-speed or miniature handpiece. A number 57 straight fissure bur or multipurpose bur will produce a smoother cut than a cross-cut fissure bur, and the surface can be finished with a multifluted carbide or ultrafine diamond bur. At least 3 mm of the apex should be removed to include most of the accessory and lateral canals, and any lesions. A 45° resection of the apex allows for better visibility of the canal, but with enhanced magnification and illumination (microsurgical attributes), there is less of a need for a beveled resection [48]. While the 45° angle may improve access, at times the medial aspect of the root may not be sufficiently removed [48]. A perpendicular resection exposes less dentinal tubules and distributes stress forces evenly [46, 59]. An elevator is used to loosen the root tip and forceps for its removal (Figure 16.13). The exposed periapical tissues should be curetted clean.

16.9.5.5 Retrograde Obturation or Filling

The type of cavity preparation for a retrograde filling is generally one of two types: a Class I cavity prep or a modified preparation known as the slot of Matzuri [46]. The Class I preparation is customarily preferred (and is always the preparation when using a piezoelectric handpiece) when location allows, as less bone and tooth structure require removal [46].

The Class I preparation is made using a small round ball bur or a coated tip on an ultrasonic handpiece [48]. The bur or piezo tip is inserted into the apical exposure of the canal to a depth of 3–5 mm (Figure 16.14). Because of the restricted space being worked in, a small piezo tip with 90° angle or a microhead handpiece and microburs may be required [48]. While one evaluation minimizes the concern that an ultrasonic tip can make the apex prone to fracture, due to vibration and strain, it did show an increase in the amount of debris covering the cavity wall [60].

When root location, anatomy, or handpiece size prevents a Class I preparation, the slot of Matzuri may be applicable. The root tip is resected as previously described, although additional buccal bone may need to be removed for extension of the slot. The tip of a tapered fissure bur is placed in the apical opening of the root canal perpendicular to the long axis of the root. A 3–5 mm

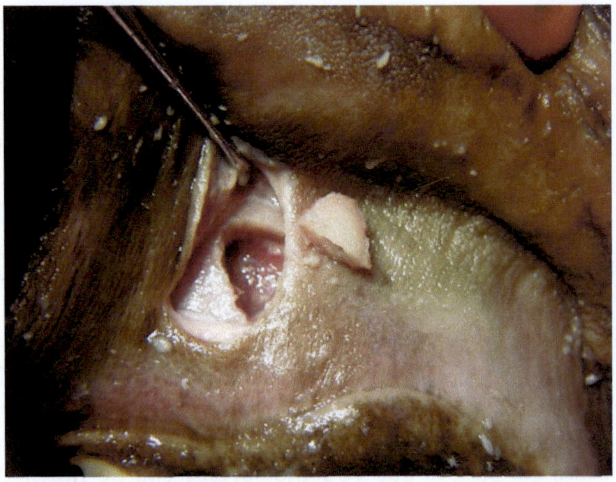

Figure 16.13 The apical tip is removed.

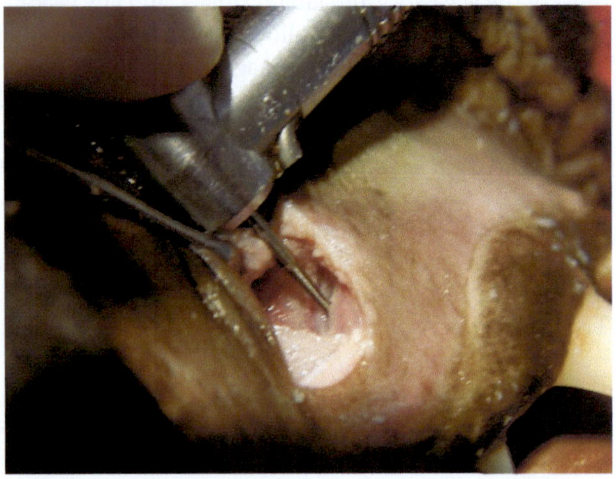

Figure 16.14 The apical opening is prepped.

long slot is then cut in the root directed coronally. A small round ball bur is placed at the apical canal opening perpendicular to the root and passed down the slot to its coronal most extent and then pulled through the lateral wall, creating an undercut and keyhole-like appearing preparation [46]. Root end conditioning to enhance fibroblast attachment can be performed, though citric acid can compromise the surrounding tissues [48]. While EDTA will be less damaging to the tissues, it can interfere with the setting of MTA, if that is to be used.

Selection of the retrograde filling material is the next consideration. Amalgam was used successfully for many years, but has been losing popularity of late to newer products. If used, generally a zinc-free, high copper is preferred, but not required [61]. Both zinc and zinc-free amalgam is well tolerated and effective, when placed and compacted in a dry preparation and environment [62]. If zinc amalgams are placed or worked in even slight moisture an expansion of 4% and more may occur

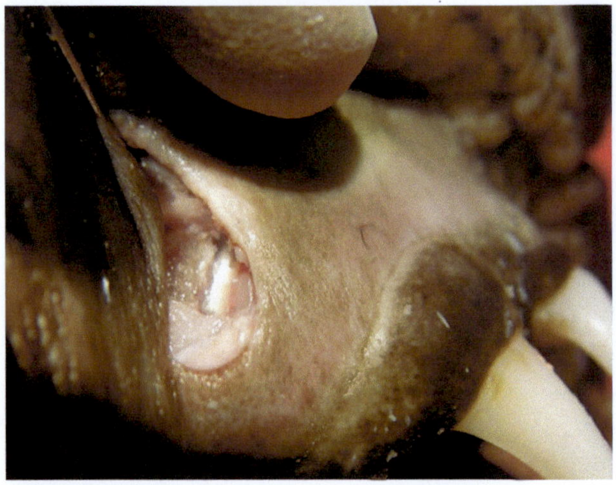

Figure 16.15 The filling material is placed and packed into the apical access.

[63, 64], which can result in creep, restorative, and root fractures, loss of the apical seal, and failure of the procedure. Regardless of the type of amalgam used, a good undercut and the use of a cavity varnish in a dry environment greatly improves apical seal and long-term success [65, 66].

Other products that have been used include zinc oxide eugenol cements and combinations, glass ionomer cement, composite resins, resin–glass ionomer hybrids, and MTA [48]. At this time, the zinc oxide cements or MTA are currently the recommended products for retrograde filling in veterinary dentistry [56, 57, 67]. MTA is composed primarily of tricalcium silicate, tricalcium aluminate, tricalcium oxide, and silicate oxide. In numerous studies, MTA has shown to have less marginal gap formation, less leakage, and better biocompatibility and less cytotoxicity than amalgam, Super EBA, or IRM [31]. Once placed and compacted into cavity preparation (Figure 16.15), excess material is removed with dry or lightly moistened cotton pellets and a dental radiograph is taken to evaluate the retrograde filling (Figure 16.16). MTA sets in the presence of moisture and has a hardening time of three to four hours [46]. CEMs have a shorter setting time and have been associated with a regenerative periapical tissue response, similar to MTA [68].

Closure begins with cleaning of the osseous access site. If bone wax, cotton pellets, or gauze where properly placed, their careful withdrawal typically removes all debris. Gentle lavage with sterile saline should remove any small loose particles. Regenerative materials can be placed at this time, if deemed necessary [48]. The mucosal/gingival flap is sutured closed, apposing the cut mucosa with 4-0 or 5-0 absorbable sutures in a simple interrupted pattern and closing the dermal layer for a mandibular canine.

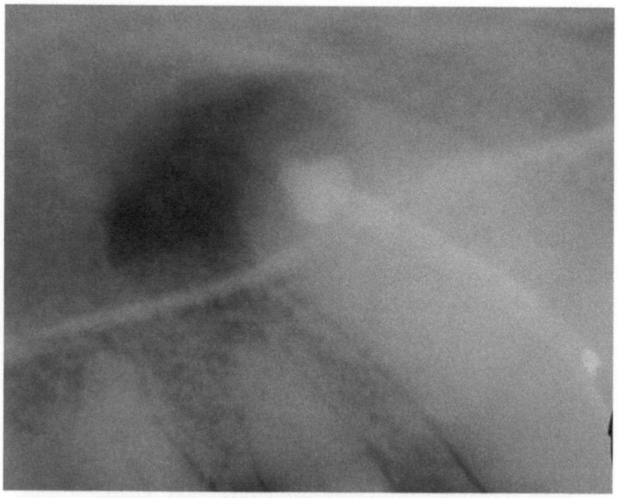

Figure 16.16 Radiograph of completed apicoectomy and fill.

16.10 American Veterinary Dental College (AVDC) Resource – Abbreviations

See Table 16.1.

Table 16.1 AVDC abbreviation list for advanced endodontic therapy (https://www.avdc.org/traineeinfo.html; accessed March 3, 2018).

	Definition
FX	Fracture (tooth or jaw; see T/FX for tooth fracture abbreviations)
HS	Hemisection
PCD	Direct pulp capping
PCI	Indirect pulp capping
RCT	Standard root canal therapy
RCT/S	Surgical root canal therapy
RO/X	Root resection/amputation

References

1 Kuntsi-Vaattovaara, H., Verstraete, F.J.M., and Kass, P.H. (2002). Results of root canal treatment in dogs: 127 cases (1995–2000). *J. Am.Vet. Med. Assoc.* 220 (6): 775–780.
2 Gutmann, J.L. and Lovdahl, P.E. (2006). Problems encountered in access to the pulp chamber space. In: *Problem Solving in Endodontics*, 4e (ed. J.L. Gutmann, T.C. Dumsha and P.E. Loudahl). St. Louis, MO: Elsevier.
3 Wiggs, R.B. (1993). Problem solving in veterinary endodontics. *J. Semin. Vet. Med. Surg. (Small Anim.)* 8 (3): 165.
4 Marretta, S.M., Golab, G., Anthony, J.M. et al. (1992). Development of a teaching model for coronal access to the canine dentition. *J. Vet. Dent.* 9 (4): 7–11.
5 Eisner, E.R. (1990). Transcoronal approach for endodontic access to the fourth maxillary premolar in dogs. *J. Vet. Dent.* 7 (4): 22.
6 Vertucci, F.J. and Haddix, J.F. (2011). Tooth morphology and access. In: *Cohen's Pathways of the Pulp*, 10e (ed. K.M. Hargreaves and S. Cohen), 136–222. St. Louis, MO: Mosby-Elsevier.
7 Gioso, M.A., Knobl, T., Venturini, M.A., and Correa, H.L. (1997). Non-apical root canal ramifications in the teeth of dogs. *J. Vet. Dent.* 14 (3): 89–90.
8 Wiggs, R.B. (1987). Pulpotomy: a case report. *J. Vet. Dent.* 4 (2): 6.
9 Wiggs, R.B. (1991). Endodontic instrumentation. *J. Vet. Dent.* 8 (4): 11.
10 Kerns, D.G. and Glickman, G.N. (2011). Endodontic and periodontic interrelationships. In: *Cohen's Pathways of the Pulp*, 10e (ed. K.M. Hargreaves and S. Cohen), 655–670. St. Louis, MO: Mosby-Elsevier.
11 Roda, R.S. and Gettleman, B.H. (2011). Nonsurgical treatment. In: *Cohen's Pathways of the Pulp*, 10e (ed. K.M. Hargreaves and S. Cohen), 890–953. St. Louis, MO: Mosby-Elsevier.
12 Chenail, B.L. and Teplitsky, P.E. (1987). Orthograde ultrasonic retrieval of root canal obstructions. *J. Endod.* 13 (4): 186–190.
13 Reiter, A.M., Lewis, J.R., Rawlinson, J.E., and Gracis, M. (2005). Hemisection and partial retention of carnassial teeth in client-owned dogs. *J. Vet. Dent.* 22 (4): 216–226.
14 Peters, O.A. and Peters, C.J. (2011). Cleaning and shaping of the root canal system. In: *Cohen's Pathways of the Pulp*, 10e (ed. K.M. Hargreaves and S. Cohen), 283–349. St. Louis, MO: Mosby-Elsevier.
15 Waterhouse, P.J., Whitworth, J.M., Camp, J.H., and Fuks, A.B. (2011). Pediatric endodontics. In: *Cohen's Pathways of the Pulp*, 10e (ed. K.M. Hargreaves and S. Cohen), 808–858. St. Louis, MO: Mosby-Elsevier.
16 Emily, P. (1990; 2(1)). Problems associated with the diagnosis and treatment of endodontic disease. In: *Problems in Veterinary Medicine, Dentistry* (ed. S.M. Marretta), 152. Philadelphia, PA: JP Lippincott Co.
17 Asgary, S., Parirokh, M., Eghbal, M.J., and Ghoddusi, J. (2007). SEM evaluation of pulp reaction to different pulp capping materials in dogs' teeth. *IEJ* 1 (4): 117–123.
18 Tziafa, D., Belibasakis, G., Veis, A., and Papadimitriou, S. (2001). Dental regeneration in vital pulp therapy: design principles. *Adv. Dent. Res.* 15: 96–100.

19 Clarke, D.E. (2001). Vital pulp therapy for complicated crown fracture of permanent canine teeth in dogs: a three-year retrospective study. *J. Vet. Dent.* 18 (3): 117–121.

20 Niemiec, B.A. (2001). Assessment of vital pulp therapy for nine complicated crown fractures and fifty-four crown reductions in dogs and cats. *J. Vet. Dent.* 18 (3): 122–125.

21 Luotonen, N., Kuntsi-Vaattovaara, H., Sarkiala-Kessel, E. et al. (2013). Vital pulp therapy in dogs: 190 cases (2001–2011). *J. Am. Vet. Med. Assoc.* 244 (4): 449–459.

22 Schuurs, A.H.B., Gruythuysen, R.J.M., and Wesselink, P.R. (2000). Pulp capping with adhesive resin-based composite vs calcium hydroxide: a review. *Endod. Dent. Traumatol.* 16: 240–250.

23 Torabinejad, M., Hong, C.U., McDonald, F., and Pitt Ford, T.R. (1995). Physical and chemical properties of a new root-end filling material. *J. Endod.* 21 (7): 349–353.

24 Asgary, S., Eghbal, M.J., Parirokh, M. et al. (2006 April). SEM evaluation of neodentinal bridging after direct pulp protection with mineral trioxide aggregate. *J. Aust. Soc. Endod.* 32(1): 26–32(1): 30.

25 Asgary, S., Eghbal, M.J., Parirokh, M., and Torabzadeh, H. (2006). Sealing abilities of three commercial mineral trioxide aggregates and an experimental root-end filling material. *IEJ* 1 (3): 101–105.

26 Cvek, M. et al. (1982). Pulp reactions to exposure after experimental crown fracture or grinding in adult monkey. *J. Endod.* 8: 391.

27 Heide, S. (1983). Pulp reactions to exposure for 4, 24 and 168 hours. *J. Dent. Res.* 59: 1910.

28 Sigurdsson, A.M., Trope, M., and Chivian, N. (2011). The role of endodontics after dental traumatic injuries. In: *Cohen's Pathways of the Pulp*, 10e (ed. K.M. Hargreaves and S. Cohen), 620–654. St. Louis, MO: Mosby-Elsevier.

29 Cvek, M. (1978). A clinical report on partial pulpotomy and capping with calcium hydroxide in permanent incisors with complicated crown fractures. *J. Endod.* 4: 232.

30 Andreasen, J.O., Farik, B., and Munksgaard, E.C. (2002). Long-term calcium hydroxide as a root canal dressing may increase risk of root fracture. *Endod. Dent. Traumatol.* 18: 134–137.

31 Gatewood, R.S. (2007). Endodontic materials. *Dent. Clin. North Am.* 51 (3): 705–706.

32 Torneck, C.D. (1982). Effects and clinical significance of trauma to the developing permanent dentition. *Dent. Clin. North Am.* 26 (3): 481–504.

33 Juriga, S., Manfra Maretta, S., and Weeks, S.M. (2008). Endodontic treatment of a non-vital permanent tooth with and open apex using mineral trioxide aggregate. *J. Vet. Dent.* 25 (3): 189–195.

34 Felippe, M.C.S., Felippe, W.T., Marques, M.M., and Antoniazzi, J.H. (2005). The effect of the renewal of calcium hydroxide paste on the apexification and periapical healing of teeth with incomplete root formation. *IEJ* 38: 436–442.

35 Banchs, F. and Trope, M. (2004). Revascularization of immature permanent teeth with apical periodontitis: new treatment protocol? *J. Endod.* 30 (4): 196–200.

36 Chueh, L.H. and Huang, G.T. (2006). Immature teeth with periradicular periodontitis or abscess undergoing apexogenesis: a paradigm shift. *J. Endod.* 32 (12): 1205–1213.

37 Iwaya, S.I., Ikawa, M., and Kubota, M. (2001). Revascularization of an immature permanent tooth with apical periodontitis and sinus tract. *Dent. Traumatol.* 17 (4): 185–187.

38 Shah, N., Logani, A., Bhaskar, U., and Aggarwal, V. (2008). Efficacy of revascularization to induce apexification/apexogenesis in infected, non-vital, immature teeth: a pilot clinical study. *J. Endod.* 34 (8): 919–925.

39 Tawfik, H., Abu-Seida, A.M., Hashem, A.A., and Nagy, M.M. (2013). Regenerative potential following revascularization of immature permanent teeth with necrotic pulps. *Int. Endod. J.* 46 (10): 910–922. Epub 2013 Mar 11.

40 Ostby, B.N. (1961). The role of the blood clot in endodontic therapy: an experimental histologic study. *Acta Odontol. Scand.* 19: 324–353.

41 Hargreaves, K.M. and Law, A.S. (2011). Regenerative endodontics. In: *Cohen's Pathways of the Pulp*, 10e (ed. K.M. Hargreaves and S. Cohen), 602–619. St. Louis, MO: Mosby-Elsevier.

42 Rodríguez-Benítez, S., Stambolsky, C., Gutiérrez-Pérez, J.L. et al. (2015). Pulp revascularization of immature dog teeth with apical periodontitis using triantibiotic paste and platelet-rich plasma: a radiographic study. *J. Endod.* 41 (8): 1299–1304. Epub 2015 Jun 14.

43 Chalisserry, E.P., Nam, S.Y., Park, S.H., and Anil, S. (2017). Therapeutic potential of dental stem cells. *J. Tissue Eng.* 8: 1–17.

44 Moradi, S., Talati, A., Forghani, M. et al. (2016). Immunohistological evaluation of revascularized immature permanent necrotic teeth treated by platelet-rich plasma: an animal investigation. *Cell J.* 18 (3): 389–396. Epub 2016 Aug 24.

45 Laureys, W.G., Cuvelier, C.A., Dermaut, L.R., and De Pauw, G.A. (2013). The critical apical diameter to obtain regeneration of the pulp tissue after tooth transplantation, replantation, or regenerative endodontic treatment. *J. Endod.* 39 (6): 759–763.

46 Hennet, P. and Gomez, N. (2005). Surgical endodontics in dogs: a review. *J. Vet. Dent.* 22 (3): 148–158.

47 Fulton, A., Fiani, N., Arzi, B. et al. (2012). Outcome of surgical endodontic treatment in dogs: 15 cases (1995–2011). *JAVMA* 241 (12): 1633–1638.
48 Johnson, B.R. and Fayad, M.I. (2011). Witherspoon. Periradicular surgery. In: *Cohen's Pathways of the Pulp*, 10e (ed. K.M. Hargreaves and S. Cohen), 720–776. St. Louis, MO: Mosby-Elsevier.
49 Luukko, K., Kettunen, P., Fristad, I., and Berggreen, E. (2011). Structure and functions of the dentin-pulp complex. In: *Cohen' Pathways of the Pulp*, 10e (ed. K.M. Hargreaves and S. Cohen), 452–503. St. Louis, MO: Mosby-Elsevier.
50 Metzger, Z., Huber, R., Tobis, I., and Better, H. (2009). Enhancement of healing kinetics of periapical lesions in dogs by the Apexum procedure. *J. Endod.* 35 (1): 40–45.
51 Serrano-Gimenez, M., Sanchez-Torres, A., and Gay-Escoda, C. (2015). Prognostic factors on periapical surgery: a systematic review. *Med. Oral Patol. Oral Cir. Bucal* 20 (6): e715–e722.
52 Von Arx, T. (2011). Apical surgery: a review of current techniques and outcome. *Saudi Dent. J.* 23: 9–15.
53 Rosenberg, P.A. and Frisbie, J.C. (2011). Case selection and treatment planning. In: *Cohen's Pathways of the Pulp*, 10e (ed. K.M. Hargreaves and S. Cohen), 71–87. St. Louis, MO: Mosby-Elsevier.
54 Lin, L.M. and Huang, G.T.J. (2011). Pathobiology of the periapex. In: *Cohen's Pathways of the Pulp*, 10e (ed. K.M. Hargreaves and S. Cohen), 529–558. St. Louis, MO: Mosby-Elsevier.
55 Manfra Marretta, S., Eurell, J.A., and Klippert, L. (1994). Development of a teaching model for surgical endodontic access sites in the dogs. *J. Vet. Dent.* 11 (3): 89–93.
56 Luskin, I.R. and Smith, M.M. (2004). Step by step: surgical endodontics of the maxillary canine tooth. *J. Vet. Dent.* 21 (1): 53–58.
57 Niemiec, B.A. (2006). Step by step: surgical endodontic therapy of the mandibular canine tooth. *J. Vet. Dent.* 23 (1): 62–66.
58 Vy, C.H., Baumgartner, J.C., and Marshall, J.G. (2004). Cardiovascular effects and efficacy of a hemostatic agent in periradicular surgery. *J. Endod.* 30 (6): 379–383.
59 Mauger, M.J., Schindler, W.G., and Walker, W.A. (1996). An evaluation of canal morphology at different levels of root resection in mandibular incisors. *J. Endod.* 24 (9): 607–609.
60 Brent, P.D., Morgan, L.A., Marshall, G., and Baumgartner, J.C. (1999). Evaluation of diamond-coated ultrasonic instruments for root-end preparation. *J. Endod.* 25 (10): 672–675.
61 Arens, D.E. (1991). Surgical endodontics. In: *Pathways to the Pulp*, 5e (ed. S. Cohen and R.C. Burns), 574. Philadelphia, PA: Mosby Year Book.
62 Kimura, J. (1982). A comparative analysis of zinc and non-zinc alloys in retrograde endodontic surgery, 1: Apical seal and tissue reaction. *J. Endod.* 8 (8): 359.
63 Liggett, W.R. et al. (1980). Light microscopy, scanning electron microscopy, and microprobe analysis of bone response to zinc and non-zinc amalgam implants. *Oral Surg.* 49: 263.
64 Zartner, R., James, G., and Birch, B. (1976). Bone tissue response to zinc polycarboxylate cement and zinc-free amalgam. *J. Endod.* 2: 203.
65 Abdal, A.K., Retief, H.D., and Jamison, H.C. (1982). The apical seal via retrosurgical approach, II, an evaluation of retrofilling materials. *Oral Surg.* 54: 213.
66 Tronstad, L. et al. (1983). Sealing ability of dental amalgam as retrograde fillings in endodontic therapy. *J. Endod.* 9: 551.
67 Eisner, E.R. (2012). Apicoectomy techniques. In: *Oral and Maxillofacial Surgery in Dogs and Cats*, 221–232. St. Louis, MO, Saunders Elsevier.
68 Asgary, S., Eghbal, M.J., and Ehsani, S. (2010). Periradicular regeneration after endodontic surgery with calcium-enriched mixture cement in dogs. *J. Endo.* 36 (5): 837–841.

17

Restorative Dentistry

Anthony Caiafa[1] and Louis Visser[2]

[1] School of Veterinary and Biomedical Sciences, James Cook University, Townsville, Queensland, Australia
[2] Arizona Veterinary Dental Specialists, Scottsdale, AZ, USA

17.1 Introduction

Operative dentistry is that field of dentistry concerned with restoring defective areas of vital and non-vital teeth back to normal masticatory function, periodontal health, and esthetics. Defects can be due to disease, infection, trauma, or abnormal development. Operative dentistry includes the application of material and instrument science in the treatment planning and restoration of the teeth.

17.2 Restorative Terminology

Many areas and concepts of restorative and prosthodontic therapy overlap (see Chapter 18 – Crowns and Prosthodontics), with other basic terminology covered in Chapter 1 (Oral Anatomy and Physiology). Specific terms relevant to restoration are covered here:

- *Enamel prisms.* Basic keyhole-shaped enamel units running from the dentinoenamel junction to the surface of the tooth.
- *Contact point.* The point or area of contact between the proximal surface of one tooth to the proximal surface of the neighboring tooth. For incisor teeth, the contact point tends to be closer to the incisal margin, whereas in caudal teeth, the contact point is more apical.
- *Embrasures.* V-shaped spaces located between the proximal surfaces of adjacent teeth and located both incisally/occlusally and apical to the contact point of two teeth. Applicable to incisors and caudal teeth.
- *Biologic width* [1]. The combined width of the connective tissue and the epithelial attachment to the tooth above the crestal alveolar bone.
- *Undercut.* A designed feature of a restorative preparation created by removing a portion of the dentin within the preparation for the intention of providing retentive qualities to a restoration. Often used for retention of amalgam restorations.
- *Overhang.* An excess of restoration projecting beyond the parameters of a preparation margin resulting in a projection or shoulder. Overhangs can lead to accelerated periodontal disease.
- *Flashing.* Restorative that extends beyond the preparation outline, but when initially placed does not cause an overhang.
- *Sealer.* A cavity sealer is a material that seals the dentinal tubules and provides a protective coating for the freshly cut tooth structure of the prepared cavity.
- *Liner.* A cavity liner is an aqueous or volatile organic suspension or dispersion of zinc oxide or calcium hydroxide that can be applied to a cavity surface in a relatively thin film. Glass-ionomer cement (GIC) and resin-modified glass ionomer cement (RMGIC) are also suitable for use as lining materials.
- *Base.* A cavity base is a material, usually a type of cement, used to base a prepared cavity before the insertion of a permanent restoration, to protect the pulp and act as a dentine replacement. RMGICs are popular choices here.
- *Pin.* A metal pin or wire cemented or threaded into the dentin at a preparation site to aid in retention of a restoration.
- *Post.* A cylindrical metal or fiber rod cemented or threaded into the root canal system as a retentive device for a core or post and crown. Posts are used to support the crown core.
- *Core.* A direct or indirectly made substructure for a crown, which may be part of a post and core system.

Wiggs's Veterinary Dentistry: Principles and Practice, Second Edition. Edited by Heidi B. Lobprise and Johnathon R. (Bert) Dodd.

17.2.1 Surfaces of Teeth [2]

When describing a cavity or restoration, the location can be described by the surfaces of the tooth that are involved. These are as follows:

- *Mesial.* Nearest to the midline of dental arch
- *Distal.* Further from the midline of dental arch
- *Labial.* Next to lips (anterior teeth)
- *Buccal.* Next to cheeks (posterior teeth)
- *Lingual.* Next to tongue (lower teeth)
- *Palatal.* Next to palate (upper teeth)
- *Incisal.* Cutting edge of anterior teeth
- *Occlusal.* Chewing surface of posterior teeth.

17.2.2 Classifications of Cavities and Restorations

In order to properly treat lesions, they are best classified as to the tooth involved, type, and extent of lesion. Individual tooth identification systems can be found in the chapter on oral examination (see Chapter 2 – Oral Examination and Diagnosis). The following are some of the more common tooth pathology classifications dealing with type and extent. Classification by location includes the G.V. Black Modified Cavity Preparation Classification system (Table 17.1 and Figure 17.1), the Elementary Cavity Class, and the Practical Cavity Classifications.

Table 17.1 G.V. Black modified cavity preparation classification system.

Class I	I, PM, M	Beginning in structural defects, such as pit or fissure, commonly found on occlusal surfaces (occlusal lesions)
Class II	PM, M	Proximal surfaces; when a tooth with a class 2 lesion includes a class 1, it is still considered as class 2 (proximal surfaces posterior/caudal teeth)
Class III	I, C	Proximal surfaces, incisal angle not included (proximal surfaces anterior/rostral teeth)
Class IV	I, C	Proximal surfaces, incisal angle included (proximal surfaces anterior/rostral teeth involving the incisal angle)
Class V	I, C, PM, M	Facial or lingual, gingival third; excluding pit or fissure lesions (cervical surfaces)
Class VI	I, C, PM, M	Defect of incisal edge or cusp; not included in Black's original classification.

Note: There may also be two separate lesions present on the same tooth (i.e., Class II, Class V) or a combination lesion where two locations are present and contiguous (i.e., Class II/V).

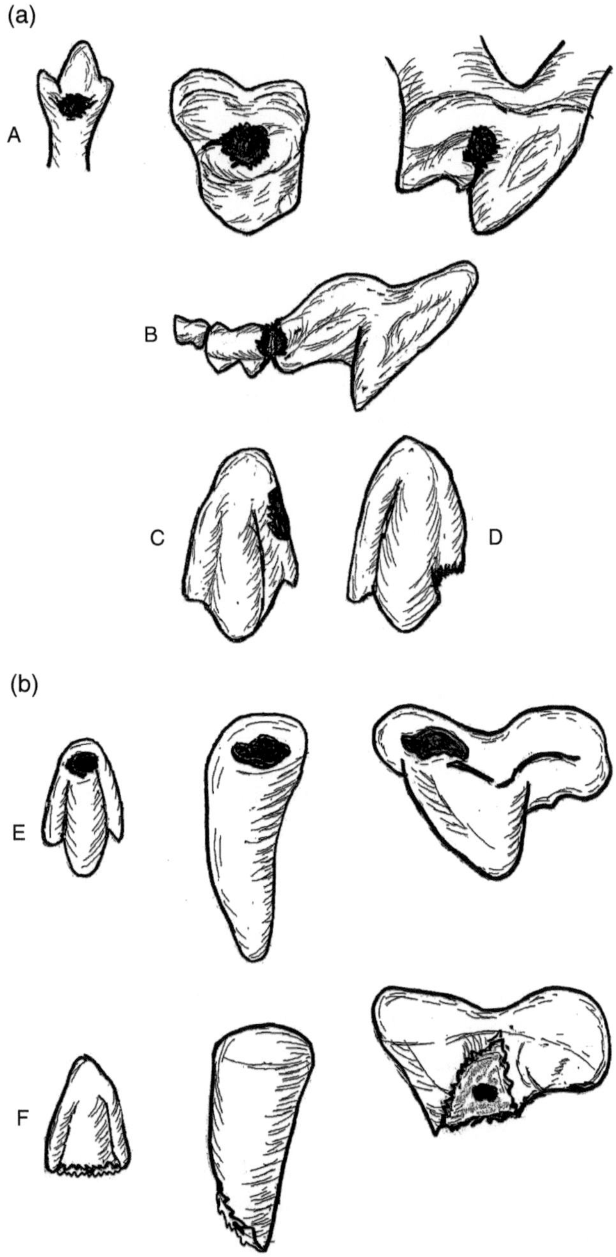

Figure 17.1 (a) The modified G.V. Black lesion and cavity preparation classification system (illustration by Anthony Caiafa adapted from the First Edition). A: Class I – lesions beginning in pits, fissures, or developmental grooves of teeth (from left to right): developmental groove on the lingual surface of an incisor; pits and fissures on occlusal surfaces of premolar and molars; buccal surface developmental groove of maxillary fourth premolar. B: Class II – lesions of the proximal surfaces of premolars and molars. C: Class III – lesions of the proximal surface of an incisor or canine tooth. D: Class IV – lesions at the proximal surface of an incisor or canine tooth that involves an incisal edge. (b) E: Lesions on labial, buccal, or lingual surfaces of an incisor, cuspid, premolar, or molar. F: Lesions of the incisal edge or cusp tip (illustration by Anthony Caiafa adapted from the First Edition).

17.2.2.1 Elementary Cavity Class [3]

- *Simple.* Involving only one tooth surface.
- *Compound.* Involving two tooth surfaces, when prepared.
- *Complex.* Involving three or more tooth surfaces, when prepared.

Practical Cavity Classification [3] (Note that descriptions with "facial" are more appropriate for human dentistry):

- O – Occlusal
- MO – Mesio-occlusal, or the mesial and occlusal surfaces
- DO – Disto-occlusal
- MOD – Mesio-occluso-distal
- B – Buccal
- L – Lingual
- F – Facial (labial or buccal)
- I – Incisal
- DI – Distoincisal
- MI – Mesioincisal
- MID – Mesioincisodistal
- DL – Distolingual
- ML – Mesiolingual
- MLD – Mesiolingodistal
- MF – Mesiofacial
- DF – Distofacial
- MFD – Mesiofaciodistal.

17.2.3 Dental Fracture Class

The American Veterinary Dental College (AVDC) Nomenclature classification of dental fractures can be found in Chapter 6 (Traumatic Dentoalveolar Injuries – TDI), along with discussion of expanding these descriptions to include root fractures, luxation, and alveolar injuries [4]. A previously used staging classification is listed below, but it is recognized that a more complete nomenclature listing may be needed. This more inclusive system would identify fractures into the enamel (Stages 1 and 8 below), enamel–dentin fracture (Stages 2 and 8), enamel-dentin-pulp fracture (Stages 3, 4, and 9), root fractured and displacement/avulsion (see Chapter 6 – TDI). Additional classification of tooth resorption (TR) can be found in Chapter 20 – Domestic Feline Oral and Dental Diseases. Generally, these TR lesions are not restored.

17.2.4 Staging of Tooth Injuries [5, 6]

These are generally referred to as stages and are used in combination with Black's Modified Classification of tooth lesion locations (classification by extent of pathology).

Stage:

1) Simple fracture of the enamel.
2) Fracture extends into the dentin.
3) Fracture extends into the pulp chamber; pulp vital.
4) Fracture extends into the pulp chamber; pulp non-vital.
5) Tooth displaced.
6) Tooth avulsed.
7) Root fracture; no coronal involvement; tooth stable.
8) Root fracture; combined with stages 1–2 coronal fracture; tooth stable.
9) Root fracture; combined with stage 3 coronal fracture; tooth stable.
10) Root fracture; in combination with stages 1–4; unstable tooth.

17.2.5 AVDC Dental Abbreviations – Restorative AVDC Nomenclature

See Table 17.2.

Table 17.2 AVDC abbreviations – restorative (https://www.avdc.org/traineeinfo.html; accessed 25 October 2017).

AB	Abrasion
AT	Attrition
C	Caries
DP	Defect preparation (prior to filling a dental defect)
E	Enamel
E/D	Enamel defect
E/H	Enamel hypoplasia
E/HM	Enamel hypomineralization
PCB	Post-and-core buildup
PCD	Direct pulp capping
PCI	Indirect pulp capping
R	Restoration (filling of a dental defect)
R/A	Filling made of amalgam
R/C	Filling made of composite
R/CP	Filling made of compomer
R/I	Filling made of glass ionomer
T/FX	Tooth fracture
T/NE	Tooth near pulp exposure
T/PE	Tooth/pulp exposure
Other abbreviations that may be found:	
DB	Dentin bonding agent
P&F	Pit and fissure
P&FS	Pit and fissure sealer
SI	Staining, intrinsic (blood, tetracycline, etc.)
SE	Staining, extrinsic (metal, food etc.)
VBL	Vital bleaching
NVBL	Non-vital bleaching
VER	Veneer

17.3 Dental Defense Mechanisms

In human dentistry, dentinal and pulpal inflammation and pain responses are considered to be some of the first diagnostic indicators of pathology and initiators of the dentinal defense mechanism [7]. In animal patients the pain response is not as useful due to the fact that responses may be challenging to elicit.

17.3.1 Successful Dental Defense Mechanism Sequence

1) Pain (sensible dentin).
2) Pulpitis (reversible).
3) Blockage of tubule with material from dentinal fluid or odontoblast.
4) Mineralization of material at exposed dentinal tubule surface and apertures.
5) Formation of sclerotic or tertiary (reparative) dentin at the site.

17.3.1.1 Pain

In order to understand the pain response of the tooth and its defense mechanism, a fundamental knowledge of the dentinal tubules and pulp is required. There are approximately 30 000–40 000 dentinal tubules per square millimeter of surface dentin [7]. In most domestic animals the odontoblastic process extends 0.2–1.5 mm into the dentinal tubule. In addition, there may be an afferent nerve fiber extending into the tubule 0.1–0.4 mm from the pulp. These fibers are sensory nociceptors, either A-delta or C-type fibers. A-delta fibers are larger in diameter, are myelinated, and conduct nerve impulses more rapidly. They typically cause a rapid, sharp type of pain, often associated with a level of pulpitis that is still reversible. C-type fibers are myelinated, have a smaller diameter, conduct impulses more slowly and elicit dull aches, as found in late pulpitis. As the response to thermal stimuli intensifies, the pain lasts well after the stimulus is removed. This inflamed pulp undergoes an irreversible change (irreversible pulpitis leading eventually to pulp necrosis). The tooth then will respond markedly to hot stimuli with cold stimuli potentially having a soothing effect on the tooth (an ice pack now relieves the pain).

If a tooth responds to pain, it is said to have sensible dentin, which can provoke pulpal inflammation or pulpitis. While the presence of sensible dentin implies that a tooth is still vital, it does not necessarily indicate if the pulpitis is reversible or irreversible. Insensible dentin is generally indicative of a non-vital tooth [8], though there can be areas of dentin in which there are no neural fibers in the tubules to elicit a pain response [9]. This can result in an insensible dentin response in a healthy vital tooth.

It is interesting to note that while the afferent nerve endings respond to a variety of stimuli (temperature, pressure, etc.), the perceived sense is one of pain.

In addition to the fibers, a dentinal tubule is filled with dentinal fluid, making it a hydrodynamic organ. Capillary permeability and blood pressure in the pulp results in intrapulpal pressures of 15–30 mmHg. The outwardly directed pressure gradient of the pulpal fluid gently drives it into the dentinal tubules, around the odontoblasts and nerve fibers, to become dentinal fluid. A slow outward flow of water and small molecules occurs through the dentinal tubules, even in areas covered with intact enamel or cementum, as these structures are permeable. If a dentinal tubule's surface is exposed, the flowrate could be around 1 mm per hour [9].

A series of studies described by Brannstrom provided evidence that the main cause of dentinal pain is a rapid outward flow of fluid in the dentinal tubules that is initiated by strong capillary forces [10]. Cold stimulus caused a rapid outward flow of fluid at the pulpal end of the dentinal tubule, whereas heat stimulus caused a rapid inward flow of fluid. Rapid capillary action can also be caused by surface dehydration, friction (venturi effect), or fluid contraction. This fluid flow, although being insufficient to displace odontoblastic processes within the dentinal tubules, was sufficient enough to stimulate the sensory nerve endings in the underlying pulp dentin border zone [10].

Within the pulp are distinct cell zones, each with a specific function in healing. The cell layer closest to the tubules is the odontoblastic cell layer or primary cell layer. Next, there is a cell free zone, followed by a subodontoblastic cell-rich zone or secondary cell zone (layer of Höhl) [7].

The primary layer of odontoblasts is a highly differentiated group of sensitive cells. These cells can be easily killed by toxins defusing through open tubules or from aspiration during rapid capillary action. A new generation of odontoblasts can come from the subodontoblastic cells, fibroblasts, undifferentiated mesenchymal cells from the pulp core, and vascular-derived pericytes. These cells are more tolerant of toxins and can traverse the cell-free zone to differentiate into odontoblasts. These newly differentiated cells can lay down new layers of reparative (tertiary) dentin to block the apertures of the dentinal tubules [11].

17.3.1.2 Pulpitis

Pulpal inflammation, in association with sensible dentin, is the early defense mechanism for the tooth's endodontic system [12]. In slight pulpitis, symptoms may not be apparent, but as the reactions increase, the healing sequence may be stimulated. Severe pulpitis may develop when profuse amounts of toxic products reach the pulp, accompanied by an excessive immunologic reaction, ultimately leading to pulpal necrosis [7]. Additionally, if the inflammatory or immune response is too weak or absent, the subsequent infection may result in liquefaction necrosis and pulpal death [12]. In mature teeth the pulp cavity is more narrow with a limited blood supply, with few, if any, undifferentiated mesenchymal cells left in a depleted cell-rich zone of the pulp. These can limit the pulp's ability to respond to disease [7].

17.3.1.3 Reparative Dentin

When tubules are exposed on the surface due to injury, disease, abrasion, attrition, scaling, or root planing, material may accumulate at the surface aperture and eventually mineralize [8]. Materials such as dentinal fluid, salivary substances, fluorides, some lithotropic bacteria, and other substances accumulate at the aperture and then mineralize in a fashion similar to that of plaque mineralizing into calculus [7, 13]. However, in some cases, continued attrition or abrasion may prevent the tubules from being protectively sealed in this fashion. In these cases, removal of the continued source of wear and some form of dentinal sealer can be used to rectify the problem, or more advanced restorative procedures performed (inlays, onlays, crowns, etc.).

Sclerotic dentin is more highly mineralized, with tubules being obliterated as they are filled with additional mineralization [7]. This process is similar to the surface mineralization, but extends well down into the tubule. For this to occur the odontoblast must have been lost, leaving a dead tract (unoccupied tubule). Tertiary (reparative or irregular secondary) dentin then forms at the tubule access, after which the sclerotic dentin can form [12]. Sclerotic dentin can also form in pulpless non-vital teeth, although it may take more time [7]. It is seen in many older patients on exposed root surfaces as a highly translucent root dentin. Clinically, it is more difficult to bond a composite resin restoration to this type of dentin.

Tertiary dentin is of two types, either reactionary, where dentin is formed from a pre-existing odontoblast, or reparative, where newly differentiated odontoblast-like cells are formed due to the death of the original odontoblasts, from a pulpal progenitor cell [11]. Tertiary dentin is deposited rapidly, often with a sparse and irregular tubular pattern. It sometimes contains cellular inclusions within its structure (osteodentin). This provides a positive effect to seal the pulp cavity from invasion by toxins and microbes. However, it should also be realized that reparative dentin can also have negative effects [14]. To begin with, it can result in a response that causes no pain, therefore not stimulating the endodontic immune system to mount a response to impending disease. Second, it can result in a reduced pulp canal, which can cause problems when accessing, or in instrumentation of the pulp chamber and canal when performing endodontic procedures.

17.4 Basic Concepts of Restorative Procedures

When a defect occurs in the hard tissues of the tooth (enamel, dentin), optimally it is best to preserve the function and structure of the object by restorative means. It is essential to know basic components of restorative efforts before undertaking therapy, including knowledge of cavity preparation, from skills involved to the final preparation that is required. These rules include conservation, esthetics, contours and contacts, cavity preparation, and identification with resolution of the cause.

17.4.1 Conservation of Natural Tooth Structure

The conservation of natural tooth structure is the first rule of operative dentistry [3]. Conservation of tooth structure is essential for protection of the vital pulp. However, not only must the depth of preparationbe considered but also the size of the area. There are 30 000–40 000 odontoblasts per millimeter of dentinal surface area [7]. Therefore, a one-centimeter squared preparation into the dentin will injure between three and four million odontoblasts in the pulp cavity, by severing off some degree of their processes or Tomes fibers. The degree of injury determines whether the individual odontoblasts become non-vital. Crown preparation for a full coverage on a vital tooth will injure and irritate all of the odontoblasts in the crown pulp chamber. The more odontoblasts irritated, the more the pulp will be irritated.

17.4.2 Esthetics

Natural, healthy, unmarred enamel that is supported by health dentin, pulp, and periodontium is the most esthetically pleasing. Therefore, the conservation of these healthy tissues is the best esthetic outcome possible. However, when tooth structure fails, esthetic restorative procedures come into play. The functional and esthetic outcome desired by the owner will then dictate the design of the operative preparation.

17.4.3 Contours and Contacts

A good general knowledge of dental anatomy is required to understand the physiology and function of tooth crown contours (see Chapter 1 – Oral Anatomy and Physiology). Contact areas, marginal form, and the buccal and lingual contours must be properly designed to reduce food impaction during mastication. Typically, contact areas should be restored to the condition that was present when the tooth was young and healthy. Restoration of the axial contours (buccal bulge, etc.) should be performed to protect periodontal health.

17.4.4 Cavity Preparation

See later in the chapter.

17.4.5 Identification and Resolution of Cause

If the cause of the disease can be ascertained, steps should be taken to relieve it and prevent it from recurring. Long-term success of any restoration will be in doubt if the cause cannot be identified and resolved. This is important when dealing with pets that have habits such as chewing on cages, rocks, or sticks. In police, military, and protection trained dogs the source of the trauma can usually be identified, but not removed. In the required continuing bite training, the reinforced bite sleeve can sometimes cause damage, as well as actual on-duty activity. If the bite sleeve caused an injury, it should be examined to determine if it can be modified or improved to reduce the probability of a recurrence of the injury. Dogs with a strong grip and rotational apprehension methods can break the teeth subgingivally.

Abrasion patterns of incisors can be seen with atopic dogs, so dermatologic interventions may be needed. Any object that is non-compressive or non-bendable can cause tooth fractures with heavy chewing, especially of the carnassial teeth. Items with cloth or fibrous coverings can be extremely abrasive, especially if allowed to collect dirt or sand on surfaces. Play (or serious) fighting with other dogs or games of tug-of-war can also cause injuries to incisors and canine teeth

17.5 Treatment Planning

Treatment planning requires a systematic approach to assess the structures and associated problems that may challenge treatment success. A close study of existing conditions that have led to the problem is required. It should be determined if modification in behavior, environment, or a combination of both is required. Additionally, the patient's occlusion and periodontal health must be taken into consideration to optimize success [3]. The tooth structure must be evaluated for the ability to sustain a load, its relative retentive qualities, and esthetic requirements.

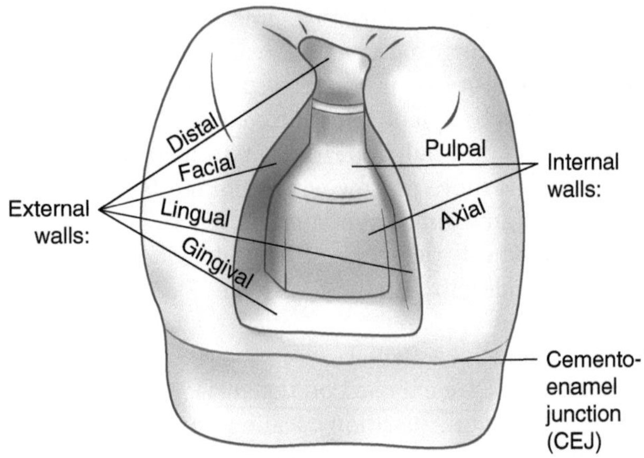

Figure 17.2 Class II cavity prep walls – the external and internal walls (floors) for an amalgam tooth preparation. From: https://pocketdentistry.com/5-fundamentals-of-tooth-preparation-and-pulp-protection. Reproduced with permission.

17.5.1 Components of Prepared Cavities

Various walls, lines, and angles are created during cavity preparation. The following terms are used to identify the various components of a cavity prepared for restoration.

An enclosing side of a prepared cavity is termed a wall. The wall is named in relation to the tooth surface of which it is formed. There are two internal walls possible, the axial and pulpal walls. The axial wall is the internal wall formed by the surface of the long axis (axial or vertical plane) of the tooth. The pulpal wall is the internal wall in the horizontal plane (Figure 17.2).

There are numerous non-internal wall surface potentials in a cavity preparation. Some of these are:

Distal wall
Mesial wall
Buccal or labial wall
Lingual wall
Incisal wall
Occlusal wall
Gingival or apical wall
Facial (buccal or labial) proximal (mesial or distal) wall
Lingual proximal (mesial or distal) wall

Additionally, there are a few subdivisions of the walls, such as the enamel and dentinal walls. The enamel wall is that portion of the preparation wall that consists of enamel. The dentinal wall is that portion of the wall that consists of dentin. The dentinoenamel junction is that juncture in the wall where the dentinal and enamel walls meet.

Where two walls meet a line angle is formed. At the point where three walls meet a point angle is produced (Figure 17.3). The cavosurface angle is the line angle formed between a wall of the prepared surface and the

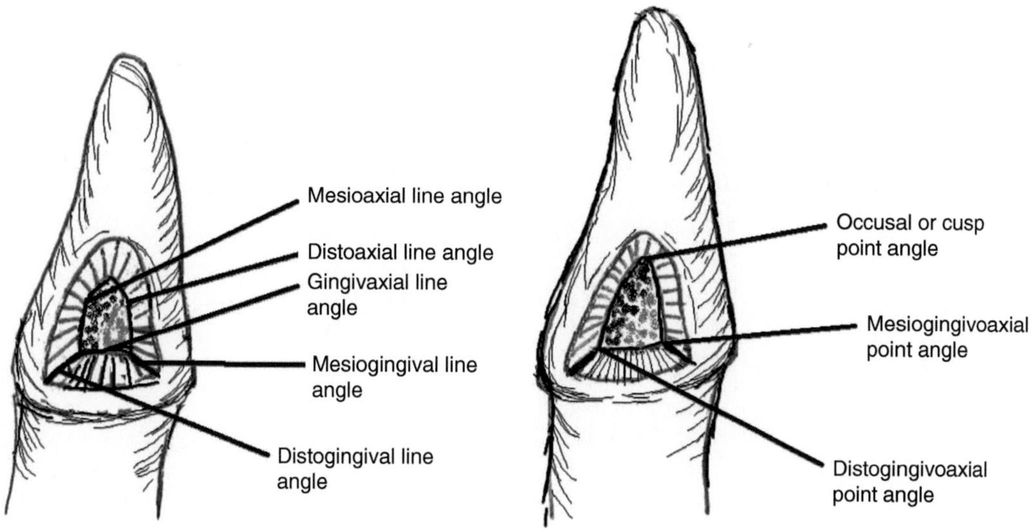

Figure 17.3 Common line and point angles in a prepared cavity (illustration by Anthony Caiafa adapted from the First Edition).

unprepared tooth surface. The cavosurface angle is also sometimes termed the preparation margin, especially once the preparation is restored. The combined peripheral extent of all of the cavosurfaces or preparation margins is termed the cavity or preparation outline. In dealing with restoratives, the restorative margin is the restorative surface that abuts the cavosurface angle or preparation margin.

17.5.2 Preparation of Cavosurface Angles or Marginal Finish Lines

Design of the cavosurface angle requires special consideration in its preparation. The preparation marginal restoration greatly affects retentive qualities of the restoration, resistance to marginal leakage, physiologic contour reactions, gingival health, and resistance to attrition, abrasion, and fracture of the restoration and restored tooth. Selection of the specific cavosurface angle treatment is dependent upon the type of restoration selected, restorative materials to be used, degree of anticipated stress demand upon the restoration, and the length and direction of the enamel prisms (Figure 17.4).

17.5.3 Modern Cavity Preparation

The mechanical cavity preparation involves the removal of defective, injured, or infected enamel and/or dentin. Affected (not infected) dentin is preserved. The cavity is then filled with a suitable restorative material that will reestablish the health, function, and often the esthetics of the tooth as well as its contour and shape. Minimal intervention dentistry has taken over from G.V. Black's old philosophy of extension for prevention. However, G.V. Black's other ideas on cavity design and tooth preparation are still relevant today [15]. Today, minimal intervention dentistry or conservative cavity preparation is designed to preserve as much healthy tooth structure as possible, only limited by access to diseased tissues and dental material requirements. This philosophy is the goal of restorative clinicians around the world.

> Modern cavity preparation and design and the evolution thereof cannot, or perhaps should not, be considered without reference to G.V. Black. Black's text *A Work on Operative Dentistry* in 1908 was the first to prescribe a systematic method of cavity preparation and the 'ideal' cavity form [15].

Multiple factors must be taken into consideration prior to the design of the preparation outline being implemented upon the tooth, including location, extent, stresses, tooth condition, and esthetics. First, the classification by location by G.V. Black or similar classification is required. This classification will then direct certain biological mechanical principles to be applied. Next, classification by extent is a necessity. This usually does not overtly affect the cavity outline, but more the depth of preparation. This in turn determines whether cavity liners, indirect pulp capping, direct pulp capping, or root canal procedures will be required. Third, the occlusal and leverage stresses that must be encountered must be carefully studied. This impacts the types of restorative materials used and whether occlusal height of the crown should be reduced to diminish occlusal and leverage stresses. Four, the general condition of the tooth, including the presence of other restoratives currently in place or to be placed, must be contemplated. Finally, the

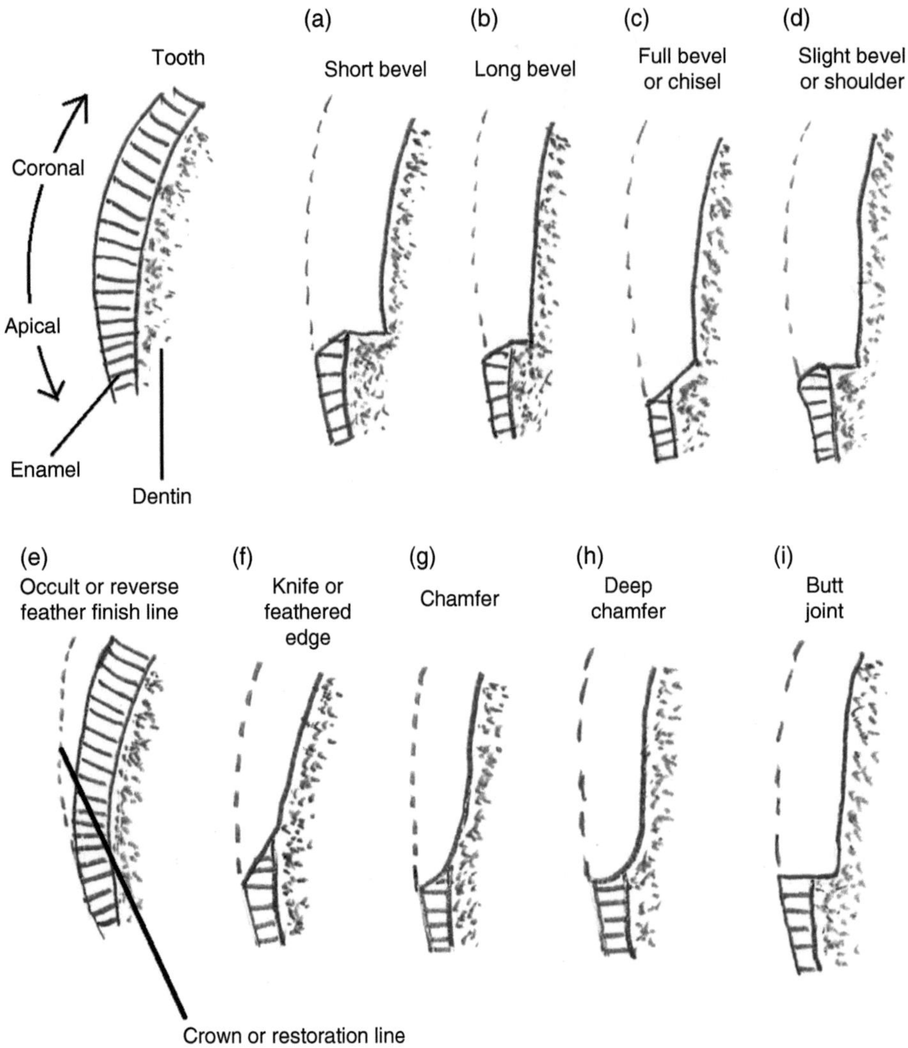

Figure 17.4 Basic types of marginal finish lines used on gingival cavosurfaces: (a) short bevel; (b) long bevel; (c) full bevel or chisel; (d) slight bevel or shoulder; (e) occult or reverse feather finish line; (f) knife or feathered edge; (g) chamfer; (h) deep chamfer; (i) butt joint (illustration by Anthony Caiafa adapted from the First Edition).

esthetic demands by the client will need assessment. For example, the use of porcelain fused to metal (PFM) for the crown will require greater tooth reduction than the use for a typical metal crown.

A more recent classification of lesions and general principles are determined by the nature and extent of the lesion, the quantity and quality of the tooth tissue remaining following preparation, functional load, and the nature and properties of the restorative system to be used [16]. In general terms, the minimal tooth substance is removed to allow access to the diseased tissues as well as allowing space for the requirements of the restorative material. For the removal of dental caries, an understanding of caries progression, tooth anatomy, including the position of the pulp (often based on an intraoral radiograph) and dental material science, is essential before starting.

17.6 Steps of Cavity Preparation

Preparation of a tooth to accept any form of restorative material requires specific steps, requiring planning, instrumentation skills, and an attention to detail. Dr. G.V. Black, almost a 100 years ago, set forth the basic sequence of tooth preparation for restoration [17]. This sequence included: outline form, resistance form, retention form, convenience form, pathology removal form, wall form, and preparation cleansing form. In addition to these, marginal placement and pulpal protection are also closely observed.

17.6.1 Outline Form

Outline form consists of the external and internal pattern boundaries of the preparation. This includes consideration of the area of pathology, all undermined enamel, and adjacent pathology, tooth contours, and anomalous anatomy. The preparation margins are placed in areas least susceptible to pathology, where visualization and finishing are suitable for the operator, and where access for warranted hygiene by the client is adequate. In addition, the outline form must take into consideration access to the pathology, type of restorative material used, functional needs of the patient, and esthetic requirements. It is generally necessary to gain access using a friction-retained, water-cooled, diamond bur held in an air turbine handpiece. Diamond burs cut enamel very efficiently and would be the bur of choice for accessing caries through the enamel. The original tooth contour should be reestablished where possible and the reproduction of the contact point, if present, is important in preventing food impaction problems, which can lead to periodontal disease.

17.6.2 Resistance Form

Resistance form is the shape formulated for the preparation to resist fracture of the tooth and restoration, both during insertion and function. This would encompass the functional needs of the restorative material selected, by adequate reduction preparation for the volume of restorative material required and the correct angulation form of the walls to withstand the functional forces of occlusion. Any preparation will weaken a tooth and predispose it to fracture. To minimize this effect, all internal line angles should be rounded.

Any increase in cavity depth can lead to flexure of cusp walls, which may predispose them to fracture. Rounding or curving the floor of the preparation can assist in minimizing this flexure. If a cusp has been totally undermined with no supporting dentin, then the operator should consider cusp reduction and a cusp overlay with a restorative material to minimize cusp fracture.

17.6.3 Retention Form

Retention form is the shaping of the internal aspects of the preparation to assist in the prevention of the displacement of the restoration. This includes retentive undercuts, groove cuts to prevent rotation, dovetails, pins, posts, and the internal wall angle form. Today, with the use of adhesive materials, the need for pins, grooves etc. are less warranted. However, if a substantial amount of tooth structure has been lost, then an indirect type of restoration may need to be considered. In summary, the choice of material will influence the final form of the preparation, especially with the need for undercuts for non-adhesive restorations such as amalgam.

17.6.4 Convenience Form

Convenience form is the shaping of the preparation in order to provide adequate visualization, suitable accessibility, and reasonable ease in placement of the restoration and its finishing.

17.6.5 Pathology Removal Form

Pathology removal form is the shaping of the preparation that is necessary to remove or compensate for diseased, injured, or esthetically unpleasing dental tissue. The extent of pathology removal many times determines the need for the use of materials or agents to protect vital pulps. This may also result in the need for specific endodontic procedures.

In the case of caries removal, caries should be initially removed from around the amelodentinal junction and then, working apically, toward the areas overlying the pulp. If caries extends down to the pulp, the operator will need to make a decision on whether to leave affected dentin or slightly soft dentin behind, so as not to enter the pulp. The use of caries detecting solutions may or may not assist the operator in identifying infected versus affected dentin. Affected dentin can be remineralized with the use of a therapeutic liner. The area of the amelodentinal junction must always be made completely caries-free.

17.6.6 Wall Form

Wall form is the refinement in the shaping of the preparation. This is typically required to eliminate unsupported enamel rods at the margin, or the smoothing of an irregular or rough outline form.

17.6.7 Preparation Cleansing Form

Cleansing form is typically the final shaping of the preparation prior to restoration placement. It is generally accomplished with explorers, air, water, spray, cotton pellets, and other agents to remove debris from the preparation.

17.6.8 Margin Placement

G.V. Black originally proposed that margins should be placed well into the embrasures in cleansable areas and sometimes subgingivally. It is now accepted that margins should be kept free of the gingivae where possible to avoid periodontal problems and that incidence of overhangs and marginal gaps must be avoided. Any encroachment of the biologic width (approximately 2.5 mm from the margin of restoration to the crestal bone) will lead to periodontal inflammation. If the margin does violate biologic width, then a crown lengthening procedure will need to be performed prior to placing the restoration.

17.6.9 Pulpal Protection

As younger patients tend to have larger pulp chambers than older patients, inadvertent pulp exposure during the restorative procedure is a risk in the younger patient. A diagnostic radiograph showing the size and position of the pulp is mandatory. Where the operator gets within 0.5 mm of the pulp, pulpal protection is required in the form of a pulp capping material such as calcium hydroxide or mineral trioxide aggregate (MTA). Deep cavities may also require the need for a liner or base prior to restorative placement (see Chapter 16 – Advanced Endodontic Therapy).

17.7 Operating Fields

During operative procedures, various isolation schemes are used to enhance visualization, instrumentation, control moisture contamination from instruments, reduce salivary interference, and protect the patient from instrument or chemical injury. The isolation may be either for single teeth or entire arches. There are many methods for isolation, but the type and extent of isolation selected is determined by the type of procedure, length of procedure, area anatomy, and operator requirements. Moisture contamination including blood or saliva can interfere with the bonding of unfilled resins (bonding agent) to tooth structure as well as the cohesive bond between the composite resin and the unfilled resin. Blood contamination can also stain or discolor the restoration. Saliva may also contaminate the site with bacteria, especially when performing endodontic therapy on a tooth.

17.7.1 Mouth Mirror and Suction

The mouth mirror in combination with suction can be a highly expedient tool for isolation of an area. The mirror can be used as a lip or soft tissue retractor, an indirect visual aid, and to redirect light to an area to improve visualization. Suction can provide moisture and debris control for a clear field of view.

17.7.2 Cotton Rolls

Cotton rolls are tubes of absorbent material used to help control moisture at a site. They may improve or hinder visualization and access when in place and come in an assortment of diameters and lengths. Cotton rolls and hybrid cotton can be used to help isolate teeth, absorb excess moisture, occlude salivary duct openings, to aid in cheek retraction, or to apply medicaments. Rolls are used for tooth isolation for restorations and topical treatments, such as fluoride. They are placed in the buccal or lingual vestibule to aid in the control of moisture, being replaced as they become saturated. In the lower arch, cotton rolls and holders are sometimes used to provide retraction for access and improved visualization.

17.7.3 Retractors and Shields

Lip retractors are useful when working on the maxillary teeth to help prevent moisture contamination when placing a restoration. An atraumatic retractor can lift the upper lip out of the way, especially when working on rostral teeth. Cheek retractors can be made of metal or plastic and be single or double ended. They are used primarily to displace the cheeks away from the caudal teeth, either for dental visualization or shielding of soft tissues in dental procedures or for visualization during photography. Most tongue retractors are made of metal with rubberized tongue grips, and tongue shields are typically made of plastic or metal. Tongue retractors are used to move the tongue out of the way for procedures, while shields or guards generally partially cover the tongue for its protection.

17.7.4 Rubber Dam

A rubber dam is a thin sheet of rubber or latex used to isolate an operating field in the oral cavity. The rubber dam is by far the most effective method of tooth isolation and moisture control (Figure 17.5). However, it may be difficult to place in dogs and cats due to a lack of customized rubber dam clamps. It can provide an area that is

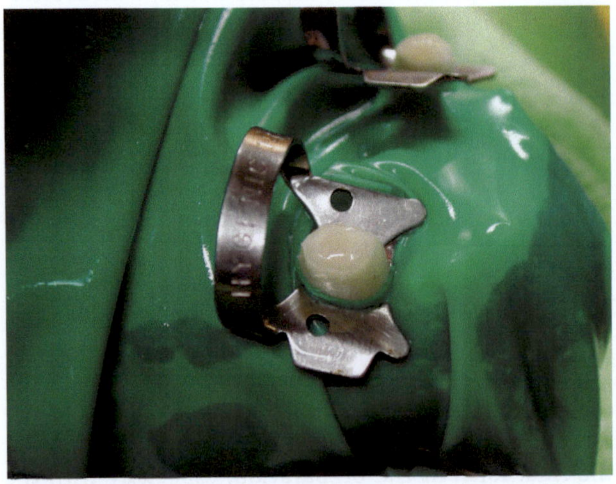

Figure 17.5 Use of a rubber dental dam and clamp to isolate the surgical site.

easier to maintain asepsis, a dry field, retraction of soft and hard tissues during oral treatments, and also allows for better visualization of the operative field. Latex gloves with holes punched into them can be used as rubber dams in animals, as they can be easily slipped over the muzzle and hold their position more naturally, particularly when working on canine teeth. True rubber dams come in various thicknesses and sizes for use according to the size of the oral cavity and teeth. The heaviest thickness that can be managed for an area is generally best. Some form of stabilization is needed to maintain the placement, with rubber dam holders, clamps, ligatures, interproximal devices, and tooth attachments. Care should be taken to avoid damage to surrounding gingiva.

17.7.5 Astringents and Retraction Cord

These may be applied to control gingival hemorrhage. A retraction cord can be placed, especially when restoring Class V lesions at the gingival margin. The retraction cord comes in various thicknesses. It can be soaked in astringent such as ferric sulfate to assist in the control of bleeding. The retraction cord also slows down the flow of gingival crevicular fluid from the gingival sulcus. The infiltration of a local anesthetic agent with adrenaline may also aid in the control of bleeding.

17.7.6 Lesion and Caries Detection

Detection of lesions, such as caries, TR, and enamel defects is commonly performed with a sharp explorer, mouth mirror, good lighting, air syringe, and intraoral radiographs. Early detection of enamel disease is most reliant upon visualization and tactile inspection of the teeth. Incipient carious lesions of enamel may appear as rough or chalky white in good light, when air is blown across it. Sharp explorers, when pressed into a dental disease lesion, will ordinarily stick or catch on withdrawal. In moderate to advanced carious lesions of enamel, a brown to black appearance may develop in the pit, fissure, or developmental grooves, but must be differentiated from staining. In moderate to advanced resorptive and carious lesions, lucent areas may be detected radiographically. Laser caries detectors using laser fluorescence are now being used in human dentistry to detect early occlusal caries where radiographs and probing are equivocal.

Once lesions have been detected, both the extent of involvement must be ascertained, as well as the relationship to the pulp cavity and pulp vitality. Near-pulpal exposures can typically be visually detected by the pink hue of the dentin. This will usually be an indication for an indirect pulp capping procedure (see Chapter 16 – Advanced Endodontic Therapy). If the pulp has been exposed, but is still vital, a direct pulp capping or possibly a complete root canal procedure may be warranted. If the canal is exposed and the pulp is non-vital, or is expected to become so, then a complete root canal procedure prior to restoration would be the treatment of choice.

17.8 Restorative Materials

Operative chairside restorations generally involve the use of one, or more, of three basic restorative materials: composite resins, GIC, and amalgam. These products are held in place by micromechanical retention, chemical crystal formations, or macromechanical retention. Micromechanical retention is obtained by the use of bonding agents that microscopically interlock in enamel porosities, dentinal tubules, or other microscopic anatomy. This is used primarily with light cured composites and bonded amalgam restorations. Chemical crystal formations occur with glass ionomers as they form a crystal between the ionomer and the minerals within the enamel and dentin. Macromechanical retention are undercuts in the dentin and are used with non-bonded amalgams and self- or autocure composites.

17.8.1 Composites

The potential for the use of acrylic resins for permanent restorations in dentistry first began to be realized in 1955, when Buonocore reported upon the use of phosphoric acid on the tooth surface. He found that etching enamel dramatically enhanced the bonding of acrylic to the surface [18]. In 1962, Bowen introduced the new resin we today call composite, a reaction product of bis-phenol A and a glycidyl methacrylate, commonly abbreviated to bis-GMA [19]. The original formula was marketed as a powder–liquid system and a paste–paste form, both of which were self- or chemical-cured products. In 1972, the first light-cured composite resins were developed, which used an ultraviolet 365 nm curing light source [20]. This resulted in a controlled working and setting time. Most clinically used composites today use the visible light range of 460–480 nm, which provides a more controlled curing in a clinical setting. Today's composites can be bonded to enamel, dentin, cementum, metals, porcelain, glass ionomers, and of course to other composites [20].

The composite resins on the market today come as a chemical cure, visible light cure, and ultraviolet light cured. The ultraviolet light cured resins are used mostly for indirect techniques using dental laboratories, while the chemical and visible light cured products are used predominately in clinics. The chemically activated resins normally use benzoyl peroxide as an activator. With the light cured products, most ultraviolet systems use benzoin methyl ether, while visible light systems use camphoroquinone [20].

There are four major components that make up a composite resin (CR): inorganic fillers (mainly quartz/glass particles), organic resins (the glue), coupling agent (the link or bond between the glue and the glass), and the initiator–accelerator system.

The dispersed inorganic filler particles may consist of one or more inorganic materials, such as finely ground quartz or glass, sol–gel derived ceramics, microfine silica, or more recently nanotechnology derived particles. These fillers act to strengthen the matrix (increase hardness, reduce wear, and offer acceptable strength) and reduce volumetric shrinkage (too much matrix increases the shrinkage) and thermal expansion. The fillers also improve the handling characteristics by making it thicker as well as increasing the radiopacity of the CR (important for identifying the restoration on radiographs).

The coupling is the coating on the filler particles (usually silane) that allows the glass to attach or couple with the resins [20]. Silane is a synthetic hybrid inorganic–organic compound, and is applied to the surface of the glass particles by the manufacturer (silanization). Silane acts as a surface conditioner or coupling agent, producing a stable bond between the inorganic filler and the organic resin when polymerized. Silane is also used as a coupling agent for ceramic restorations.

The role of the initiator–accelerator system is to polymerize and cross-link the system into a hardened mass. The polymerization reaction can be triggered by light-activation, self-curing (chemical activation), and dual-curing (chemical and light-curing).

The CR is usually composed of an organic polymer matrix of high molecular weight [21, 22], usually a bis-GMA (bisphenol A glycidyl methacrylate), TEGDMA (triethylene glycol dimethacrylate) or UDMA (urethane dimethacrylate) resin, with or without fillers. bis-GMA resin was first introduced in the 1960s, but polymerization shrinkage has always been a problem with methacrylate types of resin matrix; the restoration can pull away from the bonded tooth surface allowing for microleakage (bacterial ingress) or even loss of the restoration itself. There is also the risk of cusp deformation, especially in molars causing pain in the patient.

A new resin monomer system called silorane (introduced in 2007) was developed to reduce shrinkage and internal stress buildup resulting from polymerization seen in the older methacrylate CRs. Silorane consists of siloxane and oxirane. By using a cationic ring-opening polymerization reaction (silorane) instead of a free radical type of polymerization (methacrylate), polymerization shrinkage has been substantially reduced with the newer silorane-based CRs. Newer silorane-based adhesives have also been developed for bonding the silorane CRs to tooth structure. However, be wary as two different resin monomer systems should not be mixed.

As with any technology today, dental restorative manufacturers are looking for new composite resins that offer better wear characteristics as well as less shrinkage, but delivering better esthetic outcomes as well. With the advent of newer products, the silorane composite resins will soon be phased out with nanoparticle composite technology continuing advancements in restorative dentistry.

Composites require acid etching of the enamel (at least) to create microporosities that the unfilled resin (bonding agent) can flow into, while keeping a very thin film of the material to which the filled resin will bind. Composite resins are hydrophobic and can fail when there is moisture contamination while placing the restoration. Good moisture isolation is imperative when placing the composite. Even manipulating composite resins with ungloved hands can cause premature failure of the restoration through oil and moisture contamination.

Fillers are added to increase hardness, strength, resistance to temperature, ability to withstand wear, and control shrinkage during polymerization [23]. Fillers can also provide a lower coefficient of thermal expansion, lower water sorption, greater wear resistance, alter polishability, and, depending on the material, a variety of colors [24]. The inorganic filler portion is typically 70–80% of the material by weight, primarily in the form of crystal quartz, silica, lithium, and other particles [25].

Composite resins come in radiopaque and radiolucent forms. In Class II and III lesions, with lesions in proximal surfaces, radiopaque composites help to define the extent of the restorative in an area of difficult physical visualization with little interference to radiographic visualization of the remainder of the tooth. However, in Class V and veneers the radiopacity can obscure visualization of the entire tooth radiographically, thereby camouflaging other lesions that may develop.

In addition, composite resins come as macrofilled, intermediate filled or small particle, microfilled, hybrids, microhybrids, and nanohybrids. The names refer to the size of the filler particles or combination of sizes used in the resin.

Microfilled composites have particles less than or equal to 0.04 μm (microns), usually a colloidal silica. The filler content may only be 35–50%, so there will be a higher coefficient of thermal expansion, potentially increased shrinkage during polymerization (making acid-etching and dentinal bonding vital), may absorb more water [21], and are less fracture and wear resistant. With the small particle size, however, it is extremely polishable, so esthetically is advantageous in non-stressed areas such as Class III and Class V restorations.

The hybrid composites consist of two types of fillers that are blended together: (i) fine particles of average particle size 2–4 μm and (ii) 5–15% of microfine particles, usually silica, of particle size 0.04–0.2 μm. In microhybrid composites, the fine particles of a lower average particle size (0.04–1 μm) are blended with microfine silica. They possess a chameleon-like property that makes them blend in well with the surrounding natural tooth structure. They are often used for anterior teeth and are highly polishable.

Nanotechnology is the production of functional materials and structures in the range of 1 to –100 nm (0.001–0.1 μm). At present there are two distinct types of dental composite resins available that contain nanoparticles:

a) *Nanofills.* These contain nanometer-sized particles (0.001–0.1 μm) throughout the resin matrix. Larger primary particles are not present.
b) *Nanohybrids.* These consist of large particles (0.4–5 μm) with added nanometer-sized particles. Thus, they are hybrid materials, not true nanofilled composite resins.

The uniqueness of the nanofilled composite is that it has the mechanical strength of a microhybrid but at the same time retains the polishability of a microfill. The particles in nanohybrids are more spherical, which gives them good wear characteristics. They have been marketed to clinicians as the universal composite resin for both posterior and anterior teeth use. Today, most composite resin materials in the market use some form of nanoparticles within the material (Table 17.3).

A recently introduced flowable composite resin material is self-adhering, requiring no bonding agent at all (the bonding agent is incorporated into the composite resin itself). The cavity is simply prepared and then the flowable composite is placed and visibly light cured. There is also a new sonic-filled composite resin material that can be built up in bulk (up to 5 mm increments before light curing) without the issues of polymerization shrinkage or undercuring. The material becomes 90% less viscous with sonic energy activation. A special gun is used to deliver the material into the prepared cavity.

A flowable composite's particle sizes range between 1 and 2 μm. The filler is reduced by 50% by weight and the unfilled resin component is increased. They display greater shrinkage than other types of composite resins and should only be built up in small increments to avoid this increased shrinkage. They also have a tendency to trap air bubbles when applied to the tooth and have poor wear characteristics. They may be suitable as a base under a conventional composite resin or in Class V restorations.

For high stress-bearing areas, bulk fill and short glass fiber reinforced composite resins have been introduced.

17.8.1.1 Visible Light Curing Equipment

Light-initiated composites require a light-activation unit to begin the reaction. Most modern materials need light of a wavelength close to 475 nm. Laser, plasma arc, and halogen curing units are available. Although the more expensive plasma arc and laser units are faster, at this time there is no compelling evidence that they are clinically superior to the halogen or LED units that are less expensive. The unit should be capable of generating light of an intensity of at least 600 mW/cm^2. Light gun output should be tested regularly, as the efficiency of lights diminishes with time due to contamination of the curing tip, degeneration of the filament, and changes in the transmitting ability of the light guide. There are some composite resins available today that use different

Table 17.3 Characteristics of various composite resins – handling characteristics and properties.

Type of composite	Size of filler particles (μm)	Volume of inorganic filler (%)	Advantages	Disadvantages
Hybrids	0.04–0.2, 2–4 μm	60–70	High strength, high modulus	
Nano-composites Nanofill	0.001–0.1 μm	78.5	High polish, high strength, high modulus	
Nanohybrid	0.001–0.1 μm 0.4–5 μm			
Microfilled	0.04 μm	32–50	Best polish, best esthetics	Higher shrinkage
Packable	0.04, 0.2–20 μm	59–80	Packable, less shrinkage, lower wear	Low polish
Flowable	0.04, 0.2–3.0 μm	42–62	Syringeable, lower modulus	Higher wear Higher shrinkage
Laboratory	0.04, 0.2–3.0 μm	60–70	Best anatomy and contacts, lower wear	Lab cost, special equipment, requires resin cement

photoinitiators that require multiwavelength visible light curing (VLC) guns.

17.8.1.2 Composite Polymerization and Shrinkage

Composite resins shrink approximately 3% linearly and 1.5% volumetrically during the curing process [26]. Flowable composite resins shrink a little more due to a low filler content. Shrinkage can result in problems with bond strength and marginal leakage. When the shrinkage occurs, some bonding points must suffer. The two weakest points of the bond are at the dentin interface and the cervical enamel cavosurface. This results in the composite resin pulling away from parts of the dentinal surface, and with the cervical enamel surfaces, either having the bond break or the enamel rods being pulled out of the tooth. With time, some of the shrinkage is counteracted by expansion of the composite resin due to its absorption of oral moisture. However, areas of bonding may have been permanently disrupted and some degree of marginal leakage may already have occurred. This problem cannot be solved with stronger bonding agents, as the shrinkage contraction is so strong that either tooth or restoration must give. Only improved composite resins that are not susceptible to volumetric change can solve this obstacle.

17.8.2 Glass Ionomer Cements (GICs)

While glass ionomer products typically do not bear up to stress and wear as well as composites or amalgam, when placed in non-occlusal areas (Classes III and V, Modified Black Classification), these compounds can be very useful. The basic composition of glass ionomers is an aluminosilicate glass powder (calcium or strontium fluoroaluminosilicate (FAS) glass) mixed with a polyalkenoic acid (polyacrylic acid), with additional components (water, tartaric acid) [21]. They chemically bind to enamel and dentin by ions forming salts that bond to the calcium in the tooth [27], even if slight moisture is present (hydrophilic). This can be an advantage, especially when mechanical retention procedures of undercutting and acid-etching are best avoided in small or delicate teeth. As mentioned before, another advantage of glass ionomer is that they slowly release fluoride over time, helping to retard decay and decrease sensitivity, while being biologically compatible with the pulp, negating the need for cavity liners in most cases [21]. GICs have a coefficient of thermal expansion closely approximating that of the tooth structure, so a tight marginal seal is maintained. Some products have silver added to enhance the strength, with decreased setting time, but the darker color is not as esthetically pleasing.

The longer setting time of some glass ionomer products, along with moisture restrictions in the area (should not be desiccated, but not wet), can make them more technique-sensitive at times [28]. Although relatively easy to work with, there are certain common guidelines for success. When used as liners or bases, the powder-to-liquid ratio should be carefully measured, and it is essential to incorporate all the powder into the mix for best results [20]. Insufficient powder into the mix substantially reduces the ionomer's strength, results in a slower setting time, and increases its susceptibility to dissolution [29]. Most glass ionomers should be mixed in under 45 seconds, in order to ensure that all of the powder is incorporated into the mix prior to placement and commencement of the setting reaction. Working time is the time from completion of mixing until the setting reaction begins. With glass ionomers, the working time ends once the surface sheen is gone from the mix. At this point the setting reaction has begun and the material becomes spongy and will not adapt or adhere well to the tooth surface. The use of a cool glass slide for mixing will extend the working time [20].

Fluoride release varies greatly between products. However, in all glass ionomers the initial setting reaction creates a reservoir of excess fluoride that is slowly released from the mature restoration by a leaching process [30].

Polyacrylic acid dissolves the aluminosilicate GIC particles (dissolution zone). Fluoride is absorbed more readily by the enamel than the dentin or cementum surfaces and forms a fluorapatite complex [31]. The fluoride release aids in the prevention of carious lesions, not only at the immediate site of the restoration but also at a moderate distance from it [32]. Due to the nature of GICs, they lend themselves to atraumatic restorative techniques (ARTs), where infected dentin is removed but affected dentin can be left behind to be remineralized by the GICs.

The mild bond created by glass ionomer cements to the tooth structure is created by an ion exchange adhesion reaction. When the powder (FAS glass) and liquid (polyalkenoic acid) of the GIC are mixed, there is an acid–base reaction. The acid in the liquid dissolves some of the glass particles, releasing alumina, strontium, and fluoride. A silica gel is also formed around the unreacted glass particles. The initial setting reaction takes about four to six minutes but continues for hours after this as the material matures. Barium, zinc oxide, and other metals are added to the GIC to provide radio-opacity. The final set material consists of undissolved glass particles, surrounded by silica gel and a matrix of polyions cross-linked by ionic bridges.

The setting reaction involves an attraction between the calcium of the tooth and the aluminosilicate of the glass [33]. There is an ionic interaction with the exchange of calcium and/or phosphate ions from the surface of the enamel or dentin (hydroxyapatite component). The main ions released from the GIC are strontium, silica, aluminum, and fluoride. Calcium ions increase within the GIC material. Therefore, there is an ion exchange between the GIC and the enamel/dentin, leading to a chemical bond between the tooth and the restorative material. Due to the higher calcium content of enamel, the bond of the GIC is stronger to enamel than to dentin. However, the bond of glass ionomer to enamel is only about one-third of that of composite resin to enamel [34]. Most GICs make use of a 10 second application of a 10–25% polyacrylic acid or a mild citric acid product to the dentin, which is then rinsed off. It is used to remove the smear layer on the dentin to enhance the bonding to the dentin [34].

Products with more rapid setting times and even combination products that allow for light curing are sometimes preferred. Light cured resin modified (RM) GIC restorative materials (see later) have a resin incorporated within them that is set during curing, which eliminates the separate application of a barrier. The light cured RMGICs have been shown to be more useful as a restorative material than barriers such as oils or varnishes over self-cure GICs [35].

All glass ionomers bond to dentin better than some composite resins combined with their bonding agents [20]. For this reason glass ionomers (including RMGICs) are occasionally used as a laminate with composite resins, in what is sometimes referred to as a "sandwich technique" [36, 37]. The glass ionomer is placed against the dentinal walls. It is then acid etched for 15–20 seconds with 37% phosphoric acid, rinsed, and dried. A composite resin is then bonded to the glass ionomer and the enamel of the cavity preparation.

17.8.2.1 Classification of Glass Ionomers

Type I Luting cements
Type II Esthetic restorative
Type III Bases and liners
Type IV Admixtures

Type I luting cements are finely ground ionomers that achieve a film thickness of less than 25 µm. They are commonly used for cementation of orthodontic bonds and metal and veneered crowns. Type II glass ionomers are used for restorations when fluoride release is desired but esthetics and strength are not as critical. Type III glass ionomers are base and liner materials. These can be used even in deep cavity preparations due to their enhanced pulpal compatibility [38]. However, this does not negate the need for proper use of calcium hydroxide or MTA liners. Type IV materials are admixtures or have a substantial metallic component. The admixtures are usually gold, silver, or amalgam alloy. They are most commonly used for temporary restorations or buildups and cores, but are much weaker than more conventional materials and are contraindicated in stress-bearing areas [20]. Composite resins are from three to eight times and amalgam four to ten times more fracture resistant than glass ionomers [39]. Therefore, buildups with composite or amalgam for cores would ordinarily be preferred over glass ionomers.

17.8.2.2 Resin Modified Glass Ionomer Cements (RMGICs)

To create a longer working time yet quick setting time so that immediate finishing can take place, the concept of RMGIC was introduced in the late 1980s. The essential components are similar to those in conventional GICs in which an aqueous polyalkenoic acid undergoes an acid–base setting reaction with fluoroaluminosilicate glass. To this methacrylate, components are added in limited amounts so a photo-initiated curing reaction can also occur. Although commercial materials vary widely in composition, the essential components of true RMGICs are as follows:

- Polyalkenoic acid polymer
- Fluoroaluminosilicate glass
- Water
- Hydrophilic methacrylate monomer.

The resin-modified glass ionomers contain some methacrylate components common in resin composites. Two distinct types of curing reactions take place in a true light-cure glass ionomer, the traditional acid–base glass ionomer reaction, and the free radical methacrylate polymerization.

Traditionally GICs and RMGICs were in a powder and liquid formulation that was hand mixed. To aid in the dispensing and mixing, the glass ionomers are also supplied in a single-unit encapsulated version. The powder and liquid are kept separated in the capsule for shelf-stability. Prior to clinical use the capsule is activated and then triturated in an amalgamator to mix the two components. An applicator is provided that pushes the mixed material through a narrow tip so that it can be directly placed into the prepared cavity.

Recently, the RMGICs (type III) have been formulated in a paste liquid or two-paste system. This system eliminates uneven measures of powder and liquid, provides less waste, as well as being a more time-effective method of mixing. The GIC liner or base is usually applied to the cavity floor with a calcium hydroxide applicator. The material then can be polymerized with a curing light for approximately 20 seconds.

Clinically, both conventional (self-cure) and resin-modified glass ionomers are used for a variety of restorative applications, particularly in situations of high caries activity or where caries are likely to recur. In veterinary dentistry, GICs tend to be used as a base under composite resin restorations, especially in pulpotomy and pulpectomy procedures [27].

17.8.3 Compomers

Compomers (polyacid modified resin composites) need to be bonded to a tooth structure, similar to composite resins, and have similar glass filler particles as GICs. They are not as hard wearing as regular composite resins. Compomers can release some fluoride into the tooth and have been used in human dentistry mainly as restorations in deciduous teeth. They are not used very much in veterinary dentistry.

17.8.3.1 Giomers

To overcome the disadvantages of compomers, a new category of bioactive esthetic restorative material which differs from both resin modified glass ionomer and composite resin has been introduced by Shofu Inc. (Kyoto, Japan). Giomer is a fluoride-releasing, resin-based dental adhesive material that comprises pre-reacted glass ionomer filler technology, which allows the release of high levels of fluoride ions as well as being more moisture resistant, which greatly improves the long-term durability of the restoration in the mouth.

17.8.4 Amalgam

The initial advocation of the use of dental amalgams is credited to M. Traveau in Paris, France, in 1826. It was promoted in the United States by the Crawcour brothers in 1933, as the "Royal Mineral Succedaneum" or the successor of gold. Its less expensive basic combination of mercury and silver made dental restorations more affordable. However, toxicity concerns and esthetic image have greatly reduced its use, even in veterinary dentistry. The concerns over mercury hygiene as related to the patient, dental professionals, and the environment are valid [20]. Prudent care when working with amalgam is simply common sense.

Clinical properties of amalgam include setting time, plasticity, setting strength, tensile strength, tarnish and corrosion resistance, dimensional stability, and creep [3]. With setting time, the main concern is adequate time to compact the material before setting, otherwise strength and marginal adaptation will be compromised [40]. The faster the setting of the alloy selected the more rapidly and forcefully it must be compacted. Plasticity is the malleability or moldability of freshly mixed amalgam as related to the technique used to compact the material into a prepared cavity site. The higher the plasticity rating of an amalgam, the easier it is to compact and accomplish acceptable cavity and marginal adaptation. However, to achieve greater plasticity, higher percentages of mercury must typically be incorporated into the amalgam. Setting strength is affected by the quality of compaction and amalgam formula. At about 24 hours following mixing regular amalgam reaches its highest setting strength, although rapid setting amalgams may reach that point much earlier [3]. Tensile strength relates to the strength of the final restoration and its resistance to cracking and chipping. Mercury can also adversely affect tensile strength, when the content is greater than 52% in the final restoration [41]. High percentages of mercury in the final restoration are usually a result of improper mix ratios, poor trituration (mixing or amalgamating), or inadequate compaction. In addition, the finer the lathe cut (ultrafine as compared to fine) of the alloy, typically the lower the tensile strength [42]. Deterioration of the surface and margin by corrosion and tarnishing is dependent upon the alloy combination selected, proper trituration, effective compaction, freedom from moisture during placement, smoothness of the final finish, and the oral hygiene levels. However, research has shown that a limited amount of marginal corrosion can benefit the restoration by improving the marginal seal [40, 41]. Dimensional stability relates to the expansion or contraction of the amalgam upon setting. A formulation to provide a very slight expansion is typically used to improve the marginal seal. Nevertheless, excessive expansion, as great as 5%, can be caused by moisture contamination during mixing or placement [3]. This can result in post-operative pain, extrusion of the amalgam, cracking of the amalgam, cracking of the tooth, decreased tensile strength, and increased corrosion. Following proper placement and compaction of the amalgam, moisture does not affect the amalgam's dimensional stability [40]. Creep is a term used to denote the slow flow or change in shape of amalgams due to chronic pressures. Creep can eventually result in marginal leakage.

Amalgams are indicated for restorations that are only small to moderate in size and must be supported by sound tooth structure. It is used as a restoration in pits and fissures, interproximal lesions, gingival third restorations, and distal surface of the canine teeth. It is used in deciduous teeth in preference to gold, since it will be lost. Amalgam is used in bases, foundations, and cores to help support or retain cast restoration. In endodontics it is used as root end fillings and for access closures. The use of amalgam is generally governed by size of the area to be restored, esthetic demands by the owner, availability of other restorative materials and equipment, and economic restraints. It should not be used in extensive restorations that are subject to excessive stress in occlusion from mastication or bite work.

17.8.4.1 Trituration

Trituration is amalgamation, or the mixing of the dry dental alloys and mercury into an amalgamated mass, or

Table 17.4 Comparison of restorative materials.

Property	RMGIC	GIC	CR	Amalgam
Ease of handling	Good	Average to good	Good	Average
Type of bonding	Chemical	Chemical	Micromechanical	No bond-mechanical retention
Fluoride release	Medium	Medium to high	None	None
Moisture tolerance	Average	Good	Very poor	Good
Visible light curing (VLC)	Yes	No	Yes	No
Self-setting	Yes (polymerization can still occur without VLC)	Yes	Yes (self-curing CRs only)	Yes
Polishability	Average	NA	Good to excellent	Good
Compressive strength	Medium	Low to medium	High	High
Flexural strength	Medium	Low to medium	Medium to high	High
Wear resistance	Medium	Low	High	High
Setting Shrinkage	Low to medium	Low	Medium	Low
Esthetics	Good	Average	Good to excellent	Poor
Clinical application	Classes III, V or provisional or temporary restoration, fissure sealant Orthodontic brackets or bands	Provisional or temporary restoration or as liner/base Fissure sealant Orthodontic brackets or bands	Classes I–VI Fissure sealant Orthodontic brackets	Classes I–VI

amalgam. Hand trituration with a mortar and pestle is past its usefulness, with present new improved alloys. In fact, many older amalgamators, mechanical mixers, cannot mix the newer alloys properly. Mechanical trituration with an amalgamator provides a superior mix with uniform consistency of the amalgam.

Most amalgams are provided in a sealed capsule. The duration of amalgamation (trituration) is dependent upon the alloy combination used, the amount of material to be mixed (single or double spill), the amalgam setting time, and the amalgamator used. Most are mixed for between 10 and 20 seconds, but the manufacturer's recommendations should always be used as a general guideline, and then the time should be refined by experimenting for your individual machine.

Inadequate trituration results in failure to wet the alloy particles with mercury. The mix may still be in a separate powder and liquid form when spilled into an amalgam well or simply powdery looking. An amalgam well is a holding dish for the amalgam with tapered sides that concentrates the material into the bottom of the well. Undertrituration results in increased expansion, high susceptibility to corrosion and tarnish, a decrease in strength, and a greater failure rate of the restoration [43]. Overtrituration results in a contraction of the amalgam, poor flow, and difficultly in complete filling of the preparation (Table 17.4).

17.9 Additional Materials

17.9.1 Varnishes, Liners, Bases, and Cements

With many of the restoratives, additional materials are required beneath or over the material to protect the pulp from thermal or bacterial insult, as well as protecting the restorative material from moisture or dehydration during the material's maturation phase.

- *Varnish.* A cavity varnish is a liner used to seal the dentinal tubules to help prevent microleakage and is placed into cavities that will receive an amalgam restoration. A base may or may not be placed underneath the varnish. Varnishes can also be used to protect a glass ionomer restoration from dehydration or moisture uptake (see below). Varnishes are rarely used today.
- *Liner.* A cavity liner is an aqueous or volatile organic suspension or dispersion of zinc oxide or calcium hydroxide that can be applied to a cavity surface in a relatively thin film. GIC and RMGIC are also suitable for use as lining materials.
- *Base.* A cavity base is a material, usually a type of cement, used as a base for a prepared cavity before the insertion of a permanent restoration. They protect the pulp and act as a dentine replacement. RMGICs are popular choices here.

Waterproof varnishes helped contain moisture contamination after glass ionomer restoration placement by first protecting the material from excessive moisture during its setup time and then protecting the completed restoration from dehydration [21, 44]. Varnishes do not provide thermal insulation and nor can they stimulate the production of reparative dentin. Today, unfilled resins have taken the place of varnishes in protecting GIC restorations from dehydration or overwetting.

There are several different types of materials that can be used as liners, bases, or cements, depending on the formulation, thickness, and application [25]. Cavity liners help protect the pulp and decrease dentinal sensitivity like varnishes, but can also provide other advantages, especially if the pulp is exposed or near exposure. While providing a physical support for the final restoration when replacing structural loss, bases can also help protect the pulp from irritating substances and thermal changes. Liners listed earlier may be placed in several layers to achieve the same bulk, but do not have the strength of some materials specifically used as bases, such as reinforced zinc oxide eugenol (ZOE) products and other cements. Cements are used to apply orthodontic brackets, appliances, and crowns or other prosthodontics devices.

Calcium hydroxide liners are used primarily to induce reparative dentin bridge formation (through its high pH and stimulation of the subodontoblastic layer to form odontoblasts). This will protect the pulp, which is especially important when 0.5 mm or less of dentin is left.

ZOE products can be used as liners to protect the dentinal surfaces from sensitivity, as the pH of 7–8, even of the reinforced ZOE cements, help to sedate the pulp, in contrast to zinc phosphate or other restoratives. Direct placement over exposed pulp can cause inflammation, so with exposed pulp, or near exposure, it is still recommended to use a calcium hydroxide liner or MTA under the ZOE base.

ZOE cements can have a detrimental effect on the setting of some resin systems used in composite materials and have the potential to contaminate tooth surface prior to using bonding agents. It does not have the strength of the zinc phosphates, although the reinforced products are useful as intermediate or temporary restoratives. ZOE products are used in dentistry to cement provisional crowns after a crown preparation procedure. ZOE is also used in human pediatric dentistry as a deep base in pulpotomy procedures.

Glass ionomers can be used as liners, particularly some of the newer light-cured products. The benefits of bonding to the dentin and releasing fluoride are complemented by the fact that it has greater tensile and compressive strength than calcium hydroxide [44], and even comparable to or higher than zinc phosphate, making them very useful bases. Placed over an endodontically treated tooth, it bonds to the internal dentin and can be acid-etched to facilitate the placement of composites [44]. The cariostatic effects of its fluoride are also beneficial when used to cement on orthodontic brackets and bands. All these advantages, plus the low viscosity of type I, or luting, glass ionomers make them a good choice for post and crown cementation as well. Generally, they have been found to retain complete coverage castings better than zinc phosphate or polycarboxylate cements [45].

Some sensitivity may be experienced after crown cementation with GICs, for various reasons, and, of course, any near pulpal exposure should be treated appropriately prior to any crown placement. Removal of the smear layer has been debated (increased binding versus potential sensitivity) and dentinal desiccation should be avoided.

Zinc phosphate cement has been regulated by ADA Specification No. 8, Zinc Phosphate Cements, since 1935 (http://JAmDentAssoc.ada.org/article/S0375-8451(37)12022-7/abstract). It is sometimes incorrectly termed zinc oxyphosphate cement, but no study has proven oxyphosphate formation during setting. It is supplied in powder/liquid kits for mixing. It is used as luting cement. Type I zinc phosphate cements have fine grain particles used for seating precision appliances, inlays, onlays, crowns, and bridges. Type II is of a medium grain particle size and used as an insulating base under restorations. Zinc phosphate cement usage has declined dramatically over the past 20 years.

The polycarboxylate cements are regulated by ADA under Specification No. 61, Polycarboxylate Cements (http://JAmDentAssoc.ada.org/article/S0002-8177(80)14031-9/pdf). They form a good adhesive bond to enamel, dentin, and stainless steel, but a very weak bonding to gold and almost negligible attachment to porcelains. Polycarboxylate cements were used for cementation of cast crowns, bridges, and orthodontic bands or as a base under amalgams. Again, there are much better cement material options available today including the GICs and composite resin adhesives.

Cements made either of composites or acrylic resins are useful in bracket cementation due to their lack of solubility in water. Whether a two-paste system or a single-filled resin is used with a liquid activation on the bracket, the tooth should first be cleaned, polished with flour pumice, rinsed, dried, and acid-etched. They tend to be thinner preparations than the typical restorative composites, to allow a minimal thickness of the material to obtain better retention. With posts and crowns, use of a light cured bonding agent will also increase adherence. Newer products that bond to sandblasted base or noble metals are extremely useful in crowns, though oxygen inhibition is necessary for the chemical cure and it is an expensive material. The latest self-adhesive composite resin cements are popular choices for the permanent cementation of crowns, bridges, inlays, onlays, and Maryland bridges. These cements require no etching and are dual cured.

17.9.2 Acid Etching

Acid etching is used to selectively dissolve some of dental or restorative surfaces. This leaves a surface with more microporosities in which resins can enter to provide a greater micromechanical interlock or bond. In bonding a composite resin to a dental cavity preparation, the acid etching provides greater bonding strength and margins that are a great deal more resistant to leakage.

The acid etchant most commonly used currently is phosphoric acid. A 35–38% gel or solution is used on enamel and on dentin. Dentin requires a shorter application time for etching.

In etching the tooth surface, the first step is to clean the surface to be etched by scaling, followed by polishing with flour of pumice and water. Non-fluoride prophy pastes can be used for this purpose only if they are completely water soluble, which many are not. Fluoride in the paste is contraindicated as it may make the enamel more resistant to the acid. Acid conditioning of the enamel causes enamel prisms and interprismatic enamel to dissolve and a micro retentive surface is created.

Following etching, water can be used for rinsing [18]. Moisture contamination can inhibit proper bonding of the resin to the surface. Therefore, adequate dry field isolation should be used. Generally, etching with a 30–38% phosphoric acid for about 30 seconds on enamel and 15 seconds on dentin is sufficient. Research has shown that the shorter etching periods on enamel are generally as effective as the longer 60 second etchings in humans [46]. Prolonged etching of 120 seconds or longer only creates an insoluble calcium precipitate on the surface, which reduces the strength of the bond [20]. The etchant should be applied in a fashion that will not allow the tooth to dry out while being etched. This may mean reapplication of the etchant. Some research has indicated that light agitation of the acid while on the enamel surface can improve the etch pattern and possibly the resin retention effect [47].

Thicker acid gel excesses can be gently removed with a cotton swab. Acid solutions and remaining gel on the tooth should then be rinsed off the surface. Rinsing should last for at least 10 seconds, but not exceed 20 seconds [48]. Spraying water for more than 60 seconds has shown to damage the etched surface, resulting in a decreased bond strength [49]. When properly etched and the enamel is air dried, the surface will appear to have a light chalky appearance. If the surface is still shiny, the etching was unsuccessful. This is usually an indication of either a failure to properly clean the tooth prior to etching or a failure in preventing moisture contamination. If old resin is still on the tooth surface it will inhibit etching. It should be scaled off, or in some cases the light use of a diamond bur may be required for its removal.

17.9.3 Enamel Bonding

Enamel bonding agents are liquid unfilled or lightly filled resins. Bonding agents improve restoration retention, while aiding in the prevention of marginal leakage. Marginal leakage is more common along cavosurface margins in cervical enamel than the other parts of the enamel [26]. This is due to the fact that the bond between the composite resin and the tooth is weakest with cervical enamel, as a result of its anatomical makeup [50]. Gently brushing the bonding resin into a thin coverage rather than using air to blow the layer thin may be better [20]. The aggressive use of air may blow air into the resin layer, which can inhibit curing. The use of a gentle air stream angled across the cavity can avert air being blown into the resin. On etched enamel, a low-viscosity bonding agent disperses easily, penetrates the microporosities of the treated enamel surface, and thus provides for microretentive bonding of the composite. Bonding composite resins to enamel is considered very predictable.

17.9.4 Dentin Bonding

The benefits of "adhesive" dentistry are now well accepted. Cavity preparations can be much smaller as macromechanical retention is not required as it is with materials such as amalgam alloys. When dealing with dental caries or other bacterial ingress into the tooth, the cavity "seal" is enhanced with micromechanical adhesion.

The adhesive systems used today offer satisfactory bond strengths for both enamel and dentin. The problem with most systems is their method of use, since dentin bonding can be characterized by a complex series of steps. Operator error in following these steps can lead to premature failure of the restoration.

Since the introduction of resin bonding to enamel in 1955, many attempts have been made to achieve a similar quality of bond to dentin [20]. This is due to the need for additional retention in some restorations that have significant amounts of exposed dentin, cavosurfaces of dentin or cementum, and the fact that certain restorations are under greater stress patterns. There are several reasons for the poorer quality of bond to dentin as compared to enamel in the past. Enamel has approximately a 96% inorganic composition, while dentin has approximately only a 70% composition, with the remaining 30% being principally water and collagen fibers (see Chapter 1 – Oral Anatomy and Physiology). In addition, during cavity preparation a smear layer is created on the exposed dentinal surface by the instrumentation, which blocks entrance of the potential bonding surfaces within the tubules.

With composite resins restorations, dentin bonding agents are indicated for all exposed dentin surfaces. Additionally, they are indicated for dentin and cementum cavosurfaces. They help control marginal leakage, marginal discoloration, pulpal sensitivity, and recurrence of caries. Dentin bonding agents should be used as an adjunct to enamel bonding, dentinal undercuts, dovetails, pinholes, grooves, or pins. On Class V lesions enamel surfaces should be beveled, but if a dentin or cementum cervical cavosurface is present, a light undercut along that surface in the dentin would be recommended.

Due to the variety of dentinal bonding agents on the market, their differences in technique of mixing and application, and their sensitivity to some techniques, the manufacturer's recommendations should be followed closely for each individual product. Research into dentin bonding agents will eventually provide the practitioner with agents that have ease of placement, high-quality bonding, marginal security, biocompatibility, are non-irritating or even soothing to the pulp, and have long-term stability in the oral cavity.

17.9.4.1 History of Dentin Bonding Systems

Dentin bonding has evolved through what may be classified as eight generations. In the late 1950s and early 1960s, the first generation of dentinal bonding agents came on the market, which were cyanoacrylics, polyurethanes, glycerophosphoric acid dimethacrylate, and *N*-phenyl glycine with glycidylmethacrylate. These had poor clinical success as they achieved only a 10–20 kg/cm^2 bond strength, with shear type tests [51].

In the mid 1970s, the second generation of bonding agents were mostly halophosphorous esters of bis-GMA. These undertook to form a phosphate–calcium bond with the inorganic part of the dentin. The bond strength varied widely with the product and skill of the operator, but 30–90 kg/cm^2 was reported [52]. However, the oral cavity environment resulted in the bond being hydrolyzed with time. With a bond strength that only rated from poor to fair to begin with, the hydrolization and failure of that with time resulted in unpredictable and unsatisfactory clinical performance [53, 54].

In 1982, the third generation of bonding agents was introduced [55]. These were the oxalate systems, which originally had elaborate and time consuming procedures for mixing and application by the operator, which resulted in unpredictable results. In addition, frequently a light brown marginal discoloration was encountered, which was thought to be due to the acidified ferric oxalate used in the system. However, these systems did demonstrate a bond strength of 100–150 kg/cm^2 [55].

The fourth generation of bonding agents evolved in the early 1990s with improved handling qualities and bonding strength. There were still some inconsistencies with their application and they were technique sensitive, but they were reported to have bond strengths of 200–220 kg/cm^2, which approaches 210–250 kg/cm^2 bond strength of resins to enamel [20]. However, standardized testing and research protocols were not used [56], and direct extrapolation of *in vitro* tests to the complex environment of the oral cavity has not been possible [57].

The accepted concept of wet dentin bonding, using adhesive systems containing hydrophilic primer dissolved in acetone or ethanol, was found to produce higher bond strengths when acid-conditioned dentin was left visibly moist prior to bonding [58]. Micromechanical retention was achieved by means of resin infiltration into the conditioned collagen matrix to form a hybrid layer of resin impregnated dentin. The benefit of moist bonding is derived from the ability of water to keep the interfibrillar channels within the collagen network from collapsing during resin infiltration.

The fifth generation in the mid 1990s combined primer and adhesive in the one bottle and the enamel and dentin was etched prior to bond application. Bond strengths to dentin were still good [59, 60]. The one-bottle systems consisted of hydrophilic and hydrophobic resins simultaneously dissolved in a solvent like alcohol or acetone, displacing water and achieving an intimate contact to dentinal structures. These materials also generally rely on residual moisture in the dentin and hydrophilic water chasing compositions to effect resin penetration into the dentin. Given the relatively high percentage of solvent, these formulations may be less forgiving to small changes in the dentin moisture content and may also require multiple application of primer/adhesive combination for successful bonding.

The sixth generation of agents came in the late 1990s and early 2000s. They were split into Type I, which had self-etching primers plus a separate bottle of adhesive, and type II self-etch adhesive, where products were mixed prior to applying it to the tooth. Type I were the self-etch primers, where a weak acid and the primer were in the same bottle, followed by a separate bottle for the dentin bond. The second type or type II include two bottle systems, or a single applicator system where wells were compressed together to mix the products (3M Espe Adper Prompt L-Pop self-etch adhesive). In humans, these systems tended to reduce post-operative sensitivity. However, the bond strength to enamel and dentin was lower than fourth or fifth generation bonding agents.

The seventh generation, or "all in one" products, combine etch, primer, and bond in the one solution. This made application more user friendly without worrying about how dry or wet the tooth surface needed to be. They can be purchased in a bottle or single applicator forms. Eighth generation bonding agents have a stable nanofiller component in the single bottle and can be used for direct or indirect restorations.

17.9.4.2 Current Bonding Systems

There are currently four recognized dentin bonding system types. When using any system, be sure to read the instructions thoroughly. Some systems require more than one application of the bonding agent. Also do not mix systems, due to compatibility issues. Examples provided are not meant to be an endorsement and the list of available products is constantly expanding.

1) "Three-step" systems (fourth generation) consist of etching the enamel and dentin, usually with 37% phosphoric acid, washing and then lightly drying the dentine (be careful not to over-dry and collapse collagen fibers), and then placing a primer (usually hydroxyethyl methacrylate or HEMA), which can be thinned out with air from an air–water syringe to evaporate the solvent (water, acetone, or alcohol). The bonding agent (usually consisting of bis-glycidyl-methacrylate or bis-GMA, urethane dimethacrylate or UDMA plus photo-initiators that react at a certain wavelength of light) is then placed and agitated, thinning it out with air prior to photo-curing the bond. A composite resin is then placed on to the bonded enamel and dentine.
2) The phosphoric acid etch followed by a combination of the primer/bonding agent in the one bottle and a single-step – the so-called "two-step" – total etch or etch and rinse systems. Alternatively, the etch and primer can be in the one bottle, followed by the bonding agent in another bottle– the so-called "self-etching primer" system (sixth generation). There is no washing involved with this system, which limits the chance of over- or underhydrating the collagen fibers in the dentine. Usually the acid used is a weak acid such as 10% maleic acid, which may compromise bond strengths to enamel.
3) The "all-in-one" system (seventh and eighth generation) is where the etch, primer, and bonding agent are all in the one container. The solution is applied to the tooth, thinned out with air, and then photocured and a composite placed. Again, there is no washing of the tooth.

17.10 Principles of Cavity Preparation Design

The design of the cavity preparation for a restoration is dictated by the lesion and characteristics in the intended material's physical properties. For amalgam, the major properties of concern are its low edge and tensile strength, creep or distortion under physical stress, inability to materially bond to the dental structure, and high thermal conductivity [3, 43]. Characterizations of composites and glass ionomer material will be discussed in applicable sections. In general, the following ideals should be contemplated:

1) Cavosurface angles should be at a 90° angle to the surface or parallel to the enamel rods.
2) The cavity preparation should be designed so the dentinal tooth structure supports the restoration.
3) Preparation should be complete, but conservative in nature.
4) For amalgam retention in the form of dentinal undercuts, pin ledges, pins, or posts are typically incorporated. Undercuts are not needed for glass ionomers, due to natural bonding to tooth structures. Bonding agents used with composites also make additional retention usually unnecessary.
5) In preparations approaching the pulp, a protective insulation layer should be placed between the restoration and pulp.
6) In areas where stress will be a factor (occlusal surfaces, etc.), sufficient bulk for strength will be necessary.

17.10.1 Cavity Preparation

17.10.1.1 Class I Caries Prevention

Class I cavities of the pits and fissures are some of the most common carious lesions of humans, non-human primates, and the dog (Figure 17.6). When tooth anatomy is of sufficient depth or irregular shape to be predisposed to the development of caries or other pathology, preventive means can be performed. For caries prophylaxis, a heavy fluoride treatment, prophylactic odontomy, or placement of a pit and fissure sealant are the choices from which to select. Prophylactic odontomy is the removal of disease-prone dental tissue that is then restored to a normal form, but is rarely used in human dentistry, as the use of pit and fissure sealants is now considered standard practice.

The pit and fissure sealants allow for a more conservative, yet highly effective, approach to treatment.

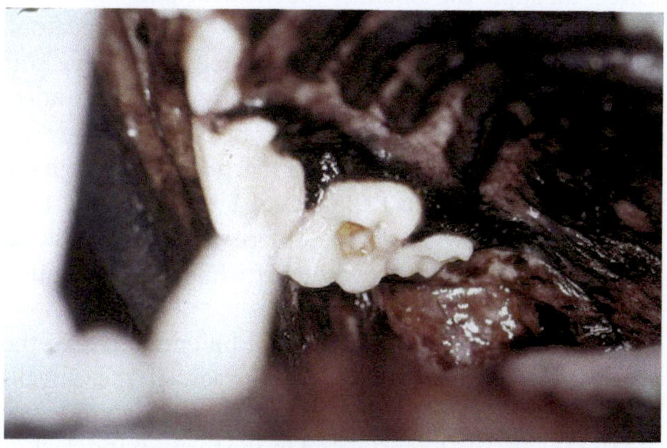

Figure 17.6 109 occlusal cavity prep.

The tooth is cleaned meticulously within the pit and fissure region. The structure is then polished with a flour of pumice and water, and rinsed clean. An acid etch material is applied to the area, according to the manufacturer's recommendations, and rinsed. The tooth is air-dried, an unfilled resin applied and light cured, followed by application of the pit and fissure sealant. Most pit and fissure sealants are thinly filled composite resins that are commonly fluoride-impregnated. Only light cure products are available today. There are also glass ionomer pit and fissure sealants available, used when moisture control is difficult. However, in humans, some concerns arise about trapping the cariogenic bacteria under the restoration if not thoroughly disinfected.

17.10.1.2 Classes I, II, III, and V Restorations

In cutting the cavity preparation, the outline form can be established with a high-speed air-driven dental handpiece, with adequate water flow, using a straight, tapered, or round bur [3] of a size suitable to the dimensions of the tooth. The No. 1/2 round and 699L taper burs have been used in veterinary dentistry for a number of years. The bur size can be increased according to the tooth and lesion dimensions. When using round burs to establish outline form, the margins must be checked more carefully for undermined or unsupported enamel. Diamond friction grip (FG) burs are becoming popular in veterinary dentistry for cavity preparation. ISO 109-010 is a 1 mm wide, flat-end cylinder diamond-encrusted bur that cuts through enamel and dentine rapidly. FG diamond burs come in various levels of grit coarseness with extra coarse grit (black banded), coarse grit (green banded), medium grit (blue banded), fine grit (red banded), and extra fine grit (yellow banded). The finer grit burs are often used for polishing and smoothing over restorations.

Once the general outline form is established, a straight or tapered bur can be used to further develop the outline form, while avoiding undermining the enamel. Once through the enamel, mechanical pear or round burs, or hand instruments including spoon excavators, Wedelstaedt chisels, etc., can be used to remove soft carious dentin as well as to create any required undercuts in the dentinal walls. Inverted cone burs are no longer used because they leave a sharp angle between the axial and pulpal walls. The use of RA burs (latch type shank) in a slow-speed handpiece limits the risk of removing too much tooth structure while also preventing iatrogenic pulp exposures.

The axial or pulpal walls should be contained to the natural curvature of the tooth surface. If these walls approach or contact vital pulp tissue, then endodontic treatment should be instigated in the form of indirect or direct pulp capping, a root canal procedure, or other appropriate procedures.

17.10.1.3 Classes IV and VI Restorations

Classes IV, VI, or extensive lesions are generally best managed with cast or milled restorations. However, amalgam and composite are frequently used for the treatment of these lesions with a reasonable degree of success when skillfully constructed in the correct patient and if the cause of the defect has been identified and eliminated. Chairside restoration of these lesions is generally not recommended for working dogs as it may aggressively stress the region. Additionally, if the lesion is related to behavioral issues, they must be well managed, otherwise long-term success will be at risk.

When restorations cannot be contained within four walls of a sound tooth structure, an optimum resistance form cannot be provided. When possible, to compensate for this deficiency, the restorations bulk may be increased. In lesions where missing cusps must be replaced by an overlay or onlay, the bulk of the restorative must again be increased to prevent occlusal forces from easily fracturing it away from the tooth. This ordinarily means that the overlay area should have a 2.5–3 mm depth of restorative material against the walls that are perpendicular to the lines of occlusal force (pulpal and gingival walls). In addition to undercuts, some cases may require dovetails, pinholes, or pins to provide needed retention or resistance form.

17.10.2 Considerations for Amalgam Restorations

Due to the lack of tensile strength of amalgam at margins, the cavosurface margins should be structured to result in no unsupported enamel, while providing approximately a 90° cavosurface angle. However, occlusal margins can be modified by beveling to an angle of up to 70° when required, and if no unsupported enamel rods are created. Greater than a 70° modification would predispose the restorative marginal edge to chip and break.

Undercuts are used in the dentinal portion of certain walls to provide the mechanical retention required for amalgam. Many times in following the angle of the enamel rods, a natural angle of undercut is developed in pits, fissures, and occlusal surfaces (Class I, Class II), but the opposite is typically true on walls in the axial plane (Class II, Class III, Class IV, Class V) and cusp (Class VI). According to the cavity preparation being performed, undercuts should be placed in the dentin of the gingival and coronal (incisal or occlusal) walls, and the distal aspect of the buccal and lingual walls [4]. Undercutting all walls is unnecessary and violates "Rule No.1 of Restoration," which is conservation of dental structure. Amalgam is not highly advisable in Class IV and Class VI lesions, due to the occlusal stress and pressures. Occasionally, dovetailing the distal and lingual walls is used to improve retention [3]. Amalgam is still a popular choice for restoring the occlusal surfaces (Class I) of caries-affected maxillary molar teeth in the dog. It has good tensile strength and can withstand the masticatory forces applied to these teeth.

17.10.3 Considerations for Composite Resins

Beveling of the tooth's cavosurface margins in cavity preparations for composite resins has several positive effects for Classes III, IV, V, and VI restorations, but is not recommended in Classes I and II occlusal surfaces [20, 26]. In the former groups, beveled enamel preparations can provide greater retention strength, due to the greater enamel surface area, and improved esthetics provided by the gradual transition from composite to enamel. In a properly beveled cavity preparation, in concert with accurate composite color matching and finishing, an almost invisible restoration can be accomplished (Figure 17.7).

Beveling of the occlusal cavosurface margins in Classes I and II restorations is not beneficial because of the direction of the enamel rods (exposed rods are already present) on the occlusal surface of the tooth. First, this would enlarge the surface area of composite in occlusion. Composite resins are not as strong as enamel and wear faster, which can result in the need for early restoration replacement. Additionally, the thinned areas of composite along the margins are more prone to fracture from occlusal stress, which could result in marginal leakage and deficit areas in the restoration where food and debris can accumulate. These factors can easily result in failure of the restoration. Therefore, occlusal enamel should not be sacrificed for beveling. However, beveling of non-occlusal cavosurfaces in these classes is typically recommended [20].

In Class V and other classes of restoration where the cementoenamel junction is being approached, beveling should not be undertaken if a non-beveled margin would maintain the enamel margin, while still completing the cavity preparation. The bond strength to enamel and its marginal leakage integrity is greater than that of cementum or dentin. [50, 61] Therefore it would be preferred to end the margin in enamel rather than cementum or dentin (Figure 17.8).

In beveling the cavosurface, the choice of instrument or bur is generally the operator's preference in most cases. When additional bond strength is desired on enamel or dentin, the use of a coarse diamond can dramatically increase the surface area and the potential bonding surface, as well as provide a huge number of miniature interlocking surfaces [26]. A good bur choice for beveling the enamel would be a coarse grit flame diamond bur.

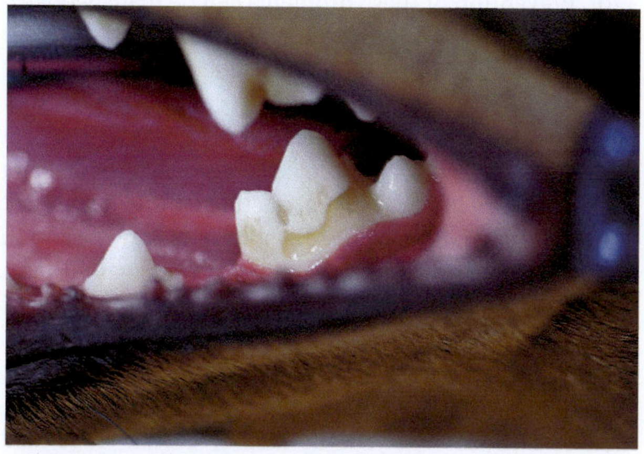

Figure 17.8 Class V lesion – 309; beveling at the apical extent would not be recommended if the bevel extended the finish line on cementum instead of enamel.

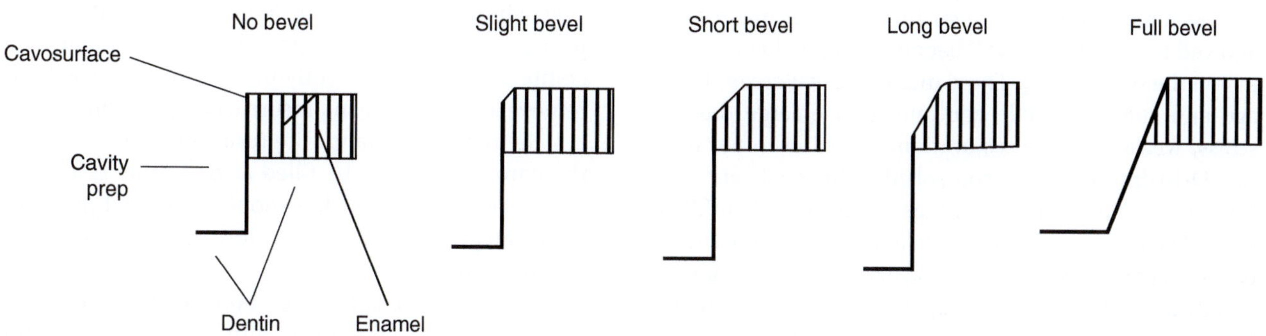

Figure 17.7 Basic types of marginal finish lines used on non-gingival cavosurfaces (illustration by Anthony Caiafa adapted from the First Edition).

If the bonding procedure before composite placement is not performed precisely, tiny air bubbles can be trapped between the tooth and bonding material. This can act to prevent the bonding agent from making contact with portions of the dental surface, inhibit resin curing, cause porosities that may lead to discoloration of the resin, and generally lead to a poor retentive bond and marginal leakage [62]. Usually the bond is thinned out with either a cotton pellet or a gentle stream of moisture-free air from the three-way syringe, angled obliquely across the preparation and not directly into the cavity.

17.10.4 Considerations for Glass Ionomers

Traditional glass ionomers are highly sensitive to moisture contamination during working, setting time, and maturation. Excess moisture is readily taken into the restorative. Early contamination results in a restorative that easily dissolves and can be washed out of the cavity preparation. Moisture contamination during setting results in cloudy spots at the points of contamination, which is due to crazing or microcracks in the restoration [20]. Prevention of these problems can be managed with a proper dry field isolation technique and if close to the gingiva, control of gingival crevicular fluid by use of astringents or open gingival flap techniques. The mild bond created by glass ionomer as it cements to the tooth structure is created by a chelation process. The setting reaction of material has an attraction to the calcium of the tooth as well as that in the silicate of the glass [63]. This means that the bond is stronger to enamel than dentin, since it is richer in calcium. However, the bond of glass ionomer to enamel is only about one-third of that of composite resin to enamel [34]. Some, but not all, glass ionomer cements make use of a 10 second application of a 10–25% polyacrylic acid or a mild citric acid product to the dentin, which is then rinsed off and the surface air-dried (not dessicated). It is used to remove the smear layer on the dentin in an attempt to enhance the ionomers bonding to the dentin [34]. Once set, but not hard, the glass must be prevented from dehydrating during maturation for several hours. If the material is allowed to dehydrate it will become opaque due to crazing on the surface [45]. These microcracks increase leakage and staining, while continuing to enlarge due to stress, weakening the restoration toward eventual failure. Dehydration can be controlled by the application of a moisture barrier [56], such as a light-cured unfilled resin. The ionomer should be coated as soon as the sheen is lost. Light-cured RMGICs have a resin incorporated within them that is set during curing, which eliminates the separate application of a barrier. The light-cured resins have been shown to be more effective than oils and varnishes [35].

Finishing can be done with simple hand instruments such as a gingival curette. The carving should be done as quickly as possible and a protective coat reapplied to prevent desiccation of the material. Bladed rotary instruments should be used very carefully as they have a tendency to disrupt the mild bonding effect the restorative has to the dental structure [57]. Once the restorative has been set up well, gross reduction and light finishing can be done with an aluminum oxide rotary stone point with a water spray, although some matrix dissolution may occur from the water in chemical cure products [57]. Final polishing can be done with a prophy angle, a rubber prophy cup, and a composite polish. The polishing should be done at a very slow speed and in chemical cure products it needs to be done quickly to avoid dehydration at this point when the restorative is stripped of a protective layer. Light-cured glass ionomers need no further treatment, but chemical-cured products should receive an additional protective coating at this point.

17.11 Steps Involved in Placing the Composite Restoration

- Clean the tooth with a scaler and pumice, and rinse clean. Maintain a dry field by the use of cotton rolls or pellets and astringents, as previously described. Place a liner or base if required.
- Etch the enamel for 30 seconds and the dentin for 15 seconds with 33–38% phosphoric acid. Rinse with a clean water spray for 10–20 seconds.
- Dry with a moisture/oil-free air source to see if the enamel is frosted. If not, re-clean the surface and repeat the acid etching (see Acid Etching for additional information).
- Apply the dentin bond/enamel bond depending on which system is used. Follow the manufacturer's recommendation on the dentin and enamel bonding agents.
- A flowable composite can then be used on the dentin.
- The hybrid composite resin can be placed with a composite carrier or with a coated plastic instrument. The composite should be lightly packed into the cavity to remove any air voids and insure a complete fill.
- If a chemical cure composite resin is being used, then the entire cavity can be filled at one time. If a light-cured composite is used, it should be placed in increments no greater than 2 mm before curing (this applies to most composite resins).
- New composite resin can be applied to pre-existing uncontaminated composite within five minutes and the bond between the two will be as strong as if they had been placed simultaneously [64].

- Cure the composite for the time recommended by the manufacturer, typically between 20 and 30 seconds.
- Continue placement of material until the preparation is filled to the desired level.
- Check the occlusion, using articulation paper, if needed, to indicate areas that need adjustment.
- The restorative can be adjusted and finished with a rotary white stone point or a sanding disk to remove any gross excess of material and obtain a smooth margin.
- Fluted finishing burs or diamond polishing burs can also be used for this purpose, but are highly aggressive and sometimes produce a washboard effect on the surface if not used correctly.
- Polish with a composite polishing paste with a prophy cup used on a low speed.

With light-cured products, the greatest polymerization and hardness occurs at the site closest to the light source. If this was an occlusal surface, much of the hardest composite may have been removed during finishing. Additionally, the surface may have some remaining microporosities not corrected by polishing and some marginal integrity may have been lost due to shrinkage. To counteract these factors, an additional layer of an unfilled resin-bonding agent should be applied and cured. All surfaces that were etched should be coated with the bonding agent. Uncoated areas may take as long as two to three months to remineralize [62], may stain or discolor, and allow a more rapid attachment of plaque and calculus.

17.12 Steps Involved in Placing the Glass Ionomer Restoration

- Maintain a dry field by the use of cotton rolls or pellets and astringents, as previously described.
- Follow the manufacturer's recommendation as to whether citric acid or polyacrylic acid is used for removal of the dentinal smear layer.
- Dry the cavity prep lightly, but do not desiccate.
- Measure out the required powder-to-liquid ratio on a glass slab.
  - Divide the powder into quarters.
  - Rapidly, using a W3 plastic instrument, mix one of the quarters of powder into the liquid and then as quickly as possible add the other three quarters.
  - The mixing should be completed within 45 seconds, to allow for sufficient working time for placement.
- With the tip of the instrument pick up a drop of the material and transfer it to the cavity prep and smooth it into place.
- The base liner type materials commonly flow well into preparations.
- Continue placement of material until the preparation is filled to the desired level.
- If using a light-cured GIC material, these can be applied to the cavity with an applicator gun after trituration.
- Light cure for the amount of time recommended by the manufacture, approximately 20–30 seconds.
- If using a chemical cure product, wait for the sheen to dull and apply a protective coating of an oil, varnish, or light-cured resin.
- Once the restorative has hardened, check the occlusion. If needed, articulation paper can be used to identify areas that need adjustment.
- Use a hand curette or rotary white stone point to remove any gross excess of material and obtain a smooth margin.
- Polish quickly with a composite polishing paste with a prophy cup used on a low speed.
- Light-cured products would be finished at this point, but chemical cure ionomers will need an additional protective coating quickly applied.

17.13 Steps Involved in Placing the Amalgam Restoration

- Class II and Class III lesions – place a matrix band to retain the material within the preparation during placement.
- Select amalgam and spill size.
- Place cavity liner/base (RMGIC) if required.
- Remove any excess base from the walls of preparation.
- Place an amalgam bonding agent if required (Amalgambond®, Parkell Co., Farmingdale, NY). Most amalgam bonding agents must still be fresh and moist when amalgam is applied.
- Triturate amalgam.
- Empty amalgam into the amalgam well.
- Pick up amalgam from the well by loading an amalgam carrier and pressing it into the amalgam ball.
- Place the tip of the amalgam carrier into the floor of the preparation and press the carrier lever to deliver the amalgam into the cavity.
- Use a small amalgam plugger to compact the amalgam into all the angles and details of the preparation. Then go to a larger plugger for heavier compaction.
- Repeat steps placement and plugging until the cavity is slightly overfilled.
- Use an amalgam or ball burnisher to remove any excess mercury from the restoration. Newer pre-filled amalgam capsules are very well proportioned in their alloy-to-mercury ratio and rarely have excess mercury that can be burnished out.

- Check the occlusion, using articulation paper if needed (may require extubating the patient). Adjustments can be made with a large discoid carver to remove excess bulk and a cleoid carver to fashion anatomy. It is helpful to partially rest the carver on the tooth surface and carve toward the amalgam.
- Remove the matrix band, if applied.
- Examine the wall covered by the matrix band and use a sanding disk or strip to remove remote proximal excesses.
- The side of an explorer can be used to remove excess material from the margins.
- The material can now be burnished lightly to provide some degree of finish or polish. Under normal circumstances amalgam should be allowed to set for 24 hours before polishing. However, in veterinary dentistry it is not always possible or prudent to place an animal under anesthesia a second time within 24 hours. However, highly finished and polished amalgam margins are more resistant to tarnish and corrosion.
- When polishing is possible, rubber abrasive points and disks are highly effective on a slow-speed contra-angle handpiece (Figures 17.9 and 17.10).

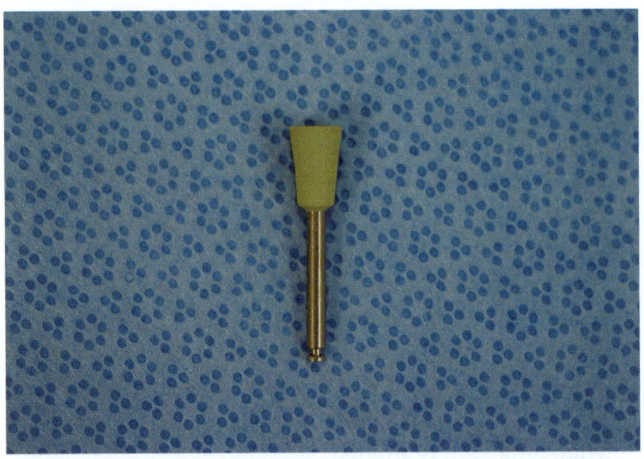

Figure 17.9 Finishing rubber abrasive points.

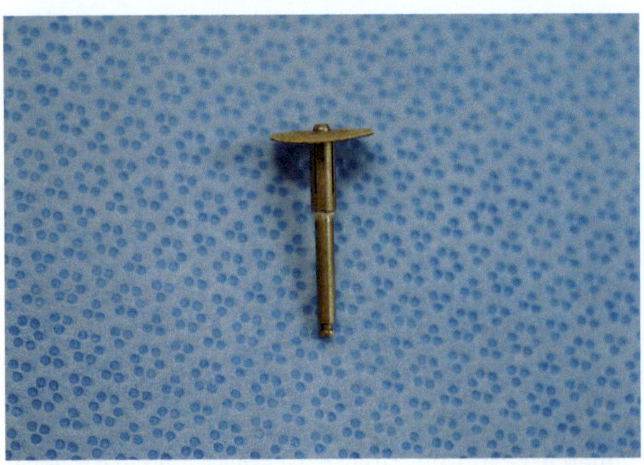

Figure 17.10 Finishing disk.

17.14 Retentive Aids for Restorations

17.14.1 Pots, Slots, Retentive Grooves, and Channels

"Pots and slots" are mechanical features cut into the dentin that are incorporated into a cavity preparation that helps to support and maintain the final restoration, primarily for amalgam. For dentinal pots and slots to be effective, they need to be placed 0.5 mm from the dentinoenamel junction. Unfortunately, these retentive aids remove healthy tooth structure and today are rarely used for mechanical retention of the restoration [65].

17.14.2 Pinholes and Pin Ledging

Pinholes are holes drilled into the dentin for the restorative to be packed into to provide retention or resistance for the restorative, or for pins to be inserted to provide the same. When a ledge is created on which the pinhole is placed, it is commonly called pin ledging.

17.14.3 Restoration Pins

Pins are used to provide either a resistance form or a retentive form, and extend both into the tooth and restoration. However, they actually weaken the tooth and restorative into which they are inserted, by making voids and reducing structure. Pins should only be used if the additional support is needed and the risk of restoration failure is increased by not using them.

17.14.3.1 Tooth Considerations for Pins

There are many biological and physiological factors that must be considered when considering the use of pins. Dentin in non-vital and older teeth loses elasticity provided by the organic structures and organs that fill the dentin in a vital tooth. Posts and pins that rely upon induced stress to provide retention may cause crazing in teeth with reduced elasticity [65]. For friction locked or threaded pins where the drill hole is smaller than the pin, stresses within the tooth and cracks can appear. Dental crazing is the formation of microscopic cracks in the tooth structure induced by stress factors. Crazing under continued stress may eventually result in cracks and structural failure of portions of the tooth, with cracks even traveling toward the pulp. Drilled holes and cemented posts or pins are a more prudent choice in non-vital or older teeth. Self-threading and friction-retained pins are best used in vital teeth with their greater elasticity.

Pulp location becomes important in pin placement. Vital teeth should not have pins inserted into the pulp cavity to insult the vital structures. This can lead to pulpitis and eventually pulp necrosis. In non-vital teeth the pulp cavity can be used conveniently for endodontic dowels (a pin placed in an endodontic cavity), while reducing the need for the removal of additional tooth structure for a pinhole site.

Morphology of the crown, root, and endodontic cavity becomes important in determining pin placement, as well as the extent of dentinal wall. Insufficient dentinal bulk may preclude the use of a pin at a site, so tooth size becomes a problem in many animals. Additionally, the occlusal stress (compression, shearing, leverage, and rotation) must be taken into consideration. In most carnivores there are considerable leverage and rotational forces placed upon the canine teeth, and compression and shearing force upon the carnassial teeth.

17.14.3.2 Pin Selection

Most pins are designed as threaded, cemented, or friction-retained (locked). With cemented pins, a pinhole is drilled and cleaned. Cement is then placed either in the hole or on the pin and it is inserted into the hole. Friction-retained pins also require a guide hole to be drilled, but will be undersized for the pin. Cement is then placed upon the pin or in the hole and the pin is pressed or tapped into place. Self-threading pins also make use of an undersized guide hole. The pin is then screwed into place with a small driver, or some pins are designed for use with a reduced (1:10 ratio) slow-speed contra-angle, as they have a latch attachment base. No cement is used with self-threading pins unless the hole is oversized in drilling or stripped out by too rapid a placement with the slow-speed contra-angle.

The threaded and friction retained pins can both cause stress resulting in crazing in brittle dentin (see Crazing). Newer designs of threads and placement have reduced but not eliminated these stresses. Generally, self-threading and friction-retained pins are best used in young vital teeth [66]; however, retentive demands with animals many times dictate their use in old and non-vital teeth. Cemented pins can be used in almost any case, young or old, vital or non-vital [67].

Considerations for pin size depend on the amount of retention required and the amount of structural weakness that is likely to be caused to the tooth from the pin. The larger the pin used, the more natural tooth structure must be removed for placement, increasing tooth weakness. Cemented pins, generally, have less retentive ability than self-threaded pins. A 0.025 inch diameter cemented pin has about 18 lb tensile load strength, while a 0.023 inch diameter self-threading pin has closer to 34 lb. Also, the larger the pin used, the greater the retention strength, as a 0.031 inch diameter self-threading pin has almost 59 lb tensile strength to resist failure [67]. Newer resin cements are improving the retentive strength of cemented pins and posts.

17.14.3.3 Pin Placement

Depth of pin placement into the dentin is dependent upon the type of pin used. Self-threading pins achieve their optimum practical retention at 2 mm into the dentin. The clinically practical depth for cemented pins is usually about 3 mm into the dentin [3].

Pins increase the retention of a restoration. However, they do not reinforce or strengthen the restoration, but actually weaken them [3]. Fracture tests have shown that the weak spots in the restoration are around the pins [67]. Research indicates the optimum length of pin into the restoration to be approximately 2 mm, as increased length further weakens the restoration, without increasing retention [67]. The pin can be cut off to the desired length using a No. 1/4 round bur, but many pins are designed with a shear point near the normal desired lengths. Location of pin placement is primarily dependent upon tooth morphology and the restorative design. Pins should not be placed closer than 0.5 mm to the dentinoenamel junction or crazing of dentin or enamel may occur, resulting in pin failure. In vital teeth all pins should be placed to avoid injury to the pulp, and in all teeth the periodontal ligament should be spared. Furcation and fluted root areas should be avoided unless there is sufficient dentinal depth to support a pin and be placed without perforation into the periodontal structures, as this may result in complications and even tooth loss. When two or more pins are used, they should be separated as far as morphology will allow for best structural integrity, but typically no closer than 1–2 mm apart [3].

The number of pins used is a clinical decision based upon the amount or retention or resistance required and the morphology and size of the tooth. To resist rotation at least one pin is required. When a restoration will overlay cusps, a general rule is one pin for each missing cusp. When retention is the prime requirement, self-threading pins provide greater retentive strength than cemented pins, and therefore fewer self-threading pins would be required [67].

The direction of pin placement is based upon the type of pin and number. For amalgam and resins, greater retention is derived when the pins are not parallel, but divergent to each other. However, in cast restoration placement of a single pin, it must be parallel to the line of draw. The line of draw is the direction the restoration must follow to be correctly placed upon the tooth, without binding. When two or more pins are used for cast restorations the pinholes need to be parallel to the line of draw and to each other in order to allow placement or the restoration, especially in crown and bridge work [3]. Generally, it is safest to place pins 0.5 mm from the dentinoenamel junction along the buccal line angles of the canine tooth. Due to the distal curvature of the crown and root canal, distal placement increases the chance of entrance into the canal and fracturing the overlying dentinal surface. This may also result in the pin being exposed to the surface during finishing. Mesial placement in the canine should be checked carefully, as the pin may perforate into the periodontal tissues.

In standard pins of normal cavity preparations, the optimum pin placement is customarily in alignment with the long axis of the tooth or parallel to the outside surface [68]. However, cleat-type pins are always placed at a 90° angle to the surface to which it is applied. In slab fractures of maxillary fourth premolars, this may mean that a cleat-type pin is placed at an angle to the tooth axis.

17.14.4 Endodontic Dowels or Root Canal Posts

The basic information for pin types or design also applies to endodontic posts or dowels [3]. Threaded pins and posts make use of friction and wall stress for retention, which increase the possibility of creating internal stress that may eventually result in tooth fracture [66]. Many of the threaded pins have a complex superstructure portion for retention of the restorative to the post known as a "Christmas tree." This superstructure is in alignment with the straight axis of the post. Most carnivore cuspids have a natural distal curvature of the crown. Typically, the post cannot be pre-curved and screwed into place, due to interference of the superstructure or exposed post with the surrounding structures. Once placed, they should not be bent, as this places severe stress on the root structure causing crazing, increasing the possibility of splitting the root structure, and the eventual loss of the tooth.

Standard posts usually require bending to allow them to conform to the gentle curvature of the cuspid root canal. For proper retentive and resistance form, these posts should extend into the canal a distance equal to as high as the eventual restoration will be. This generally correlates to twice as much post in the canal as is exposed, prior to restoration. Few posts are of a length suitable for this purpose in the dog. For this reason, metal intramedullary bone pins are commonly used, being bent and cut to need. In order to improve their retentive qualities for cementation and restorative placement, these customized posts should be scarified on the surface with a bur. Another alternative is to use Markley Threaded Wire™ (Almore Intl, Portland, OR), which comes in one-foot lengths. The wire can be cut to the desired lengths and cemented in place without engaging the threads in a screw fashion, but only using the threads for cement retention. Additionally, posts do not counteract rotational forces well. For this reason, one or more pins should be strategically placed around the post as a resistance to rotation.

17.15 Bleaching Teeth

In the previous edition, a discussion of bleaching vital and non-vital teeth for esthetic reasons was discussed. It has been removed from this edition.

References

1 Nagala, B., BB, K., Sahitya, S., and Krishna, P.M. (2012). Biological width and its importance in periodontal and restorative dentistry. *J. Conserv. Dent.* 15 (1): 12–17.

2 AVDC Nomenclature: Surfaces of Teeth. https://www.avdc.org/Nomenclature/Nomen-Dental_Anatomy.html#surfaces; accessed 25 October 2017.

3 Howard, W.W. and Moller, R.C. (1981). *Atlas of Operative Dentistry*, 3e. St. Louis, MO: The CV Mosby Co.

4 AVDC Nomenclature: Classification of Tooth Fractures. https://www.avdc.org/Nomenclature/Nomen-Teeth.html#fracture; accessed 25 October 2017.

5 Basrani, E. (1985). *Fractures of Teeth: Prevention and Treatment of the Vital and Non-vital Pulp*. Philadelphia, PA: Lea & Febiger.

6 Robinowich, B.Z. (1956). The fractured incisor. *Pediatr. Clin. N. Am.* 3: 979.

7 Brannstrom, M. (1982). *Dentin and Pulp in Restorative Dentistry*. Castelnovo, Italy: Wolf Med Pub.

8 Brannstrom, M. (1963). A hydrodynamic mechanism in the transmission of pain-producing stimuli through dentine. In: *Sensory Mechanism in Dentine* (ed. D.J. Anderson), 73. Oxford: Pergamon Press.

9 Berggren, G. and Brannstrom, M. (1965). The rate of flow in dentinal tubules due to capillary attraction. *J. Dent. Res.* 44: 415.

10 Brannstrom, M. (1986). The hydrodynamic theory of dentinal pain: sensation in preparations, caries, and the dentinal crack syndrome. *J. Endodont.* 12 (10): 453–457.

11 Sveen, O.B. and Hawes, R.R. (1968). Differentiation of new odontoblasts and dentine bridge formation in rat molar teeth after grinding. *Arch. Oral Biol.* 13: 1412.

12 Symons, N.B.B. (ed.) (1968). *Dentine and Pulp: Their structure and reactions, A Symposium*. Edinburgh: UK; University of Dundee. E&S Livingstone Ltd.

13 Streckfuss, J.L. et al. (1979). Calcification of selected strains of streptococci. *J. Dent. Res.* 58: 1917.

14 Gottlieb, B. (1946). The formation of secondary dentin and related problems. *J. Dent. Res.* 25: 34.

15 Qualtrough, A.J.E. (2005). *Principles of Operative Dentistry*. Oxford, UK, Ames, IA, or Carlton, Victoria, Australia. Blackwell Munksgaard.

16 Mount, G.J., Tyas, J.M., Duke, E.S. et al. (2006). A proposal for a new classification of lesions of exposed tooth surfaces. *Int Dent J.* 56 (2): 82–91.

17 Black, G.V. (1920). *Operative Dentistry*, 4e. Chicago, IL: Medico-Dental Pub Co.

18 Buonocore, M.G. (1955). A simple method of increasing the adhesion of acrylic filling materials to enamel surfaces. *J. Dent. Res.* 34: 849.

19 Bowen, R.L. (1962). Dental filling material comprising vinyl silane treated fused silica and a binder consisting of the reaction product of bis-phenol and glycidyl acrylate. US Patent 3,006,112.

20 Dale, B.G. and Ascheim, K.W. (1993). *Esthetic Dentistry a Clinical Approach to Techniques and Materials*. Philadelphia, PA: Lea & Febiger.

21 Craig, R.G. (1985). *Restorative Dental Materials*, 7e. St. Louis, MO: CV Mosby Co.

22 Macchi, R.L. and Craig, R.G. (1969). Physical and mechanical properties of composite restorative materials. *J. Am. Dent. Assoc.* 78: 328.

23 Zwemer, T.J. (1982). *Boucher's Clinical Dental Terminology*, 3e, 228. St. Louis, MO: CV Mosby.

24 Wiggs, R.B., and Lobprise, H.B. (1991). Dental materials. In: *AVDC/AVD Forum Proceedings*. 27.

25 (1983). *Dentists' Desk Reference, Materials, Instruments and Equipment*, 2e. Chicago, IL: American Dental Association.

26 Jensen, M.E. and Chan, D.C.N. (1985). Polymerization shrinkage and microleakage. In: *International Symposium on Posterior Composite Resin Dental Restorative Materials* (ed. G. Vanherle and D.C. Smith), 243. Netherlands: St. Paul, MN; Peter Szulc Co.

27 Oilo, G. (1981). Bond strength of new glass ionomer cements to dentin. *Scand. J. Dent. Res.* 89: 344.

28 Braswell, L.D. and Smith, J.S. (1989). Veterinary dental materials. *J. Vet. Dent.* 6 (4): 8.

29 Crisp, S., Lewis, B.G., and Wilson, A.D. (1976). Characterization of glass ionomer cements. Effect of the powder: liquid ratio on the physical properties. *J. Dent. Res.* 4: 287.

30 Forsten, L. (1977). Fluoride release from glass ionomer cement. *Scand. J. Dent. Res.* 85: 503.

31 Retief, D.H., Bradley, E.L., Dentin, J.C., and Switzer, P. (1984). Enamel and cementum fluoride uptake from glass ionomer cement. *Caries Res.* 18: 250.

32 Hicks, M.J., Flaitz, C.M., and Silverstone, L.M. (1986). Secondary caries formation in vitro around glass ionomer restorations. *Quintessence Int.* 17: 527.

33 Wilson, A.D. and Prosser, H.J. (1983). Mechanism of adhesion of poly electrolyte cements to hydroxyapatite. *J. Dent. Res.* 62: 590.

34 Powis, D.R., Folerars, T., Merson, S.A., and Wilson, A.D. (1982). Improved adhesion of a glass ionomer cement to dentin and enamel. *J. Dent. Res.* 61: 1416.

35 Earl, M.S.A., Hume, W.R., and Mount, G.J. (1989). Effect of varnishes and other surface treatments on water movement across the glass ionomer surface II. *Aust. Dent. J.* 34: 326.

36 McClean, J.W., Powis, D.R., Prosser, H.J., and Wilson, A.D. (1985). The use of glass-ionomer cements in bonding composite resins to dentine. *Br. Dent. J.* 158: 410.

37 Mount, G.J. (1989). Clinical requirements for a successful "sandwich" - dentine to glass ionomer cement to composite resin. *Aust. Dent. J.* 34: 259.

38 Smith, D.C. (1979). Composition and characteristics of glass ionomer cement and its relationship to the setting process. *J. Dent. Res.* 58: 1072.

39 Osman, E. et al. (1986). Fracture toughness of several categories of restorative materials. *J. Dent. Res.* 65: 220.

40 Phillips, R.W. (1957). Research on dental amalgam and its application in practice. *J. Am. Dent. Assoc.* 54: 309.

41 Mahler, D.B. (March 1967). Physical properties and manipulation of amalgam. *Dent. Clin. North Am.* 228.

42 Mahler, D.B., Terkla, L.G., Van Eysden, J., and Risbeck, M.H. (1970). Marginal fractures vs. mechanical properties of amalgam. *J. Dent. Res.* 49: 1452.

43 Healy, J.H. and Phillip, R.W. (1949). A clinical study of amalgam failures. *J. Dent. Res.* 28: 439.

44 Going, R.E. (1972). Status report on cavity liners, varnishes, primers and cleansers. *J. Am. Dent. Assoc.* 85: 654.

45 Phillips, S. et al. (1985). An *in vitro* study of the effect of moisture on glass ionomer cement. *Quintessence Int.* 16: 175.

46 Barkemeier, W.W. et al. (1986). Effects of 15 versus 60 second enamel acid conditioning on adhesion and morphology. *Oper. Dent.* 11 (3): 111.

47 Baharav, H. et al. (1988). The efficiency of liquid and gel etchants. *J. Prosth. Dent.* 60 (5): 545.

48 Mixson, J.M. et al. (1988). The effects of variable wash times and techniques on enamel composite resin bond strength. *Quintessence Int.* 19 (4): 279.

49 Schulein, T.M. et al. (1986). Rinsing times for a gel etchant related to enamel/composite bond strength. *Gen. Dent.* 345.

50 Crim, G.A. and Mattingly, S.L. (1980). Microleakage and the Class V composite cavosurface. *J. Dent. Child.* 47: 333.

51 Asmussen, E. (1985). Clinical relevance of physical, chemical and bonding properties of composite resins. *Oper. Dent.* 10: 61.

52 Fan, P.L. (1987). Dentin bonding systems. An update. *J. Am. Dent. Assoc.* 114: 91.
53 Doering, J.V. and Jensen, M.E. (1986). Clinical evaluation of dentin bonding materials on cervical abrasion lesions. *J. Dent. Res.* 65: 173.
54 Dennison, J.B., Ziemiecki, T.L., and Charbeneau, G.T. (1986). Retention of unprepared cervical restorations utilizing a dentin bonding agent. Two-year report. *J. Dent. Res.* 65: 173.
55 Bowen, R.L., Cobb, E.N., and Raapson, J.E. (1982). Adhesive bonding of various materials to hard tooth tissues. Improvement in bond strength to dentin. *J. Dent. Res.* 61: 1070.
56 Kim, K.C. (1988). The microleakage of a glass cement using two methods of moisture protection. *Quintessence Int.* 18: 835.
57 Pearson, G.J. (1983). Finishing of glass ionomer cements. *Br. Dent. J.* 155: 226.
58 Kanca, J. (1992). Resin bonding to wet substrates. 1: Bonding to dentin. *Quintessence Int.* 23: 39–41.
59 Mason, P.N., Ferrari, M., Cagidiaco, M.C., and Davidson, C.L. (1996). Shear bond strength of four dentinal adhesives applied *in vivo* and *in vitro*. *J. Dent.* 24 (3): 217–222.
60 Kanca, J. (1996). Improved bond strength through acid etching of dentin and bonding to wet dentin surfaces. *J. Am. Dent. Assoc.* 123: 35–43.
61 Davidson, C.L. and Kemp-Scholte, C.M. (1989). Shortcomings of composite resins in Class V restorations. *J. Esthet. Dent.* 1 (1): 1.
62 Albers, H.F. (1985). *Tooth Colored Restoratives*, 7e. Cotati, CA: Alto Books.
63 Wilson, A.D. et al. (1986). The release of fluoride and other chemical species from a glass ionomer cement. *Biomaterials* 6: 431.
64 Boyer, D.B. et al. (1984). Buildup and repair of light cured composites: bond strength. *J. Dent. Res.* 63 (10): 1241.
65 Vaught, R.L. (2007). Mechanical versus chemical retention for restoring complex restorations: what is the evidence? *J. Dent. Educ.* 71 (10): 1356–1362.
66 Markley, M.R. (March 1967). Pin retained and reinforced restorations and foundations. *Dent. Clin. North Am.* 229.
67 Moffa, J.P., Rozzano, M.R., and Doyle, M.G. (1969). Pins – a comparison of their retentive properties. *J. Am. Dent. Assoc.* 78: 529.
68 Dilts, W.E. and Mullaney, T.P. (1968). Relationship of pinhole location and tooth morphology in pin-retained restorations. *J. Am. Dent. Assoc.* 76: 1011.

18

Crowns and Prosthodontics

Curt Coffman[1], Chris Visser[1], Jason Soukup[2], and Michael Peak[3]

[1] *Arizona Veterinary Dental Specialists, Scottdale, AZ, USA*
[2] *School of Veterinary Medicine, University of Wisconsin-Madison, Madison, WI, USA*
[3] *Tampa Bay Veterinary Specialists, Largo, FL, USA*

18.1 Introduction

Prosthodontics is the dental specialty pertaining to the diagnosis, treatment planning, rehabilitation and maintenance of oral function, comfort, appearance, and health of patients with clinical conditions associated with missing or deficient teeth and/or oral and maxillofacial issues (American Dental Association, Specialty Dentistry Definitions: http://www.ada.org/en/education-careers/careers-in-dentistry/dental-specialties/specialty-definitions; accessed 5 November 2017). According to the American College of Prosthodontists, a Prosthodontist is a dentist who specializes in the esthetic (cosmetic) restoration and replacement of teeth, including the treatment planning and restoration of implants, temporomandibular joint disorder, and rehabilitation of occlusion with prostheses. Prosthodontic treatment in veterinary dentistry involves restoration of tooth structure lost to trauma, wear, or disease. Prosthodontic treatment is used most frequently in veterinary patients to restore fractured, worn, or decayed teeth and following endodontic treatment. Less common prosthodontic treatments for veterinary patients include inlays, onlays, partial crowns or veneers, bridges, and dental implants. The majority of the topics contained in this chapter pertain to treatments and materials commonly used in veterinary patients. While some of the information discussed may be more pertinent to human dentistry, these items are presented to expand the general knowledge base for veterinary dentists.

18.2 Definitions of Prosthodontic Terms

- Axial grooves. Grooves placed in a tooth preparation that provides improved retention of a restoration.
- Biologic width. The distance physiologically maintained by the body's defense mechanisms between the restorative and the base of the sulcus.
- Cast dowel core. A metal casting of a fully integrated endodontic dowel and core material.
- Cast dowel crown. A metal casting of a fully integrated endodontic dowel and crown.
- Cast restoration. A restoration that is fabricated by introducing a molten alloy into a mold in a process referred to as casting.
- Convergence angle. The angle between two opposing axial walls of a preparation.
- Core. The foundational replacement of a missing clinical crown whose purpose is to provide a rigid base for retention of a cast crown restoration.
- Crown. A cemented extracoronal restoration that covers the entire outer surface of the clinical crown.
- Crown lengthening. The exposure of a root (and/or crown) structure for use as a clinical crown for restorative coverage.
- Dowel. A cylindrical rod cemented or threaded into the root canal system as a retentive device for a core, cast dowel core, or cast dowel crown.
- Ferrule. A circumferential ring of metal around a natural tooth structure used to join a cast metal crown.
- Flashing. Restorative that extends beyond the preparation outline, but when initially placed does not cause an overhang.
- Full crown. A crown that covers the tip and all sides of the clinical crown (i.e., a full metal crown).
- Full veneer crowns. A restoration that covers the entire clinical crown (i.e., full coverage veneer).
- Inclination. The angle of deviation from a particular line or plane of reference.
- Inlay. A restoration made to fit into a cavity in a tooth.

Wiggs's Veterinary Dentistry: Principles and Practice, Second Edition. Edited by Heidi B. Lobprise and Johnathon R. (Bert) Dodd.

- Limiting average convergence angle. The point at which resistance is lost is recognized as a minimally acceptable convergence angle.
- Onlay. A restoration made to fit over or replace an incisal edge or occlusal cusp, either partially or completely.
- Overhang. An excess of restoration projecting beyond the parameters of a preparation margin, resulting in a projection or shoulder.
- Partial crown. A crown that covers only a portion of the clinical crown (½, ¾, etc.), where ¾ crowns are a type of partial veneer crown sometimes employed in the treatment of distal abrasion of the canine tooth in dogs.
- Partial veneer crown. A restorative crown that covers only a portion of the clinical crown.
- Pin. A metal pin or wire cemented or threaded into the dentin at a preparation site to aid in retention of a restoration.
- Porcelain fused to metal (PFM). A cast metal crown to which porcelain is bonded.
- Post. A cylindrical metal rod cemented or threaded into the root canal system as a retentive device for a core or post and crown. Can also be prefabricated as part of a post crown.
- Post and core. A substructure for a crown, which is retained by a post set into the root canal system. Can be a one-piece cast post and core or a post and core buildup made from a prefabricated post surrounded at its exposed part by a core buildup of a restorative material such as composite.
- Resistance. The ability of a restoration to resist dislodgement when apical or oblique forces are applied.
- Retention. The ability of a restoration to be retained on the tooth when subjected to tensile forces along the long axis of the tooth preparation.
- Stress riser. A mechanical defect or feature in a material, which concentrates stress in the area and increases the risk of failure of the material at that site.
- Taper. The angle between one axial wall of the preparation and the long axis of the preparation.
- Tooth preparation. The mechanical alteration of a defective, injured, or diseased tooth receives a restorative material that reestablishes a healthy state. This term may also be used as a noun to describe the prepared tooth.
- Undercut. A designed feature of a restorative preparation created by removing a portion of the dentin within the preparation for the intention of providing retentive qualities to a restoration.
- Veneer. A thin restorative covering; generally used to conceal or repair a discoloration, malformation, attritional wear, typically made from acrylic, resin, glass, or porcelain.

18.3 Classifications of Lesions in Teeth

Many of the elemental principles as well as materials and equipment used in prosthodontics are also integral to operative dentistry. Describing defects in tooth structure using modifications of human cavity classification systems (see below) can be useful in treatment planning. However, use of American Veterinary Dental College (ADVC) nomenclature found at www.avdc.org is advised (AVDC Nomenclature Committee: www.avdc.org/nomenclature; accessed 5 November 2017). Additional discussion of operative dentistry techniques is included later in this chapter and also in Chapter 17 – Restorative Dentistry.

18.3.1 The AVDC Tooth Fracture Classifications

- Enamel infraction (EI). An incomplete fracture (crack) of the enamel without loss of tooth substance.
- Enamel fracture (EF). A fracture with loss of crown substance confined to the enamel.
- Uncomplicated crown fracture (UCF). A fracture of the crown that does not expose the pulp.
- Complicated crown fracture (CCF). A fracture of the crown that exposes the pulp.
- Uncomplicated crown–root fracture (UCRF). A fracture of the crown and root that does not expose the pulp.
- Complicated crown–root fracture (CCRF). A fracture of the crown and root that exposes the pulp.
- Root fracture (RF). A fracture involving the root.
- Tooth fracture (T/FX).

When used in dental charting and AVDC case log entries, the tooth fracture abbreviations noted above are stated as T/FX/(specific abbreviation) (e.g., T/FX/CCF). This tooth fracture classification can be applied for brachydont and hypsodont teeth, which covers domesticated species and many wild species. Fractures of teeth in some wild species may not fit into this classification because of differences in the tissues present in the teeth. Other abbreviations used for restorative terms can also be found on the AVDC website (https://www.avdc.org/traineeinfo.html) (see Table 18.1). The G.V.Black cavity preparation classification system can be found in Chapter 17 – Restorative Dentistry [1].

18.4 Dental and Periodontal Anatomy Concerns

A working understanding of dental anatomy is essential when considering extensive prosthodontic restorative work such as crown restoration. While most teeth

Table 18.1 AVDC nomenclature abbreviations (https://www.avdc.org/traineeinfo.html; accessed 5 November 2017).

CR		Crown
	CR/M	Crown metal
	CR/PFM	Crown porcelain fused to metal
	CR/P	Crown preparation
CRA		Crown amputation
CRL		Crown lengthening
CRR		Crown reduction
CBU		Core buildup
IM		Impression and model
IMP		Implant
R		Restoration of tooth
	R/A	Restoration with amalgam
	R/C	Restoration with composite
	R/CP	Restoration with compomer
	R/I	Restoration with glass ionomer

requiring prosthodontic restoration in veterinary patients are non-vital and have received standard endodontic therapy, some vital teeth require attention as well. Crown preparation on vital teeth commonly leaves many open dentin tubules, resulting in dental pain, and possible pulpitis. A temporary crown may be placed to protect the tubules and pulp, knowing that these can sometimes be difficult to maintain on the animal. Alternatively, the tubules should be sealed with a bonding agent temporarily, until the permanent restoration is placed. When restoratives are placed upon vital teeth, it is extremely important to perform follow-up examinations to reassess and confirm continued tooth vitality.

Restorative dentistry not only concerns itself with the crowns of teeth but also with the teeth as anchorage units with the alveolar bone. In a simplified sense, teeth with a large amount of root inside the bone are considered to have favorable crown-to-root ratio [2]. When alveolar bone support is lost the ratio becomes less favorable. This basic concept of anchorage should be considered in treatment planning for restorations, but also underscores the importance of maintaining proper periodontal health and attachment in all restored teeth. Because periodontal disease is a common cause of tooth loss in veterinary patients, the clinician must be aware of each patient's periodontal health status when planning prosthodontic treatment. The patient's current periodontal health as well as the pet owner's ability and willingness to perform necessary future oral hygiene are vital to the long-term success for any restored tooth. The clinician planning a prosthodontic restoration must identify and institute effective periodontal treatment before completing definitive restorative treatment. It is a major disappointment to lose a properly restored tooth as a result of uncontrolled periodontal disease.

18.5 Treatment Planning

If the cause of tooth trauma or disease can be determined, steps should be taken to resolve the problem when possible. Any traumatic injury to the head or face can cause accompanying tooth fractures in dogs and cats. A common cause of tooth fracture in pet dogs is chewing on hard bones, objects, or toys, but any traumatic injury to the head or face may potentially cause accompanying tooth fractures in dogs and cats [3]. Many products marketed as chew toys are hard enough to cause tooth fracture and abrasion from a dog's normal chewing forces. Working dogs may injure teeth during training, patrol, or protection work. Cage biting, tug of war games, and uncontrolled dermatologic problems are also common causes of tooth wear and injury. The long-term success of any planned restorative treatment can be compromised if the initial problem cannot be identified and resolved.

18.5.1 Material and Design

The selection of the material and design of the restoration should be based on several factors [4]:

1) Amount of destruction of the tooth structure
2) Esthetics and function
3) Plaque control
4) Financial considerations
5) Retention.

If the degree of tooth destruction from the original injury requires the restoration to add strength and protection, a cast metal or ceramic crown may be indicated over composite resin restoration. Esthetic considerations may not be as important for pets as in people. However, many pet owners consider their pets to be a family member and may request a tooth colored restoration over cast metal. Recent advances in ceramic technology allow some tooth colored restorations to approach the strength of cast metal restorations, but cast metal must be considered the "gold standard" for veterinary restorations until solid research proves otherwise. Plaque control and the health of the periodontal tissues are critical concerns when planning a restoration. If the supporting tissues of the tooth are diseased, the periodontal disease must be treated and controlled before placement of definitive restorations. The pet owner must be willing to commit to routine oral hygiene at home and be willing to present the pet for proper follow-up in the veterinary office.

The clinician must consider the source of the original trauma to the tooth and the goal for protection weighed with preservation of a tooth. In some dogs that are "cage biters," reduction of less coronal structure with a ¾ crown onlay may help prevent further abrasion of the distal aspects of the canine teeth [5]. However, full coverage crowns are generally accepted to be the most retentive restorations when compared to ¾ crowns and other types of partial coverage crowns [4].

Designing a restoration for a tooth that has been previously treated endodontically is dependent primarily on the amount of remaining tooth structure. Often in veterinary patients, the amount of tooth structure lost to the original injury precludes restoration of teeth to their original height and contour. The remaining tooth structure must be evaluated for its ability to sustain normal occlusal load and stress, its retentive qualities, and the esthetic requirements of the restoration. Because of the size variability of veterinary patients, there is no easy rule of how much remaining crown structure is required to support a successful crown restoration. In general, the greater the amount of remaining sound tooth structure, the more retentive and resistant the final crown restoration will be. If the amount of remaining tooth structure is deemed insufficient, a crown lengthening procedure can be considered. The encirclement of the axial tooth structure within the walls of a full crown creates a ferrule effect that will protect the tooth from fracture. In humans approximately 2 mm of a sound vertical tooth structure must be present to achieve this effect [4].

18.6 Materials Used for Crown Restorations

When contemplating crown restorations, some considerations for the crown and preparation design include: material, preparation type (for full crown coverage or partial crown coverage either inlay or onlay), the supragingival or subgingival margin, the need for additional retentive designs and tooth preservation.

The material used for the crown should be based on the needs of the patient and the desires of the owner. If strength and maximum protection is needed, then a full metal crown is the best choice. If esthetics are the primary concern, then other crown restorative materials such as ceramic, PFM, or composite may be more appropriate. Each of these materials has its advantages and disadvantages as well as preferred methods for preparation of the tooth. The clinician should be familiar with all these crown substrates and their requirements. While the general focus of the clinical techniques described in this chapter pertains to metal crown restorations, veterinary dentists may occasionally choose materials other than metal at the pet owner's request.

18.6.1 Metals

Metal, in general, can be classified as either ferrous or non-ferrous based on the content of iron. Ferrous metals include metals such as iron or steel. Non-ferrous metals can be further broken down into noble metals, base metals, and light metals [6]. Prosthodontic crowns are usually made from non-ferrous metals. Noble metals contain gold and the platinum group of metals: platinum, palladium, ruthium, rhodium, iridium, and osmium. Gold has long been used for metal crown restorations. It has the advantage of being relatively non-reactive and resists corrosion in the oral cavity. It is very malleable which helps in finishing the margins and allows for a good marginal fit. The disadvantages of gold include its hardness (gold is relatively soft), its cost, and its color when considering esthetics. Noble metals are relatively non-reactive and resistant to corrosion and tarnishing. Silver is not considered a noble metal in dentistry since it does corrode in the oral cavity. All of the noble metals plus silver can be grouped together as precious metals. Other metals are considered "non-precious" or "base" metals. A combination of several of metals is known as an alloy.

The vast number of alloy systems requires greater reliance upon laboratory guidance. However, some of the new non-precious alloys often provide very good results more economically than the costlier precious alloys. Casting alloys are typically classified into two broad groups based upon their fusion temperatures [7]. The normal fusing alloys are formulated for all metal restoration, while high fusing alloys are designed for PFM restorations [8]. However, high fusing metals are sometimes used for all metal restorations. A high fusing metal must be used for the metal layer of PFM restorations, so that they do not melt or creep during the repeated heating required to bake on the porcelain layers [9]. When cost is not a concern, gold alloy is a good overall selection. However, there are many newer precious metal alloy combinations that provide good results more economically than gold. The base metals, although highly durable and inexpensive, have disadvantages that must be taken into consideration [10–12]. The gold–palladium alloys have many good characteristics for PFM use and are considered a good choice by many human clinicians. High palladium alloys are a combination primarily of palladium, with a moderate amount of base metal and a small amount of gold and silver. They are very hard and compatible with most porcelain systems, but are more technique-sensitive and more difficult to cast well [9].

Table 18.2 Revised classification system for alloys for fixed prosthodontics (ADA) (http://www.ada.org/en/about-the-ada/ada-positions-policies-and-statements/revised-classification-system-for-alloys-for-fixed-prosthodontics).

Classification	Requirement
High noble alloys	Noble metal content ≥60% (gold + platinum group[a]) and gold ≥40%
Titanium and titanium alloys	Titanium ≥85%
Noble alloys	Noble metal content ≥25% (gold + platinum group[a])
Predominantly base alloys	Noble metal content ≤25% (gold + platinum group[a])

[a] Metals of the platinum group are platinum, palladium, rhodium, iridium, osmium. and ruthenium.

Base alloys contain less than 25% noble metal and have a place in veterinary dentistry due to their lower cost, hardness, and strength. They are used for full-cast restorations as well as PFM restorations. As a group they are much harder, stronger, and have twice as high an elastic modulus as do the high noble and noble metal alloys. This latter property is advantageous because casting can be made thinner and still retain rigidity.

The ADA Council revised the classification system in 2003 with regard to the use of titanium and titanium alloys in dentistry (http://www.ada.org/2190.aspx). Titanium and titanium alloys have been added between high noble and noble alloys because of their excellent biocompatibility in the revised classification system (Table 18.2).

18.6.2 Composites

The indirect composite resin technique requires the composite restoration to be fabricated on a model rather than directly upon the tooth. Indirect techniques do have some advantages over direct applications. Composite resins, both direct and indirect, when cured have shrinkage in the resin matrix during polymerization. With directly applied composites, this can result in gaps in the marginal seal and possible marginal leakage. With indirect technique the shrinkage occurs prior to placement, which is chiefly offset with the luting or bonding agent at the time of placement. This results in less marginal gapping and a decreased risk of marginal leakage [9]. In addition, laboratories can use ultraviolet light (direct composites normally use visible light curing composites), heat, and vacuum to provide a superiorly cured composite resin restorative [13]. This results in a composite resin that may be harder and have greater tensile strength, which would then be a stronger, longer lasting restoration [14].

Composite resins are softer than porcelain, do not generally accelerate wear of the opposing natural tooth structure, and are easy to re-polish following adjustment. These advantages, along with continued improvement in composite technology, have resulted in direct composite resin becoming one of the most commonly used types of restoration in both human and veterinary dentistry.

18.6.3 Ceramics

Dental ceramics are man-made, inorganic, non-metallic materials produced by the heating of raw minerals at high temperatures [15]. Ceramics are widely used in prosthetic dentistry because they are aesthetically pleasing in color, shade, and luster, and they are chemically stable. The main constituents of dental ceramic are silicon-based inorganic materials, such as feldspar, quartz, and silica [16] (Table 18.3). Traditional feldspar-based ceramics are also referred to as "porcelain." Ceramics are generally considered brittle, which means that they display a high compressive strength but low tensile strength and may be fractured under very low strain (0.1%, 0.2%). As restorative materials, traditional dental ceramics have disadvantages mostly due to their inability to withstand functional forces that are present in the oral cavity. Hence, initially, they found limited application in the premolar and molar areas, although further development in these materials has enabled their use as posterior prosthetic restorations and structures over dental implants in people [17]. All dental ceramics display relatively lower fracture toughness when

Table 18.3 Types of dental ceramics.

Restoration type		
All ceramic		
	Traditional dental ceramics	Silica-based ceramics
	Glass ceramics	Leucite-feldspar ceramics
		Fluormica ceramics
		Lithium disilicate ceramics
Porcelain fused metal (PFM)–high-strength core ceramics	Glass-infiltrated ceramics	
	Metal oxide ceramics	Alumina-based ceramics
		Zirconia-based ceramics

Source: Adapted from reference [16].

compared with dental alloys [18]. The main difference between a regular ceramic and a dental ceramic is the proportion of feldspar, quartz, and silica contained in the ceramic. A dental ceramic is a multiphase system, containing a dispersed crystalline phase surrounded by a continuous amorphous phase (a glassy phase). Modern dental ceramics contain a higher proportion of the crystalline phase that significantly improves the biomechanical properties of these ceramics.

The so-called cast-glass ceramics are different from traditional feldspar-based (porcelain) ceramics because of the larger crystalline phase that helps stop crack growth. Examples of these high crystalline ceramics include lithium disilicate and zirconia. These infiltrated ceramics such as In–Ceram (Vita) are made through a process called slip-casting, which involves the condensation of an aqueous porcelain slip on a refractory die [19]. This fired porous core is later glass infiltrated, a process by which molten glass is drawn into the pores by capillary action at high temperatures. Materials processed in this way exhibit less porosity, fewer defects from processing, greater strength, and higher toughness than conventional feldspathic porcelains [20]. These are made of a glass-infiltrated core that is later veneered with a feldspathic ceramic for final esthetics. The Vita In-Ceram slip-casting system makes use of three different materials to gain a good compromise between strength and esthetics. Three variations of In-Ceram are spinell, alumina, and zirconia.

Solid-sintered ceramics have the highest potential for strength and toughness but, because of high firing temperatures and sintering shrinkage techniques, they were not available to use as high-strength frameworks for crowns and fixed partial dentures until recently. Solid-sintered monophase ceramics are materials that are formed by directly sintering crystals together without any intervening matrix to form a dense, air-free, glass-free, polycrystalline structure [21]. There are several different processing techniques that allow the fabrication of either solid-sintered aluminous oxide or zirconia oxide frameworks. Examples of these systems include Procera (Nobel Biocare), Lava (3M ESPE), and Cercon (Dentsply). Cast glass ceramics or solid sintered ceramics can be considered for esthetic repairs of canine teeth of non-working dogs. However, even these newest ceramics may still be vulnerable to the complex shearing forces of animal carnassial teeth, where metal restorations are generally better suited.

18.6.4 Porcelain – Porcelain Fused to Metal (PFM)

Traditional feldspar porcelain is infrequently used as a singular restorative material in veterinary patients because of its tendency to fracture under strain. Porcelains with a higher coefficient of thermal expansion were developed in the early 1960s [9]. This allowed the compatible fusing of porcelains to that of casted metal dental alloys, and the acceptable fabrication of the PFM restoration. While the outer porcelain coating of PFM restorations remain relatively brittle compared to ceramic and full metal restorations, the metal interior of PFM restorations provide a strong inner core to protect the tooth structure. Porcelain fuses to the metal by both a chemical and mechanical bonding. The chemical bond occurs as the porcelain forms a crystalline attachment to oxides on the surface of the metal alloy. The mechanical interlock occurs both on a gross level from the design and on a micromechanical level from the abrasive treatment of the metal, which forms a surface texture for bonding [22].

The metals for the substructure must be able to take repeated firing for the application of the various layers of porcelain without deformation or creep. This means that the substructure metal of a PFM should be a high fusing alloy (see Section 18.6.1 – Metals, above) [23]. The porcelain must be able to resist slumping and devitrification. Slumping results in slow deformation of porcelain from repeated heating. Devitrification is the crystallization that occurs from the repeated firings, resulting in a clouding of the porcelain and an opaque, non-vital appearance to the restoration [22].

The axial reduction with PFM needs to be in the range of 1.5 mm to allow for a 0.5 mm metal substructure and the 1 mm of porcelain needed to cover the metal esthetically. The incisal reduction should be in the 2.0 mm and occlusal 1.5 mm range [9]. Failure to provide sufficient reduction will result in poor esthetics, a weak restoration, or an oversized restoration [24]. In addition, the porcelain layer should not generally exceed 2 mm in thickness, as it is not required for esthetics and the porcelain is the weak link in the restoration. Therefore, the metal substructure should be designed to prevent overlayering of the porcelain [25]. The esthetic outer structure of PFM crowns is certainly susceptible to chipping in veterinary patients, but the inner metal core will provide circumferential protection for the tooth identical to a full metal veneer, so PFMs can be considered if the pet owner understands the risk of damage to the porcelain.

18.7 Operative Equipment Required

Preparation of teeth for crown restoration does not require an extensive armamentarium. Most preparations require a selection burs and a high-speed air turbine handpiece. Small pointed diamond burs used with a water–air spray will allow precise removal of tooth structure. Gross reduction of the tooth is accomplished with coarse diamond burs. In order to leave a smooth finish line at the margin, a fine diamond or other finishing bur should be used to smooth the preparation margin [25]. This will facilitate fabrication of the restoration and allow for a smooth, continuous finish line and a well-adapted margin. Cementation of the restoration requires simple restorative materials for use with adhesive cements. A basic list of equipment and materials for prosthodontics includes:

High-speed dental handpiece
Air/water source
Various dental burs (carbide and diamonds, fine to coarse grits)
Medium and coarse grit round-end taper cylinder
Medium and coarse grit round/ball, sizes 012–016
Impression materials and trays
Dental loupes/magnification
Adjustable lighting for the operative field
Adhesive cements.

18.8 Tooth Preparation

18.8.1 General Concepts for Restorative Procedures

When a defect occurs in the hard tissues of the tooth (enamel, dentin), optimally it is best to preserve the function and structure of the object by restorative means. It is essential to understand the basic components of restorative dentistry, including cavity preparation, as well as skills involved in shaping the final preparation. The clinician should be familiar with the basics concepts of restorations including conservation, esthetics, contours and contacts, extension for prevention, cavity preparation, and identification and resolution of the cause of the tooth defect (see Chapter 17 – Restorative Dentistry).

18.8.2 Components of Prepared Cavities

Various walls, lines, and angles are created during cavity preparation (see Chapter 17 – Restorative Dentistry) In crown and bridge preparation the primary walls of concern are the pulpal, axial, and gingival. Additionally, there are a few subdivisions of the walls, such as the enamel and dentinal walls. The enamel wall is that portion of the preparation wall that consists of enamel. The dentinal wall is that portion of the wall that consists of dentin. The dentin–enamel junction is that juncture in the wall where the dentinal and enamel walls meet.

Where two walls meet, a line angle is formed. At the point where three walls meet a point angle is produced. The cavosurface angle is the line angle formed between a wall of the prepared surface and the unprepared tooth surface. The cavosurface angle is also sometimes termed the preparation margin, especially once the preparation is restored. The combined peripheral extent of all of the cavosurface or preparation margins is termed the cavity or preparation outline. In dealing with restoratives, the restorative margin is the restorative surface that abuts the cavosurface angle or preparation margin.

18.8.3 General Concepts of Prosthodontic Preparations

Design of the cavosurface angle requires special consideration in its preparation. The preparation margin greatly affects retentive qualities of the restoration, resistance to marginal leakage, physiologic contour reactions, gingival health, and resistance to attrition, abrasion, and fracture of the restoration and the restored tooth. Selection of the specific cavosurface angle for the margin is dependent upon the type of restoration selected, restorative materials to be used, and the degree of anticipated stress demand upon the restoration. The preparation margin comprises two components: the recess and the finish line. The recess is the depth of tooth structure removed and must provide enough room for the intended restoration. The finish line delineates the most apical border of the preparation. An optimal finish line should be well-defined and crisp [26].

Historically many configurations and variations of finish lines have been used for margins of cemented crown restorations and onlays. The basic preparation margins commonly used with current restorative materials in veterinary patients (chamfer, shoulder, and heavy (deep) chamfer) are discussed further below. Shoulders and heavy chamfers may be provided with a bevel, which is an oblique cut into the external angle of the recess. The potential benefit to adding a bevel is that it will decrease the thickness of the cement interface at the restoration margin [1].

The use of occult finish lines or very steep bevels may leave a stronger tooth substructure to support the crown, but also results in an oversized restoration. Theoretically, an occult finish line may benefit cases where additional foundation strength is required (i.e., military working dogs), but there are no published studies to support this idea. Additionally, these finish lines are clinically more difficult to prepare and reproduce in the dental laboratory.

18.9 Principles of Tooth Preparation for Cast Restorations

In order to place a cast restoration on a tooth, some tooth structure must be removed. This process is termed tooth preparation. The guiding principles of tooth preparation in humans, although only studied to a small degree in dogs, are likely to be applicable in companion animals. However, continued research in this field of veterinary dentistry is highly encouraged in order to promote evidence-based tooth preparations. There are five governing principles for the design of a tooth preparation: preservation of tooth structure, retention and resistance, structural durability, marginal integrity, and preservation of the periodontium.

18.9.1 Preservation of Tooth Structure

Tooth preparation is a balance between removing the appropriate quantity of tooth material to place and maintain a restoration and maintaining the appropriate quantity of tooth material to preserve tooth strength and pulpal health. Efforts should be made to maintain as much normal tooth structure as possible. If a partial veneer crown achieves the clinical goal while respecting the other governing principles, especially retention and resistance, it may be chosen to minimize removal of the tooth structure. Partial veneer crowns (¾ crowns) have been advocated for the management of distal abrasion of canine teeth in dogs [4]. However, studies have shown that full veneer crowns are generally more retentive than partial veneer designs [26–28] (Figure 18.1). Therefore, the operator must weigh the pros and cons of each design for their patient's unique clinical presentation.

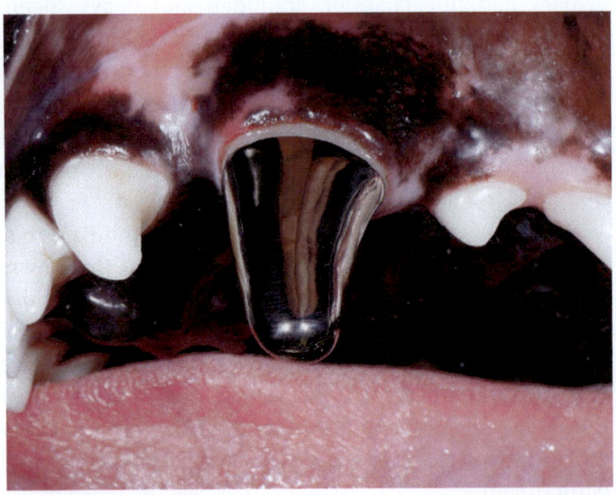

Figure 18.1 Full metal crown.

While subgingival finish lines may increase clinical crown height, there are many disadvantages to their use in companion animals in regard to periodontal health. When not dictated by a client's esthetic preferences, the use of subgingival finish lines should be avoided in order to maintain as much tooth structure as possible.

Excessively tapering the axial walls of a tooth crown during preparation or removing large amounts of tooth structure during occlusal reduction will weaken the remaining tooth structure. In addition, in the vital tooth, there may be an increased risk of causing pulpitis and pulpal necrosis.

However, in some cases removal of larger amounts of sound tooth structure is needed in order to preserve the remaining tooth structure. When the removed tooth structure is replaced by a sufficient bulk of metal alloy, the underlying tooth structure is protected from normal occlusal loads. This concept applies to areas that are placed under higher occlusal loads such as maxillary fourth premolars and maxillary and mandibular molars.

18.9.2 Retention and Resistance

A restoration cannot be held in place based solely on the adhesive properties of currently available luting cements [29]. Therefore, the geometric design of the tooth preparation must support crown retention and resist crown dislodgement. Retention is the ability of a restoration to be retained on the tooth when subjected to tensile forces along the long axis of the tooth preparation [30]. Resistance is the ability of a restoration to resist dislodgement when apical or oblique forces are applied [30]. Although we speak of the two terms independently, retention and resistance are inherently interrelated. There are four operator-controlled factors in tooth preparation that influence retention and resistance in companion animals: convergence angle, crown height, auxiliary features, and freedom of displacement [30].

18.9.2.1 Convergence Angle

In order for a cast restoration to be placed on a preparation, some degree of axial wall inclination must exist to permit the restoration to seat. Axial wall inclination is best expressed as the preparation convergence angle, which is the angle between two opposing axial walls (Figure 18.2). The appropriate inclination has been the subject of much research and discussion since it was first demonstrated experimentally that retention increases as convergence angles decrease [31]. Theoretically, a tooth preparation with parallelism of opposing axial walls would provide a maximal degree of retention and resistance. However, operators who have been instructed to achieve parallelism inevitably create undercuts [32]. In addition, precise parallelism of opposing axial walls leads to poor

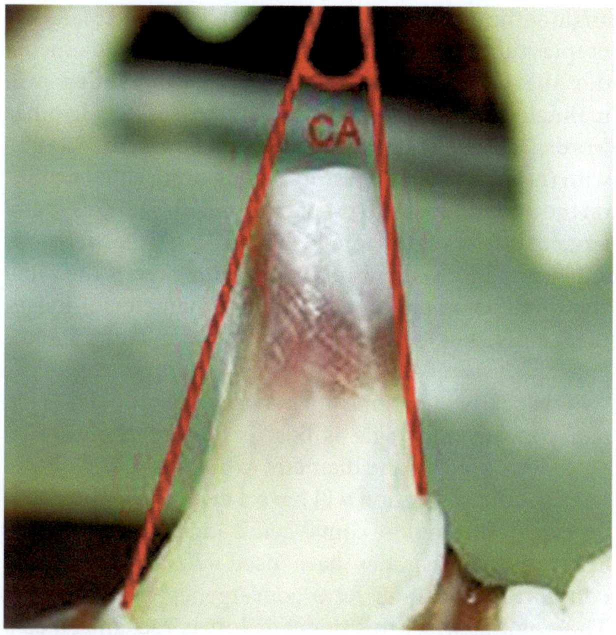

Figure 18.2 Illustration depicting the convergence angle between two opposing axial walls of a tooth preparation.

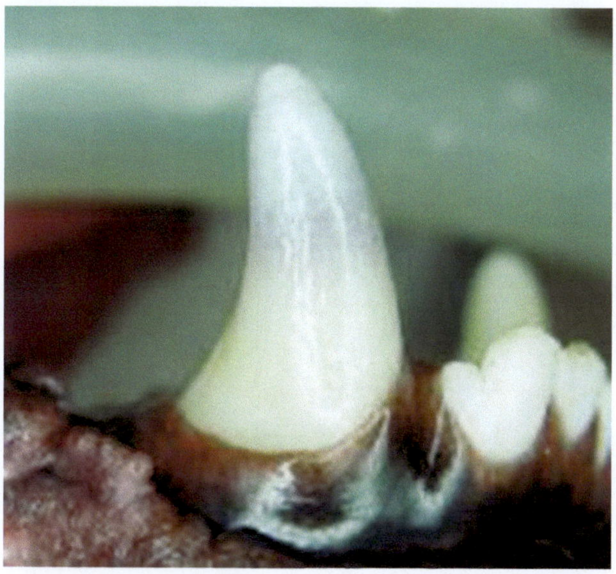

Figure 18.3 Photograph of a discolored canine tooth highlighting the dynamic curvature of the distal aspect of the crown.

seating of cast restorations [33]. Thus, recommended convergence angles have historically been between 3° and 15° [31, 34–43].

Due to the dynamic curvature and steep inclination of the distal axial wall, the canine teeth and carnassial teeth of dogs have a naturally unfavorable convergence angle [30, 44] (Figure 18.3). In addition, when tooth structure has been lost from a traumatic injury, the convergence angle becomes even less favorable [30]. The clinically achievable convergence angle of canine teeth that have been traumatically shortened may be as high as 70° [30]. Thus, achieving the recommended convergence angle is nearly impossible. In one study, the mean achievable convergence angle of canine teeth in dogs was 35.5° in the mesial to distal plane and 18.48° in the facial to lingual plane [30]. The natural convergence angle of the mandibular first molar tooth and the maxillary fourth premolar tooth have recently been reported to be 36° and 43°, respectively [44]. In addition, the ideal convergence angle is rarely clinically achieved in dogs and humans. Recently, studies have also shown that the recommended convergence angles are only achieved 0.4–13% of the time in humans [45, 46].

Despite large convergence angles, dog studies have shown crown adhesion/cohesion failure rates of only 2.6–9.7% in canine teeth [30, 47]. This is probably explained by two important factors. The first is the interrelationship between the convergence angle, crown height, and crown diameter, which is discussed in greater detail under the section on height below. The other factor is related to the fact that most veterinary dentists use resin-based cements. Luting cements appear to play a pivotal role in the retention of a cast restoration [48, 49]. Restorations cemented with a resin-based cement on to a preparation with a 70° convergence angle have been shown to have higher retention compared to restorations cemented with zinc phosphate cement on to a preparation with a 24° convergence angle [48]. Preparations with convergence angles greater than 24° should be cemented with resin-based cements to improve retention [49].

Given the large convergence angles seen in the canine tooth of dogs, the operator may consider additional design features to decrease the effective convergence angle, which may be achieved by one of two fundamental approaches. The first approach is the use of a tiered design in which "stair-steps" are created within the distal axial wall of the tooth [43] (Figure 18.4). However, the potential gain in resistance from a tiered design has not been evaluated in dogs. In addition, the introduction of tiers with 90° internal line angles introduces stress risers that may lead to biomechanical weakening and fracture of the tooth [50, 51]. The second is the implementation of auxiliary features, which are described in more detail below [52].

18.9.2.2 Height

Resistance and retention is not dictated by the convergence angle alone. The height of the crown contributes substantially to the retentive features of a tooth preparation. This is mediated primarily by the interference of the axial wall occlusal to the finish line with the path of displacement and is also dependent on the diameter of the preparation at the finish line and the convergence

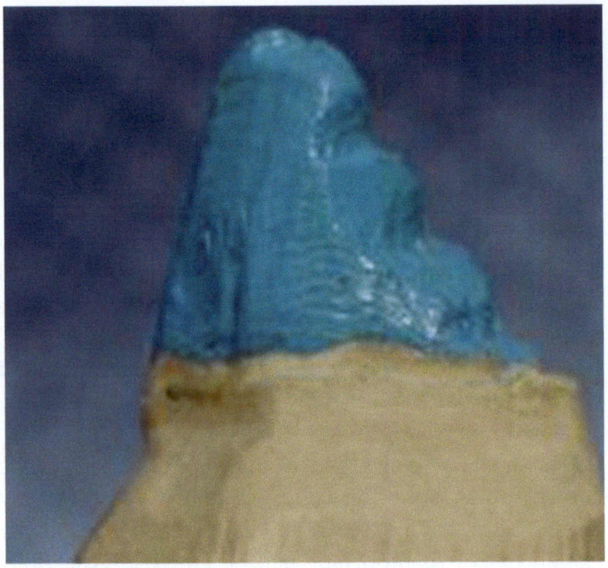

Figure 18.4 Photograph of a stone die of mandibular canine tooth with a tiered preparation design.

angle of the opposing axial walls [53] (Figure 18.5). As the preparation height increases, for a given base diameter, the maximal allowable convergence angle that will maintain adequate resistance also increases [53]. In other words, the preparation must be tall enough to interfere with the arc of the cast restoration pivoting about a point on the finish line. Tooth preparations with short walls and large diameters rely more heavily on a low convergence angle for dislodgement resistance. However, if the same short-walled preparation has a small diameter, dislodgement resistance is improved and is less reliant on a low convergence angle.

Perhaps the relationship between height, diameter, and convergence angle is best expressed clinically by considering height and diameter as a ratio (*H*/*D*) [30, 53]. Each tooth preparation will have a distinct *H*/*D* that can be used to determine a convergence angle that is clinically acceptable. Researches have used *H*/*D* to investigate conceptual guidelines for a convergence angle [30, 54]. The point at which resistance is lost is recognized as a minimally acceptable convergence angle and is denoted

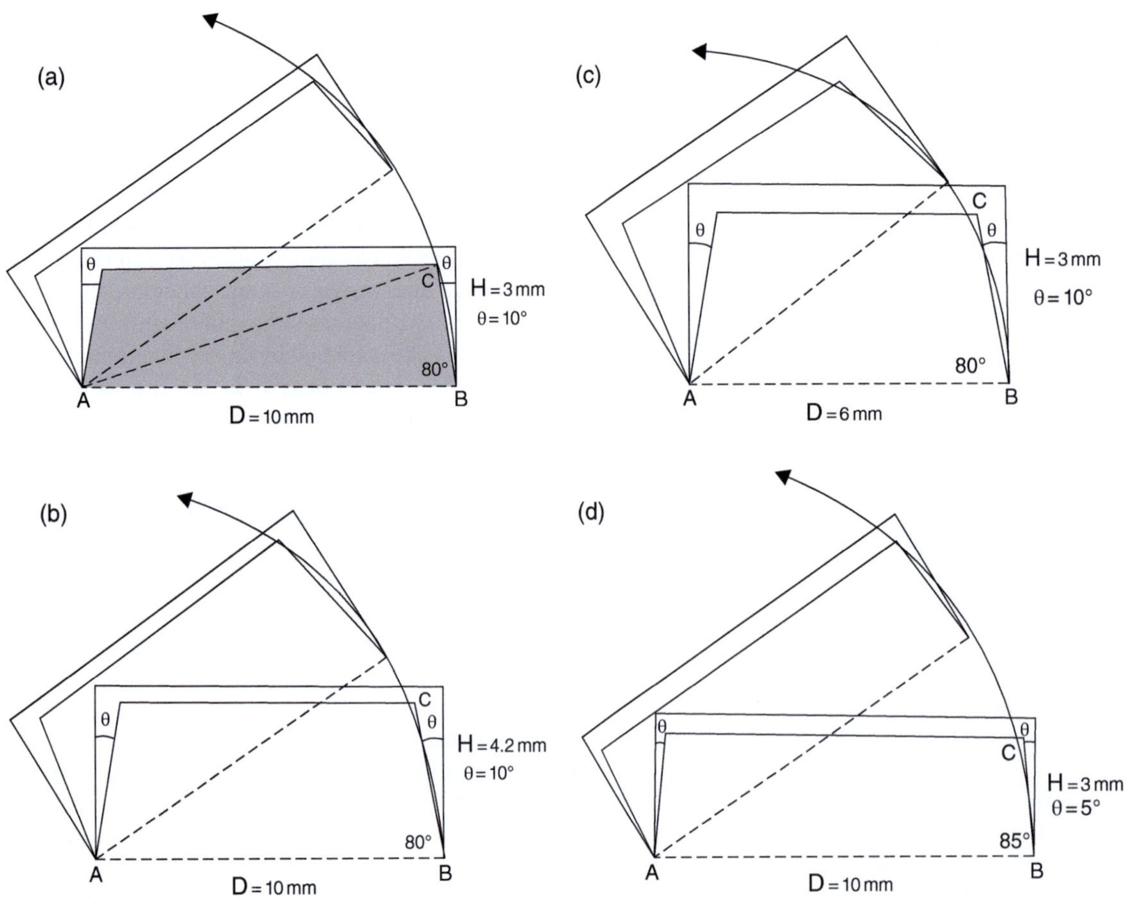

Figure 18.5 Illustration of the interdependency of convergence angle, crown height, and crown base diameter in the determination of resistance/retention form. *Source*: Adapted from reference [53].

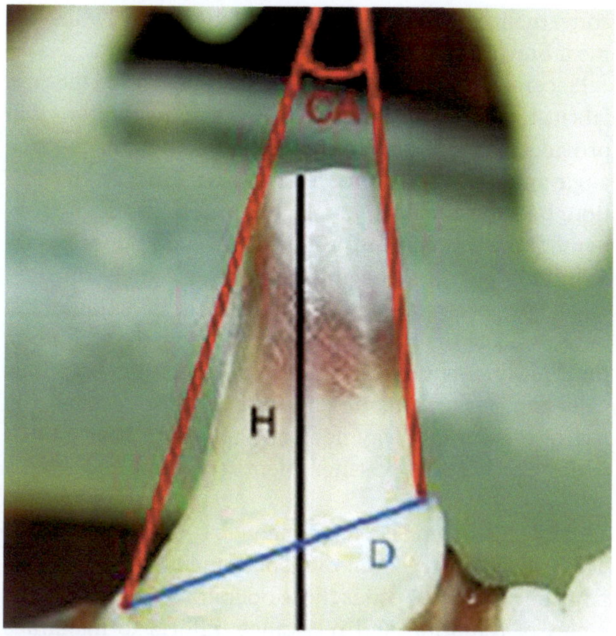

Figure 18.6 This shows how the formula $CA_{lim} = arc_{isn} (H/D)$ can be use in clinical practice to guide tooth preparation design. In this example, if $H = 10$ mm and $D = 7.5$ mm, then $H/D = 1.33$. The arcsin of 1.33 = infinity. Therefore, theoretically there is no limiting CA and any CA would provide the appropriate resistance form. However, if the crown were significantly shorter and $H = 5$, then $H/D = 0.66$. The arcsin of 0.66 = 41.3°. Therefore, the clinically achieved CA would need to be below 41. 3° in order to have an appropriate resistance form.

as the limiting average convergence angle. Tooth preparations with a convergence angle lower than this value do have resistance and those greater do not have resistance. The limiting average convergence angle (CA_{lim}) can be calculated with the formula CA_{lim} = arcsin (H/D) (Figure 18.6). In one clinical study, canine tooth preparations with a convergence angle that exceeded the CA_{lim} were 2.7 times more likely to be dislodged compared to those that did not [30]. Because the arcsin of 1.0 is infinity, theoretically, any tooth preparation with an $H/D \geq 1.0$ should always have positive retention features regardless of the convergence angle. This concept should serve as a clinical guideline rather than an absolute fact. Not all tooth preparations with $H/D \geq 1.0$ will have a sufficient resistance form [30, 54]. Dogs with tooth preparations possessing H/D ratios < 1.6 may be more likely to be dislodged [30]. When the clinically achieved convergence angle is higher than the calculated CA_{lim}, the operator may consider taking additional measures to help improve the resistance features.

The tooth preparation height is directly proportional to the preparation surface area. A positive correlation exists between an increased surface area and an increased unseating force in humans [35]. In addition, a positive correlation between the tooth preparation surface area and the clinical retention of crowns in dogs has been suggested [29]. The surface area will change with alterations of the underlying operator-controlled design features because of the interdependency of height, diameter, and convergence angle.

Although height alone does not determine the resistance and retention features of a tooth preparation, in most cases efforts should be made to maintain height. In some cases where significant clinical crown damage has occurred, efforts to increase height may be needed. Height can be gained by building up the tooth preparation with a pin- or dowel-retained core, performing crown lengthening, or by utilizing a subgingival margin. A discussion on the negative consequences of subgingival margins can be found later in this chapter.

A core of composite or amalgam can be used after endodontic therapy when significant tooth structure has been lost. If not firmly anchored to the remaining tooth structure, the core material will offer no substantial advantage over allowing the bulk of the casting to occupy the space [55]. The core may be anchored with prefabricated pins or dowels (i.e., post). Pin and dowel placement is discussed in greater detail in Chapter 17 (Restorative Dentistry). After the core buildup is performed, it is treated similarly to a normal tooth during tooth preparation. The operator should be cognizant of the need to extend the preparation finish line into the normal tooth structure. This will provide a protective circumferential ring of metal (ferrule) around the natural tooth structure that will help maximize retention of the cast restoration and minimize the chance of future tooth fracture, especially when the core is supported by an endodontic dowel [56].

Height may also be gained by utilizing a cast dowel core or a cast dowel crown. However, any system that utilizes a dowel, especially when a ferrule is absent, will gain most of its retention and resistance features from the dowel anchored within the canal, rather than on the preparation design of the clinical crown or core material. Therefore, significant load will be transferred into the root, which may overcome the root dentin strength and lead to catastrophic failure of the tooth and require tooth extraction [57].

The height of the clinical crown may also be increased with crown lengthening. Crown lengthening is the exposure of the root structure for use as a clinical crown for restorative coverage [9]. If combined with a dowel, the amount of additional tooth material needed to be gained from crown lengthening may only need to be enough to produce a ferrule effect, the 1.5–2 mm of natural tooth structure to be encircled by a band of metal crown [55].

Prior to considering crown lengthening procedures, the operator must have an understanding and respect for the physiologic principles of biologic width [9]. Biological width is the distance physiologically maintained by the body's defense mechanisms between the restorative and the base of the sulcus. The commonly understood biologic width in the dog is approximately 2 mm, which is the combination of approximately 1 mm of supracrestal connective tissue and 1 mm of junctional epithelium. Restorations that impinge upon this biologic width can cause a response to reestablish the biologic width. The body reacts with an inflammatory response that results in crestal bone resorption and apical migration of the periodontal soft tissues. The inflammatory response will only cease once the biologic width has been reestablished, which may take years.

There are three types of crown lengthening procedures: Type I (gingivectomy), Type II (apically repositioned flap with osseous recontouring) and Type III (orthodontic extrusion). In individual teeth where there is sufficient attached gingiva, a Type I crown lengthening procedure may provide additional height [58]. In order to provide additional clinical crown height, without effecting a response to biologic width physiology by placing the restorative margin too close to the alveolar crest, an apically repositioned flap with subsequent osseous recontouring may be performed [9, 59]. This procedure is considered as Type II crown lengthening (Figure 18.7a–c). Type III crown lengthening is the orthodontic extrusion of a tooth to increase the clinical crown height. This procedure may be involved and time consuming to reach a satisfactory clinical crown height.

18.9.2.3 Auxiliary Features

It may not always be possible to rely on opposing axial walls for retention. For example, when a traumatic injury to a canine tooth results in the loss of significant crown height, the convergence angle becomes quite unfavorable. In such instances the addition of auxiliary features into the tooth preparation design may be beneficial [60–62].

Human studies have shown that axial grooves placed in opposing axial walls of dies with unfavorable preparation design features (height of 3–4 mm or H/D of 0.25 and convergence angles of 20–35°) provide improved resistance to dislodgement when compared to teeth without the addition of axial grooves [60, 61]. Two recent studies in dogs revealed a statistically significant increase in the force required to dislodge metal crowns in the canine tooth and the maxillary fourth premolar tooth when axial grooves were included in the preparation design [63, 64]. Axial grooves provide two primary means of improving resistance form. The grooves increase the overall tooth surface area, which may reduce the chance of crown dislodgement in clinical patients [29]. In addition, the grooves provide for an engagement of the cast restoration with the tooth in a way that improves the effective convergence angle [65, 66] (Figure 18.8). The convergence of an axial groove approximates the convergence of the bur that created the groove, which for most burs is 8° to 12°.

Placement of internal grooves to receive pins that are fabricated as an integral part of a cast restoration will provide the same improvement in effective convergence angle and, thus, resistance form as axial grooves. In addition, because they can be placed deep to the cementoenamel junction and into the root, they do not rely on a minimum degree of height. However, pin holes must be placed perfectly parallel with the path of insertion of the outer walls of the preparation. In addition, the technique for reproducing the pin hole in the impression is technically demanding. Possibly because of these reasons, the use of pins in this way does not appear to have gained widespread use in veterinary dentistry.

18.9.2.4 Freedom of Displacement

The concept of freedom of displacement is dictated to a large degree by the other three operator-controlled principles of retention and resistance. Efforts to maximize parallelism of opposing axial walls, maintaining preparation height, and utilizing auxiliary features all combine to geometrically limit the number of paths along which a restoration can be removed. A tooth preparation that maximizes all of the retentive features discussed above will limit the potential paths of displacement.

Freedom of displacement from rotational forces must also be considered for tooth preparations that take on a more cylindrical geometrical form. Fortunately, the basic geometrical shape of the teeth most commonly treated with cast restorations in veterinary species is elliptical (canine and carnassial teeth) or triangular (maxillary molars), which provides a natural freedom of displacement against rotational forces. Efforts should be made to preserve these natural features when possible.

18.9.3 Structural Durability

Structural durability refers to the idea that a sufficient bulk of cast restorative material must be present in order to resist the normal forces of occlusion and prevent overcontouring of the cast restoration. Therefore, sufficient tooth material must be removed on all surfaces of the tooth.

Significant occlusal forces are primarily present in the premolar and molar teeth of dogs. Insufficient reduction of the occlusal table of the molar teeth may result in overcontouring of the cast restoration by the lab. As a result, premature contact of opposing teeth with subsequent temporomandibular joint (TMJ) stress and acute apical periodontitis may develop. If the lab does not overcontour the restoration, there will be thin areas of cast material that are susceptible to wear and perforation.

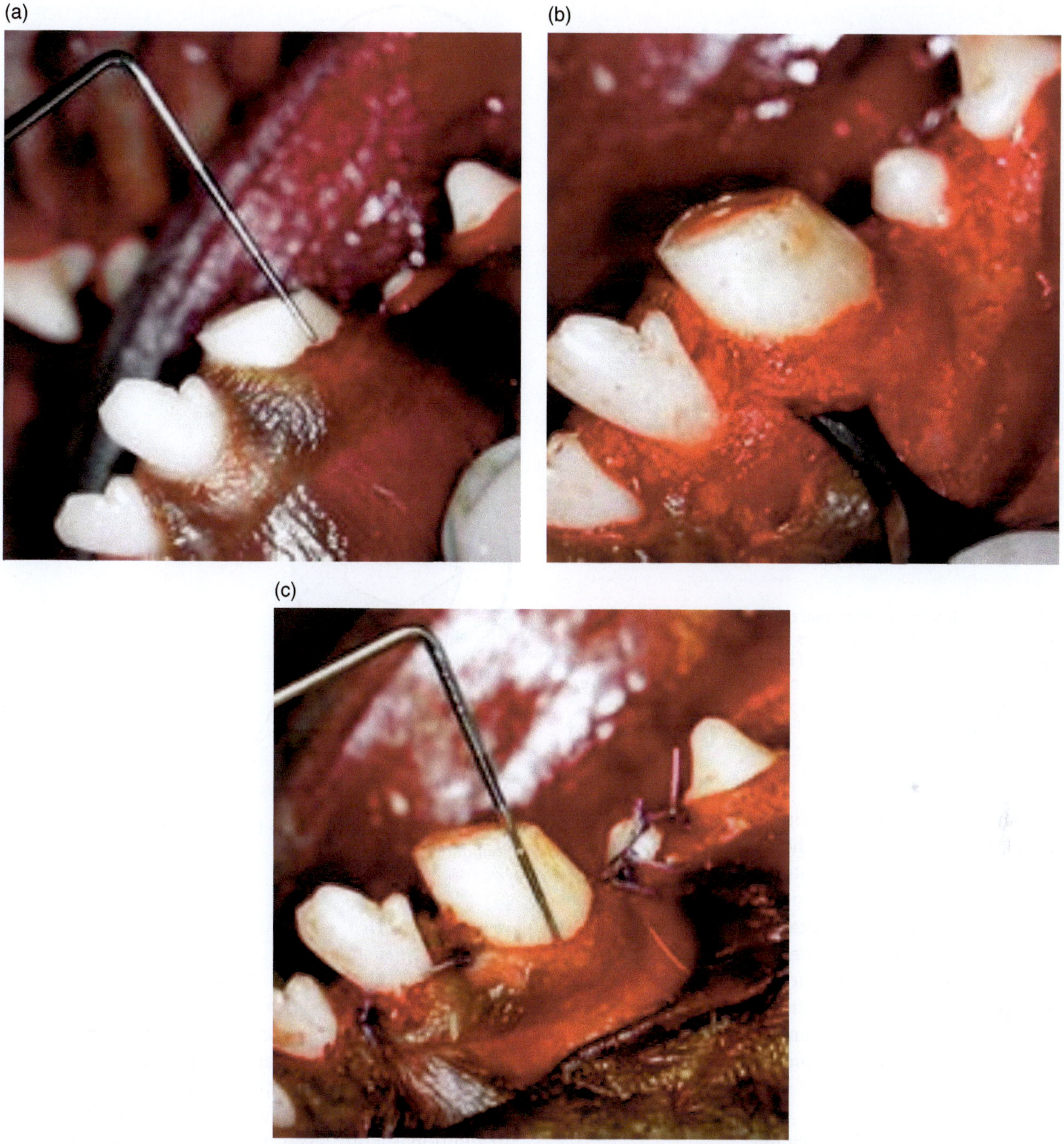

Figures 18.7 Photograph of a canine tooth receiving type II crown lengthening: (a) prior to surgery, (b) during osseous resection and recontouring and (c) after apical positioning of the mucoperiosteal flap. *Source*: Adapted from reference [59].

If sufficient material is not removed from the axial walls during tooth preparation, the cast restoration may be thin and prone to dimensional distortion prior to cementation on the preparation [4]. A lab technician may compensate for this by overcontouring the restoration, which will be detrimental to periodontal health.

18.9.4 Marginal Integrity

Good adaptation of the interface between the tooth and the restoration, commonly referred to as the margin, is crucial for long-term success of the restoration. Instrumental in the determination of marginal adaptation is the operator's choice of finish line configuration.

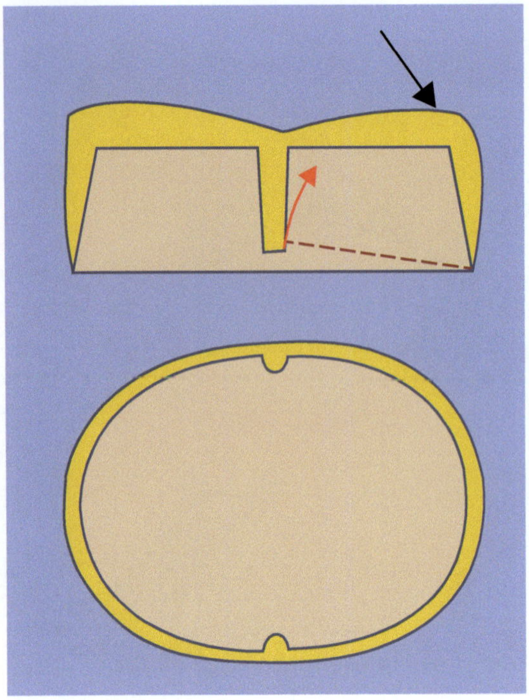

Figure 18.8 Internal grooves placed in a crown preparation with poor resistance/retention features. Note the wall of the internal groove intersects with the path of rotation (red arrow) reducing the "effective" convergence angle of the preparation and prevents dislodgement of the crown when an oblique occlusal force (black arrow) is delivered. *Source*: From reference [66]. Reprinted with permission.

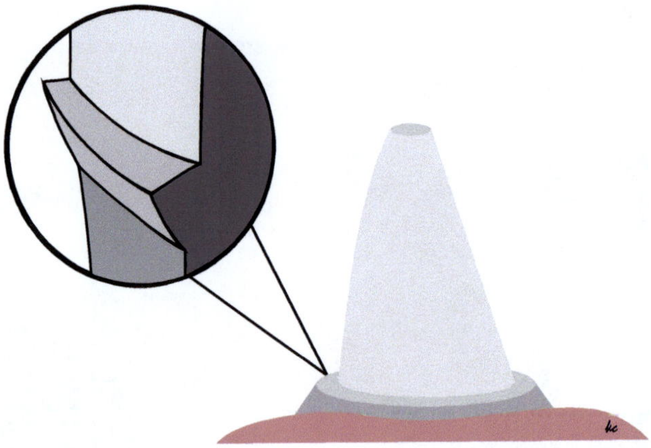

Figure 18.9 Illustration of a shoulder finish line configuration.

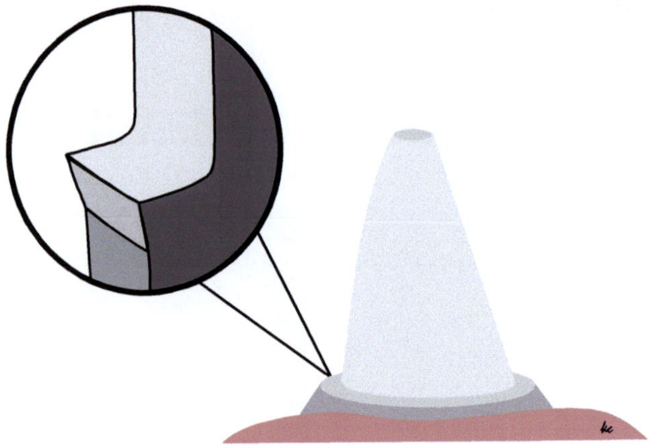

Figure 18.10 Illustration of a radial shoulder finish line configuration.

Finish line configurations with wide bevels, such as long bevel, full bevel, knife (feather), and occult, have been advocated in veterinary dentistry in the past. However, they invariably lead to overcontouring that can have disastrous effects on periodontal health [4, 56]. Therefore, they should be avoided when possible. The operator's choice of finish line configuration should be guided by two primary principles: (i) the margin should be easily identifiable to the lab technician and (ii) the margin should allow for a restoration with an acute edge with a nearby bulk of metal [4, 56].

18.9.4.1 Finish Line Configurations

18.9.4.1.1 Shoulder

With a 90° cavosurface angle, the shoulder configuration is considered to provide the ideal finish line for all ceramic restorations (Figure 18.9). It may also be used for PFM and all metal restorations. However, it requires significantly more removal of tooth structure compared to any other configuration. In addition, the 90° internal line angle creates a stress riser, making the tooth more susceptible to fracture [50, 51]. Therefore, the shoulder configuration should be reserved for all-ceramic restorations and PFM restorations exposed to high occlusal load.

18.9.4.1.2 Radial Shoulder

The radial shoulder can be considered a modified form of the shoulder finish line. Like the shoulder finish line, it has a 90° cavosurface angle with an adjacent ledge. However, the internal line angle is rounded off to prevent stress concentration and still maintains enough support for the walls of an all-ceramic restoration (Figure 18.10). In addition, slightly less tooth structure is removed when compared to the shoulder finish line.

18.9.4.1.3 Chamfer

The chamfer finish line is the preferred configuration for veneer metal restorations [4, 56, 67]. Because veneer metal restorations are the most common cast restorations utilized in veterinary dentistry, the chamfer finish line is the configuration most commonly instituted. Stress risers are minimized and the chance of failure of the underlying luting cement is reduced by rounding of the internal line angle (Figure 18.11). In addition, the

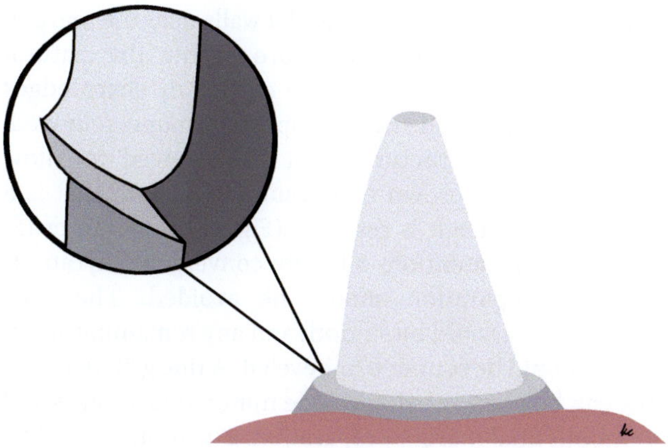

Figure 18.11 Illustration of a chamfer finish line configuration.

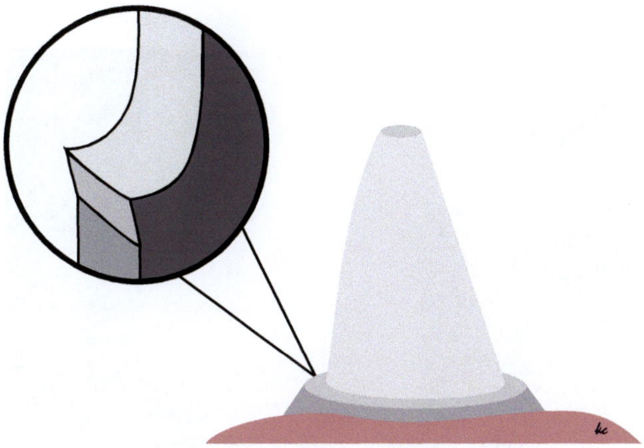

Figure 18.12 Illustration of a heavy chamfer finish line configuration.

total quantity of tooth material removed is reduced in comparison to shoulder configurations.

18.9.4.1.4 Heavy Chamfer

The heavy chamfer combines the 90° cavosurface angle of the shoulder finish line with the rounded internal line angle of the chamfer finish line (Figure 18.12). Because this configuration provides for a small ledge between the cavosurface angle and the internal line angle, this configuration is better suited to support a ceramic restoration than a regular chamfer configuration. However, caution must be exercised to avoid creating a lip of unsupported tooth structure at the cavosurface angle [4, 56]. This fragile lip of tooth structure can fracture and add to marginal discrepancy.

Even the most precise finish line will have some degree of inconsistency between the margin of the preparation and the margin of the restoration. This marginal discrepancy

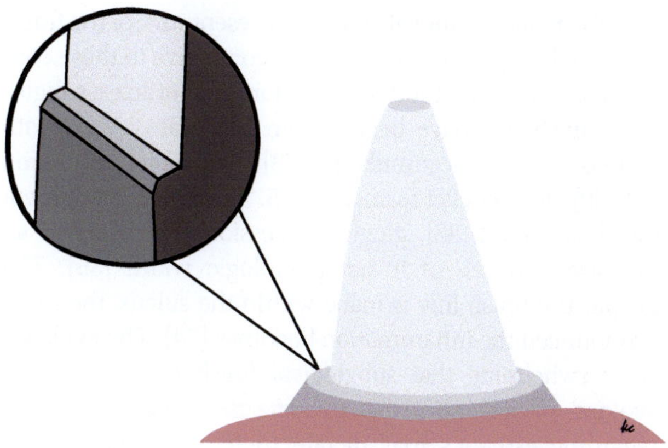

Figure 18.13 Illustration of beveling added to a shoulder finish line configuration.

becomes more prevalent as the convergence angle increases. Minimal amounts of marginal discrepancy are seen with convergence angles between 2° and 20° but can be quite significant above 20° [33]. Tooth preparations of canine teeth in dogs generally possess convergence angles higher than 20° and, thus, may be prone to a clinically significant decrease in marginal integrity [30].

Beveling of the finish line has been advocated as a means to improve the integrity of the margin [68] (Figure 18.13). A bevel can be added to any of the finish line configurations discussed above. However, the theoretical benefit of adding a bevel to a finish line as it relates to marginal integrity is potentially lost when considering the addition of cement between the preparation and the cast restoration [69]. The hydrodynamic properties and quantity of cement used during the clinical seating of the restoration directly impacts the degree to which a restoration can be seated on a preparation [33]. Thicker cements lead to larger degrees of marginal discrepancy [70]. Resin-based cements have been shown to create the highest degree of marginal discrepancy compared to other common luting cements [71]. Therefore, the addition of a bevel to the finish line configuration cannot fully counteract the marginal discrepancy introduced by cements. When using a cast metal restoration, many advocate the use of a 30° to 45° bevel at the finish line. However, the cast restoration will be likely to need to be burnished after cementation to improve its marginal adaptation [4, 72].

18.9.5 Preservation of the Periodontium

To improve the chance of long-term periodontal health after placement of a cast restoration, the gingival finish line should be placed where the operator can ensure smooth, well-adapted margins that are easily cleaned by the pet owner. A key factor in the establishment of a well-adapted margin is the ability to obtain impressions that do not tear or deform upon removal and are representative of the finish line. A subgingival finish line is not conducive to these conditions. As a result, tooth preparations that utilize a subgingival finish line have been shown to be associated with increased plaque accumulation [73], gingival inflammation [74–80], deep pocket formation [75, 76, 79, 81], attachment loss [75, 76, 82, 83], gingival recession [74, 84], and an increased chance of invading biologic width [85]. The deeper the finish line is made within the sulcus, the more pronounced the inflammation becomes [74]. The evidence is overwhelming that subgingival finish lines should be avoided whenever possible. In some cases, owner concerns regarding esthetics may dictate their use. However, the owner should be dedicated to daily oral hygiene. The reality is that oral hygiene efforts by most pet owners are moderate at best [86].

18.10 Clinical Technique for Tooth Preparation for a Full Metal Crown

The clinical steps used for preparing a tooth for full crown restoration are often a matter of personal preference and may be conducted in several ways. Thus, many clinicians have developed their preferred set of burs and sequence of steps in tooth preparation. As with all clinical procedures, it is not the specific sequence that matters but that the clinician establishes a logical clinical sequence he or she is comfortable with. This will help ensure an efficient and successful outcome. The steps below detail one of many potential tooth preparation sequences [87].

18.10.1 Margin Preparation

A round, coarse diamond bur (size 012) on a high-speed water-cooled handpiece is swept around the cervical aspect of the tooth, from facial to lingual, cutting a grove into the enamel to a depth of 0.5–1.0 mm (the diameter of a 012 round diamond bur is approximately 1.2 mm). The round bur head will create a chamfer-type margin, which is the preferred margin prep for metal crowns. The margin should have the smoothest finish possible. Smoothing the margin can be accomplished with a similar sized fine grit diamond bur. Rough surfaces at the margin can lead to poor margin adaptation, tooth fractures, or improper seating of the crown. Variations include using a smaller round-end diamond bur or a finer round-end tapered bur for small and toy breeds and a flat-end cylinder diamond for creation of a shoulder joint for PFM restorations.

18.10.2 Bulk Tooth Reduction

Using a coarse, round-end tapered diamond bur the axial walls of the tooth are reduced to a depth equal to the margin. The bur is held nearly parallel to the long axis of the tooth to create parallel walls near the margin. The reduction angles therefore follow the natural taper of the crown toward the cusp. Any sharp edges should be smoothed and unsupported enamel removed. Enough tooth structure must be removed to allow fabrication of a crown that results in a tooth that is a normal size once it is restored (Figure 18.14). In order to maximize retention, a highly convergent (pyramid-shaped) preparation should be avoided. The final preparation should be smooth and any remaining sharp edges should be rounded or beveled. A fine grit diamond bur can be used to help provide minor adjustments and a smooth final margin preparation. The tooth should be viewed from all angles to ensure there is a smooth taper toward the cusp and no undercuts in the preparation (Figure 18.15).

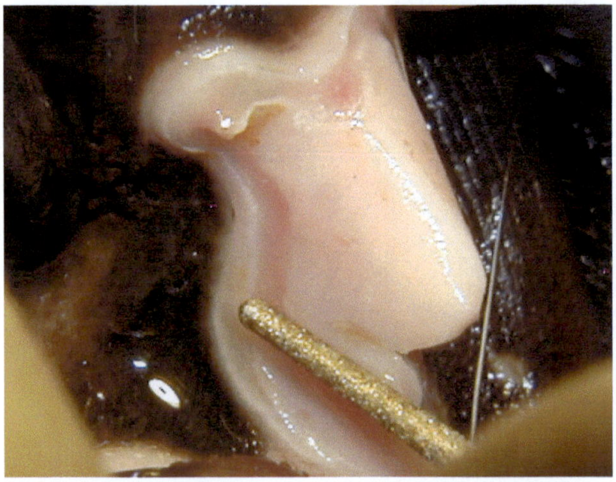

Figure 18.14 Axial reduction using a round end taper cylinder diamond bur.

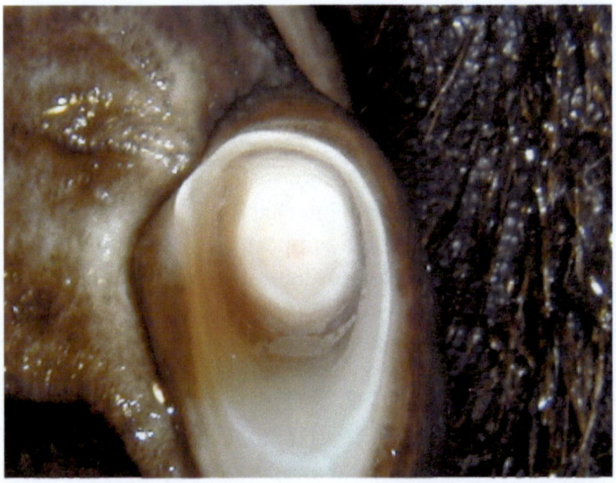

Figure 18.15 Final appearance of a crown preparation for a full metal crown with a chamfer margin–maxillary canine.

18.11 Impressions

18.11.1 Materials and Necessary Equipment

An impression is an imprint of the tooth preparation made by placing a soft, semi-fluid material in the mouth and allowing it to set and then removed. From this negative form of the teeth a positive reproduction or cast (model) is made. This indirect technique for fabricating the restoration allows the crown to be made away from the patient at the dental lab. In order for the crown restoration to fit precisely, the cast model must be a nearly exact replication of the prepared tooth in the mouth. Thus, an accurate, undistorted impression is vitally important. CAD/CAM (computer-aided design and computer-aided manufacturing), an alternative to the traditional impression-model system used for lab manufacturing of cast metal and ceramic restorations, is discussed later in this chapter.

A proper impression should show an exact duplicate of the prepared tooth and enough area around the preparation to allow the clinician and lab technician to be certain of the configuration and location of the restoration margin on the prepared tooth. Adjacent teeth and tissue should also be reproduced to allow proper articulation of the model and contouring of the restoration, and it should be free of bubbles, especially in the area of the margin. Many different materials are available for impression, but the ideal impression material for crown restorations is polyvinylsiloxane (PVS). These materials are also called addition reaction silicones and, occasionally, vinyl polysiloxane or vinylpolysiloxane [88]. Polyvinylsiloxane or the abbreviation "PVS" will be used in this chapter.

PVS is accurate and has a medium to long working time, high tear strength, and excellent reproduction of detail. PVS impressions have a very high resistance to deformation and excellent dimensional accuracy. PVS is usually packaged as two pastes (base and catalyst), and mixing equal quantities of each results in a reaction that yields a stable material once set. PVS provides excellent detail and has been described for use in veterinary patients [56, 87]. Because of its good dimensional stability after removal from the mouth the impression can be transported to the dental lab for pouring of the stone model and eventual fabrication of the crown. The PVS materials are further grouped by their viscosity and working time. The viscosity of a material is sometimes described as its "body." A "wash" PVS material has a very thin viscosity, which flows well into anatomic details. Other descriptions include light body, medium body, and firm body. The heavy-bodied "putty" form can be used to fabricate a custom tray chairside. These materials also have varying working times based on the chemical makeup of the reacting chemicals within each.

Once the clinician is satisfied with the tooth preparation and no further changes are to be made, the tooth is ready for the impression. An accurate impression allows the laboratory technician to make an optimal-fitting crown [87]. In the two techniques described below PVS putty and wash are used to create a detailed impression. The contralateral tooth can be included in the impression to provide the dental lab with an example of normal tooth anatomy for the crown fabrication.

18.11.2 Two-Step PVS Impression Technique

The two-step overimpression changes a basic tray into a custom tray in this putty-wash technique, which reduces the large-dimensional change that occurs when injection materials are used in a full-arch tray. Using a proper sized impression tray will allow impressions of the prepared tooth and the contralateral tooth. The PVS putty is mixed by hand to a homogenous consistency (equal amounts of base and catalyst). Latex gloves can affect the setting of some PVS materials. The individual mixing of the material should insure that their hands are clean and dry before mixing the putty and placing it in the tray. This problem can also be avoided by using vinyl gloves [88]. The putty is set to create an enlarged impression. The tray is removed while the putty is still soft and the impression is further enlarged at the space around the prepared tooth to create room for the light-bodied wash. Once the putty has set, this creates a customized tray for the final, detailed impression of the preparation.

The light bodied wash is next used to make the final, detailed impression. The set putty should be checked to make sure it is clean and dry. The teeth and adjacent tissues should also be clean and completely dry. When a dry field is achieved, the automixing syringe is used to apply a thin layer of the PVS light-bodied wash around the prepared tooth and over all remaining teeth to be included in the impression. Before placing the mixing tip on automixing devices, extrude some material from the cartridge to ensure that both sides flow freely and to remove any material that might have set. An air syringe can be used to lightly blow the impression material into the sulcus of the prepared tooth. Alternatively, the wash can be rubbed gently into the sulcus. The putty tray is then filled with the PVS light-bodied wash (Figure 18.16). When placing the wash material keep the mixing tip down to avoid trapping air bubbles. The PVS-filled impression tray is then placed into the mouth with passive pressure until the PVS has reached a full set. Excessive pressure should be avoided as it can cause an inaccurate impression. The wash material should not be placed over the palate. The impression material on the palate shrinks because of the bulk and distorts the lingual margins of prepared teeth.

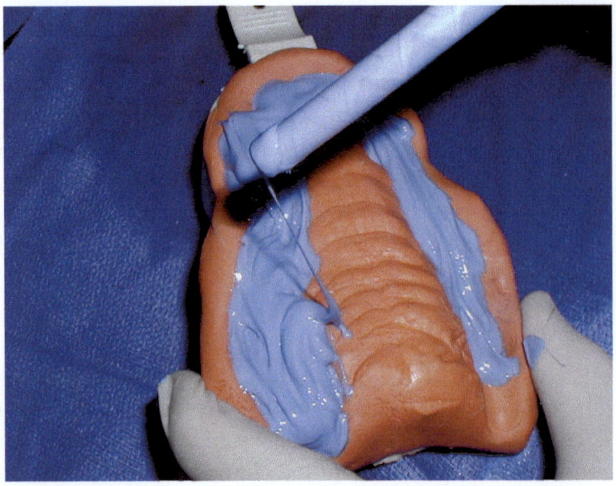

Figure 18.16 Light bodied wash added to the underimpression using the two-step PVS putty–wash technique.

Once the impression material has reached its specified setting time, the tray is removed along the original path of insertion in one quick motion. The impression should be checked for accuracy and with special attention given to the preparation margin, making sure there are no bubbles or defects. If any putty shows through in the putty preparation area, the impression should be taken again. Exposed set putty creates a pressure spot that rebounds when the impression is removed and results in too small a casting; thus the underlying putty should not be visible through the final impression with this technique. The impression should be rinsed and dried to prepare it for transport to the dental lab. An alginate impression of the opposing arch can be taken to provide a low detail model used for checking occlusion. A bite registration should be taken once the animal is extubated. A PVS bite registration wash can be used as an alternative material to pink a wax sheet for bite registration (see below).

18.11.3 One-Step PVS Impression Technique

The one-step or "one-step, double-mix" technique [25] is similar to the two-step technique in that both putty and a wash are used. However, with the one-step technique the putty and wash are applied in the mouth simultaneously on or around the prepared tooth or teeth. Since the putty and wash are applied and allowed to set simultaneously, timing is critical, making at least two assistants preferable.

When performing the one-step technique using a regular setting putty material will help ensure enough working time. In the impression tray, prior to taking the impression try to ensure that the tray adequately covers the tooth or teeth to be impressed. Properly dry the teeth and ensure that the teeth are not contaminated with blood, saliva, or debris. Mix the putty as directed and load the putty material into the tray. Before the putty has set, using a mixing tip, place the wash and ensure that all the teeth desired to be impressed are covered properly. Insert the still soft, putty-filled impression tray straight and evenly into the mouth over the wash covered teeth. Immobilize the tray using passive pressure. Use a timer to help follow the recommended setting time in the mouth. Remove the tray from the mouth and inspect the impression. With this technique, it is acceptable to have putty showing through the light bodied wash once the impression has set.

18.11.4 Impression-Taking Technique for Alginate

Alginate, also known as an irreversible hydrocolloid, is inexpensive, easy to pour, easy to remove, and ideal for less accurate stone models. Alginate displaces blood and tissue fluid, is hydrophilic, and pours well with stone. Full-mouth alginate impressions will provide stone models that assist in proper articulation of the crown restoration.

Teeth included in the impression should be clean and free of debris. Excessive saliva and dental calculus should be removed if present. A final rinse and dry should be done immediately before the impression is taken. The correct size of tray should be used to get an exact impression. The tray should fit the animal's mouth properly, allowing room for all the teeth, without making contact with the impression tray.

The amount of alginate needed for the size of the tray is measured. One measure of tepid water is placed into the bowl for each scoop of alginate powder. Note that the cold water slows down the set of the alginate and, therefore, increases the working time, and that warm water speeds up the set and decreases the working time. The water is poured into the pre-measured powder and is stirred slowly with the spatula. Once the powder is wet, it is vigorously stirred against the sides of the bowl until no lumps of powder are left in the mixture. This process should be completed in less than one minute. The impression tray is loaded with the alginate, being careful not to create air bubbles or voids. The surface is smoothed, making the alginate level with the sides of the tray.

An assistant should hold the jaw level, open the mouth, and retract the animal's lips. The tray can then slide easily into the patient's mouth. The tray is seated in the distal portion of the mouth and then in the anterior portion. The tray is held steady until the alginate has set. The alginate sets in approximately 3–7 minutes, depending on the type of alginate used. Touching the alginate around the top of the impression tray periodically can help determine when the alginate has set. To remove the tray, the front of the tray is gripped and is firmly snapped off the teeth while discrepancies are checked for. Once the desired impression is obtained, the stone can be poured immediately. If the stone is not poured immediately, the impression should be wrapped in a dampened paper towel and refrigerated. The alginate is sensitive to air, heat, and loss of moisture, so the stone should be poured within 30 minutes.

The full-mouth alginate impressions should be poured with a good-quality dental stone or should be kept cool and moist until they are picked up by the lab. After the stone is poured, the stone model should be left to set for two hours. The alginate is loosened around the edges of the tray, and the stone model and alginate are lifted from the tray.

18.11.5 Bite Registration

Capture of a bite registration is an important aspect of replication of the overall dental anatomy and how the teeth occlude with each other. This is of particular importance when the canine teeth are to be restored, especially if there is tight occlusion of the opposite arch teeth. After the crown is made, it should be applied to the full mouth model and the models placed into proper articulation. Using the bite registration will give the most accurate representation of how the restorative will fit in occlusion. In order to quickly obtain a bite registration a super-fast setting bite registration PVS material that sets in less than one minute can be utilized. The patient is extubated and the bite registration is quickly made by pressing the teeth together into the PVS material. The patient can either be recovered or intubated again if required.

The specific area must be determined that is best for registration. For example, if the restorative is at the canine teeth, the registration should be taken at the premolar teeth so the registration material does not interfere with the occlusion once the final restorative is placed on the full mouth stone model. If the final restoration is on premolar or molar teeth, the registration should be taken more rostrally or on the contralateral side.

18.11.6 Lab Instructions

The impressions and stone model of the opposing arch should be packaged carefully and submitted to the dental laboratory for fabrication of the crown. A submission form for the dog and cat dentition should be developed with the dental lab technician. This form can be used to indicate which tooth, materials, and any special requests are required for the crown fabrication. Working closely with a selected dental laboratory will help prevent confusion and improve the final results of the crown fabrication.

18.12 Try-in and Cementation

When the crown is returned from the dental lab it should be closely examined to ensure it has been accurately cast. Trial-fit the restoration on the tooth before cementation. The restoration should be verified to fit contour and occlusion. Use an explorer to evaluate marginal integrity of the crown and ensure that the margins are closed and the crown is properly seated. Minor adjustments to the crown can be made. A spray articulation marking material can be used on the inside of the crown to indicate areas for minor adjustments. However, if the crown does not seat properly or the shape and contour are incorrect, the preparation should be corrected and a new impression taken.

18.12.1 Cementation

Once the clinician is satisfied that the crown is properly adapted to the preparation, the tooth surface should be cleaned with pumice and water to remove any plaque and debris. Resin-based cements are generally advised for animals as they provide a stronger bond than other cements [29, 30, 52]. The tooth surface and crown are prepared and conditioned according to the cement manufacturer's instructions. The cement is mixed according to manufacturer's directions and evenly applied to the inside of the metal crown surface. The crown is then immediately placed over the prepared tooth and pressed firmly into place until the margins are completely seated. Excess cement should be wiped away from the crown margin and firm pressure should be held on the crown. The margin is cured with a curing light or an oxygen barrier applied to allow the cement to cure depending on manufacturer's directions. Specific directions will vary between different brands of resin cement. Resin-based cements such as Panavia 2.0 (Kuraray) and C&B Metabond (Parkell) are commonly used in veterinary patients.

18.12.2 Follow-up and Recheck

Pet owners should be instructed to avoid all hard bones, chews, or toys that could damage the restoration. Follow-up dental radiographs must be obtained annually to evaluate the vitality of the tooth or the success of previously performed endodontic treatment. Daily oral hygiene in the form of tooth brushing should be advised. Daily brushing along with regular professional teeth cleaning in the veterinary office is the best defense against periodontal disease. During professional dental cleaning the prosthetic crowns can be hand-scaled and polished to remove surface stain, plaque, and calculus. Ultrasonic scalers should be avoided as the vibration can damage the cement bonding and results in de-bonding to the restoration. Minor scratches or imperfections in metal crowns can be removed with silicon polishing points using a dental handpiece [72].

18.13 Other Prosthodontic Treatments

Bridges and prosthetic dental implants are not commonly utilized in veterinary patients. While some pet owners may feel the need to replace lost teeth in their pets, the involved methods required for application of dental bridges and implants make their use questionable. A basic discussion of these prosthetic treatments is included here to provide a general knowledge base for veterinary dentists.

18.13.1 Bridges

A bridge is a fixed dental prosthesis used to replace a missing tooth (or several teeth) by joining an artificial tooth permanently to adjacent teeth or dental implants. Types of bridges may vary, depending upon how they are fabricated and the way they anchor to the adjacent teeth. Conventionally, bridges are made using the indirect method of restoration. However, bridges can be fabricated directly in the mouth using such materials as composite resin.

The portion of a bridge replacing a missing tooth is termed the pontic. The abutment is a tooth, crown, or portion of an implant used to support, stabilize, and/or anchor a bridge. A pier is any abutment other than the terminal abutment. The portion of the bridge restoration that rebuilds the prepared abutment and pier tooth is known as the retainer. The joint or connector is that part of a bridge or prosthetic device that connects the retainer with the pontic. The portion of the bridge that is suspended between the abutments is termed the span. A resin bonded bridge (Maryland Bridge) relies on metal wings, which are cemented on to one or two abutment teeth, also supporting the pontic.

Ideally the root surface area of the abutment teeth should be equal to or greater than the root surface area of the tooth or teeth being replaced by the pontic(s). In human dental practice, a bridge has historically been a common way of esthetically replacing missing teeth. Bridges are not commonly used in veterinary patients due to the need for a more functional prosthesis.

18.13.2 Dental Restorative Implants

A dental implant (also known as an endosseous implant) is a surgical component that interfaces with the bone of the jaw or skull to support a dental prosthesis such as a crown, bridge, denture, or facial prosthesis. Most implants connect with other components in order to function. A common component is an abutment, which can provide the connection to a dental prosthetic crown. Initial studies in dogs demonstrated that titanium implants could be anchored directly to bone. This process of using metal oxides coated implants is known as osseointegration or functional ankylosis.

Implant restorations generally consist of three major parts: the implant itself, which integrates into the jaw bone, the abutment, which attaches to the implant with an abutment screw, and the restoration. The restoration is formed around a central cylinder, which also acts as the interface with the abutment. The restoration is then held in place on the abutment by a prosthetic retaining screw. There are many types of implants, each varying to some degree on the component parts.

For osseointegration to be successful in the long term, the implant must be biocompatible, osseointegrate, and the integration hold up in the long term. Titanium is used for most implants, due to its documented biocompatibility, osseointegration, and long-term success [89, 90]. Implant surgery is typically a two-stage procedure [91]. The first stage is the placement of the implant and the second stage covers its exposure. In Stage I, the surgical technique of opening the recipient site must be sterile, precise, low trauma, and non-heating. The site should be prepared as close to the design of the implant as possible. This should be done in a highly sterile fashion, while not traumatizing tissues any more than is necessary. Heat damage to the bone during cutting must be avoided by using a slow-speed drill. The implant must be placed in a stable and protected position in relationship to the bone in order to encourage osseointegration. To protect the implant, it is submerged by covering the exposed top with a gingival flap. This aids in the prevention of bacterial migration around the implant, while adding in its stability.

In Stage II, the implant is uncovered and loaded (restorative crown attached). This step should not be performed until osseointegration of the implant has occurred. This usually requires three to five months following implantation. Once osseointegration has occurred the implant is uncovered and an abutment or temporary abutment is placed. A temporary screw is placed in the abutment to protect it and prevent debris from falling inside. Once the tissue surrounding the abutment has healed the prosthetic restoration can be applied [91].

In the dog, dental implants have been reportedly used for the replacement of single teeth, but have not shown long-term success as functional teeth for bite work. In the dog, implants for canine and carnassial teeth are not generally recommended, due to the tremendous functional stresses involved. Areas with poor supporting bone are contraindicated for implant placement. Additionally, unless the owner is committed to good home oral hygiene care of the animal, complicating periodontal disease should be expected. There have also been ethical discussions regarding their placement in companion animals [91]. Consideration of a dental implant in an animal should be carefully considered and discussed with the pet owner. The procedure should be considered experimental and carry a guarded long-term prognosis for success.

18.14 CAD/CAM Techniques

CAD/CAM methods are changing the way prosthodontic restorations are being designed and made [23]. An integrated chairside–laboratory technique using CAD/CAM can still require two visits but are also being used to manufacture single-visit restorations in people. The clinician can either scan the preparation directly and then send the scan to the laboratory or can take a traditional impression, after which a stone model is poured and the laboratory scans the stone model. In the first case, the patient still does not require an impression, removing a source of discomfort for people and a potential source of inaccuracy for the clinician. CAD/CAM has become somewhat synonymous with zirconia, but systems are available that can machine any type of ceramics (i.e., glass ceramics, interpenetrating-infiltration ceramics materials and solid-sintered monophase ceramics such as zirconia.

The CEREC system uses CAD/CAM technology to provide a single visit in-office alternative for porcelain/ceramic restorations. The tooth preparation is sprayed and bonded to titanium dioxide contrast powder in the patient's mouth. An infrared camera records the powder and creates a three-dimensional optical impression on the computer. This image can be manipulated by the dentist to recreate ideal anatomy before processing. The shade of dental ceramic is selected by the dentist and then entered into the computer. The computer then tells the dentist what block of ceramic or composite is to be used. This block is then milled in-office according to the computer design. The restoration comes out of the milling machine with a ceramic sprue that must be removed and the restoration is then tried in the patient's mouth. In humans, proximal contacts may need to be adjusted and flash may need to be removed, but if the restoration is adequate and esthetic, it can be immediately cemented.

18.15 Summary

This chapter is meant to serve as a reference for veterinarians performing prosthodontic dental treatment. The clinician's choice of materials and techniques for placing a final restoration will depend ultimately on multiple factors for each patient. No single technique or material will ensure a successful restoration for each patient. A thorough understanding of restorative materials combined with the clinical skills to apply them will help ensure an optimal outcome for each restored tooth.

References

1 Black, G.V. (1917). *A Work on Operative Dentistry, The Technical Procedures in Filling Teeth*, vol. 5. Chicago, IL: Medico-Dental Publishing.

2 Wiskott, H.W. (2011). *Fixed Prosthodontics Principles and Clinics*, vol. 22. London, UK: Quintessence Publishing.

3 Soukup, J.W., Mulherin, B.L., and Snyder, C.J. (2013). Prevalence and nature of dentoalveolar injuries among patients with maxillofacial fractures. *J. Small Anim. Pract.* 54: 9–14.

4 Shillingburg, H.T., Sumiya, H., Whitsett, L.D. et al. (1997, 1997). Principles of tooth preparation. In: *Fundamentals of Fixed Prosthodontics*, 3e, vol. 73. Chicago, IL: Quintessence Publishing Inc.

5 Luskin, I.R. (2001). Three-quarter crown preparation. *J. Vet. Dent.* 18: 102–105.

6 Givan, D.A. (2007). Precious metals in dentistry. *Dental Clin. of N. Am.* 51 (3): 591–601.

7 American Dental Association (1989). Revised ANSI/ADA Specification No. 5 for dental casting alloys. *J. Am. Dent. Assoc.* 118: 379.

8 Bertolotti, R.L. (1990). Casting metals, Part I. *Compend. Cont. Ed. Dent.* 11 (5):3 00.

9 Dale, B.G. and Ascheim, K.W. (1993). *Esthetic Dentistry a Clinical Approach to Techniques and Materials.* Philadelphia, PA: Lea & Febiger.

10 Van Loon, L.A.J., Van Elsas, P.W., Van Joost, T. et al. (1984). Contact stomatitis and dermatitis to nickel and palladium. *Contact Dermatitis.* 11: 294–297.

11 Magnusson, B., Bergman, M., Bergman, B. et al. (1982). Nickel allergy and nickel containing dental alloys. *Scand. J. Dent. Res.* 90: 163–167.

12 Bruce, G.J. and Hall, W.B. (1995). Nickel hypersensitivity-related periodontitis. *Compend. Cont. Ed. Dent.* 16 (2): 178–184.

13 Berge, M. (1989). Properties of prosthetic resin-veneer materials processed in commercial laboratories. *Dent. Mater.* 5: 77.

14 Lappalainen, R., Yll-Urpo, A., and Seppa, L. (1989). Wear of dental restoratives and prosthetic materials *in vitro*. *Dent. Mater.* 5: 35.

15 Rosenblum, M.A. and Schulman, A. (1997). A review of all ceramic restorations. *J. Am Dent. Assoc.* 128: 297–307.

16 Ho, J.W. and Matinlinna, J.P. (2011). Insights on ceramics as dental materials. Part I: Ceramics material types in dentistry. *Silicon* 3 (1): 109–115.

17 Rizkalla, A.S. and Jones, D.W. (2004). Mechanical properties of commercial high strength ceramic core materials. *Dent. Mater.* 20: 207–212.

18 Rizkalla, A.S. and Jones, D.W. (2004). Indentation fracture toughness and dynamic elastic moduli for commercial feldspathic dental porcelain materials. *Dent. Mater.* 20: 198–206.

19 Probster, L. and Diehl, J. (1992). Slip casting alumina ceramics for crown and bridge restorations. *Quintessence Int.* 23: 25–31.

20 Shenoy, A. and Shenoy, N. (2010). Dental ceramics: an update. *J. Conserv. Dent.* 13 (4): 195.

21 Craig, R.G. (1985). *Restorative Dental Materials*, 7e. St. Louis, MO: The CV Mosby Co.

22 Bertolotti, R.L. (1990). Casting metals, Part II. *Compend. Contin. Ed. Dent.* 11 (6): 370.

23 Eissman, H.S., Rudd, K.D., and Marrow, R.M. (1980). *Dental Laboratory Procedures in Fixed Partial Dentures*, vol. 2. CV Mosby Co.: St. Louis, MO.

24 Schillingberg, H.T., Hobo, S., and Whitsett, L.D. (1981). *Fundamentals of Fixed Prosthodontics*, 2e. Chicago, IL: Quintessence Publishing Inc.

25 Wiskott, H.W. (2011). *Fixed Prosthodontics Principles and Clinics*, vol. 422. London, UK: Quintessence Publishing.

26 Lorey, R.E. and Myers, G.E. (1968). The retentive qualities of bridge retainers. *J. Am. Dent. Assoc.* 76: 568–572.

27 Reisbick, M.H. and Shillingburg, H.T. (1975). Effect of preparation geometry on retention of cast gold restorations. *J. Calif. Dent. Assoc.* 3 (4): 51–59.

28 Potts, R.G., Shillingburg, H.T., and Duncanson, M.G. (1980). Retention and resistance of preparations for cast restorations. *J. Prosthet Dent.* 43: 303–308.

29 Riehl, J., Soukup, J.W., Collins, C. et al. (2014). Effect of preparation surface area on the clinical outcome of full veneer crowns in dogs. *J. Vet. Dent.* 31 (1): 22–25.

30 Soukup, J.W., Snyder, C.J., Karls, T.L. et al. (2011). Achievable convergence angle and the effect of preparation design on the clinical outcome of full veneer crowns in dogs. *J. Vet. Dent.* 28 (2): 72–82.

31 Jorgensen, K.D. (1955). The relationship between retention and convergence angle in cemented veneer crowns. *Acta. Odontol. Scand.* 13: 35–40.

32 Mack, P.J. (1980). A theoretical and clinical investigation into the taper achieved on crown and inlay preparations. *J. Oral Rehabil.* 7: 255.

33 Chan, D.C.N., Wilson, A.J., Barbe, P., and al, e. (2005). Effect of preparation convergence on retention and seating discrepancy of complete veneer crowns. *J. Oral Rehabil.* 32: 58–64.

34 Ward, M.L. (1926). *The American Textbook of Operative Dentistry*, 6e, 381–395. New York: Lea & Febiger.

35 Kaufman, E.G., Coelho, D.H., and Colin, L. (1961). Factors influencing the retention of cemented gold castings. *J. Prosthet. Dent.* 11: 487–502.

36 Dykema, R.W., Goodacre, C.J., and Phillips, R.W. (1986). *Johnston's Modern Practice in Crown and Bridge Prosthodontics*, 4e, vol. 24. Philadelphia, PA: WB Saunders Co.

37 Shillingburg, H.T., Hobo, S., and Fisher, D.W. (1974). *Preparations for Cast Gold Restorations*, vol. 16. Chicago, IL, Quintessence Publishing Inc..

38 Tylman, S.D. and Malone, W.F.P. (1978). *Tylman's Theory and Practice of Fixed Prosthodontics*, 7e, 103. St. Louis, MO: CV Mosby Co.

39 El-Ebrashi, M.K., Craig, R.G., and Peyton, F.A. (1969). Experimental stress analysis of dental resotrations. Part IV. The concept of parallelism of axial walls. *J. Prosthet Dent.* 22: 346–353.

40 Holmstrom, S.E. and Gammon, R.L. (1989). Full crown restorations. *J. Vet. Dent.* 6 (1): 8.

41 Grove, T.K. (1990). Functional and esthetic crowns for dogs and cats. *Vet. Med. Rep.* 2: 409–420.

42 Harvey and Emily (1993). Restorative dentistry. In: *Small Animal Dentistry*, 1e (ed. C.E. Harvey and P.P. Emily), 213–265. St. Louis: Mosby.

43 Holmstrom, S.E., Fitch, P.F., and Eisner, E.R. (2004). Restorative dentistry. In: *Veterinary Dental Techniques for the Small Animal Practitioner*, 3e (ed. S.E. Holmstrom, P.F. Fitch and E.R. Eisner), 415–497. Philadelphia, PA: Saunders.

44 Zimmerman, C. and Soukup, J.W. (2015). Evaluation of the natural crown convergence angle of dog carnassial teeth. *J. Vet. Dent.* 32 (4): 222–225. PubMed PMID: 27012059.

45 Noonan, J.E. and Goldfogel, M.H. (1991). Convergence of the axial walls of full veneer crown preparations in a dental school environment. *J. Prosthet Dent.* 66: 706–708.

46 Patel, P.B., Wildgoose, D.G., and Winstanley, R.B. (2005). Comparison of convergence angle achieved in posterior teeth prepared for full veneer crowns. *Eur. J. Prosthodont. Rest. Dent.* 13: 100–104.

47 van Foreest, A. and Roeters, J. (1998). Evaluation of the clinical performance and effectiveness of adhesively-bonded metal crowns on damaged canine teeth of working dogs over a two- to 52-month period. *J. Vet. Dent.* 15 (1): 13–20.

48 El-Mowafy, O.M., Fenton, A.H., Forrester, N. et al. (1996). Retention of metal ceramic crowns cemented with resin cements: Effects of preparation taper and height. *J. Prosthet. Dent.* 76: 524–529.

49 Zidan, O. and Ferguson, G.C. (2003). The retention of complete crowns prepared with three different tapers and luted with four different cements. *J. Prosthet. Dent.* 89: 565–571.

50 Pilkey, W.D. and Pilkey, D.F. (2008). Shoulder fillets. In: *Pilkey's Stress Concentration Factors*, 3e (ed. W.D. Pilkey and D.F. Pilkey), 135–175. Hoboken, NJ: Wiley.

51 Anusavice, K.J. (2003). Mechanical properties of dental materials. In: *Phillips' Science of Dental Materials*, 11e (ed. K.J. Anusavice), 73–101. St. Louis, MO: Elsevier.

52 Soukup, J.W. (2013). Crown preparation design: An evidence-based review. *J. Vet. Dent.* 30 (4): 214–219.

53 Weed, R.M. and Baez, R.J. (1984). A method for determining adequate resistance form of complete cast crown preparations. *J. Prosthet. Dent.* 52: 330–334.

54 Parker, M.H., Calverley, M.J., Gardner, F.J. et al. (1993). New guidelines for preparation taper. *J. Prosthodont.* 2: 61–66.

55 Shillingburg, H.T., Hobo, S., Whitsett, L.D. et al. (1997). Preparations for extensively damaged teeth. In: *Fundamentals of Fixed Prosthodontics*, 3e (ed. H.T. Shillinburg, S. Hobo, L.D. Whitsett, et al.), 181–209. Chicago, IL: Quintessence Punlishing Inc.

56 Visser, C.J. (1998). Restorative dentistry: crown therapy. *The Vet. Clin. N. Am. Small: Canine Dentistry.* 28: 1273–1284.

57 Bladowski, M., Kotowicz-Gears, A., and Choszcz, D. (2013). et. al. Prosthetic reconstruction of broken canine teeth in dogs with use of cast metal posts. *Pol. J. Vet. Sci.* 16 (2): 399–402.

58 Shillingburg, H.T., Hobo, S., Whitsett, L.D. et al. (1997). Fluid control and soft tissue management. In: *Fundamentals of fixed prosthodontics*, 3e (ed. H.T. Shillinburg, S. Hobo, L.D. Whitsett, et al.), 257–279. Chicago, IL: Quintessence Publishing Inc.

59 Hale, F. (2001). Crown lengthening for mandibular and maxillary canine teeth in the dog. *J. Vet. Dent.* 18 (4): 219–221.

60 Proussaefs, P., Campagni, W., Bernal, G. et al. (2004). The effectiveness of auxiliary features on a tooth preparation with inadequate resistance form. *J. Prosthet. Dent.* 91: 33–41.

61 Goldschmidt, S., Collins, C.J., Hetzel, S. et al. (2016). The influence of axial grooves on dislodgment fesistance of prosthetic metal crowns in canine teeth of dogs. *J. Vet. Dent.* 33 (3): 146–150. doi: 10.1177/0898756416676558 PubMed PMID: 28327073.

62 Goldschmidt, S., Collins, C.J., Hetzel, S. et al. (2016). The influence of axial grooves on dislodgment resistance of prosthetic metal crowns in maxillary fourth premolar teeth of dogs. *J. Vet. Dent.* 33 (3): 151–156. doi: 10.1177/0898756416674379 PubMed PMID: 28327065.

63 Woolsey, G.D. and Matich, J.A. (1978). The effect of axial grooves on the resistance form of cast restorations. *J. Am. Dent. Assoc.* 97: 978–980.

64 Roudsari, R.V. and Satterthwaite, J.D. (2011). The influence of auxiliary features on the resistance form of short molars prepared for complete cast crown. *J. Prosthet. Dent.* 106: 305–309.

65 Kent, W.A., Shillinburg, H.T., and Duncanson, M.G. (1988). Taper of clinical preparations for cast restorations. *Quintessence Int.* 19: 339–345.

66 Blair, F.M., Wassell, R.W. et al. (2002). Crowns and other extra-coronal restorations – preparations for full veneer crowns. *Br. Dent. J.* 192: 561–571.

67 Coffman, C.R., Visser, L., and Visser, C.J. (2007). Tooth preparation and impression for full metal crown restoration. *J. Vet. Dent.* 24 (1): 59–65.

68 Rosner, D. (1963). Function, placement and reproduction of bevels for gold castings. *J. Prosthet. Dent.* 13: 1160–1166.

69 Ostlund, L.E. (1985). Cavity design and mathematics: Their effect on gaps at the margins of cast restorations. *Oper. Dent.* 10: 122–137.

70 Wilson, P.R. and Stankiewicz, N.R. (1998). Effect of cement space and delayed placement on the seating of crowns luted with Vitremer, Fuji Duet and Dyract Cem. *Am. J. Dent.* 11 (5): 240–244.

71 Proussaefs, P. (2004). Crowns cemented on crown preparations lacking geometric resistance form. Part II: effect of cement. *J. Prosthodont.* 13 (1): 36–41.

72 Crowder, S.E. (2010). Care of metal crown restorations. *J. Vet. Dent.* 27 (3): 191–196.

73 Kosyfaki, P., del Pilar Pinilla Martin, M. et al. (2010). Relationship between crowns and the periodontium: a literature update. *Quintessence Int.* 41: 109–122.

74 Karlsen, K. (1970). Gingival reactions to dental restorations. *Acta. Odontol. Scand.* 28: 895–904.

75 Valderhaug, J. and Birkeland, J.M. (1976). Periodontal conditions in patients 5 years following insertion of fixed prostheses. Pocket depth and loss of attachment. *J. Oral Rehabil.* 3: 237–243.

76 Valderhaug, J. (1980). Periodontal conditions and carious lesions following the insertion of fixed prostheses: a 10-year follow-up study. *Int. Dent. J.* 30: 296–304.

77 Gemalmaz, D. and Ergin, S. (2002). Clinical evaluation of all-ceramic crowns. *J. Prosthet. Dent.* 87: 189–196.

78 Bader, J.D., Rozier, R.G. et al. (1991). Effect of crown margins on periodontal conditions in regularly attending patients. *J. Prosthet. Dent.* 65: 75–79.

79 Kancyper, S.G. and Koka, S. (2001). The influence of intracrevicular crown margins on gingival health: preliminary findings. *J. Prosthet. Dent.* 85: 461–465.

80 Larato, D.C. (1975). Effects of artificial crown margin extension and tooth brushing frequency on gingival pocket depth. *J. Prosthet. Dent.* 34: 640–643.

81 Orkin, D.A., Reddy, J. et al. (1987). The relationship of the position of crown margins to gingival health. *J. Prosthet. Dent.* 57: 421–424.

82 Parma-Benfenati, S., Fugazzotto, P.A. et al. (1986). The effect of restorative margins on the postsurgical development and nature of the periodontium. Part II. Anatomical considerations. *Int. J. Periodont. Rest.* 6: 65–75.

83 Tal, H., Soldinger, M. et al. (1989). Periodontal response to long-term abuse of the gingival attachment by supra-crestal amalgam restorations. *J. Clin. Periodontol.* 16: 654–659.

84 Padbury, A. Jr., Eber, R. et al. (2003). Interactions between gingiva and the margin of restorations. *J. Clin. Periodontol.* 30: 379–385.

85 Nevins, M. and Skurow, H.M. (1984). The intracrevicular restorative margin, the biologic width, and the maintenance of the gingival margin. *Int. J. Periodont. Rest.* 3: 31–49.

86 Miller, B.R. and Harvey, C.E. (1994). Compliance with oral hygiene recommendations following periodontal treatment in client-owned dogs. *J. Vet. Dent.* 11 (1): 18–19.

87 Coffman, C.R. and Visser L Visser, C.J. (2007). Tooth preparation and impression for full metal crown restoration. *J. Vet. Dent.* 24 (7): 59–67.

88 Shillingburg, H.T., Sumiya, H., Whitsett, L.D. et al. (1997). Impressions. In: *In: Fundamentals of Fixed Prosthodontics*, 3e, 299. Chicago, IL: Quintessence Publishing Inc.

89 Adell, R., Lekholm, U., Rockler, B. et al. (1981). A 15-year study of osseointergrated implants in the treatment of the edentulous jaw. *J. Oral Surg.* 10: 387.

90 Branemark, P.I., Zarb, G.A., and Albrektsson, T. (1985). *Tissue-integrated prothesis*. Chicago, IL: Quintessence Publishing Inc.

91 Tannenbaum, J., Arzi, B., Reiter, A.M., and al, e. (2013). The case against the use of dental implants in dogs and cats. *J. Am. Vet. Med. Assoc.* 243: 1680–1685.

19

Occlusion and Orthodontics

Heidi B. Lobprise

Main Street Veterinary Dental Clinic, Flower Mound, TX, USA

19.1 Introduction

The term orthodontics comes from the Greek language of *ortho* meaning correct and *odontics* meaning tooth. From early goals of having ideal dental occlusion and jaw relationships, modern treatment goals now involve a soft tissue paradigm in human dentistry. With an increased focus on clinical examination to obtain diagnostic information, there is emphasis on soft tissue relationships and adaptations for optimal facial appearance, as well as functional occlusion [1]. As the functional dentition and oral support tissues are at risk when the animal's occlusion is abnormal, the assessment of the best course of treatment and whether or not to consider treatment or genetic counseling is one of the most critical points in veterinary orthodontics.

19.2 Ethical Standard of Orthodontics

Every animal both deserves and has the medical right to an occlusion that is functional and free from discomfort, as can be reasonably provided by therapy. In some dogs, and to a lesser degree in the cat, human intervention has perpetuated some occlusal aberrations. The American Veterinary Dental College (AVDC) has a position statement: "The goal of orthodontic procedures in companion animals is to provide pets with a healthy and functional occlusion. The AVDC supports the AVMA policy regarding cosmetic procedures that enhance the appearance of show or breeding animals" (http://www.avdc.org/statements.html – Orthodontic Procedures). The Principles of Veterinary Medical Ethics of the AVMA (Section I.e.) states: "Performance of surgical or other procedures in all species for the purpose of concealing genetic defects in animals to be shown, raced, bred, or sold, as breeding animals is unethical. However, should the health or welfare of the individual patient require correction of such genetic defects, it is recommended that the patient be rendered incapable of reproduction" (Section VII, Genetic Defect) (https://www.avma.org/KB/Policies/Pages/Principles-of-Veterinary-Medical-Ethics-of-the-AVMA.aspx). The American Kennel Club disqualifies a dog from competition if its appearance has been changed by artificial means due to procedures, substances, or drugs that can obscure, disguise, or eliminate any congenital or hereditary abnormality or undesirable characteristic, even if absolutely necessary to the health and comfort of the dog. This includes correction of harelip, cleft palate, restorative dental procedure, the use of bands or braces on teeth, or any alteration of the dental arcade (amongst other named procedures) (http://images.akc.org/pdf/rulebooks/RREGS3.pdf).

When there are reasonable indications of hereditary involvement the owner should be informed as to the possibility and, should treatment be considered, the owner or agent should acknowledge their responsibilities prior to treatment and genetic counseling should be advised. One of the major obstacles in advising clients as to dental hereditary involvement is the lack of definitive studies to distinguish hereditary from non-hereditary conditions. It is generally conceded that orofacial skeletal length variations are hereditary, with the exception of those caused by local oral or systemic influences, and there is reasonable research on the dog to support it.

19.3 Etiology

When etiology can be determined, the client should be counseled as to preventive measures that may be able to be taken to help control the condition, and of the likelihood of the dentofacial deformity being passed on

Wiggs's Veterinary Dentistry: Principles and Practice, Second Edition. Edited by Heidi B. Lobprise and Johnathon R. (Bert) Dodd.

to offspring. Dentofacial deformity refers to abnormalities of the teeth in morphology or location, and/or of the facial support structures. These deformities typically fall into one or more of three general categories involving *heredity, systemic influences,* or *local influences.* It is not unusual for some influences to fall within several categories, or fall within one yet also cause influence within another.

19.3.1 Heredity

Heredity is concerned with traits and characteristics that are transmitted from parents or other ancestors to offspring. This can be of great concern in breeding lines and influences the determination of removing an animal from the genetic pool. Interference, including genetic and developmental ones, with neural crest cells migrating to branchial arches can result in craniofacial abnormalities. While odontoblasts also develop from the neural crest, the ectoderm of the first pharyngeal arch is also involved, so a wide variety of abnormalities may arise [2]. These may include variations in size, number, length, shape, or lack of development of the teeth, jaws, periodontium, or orofacial supporting tissues. Defects in any of these components may affect occlusion or their presence may not affect occlusal function at all.

Numbers of teeth, either too few or too many, can all have effects on the occlusal pattern. With the jaws, the length, size, and development can all affect occlusion. Almost any alteration in morphology of the teeth, jaws, or supportive tissues, pattern or chronology of primary tooth exfoliation, lack of primary tooth exfoliation, and pattern, direction, or chronology of eruption of primary or permanent teeth may result in some form of orthodontic disturbance. Brachycephalic dogs with chondrodystrophy results in the underdevelopment of the base of the skull and tooth crowding is frequently found [3].

Macroglossia, a tongue that is too large, may place pressures on the lingual surface of the teeth, forcing them facially and out of position, while microglossia, a tongue that is too small, may allow the dental arch to collapse lingually. A short frenulum may lead to altered tongue posturing, which may release or apply pressures to lingual tooth surfaces.

Excessively loose lips may fail to place appropriate pressures to the facial surfaces of the teeth, thereby allowing a facial or even a mesial drift of the teeth [4]. On the other hand, a tight lip, a condition of lip attachment too close to the dentition, can place excessive facial surface pressures on the teeth and jaw, resulting in linguoversion of teeth and even a shortened jaw in the effected arch [5].

19.3.2 Systemic Influences

Systemic influences include two groups, pre-natal (congenital) and post-natal (developmental). Pre-natal problems differentiate from hereditary ones in that heredity implies a genetic origin, whereas congenital ones can be caused by various influences during pregnancy. Post-natal problems encompass defects that develop from exposure to a systemic influence after birth, including nutritional disturbances, infectious diseases, endocrine imbalances, radiation effects, and chemical exposures. Any of these factors may alter development of the teeth or the orofacial complex.

19.3.3 Local Influences

Local influences are those stimuli that may affect the orofacial complex, such as an injury that causes loss of teeth, in that the loss of the teeth allows changes in the orofacial complex to occur. Early loss of any primary or permanent tooth may allow migrational changes. Delayed loss of primary teeth can result in impactions and/or crowding. The local influence of periodontal destruction and tooth loss can affect surrounding tissues. Cysts, tumors, and other growths also can have a dramatic impact on the area [6]. Behavioral habits from cage biting, bruxing, chewing habits, and suckling habits may all likewise alter the complex [7]. Management of the local influences is necessary for successful orthodontic management.

19.4 Sequelae of Malocclusion

There are many pathologic possibilities, both short and long range, that may develop from untreated malocclusions. These unfavorable consequences vary with species, but include problems with mastication, temporomandibular joint (TMJ) function, caries formation, incidence of periodontal disease, effects on dentofacial growth and development, soft tissue trauma, traumatic dental fractures, and dental attrition. Each of these is a legitimate reason to initiate orthodontic treatment. Orthodontic treatment should be biologically based for a harmonious occlusion, rather than cosmetic orientation of teeth.

19.5 Evaluation of Occlusion

Before attempting to assess animal occlusions, a basic understanding of the establishment of normal standards for species and breeds, as well as the nature of malocclusions, is necessary. There are three basic skull and jaw types dealt with, which may be either breed or individual specific. Dolichocephalics are individuals with long narrow facial profiles, such as Collies and Grayhounds. The brachycephalics have a short broad facial profiles, such as Boxers and Bulldogs. The mesocephalics have a more balanced facial profile somewhere between the two previously mentioned, such as in the Beagle and German Shepherd. Certain breeds (i.e., Boxers, Bulldogs, etc.) have a pronounced mandibular mesioclusion (Class III) according to dental and medical standards, but according to breed standards their occlusion is acceptable, within a certain range.

19.6 Occlusion Terms

When discussing occlusions there are some terms of which a general understanding may be needed at times.

Occlusion. The contact of the teeth of the maxillary arch with those of the mandibular.

Centric occlusion. The position of the arches to each other when the teeth are in maximum occlusal contact.

Static occlusion. The relationship of the teeth when the jaws are closed in centric occlusion. Static occlusion can be studied in the actual patient or on an occluded study cast or model, and it is based on this that most occlusions are classified.

Centric relation. This is the most functional, unrestrained, anatomically retruded position of the heads of the condyles of the mandible in the glenoid fossae of the TMJ.

Functional or dynamic occlusion. Refers to the active tooth contacts during mastication and swallowing.

Malocclusions. Any deviation from normal occlusion.

19.6.1 AVDC Occlusion Nomenclature

The American Veterinary Dental College has provided distinct definitions and examples of malocclusions on the website: http://avdc.org/nomenclature.html#occlusion. The abbreviations concerning occlusion and orthodontics can be found in Table 19.1.

An ideal occlusion can be described as perfect interdigitation of the maxillary and mandibular teeth. In the dog, the ideal tooth positions in the arches are defined by the occlusal, interarch and interdental relationships of the teeth of the archetypal dog (i.e., wolf). This ideal relationship with the mouth closed can be defined by the following.

The maxillary incisor teeth are all positioned rostral to the corresponding mandibular incisor teeth (Figure 19.1). The crown cusps of the mandibular incisor teeth contact the cingulum of the maxillary incisor teeth. The mandibular canine tooth is inclined labially and bisects the interproximal (interdental) space (diastema) between the opposing maxillary third incisor tooth and canine tooth. The maxillary premolar teeth do not contact the mandibular premolar teeth (Figure 19.2). The crown cusps of the mandibular premolar teeth are positioned lingual to the arch of the maxillary premolar teeth. The crown cusps of the mandibular premolar teeth bisect the interproximal (interdental) spaces rostral to the corresponding maxillary premolar teeth. The mesial crown cusp of the maxillary fourth premolar tooth is positioned lateral to the space between the mandibular fourth premolar tooth and the mandibular first molar tooth.

19.6.2 Terms of Malocclusion

19.6.2.1 Skeletal Malocclusions (Symmetrical)

Neutroclusion (Class 1 malocclusion; MAL/1). A normal rostral–caudal relationship of the maxillary and mandibular dental arches with malposition of one or more individual teeth.

Mandibular distoclusion (Class 2 malocclusion; MAL/2). An abnormal rostral–caudal relation relationship of the maxillary and mandibular dental arches in which the mandibular arch occludes distal to its normal position relative to the maxillary arch (Figure 19.3a and b).

Mandibular mesioclusion (Class 3 malocclusion; MAL/3). An abnormal rostral–caudal relation relationship of the maxillary and mandibular dental arches in which the mandibular arch occludes rostral to its normal position relative to the maxillary arch (Figure 19.4a and b).

19.6.2.2 Asymmetrical Skeletal Malocclusions

Maxillary–mandibular asymmetry describes skeletal malocclusions that can occur in a rostrocaudal, side-to-side, or dorsoventral direction.

Maxillary–mandibular asymmetry in a rostrocaudal direction occurs when mandibular mesioclusion or distoclusion is present on one side of the face while the contralateral side retains normal dental alignment.

Maxillary–mandibular asymmetry in a side-to-side direction occurs when there is loss of the midline alignment of the maxilla and mandible.

Maxillary–mandibular asymmetry in a dorsoventral direction results in an open bite (OB), which is defined as an abnormal vertical space between opposing dental arches when the mouth is closed.

The expression "wry bite" is a layman term that has been used to describe a wide variety of unilateral occlusal abnormalities. Because "wry bite" is non-specific, its use is not recommended.

Table 19.1 AVDC nomenclature abbreviations (http://avdc.org/nomenclature.html#occlusion).

CB		Crossbite
	CB/C	Caudal crossbite
	CB/R	Rostral crossbite
CR		Crown
	CR/A	Crown amputation
	CR/XP	Crown reduction
D		Diastema
	D/O	Open diastema
DC		Diagnostic cast
	DC/D	Die
	DC/SM	Stone model
DT		Deciduous tooth
	DT/P	Persistent deciduous tooth
IM		Detailed imprint of hard and/or soft tissues (e.g., individual teeth or palate defect)
	IM/F	Full-mouth impression (i.e., imprints of teeth of upper and lower dental arches)
IP		Inclined plane
	IP/AC	Acrylic inclined plane
	IP/C	Composite inclined plane
	IP/M	Metal (i.e., lab-produced) inclined plane
MAL		Malocclusion
	MAL1	Class 1 malocclusion (neutroclusion; dental malocclusion with normal upper/lower jaw length relationship)
	MAL1/BV	Buccoversion
	MAL1/DV	Distoversion
	MAL1/LABV	Labioversion
	MAL1/LV	Linguoversion
	MAL1/MV	Mesioversion
	MAL1/PV	Palatoversion
	MAL2	Class 2 malocclusion (mandibular distoclusion; symmetrical skeletal malocclusion with the lower jaw relatively shorter than the upper jaw)
	MAL3	Class 3 malocclusion (mandibular mesioclusion; symmetrical skeletal malocclusion with the upper jaw relatively shorter than the lower jaw)
	MAL4	Class 4 malocclusion (asymmetrical skeletal malocclusion in a caudoventral, side-to-side, or dorsoventral direction)
	MAL4/DV	Asymmetrical skeletal malocclusion in a dorsoventral direction
	MAL4/RC	Asymmetrical skeletal malocclusion in a rostrocaudal direction
	MAL4/STS	Asymmetrical skeletal malocclusion in a side-to-side direction
OA		Orthodontic appliance
	OA/A	Orthodontic appliance adjustment
	OA/AR	Arch bar
	OA/BKT	Bracket, button, or hook
	OA/CMB	Custom-made OA/BKT
	OA/EC	Elastic chain, tube, or thread
	OA/I	Orthodontic appliance installment
	OA/R	Orthodontic appliance removal
	OA/WIR	Orthodontic wire
OR		Orthodontic recheck
OS		Orthognathic surgery

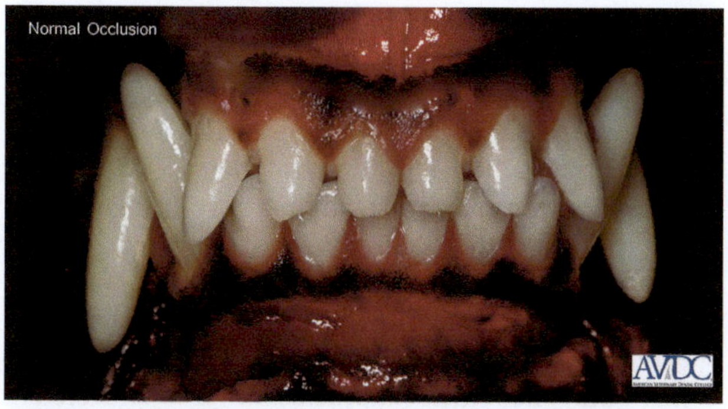

Figure 19.1 Normal occlusion in a dog – rostral view. *Source:* Copyright AVDC®, used with permission from https://www.avdc.org/Nomenclature/Nomen-Occlusion.html; accessed November 2017.

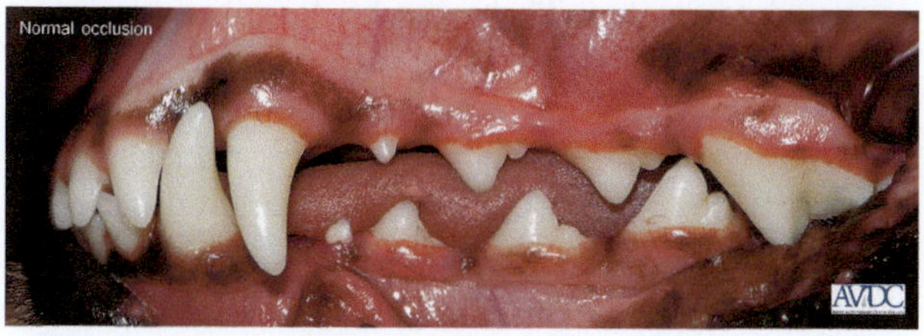

Figure 19.2 Normal occlusion in a dog – buccal view. *Source:* Copyright AVDC®, used with permission.

19.6.2.3 Dental Malocclusions

Distoversion (DV) describes a tooth that is in its anatomically correct position in the dental arch, but which is abnormally angled in a distal direction.

Mesioversion (MV) describes a tooth that is in its anatomically correct position in the dental arch, but which is abnormally angled in a mesial direction.

Linguoversion (LV) describes a tooth that is in its anatomically correct position in the dental arch, but which is abnormally angled in a lingual direction.

Labioversion (LABV) describes an incisor or canine tooth that is in its anatomically correct position in the dental arch, but which is abnormally angled in a labial direction.

Buccoversion (BV) describes a premolar or molar tooth that is in its anatomically correct position in the dental arch, but which is abnormally angled in a buccal direction.

Crossbite (CB) describes a malocclusion in which a mandibular tooth or teeth have a more buccal or labial position than the antagonist maxillary tooth. It can be classified as rostral or caudal.

In rostral crossbite (CB/R, similar to anterior crossbite in human terminology) one or more of the mandibular

(a) (b)

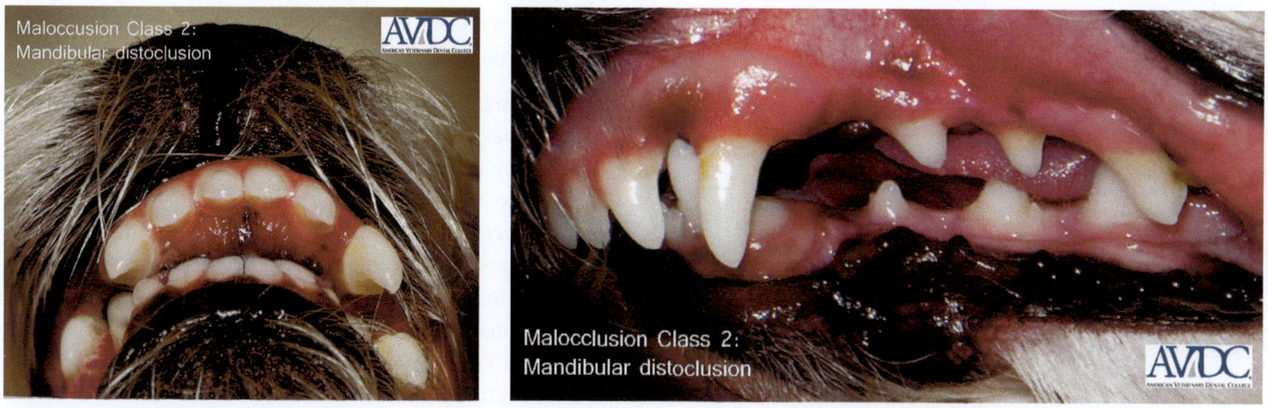

Figure 19.3 Mandibular distoclusion (Class 2) in a dog: (a) ventral view; (b) buccal view. *Source:* Copyright AVDC®, used with permission.

(a) (b)

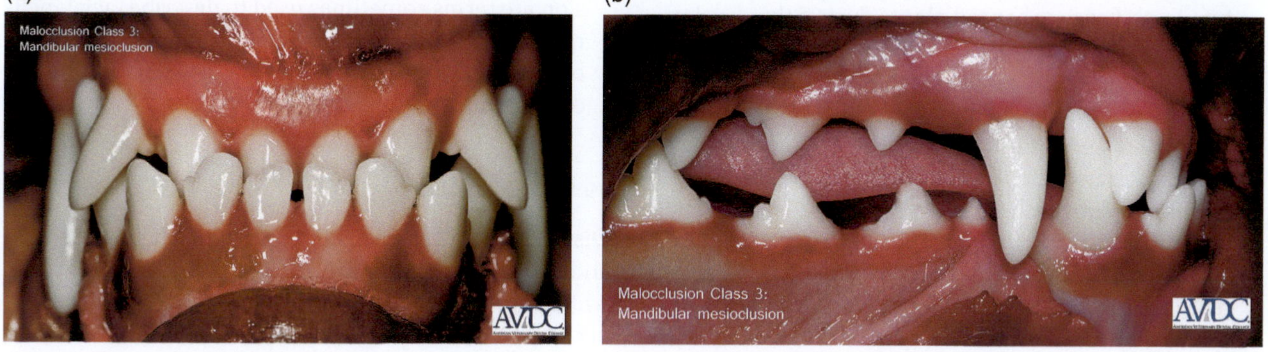

Figure 19.4 Mandibular mesioclusion (Class 3) in a dog: (a) rostral view; (b) buccal view. *Source:* Copyright AVDC®, used with permission.

incisor teeth is labial to the opposing maxillary incisor teeth when the mouth is closed. In caudal crossbite (CB/C, similar to posterior crossbite in human terminology) one or more of the mandibular cheek teeth is buccal to the opposing maxillary cheek teeth when the mouth is closed.

19.6.3 Additional Terminology

Scissors bite is the normal relationship of the maxillary incisors overlapping the mandibular incisors whose incisal edges rest on or near the cingulum on the lingual surfaces of the maxillary incisors.

Overbite or vertical overlap is the extension of the maxillary teeth over the mandibular in a vertical direction, when opposing teeth are in contact and in centric occlusion.

Overjut, overjet, and horizontal overlap are also all basically the same thing. They are the facial projection of the maxillary teeth anterior or posterior teeth beyond their antagonist in a horizontal direction.

Level bites are when the incisor teeth meet edge to edge (edge to edge bite) or the premolars or molars occlude cusp to cusp (end to end bite). This is a traumatic occlusion for the teeth, which can cause attritional wearing down of the teeth into a closed bite.

Open bites are when a part or all of the teeth are prevented from closing to normal occlusal contact. Rostral open bites in the incisal region are the most universal and are seen commonly in association with unilateral occlusal abnormalities. Caudal open bites are seen most commonly in association with traumatic CB/Cs. Full open bites are seen most often in traumatic conditions of partially avulsed caudal teeth or CB/Cs.

Closed bites are those that when the bite is in static occlusion the dental arches close too far. This typically is seen when excessive wear of the teeth occurs allowing excessive closure of the occlusion.

19.6.4 Malpositioning of Teeth Terms

Transposition. Term used to describe a condition where two teeth have exchanged places during the development of the occlusion.

Embrication. Irregular arranged teeth within an arch due to a lack of space (crowding), typically seen in mandibular incisors and maxillary premolars in brachycephalic breeds. Rotated, tipped, supraerupted (supraclusion), infraerupted (infraclusion), and displaced teeth are not uncommon in embrication.

Infraclusion or shortened tooth. Terms used to describe teeth in which the occlusal surface or incisal edge has not reached the same or appropriate level of other teeth of the same type. This is typically seen in teeth that have failed to fully erupt (partially impacted) or that have been intruded by force or injury.

Supraclusion or supraocclusion. Terms used to describe teeth that are above their appropriate occlusal level. Seen most commonly in teeth that have been extruded due to injury or disease, or have overerupted due to a lack of occlusal contact.

Supereruption. Term used to describe teeth that have the cementoenamel junction (CEJ) erupted above the normal. May be either supraclusion or supraversion. Additionally, these teeth may be in supraclusion or may not be due to clinical removal or traumatic loss of a portion of the crown. Commonly seen in older cats.

Rotations, torsiversion, or torsoversion. Teeth that are turned or rotated. These can be described by one of two terms: mesiolingual and distolingual rotations. A mesiolingual rotation describes a tooth that is rotated on its long axis so that the mesial aspect is moved towards the tongue. Distolingual rotation describes a tooth that is rotated on its long axis so that the distal aspect is moved towards the tongue.

19.6.5 Version Terms

Tipping, inclinations, and versions: describes a tooth in which the crown is tipped or inclined in an abnormal position. Version is a term that can also be used to describe malposition of one or more teeth.

Mesial inclination, mesial tipping, and mesioversion. Describes a tooth in which the crown leans in a mesial direction (i.e., mesial inclination of a maxillary canine in a Sheltie, sometimes incorrectly termed rostroversion).

Distal inclination, distal tipping, and distoversion. Describes a tooth in which the crown leans in a distal direction.

Lingual inclination, lingual tipping, and linguoversion. Refers to a tooth tilted so that its crown leans towards the tongue.

Facial or vestibular inclination, or tipping, and facioversion. Refers to a tooth that is leaning away from the tongue. Labial inclination, labial tipping, and labioversion are terms sometimes used to describe facial inclination of the rostral teeth, and buccal inclination, buccal tipping, and buccoversion for facial inclination of the caudal teeth.

19.6.6 Displacement Terms

Displacement describes a tooth in which both the crown and root have moved principally in the same direction, which is sometimes described as an occlusion (i.e., mesial occlusion).

Mesial displacement, mesial occlusion, mesioclusion. Refers to a tooth which is bodily displaced mesially or towards the midline of the arch.

Distal displacement, distoclusion. Refers to a tooth which is bodily displaced distally or away from the midline of the arch.

Lingual displacement, linguoclusion. Describes a tooth bodily displaced towards the tongue.

Facial displacement, facioclusion. Describes a tooth bodily displaced away from the tongue. Labial displacement and labioclusion can be used to describe this effect in the rostral teeth and buccal displacement and buccoclusion in the caudal teeth.

19.6.7 Deciduous Malocclusions and Orthodontics

Malocclusions in young dogs and cats with deciduous dentitions, which are best termed deciduous malocclusions, are not unusual. Fairly mild malpositioning of the jaw positions could be due to a temporary disproportionate relationship caused by an independent jaw growth surge. If left on its own, there is a chance that the opposing jaw will soon experience its own surge in growth to return it to the correct relationship, if genetically coded to do so. Maturation usually evens out this unique growth pattern between the jaws, with the mandible typically experiencing the later growth of the two. One problem that can result in the interim, however, is the abnormal or malevolent interlocking of deciduous teeth in a relationship opposite to their norm, or having impingement on soft tissue. One of the most common deciduous malocclusions is where the mandible grows excessively and the incisors become rostral (labial) to the maxillary incisors. While this is certainly anticipated in brachycephalic breeds, in others this interlock may have serious consequences. With a mechanical interference such as this, maxillary growth could be hindered, keeping the jaw relationship abnormal. If still in this position when the permanent maxillary incisors begin to erupt, especially if the maxillary deciduous incisors are retained, they will come in even further lingually.

Deciduous mandibular canines that are contacting or indenting into the palate or other soft tissue should have treatment as soon as the condition is identified (linguoversion). With a firm holding indentation into the palate, not only can these teeth interfere with the forward growth of the mandible (even to the point of the mandible "bowing" downward) but they can also disrupt the normal lateral growth, exacerbating the width discrepancy problem (Figure 19.5).

Grossly abnormal dentitions may require exodontia just to provide the patient with a functional or comfortable malocclusion. This is typically either genetic or the result of facial trauma effecting bone growth. Trauma problems vary greatly, but facial bites by the mother or littermates have been seen to cause this problem.

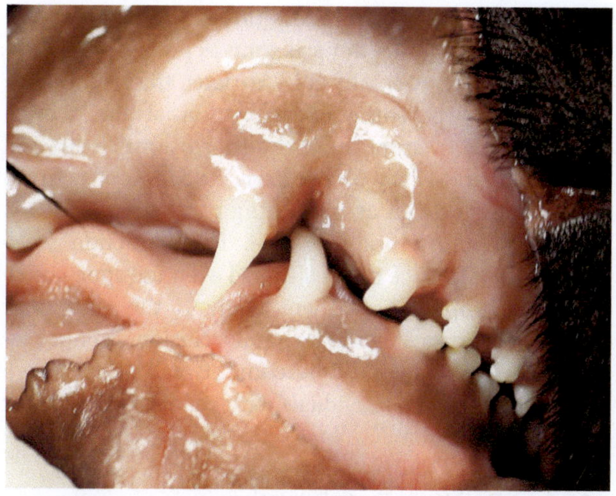

Figure 19.5 Deciduous malocclusion – linguoversion mandibular canines that are contacting the palatal mucosa.

19.7 Aims of Orthodontic Treatment

The aims of orthodontic treatment are to provide a reasonably functional, esthetic, stable, and harmonious occlusion by altering the position or presence of the natural teeth. To attain these aims, in veterinary orthodontics there are four goals to strive to accomplish. These are:

1) Proper assessment and supervision of the occlusion.
2) Removal of etiological factors that may disrupt normal growth patterns of the dentofacial complex, when possible, in an interceptive action.
3) To correct conditions that may allow the occlusion to deteriorate, by preventive measures.
4) By corrective acts, to establish and maintain as functional and as close to normal an occlusion as is reasonable.

19.8 Categories of Orthodontic Treatment

19.8.1 Interceptive

Interceptive orthodontics is generally considered to be the extraction or recontouring (crown reduction) of primary or permanent teeth that are contributing or will contribute to alignment problems of the permanent dentition. Interceptive measures are not always successful due to time interval limitations and/or hereditary influences that cannot be overcome. In these situations, interceptive orthodontics or selective extraction of the deciduous teeth that are "caught" will help to relieve this interlock and not impede any future jaw growth. The extractions ideally are done as soon as possible, between four and eight weeks of age (no later than 12 weeks), to allow any potential normalization of the growth pattern prior to eruption of the successional teeth and re-interlocking of the bite pattern. Selection of teeth to be extracted as well as the timing of the extractions is crucial to the occlusal outcome. The extraction technique may influence the health and eventual appearance of the unerupted permanent teeth. If the hereditary influence is for a specific jaw malocclusion, this procedure will not change the outcome. It will only make a difference in those individuals with genetic potential for a normal occlusion.

19.8.1.1 Deciduous Tooth Extraction

Particularly in younger animals, the process of exodontia should be carried out with extreme caution to minimize the potential damage to the adjacent permanent tooth buds. Gingival flaps or epithelial attachment severing are best performed gently. Elevators used to fatigue the periodontal ligament (PDL) should be small and delicate, and utilized with minimal pressure, preferably on the sides of the tooth that are furthest from the permanent bud. Excessive force or gouging should be avoided and extraction forceps should only be used to remove an extremely loose tooth from its attachment. Any fractured or retained roots tips should be retrieved if possible, especially in interceptive orthodontic cases, as the root can still deflect the permanent tooth's eruption. Extraction of retained deciduous teeth usually occurs once the permanent tooth has begun eruption, so damage to its formative stages is less likely.

When considering deciduous extraction, the owner should always be informed that while reasonable precautions are being taken to minimize potential damage to the developing permanent teeth, problems may still occur. These vary from minimal pitting of the enamel to major structural defects (gouging, disruption of the crown/root junction) to complete relocation of the tooth [8]. With skillful care and appropriate protocol the risk and degree of complications can be greatly reduced.

19.8.2 Preventive

Preventive orthodontics is the evaluation and elimination of conditions that may lead to irregularities in the developing or mature occlusal complex. Preventive orthodontics basically break down into three categories: occlusal assessment and supervision, space control, and behavioral control. Occlusal assessment and supervision includes the supervision of timely primary dental exfoliation and permanent dental eruption. Even though exfoliation and eruption supervision is considered preventive, the actual act of assisting exfoliation or eruption is an interceptive orthodontic action. The act of occlusal assessment and supervision is classified as a part of preventive orthodontics, but the treatment of the assessed problem may fall into interceptive, preventive, or corrective categories. Space control includes treatment of traumatic, congenital, or hereditary anomalies, as well as dentally destructive diseases (caries, dental resorption, periodontal disease, etc.) and maintenance of dentally voided spaces. Behavioral control deals with therapy to manage deportment, which can affect occlusion.

19.8.3 Corrective

Corrective orthodontics has two stages: active treatment and retention. The active treatment refers to the application of devices to restore dental occlusion to a reasonably functional and esthetics state. Prior to undertaking such an action the animal's occlusion should be evaluated, as well as the effects of various apparatuses that may be selected on the dentofacial complex. Once the active treatment stage is completed, it is necessary to have the teeth stabilized in their new position to allow a harmonious state to develop, which is termed the retention stage. During active treatment the alveolar bone is induced into a state of accelerated resorption and deposition. The retention stage allows this bone to return to a more normal physiologic state, while hopefully allowing the bone to eventually provide a sound harmonious tooth support structure. The device that provides the retention is called the retainer. Retainers can be either fixed or removable, but in veterinary orthodontics the fixed retainer is more typical. Occasionally mild cases of Class II or III malocclusions are treated for cosmetic reasons, which is termed orthodontic camouflage treatment.

19.9 Diagnostic Aids

Diagnosis and treatment planning is principally based upon visual assessment accompanied by certain aids [3]. These aids help to improve the evaluation to reduce the chance of unexpected and possibly disastrous consequences. There are five basic diagnostic tools in veterinary orthodontics. These are history, physical and oral examination, photographs, dental models and bite registrations, and radiographs.

Written records and history is always important, but in orthodontics they are essential in the determination of progression and response to treatment. History provided by the owner can be helpful, but must be screened carefully due to their lack of understanding of terminology and dental normals. All aspects of previous illnesses and accidents and their treatment are important. Information concerning the line and family can be extremely useful in attempting to classify an anomalous condition as hereditary.

Nothing can take the place of a good physical and oral examination in assessment of occlusion. Only first-hand viewing of the true dental articulation can give a reasonable evaluation of the range of motion, potential attritional wear, and interferences to tooth movement. Many TMJ dysplasias can be felt or heard. Oral soft tissue health is best evaluated by visual and tactile senses. Photographs provide records of before and after treatment.

Dental models and bite registrations of a patient's dental arches and supporting tissues are an excellent source for study of abnormalities and treatment planning. The bite registration allows for a reasonable articulation of the models. With these models, orthodontic appliances can be deliberated, designed, and fabricated.

Radiographs allow analysis of potential complications to treatment and from treatment. Abnormalities and lesions must be considered prior to treatment. Resorptive lesions, caries, periodontal disease, missing teeth, unerupted teeth, root abnormalities, degree of root maturity, quality of alveolar bone, etc., must all be taken into consideration, and radiology is the best tool to address many of these.

Cephalometrics and computer treatment simulations are very impressive. However, the lack of cephalometric standards in animals makes this tool unreliable. Computerized treatment simulations in animal dentistry is at this time more of a toy than a tool, but will eventually be an important diagnostic device.

19.10 Age, Timing, and Treatment

Ideally, orthodontic treatment should be initiated as soon as possible, once favorable conditions exist for assisting orthodontic procedures. Young bone is less resistant to tooth movement, young tissues are generally more forgiving, and young animals typically accept placement of oral appliances more easily than mature animals. Tooth movement is easier to produce in younger animals due to the fact that their cells are in an active growth phase and readily adapt to changes, whereas there is a more sluggish cellular response in older individuals. Also, with interceptive orthodontic procedures involving deciduous extractions, early institution of treatment is essential for optimal effect. However, the advantages are offset to a degree due to the fact that making an accurate diagnosis becomes more difficult the younger the animal. Additionally, treatments to animals with deciduous or mixed dentition may have to be repeated for the permanent dentition, and adjustments to young permanent dentition may require prolonged supervision for retention or retreatment due to drift or recoil. Most interceptive extractions must be delayed until the teeth have erupted or until adjacent teeth will not be injured in the process.

A complete treatment plan must include the control of any active dental or oral disease [9]. Periodontitis or active periodontal disease must be controlled prior to orthodontic treatment, as orthodontic tooth movements (OTMs) superimposed on periodontitis can lead to the inevitable destruction of the periodontium [10, 11]. Once controlled, the disease should continue to be treated even during orthodontics, as research in humans has shown that regular professional treatment can halt or even reverse attachment destruction [12, 13]. Clinical research has shown that orthodontic treatments in both normal and compromised periodontal tissues can be completed without loss of attachment, providing that appropriate treatment and optimal oral hygiene had been initiated prior to and during tooth movements [11, 14].

19.11 Physiologic and Histologic Aspects of Tooth Movement

The changes that allow OTM is a biological response that is primarily a PDL process impacting a bony response, but also including growing areas distant from the dentition [15]. It is the external forces that can be managed by the practitioner, by providing the least amount of force needed to result in appropriate treatment with the lowest levels of complications or discomfort for the patient [16].

Cellular response depends upon the degree and duration of applied force. Estimation of the root surface area is important in determining anchorage and force application. In the dog some research has been done on root surface areas of the maxillary fourth premolar and mandibular first molar [17, 18], but there are variations within breeds and from individual to individual. In the first edition the authors attempted to provide some approximations of the dog root surface area to act as a general guide (Table 19.2). While these values are just approximations, they correlate with the two studies that showed a mean root surface area for a maxillary fourth premolar was $562.8 \pm 124.9\,mm^2$ and for the mandibular first molar was $497.1 \pm 116.2\,mm^2$ [17, 18], which are similar to the values for a dog up to 50 pounds in the table. When a light to mild force is applied, it acts as a stimulus to initiate cellular activity resorption and deposition of bone, which is termed the physiologic movement. When these pressures are exceeded with a heavy force there will be necrosis of periodontal tissues on the pressure side and poor to no deposition of bone on the traction side, which is labeled pathologic movement.

Table 19.2 Approximate tooth root surfaces of the dog in square centimeters in relation to the relevant weight of dog.

	<10 lb	<25 lb	<50 lb	<90 lb
Maxillary				
First incisor	0.7	1.0	1.3	1.7
Second incisor	0.8	1.2	1.5	1.9
Third incisor	1.2	1.6	2.25	2.6
Canine	3.4	5.4	7.8	9.5
Fourth premolar	2.5	4.15	5.25	6.75
First molar	1.5	2.25	3.25	4.25
Mandibular				
First incisor	0.6	0.9	1.2	1.6
Second incisor	0.7	1.2	1.5	1.8
Third incisor	0.9	1.4	1.7	2.0
Canine	3.3	5.25	7.65	9.25
Fourth premolar	1.3	1.9	3.25	3.75
First molar	2.6	3.8	4.75	6.00

Much discussion and study has centered around the concept of the optimal force magnitude, to the extent that wide variations in the data collected have resulted in the conclusion that the optimal force may differ for each tooth and individual patient [19]. There are several proposed models for the relationship between the magnitude of applied force and rate of OTM, including an "on–off switch" model where movement occurs once a certain level of force is reached and continues at the same level of movement beyond that point [20]. Another scenario includes reaching the threshold at some point, but with a linear increase in movement with a force increase or a decrease in movement after higher forces are reached. The most accepted model shows an initial dose–response increase in movement after an initial threshold, with a plateau and no further increases in movement with increases in force [20]. It has been shown that in the very low force range there is a dose–response relationship, but it is not a linear response, and the increased movement does plateau with higher force magnitudes [16]. In a mathematical model, it was shown that the force velocity curves are similar for dogs and humans, but that no threshold can be defined as the switch-on point for tooth movement, so optimal forces cannot be calculated [21].

19.11.1 Pressure Side and Tension Side

The classical theory of the pressure–tension concept states that the application of an orthodontic force generates a pressure side and a tension side within the PDL. This change in tissue pressure approximates the capillary vessels blood pressure, with an optimal level high enough to cause change, but not excessive enough to cause necrosis. On the pressure side (direction of tooth movement), the periodontal membrane is compressed with an increase in the capillary pressure and blood supply at pressure points, initially the alveolar crest. This results in an increased mobilization of fibroblasts, cementoblasts, osteoblasts, and osteoclasts to the area. These activated cells are responsible for the resorption and remodeling of bone and periodontal tissues. With the bone it will take several days for the needed influx of osteoclasts to become established. The initial bone absorption typically occurs within the tooth socket along the wall near the crest. The osteoblasts will be found in crescent-shaped excavations known as Howship's lacunae. Within a few weeks osteoblasts and osteoclasts will be found within the cancellous bone where it is being reoriented by absorption and apposition. The trabecular pattern, which is normally primarily vertically oriented, reorganizes in a more horizontal fashion. The original pattern will gradually be reestablished once tooth movement is terminated.

On the tension side (away from the direction of tooth movement), the PDL is stretched, resulting in a widening of the periodontal membrane space. In response the capillary blood flow and cellular activity increases. This results in the deposition of new bone along the traction areas of the lamina dura.

19.11.2 Biomechanical Process

Current thoughts on the biological mechanisms of OTM have a focus shifted to the effect of initial matrix strain and fluid changes in the PDL and bone, which leads to cellular deformation and strain and the subsequent cell biological processes [16, 19, 22], resulting in resorption and apposition sides [23]. The OTM depends largely on the biomechanical properties of the PDL [24], as the orthodontic forces applied are far below typical thresholds needed for osseous remodeling [25].

The first phase of OTM, or the initial movement of the tooth within the socket (24 hours to 2 days), has a rapid transpositional movement that is followed by a slower "creep" movement [24]. A halt in tooth movement is due to the hyalinization of the PDL caused by vascular obliteration and subsequent local necrosis. This second, or lag, phase can last from 20 to 30 days [26]. The acellular, avascular, homogeneous (glass-like) layer must be removed by macrophages and replaced with new connective tissue before extracellular matrix and osseous remodeling can occur. After the removal of the necrotic tissue, the post-lag phases (3 and 4) comprise the periods of real tooth movement.

The cellular responses seen in OTM have further been evaluated with the identification of many factors that play an intricate role, proinflammatory cytokines that initiate osteoclastic activity (IL-6, CCL2, CCL3, CD40) to osteoblastic progenitors. Regulation of bone activity by the parathyroid hormone (PTH) and calcitonin may also play a role [27, 28].

There can be a high variability in individual tooth movement due to factors ranging from variation in bone density and metabolism to levels of cytokines and growth factors [26]. The presence of even focal hyalinized tissue can impact the rate of movement [24, 26] and while finite element (FE) models can help approximate responses to varying forces [25, 29], there is still great variability and challenges in addressing all factors.

Most orthodontic movements are simple tipping, resulting in the greatest amount of changes occurring near the alveolar crest, less as the fulcrum point is approached, and then increasing again as the apex is approached. In correction of infraclusion with extrusion, deposition of bone normally occurs at the alveolar crest, along the socket walls, and at the socket apex. In treating supraclusion with intrusion, resorption of bone along the walls and apex occurs initially. This may be the most potentially hazardous movement, in that damage to the PDL and possible pulpal necrosis may occur due to compression of the apical blood supply. Rotation holds its own risks, especially in movements greater than 45°. If performed too quickly, osteoblastic activity will not be able to maintain pace with the osteoclastic activity. This can result in poor support and an unstable position. Rotation movements are best accomplished by light forces for slow transition, and use of intermittent force application. Teeth should be either overrotated to help compensate for recoil or stabilized securely in position with a retainer for an extended period of time.

19.11.3 Changes in Other Tissues Associated with Tooth Movement

Gingival tissues eventually adapt to the tooth's new positioning. However, these changes are commonly less rapid than that of the alveolar bone. In cases where rapid movement is achieved, this may result in tissue mounding or wrinkling up on the pressure side and being stretched tight on the tension side until the gingival tissue compensates. This tissue can easily become irritated and inflamed if appliances are allowed to impinge upon it. Additionally, the elasticity of the gingival tissue in this condition can act to cause recoil of the tooth back towards its original position, especially in rotation movements [30].

Changes in the TMJ may also occur during occlusal adjustments from orthodontics, though a literature review indicates that orthodontic treatment did not provide a significant risk to the joint [31]. Some human studies show a potential improvement in temporomandibular disorders, but not at a significant level [31].

19.12 Types of Tooth Movements

In order to perform orthodontics teeth must generally be moved and/or removed. There are six basic tooth movements that are utilized or occur in orthodontics, which are tipping, radicular (root), translation (bodily), rotation (torsion), extrusion, and intrusion [15].

19.12.1 Tipping

Tipping movements occur when the crown of the tooth carries the primary movement. When compression or tension (traction) is applied to a tooth the force is transferred through the PDL to the alveolus, and the alveolar crest usually attempts to act as a pivotal point. However, the true center of rotation, or fulcrum, created in tipping occurs approximately at the junction of the middle and apical thirds of the root. In tipping, both crown and root typically move, but in opposite directions. The crown and root that is coronal to the fulcrum point move the greater distance, as compared to the apex to the tooth. Lighter forces generally provide the best tipping movements, as the lighter the force applied the more apical will be the fulcrum. This is the most common movement made use of in veterinary orthodontics.

19.12.2 Radicular

Radicular or root movements occur when the apex of the tooth carries the primary or greatest distance of movement, in comparison to the crown. Radicular movement is basically tipping from the opposite end of the tooth. The fulcrum is found approximately at the junction of the middle and cervical thirds of the root. The movement is sometimes used in teeth where the crown cusp or incisal edge is in the correct position but the neck of the tooth is not. Typically the coronal tip of the tooth is held stationary, while compression or tension is applied near the cervical region of the tooth.

19.12.3 Translation/Bodily

Translation or bodily movement occurs when the crown and apex both travel in the same direction. To move a tooth bodily typically requires a fixed attachment to the crown as a great deal more resistance is encountered from the periodontium than with tipping movements, and therefore is more difficult. Lighter forces are initially used for this type of movement, but moderate pressures are typically required to complete the movement, in animals, within a reasonable period of time.

19.12.4 Rotation or Torsion

Rotation or torsion movements are when the tooth is rotated on its long axis in one direction or the other. In this movement all of the PDL fibers are stretched in the same spiral direction around the tooth. This makes recoil a serious problem in this type of movement. Several things can be done to help to counteract recoil from torsion movements. The first is that when teeth are rotated with a lighter pressure over a longer period of time, less recoil occurs. Second, use of alternating periods of movement and stabilization can reduce the recoil effect. Third, and most importantly, the teeth should have some type of retainer applied for several months.

19.12.5 Extrusion

Extrusion is actually movement of the tooth further out of the alveolus, typically in the same direction as normal eruption. If there is no occlusal interference to be dealt with and an appropriate appliance designed, extrusion is the easiest movement to accomplish in theory. However, in carnivores, the canine teeth with their tremendous root structure and greater occlusal height can sometimes be a challenge. In extrusion, light forces are used to reduce the chance of accidentally avulsing the tooth. Once extruded, realignment of the biological width is essential to support optimal periodontal health.

19.12.6 Intrusion

Intrusion is the movement of the tooth further into the alveolus. The forces required are applied in the same direction as the forces of occlusion. Therefore, the periodontium is best suited to resist this type of movement, making it the most difficult movement to accomplish. However, once attained, coronal recoil is seldom seen, though in humans relapse is common and the use of implant anchors and orthognathic surgery may be needed [32]. Light forces are best used in order to reduce the chances of apical resorption.

19.13 Anchorage

In tooth movements there must be a stable foundation that acts as the point of resistance for the appliance to be attached to. This site of delivery from which force is exerted is known as the anchorage [15]. The resistance of the anchorage must be greater than the target. The less the anchorage is able to move, the greater the anchorage-to-target ratio of resistance must be, so it is common to make use of multiple teeth in anchorage. These teeth are referred to as the anchorage unit.

Resistance to movement is complex, with the root surface area (anchorage value), quality of root, alveolus surface area, quality of alveolus, leverage of appliance, type of movement, and direction of force all being factors. Appliance leverage is used to help counteract target resistance. By applying the anchorage near the cervical region and the target attachment near the coronal tip of the teeth, a leverage advantage for the anchorage can be obtained. Additionally, the type of movements involved can affect resistance. Bodily movement provides greater resistance than tipping. Direction of movement also plays a role in resistance. There is greater resistance to distal movement in the distal teeth, due to the outward growth patterns of the jaw and the distal inclination of roots. For the rostral teeth there is greater resistance to lingual movement, due to tongue pressures, growth patterns of the jaw, and the lingual inclination of the roots.

There are several situations of orthodontic anchorage beyond simple anchorage: reciprocal, reinforced (stationary), cortical, skeletal, and differential effect of very large forces [15].

19.13.1 Simple Anchorage

Simple anchorage occurs when a greater tooth resistance to movement is used in association with an appliance than that of the target of movement in the same dental arch. Keeping in mind the factors of resistance, an advantage of at least two to one of anchorage to target teeth is preferred. Typically, but incorrectly, this is generally thought of as root surface ratios.

19.13.2 Reciprocal Anchorage

Reciprocal anchorage is when two teeth or tooth groups are moved to an extent in opposite directions and more or less to an equal extent, either away from each other or towards each other. For this to work properly, each group must provide a similar resistance.

19.13.3 Reinforced Anchorage

Reinforced anchorage (planes and stationary) is used when on occasion the action of a force with simple anchorage will be insufficient to resist the reaction of the movement target. In these cases the anchorage may be augmented for stabilization in one of several ways. These are the addition of more resistance units (teeth), use of planes, and stationary anchorages. Planes are reinforcements to the anchorage that allow a part of the resistance to be transferred from the teeth to paradental tissues, such as the palate. Stationary reinforcement is the use of fixed anchorage attachment that is designed so that only bodily movement of the anchorage teeth can occur.

19.13.3.1 Intermaxillary Anchorage

Intermaxillary anchorage is when an appliance anchorage is placed in the opposing jaws or in both the mandible and maxilla. This is a form of reinforcement, but due to its uniqueness is placed in its own category.

19.13.4 Cortical Anchorage

Torquing movements may adjust the tooth to be positioned against the cortical bone, which is more resistant to remodeling. However, root resorption (RR) is likely and the cortical bone may even be penetrated, so this anchorage could be challenging.

19.13.5 Skeletal Anchorage

Application of screws and plates for skeletal anchorage has become fairly routine. Complete osseointegration is not necessary for these temporary attachments and they will not move unless there is degeneration around the bone.

19.13.5.1 Extraoral Anchorage

Extraoral anchorage is when anchorage is sought outside the mouth. This is typically done in people using a variety of head and neck harnesses. The heavy intermittent force is not optimal in people and is not applicable to most veterinary patients.

19.14 Application of Force

19.14.1 Intermittent Force

Intermittent force is where the drive or energy is applied in incremental steps with periods of rest in between. Force application of this type is generally preferred with tooth movements in which recoil is an expected problem. Intermittent force is most commonly applied using orthodontic appliances with screw-type drives and inclined planes. With inclined planes the force is self-regulated by the discomfort of the periodontal membranes. With screws, the limiting factor is the adjustment. Most are designed to provide 0.18 to 0.20 mm of movement per quarter turn (see expansion screws).

19.14.2 Continuous Force

Continuous force is where the drive or energy is applied in a constant fashion until the target tooth is moved to its new target site. This type of force application customarily provides a more rapid movement of the target tooth to the target site than intermittent force. Orthodontic appliances with elastics and springs are most commonly used to provide this type of force application. In order to maintain continuous force, springs and elastics are readjusted prior to their becoming totally relaxed or dead. Springs and elastics can be used in an intermittent force concept, just as some screws have internal spring devices and can be used in a continuous force manner. To prevent damage to the periodontium or tooth, the force should be limited to remain below that of capillary blood pressure: 20–26 g/cm^2 of tooth root surface.

19.15 General Types of Orthodontic Appliances

19.15.1 Removable

Removable appliances are those that are designed to be easily and routinely removed, and then reinserted. These appliances are preferred in those cases in which, due to oral or dental disease, intensive oral hygiene is required, or when other dental treatments must be carried out simultaneously. This allows all food debris to be removed, the teeth to be brushed, periodontal infections to be treated, the appliance to be cleaned, and other dental problems to be treated as necessary. In addition, repairs can be made at leisure or by a technician while the appliance is out of the oral cavity. In veterinary orthodontics most of these appliances consist of three parts: a removable base, an active force attached to the base, and a fixed anchorage. The base of the appliance may be made of acrylic or metal, and serves as a platform for the active force. The active force is usually provided by screws, springs, or elastics. The anchorage most often consists of brackets bonded to teeth that allow elastics to attach the base in place for activation. Its main disadvantages are that they are frequently more bulky, which may sometimes interfere with normal occlusion, and in some astute pets they may learn to remove the appliance themselves, which may then be swallowed, becoming an intestinal foreign body. Newer sequential alignments have been adapted from human dentistry for veterinary patients.

19.15.2 Fixed

Fixed appliances are typically attached to provide a center for a movement force without removal until the tooth attains its target site. Fixed appliances customarily provide greater security of the applied force, are less bulky, have improved precision, and enhanced gentleness, when properly applied and supervised. Its main disadvantage is the need for greater hygiene care, as food and debris may accumulate beneath its recesses, and visual monitoring for disease or trauma may be hampered by the appliance. Additionally, any repairs must generally be made chairside with a sedated patient. Fixed appliances ordinarily consist of three parts: base plates or bands for anchorage, a framework or bracket for force attachment, and the active force. The active force may consist of wires, springs, screws, or elastics.

19.16 Orthodontic Appliances and Materials

19.16.1 Wires

Orthodontic wire is commonly used in a large variety of orthodontic appliances. Bending and forming wires is not beyond the abilities of the average practitioner, but is time consuming and requires careful consideration, technique, and knowledge. For these reasons a laboratory is best used by most.

There are three basic types of orthodontic wire: round, rectangular, and braided. Round wire is the simplest to handle and work with, but when torque is required, specially designed auxiliary parts must be added to achieve a torqueing force. Rectangular wire, when used with rectangular brackets or tubes, can apply torqueing forces with the greatest accuracy. Braided wires are made of multiple strands of thinner wires that are twisted or braided together and provide the most flexibility of the three types. The physical properties and mechanical behavior of wire depends to a great deal on the type of metals employed within them. Stainless steel and cobalt–chromium wires are most commonly used, with nickel titanium (martensitic and austenitic) and beta-titanium wire for increased springiness [33].

Simple stainless steel appliance bends can be performed with bird beak, square, Howe, three-prong, and wire cutter pliers. Bends are basically classified according to the direction of force. There are three basics bends, which are the primary or first-order, secondary or second-order, and tertiary or third-order. First-order bends are in the horizontal plane, and are in and out bends. Second-order bends are in the vertical plane, and are up and down bends. Third-order bends are bends that produce a torque force. There are three types of third-order bends, which are single tooth torque, anterior torque, and posterior torque.

19.16.2 Springs

Springs, kick and coil, can easily be incorporated into appliances to provide either traction or compression. Open coil springs are used for compression and closed coil springs for traction. The longer the wire and the more helix loops applied to the spring, the gentler will be the force and the better the maintenance of direction [34]. The main disadvantage of the kick spring in tilting movements has been that as the tooth tilts, the spring has a tendency to ride up the lingual surface and possibly over it, disrupting its function. This is best controlled by designing the spring to engage the tooth as close to the cervical area as possible, or in acrylic appliances, placing the spring into a recessed box cavity. The W-spring is most commonly used in veterinary orthodontics with banding for spreading both mandibular canines when they are base narrow.

19.16.3 Arch Bars

Arch bars, wires and cast with their various types and auxiliaries, are possibly the most versatile of the orthodontic appliances [35]. These can be either labial or lingual to the teeth and are used in the maxilla or mandible. The anchorage attachment is often either bands or brackets. The bands can be matrix or cast. The actual arch wire or bar can also be either prefabricated wire or a casted metal. The cast metal arch bars have the greater strength, but are relatively non-flexible. This inflexibility can lead to problems if not compensated for in young or growing animals. Therefore in young animals, where the use of a flexible wire is soldered to the anchor bands or in cast bars, the placement of a telescoping central joint alleviates most of these problems. The canine teeth are possibly the most commonly banded teeth for anchorage. These teeth must be carefully examined for paralleling or a lack of it. If the two teeth flare or converge to any degree, a solid cast appliance cannot be placed, unless a joint or flexibility is built into the arch bar.

19.16.4 Orthodontic Band

An orthodontic band is a flattened piece of metal constructed as a ring to fit around the clinical crown of a tooth and be cemented in place. Bands can be prefabricated on models or formed by an operator with strips of band metal material for a custom fit. Various brackets are welded or soldered to the bands to provide the type of force or anchorage required by the design. Custom fits are generally made by the "pinch band technique," where a roll of band material is fitted around a tooth and the ends pinched together with a pair of Howe pliers. The metal is welded at the pinch, the loose ends trimmed, folded over, and welded, thus forming a band.

19.16.5 Base Plates

Base plates are the foundation that provide a surface for direct bonding to the tooth surface. Various brackets and tubes can be attached to the base plate to provide anchorage or movement sites. Base plates typically have a wire mesh or patterned imprint on the side facing the tooth, which allows for greater adherence by the cement. Base plates can be made from plastics, ceramics, or metals. Metals provide the greatest strength, but plastics and ceramics give a better cosmetic appearance during treatment.

19.16.6 Brackets and Tubes

Orthodontics brackets and tubes are devices that are attached to base plates or bands and provide attachment for wires, springs, and elastics. Tubes can be round or rectangular according to the needs of the appliance. There is a wide variety of brackets available: slotted, cleats, hooks, and buttons. Buttons are currently the most widely used bracket in veterinary orthodontics.

19.16.7 Elastics

Many forms of orthodontic elastics are available. These are used as the source of force for many appliances. Gum rubber and elastomeric plastics deteriorate in the mouth, losing elasticity, while latex elastics have a longer useful performance [34]. Generally, four forms are in common use: rings, ligatures, tubes, and chains. Elastic rings, which come in various sizes and strengths, can be used as the actual force, but are also used as the attachment for removable appliances. Ligatures are strings of elastic that come in various sizes, which affects their strength. Elastic tubes are a form of hollow elastic ligature. The tubes have greater strength than the ligature, but a shorter stretch distance and are more bulky. Chains are flattened elastics with an arrangement of holes to allow their attachment to buttons or similar brackets. The spacing of the holes comes in three patterns: long filament, short filament, and continuous filament. The continuous filament is the most practical in veterinary work. "K" modules are individual filaments with only two attachment sites, which provide a continual gentle force for long periods of time.

19.16.8 Acrylics

Orthodontic acrylics are used to form a framework or base structure from which various inclines, springs, arch wires, or expansion devices can be attached. Most are made from heat-cured acrylics in laboratories, but many are made with cold-cure acrylics in the clinic by the operator. Direct construction in-house in the animal's mouth requires good ventilation and a slow application to minimize exothermic heat that can build up when forming. Its advantages are that it does not require a second anesthesia for installation and treatment can be initiated more quickly.

19.16.9 Expansion and Contraction Devices

Expansion and contraction screw devices are most commonly used for intermittent movement pressures. They are available in a variety of types designed for single or multiple tooth movements. The normal expansion screw operates by the use of a small wire key that, when used to turn the central screw properly, separates the halves of the unit. With screws, the limiting factor is the adjustment. Most are designed to provide 0.18–0.20 mm of movement per quarter turn. Most periodontal membrane spaces are between 0.15 and 0.30 mm, with the smaller space seen in smaller breeds and older animals. Typically younger animals have a larger PDL space due to eruptive demands. Therefore application of force should be calculated to no more than 65% of the PDL space to aid in prevention of pathologic injury to the periodontium or tooth. Excess pressure on a palatal expansion device could cause a midline sutural opening. The piston screw is for the movement of a single tooth and, when advanced, has a spring that can maintain a continuous pressure for a movement up to 0.5 mm before requiring readjustment. It is activated with the use of a miniature screwdriver. Specific instructions must be given to owners so that adjustments are made in the correct direction.

19.16.10 Incline Planes

Incline planes (IP) are appliances designed to make contact with the cusps or incisal edges of the teeth of the opposing occlusion to stimulate tooth movement. Inclines have no active movement device, but rather rely upon the muscles of mastication to provide the movement force. When the incline is designed to prevent occlusal closure it is called a bite plane. When the incline covers a tooth it is known as incline capping. Half capping is when the lingual and occlusal surface of the tooth is covered, but if the coverage extends over to the facial surface it is known as full incline capping. Incline planes can be made as removable or fixed appliances and consist of acrylics or cast metals. When making use of fixed incline planes one major consideration is allowance for growth. The Mann incline plane is a cast fixed appliance that is anchored to the maxillary canine teeth with a telescoping support bar between the two, which allows for skeletal growth. It has one or two spoon-shaped incline planes that engage the mandibular canines to move them labially [36]. Crown extensions of composite built directly on to the mandibular canines are also a form of incline plane.

19.17 Conditions Treatable by Orthodontics

When considering an appliance, there are certain things that can help guide the clinician. First, select or design the appliance to achieve the desired results in the simplest manner, as complex appliances have complex flaws. The pattern of the appliance should fit the patient with reasonable comfort, by insuring a proper fit. Refrain from overextending the appliance coverage, which may irritate the periodontium. Avoid occlusal interference, except in incline planes where it should be the minimum necessary. Custom fit brackets and bands for best comfort and adhesion. Always check to make sure brackets and arch wires will be at the level most appropriate for treatment. Select the designs that best accomplish the movements, but always take into consideration hygiene and ease of cleaning for the owner. Do not attempt too many movements simultaneously, but rather stage the treatment. The appliance should be as versatile as possible, so that as many stages as possible can be accomplished with it.

19.17.1 Class I Malocclusions – Individual Tooth or Teeth

19.17.1.1 Rotation or Torsion Movements

Rotation or torsion movements are when the tooth is rotated on its long axis in one direction or the other. It is most commonly encountered in incisors and premolars. The simplest approach to treatment is the use of button brackets and elastic chains. Attach the movement brackets to the facially deviated portion of the facial surface and the most lingually deviated part of the lingual surface of the tooth. One to two simple anchorage brackets should be placed mesially and distally as dictated by root surfaces. The anchor bracket should be placed on the facial or lingual surface towards which the mesial or distal surfaces of the tooth are to be rotated, customarily opposite the movement bracket. Once the appliance is in place, tighten the elastic chain only one notch to begin with. Allow the tooth to move to the point at which the stretch of the elastic is lost. Then tighten one notch again, repeating the process until the tooth has properly rotated. In this type of movement all of the PDL fibers and the gingival collar are stretched in the same spiral direction around the tooth, making recoil a possible problem.

19.17.1.2 Teeth with Infraversion

Teeth with infraversion are those in which their crowns have failed to completely erupt, and are frequently either ankylosed or impacted. The first step is to determine the status of the root structure. If the root apex is still vital and open, and the impaction cause is relieved, the tooth may continue to erupt on its own [37]. If the apex is closed, it is most likely that extrusion orthodontics will be required. When teeth are ankylosed there is an area of root cementum and alveolar bone that has fused, which must be relieved prior to extrusion orthodontics, if attempted at all. If the impaction is soft tissue, it should be excised. If the impaction is of a bony nature, then soft tissue and bone must both be resectioned. Once the crown tip is exposed a bracket can be attached to attempt orthodontic movement, with other buttons on the adjacent or opposing teeth for sufficient reinforced anchorage. Extrusion typically goes quickly once the impaction cause is relieved, but some precautions should be taken (see Extrusion Movements).

19.17.1.3 Rostral Crossbites

Rostral crossbites are conditions where one or more incisors are in version to their counterparts in the opposing jaws. Ordinarily, tipping movements will be used to correct the condition. There are three basic things that must be examined for: crowding, open bite, and whether the incisal version or inclination is in the maxillary or mandibular teeth. If crowding or embrication is a problem, either odontoplasty (stripping) to reduce the tooth size or selective interceptive extractions may be required to make room. When moving teeth facially, a natural expansion of the arch normally occurs, which may correct the spacing problem. Odontoplastic stripping is the process of reducing the interproximal contacts, using various abrasives strips or thin fluted burs. Stripping reduces the mesiodistal width of the teeth, thus reducing the space required for alignment. It also flattens the interproximal contacts, making that area of the arch more stable.

Next, observe the rostral occlusion closely for partial open bites. It is not uncommon to find that the maxillary incisors will not cover the mandibular teeth when the mouth is closed and a small freeway space between the maxillary and mandibular teeth exists. If there is a partial rostral open bite, then correction will require not only facial or lingual movement but also extrusion to obtain a bite that will not recoil. Lastly, try to determine whether the principle problem is linguoversion of maxillary incisors or labioversion of the mandibular.

For the mandibular labioversion, the general appliances used are elastic ligature ties (for a simple single incisor movement), maxillary incisal capping incline planes (blocks the bite open), and mandibular brackets and elastic chains to move the mandibular incisors lingually and back into a scissors bite. Buttons can be bonded to all mandibular incisors on the cervical third of the crown to avoid the possibility of occlusal trauma from the maxillary incisors. This is less favorable from a leverage standpoint, so appropriate anchorage (rostral on the canines or caudal on the fourth premolars and first molars) is critical. The rostral anchor on the canines can force them to tip lingually or may not provide enough room if the third incisors need significant lingual movement. In this case, the elastic can be brought interproximally between the incisor and canine, around the lingual and distal aspects of the canine, and then attaching to the bracket.

For the linguoversion of the maxillary incisors the appliances most commonly used are elastic ligature ties, lingual maxillary arch bar with kick springs, mandibular incisal incline plane, maxillary expansion screw appliance, and labial maxillary arch bar with elastics. The labial maxillary arch bar (telescoping for young patients) and elastics can also provide extruding movements if the bite is open [35]. The arch bar is anchored to full or partial bands around the canine teeth, with small buttons or hooks at intervals to apply individual elastics to the buttons (lingual) on the maxillary incisors. A lingual maxillary arch bar incorporates canine bands that are lightly cemented (allows for regular adjustment) and one or more kick springs aligned to press the selected incisors facially. The springs can be bent out of shape with inappropriate chewing habits, and in growing patients, the appliance should be telescoping or more flexible to allow for growth. Maxillary expansion screw appliances, made of either acrylic or metal, also apply force to the palatal surfaces of the maxillary incisors, using a screw device that is adjusted to move the rostral portion of the device forward.

19.17.1.4 Caudal Crossbites

Caudal crossbites can be seen in almost any breed, though the Collie appears to be the most commonly affected breed. If caught in a deciduous occlusion, interceptive orthodontics should be instigated and the inclined teeth extracted, in the hope that the permanent teeth will not follow suit. In most cases presented in permanent occlusion, if the bite is functional, no treatment should be undertaken, unless individual teeth are damaged [38]. In cases of bite interference where the occlusion is being forced into an abnormal position, preventive orthodontics should be undertaken with selective extraction of the teeth causing the most disruption. Should corrective orthodontics be undertaken, an inclined bite plane will be required to block the bite open to allow the teeth to pass each other during treatment. An expansion screw appliance can be used on the maxillary fourth premolar to force the tooth buccally, while a lingual arch bar with elastics or a similar device will be required to pull the mandibular molar lingually. The bite will be required to be held open for two to three weeks during this movement. Corrective treatment should be discouraged as many problems may arise from treatment, as the open bite can allow teeth to drift or supererupt, problems with the TMJ may arise, and the mastication interference can require special dietary care.

19.17.1.5 Linguoversion Mandibular Canines

The linguoversion of mandibular canine teeth (base narrow) can be handled in many ways according to the location of the tooth in relationship to the maxillary teeth. With Class I occlusions the base of the tooth is in a normal mesiodistal relationship. Those that are involved with mesiodistal discrepancies, especially of the jaw, may be classified as Class II, III, or IV malocclusions, and are discussed under those categories. Any attempts at movement require adequate space in the diastema between the mandibular third incisors and canines in order to be successful, unless final mandibular tooth position will be in occlusion distal to the maxillary canine (some Class II patients)

When caught early in deciduous dentitions, interceptive orthodontics may be performed. Early management of uncomplicated cases with permanent teeth (sufficient diastema, no jaw length discrepancies) may include the use of a round or oval hard rubber device (ball) and training the dog to play with it for 15 minutes three times daily. The device should sit in between and just behind the canines, just larger than the distance between them. Twenty-six out of thirty-eight dogs corrected in 2–12 weeks, with the more complicated cases needing additional therapy [39].

In very mild cases, where the mandibular canine only lightly impales the maxillary diastema gingival margin, preventive orthodontics of a simple gingivoplasty may correct the problem [40]. The gingiva is beveled with a diamond point or fluted bur to a depth that obliterates any impression in the gingival margin, in an hour-glass configuration. Tissue hemorrhage can be controlled with a gingival hemostatic solution and then coated with Tincture of Myrrh and Benzoin. This should move the tip of the tooth free of gingival cusp impaction, and the natural incline plane will help to continue the tooth's movement labially.

If the diastemal space is insufficient, or the mandibular canine occludes with the maxillary third incisor, odontoplasty of the distal edge of the incisor, or even extraction of the incisor, may provide the space that is needed for a more comfortable occlusion. With incisor extraction, the alveolar margin can also be contoured (osteoplasty) to accommodate the mandibular canine crown [40].

Corrective orthodontic treatments may involve any one of several types of appliances. Expansion screws and

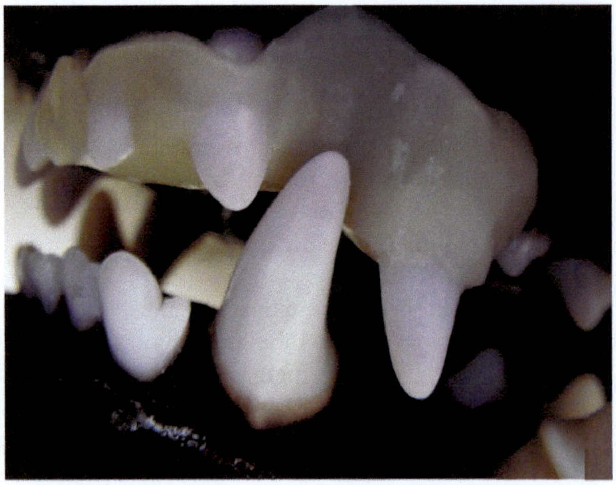

Figure 19.6 Palatal composite incline plane to treat the linguoversion of mandibular canine with sufficient diastemal space.

W-springs that apply pressure to the lingual surfaces of the mandibular canines may result in bodily movement, or even a spreading of the mandibular symphysis.

Palatal incline planes can be cast metal appliances that are inserted, or directly applied devices constructed of acrylic or composite (Figure 19.6). The target locations of incline of the crest are the points at which the mandibular canine teeth make initial contact with the device. This should be the highest point of the incline, with a sloping angle of approximately 60° toward its target site (diastema). If uncertain as to the exact incline crestal target locations, articulation or carbon paper can be placed on the acrylic base and the occlusion closed and the canines tapped against the paper to place marks on the base indicating their position. Once cured, an acrylic white stone or a laboratory acrylic bur can be used to refine the incline's path. The incline can be smoothed with an unfilled resin or polished with pumice and water. The appliance can also be initially formed in the mouth, removed, and adjusted outside the mouth, then bonded to the teeth [41]. Concerns for continued maxillary growth can be accommodated by fabricating two separate devices [42–44], incorporating a telescoping device between the two sides [45] or having a metal telescoping device fabricated.

An incline plane may also be fabricated as a crown extension of the mandibular canines, for movements of short distances and small angles (maximum 20°). Placement of a temporary composite to extend the height of the crown (bilaterally), with a deliberate slant to the extension to allow it to occlude lateral to the maxillary gingival margin, provides forces to tip the teeth into the correct position (Figure 19.7a to c). Once the teeth are in place, the composite extensions can be removed and the tooth positioning will provide its own retention. In a reported case of a cat with persistent linguoversion after deciduous canine extraction and attempts at crown extenders, the use of thermoplastic aligners (five incremental removal IPs) provided success [46].

Extraction or crown reduction of the mandibular canine may be performed if orthodontic therapy is declined or discouraged [47] (Figure 19.8a and b). Any goal should result in a patient that now has a comfortable bite. Any teeth that have been damaged extensively by an undiscovered malocclusion may also need extraction.

19.17.1.6 Rostromesial Inclination of Maxillary Canine Teeth

Rostromesial inclination of maxillary canine teeth is most commonly seen in the Shetland Sheep Dog. The simplest approach to treatment is with bonded brackets and elastic chains. The number and placement of the brackets and initial tension of the elastic chain are very important for reasonable results with diminished possibility of complications. The maxillary fourth premolar and first molar can be used for anchorage, with the anchorage brackets placed on the buccal surface near the cervical third of the crowns. Use of acrylic or twisted wire to connect the two brackets/buttons provides a single anchorage unit. Careful placement of a figure-of-eight 24 gauge wire looped around the fourth premolar and molar can be covered with acrylic and twisted at the mesial aspect to make a hook for placement of the elastic chain [47].

The location of the attachment of the movement brackets on the maxillary canine should be on the labial surface at the middle to coronal thirds of the tooth, with a slight mesial shift to prevent ease of chain loss due to slippage. If the canine is crowded against the corner incisor preventing placement of the bracket at the desired location, either the initial bracket can be placed lingually until the tooth clears the incisor, a slight gingivoplasty performed, or a dental wedge can be gently forced between the two teeth to allow space for placement. Alternate placement of a twisted wire placed on the coronal aspect of the crown with a hook formed at its distal aspect provides a direct caudal force without rotation [47]. Use of a composite "snowman" shaped knob on the coronal aspect of the canine can decrease the amount of force that needs to be applied for movement [48] (Figure 19.9). Applying a composite incline plane to the mesial aspect of the palatal canine tooth (but not attached to the third incisor to prevent it acting as an anchor) can begin lateral movement of the mandibular canine once the diastema is wide enough to accept it [49] (Figure 19.10).

The elastic chain is then applied. For an initial period of a week to 10 days, the chain should be tightened lightly to stimulate physiologic movement. As the tooth begins movement, up to adjustments of 80–75% of the masel chain length can be applied, but excessive traction should not be attempted. Once the tooth reaches the desired position the elastic chain can be loosened so that it holds

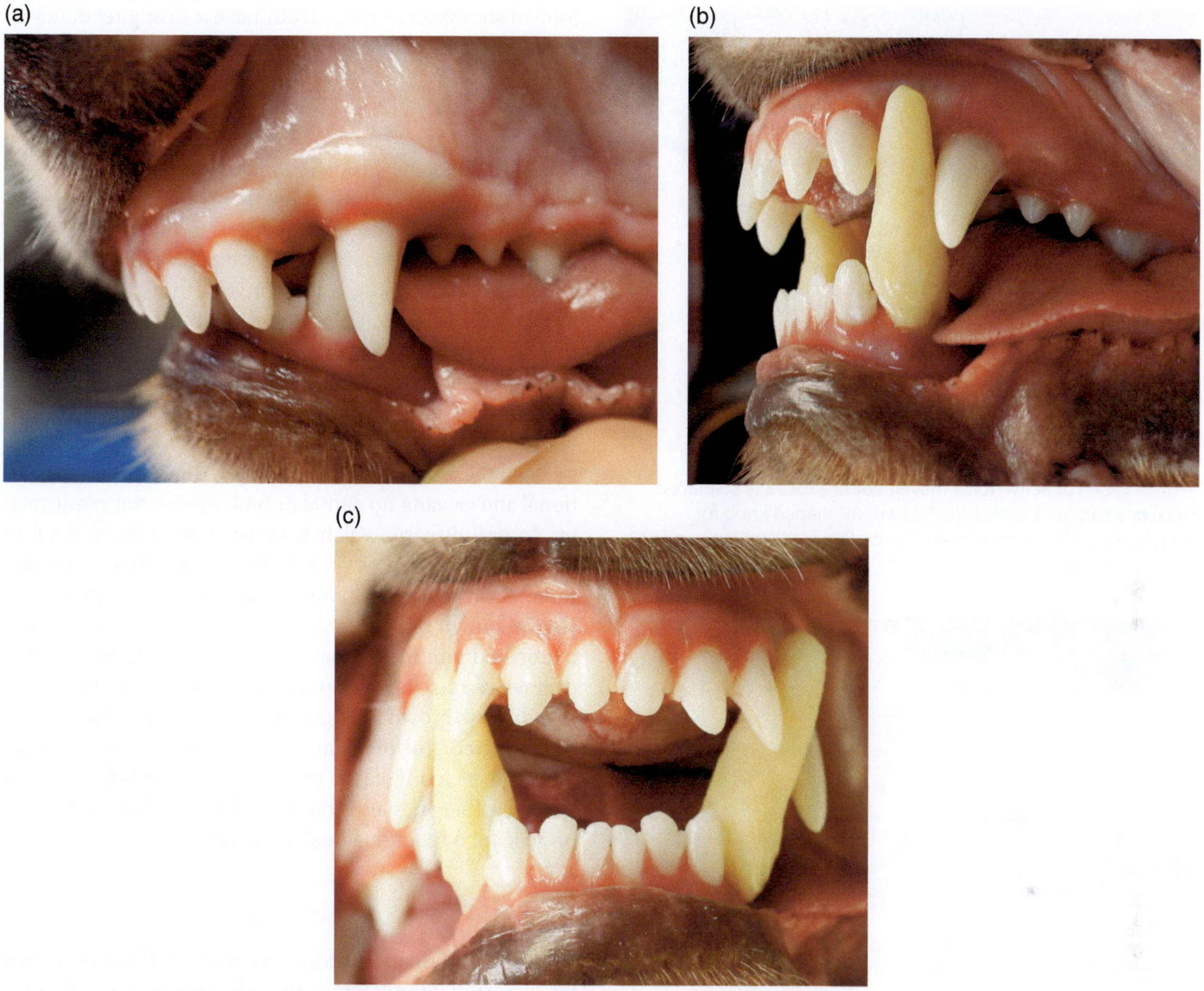

Figure 19.7 (a) Dog with slight Class 2 malocclusion and resultant linguoversion of mandibular canines; (b) composite crown extensions are built on the mandibular canines to tip the teeth mesially and then buccally to reposition them to occlude into the maxillary diastema; (c) rostral view of bilateral crown extensions (incline planes).

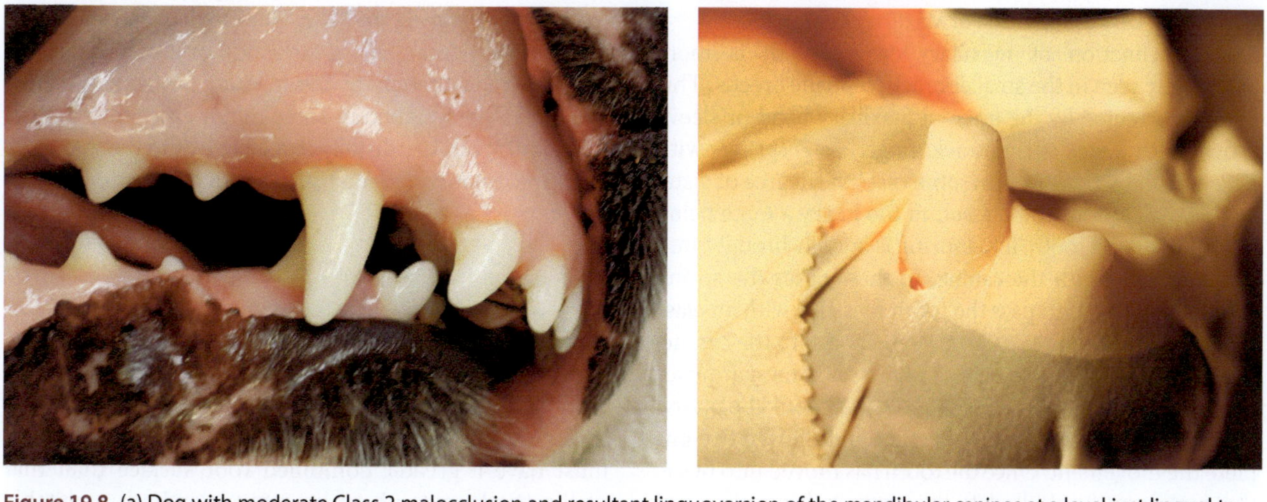

Figure 19.8 (a) Dog with moderate Class 2 malocclusion and resultant linguoversion of the mandibular canines at a level just lingual to the maxillary canines; (b) crown reduction and vital pulp therapy was elected in place of orthodontic movement.

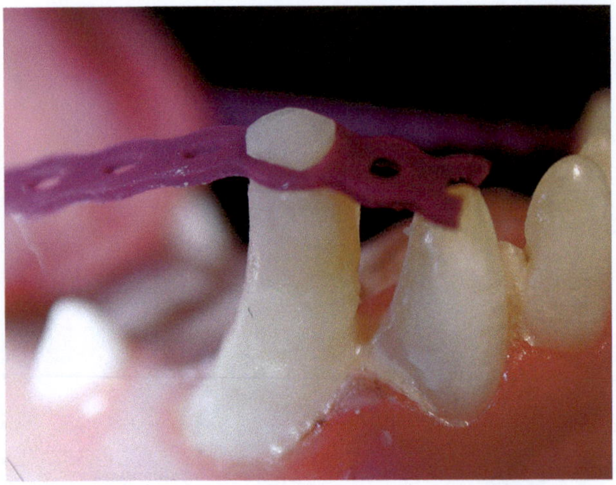

Figure 19.9 For active force movement of a rostrally displaced maxillary canine, a composite "snowman" shaped knob for attachment of the elastic chain. *Source:* Reprinted with permission from reference [48].

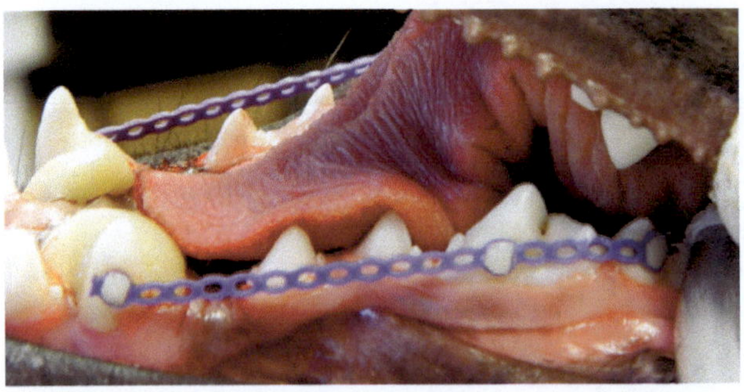

Figure 19.10 Composite buttons and elastic chain have been applied to the 104, 108, and 109 teeth. An inclined plane has been created on teeth 104 (not 103). *Source:* Reprinted with permission from reference [49].

the tooth in place during the retention period, or a wire can be placed [50].

19.17.1.7 Distal Inclination of Maxillary Canine Teeth

Distal inclination of maxillary canine teeth is more commonly seen in the smaller brachycephalic breeds. This can be corrected by the use of a maxillary band or sleeve crown with a kick spring. Kick, finger, or Z springs with helixes usually work well. In some cases the degree of distal canine inclination would result in too heavy a force being placed upon the tooth, if the spring is initially brought into direct contact with the canine. In these cases the spring should be allowed to pass the tooth mesially, with an elastic ligature tied to the spring stretched back to the canine, tightened, and tied in a square knot. Once mesial movement is sufficient, the kick spring contact should be placed against the distal surface of the canine and allowed to complete the movement. Once the tooth has moved into place, the appliance should be left as a retainer for a period of four to six weeks as these teeth have a strong tendency to recoil towards their original position.

19.17.2 Class II Malocclusions

True Class II malocclusions cannot be corrected completely with orthodontics, since there is an underlying skeletal anomaly. Only orofacial surgery can properly contend with these conditions. In young animals with a deciduous Class II malocclusion, interceptive orthodontics may be attempted. However, corrective and preventive orthodontics can be performed to make the permanent occlusion functional and comfortable. There are cases with linguodistal mandibular canine malocclusion in which the mandibular canine teeth are not only base narrow or lingually inclined but also positioned distally. If the occlusion is functional and causing no dental or oral trauma, nor predisposing to oral disease, which is unusual, there is no need to consider corrective or preventive orthodontics. There are three basic treatment options: preventive extraction, preventive crown reduction and vital pulp therapy, or corrective orthodontic incline planes. Extraction of the mandibular canines results in a generalized weakening of the rostral mandible, so crown reduction with vital pulp therapy would be preferred. Incline planes (crown extensions) can be designed in many cases to pass the mandibular canines labially, either mesial or distal to the maxillary canines, to provide for a functional malocclusion.

19.17.3 Class III Malocclusions

True Class III malocclusions, like those of Class II, cannot be corrected completely with orthodontics, since there is an underlying skeletal anomaly. In young animals with a deciduous Class III malocclusion, interceptive orthodontics may be attempted. With a mesiolingual mandibular canine malocclusion (base narrow), extraction of the maxillary corner incisors will sometimes provide space for the mandibular canines, and is a more logical and medically sound therapy than either extraction or crown reduction and vital pulp therapy of the mandibular canine. Incline planes can be designed in some minor cases to move the mandibular canines distally and labially into the maxillary diastema, to provide for a functional malocclusion.

19.18 Band and Bracket Placement and Cementation

19.18.1 Site Selection

The tooth or combination of teeth used for the anchor must have a greater combined root surface than that of the tooth or teeth to be moved, or have a suitable leverage advantage (see Table 19.2). Sites selected on the tooth must be located so that the appliance does not obstruct normal occlusion. The position of the bracket on the tooth, apically or coronally, can provide additional leverage for movement. Generally, for a mechanical anchorage advantage, the anchorage tooth site should be near the cervical third of the tooth, and on the movement tooth at the mid to coronal thirds of the crown.

19.18.2 Selection of Brackets and Custom Fitting

The design of the appliance determines the type of brackets that will be required. Ordinarily button-type brackets use elastic chains and slotted brackets are used for arch bars. Selection is based upon the available surface space and the tooth contour at the selected site. There are plastic, ceramic, and metal brackets available. For use in animals, the more durable metal brackets are generally preferred. The base plates of the various direct bond brackets differ greatly in size and shape, with a rough imprinted surface or a wire mesh that allows the cement to attach to the bracket. If a bracket does not fit the tooth well, it can be reduced by using a diamond point on a high-speed handpiece. The base plate can be curved with a three-prong bending pliers to better fit the tooth. The bracket is then placed against the site for placement and using Howe pliers to press it against the tooth, removing unneeded curvature and providing a good customized adaption. Custom brackets can also be made with resin cements and a button template that forms the button as it is being attached to the tooth.

19.18.3 Acid Etching the Tooth

After scaling, using flour pumice to polish the teeth and drying with oil-free air, a 37% phosphoric acid solution or gel applied to the selected tooth site is customarily used to etch the enamel for about 20 seconds. If dentin requires etching, the 37% phosphoric acid can be used for 10 seconds or a 10% concentration for 15 seconds. Acid etching lightly roughens the tooth surface, allowing bonding agents, unfilled resins, and other cements to slightly penetrate the enamel or dentin and micromechanically attach. The etched tooth surface should have a chalky appearance.

19.18.4 Selection of Bonding Adhesive (See Chapter 17 – Restorative Dentistry)

For direct bond-type brackets, composite resin adhesives (light-activated filled acrylic–bisphenol A glycidyl methacrylate (bis-GMA)) are commonly used [50]. Newer self-adhesive resin cements with a self-etch primer or self-adhesive component require less preparation, but may not have as much bond strength as those with metal brackets [51]. Glass ionomer products provide fluoride release, but have less strength. Light cured products can be used on any type of bracket or band, but work best with the plastic and ceramic brackets that are clear and allow the light to penetrate well under the bracket. When using light cured adhesives on metal brackets or bands, the cement may not be fully cured under the brackets, although a proper technique can offset much of this problem. Apply the curing light source at angles that allow it to penetrate under the edges of the band or bracket and use a good-quality light cure unit. The light cure bonding agent's advantages in time and placement easily outweigh their shortcomings.

19.18.5 Application of Direct Bond Bracket to Tooth

The technique of application is to center the bracket and apply with firm gentle pressure until setting is complete. College cotton pliers or direct bond bracket pliers are routinely used to hold and place the bracket on the tooth. Bracket pliers are spring-loaded to keep a firm hold of the bracket until squeezed to release the bracket. Cotton pliers require gentle pressure to keep a hold on the bracket at all times. Should a bracket fail to attach properly, discard it.

19.18.6 Application of Cement to Bands

With bands, clean thoroughly by scaling and polishing with flour of pumice. Then repeat the entire procedure from the first step, being sure to remove all of the old cement from the tooth. Bands can be cemented by two techniques. The first is placement of the cement to the entire inner surface of the band, prior to placement. This allows the greatest security for the band. The second technique is to apply the cement after band seating, and only to a portion of the tooth just coronal to the band to hold its seating firm.

19.19 Advances in Orthodontic Therapy

In the human orthodontic field, tremendous advances have been introduced and implemented, to provide accelerated and enhanced therapy, often using dog models. Even the use of transparent, incremental aligners has been applied to the veterinary field [46]. The use of implant screws have evolved from larger implants (limited to retromolar or edentulous sites) to miniscrews, even bioabsorbable ones [52] that can be anchored on the palate, preferably in the midsagittal region [53, 54]. Considerations include the potential for bone damage, which is related to the type of device used and thickness of the cortical bone; self-drilling miniscrews implanted in the mandibular bone can be more damaging [55]. Oral hygiene must be rigorous with such implants to minimize tissue reactions and enhance the biointegration of these orthodontically loaded implants [56].

Cortical activation in dog models has been studied with both alveolar corticotomy (shallow horizontal cut line below the apices with two vertical cut lines – mesial and distal – from the alveolar margin to the horizontal line) and a grid of shallow indentations made 3 mm apart with a no. 2 round bur [57, 58]. A regional acceleratory phenomenon (RAP) with increased cellular activity (osteoclasts, fibroblasts, cementoblasts, and osteoblasts) brought about by local multicellular mediator mechanisms accelerates bone turnover, thus increasing the speed of remodeling and initial OTM. Combining selective alveolar coritcotomy and the placement of bone grafting material has been described as periodontal accelerated osteogenic orthodontics (PAOO) [59]. While the rapid alveolar bone reaction may decrease PDL hyalinization [57], a severe decrease in cellular activity six months after orthodontic therapy may also be seen [58]. Rapid tooth movement can also be accomplished with PDL distraction at the site of an extraction, making cuts in the interseptal bone with heavy forces provided by a spring [60, 61]. Applications of vibration, ultrasound, phototherapy, and photoradiation have been studied for their effects on OTM. In one study, a specific level of photoradiation may accelerate movement, while a higher dosage may decrease it [62].

19.20 Home Care Instructions

The success of an orthodontic treatment depends on supervision and care at home, as well as professional care. The appliance should be examined two to three times daily and kept clean by gently flushing it with water or oral solutions. Entangled hair or fibers should be carefully removed to avoid removing an elastic or bracket. A soft diet should be fed for the duration of the appliance and chewing devices should be avoided. Any ulceration or inflammation should be brought to the clinic's attention and regular visits for examination and adjustments are essential.

19.21 Retention Period and Retainers

Once active movement has accomplished the desired tooth movements, it is necessary to retain the teeth in their new location. The alveolar bone, gingival tissues, and PDL have been undergoing remodeling and reorganization during tooth movement. For the tooth to stabilize, the bone must transform into firm compact bone, the gingivae reorganize, and the PDL must tighten. If the teeth are not retained during this transitional period they may partially recoil or totally return to their original position. Retainers can be fixed or removable. To conserve time, materials, and anesthetics, in veterinary orthodontics it is common to let the primary corrective appliance also act as the retainer. This approach allows for a quick response by reactivation of the appliance should recoil commence. In simple movements a retainer time of two to six weeks is required. In more complex movements and those involving the torsiversion, 4–12 weeks is recommended. Occasionally, the actual scissor bite or canine interlock of the occlusion may act as a natural self-retainer. Successful retention depends upon correct diagnosis and treatment. Teeth moved to a non-harmonious position usually cannot be stabilized. While reorganization of the PDL can occur over a three to four month period, gingival fibers take longer, and can exert forces for up to a year [30]. Therefore, retention followed by an observation period is highly recommended.

19.22 Appliance Removal

Proper removal of an appliance is an intricate component in the successful final results of orthodontic treatment. A crude removal technique can result in enamel fractures and scarification. Failure to remove cements and polish the surface can easily result in plaque accumulation and possible gingivitis. If the surface appears porous, it should be sealed by bonding with an unfilled resin to help prevent discoloration from mineral absorption.

Many metal matrix sheet bands can be removed by using an ultrasonic scaler across its surface to loosen the cement, then using the tip of a scaler to hook the cervical line of the band and lift up. Others may require the use of band removal pliers. The cushioned beak is placed on the cusp and the other beak is positioned under the cervical margin of the band. The handles are then gently squeezed together.

On cast metal bands, a more aggressive approach may be needed. A crown puller may need to be used on the cervical line of the band. If excess cement is present around the band it can be removed by using a white stone point on a high-speed handpiece. Additionally, the bands may need to be cut. A cross-cut bur used carefully along the lingual surface of the band to cut it from the cervical to coronal margin can be useful. A crown splitter or small screwdriver inserted into the slot cut into the band and then rotated slightly will usually separate the band and break loose the cementation. Always make the cut on the lingual surface of the band in case damage occurs.

Brackets are usually not difficult to remove. A scaling bur or white stone can be used to remove excess cement. Band removal pliers can be used with the cushioned beak placed upon the cusp and the other beak under the cervical area of the brackets base plate, and a gentle squeeze will remove most of the cement. Additionally, needle holders can be used to grasp the bracket and then gently rotate back and forth to break the cementation. Always use a gentle force, as rapid or uncontrolled movements may fracture the enamel.

Once the appliance is removed, carefully remove all remaining cement with a scaler. Any hard to remove material may require the use of a white stone point. Inspect the oral cavity for signs of injury to the teeth or soft tissues, and treat as required. Polish the tooth with an extra-fine prophy paste and apply a fluoride treatment.

19.23 Complications from Treatment

Deleterious effects can come from an orthodontic force in four principal areas: crestal alveolar bone, root structure, PDL and alveolar attachment, and pulp. Other problems are tooth discoloration, appliance soft tissue trauma, hygiene problems, contact allergy, and elastic slippage.

Remodeling of the crestal alveolar bone as well as the rest of the alveolar bone occurs during orthodontic movement. Orthodontic movements and hygiene problems associated with appliances can contribute toward gingival inflammation, which can affect crestal bone loss. In humans, typically a slight loss of less than a 0.5 mm is seen, with loss greater than 1.0 mm being rare [63, 64]. Luckily, alveolar bone will ordinarily "travel" with the tooth, except in certain disease states, such as in cases with uncontrolled active periodontal disease. However, even patients with periodontal disease can have orthodontics, if the active disease is under control and sufficient alveolar bone is still present to stabilize the tooth following movement.

When teeth are extruded in a physiologic movement, the alveolar bone will travel with the tooth. This results in the alveolar crest height being higher in the arch following treatment, but still approximately the same in relationship to the tooth. Conversely, teeth that are intruded have a loss of alveolar height in the arch [65].

Tooth movement is only possible due to PDL activity in resorption and apposition of adjacent hard tissues, primarily the alveolar bone. However, the remodeling of hard tissues initiated by the PDL does include some to the root structures that are also contiguous with the PDL. The root cementum repairs itself during periods of quiescence of force. Areas of dentinal exposure may also undergo resorption, but repairs are also with cementum, not dentin [15]. This means root remodeling is a constant feature of active corrective orthodontics [66], but that permanent loss of root structure only occurs when cementum is not replaced. If the resorption is limited to the cementum, some degree of repair with deposition of new cementum is possible, but once the dentin is affected, it is irreversible, though it can be repaired with cementum deposition. Root structure is also affected during orthodontic treatment.

The term RR (root resorption) is used for more generalized regions, typically lateral or coronal areas, depending on the external force direction. RR can be seen in other situations as well. External apical root resorption (EARR), a permanent blunting of the apical region, may be due to the location of the center of rotation (CRot) near the apical one-third of the root [67]. When there is an excessive mechanical loading of an area and possible PDL compression [68], there will be a decrease in the bone formation rate (BFR), necessary for remodeling the alveolar bone, and increased bone resorption [66]. This can expose the root to excessive flexure, resulting in fatigue failure on the root.

The direction of force plays a role, as tipping causes periodontal peak stresses that may be three time greater than that seen in translation [69], and intrusion is associated with four times the incidence of RR than extrusion, particular in the apices and interradicular areas of multirooted teeth [70]. While there is more variation in results seen when comparing levels of force stress magnitude, many studies showed no statistical correlation with heavier forces [68, 70]. The duration of treatment more consistently shows a correlation with an increase in RR, as does the force regimen (continuous forces can cause more severe RR than intermittent forces) [68, 70] and the distance of tooth movement. One aspect has been shown to be a major factor in the occurrence of severe resorption, and this is root contact with cortical bone [71]. This most commonly occurs in cases of orthodontic camouflage treatment of mild Class II or III malocclusion. In these cases, teeth are tilted or rotated to an angle that may force root structure to make contact with the cortical plates [71]. There appears to be no increase in susceptibility to RR in teeth that have been endodontically treated [72, 73].

The only real consistency in reviewing many studies was the wide range of individual responses, including patients with low calcium levels [70]. In human studies, the presence of RR typically has low clinical significance for the patient, except in cases with short root structure, where the changes can have an impact [69, 74].

The PDL is not only responsible for alveolar remodeling but also for its own reorganization during orthodontic treatment [15]. The reorganization is necessary for the ligament to detach from the cementum or alveolar bone during movement, and then to reattach later at more harmonious locations. The PDL space widens during orthodontic movement due to resorptive activity, which can be seen in many cases radiographically. This in combination with the reorganization of the PDL itself results in a degree of tooth mobility during tooth movements. Excessive mobility is typically an indication of the use of excessive force for movement. When teeth begin to demonstrate signs of excessive mobility, all force should be removed and oral hygiene intensified until the teeth once again become stable.

The use of heavy force should be avoided if at all possible due to the possible complications. Pain during movement with this level of force is common as a result of ischemia to the PDL and pressures on the apical structures causing a pulpitis. The pain often does not occur until several hours following application of the excessive force. Should an owner call concerning a patient with signs of this type, instructions to relieve the force if possible should be given. If the appliance is such that the owner cannot disconnect the force, temporary relief may be obtained by massaging the affected teeth, which alleviates some of the pressure and allows some blood flow to the ischemic areas.

The use of corticosteroids and non-steroidal anti-inflammatory drugs (NSAIDs) help to moderate pain and inflammation by interfering with the synthesis of prostaglandins, a major participant in the development of inflammation. Corticosteroids affect this synthesis by helping to inhibit development of the prostaglandin precursor arachidonic acid. The NSAIDs work by blocking some degree of the conversion of arachidonic acid to prostaglandins, but seldom are these anti-inflammatory medications used in high enough dosages to prevent tooth movement. Bisphosphonates should be discontinued three months prior to orthodontic for optimal movement, and the rare association with its use and necrotic mandibular bone should not be an issue [15].

The ischemic episodes in the PDL can have other serious consequences. These ischemic areas may cause necrosis, leaving cementum and alveolar bone in intimate contact. This may result in ankylosis of the root and the inability to move the tooth orthodontically. In addition, the ankylosed areas may eventually undergo inflammatory resorption [75].

The pulp, under normal circumstances, should have only minimal response to light orthodontic forces. There is a transient reversible pulpitis at the initiation of treatment. This is probably due to the early response to pressures on the apical vascular and nervous supply. This response possibly contributes to the discomfort occasionally seen following activation or reactivation of the appliance, but has no long-term significance. In a review of human literature, an association between orthodontic forces and damage to the pulp has not been validated, though teeth that have undergone recent trauma may be at a higher risk for pulpitis or pulpal damage during orthodontic therapy [72, 76]. A vital pulp is not required for orthodontic movement; therefore endodontically treated teeth can be moved as long as a healthy PDL is present [72, 73].

Tooth discoloration can be caused by metal impregnation and devitalization, though devitalization is uncommon with appropriate use of forces. Metal impregnation is a result of metal ionization from the base plate or band on the tooth and its penetration into the tooth, particularly on diseased tooth surfaces [77]. Orthodontic adhesive systems, particularly etch-and-rinse and self-etch systems, can leave residual resins that irreversibly penetrate the surface, sometimes along with pigments from foods [77]. Resin-modified glass ionomer cements (RMGICs) are less likely to leave discoloration and composite burs are less likely to cause surface roughening and microscopic fractures, as compared to 12-fluted carbide burs [78].

Appliance trauma can occur from many causes. Brackets may cause physical irritation to the lingual and buccal mucosa. This can be controlled by covering them with a small amount of a rubber base impression material. Lacerations by elastics either must be endured or the elastics removed and the appliance readapted to prevent interference.

Hygiene is an owner/patient responsibility. When materials accumulate near the gingiva margins, gingivitis is sure to follow. If materials are allowed to collect under appliance bases covering the palate, a palatitis will result, which can sometimes be severe. On occasion, actual contact allergies to the materials from which the appliance is constructed may occur. In these cases the appliance must either be removed and then designed with new materials or anti-inflammatory medications started, which may impede orthodontic movements.

Elastic slippage is a problem that must be carefully monitored. Simple slippage should be corrected by either movement of the elastic or a new anchorage point designed to prevent it. Should elastics slip under the gingival margin, it can do serious damage to the epithelial attachment. Should the slippage go unnoticed for any period of time it may cut under the root of the tooth, effectively amputating the crown. Therefore, elastic placements and progress should be closely observed and recorded until removal.

19.24 Summary

Initial involvement with orthodontics should generally be made with a knowledgeable mentor for guidance, as problems or complications are not uncommon for the neophyte. It takes time, knowledge, and experience to properly assess and treat the numerous variations of malocclusions seen in veterinary dentistry.

References

1 Proffit, W.R., Fields, H.W., Sarver, D.M., and Ackerman, J.L. (2013). Malocclusion and dentofacial deformity in contemporary society. In: *Contemporary Orthodontics*, 2–14. St. Louis, MO: Mosby.

2 Proffit, W.R., Fields, H.W., Sarver, D.M., and Ackerman, J.L. (2013). The etiology of orthodontic problem. In: *Contemporary Orthodontics*, 114–145. St. Louis, MO: Mosby.

3 Hennet, P.R. and Harvey, C.E. (1992). Diagnostic approach to malocclusions in dogs. *J. Vet. Dent.* 9 (2): 21–26.

4 Moss, J.P. and Picton, D.C.A. (1967). Experimental mesial drift in adult monkeys (Macaca Irus). *Arch. Oral Biol.* 12: 1313.

5 Eisner, E.R. (2008). Vestibule deepening procedure for tight lip syndrome in the Chinese Shar Pei dog. *J. Vet. Dent.* 25 (4): 284–289.

6 Anderson, J.G. and Harvey, C.E. (1993). Odontogenic cysts. *J. Vet. Dent.* 10 (4): 5.

7 Lobprise, H.B. and Wiggs, R.B. (1993). Crown amputation and vital pulpotomy to resolve an unusual orthodontic problem in a kinkajou. *J. Vet. Dent.* 10 (3): 14.

8 Manfra Maretta, S., Patnaik, A.K., Schloss, A.J., and Kapatkin, A. (1989). An iatrogenic dentigerous cyst in a dog. *J. Vet. Dent.* 6 (2): 11.

9 Proffit, W.R., Fields, H.W., Sarver, D.M., and Ackerman, J.L. (2013). Orthodontic diagnosis: the problem-oriented approach. In: *Contemporary Orthodontics*, 151–214. St. Louis, MO: Mosby.

10 Lindhe, J. and Svanberg, G. (1984). Influence of trauma from occlusion on progression of experimental periodontitis in the Beagle dog. *J. Clin. Periodontol.* 11: 63.

11 Alfurji, S., Alhazmi, N., Alhamlan, N. et al. (2014). The effect of orthodontic therapy on periodontal health: a review of the literature. *Int. J. Dent.* 1–8.

12 Ericsson, I., Thilander, B., Lindhe, J. et al. (1991). The effect of orthodontic tilting movements on the periodontal tissues of infected and non-infected dentition in dogs. *J. Clin. Periodontol.* 18: 182.

13 Silva, V.C., Cirelli, C.C., Ribeiro, F.S. et al. (2006). Orthodontic movement after periodontal regeneration of class II furcation: a pilot study of dogs. *J. Clin. Periodontol.* 33: 440–448.

14 Artun, J. and Urbue, K.S. (1988). The effect of orthodontic treatment on periodontal bone support in patients with advanced loss of marginal periodontium. *Am. J. Orthod. Dentofacial Orthop.* 93: 143.

15 Proffit, W.R., Fields, H.W., Sarver, D.M., and Ackerman, J.L. (2013). The biologic basis of orthodontic therapy. In: *Contemporary Orthodontics*, 278–304. St. Louis, MO: Mosby.

16 van Leeuwen, E.J., Kuijpers-Jagtman, A.M., Von den Hoff, J.W. et al. (2010). Rate of orthodontic tooth movement after changing the force magnitude: an experimental study in beagle dogs. *Orthod. Craniofac. Res.* 13: 238–245.

17 Smith, M.M. and Massoudi, L.M. (1991). Potential attachment area of the fourth maxillary premolar in dogs. *Am. J. Vet. Res.* 52 (4): 626.

18 Smith, M.M. and Massoudi, L.M. (1992). Potential attachment area of the first mandibular molar in dogs. *Am. J. Vet. Res.* 53 (2): 258.

19 Ren, Y., Maltha, J.C., and Kuijpers-Jagtman, A.M. (2003). Optimum force magnitude for orthodontic tooth movement: a systematic literaure review. *Angle Ortho.* 73: 86–92.

20 Quinn, R.S. and Yoshikawa, K. (1985). A reassessment of force magnitude in orthodontics. *Am. J. Orthod.* 88: 252–260.

21 Ren, Y., Maltha, J.C., Van, t Hof, M.A., and Kuijpers-Jagtman, A.M. (2004). Optimum force magnitude for orthodontic tooth movement: a mathematic model. *Am. J. Orthod. Dentofacial Orthop.* 125: 1–7.

22 Melsen, B. (2001). Tissue reaction to orthodontic tooth movement – a new paradigm. *Eur. J. Orthod.* 23: 671–681.

23 Henneman, S., Von den Hoff, J.W., and Maltha, J.C. (2008). Mechanobiology of tooth movement. *Eur. J. Orthod.* 30: 299–306.

24 Jonsdottir, S.H., Giesen, E.B.W., and Maltha, J.C. (2012). The biomechanical behavior of the hyalinized periodontal ligament in dogs during experimental orthodontic movement. *Eur. J. Orthod.* 34: 542–546.

25 Chen, J., Li, W., Swain, M.V. et al. (2014). A periodontal ligament driven remodeling algorithm for orthodontic tooth movement. *J. Biomech.* 47: 1689–1695.

26 von Bohl, M.V., Maltha, J., Von den Hoff, H., and Kuijpers-Jagtman, A.M. (2004). Changes in the periodontal ligament after experimental tooth movement using high and low continuous forces in Beagle dogs. *Angle Orthod.* 74: 16–25.

27 Alhashimi, N., Frithiof, L., Brudvik, P., and Bakhiet, M. (2004). CD40-CD40L expression during orthodontic tooth movement in rats. *Angle Orthod.* 74: 100–105.

28 Madureira, D.F., Taddei, S.A., Abreu, M.H. et al. (2012). Kinetics of interleukin-6 and chemokine ligands 2 and 3 expression of periodontal tissues during orthodontic tooth movement. *Am. J. Orthod. Dentofacial Orthop.* 142: 494–500.

29 van Driel, W.D., van Leeuwen, E.J., Von den Hoff, J.W. et al. (1999). Time-dependent mechanical behavior of the periodontal ligament. *Proc. Inst. Mech. Eng. H.* 214 (5): 497–504.

30 Proffit, W.R., Fields, H.W., Sarver, D.M., and Ackerman, J.L. (2013). Retention. In: *Contemporary Orthodontics*, 606–617. St. Louis, MO: Mosby.

31 Leite, R.A., Rodrigues, J.F., Sakmia, M.T., and Sakima, T. (2013). Relationship between temporomandibular disorders and orthodontic treatment: a literature review. *J. Orthod.* 18 (1): 150–157.

32 Sherwood, K. (2007). Correction of skeletal open bite with implant anchored molar/bicuspid intrusion. *Oral Maxillofac. Surg. Clin. North Am.* 19: 339–350.

33 Burstone, C.J. and Goldberg, A.J. (1980). Beta titanium, a new orthodontic alloy. *Am. J. Orthod.* 77 (2): 121.

34 Proffit, W.R., Fields, H.W., Sarver, D.M., and Ackerman, J.L. (2013). Mechanical principles in orthodontic force control. In: *Contemporary Orthodontics*, 312–336. St. Louis, MO: Mosby.

35 Peak, R.M., Lobprise, H.B., and Wiggs, R.B. (1999). Fabrication of a labial maxillary arch bar from orthodontic wire, acrylic and orthodontic buttons. *J. Vet. Dent.* 16 (1): 30–32.

36 Bannon, K. and Baker, L. (2008). Cast metal telescoping inclined plane for malocclusion in a dog. *J. Vet. Dent.* 25 (4): 250–256.

37 Cahill, D.R. (1970). The histology and rate of tooth eruption with and without temporary impaction in the dog. *Anat. Rec.* 166 (238).

38 Brine, E.J. (1999). Endodontic disease of the mandibular first molar tooth secondary to caudal crossbite in a young Shetland sheepdog. *J. Vet. Dent.* 16 (1): 15–18.

39 Verhaert, L. (1999). A removable orthodontic device for the treatment of lingually displaced mandibular canine teeth in young dogs. *J. Vet. Dent.* 16 (2): 69–75.

40 Smith, M.M. (2013). Gingivectomy, gingivoplasty, and osteoplasty for mandibular canine tooth malocclusion. *J. Vet. Dent.* 30 (3): 184–187.

41 Furman, R. and Niemiec, B. (2013). Variation in acrylic inclined plane application. *J. Vet. Dent.* 30 (3): 161–166.

42 Ulbricht, R.D. and Manfra Marretta, S. (2005). Orthodontic treatment using a direct acrylic inclined plane. *J. Vet. Dent.* 21 (1): 60–65.

43 Hale, F.A. (1996). Orthodontic correction of lingually displaced canine teeth in a young dog using light-cured acrylic resin. *J. Vet. Dent.* 13 (2): 69–73.

44 van de Wetering, A. (2007). Orthodontic correction of a base narrow mandibular canine tooth in a cat. *J. Vet. Dent.* 24 (1): 22–28.

45 Legendre, L. (2010). Building a telescopic inclined plane intraorally. *J. Vet. Dent.* 27 (1): 62–65.

46 Blazejewski, S.W. (2013). Thermoplastic inclined plane aligner for correction of bilateral mandibular canine tooth distoclusion in a cat. *J. Vet. Dent.* 30 (4): 236–247.

47 Legendre, L. and Stepaniuk, S. (2008). Correction of maxillary canine tooth mesioversion in dogs. *J. Vet. Dent.* 25 (3): 216–221.

48 Gengler, W.R. (2004). Masel chain appliance for orthodontic treatment. *J. Vet. Dent.* 21 (4): 258–261.

49 Krakowski Volker, M. and Luskin, I. (2016). Management of mesioverted maxillary canine teeth and linguoverted mandibular canine teeth. *J. Vet. Dent.* 33 (3): 170–184.

50 Zachrisson, B.U. (1977). A post-treatment evaluation of direct bonding in orthodontics. *Am. J. Orthodont.* 71: 173.

51 Proffit, W.R., Fields, H.W., Sarver, D.M., and Ackerman, J.L. (2013). Contemporary orthodontic appliances. In: *Contemporary Orthodontics*, 347–394. St. Louis, MO: Mosby.

52 Aoki, T., Ogawa, K., Miyazawa, K. et al. (2003). The use of bioabsorbable implants as orthodontic anchorage in dogs. *Dent. Mat. J.* 24 (4): 628–635.

53 Wehrbein, H., Merz, B.R., and Diedrich, P. (1999). Palatal bone support for orthodontic implant anchorage – a clinical and radiological study. *Eur. J. Orthod.* 21: 65–70.

54 Asscherickx, K., Hanssens, J.L., Wehrbein, H., and Sabzevar, M.M. (2005). Orthodontic anchorage implants inserted in the median palatal suture and normal transverse maxillary growth in growing dogs: a biometric and radiographic study. *Angle Orthod.* 75: 826–831.

55 Shank, S.B., Beck, F.M., D, Atri, A.M., and Huja, S.S. (2012). Bone damage associated with orthodontic placement of miniscrew implants in an animal model. *Am. J. Orthod. Dentofacial Orthop.* 141: 412–418.

56 Gritsch, K., Larouche, N., Morgon, L. et al. (2012). A systematic review of methods for tissue analysis in animals studies on orthodontic mini-implants. *Orthod. Craniofac. Res.* 15: 135–147.

57 Iion, S., Sakoda, S., Ito, G. et al. (2007). Acceleration of orthodontic tooth movement by alveolar corticotomy in the dog. *Am. J. Orthod. Dentofacial Orthop.* 131: 448.e1-8.

58 Cho, K.W., Cho, S.W., Oh, C.O. et al. (2007). The effect of cortical activation on orthodontic tooth movement. *Oral. Dis.* 13: 314–319.

59 Amit, G., Kalra, J.P.S., Pankaj, B. et al. (2012). Periodontally accelerated osteogenic orthodontics (PAOO) – a review. *J. Clin. Exp. Dent.* 4 (5): e292–e296.

60 LV, T., Kang, N., Wang, C. et al. (2009). Biologic response of rapid tooth movement with periodontal ligament distraction. *Am. J. Orthod. Dentofacial Orthop.* 136: 401–411.

61 Chen, X., Li, N., Peng, Z. et al. (2013). Related factors and effectiveness of rapid teeth movement through

reducing resistance and distraction. *J. Cent. South Univ. (Med. Sci.)* 38 (9): 931–937.

62 Goulart, C.S., Nouer, P.R.A., Mouramartins, L. et al. (2006). Photoradiation and orthodontic movement: experimental study with canines. *Photomed. Laser Surg.* 24 (2): 192–196.

63 Kennedy, D.B., Joondeph, D.R., Osterburg, S.K., and Little, R.M. (1983). The effect of extraction and orthodontic treatment on dentoalveolar support. *Am. J. Orthod.* 84: 183.

64 Sharpe, W., Reed, B., Subtelny, J.D., and Polson, A. (1987). Orthodontic relapse, apical root resorption and crestal alveolar bone levels. *Am. J. Orthod. Dentofacial Orthop.* 91: 252.

65 Ingber, J.S. (1989). Forced eruption: alterations of soft tissue cosmetic deformities. *Int. J. Periodontics Restorative Dent.* 9: 417.

66 Wickwire, N.A., McNeil, M., Norton, L.A. et al. (1974). The effects of tooth movement upon endodontically treated teeth. *Angle Orthod.* 44: 235.

67 Deguchi, T., Seiryu, M., Daimaruya, T. et al. (2015). Decreased alveolar bone turnover is related to the occurrence of root resorption during experimental tooth movement in dogs. *Angle Orthod.* 85 (3): 386–393.

68 Maltha, J.C., van Leeuwen, E.J., Dijkman, G.E.H.M., and Kuijpers-Jagtman, A.M. (2004). Incidence and severity of root resorption in orthodontically moved premolars in dogs. *Orthod. Craniofacial Res.* 7: 115–121.

69 Oyama, K. and Motoyoshi, M. (2007). Effects of root morphology on stress distribution at the root apex. *Eur. J. Orthod.* 29: 113–117.

70 Ramirez-Echave, J.I., Buschang, P.H., Carrillo, R. et al. (2011). Histologic evaluation of root response to intrusion in mandibular teeth in beagle dogs. *Am. J. Orthod. Dentofacial Orthop.* 139: 60–69.

71 Kaley, J.D. and Phillips, C. (1991). Root resorption. *Angle Orthod.* 61: 125.

72 Walker, S., Tieu, L.D., and Flores-Mir, C. (2013). Radiographic comparison of the extent of orthodontically induced external apical root resorption in vital and root-filled teeth: a systematic review. *Eur. J. Orthod.* 35: 796–802.

73 Beck, V.J., Stacknik, S., Chandler, N.P., and Farella, M. (2013). Orthodontic tooth movement of traumatized or root-canal-treated teeth: a clinical review. *N. Z. Dent. J.* 109: 6–11.

74 Bellamy, L.J., Kokich, V.G., and Weissman, J.A. (2008). Using orthodontic intrusion of abraded incisors to facilitate restoration the technique's effects on alveolar bone level and root length. *J. Am. Dent. Assoc.* 139: 725–733.

75 Guyman, C.G., Kokich, V.G., and Oswald, R.J. (1980). Ankylosed teeth as abutments for palatal expansion in the rhesus monkey. *Am. J. Orthod.* 77: 486.

76 Javed, F., Al-Kheraif, A.A., Romanos, E.B., and Romanos, G.E. (2015). Influence of orthodontic forces on human dental pulp: a systematic review. *Arch. Oral Biol.* 60: 347–356.

77 Maijer, R., Lux, J., and Smith, D.C. (1982). Enamel staining associated with biodegradation of orthodontic bracket bases. *J. Dent. Res.* 61: 328. (Abstract #1350).

78 Boncuk, Y., Cehreli, Z.C., and Polat-Ozsoy, O. (2014). Effects of different orthodontic adhesives and resin removal technique on enamel color alteration. *Angle Orthod.* 84: 634–641.

20

Domestic Feline Oral and Dental Diseases

Alexander M. Reiter[1], Norman Johnston[2], Jamie G. Anderson[3], Maria M. Soltero-Rivera[1], and Heidi B. Lobprise[4]

[1] School of Veterinary Medicine, University of Pennsylvania, Philadelphia, PA, USA
[2] DentalVets, North Berwick, Scotland, UK
[3] Sacramento Veterinary Dental Services, Rancho Cordova, CA, USA
[4] Main Street Veterinary Dental Clinic, Flower Mound, TX, USA

20.1 Introduction

This chapter is a conglomeration of contributed topics: Tooth Resorption in Cats (Alexander M. Reiter and Maria M. Soltero-Rivera), Feline Chronic Gingivostomatitis (Norman Johnston and Jamie Anderson), with directions to feline topics covered in other chapters and additional information on miscellaneous feline oral and dental diseases.

20.2 Tooth Resorption in Cats

20.2.1 Introduction

Tooth resorption (TR) is the most common disease affecting the dental hard tissues in domestic cats [1]. It is believed that at least one-third of cats may develop TR during life, and the risk of developing TR increases with age [2]. Even though the condition may already have been present in cats living in the thirteenth century [3], it was not mentioned in the literature until 1930 and again anecdotally reported in the 1950s and 1960s [4–6]. Retrospective examinations of zoological and museum collections of feline skulls revealed a low prevalence of TR prior to the 1970s [1, 7–9]. At some point the condition was thought to be caries [10–12] until histological studies provided clear evidence of a resorptive process resulting from the destructive activity of odontoclasts [13–15]. It is important to understand that TR can develop anywhere on the root surface and not just close to the cementoenamel junction (CEJ) [15]. In the absence of dental radiography, TR will first be noted clinically at the gingival margin often when it has already become an advanced lesion [16]. While attempts at repair can be noted by production of cementum and bone-like hard tissue [17–22], TR in cats is usually progressive and continues until the roots are completely resorbed or the crown breaks off, leaving an open wound and resorbing root remnants behind [1].

20.2.2 Etiology

The etiology of TR in domestic cats remains unknown. While there are many confirmed causes of TR for individual teeth in man, the etiology of TR affecting multiple, if not all, permanent teeth of cats is not known. Periodontal disease was considered to be a possible cause because TR near the gingival attachment often occurred together with periodontal disease [19, 23, 24]. However, a significant correlation between periodontitis and TR could not be demonstrated clinically, radiographically, or histologically in a necropsy study of cats [25]. Also, the very early TR usually originates at the root surface at some distance away from the gingiva [26]. Thus, the appearance of inflammatory cells may be a secondary, and not a primary, event during development of TR in cats [27]. One study apparently found a higher incidence of TR in feline immunodeficiency virus (FIV)-positive cats; however, conclusions made in this study were vague due to the very small sample size and the lack of dental radiographs obtained [28]. Another study on an even smaller number of cats suggested a link between TR and feline herpesvirus-1 (FHV-1) [29]. Since the prevalence of TR is already high in the general cat population, it should not be surprising for cats with stomatitis to be affected at a similar or higher degree compared to cats without stomatitis [30, 31]. A more recent study demonstrated that there was no association between TR and feline calicivirus (FCV) [32].

Vasodentin (vascular tissue in circumpulpar dentin) and osteodentin (cellular inclusions/remnants of odontoblasts

Wiggs's Veterinary Dentistry: Principles and Practice, Second Edition. Edited by Heidi B. Lobprise and Johnathon R. (Bert) Dodd.

between dentinal tubules) were identified in feline permanent teeth, and TR apparently was observed in areas of the tooth in which osteodentin was most typically found [19, 33]. The layer of predentin was reported to be thin or not present in cats with TR [19]. Furcation, lateral and secondary canals connecting the pulp cavity with the periodontal ligament can be observed in permanent premolar and molar teeth in cats [34–36]. Following experimental pulp injury, resorption of dental tissues and alveolar bone in the furcation area took place [36]. It was also speculated that the CEJ could be an area that favors the development of TR if the protective cementum layer fails to cover the dentin, thus attracting odontoclasts [37, 38]. A study on the elemental composition of teeth in cats revealed minimal differences in mineral content of enamel and cementum of normal and TR-affected teeth [39].

Cats with TR in some studies were more likely to be older, female, taking medications, drinking city (versus well) water, and playing less often with toys [40, 41]. A history of abscesses, dental disease, gingivitis, feeding non-commercial cat food and treats, consumption of cheese, butter and table foods, city residence, and being kept exclusively indoors were associated with an increased risk for TR [41–43]. Also, cats diagnosed with FIV and feline leukemia virus (FeLV) were reported to have an increased risk of TR [41], although another study did not find an association between FIV or FeLV and TR [44]. Owners of cats with TR reported that their pets vomited more often compared to cats without TR [45]. Some studies reported that TR was found to be associated with excessive feeding of raw liver [21, 27, 45], but there were also cats fed predominantly with raw bovine liver that did not develop TR [46]. An increased prevalence of TR was significantly associated with a calcium-deficient diet, decreased radiopacity of lamina dura and alveolar bone, and horizontal alveolar bone loss [46]. However, there is no evidence in the scientific literature that TR developed in cats with primary or secondary hyperparathyroidism [1]. A dry food diet was not found to be associated with less prevalence of TR in cats compared to feeding a soft food diet [1].

Coating the surface of dry kibbles with an acidic substance to preserve the food and enhance its palatability did not predispose teeth to TR [47]. A decreased risk for TR was found when cats were hunting prey or received a mixture of non-commercial and commercial foods or treats [42]. Cats without TR were more likely to have owners who brushed their pets' teeth and fed diets with higher magnesium, calcium, phosphorus, and potassium contents [40]. Consumption of commercial treats appeared to be protective against TR in cats [43]. Regular neutering of domestic cats was not found to be associated with TR [48, 49].

Because mechanical trauma from excessive occlusal force or traumatic occlusion can induce apical root resorption [6, 19], repeated compressive and tensile forces due to tooth flexure (e.g., from eating large dry kibbles) were suggested to cause TR in cats [23, 50, 51]. However, TR will develop on any teeth and any tooth surfaces, and not just on those exposed to occlusal or shearing forces. It was also suggested that local hypoxia [52] and local acidosis [53] could play a role in the pathogenesis of TR in cats after seeing an increase in osteoclast size and number in *in vitro* experiments.

The mRNA expression of interleukin (IL)-1 beta and IL-6 was higher in feline teeth with TR than in normal teeth [54]. Osteoprotegerin (OPG) mRNA expression was higher in gingival tissue associated with TR-affected teeth than in normal gingival tissue, whereas the reverse was true of the receptor activator of nuclear factor-kappa B ligand (RANKL) mRNA expression. The elevated expression of IL-l beta and IL-6 mRNA could play a role in the mediation of osteoclast activity in advanced TR. In contrast, OPG and RANKL might not appear to regulate osteoclasts in advanced disease. The results also suggested that OPG and RANKL mRNA play a role in mediating inflammatory responses in gingival cells and that OPG has an inhibiting effect on TR [54]. Another study found increased mRNA expression for inflammatory cytokines and the nuclear vitamin D receptor (nVDR), but not for RANKL and OPG, in tissue from TR-affected cats compared with tissue from radiologically confirmed healthy controls [55]. The mRNA expression of nVDR was positively correlated with the mRNA expression of pro-inflammatory (IL-1beta, IL-6, TNF-alpha, and IFN-gamma), anti-inflammatory (IL-10), pro-resorptive (IL-1beta, IL-6, and TNF-alpha), and anti-resorptive (IFN-gamma and IL-10) cytokines in the course of TR. The results suggested that both inflammation and an overexpression of the nVDR were likely to be involved in TR in cats [55]. One study suggested that the high number of mast cells found in gingiva of feline teeth with TR is an indication for the role of these cells in the pathogenesis of TR in cats [56].

It was hypothesized that the increase of TR recognized in the 1970s may be associated with aspects of domestication such as feeding commercial cat food [1, 6, 46]. Cats depend on dietary vitamin D intake because they are not able to produce vitamin D in the skin, but many commercial cat foods contain vitamin D concentrations in excess of current maximal allowances [57–60]. One study found that cats with TR had significantly higher serum concentrations of 25-hydroxyvitamin D (25OHD) compared to cats without TR, indicating that cats with TR must have ingested higher concentrations of dietary vitamin D. The cats with TR in that study also had significantly decreased urine specific gravity compared to cats without TR [44, 61]. It was proposed that dietary intake of excess vitamin D over several years could lead to periodontal ligament degeneration, hypercementosis, hyperosteoidosis, narrowing of the periodontal ligament space, dentoalveolar ankylosis, and replacement resorption. If such a process would occur close to the gingival attachment, an inflammatory component after lesion exposure to oral bacteria would join the disease [6]. Interestingly, when experimental animals were given excess vitamin D and vitamin D metabolites, the clinical, radiographic, and histologic changes induced resembled those found in teeth from cats with TR [6], including abnormal tooth extrusion and alveolar bone expansion [62, 63]. Other studies, however, could not demonstrate significantly higher serum concentrations of 25OHD in cats with TR compared to cats without TR [64, 65] and biochemical markers of bone turnover in the domestic cat were not different between cats with and without TR [66]. However, an increased mRNA expression of nVDR protein and the relative gene expression levels of 1-alpha-hydroxylase and the VDR-target gene, 24-hydroxylase, were indicative for the involvement of an active vitamin D signaling in the pathophysiology of TR in cats [64]. It was also suggested that more osteoclasts were formed *in vitro* from peripheral blood mononuclear cells (PBMCs) from cats with TR, compared to cats without TR, in the presence of M-CSF/RANKL with 1,25(OH)(2)D possibly due to a higher expression of VDR in TR(+) osteoclast precursors [67].

20.2.3 Prevalence

About 25–75% of domestic cats are affected by TR, greatly depending on the population of animals investigated (general practice versus dental specialist practice) and the diagnostic methods applied (observation only, exploration with an instrument, and/or dental radiography) [1]. An apparent increase of TR was recognized after the 1960s [1] and thus TR in cats is thought to possibly be associated with aspects of domestication. The prevalence of TR is underestimated without dental radiography [68] or when missing teeth are not considered to have been lost due to TR [49]. TR was demonstrated in permanent teeth of stray and feral small domestic cats [4, 7, 17, 21, 69, 70] and captive and wild small and large cats [17, 71–77]. However, the prevalence of TR in these populations generally is considered to be low compared to that in domestic cats that are kept as pets.

It was reported that TR would occur more often on the labial and buccal aspects of premolar and molar teeth and less commonly on canine and incisor teeth [9, 40, 78–80]. The maxillary and mandibular third premolar, the maxillary fourth premolar, and the mandibular first molar teeth are most commonly affected [9, 49, 81–83]. The distribution pattern of affected teeth is symmetrical in most cats [84] and there is a high statistical correlation between TR of mandibular cheek teeth (in particular the mandibular third premolar tooth) and the TR status of the whole dentition [84, 85].

The condition is rarely seen in cats less than two years of age [80, 81]. There is an increasing prevalence of TR as cats get older, with the first teeth becoming affected usually at four to six years of age [9, 25, 40, 49, 78–80, 82, 86–88]. Pure-bred cats appeared to be more commonly affected, but this finding was not statistically significant or was described for only small study samples [9, 80, 82, 89]. Persian and long-haired cats were reported to have TR at a younger age as compared with other breeds [9, 89]. Gender, neutering, and age at neutering were not found to affect the prevalence of TR [48, 49].

20.2.4 History

Most affected cats will not show distinct clinical signs, in particular when teeth are affected by replacement resorption only (which is asymptomatic) and the TR is located apical to the gingival attachment (not yet exposed to oral bacteria) [1]. Pain associated with TR may result from exposure of sensitive nerve endings in the dentinal tubules (with possible pulpal irritation) or when a replacement resorption progresses coronally, becomes exposed to oral bacteria at the gingival margin, and an inflammatory component joins the initially non-inflammatory process [6]. Cat owners may report halitosis, ptyalism, head shaking, dropping food while eating, reluctance to eat hard food, excessive tongue movements, repetitive lower jaw motions while eating, drinking, or grooming, sneezing, dysphagia, dehydration, anorexia, weight loss, and lethargy [81, 90, 91].

20.2.5 Clinical Findings

Dental deposits, hyperplastic gingiva, and granulation tissue often cover a clinically evident TR emerging at the gingival margin [17, 20, 81]. Thus, an accurate oral examination under general anesthesia must be performed for a proper diagnosis [92]. Because various degrees of oral inflammation may be present with TR [30, 93], the condition had previously been considered to be part of periodontal disease in cats [19, 87, 94]. A dental explorer can be used to detect any irregularities at the tooth surface near the gingival margin [15, 21]. Hyperplastic gingiva or granulation tissue covering a TR tends to bleed when touched [92]. The lower jaw was often reported to "chatter" or twitch when affected teeth were probed [21, 81, 93, 95]. Several studies on pain mechanisms in anesthetized cats demonstrated that reflex responses of the digastric and tongue muscles were elicited after dental stimulation, resulting in evoked licking movements of the tongue and jaw-opening reflexes [1].

Canine teeth (in particular maxillary) often appear to extrude abnormally (abnormal tooth extrusion), leading to excessive exposure of the root surface [63, 92, 95]. The crowns of the teeth seem to be longer than they should be. Thickening of alveolar bone and local osteomyelitis (alveolar bone expansion) are often associated with this phenomenon [6, 62]. There is a bulbous expansion of the alveolar bone on the labial sides of the teeth. In advanced stages of TR, the crown can fracture off, leaving an open wound and root remnants behind [96]. A small sinus tract may occasionally be observed over the site of a retained root remnant [90, 97]. When the gingiva has grown over the root remnant, a bulge underneath the gingiva can be seen or palpated [1, 98].

20.2.6 Diagnostic Imaging Findings

Without dental radiography, TR below the gingival attachment (and thus the vast majority of TR) will not be detectable [9, 25, 68, 99, 100]. A clinically evident TR emerging at the gingival margin (inflammatory resorption) will generally be visible as a notched radiolucency in the tooth with sharp or scalloped margins (type 1 resorption). The periodontal ligament space may be of normal width apical to the TR, but there will be horizontal or vertical loss of alveolar bone adjacent to the TR. Lesions on mesial and distal tooth surfaces or in the furcation area usually are more obvious on radiographs than those on labial/buccal and lingual/palatal tooth surfaces [23, 96]. Apparent pulp involvement due to TR did not appear to be associated with radiographic evidence of periapical lucencies [101]. Fusion of the root and alveolar bone (dentoalveolar ankylosis) results in focalized or generalized disappearance of the periodontal ligament space and lamina dura on radiographs. Resorbed dental tissue will gradually be replaced by bone (replacement resorption). The root will take on a striated or moth-eaten appearance ("ghost roots") and the periodontal ligament space and lamina dura will disappear on radiographs (type 2 resorption). Unlike inflammatory resorption, adjacent bone usually is not resorbed [23, 96].

Teeth with abnormal extrusion and alveolar bone expansion may display regions of hypercementosis and infrabony pocketing. A radiographic study of periodontal disease in cats also identifies the expansile lesions, with 53% of cats showing alveolar bone expansion of at least one canine tooth [87]. Even in the 12 of 41 cats with normal alveolar bone height in that study, the teeth were already displaying some degree of expansion. Of the 11 (7%) cats with moderate to severe expansion, 10 of the 11 had severe vertical bone loss associated with the affected tissue [87].

Conventional computed tomography (CT) showed a fair to poor sensitivity but good to excellent specificity with regards to detection of TR in cats [102]. An earlier study using cone-beam computed tomography (CBCT) reported that both periodontal disease and TR in cats could accurately be detected with this imaging modality [103].

20.2.7 Histological Findings

Numerous microscopic studies of the 1980s [20, 21, 45, 80, 104], 1990s [13, 17–19, 22, 105], and 2000s [26, 63, 106, 107] demonstrated that TR develops anywhere on the root surface and not just close to the CEJ [37, 38, 79], progressing through cementum into root dentin. This homogenous distribution of TR throughout the root surface has also been demonstrated radiographically [108]. Odontoclasts migrate from blood vessels in the periodontal ligament or alveolar bone toward the root surface where they resorb cementum and dentin, creating lacunae, lagoons, and canals in the dental hard tissues [13, 17, 19, 72].

One important histological study evaluated clinically and radiographically healthy teeth from cats with TR on other teeth [26]. Hyperemia, edema, and degeneration of the periodontal ligament with marked fiber disorientation, increased osteoid formation along alveolar bone surfaces, excessive formation of cellular cementum at apical and mid-root surfaces, and of acellular cementum at cervical root surfaces, gradual narrowing of the periodontal ligament space, and areas of ankylotic fusion between the tooth and alveolar bone were found, demonstrating that a majority of TR in cats may be non-inflammatory in origin [26]. Other studies confirmed that alterations in the periodontal ligament seen on histology may represent a pre-clinical stage of TR in cats [109] and demonstrated that over half of clinically healthy teeth in cats exhibit TR on electron microscopy [79]. Significant associations were found between abnormal tooth extrusion and TR (four of four canine teeth with extrusion had resorption, compared to only 1 of 5 canine teeth without extrusion in one study)[63], as well as alveolar bone expansion and TR [62].

If the condition progresses into crown dentin, the enamel could become undermined and then either gets resorbed or loses its contact with originally intact dentin and breaks off [1]. Resorption of enamel as the initial event is only rarely observed [110]. TR that emerges at the gingival margin will be exposed to oral bacteria, which results in the formation of vascular and inflamed granulation tissue [18, 20, 82, 86, 105, 107, 111] and resorption of alveolar bone adjacent to the TR [1]. Many clinically evident TRs (i.e., lesions emerging at the gingival margin) appear histologically to be in both resorptive and reparative phases simultaneously [20]. During the reparative phase, cementoblast- or osteoblast-like cells produce new hard tissue resembling cementum or bone-like material [13, 17–22, 72]. Pulp involvement in the form of pulpitis is usually not seen until late in advanced stages of TR [17, 19, 21, 72].

In an evaluation of cats with and without TR, the distance between the alveolar margin (AM) and CEJ was significantly greater in teeth with TR [63]. Thickening of cementum, beyond that considered a normal physiological aging change, was identified, with the most notable changes in the cervical region of the roots. Hypercementosis was often associated with a decreased width of the periodontal ligament space, and cementicles (extensions of cementum into the periodontal ligament space) could be found [63]. Alveolar bone expansion manifested histologically as medullary fibrosis with mild to moderate pleocellular inflammation and modest proliferation of woven bone [62]. Teeth examined in that study had a distinct rim of peripheral sclerosis, consistent with an outward compression force of expansion. Changes could also occur in premolars and molars, but with more variability in the type of osseous changes and inflammation (including gingival changes), making this region more challenging to recognize clinical alveolar bone expansion than at the canine teeth [62].

20.2.8 Classification

TR can be internal or external. In cats, TR usually originates at the external surface of the tooth, i.e., the surface facing connective tissue of the periodontium (gingival connective tissue, periodontal ligament, and alveolar bone) [1]. Its classification in the human literature is made by type (surface, inflammatory, and replacement resorption) and area (cervical, lateral, and apical resorption) (Table 20.1).

Surface resorption is confined to cementum and the outermost layer of dentin without inflammatory reaction in the periodontal ligament. It is asymptomatic and not visible on radiographs, often self-limiting, and spontaneously repaired to establish the original root contour. Inflammatory resorption is resorption of cementum and dentin associated with inflammation in the adjacent gingival connective tissue and periodontal ligament with alveolar bone resorption usually located adjacent to root resorption. Replacement resorption is usually preceded by fusion of alveolar bone and the root surface (dentoalveolar ankylosis), resulting in focalized or generalized disappearance of the periodontal ligament space and lamina dura on radiographs, decreased physiological tooth mobility, and a high-pitched sound upon tooth percussion. Resorbed root tissue is gradually replaced by bone, causing a moth-eaten appearance of the root and disappearance of the periodontal ligament space and lamina dura on radiographs. Unlike inflammatory resorption, adjacent bone is not resorbed. Dentoalveolar ankylosis and replacement resorption are considered to be asymptomatic as long as the resorption remains below the gingival attachment. Cervical resorption is resorption of the cervical portion of the root. Lateral resorption is resorption of the mid-portion of the root, and apical resorption is resorption of the apical portion of the root. Overlaps between resorption types and areas are common [1, 6].

Earlier reports used various numbers of stages and types to classify TR in cats [1, 112]. The American Veterinary Dental College currently suggests classification based on severity (stages 1–5) and radiographic appearance of the resorption (types 1–3) (https://www.avdc.org/Nomenclature/Nomen-Teeth.html#resorption; accessed October 6, 2017). (Figure 20.1a–g). Stage 1 resorption is defined as mild dental hard tissue loss (cementum or cementum and enamel). Stage 2 resorption shows moderate dental hard tissue loss (cementum or cementum and enamel with loss of dentin that does not extend to the pulp cavity). Stage 3 resorption is defined as deep dental hard tissue loss (cementum or cementum and enamel with loss of dentin that extends to the pulp cavity) with most of the tooth still retaining its integrity. Stage 4 resorption shows extensive dental hard tissue loss (cementum or cementum and enamel with loss of dentin that extends to the pulp cavity) with most of the tooth having lost its integrity; there are substages 4a (crown and root equally affected), 4b (crown more severely affected than the root), and 4c (root more severely affected than the crown). Stage 5 resorption is defined as remnants of dental hard tissue visible only as irregular radiopacities with complete gingival covering (Table 20.2).

On a radiograph of a tooth with type 1 resorption, a focal or multifocal radiolucency is present in the tooth with otherwise normal radiopacity and normal periodontal ligament space (Figure 20.2a). On a radiograph of a tooth with type 2 resorption, there is narrowing or disappearance of the periodontal ligament space in at least some areas and decreased radiopacity of part of the tooth (Figure 20.2b). On a radiograph of a tooth with type 3 resorption, features of both type 1 and type 2 resorptions are present in the same tooth (Figure 20.2c). The affected

Table 20.1 Classification of internal and external resorption by area and type.

	Internal	External
Area	Pulp chamber Root canal	Cervical Lateral Apical
Type	Inflammatory Replacement	Surface Inflammatory Replacement

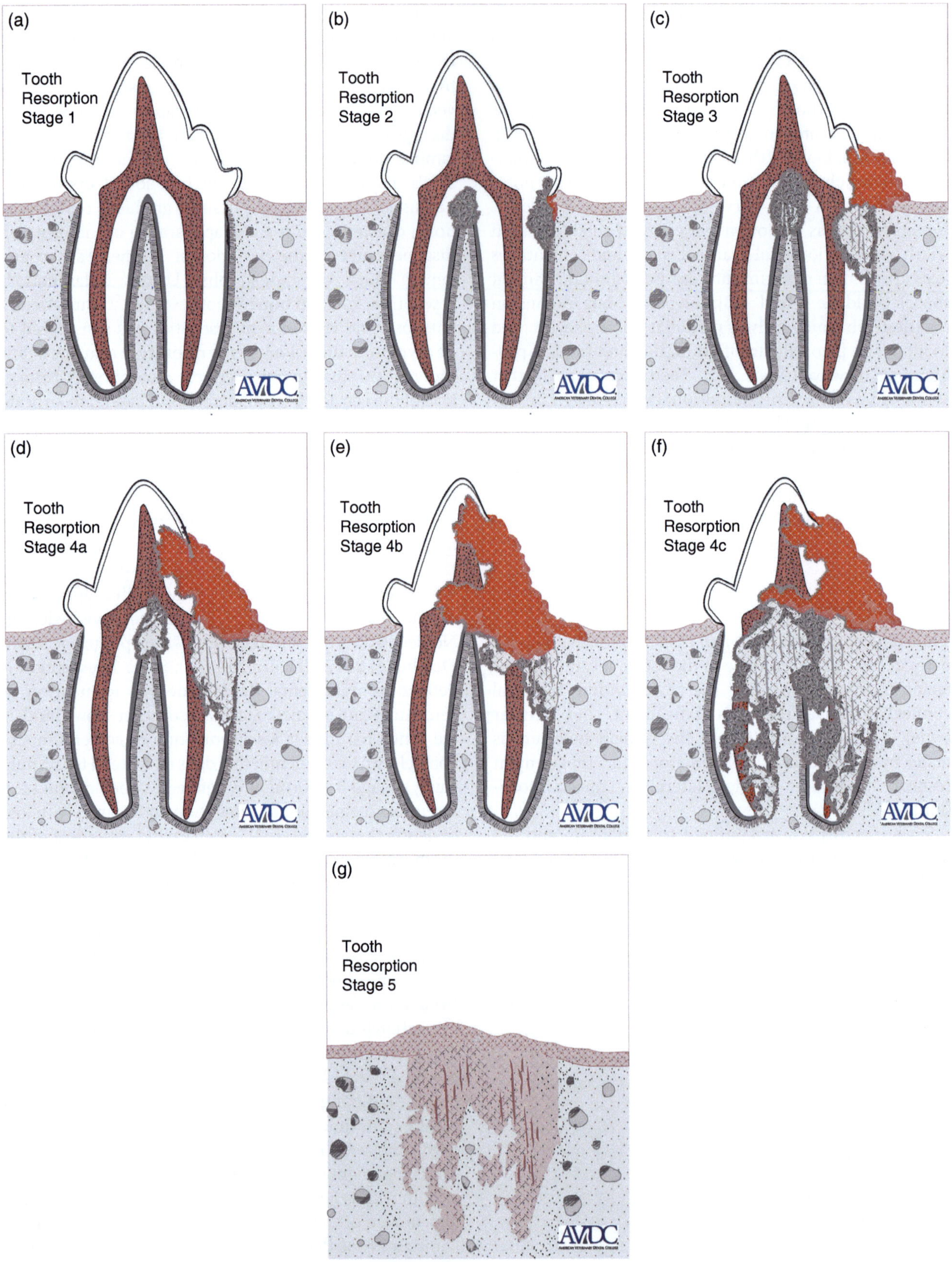

Figures 20.1 Tooth resorption – AVDC Classification of Clinical Stages. *Source:* Copyright AVDC®, used with permission. https://www.avdc.org/Nomenclature/Nomen-Teeth.html#resorption; accessed November 2017.

Table 20.2 Stages of tooth resorption (AVDC).

Stage 1	Mild dental hard tissue loss (cementum or cementum and enamel)
Stage 2	Moderate dental hard tissue loss (cementum or cementum and enamel with loss of dentin that does not extend to the pulp cavity)
Stage 3	Deep dental hard tissue loss (cementum or cementum and enamel with loss of dentin that extends to the pulp cavity); most of the tooth retains its integrity
Stage 4	Extensive dental hard tissue loss (cementum or cementum and enamel with loss of dentin that extends to the pulp cavity); most of the tooth has lost its integrity (a) Crown and root equally affected (b) Crown more severely affected than the root (c) Root more severely affected than the crown
Stage 5	Remnants of dental hard tissue visible only as irregular radiopacities; complete gingival covering

tooth shows areas of normal and narrow or lost periodontal ligament space and there is focal or multifocal radiolucency in the tooth and decreased radiopacity in other areas of the tooth (Table 20.3). There is the consideration of possibly different etiologies for type 1 and type 2 resorptions [108].

20.2.9 Treatment

Historically, a common approach for the treatment of TR included topical fluoride treatment of very early lesions, restoration with or without endodontic treatment of slightly to moderately advanced lesions, and extraction of teeth with severely advanced lesions [91, 113–117]. However, fluoride treatment remains controversial because it does not address the origin of TR (i.e., the disease apical to the gingival attachment). Furthermore, restorations with glass ionomer or composite were shown to fail in numerous studies of feline teeth with TR [82, 83, 95, 118].

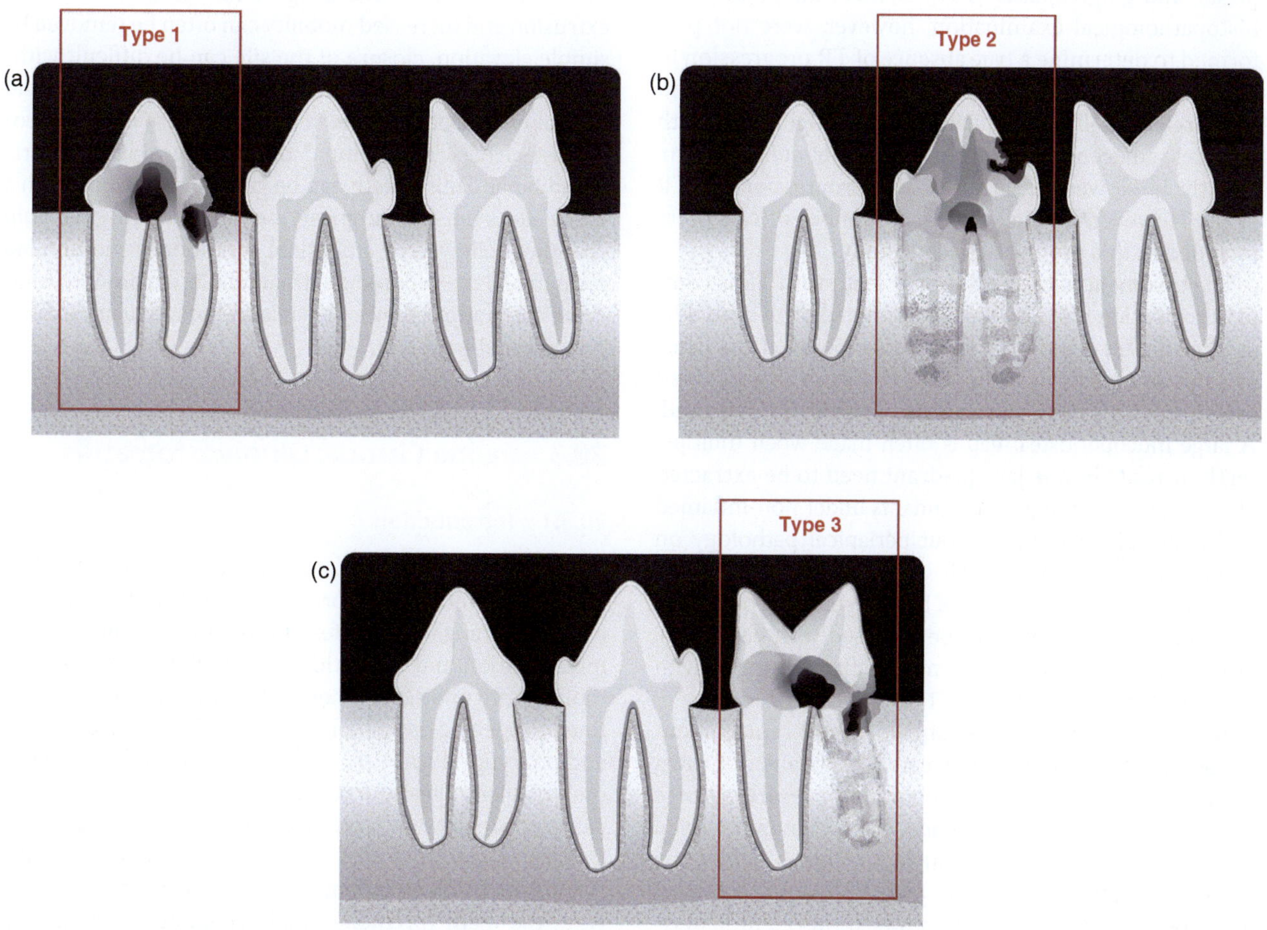

Figures 20.2 Types of resorption based on radiographic appearance: (a) Type 1 (T1); (b) Type 2 (T2); (c) Type 3 (T3). *Source:* Copyright AVDC®, used with permission. https://www.avdc.org/Nomenclature/Nomen-Teeth.html#resorption; accessed November 2017.

Table 20.3 Types of tooth resorption (AVDC).

Type 1	On a radiograph of a tooth with type 1 appearance, a focal or multifocal radiolucency is present in the tooth with otherwise normal radiopacity and normal periodontal ligament space.
Type 2	On a radiograph of a tooth with type 2 appearance, there is narrowing or disappearance of the periodontal ligament space in at least some areas and decreased radiopacity of part of the tooth.
Type 3	On a radiograph of a tooth with type 3 appearance, features of both type 1 and type 2 are present in the same tooth. A tooth with this appearance has areas of normal and narrow or lost periodontal ligament space, and there is focal or multifocal radiolucency in the tooth and decreased radiopacity in other areas of the tooth.

One author recommended supportive homeopathic treatment without providing any proof of success [119]. Another reported a very high success rate when treating feline teeth with TR with an Nd:YAG laser, enameloplasty, and gingivoplasty [120]. Dental radiography and histopathological examination, however, were not performed to determine a true absence of TR progression in that study. Alendronate, a bisphosphonate compound that preferentially accumulates in the subgingival tooth surfaces, adjacent alveolar bone, and root canal system, effectively slowed or arrested the progression of TR [121]. However, only a very small number of cats were included in this proof-of-concept study.

The treatment of choice for many teeth with TR is complete extraction [24, 122, 123]. Multirooted teeth should be sectioned after removal of the alveolar bone on the labial and buccal aspects of the roots so that each single-rooted crown–root segment can then be elevated and removed. A large mucoperiosteal flap is often made when multiple teeth or roots in one jaw quadrant need to be extracted [1, 92, 124]. Resorbing root remnants under non-inflamed and intact gingiva and without periapical pathology on dental radiographs may be left where they are [125]. They often appear as a small gingival bulge in the area of a missing tooth (which should not be confused with neoplasia). However, root remnants underneath inflamed gingiva with sinus tracts must be extracted [1, 46, 126].

Teeth with dentoalveolar ankylosis and replacement (Type 2) resorption can be treated by means of crown amputation and intentional retention of resorbing root tissue [127, 128]. A flap is made, the crown is removed with a water-cooled round bur to, or slightly below, the level of the alveolar mucosa, and the wound is rinsed and closed by suturing. Contraindications include periodontitis, endodontic, and periapical disease. Also, teeth of cats with stomatitis or that are FIV and/or FeLV-positive should not be treated with crown amputation [84, 127, 128].

The so-called "root pulverization/atomization" procedure [90, 92, 129] to crush very brittle or ankylosed root remnants into many particles with a water-cooled round bur on a high-speed dental handpiece is not recommended. Serious complications can occur with this technique, including incomplete root removal, trauma to sublingual soft tissues, alveolar bone, and neurovascular bundles, subcutaneous and sublingual emphysema, air embolus, and transportation of root remnants into the mandibular canal, infraorbital canal, or nasal cavity [95].

Canine teeth exhibiting abnormal extrusion and alveolar bone expansion should have a complete evaluation, including radiographs (from different angles to "map" the extent of changes), periodontal probing to discover any advanced vertical bone loss, and tactile evaluation of mobility. Those with mild changes and without TR could be monitored with regular clinical examinations and dental radiographs, but progression should be expected. Those with moderate to severe changes should be considered candidates for extraction, although elevating labial flaps can be very challenging. While teeth with severe extrusion and increased mobility can often be removed by simple elevation, closure of the site can be difficult without surgical reduction of the thickened alveolar bone and careful release of the periosteum at the base of the mucoperiosteal flap. The pointed tips of opposing ipsilateral mandibular canine teeth can be gently rounded off with a white stone bur (odontoplasty) without entering the pulp chamber, followed by a dentinal conditioner and unfilled resin to seal the exposed dentinal tubules, in order to minimize the trauma they can cause to the maxillary extraction site and upper lip.

20.3 Feline Chronic Gingivostomatitis

20.3.1 Introduction

Feline chronic gingivostomatitis (FCGS) is a familiar problem in small animal practice. In reality, the term covers a wide range of manifestations from the most severe inflammation and ulceration of the whole oral cavity to more focal conditions where inflammation may be confined to specific tissues and locations. It can affect all oral and pharyngeal soft tissues commonly including gingiva, oral and pharyngeal mucosa, and the tongue. Inflammation can occasionally be confined to the tissues lateral to the palatoglossal folds, known as caudal mucositis (Figure 20.3). When inflammation affects the tissues overlying the teeth (premolars/molars/canines) it is termed alveolar mucositis. The term stomatitis is generally reserved for widespread oral inflammation that is beyond

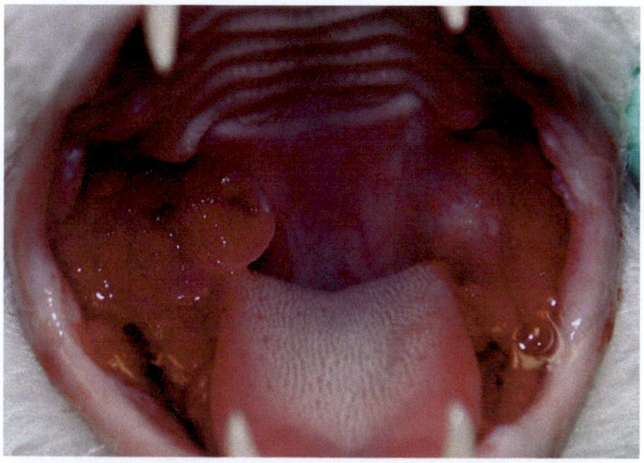

Figure 20.3 Evaluation of inflammation in the caudal mouth of cats with FCGS can be important in determining diagnosis, prognosis, and response to treatment.

gingivitis and periodontal disease and may extend into submucosal tissues (www.avdc.org; accessed October 17, 2017, and https://www.avdc.org/Nomenclature/Nomen-Oral_Pathology.html#inflammation).

This condition is reported to have prevalence of 0.7% in a study of nearly 5000 cats by 12 practices [130]. A second study [108] gave a prevalence of 5.5%. Anecdotally, the prevalence appears to be higher with lesions more intense and severe in North America and southern Europe.

20.3.2 Etiology

The actual etiology is not known but thought to be a complex result of reactions involving a number of disparate factors. It has previously been stated that environmental factors and bacterial infection (and the host response to it) acting in combination with viral infection all influence the disease process [131, 132].

One study [133] compared the oral bacterial flora in normal and FCGS diseased cats using traditional and culture independent methods (bacterial 16S rRNA gene sequencing) in order to identify novel pathogens and species that may be fastidious and challenging to cultivate. In diseased cats the oral flora was found to be less diverse, compared to normal cats, with *Pasteurella multocida* subsp. *multocida* representing more than half the identifiable flora of the oral cavity, lending credence to the theory that it may be an important factor in the etiology. Another study by the same group [134] discovered a group of novel and previously identified bacteria that have potential importance in the etiology that warrants further investigation using 16S rRNA gene sequencing. Subsequent studies have researched the oral microbiome of cats in more detail [135, 136].

The major difference between normal and diseased cats appears to be a hyperimmune response to the antigenic burden that is dental and oral plaque, though the relationship to plaque has not been definitively proven [137]. Low levels of plaque biofilm appear to initiate this abnormal response in susceptible individuals. A study of the innate immune response in both normal and FCGS cats [138] compared that response in the presence of putative pathogens previously identified. The study found a good correlation between the severity of clinical signs and the presence of several of these putative pathogens, including FCV and *Tannerella forsythia*. Complex interreactions occur in affected cats and bacteriology results suggest that opportunistic infections are likely to play a role in influencing the disease process.

The specific immunologic aberrations operating in this complex still need to be defined [139]. It is likely that immunologic mechanisms are intrinsic to the initiation and perpetuation of feline gingivitis stomatitis complex, just as they are in human idiopathic mucosal diseases such as oral lichen planus and recurrent aphthous ulceration. An early immunologic study proposed that increased immunoglobulin values in cats with chronic oral diseases were indicative of inadequate B cell function [140]. Specific evaluations of T lymphocytes, their subsets, and the cytokines secreted represent preliminary investigations into the cytokine–receptor interactions that may be aberrant in gingivitis stomatitis. Researchers have identified adequate peripheral CD_4 counts (helper T cells) and an increase in CD_8 (cytotoxic T cells and suppressor cells) [141]. Inferences from this work on potential immunopathogenic mechanisms include lack of systemic immunosuppression in affected cats and depression of T cell responses to oral antigens by the high numbers of T suppressor cells.

With regard to environmental factors, colony cats or those in multicat households appear to be more commonly affected early in life. Increased stress levels plus the closer proximity of other cats allowing transmission of viruses and other airborne microorganisms are most likely to be significant factors.

Many studies report a level of around 70% of chronically affected individuals (showing signs for over six months) testing positive to virus isolation following oropharyngeal swabbing for FCV [142–144]. The actual significance of this is not accurately known. It is possible that the virus damages cell membranes allowing easier antigenic penetration by other agents. However, other cofactors are necessary before this virus can cause disease as FCV carriage in the general cat population is around 20–30% [142, 145]. One study [146] felt that the distribution of lesions in FCV-positive cats to be more frequently associated with caudal mucositis. The relationship between FCV infection and FCGS appears strong with

70–90% of chronic stomatitis cats testing positive compared to the general cat population [142, 144].

FIV infection may also have a role to play by predisposing the cat to secondary infections. Both FIV and FeLV contribute to an aberrant immune response to oral antigens but one study [133] showed a group of FCGS cats to have only a 4% prevalence for testing positive FIV and FeLV. This is similar to the cat population as a whole. It has been reported that the relationship between FCV and FIV appears strong but the association between the two has never been established for FCGS cats [142, 147].

Pre-existing dental disease of any form can also have an exacerbating effect on FCGS. Conditions such as periodontal disease, TR lesions, or both, are important factors contributing to the overall hyperimmune response. Paradoxically the condition is often present in the absence of significant accumulation of calculus on the teeth.

20.3.3 Clinical Presentation

In the juvenile cat, there are two periods when significant oral inflammation can be found. Whether these cats eventually develop the signs of FCGS requires further study. At the time of kitten vaccinations, oral inflammation can occasionally be seen. It is not known if this is an immune response to vaccinal elements or to the eruption of the deciduous dentition and consequential increased levels in dental plaque. The inflammation is generally transient and usually resolves with improved oral hygiene and, in the presence of gingival enlargement, gingivectomy.

The second period to see an increase in oral inflammation levels is when the permanent teeth erupt. This is commonly a time when gingival inflammation levels can be severe, even in normal cats. Cats with soft tissue lesions beyond the gingiva require enhanced oral hygiene to both resolve the inflammation and prevent permanent tissue changes such as gingival recession or gingival hyperplasia.

The largest group of affected cats is seen later in life with a mean age of seven years [148]. Adult cases of FCGS present with a wide range of severity and location of clinical signs. The implication is that some cats have a very low threshold to the driving etiological factors(s) while others have a higher threshold approaching the level for normal cats.

Most cats present with dysphagia and pain due to extensive oral inflammation and ulceration of the soft tissues. In some cases, it can be hard to understand how the individual manages to eat or function normally with such extensive oral inflammation. Severely affected cats are often unkempt as grooming is hard or impossible with severe oral pain. Weight loss may also be a feature, but many cats with advanced disease do maintain a weight that is normal or overweight.

Table 20.4 Owner evaluation of cat at study entry[a].

Appetite	3	Eats only pureed food, or only when hand fed
	2	Eats wet food, cannot eat dry food
	1	Eating wet and dry food, but less than normal amount
	0	Eating normally
Activity level	3	No interest in people or other pets, spends most of time sleeping
	2	Low activity level, but will play occasionally when engaged by people or other pets
	1	Plays spontaneously, but not frequently
	0	Normal activity level (playful and active)
Grooming behavior	3	Will not groom
	2	Grooms occasionally but not at "pre-illness" level
	1	Grooming excessively
	0	Grooming normally
Perceived comfort	0–3	0 being the most comfortable, 3 being most painful

[a] The average of the scores above (total score divided by 4) is entered in the "owner evaluation" box on the initial SDAI (Stomatitis Disease Activity Index) tabulation sheet.

Inflammatory lesions may involve some or all of the oral soft tissues. Most severe cases present with inflammation and ulceration of the tissues lateral to the palatoglossal folds (caudal mucositis) in addition to the gingiva and mucosa overlying the cheek teeth (alveolar mucositis). Sublingual mucositis and contact mucositis describing lesions secondary to soft tissue contact with a tooth surface, also known previously as "contact ulcers" or "kissing ulcers," can be present. The pharynx, tongue, and linguomolar salivary glands can also be affected in severe cases. The stomatitis disease activity index (SDAI) sheet (Tables 20.4, 20.5, and 20.6) is designed to allow this to be recorded and measured as a score [139].

Halitosis is often marked and cats may drool thick, tenacious saliva. The mandibular lymph nodes are often markedly swollen and palpation is resented.

20.3.4 Diagnostic Pathway

A standard, systematic, diagnostic approach is best performed early in the case progression before irreversible changes take place, to ensure samples are collected

Table 20.5 Scoring criteria for stomatitis disease activity index (SDAI) tabulation.

Owner evaluation	0	Significant improvement
	1	Mild improvement
	2	No change
	3	Worse
Weight	0	Gain >0.5 kg
	1	Gain 0.25–0.5 kg
	2	Gain <0.25 kg
	3	Weight loss
Inflammation (specified areas as graded by clinician)	0	None
	1	Mild
	2	Moderate
	3	Severe

Table 20.6 Stomatitis disease activity index (SDAI) score tabulation.

Stomatitis disease activity index	0	1	2	3
Owner evaluation				
Weight (compared to most recent visit)				
Maxillary buccal mucosal inflammation				
Mandibular buccal mucosal inflammation				
Maxillary attached gingiva inflammation				
Mandibular attached gingiva inflammation				
Inflammation lateral to palatoglossal folds				
Molar salivary gland inflammation				
Oropharyngeal inflammation				
Lingual and/or sublingual inflammation				
Total Score (maximum = 30)				

at a time when the results are of most use. It is important to follow a step-wise approach for these cases.

- Review the general medical and specific oral history.
- Perform a full clinical examination. Cats may present initially with weight loss and poorly thriving. Although the oral cavity may be by far the most obvious reason for concern, a full examination is still required to eliminate other systemic conditions.
- Perform a full examination of the head and mouth. Many cats resent a thorough oral examination, so this may be best performed under anesthesia. Be aware that most inflammatory lesions look much less "angry" under the effect of anesthetic drugs.
- Score the oral soft tissues using the standard method (e.g., SDAI sheet and chart; (see Tables 20.4, 20.5, and 20.6) Scoring the lesions for location and severity at each examination allows the clinician to record this and assign a score. As time passes the success or otherwise of treatments can therefore be measured. The time taken is minimal, but it provides very useful prognostic information. The score sheet is based on one designed by Anderson [139].

Blood tests for hematology/biochemistry:

- Clinical pathologic abnormalities are usually limited to a polyclonal hyperglobulinemia [149, 150], and a mild basophilia [18].
- One study reported 10% of FCGS cats having chronic renal failure. Any underlying systemic disease may significantly affect the prognosis or the safety of anesthetic protocols and other drugs (e.g., long-term non-steroidal anti-inflammatory drugs (NSAIDs)).
- Other diagnostics may include ANA, Bartonella, CD4:CD8 ratios in peripheral blood and in tissues.

Virus testing. Testing for FCV/FHV assists prognosis. Additional tests for retroviruses (FIV, FeLV) are advised to ensure that there are no contraindications to subsequent therapy. Virus isolation is possible, but PCR tests provide qualitative and quantitative information of the viral burden (www.scanelis.com). At this time the significance of the quantities of viral antigen reported by PCR testing is not established, as studies are ongoing.

Bacteriology. Bacteria are a known cofactor in the etiology of this condition. Cats with FCGS have a less diverse flora than normal cats, and a high proportion of cats tested show *Pasteurella multocida* to be the dominant species [133]. In addition, *Tannerella forsythia* – if found – is considered a putative pathogen [138]. Test for both aerobic and anaerobic species. Check with your lab to find out what swab material and transport medium they might require.

Biopsy. Histopathology of affected areas often yields little useful specific information with a high proportion of lymphocytes (mixed T and B cells) and plasma cells found with fewer neutrophils and some mast cells.

- Histopathology of stomatitis is not consistent with granulomatous disease, allergic mucosal reaction (few eosinophils), desquamative gingivitis, foreign body reaction, or viral disease (no virus-induced cytopathic changes in epithelial cells or at the edge of areas of ulceration) [151].
- The pattern in most was: increased plasma cells, ulceration and loss of epithelium, or a very thin remaining epithelium with lesser lymphocyte populations and increased neutrophils.

- There is minimal basal cell layer in most cats.
- The look of the epithelium in a number of cases looks "bland" while it is being torn apart by the inflammatory infiltrate; heavy infiltrate into the epithelium is prominent in many cases. There are no microabcesses in the superficial epithelium though there are neutrophils in several cases (PAS stain negative).
- Some of the plasma cells are large with large nuclei in one study [151]; not tested for the presence of kappa and lambda IgG light chains. The underlying connective tissue was vascular with dilated, congested vascular spaces with an intense surrounding infiltrate dominated by plasma cells.
- Often a non-specific diagnosis is given by the lab. However, before treatment alters the tissue cell content it is important to eliminate neoplasms (e.g., squamous cell carcinoma (SCCa), malignant lymphoma, etc.) and other immunopathologies. This is very important if lesions are not symmetrical. It is wise to send tissue to a laboratory that is used to reviewing oral lesions.
- In a retrospective study of 75 cases of feline gingivostomatitis (FCGS), 20 cats (26%) were 12 years of age or older. In 33 cases histopathology was performed. Of those, SCCa was found in eight cases, 11%. All cases occurred in cats over twelve years of age, for a frequency of SCCA in geriatric cats with gingivostomatitis of 40%. The conclusion was made that a strong correlation exists between FCGS and SCCa in general and particularly in geriatric felines [152].

Dental chart and full-mouth dental radiographic survey. For any dental procedure the use of a chart is both useful and necessary in every case to ensure all teeth and tissues are assessed for abnormal findings with all "missing" teeth examined to locate any retained or broken root tips or those with TR lesions. The diagnostic yield of full-mouth radiographs in cats is very significant. Studies show they reveal clinically hidden pathology in 42% of cats with an otherwise "normal" mouth and additional pathology in 54% of cats in mouths with abnormal findings [68, 153]. Full-mouth radiographs are essential early in FCGS cases.

20.3.5 Clinical Management

It must be understood that the primary role of the clinician in the treatment and management of FCGS is to reduce the burden of oral antigen on a long-term basis and simultaneously improve the welfare of the patient by reducing the considerable pain that these cats endure and eliminate or improve the inflammation of the oral soft tissues.

In addition to the diagnostic tests advised above, the most important first step in all cases is to clean the teeth and remove those with no future. Some cats respond very well to routine dentistry and improved hygiene alone, while others will respond poorly to this treatment. The aim is to restore the balance between the immune response and the oral antigen burden. In effect this means zero tolerance of both existing dental disease and of oral/dental plaque.

If teeth are affected by advanced periodontal disease, they are best removed. Similarly, teeth affected by TR lesions should be removed at this stage using a technique appropriate for resorption type. Teeth affected by type 1 resorption must be removed conventionally. Teeth affected by type 2 or type 3 lesions may be suitable for crown amputation depending on radiographic diagnosis.

Antibiotics are initially useful in most cases to control excessive inflammation that can be associated with bacterial infection and to allow soft tissues to heal after surgery. Until bacteriology results are available, the initial choice should include agents with a good aerobic and anaerobic spectrum that work in the presence of purulent material and penetrate bone. For most cases, this initially means clindamycin at 11 mg/(kg/day) for up to 14 days, while minocycline has also been used. Oral treatment can be challenging for owners when the mouth is very painful. Anecdotally keeping capsules in the fridge and rolling the powder into butter balls can help the owner administer them orally. It should also be noted that some cats may culture *Pasteurella multocida*, which is clindamycin resistant. Some clinicians find cefovecin (*Convenia, Zoetis*) useful for cats that are challenging to medicate orally, as it provides 14 days of therapy from a single injection and has good activity against *Pasteurella* species.

Topical chlorhexidine provides the most effective oral antisepsis in these cases – both short- and long-term. Chlorhexidine paste or gel used once or twice daily will provide excellent post-operative plaque control and aids in reducing the overall antigenic burden. Finding a suitable product for cats can be a problem due to the bitter taste of some gels. Bright Bark & Meow (Keystone Industries, wwww.krpvet.com) or HS Petcare Chlorhexidine Paste 0.12% (Henry Schein Animal Health) seems to be acceptable to most cats. The paste can be wiped inside the lips twice daily – or brushed if the cat will allow it. Another possible alternative product from Keystone is a chlorhexidine gluconate spray. Oral disinfection with a suitable chlorhexidine product once or twice daily is one of the most important and effective measures available. Treatment may well be lifelong.

20.3.5.1 Reassessment

All cases should be reassessed in 7–10 days after professional dental cleaning:

- If improved, continue chlorhexidine up to twice daily and review in four weeks and subsequently as required. Advise the owner that more frequent scaling and polishing intervals will probably be necessary – perhaps up to 3–4 per annum. The need for professional dental cleaning is signaled when the daily use of chlorhexidine is failing to control the inflammation adequately.
- If not improved, move to elective extraction of all cheek teeth as soon as possible. The rationale is that if the tissues fail to respond (by reduction of inflammation and pain) within 2–4 weeks despite the best hygiene we can provide, elective surgical (open) extraction of all the cheek teeth should follow without delay. Although many clinicians and owners are reluctant to take this step at this time, studies over the last 18 years [154–157] consistently show the benefit of this procedure. In general, 50% of cases requiring no further treatment to resolve their signs and a further 37% need only low levels of inflammation support, but being markedly better than before. With the benefit ratio of around 9 out of 10 cases improving, it is hard to argue against this step from a welfare point of view.

Elective surgical extraction of whole cheek teeth quadrants should not be undertaken lightly. Consideration should also be made as to whether surgery should or could be performed in one session. If teeth are excessively mobile, or otherwise easy to extract, one session is preferable. On the contrary, if the surgery is challenging, it may be best to utilize two sessions out of consideration to both patient comfort and recovery as well as operator fatigue. Surgical extraction, utilizing single whole quadrant mucogingival pedicle flaps, allows removal of bone and improves access to the root furcation area. This allows sectioning of multirooted teeth and complete removal of individual roots. The surrounding alveolar bone should also be effectively curetted and debrided to remove any rough spicular or inflamed tissue (Figure 20.4). Closure of flaps in a tension-free manner improves post-operative comfort markedly.

One study [157] did not see any marked difference between full mouth extraction (including canines and incisors) and extraction of cheek teeth only.

20.3.6 Post-Operative Management

Analgesia. Morphine and methadone are powerful analgesics for pre-medication and post-operative analgesia. Some reports mention dysphoria and occasional hyperthermia in cats post-operatively, and temperature measuring is wise. Regional analgesia using mepivacaine or bupivacaine/lidocaine is also effective in a multimodal regime. An NSAID, such as meloxicam, with due regard to the dose recommendations is also useful in addition to, but not instead of, opiates. Buprenorphine is considered good for moderate to severe pain in cats at 1 ml per 15 kg (0.3 mg/ml solution) every 8–12 hours. Owners can administer this analgesic very easily by mouth for transmucosal absorption if the correct dose is dispensed, pre-filled in 1 ml syringes for up to five days post-operatively and beyond if indicated.

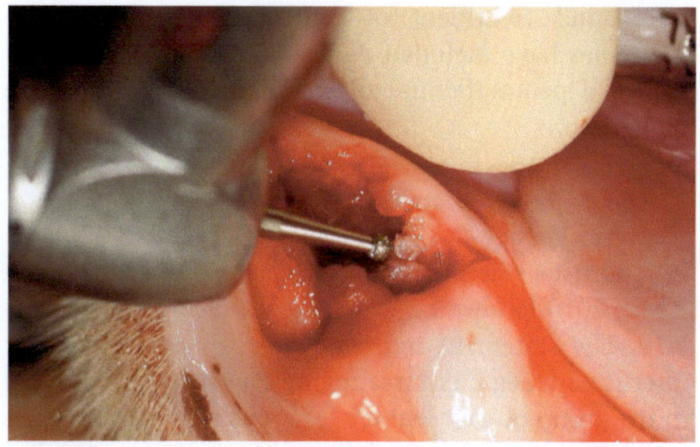

Figure 20.4 Effective alveoloplasty is an important step in removing all irritating tissues during caudal mouth extractions for FCGS.

Antibiotics. As the primary condition is a hyperimmune reaction to mixed oral antigen, antibiotics by themselves give minimal success. In the perioperative period, they will guard against opportunist infection and are often best started pre-operatively. The selected drug should have good activity in bone and on anaerobic bacteria. Clindamycin, potentiated amoxicillin, or Cefovecin (if oral administration is a problem) are the drugs of choice in most cases. Many *Pasteurella* species can be resistant to clindamycin but post-extraction it is a good choice as bone has been exposed.

Feeding. Nutritional assistance may be necessary in the short or medium term. In very severe cases it may be necessary to consider esophagostomy feeding or assisted oral feeding in the hospital. If fluid intake is suboptimal, this should also be addressed. Most cats do better at home if the owner is able to provide active help. Favorite soft and strongly flavored foods (pilchards in tomato sauce) may be necessary for three to five days post-operatively.

20.3.6.1 Other Anti-inflammatory or Immunomodulation Therapies

In the past there have been many drugs and alternative therapies advocated for this condition. Most have only anecdotal evidence to support them and/or the studies are based on very low case numbers. As a result, clinicians often find treatment of difficult cases frustrating. Therapies have included the use of minocycline, estrogen, and pentoxifylline, as well as the removal of the molar flap.

20.3.6.1.1 Feline Recombinant Interferon Omega (Virbagen, Virbac)

A consensus statement by a group of European specialists in 2010 followed a review of all the available literature. The statement indicated that feline recombinant interferon omega, as a treatment, is most effectively used in the group of cats that are FCV positive and are long-term non-responders to full mouth extraction. Studies appear to indicate that feline recombinant interferon omega equals or exceeds the potential of other treatments for this condition [158]. Long-term follow-up appears to indicate that it exceeds the potential of other treatments for this condition [159].

Results in a study of 39 cats [159] indicated that feline recombinant interferon omega is an effective treatment, particularly in the group of cats that are FCV-positive and are non-responders to elective tooth extraction. One of the author's own studies (NJ) over nine years confirm that feline recombinant interferon omega is able to reduce inflammation and improve comfort levels in the group of cats that are non-responsive to elective cheek teeth extraction[148].

Often the success of interferon allows clinicians to drop less effective treatment regimes. The trend is for oral administration by the owner in most cases. This is less expensive than injections, but it must be stressed to the owner that it may not be suitable for severe cases.

20.3.6.1.1.1 Transmucosal Oral Use Interferon given per os is believed to work by initiating a cytokine cascade when it comes into contact with cells providing an immunomodulatory effect over a long period of time. The cascade then has distant effects. It is the least expensive regime but does not work in all cases.

The contents of a 10 MU vial is reconstituted and injected into a 100 ml bag of sterile saline. Ten separate fractions of 10 ml are created, which are then frozen. When frozen they have a reported shelf life of one year. The first 10 ml fraction is used to give a dose of 1 ml per os per cat per day, resulting in a daily dose of 100 000 units of interferon. This fraction can be refrigerated normally and will have a shelf life of three weeks.

The owner continues to give 1 ml per day, alternating the side of the mouth used each day until all the fractions are used. Ideally, treatment lasts for 100 days, but longer oral administration may be required. After three months, the progress should be reassessed using the SDAI scoring system. Cats can be rechecked for FCV carriage in the oropharynx at this time.

20.3.6.1.1.2 Subcutaneous Injections In cases of severe inflammation, or when per os use has failed to provide resolution, the recommended regime by the manufacturer is subcutaneous injection. The dose is 1–2 MU/kg every other day for five doses, repeated after an interval of 21 days. This regime is much more expensive, relative to per os use, but likely to be more effective in refractive cases.

20.3.6.1.1.3 Intralesional Use The consensus statement in 2010 indicated that intralesional treatment is probably not necessary to initiate therapy. In some very severe cases, an initial treatment total dose of 5 MU injected locally into multiple sites at the junction between healthy oral mucosa and a diseased tissue can provide an initial boost to a treatment course. Using a 10 MU vial, enough saline or sterile water is drawn into the syringe to provide a reasonable volume for use – normally 1–2 ml depending on area to be injected. The contents are administered in fractions of 0.1–0.2 ml over the areas inflamed. Five injections are given in each side of 0.2 ml each.

20.3.6.2 Mesenchymal Stem Cell Therapy

There are promising reports of studies using mesenchymal stem cells (MSCs) [160]. These cells are found in fat, bone marrow, and other tissues and have a powerful ability to modulate innate and adaptive immunity by inhibition of T-cell proliferation, altering B-cell function, down-regulating MHC II, and inhibiting dendritic cell maturation and differentiation. Cells administered intravenously to a group of seven cats previously non-responsive to any treatment resulted in complete resolution of signs in five cats.

20.3.6.3 Glucocorticoids

This group of drugs are used to control inflammation in refractive cases that have had elective cheek teeth extraction and are not sufficiently controlled by feline recombinant interferon. Used as rescue therapy, their use is mainly justified on welfare grounds at the minimum effective dose rate. A short-acting molecule, such as prednisolone, at a dose rate of 5 mg twice weekly or 2 mg every other day tapering downwards, can be used in conjunction with feline recombinant interferon omega according to the manufacturer.

Transdermal prednisolone can be compounded to deliver 1 mg/kg in each 0.1 ml dose of ointment (e.g., for a 4 kg cat, each 0.1 ml will deliver 4 mg). Initially apply once daily into the inside of the pinna of the ear (alternate ears on alternate days and use gloves). Depending on the response, the dose can be decreased to an application every other day or by reducing the amount applied (from author AR).

20.3.6.4 NSAIDs

NSAIDs do not provide sufficient pain control or inflammation reduction on their own to justify their use as a monotherapy in one of the author's opinion (NJ). If used, the best option appears to be meloxicam with robenacoxib also reported as showing some promise. Any NSAID needs to be prescribed with due regard to the appropriate guidelines for use of long-term NSAIDs in cats [161].

20.3.6.5 Cyclosporine

Cyclosporine has been used to control the signs of FCGS, mainly in North America where feline recombinant interferon omega is not easily available. A study of 16 cats over 6 weeks [162] reported significant improvement in SDAI scores in most cats. The cats in this study did not receive a commercial product but a microemulsified liquid formulation compounded by a pharmacy using a tuna-flavored fish oil base. All but one owner managed to administer the medication easily.

Bioavailability of orally administered cyclosporine has been a challenge previously. In this study the microemulsified formula improved bioavailability but where trough whole blood levels of cyclosporine dropped below 300 ng/ml the oral dose had to be increased to obtain this level.

20.3.6.6 CO_2 Laser Surgery

There is not enough objective and peer reviewed data to recommend CO_2 laser use routinely in the management of FCGS. It may have a role in adjunctive pain control. One single cat case study concluded that the use of a CO_2 laser assisted recovery of soft tissues after extraction therapy but would not have been as useful as a monotherapy [163].

20.3.7 Nutritional Support

Good-quality nutritional support can encourage an effective immunological response and post-extraction healing process. Various diets and supplements have been suggested, including vitamin preparations and omega-3 polyunsaturated fatty acids (PUFA), but there is no study that has data to prove a recommendation for any specific product. Some cats receiving placebo treatment in the Lommer study showed an unexpected improvement, possibly due to the fish oil high in omega 3 PUFAs providing an anti-inflammatory and immunomodulatory effect. There is also anecdotal evidence that use of diets or supplements high in omega 3 EFAs affects platelet function and can result in excessive hemorrhage during extraction surgery.

20.4 Summary

FCGS is a poorly defined disease characterized by focal or a diffuse chronic inflammatory response involving the gingiva, oral mucosa, and frequently the pharynx, tongue, and other oral soft tissues.

The etiology is thought to be a complex result of reactions involving a number of factors including environmental, bacterial and an aberrant host response in combination with viral infection.

Studies show that bacterial population of the mouth is less diverse in affected cats and that certain bacteria (*Tannerella forsythia*) can influence the severity of the immune reaction. There is a correlation between the severity of clinical signs and the presence of putative pathogens, including FCV and *T. forsythia*. Opportunistic infections also play a role in influencing the disease process. The major difference between normal and diseased cats appears to be a hyperimmune response to the antigenic burden that is dental plaque with low levels of biofilm able to initiate a disproportionately high response in susceptible individuals.

Successful management of this FCGS requires a logical diagnostic approach. A treatment plan must start with improved oral hygiene including professional scaling, polishing, subgingival debridement, and attention to existing dental disease. The owner should be aware that aggressive home care will also be required.

Cases failing to respond to professional and high-level plaque control as a first-stage treatment should be considered for an elective cheek teeth extraction and adjunctive treatments at an early date. A systematic review of studies of FCGS management concludes that full-mouth or near full-mouth dental extractions is the current standard of care, though identifying a treatment protocol with higher remission rates is still needed [164]. Cases still non-responsive may be helped by immunomodulatory therapy, which may include daily oral interferon therapy. MSC treatment shows promise in a proof of concept study [160].

It is important that the owner is involved at an early stage with discussions as to prognosis, treatment plans, and help with home care. A highly motivated owner is a strong ally in the provision of successful treatment.

20.5 Feline Diseases Covered in Other Chapters

Chapter 5 – Periodontology. Feline inductive odontogenic tumor (FIOT), juvenile periodontitis.

Chapter 7 – Oral and Maxillofacial Tumors. FIOT, feline "epulides," primary intraosseous SCC, pyogenic granuloma, peripheral giant cell granuloma.

Chapter 8 – General Oral Pathology: Sialadenitis.
Chapter 9 – Anesthesia and Pain Management: Feline oral pain syndrome (FOPS).

20.6 Chronic Alveolar Osteitis, Alveolar Bone Expansion, and Abnormal Tooth Extrusion

In older cats, a common finding on examination may be the appearance of a bulbous expansion of the osseous tissues surrounding the maxillary canine teeth. The teeth often seem longer than normal due to abnormal extrusion. On radiographic examination, these teeth will frequently display regions of hypercementosis and replacement TR, as well as focal areas of vertical bone loss in advanced cases.

When a tooth moves beyond its normal occlusal height (extrusion), the distance between the AM and the CEJ increases. An alveolar margin and cementoenamel junction (AM-CEJ) distance of 2.5 mm or greater in the absence of horizontal or vertical bone loss will make this extrusion clinically apparent [63]. Histologically, it is thought that the alveolar bone expands by medullary fibrosis with mild to moderate pleocellular inflammation and modest proliferation of woven bone [62]. Most teeth examined had a distinct rim of peripheral sclerosis, consistent with an outward compression force of expansion [62]. Changes can also occur in premolars and molars, but with more variability in the type of osseous changes and inflammation (including gingival changes), which may make this region more challenging to recognize clinical alveolar bone expansion than at the canine teeth [63].

A more generalized syndrome encompassing alveolar bone expansion, hypercementosis with subsequent abnormal tooth extrusion, periodontal ligament degeneration, and root resorption has been proposed [63]. In an evaluation of cats with and without TR, the AM-CEJ distance was significantly greater in those with resorption. Thickening of cementum, beyond that considered normal physiological aging changes, was identified, with the most notable changes in the cervical region. Hypercementosis (cemental hyperplasia) was often associated with a decreased periodontal ligament space, and even the presence of cementicles (extensions of cementum into the PDL space) [63]. Cellular cementum was also found further coronally than previously reported [63]. A rapid and focally reparative cementum, cellular intrinsic fiber cementum, may help the tooth adjust to its new position.

Additional radiographic studies of periodontal disease in cats also identifies the expansile lesions, with 53% of cats having expansion of alveolar bone of at least one canine tooth [87]. Even in the 12 of 41 cats with normal alveolar bone height, the teeth were already displaying some degree of expansion [87]. Of the 11 (7%) of the cats with moderate to severe expansion, 10 of the 11 had severe vertical bone loss associated with the affected tissue.

Clinically speaking, each tooth should have a complete evaluation, including radiographs (from different angles to "map" the extent of changes), periodontal probing to discover any advanced vertical bone lesions in more severe cases, and tactile evaluation of mobility. Teeth with mild changes could be monitored with regular examinations and radiographs, but progression should be expected. Those teeth with moderate to severe changes should be considered for extraction, though typical labial/buccal gingival flaps can be very challenging as the soft tissues may be very thin. With the additional extrusion and possible mobility, simple elevation of the tooth is often successful. Closure of the site can be more challenging. Debridement of any marginal granulation tissue and alveolar rims, with gentle elevation of the gingiva and mucosa labially/buccally and palatally, will often provide enough release to carefully appose the edges with a cruciate suture pattern. The mandibular teeth can be gently rounded off with a white stone bur (odontoplasty with dentinal sealant) to minimize the trauma they can cause to the maxillary extraction site and upper lip.

20.7 Nasopharyngeal Polyps

Composed of fibrovascular connective tissue covered by stratified squamous or ciliated columnar epithelium, these benign, inflammatory polyps are thought to arise from the lining of the middle ear or Eustachian tube [165, 166]. If they extend into the pharyngeal region, respiratory signs such as stertor or nasal discharge may be present, while extension into the external ear canal would result in signs of otitis externa. The higher prevalence in young cats (three months) may be due to a congenital abnormality of the first pharyngeal pouch, from which the middle ear and Eustachian tube arise. Recognition of this disease in older cats (up to 15 years of age) could be the result of chronic inflammation of the middle ear, either due to respiratory inflammation or otitis [167]. Though no infectious agent has shown a consistent association with these polyps, the general inflammation is thought to result in mucociliary dysfunction and hypersecretion of mucus that give rise to a buildup of granulation tissue [167].

Respiratory signs such as dyspnea may be present and a ventral deviation of the soft palate may also be noted on oral examination in some cases. Head shaking, Horner's syndrome and even vestibular signs may be present with involvement of the middle and inner ear, with identification of a mass on otoscopic examination or ossification of the tympanic bulla evident on radiographs.

Polyps with no evidence of otic involvement may be simply retracted and avulsed, once accessed by rostral retraction of pulling of the soft palate. A midline soft palate incision is usually not necessary [168]. Gentle retraction of the polyp with Allis tissue forceps is carried out until the polyp detaches at the stalk. Minor hemorrhage may be controlled with pressure on the soft palate [169] and occasional complications of Horner's syndrome typically resolve in four weeks. Recurrence is possible (from 19 days to 9 months); prednisone given for four weeks may be helpful [170].

Polyps with evidence of otic involvement are generally best treated with ventral bulla osteotomy for better access of polyp retraction and complete removal, as well as debridement of the bulla. Horner's syndrome is even more common as a complication, but typically resolves [170], and recurrence of the polyp is decreased compared to traction/avulsion [169]. Severe cases may require total ear canal ablation, lateral bulla osteotomy, and resection or myringotomy, but this is infrequently required.

20.8 Viral Diseases with Oral Manifestations

20.8.1 Overview [171]

There are primarily three viral infections that have an impact on the oral cavity: FCV, FIV, and FeLV. FCV is a common viral respiratory disease of domestic and exotic cats characterized by upper respiratory signs, oral ulceration, pneumonia, and occasionally arthritis, or a highly fatal systemic hemorrhagic disease. FeLV is a retrovirus (Gammaretrovirus genus) that causes immunodeficiency and neoplastic disease in domestic cats. FIV is a retrovirus that causes an immunodeficiency disease in domestic cats. It is of the same genus (Lentivirus) as HIV, the causative agent of AIDS in humans.

FCV replicates primarily in the oropharynx and probably has a role in chronic gingivostomatitis and caudal mucositis [142]. Lingual ulceration in combination with nasal discharge and rhinitis is a common presentation. FHV typically affects the respiratory system and eyes. Other viruses in the cat that are more systemic and affect the immune system, such as FeLV and FIV, may predispose the individual to secondary oral infections.

20.8.2 Clinical Features Related to the Oral Cavity

FCV infection may present as an upper respiratory infection with eye and nose involvement, as an ulcerative disease primarily of the mouth, as pneumonia, as an acute arthritis, as a systemic hemorrhagic disease or any combination of these. There is typically a sudden onset and anorexia with ocular or nasal discharge with little or no sneezing. Ulcers on the tongue, hard palate, lips, tip of nose, or around claws may occur without other signs.

FeLV-infected cats may show indications of gingivitis, stomatitis, and periodontitis. Clinical signs of FeLV-induced immunodeficiency cannot be distinguished from those of FIV-induced immunodeficiency. Gingivitis, periodontitis, and stomatitis will be present in 25–50% of FIV-positive cats [172].

The American Association of Feline Practitioners classifies FHV, FPV, and FCV vaccines as core immunizations. Preventive measures include vaccinating all cats with these three agents on the initial visit (as early as six weeks of age). This is repeated every 3–4 weeks until 16 weeks of age, then boosters are given one year after that, and then every three years (AAFP Vaccination Guidelines: https://www.catvets.com/guidelines/practice-guidelines/feline-vaccination-guidelines).

There are no specific antiviral drugs that are effective against FCV, though broad-spectrum antibiotics can be given as appropriate for secondary bacterial infections. Some immunomodulatory or antiviral drugs can be used for FELV infections, but systemic glucocorticoids should be used with caution because of the potential for further immunosuppression. Cases of FIV-related gingivitis and stomatitis may be refractory to treatment. Use of antiviral, immunomodulatory, antimicrobial, and supportive therapy may be helpful. Antibacterial or antimycotic drugs may be useful for overgrowth of bacteria or fungi, though prolonged therapy or doses may be required. Management of secondary and opportunistic infections, as well as supportive care, are the primary consideration in cats infected with FeLV or FIV.

In cats with inflammatory oral disease, viral assessment is essential in determining the appropriate therapy and outcome. With FCV, oral ulcers and the acute arthritis usually heal without complications. Prognosis is excellent, unless severe pneumonia develops, though cats that recover are persistently infected for long periods and will continuously shed small quantities of virus in oral secretions. Of FeLV-infected cats, 50% succumb to related diseases within 2–3 years after infection. Within the first two years after diagnosis of FIV or 4.5–6 years after the estimated time of infection, about 20% of cats die, but 50% remain asymptomatic. In late stages of disease (wasting and frequent or severe opportunistic infections), life expectancy is about one year [172].

20.9 Eosinophilic Granuloma Complex (EGC)

Of the four syndromes within the EGC, two primary presentations may occur in the feline oral cavity, eosinophilic granulomas and indolent ulcers. These can have a genetic predisposition, thought to be a dysfunction of eosinophil regulation or due to hypersensitivity. Oral manifestations of the eosinophilic granuloma occur at the lip margin with chin swelling, giving the cat a "pouting" look, or as ulcerations of the tongue, palate, and palatal arches, which is sometimes painful [173]. Indolent ulcers are typically concave, indurated ulcers with a granular, orange-yellow color of the upper lip near the philtrum ("rodent ulcer"), and are rarely painful [173].

EGC lesions often wax and wane, and in eosinophilic granulomas with an inherited component (cats under two years of age) may spontaneously regress. An impression smear would reveal copious numbers of eosinophils, but histopathological examination is needed to distinguish between the syndromes. Atopy, flea bite, and food hypersensitivities have to be ruled out, and management may be effective. Treatment of flare-ups include immunosuppressive therapy at the lowest possible doses [173].

References

1 Reiter, A.M. and Mendoza, K.A. (2002). Feline odontoclastic resorptive lesions. An unsolved enigma in veterinary dentistry. *Vet. Clin. North Am. Small Anim. Pract.* 32: 791–837.
2 Girard, N., Servet, E., Biourge, V., and Hennet, P. (2008). Feline tooth resorption in a colony of 109 cats. *J. Vet. Dent.* 25: 166–174.
3 Berger, M., Stich, H., Hüster, H. et al. (2004). Feline dental resorptive lesions in the 13th to 14th centuries. *J. Vet. Dent.* 21: 206–213.
4 Hopewell-Smith, A. (1930). The process of osteolysis and odontolysis, or so-called "absorption" of calcified tissues: a new and original investigation. *Dental Cosmos.* 72: 1036–1048.
5 Reiter, A.M. (1998). Feline "odontolysis" in the 1920s – the forgotten histopathological study of feline odontoclastic resorptive lesions (FORL). *J. Vet. Dent.* 15: 35–41.
6 Reiter, A.M., Lewis, J.R., and Okuda, A. (2005). Update on the etiology of tooth resorption in domestic cats. *Vet. Clin. North Am. Small Anim. Pract.* 35: 913–942.
7 Dobbertin, F. (1993). Zur Pathologie der Zahn- und Zahnbetterkrankungen bei Felis silvestris forma catus. Dissertation, Hamburg University, Faculty of Human Medicine, Hamburg, Germany.
8 Gorlin, R.J., Barron, C.N., Chaudhry, A.P., and Clark, J.J. (1959). The oral and pharyngeal pathology of domestic animals. A study of 487 cases. *Am. J. Vet. Res.* 20: 1032–1061.
9 Wessum van, R., Harvey, C.E., and Hennet, P. (1992). Feline dental resorptive lesions. Prevalence patterns. *Vet. Clin. North Am. Small Anim. Pract.* 22: 1405–1416.
10 Builder, P.L. Opening paper; untitled.(1955). *Vet. Rec.* 67: 386–392.
11 Prescott, C.W. (1971). Some oral lesions in the cat. *Aust. Vet. J.* 47: 41–45.
12 Tekeli, Ö. (1973). Statistische Erhebungen über die Zahnkrankheiten bei der Katze. *Veteriner Fakultesi Dergisi.* 20: 157–167.
13 Berger, M., Schawalder, P., Stich, H., and Lussi, A. (1996). Differentialdiagnose von resorptiven Zahnerkrankungen (FORL) und Karies. *Schweiz Arch Tierheilk.* 138 (11): 546–551.
14 Kerebel, B. and Daculsi, G. (1971). Histologie et histopathologie dentaires du chat. *Science et Recherche Odontostomatologiques.* 7 (5): 29–32.
15 Harvey, C.E., Orsini, P., McLahan, C., and Schuster, C. (2004). Mapping of the radiographic central point of feline dental resorptive lesions. *J. Vet. Dent.* 21: 15–21.
16 Gorrel, C. (2015). Tooth resorption in cats: pathophysiology and treatment options. *J. Feline Med. Surg.* 17: 37–43.
17 Berger, M., Schawalder, P., Stich, H., and Lussi, A. (1995). "Neck Lesion" bei Grosskatzen; Untersuchungen beim Leoparden (*Panthera pardus*). *Kleintierpraxis.* 40: 537–549.
18 Ohba, S., Kiba, H., Kuwabara, M. et al. (1993). A histopathological study of neck lesions in feline teeth. *J. Am. Anim. Hosp. Assoc.* 29: 216–220.
19 Okuda, A. and Harvey, C. (1992). Etiopathogenesis of feline resorptive lesions. *Vet. Clin. North Am. Small Anim. Pract.* 22: 1385–1404.
20 Reichart, P.A., Dürr, U.-M., Triadan, H., and Vickendey, G. (1984). Periodontal disease in the domestic cat. A histopathologic study. *J. Periodontal Res.* 19: 67–75.
21 Schlup, D. and Stich, H. (1982). Epidemiologische und morphologische Untersuchungen am Katzengebiß. II. Mitteilung: Morphologische Untersuchungen der "neck lesions". *Kleintierpraxis.* 27: 179–188.
22 Shigeyama, Y., Grove, T.K., Strayhorn, C., and Somerman, M.J. (1996). Expression of adhesion molecules during tooth resorption in feline teeth: a model system for aggressive osteoclastic activity. *J. Dent. Res.* 75: 1650–1657.
23 DuPont, G.A. and DeBowes, L.J. (2002). Comparison of periodontitis and root replacement in cat teeth with resorptive lesions. *J. Vet. Dent.* 19: 71–75.
24 Okuda, A., Asari, M., and Harvey, C.E. (1995). Challenges in treatment of external odontoclastic resorptive lesions in cats. *Comp. Cont. Ed. Pract. Vet.* 17: 1461–1469.

25 Gengler, W., Dubielzig, R., and Ramer, J. (1995). Physical examination and radiographic analysis to detect dental and mandibular bone resorption in cats: a study of 81 cases from necropsy. *J. Vet. Dent.* 12 (3): 97–100.

26 Gorrel, C. and Larsson, A. (2002). Feline odontoclastic resorptive lesions: unveiling the early lesion. *J. Small Anim. Pract.* 43: 482–488.

27 Schneck, G.W. and Osborn, J.W. (1976). Neck lesions in the teeth of cats. *Vet. Rec.* 99: 100.

28 Hofmann-Lehmann, R., Berger, M., Sigrist, B. et al. (1998). Feline immunodeficiency virus (FIV) infection leads to increased incidence of feline odontoclastic resorptive lesions (FOLR). *Vet. Immunol. Immunopathol.* 65: 299–309.

29 Arx von, T., Schawalder, P., Ackermann, M., and Bosshardt, D.D. (2009). Human and feline invasive cervical resorptions: the missing link? Presentation of four cases. *J. Endodon.* 35: 904–913.

30 Farcas, N., Lommer, M.J., Kass, P.H., and Verstraete, F.J. (2014). Dental radiographic findings in cats with chronic gingivostomatitis (2002-2012). *J. Am. Vet. Med. Assoc.* 244: 339–345.

31 Zetner, K., Kampfer, P., Lutz, H., and Harvey, C.E. (1989). Vergleichende immunologische and virologische Untersuchungen von Katzen mit chronischen oralen Erkrankungen. *Wien Tierärztl Mschr.* 76: 303–308.

32 Thomas, S., Lappin, D.F., Spears, J. et al. (2017). Prevalence of feline calicivirus in cats with odontoclastic resorptive lesions and chronic gingivostomatitis. *Res. Vet. Sci.* 111: 124–126.

33 Okuda, A. and Habata, I. (1993). Lacunae or tubular structures in dentin of feline teeth. *J. Anim. Res. Found.* 2 (1): 7–14.

34 Negro, V.B., Hernandez, S.Z., Maresca, B.M., and Lorenzo, C.E. (2004). Furcation canals of the maxillary fourth premolar and the mandibular first molar teeth in cats. *J. Vet. Dent.* 21: 10–14.

35 Orsini, P. and Hennet, P. (1992). Anatomy of the mouth and teeth of the cat. *Vet. Clin. North Am. Small Anim. Pract.* 22: 1265–1277.

36 Winter, G.B. and Kramer, I.R.H. (1965). Changes in periodontal membrane and bone following experimental pulpal injury in deciduous molar teeth in kittens. *Arch. Oral Biol.* 10: 279–289.

37 DeLaurier, A., Boyde, A., Horton, M.A., and Price, J.S. (2005). A scanning electron microscopy study of idiopathic external tooth resorption in the cat. *J. Periodontol.* 76: 1106–1112.

38 DeLaurier, A., Boyde, A., Horton, M.A., and Price, J.S. (2006). Analysis of the surface characteristics and mineralization status of feline teeth using scanning electron microscopy. *J. Anat.* 209: 655–669.

39 Colley, P.A., Verstraete, F.J., Kass, P.H., and Schiffman, P. (2002). Elemental composition of teeth with and without odontoclastic resorption lesions in cats. *Am. J. Vet. Res.* 63: 546–550.

40 Lund, E.M., Bohacek, L.K., Dahlke, J.L. et al. (1998). Prevalence and risk factors for odontoclastic resorptive lesions in cats. *J. Am. Vet. Med. Assoc.* 212: 392–395.

41 Mestrinho, L.A., Runhau, J., Bragança, M., and Niza, M.M. (2013). Risk assessment of feline tooth resorption: a Portuguese clinical case control study. *J. Vet. Dent.* 30: 78–83.

42 Donoghue, S., Scarlett, J.M., Williams, C.A., and Saidla, J. (1994). Diet as a risk factor for feline external odontoclastic resorption. *J. Nutr.* 124: 2693S–2694S.

43 Scarlett, J.M., Saidla, J., and Hess, J. (1999). Risk factors for odontoclastic resorptive lesions in cats. *J. Am. Anim. Hosp. Assoc.* 35: 188–192.

44 Reiter, A.M., Lyon, K.F., Nachreiner, R.F., and Shofer, F.S. (2005). Evaluation of calciotropic hormones in cats with odontoclastic resorptive lesions. *Am. J. Vet. Res.* 66: 1446–1452.

45 Schlup, D. (1981). Epidemiologische und morphologische Untersuchungen am Katzengebiß. Dissertation, University of Bern, Faculty of Veterinary Medicine, Bern, Switzerland.

46 Zetner, K. (1990). Neck lesions bei der Katze. Diagnostisch-ätiologische Untersuchungen über Zusammenhänge zwischen Röntgenbefund und Fütterung. *Waltham Report.* 30: 15–23.

47 Zetner, K. and Steurer, I. (1992). The influence of dry food on the development of feline neck lesions. *J. Vet. Dent.* 9 (2): 4–6.

48 Crossley, D.A. (1991). Survey of feline dental problems encountered in a small animal practice in NW England. *Br. Vet. Dent. Assoc. J.* 2 (2): 3–6.

49 Ingham, K.E., Gorrel, C., Blackburn, J., and Farnsworth, W. (2001). Prevalence of odontoclastic resorptive lesion in a population of clinically healthy cats. *J. Small Anim. Pract.* 42: 439–443.

50 Burke, F.J.T., Johnston, N., Wiggs, R.B., and Hall, A.F. (2000). An alternative hypothesis from veterinary science for the pathogenesis of noncarious cervical lesions. *Quintessence Int.* 31: 475–482.

51 Johnston, N. (2000). Acquired feline oral cavity disease. Part 2: feline odontoclastic resorptive lesions. *In Practice.* 22: 188–197.

52 Muzylak, M., Price, J.S., and Horton, M.A. (2006). Hypoxia induces giant osteoclast formation and extensive bone resorption in the cat. *Calcif Tissue Int.* 79: 301–309.

53 Muzylak, M., Arnett, T.R., Price, J.S., and Horton, M.A. (2007). The in vitro effect of pH on osteoclasts and bone resorption in the cat: implications for the pathogenesis of FORL. *J. Cell. Physiol.* 213: 144–150.

54 DeLaurier, A., Allen, S., deFlandre, C. et al. (2002). Cytokine expression in feline osteoclastic resorptive lesions. *J. Comp. Pathol.* 127: 169–177.

55 Booij-Vrieling, H.E., Tryfonidou, M.A., Riemers, F.M. et al. (2009). Inflammatory cytokines and the nuclear vitamin D receptor are implicated in the pathophysiology of dental resorptive lesions in cats. *Vet. Immunol. Immunopathol.* 132: 160–166.

56 Arzi, B., Murphy, B., Cox, D.P. et al. (2010). Presence and quantification of mast cells in the gingiva of cats with tooth resorption, periodontitis and chronic stomatitis. *Arch. Oral Biol.* 55: 148–154.

57 How, K.L., Hazewinkel, H.A., and Mol, J.A. (1994). Dietary vitamin D dependence of cat and dog due to inadequate cutaneous synthesis of vitamin D. *Gen. Comp. Endocrinol.* 96: 12–18.

58 Morris, J.G. (1996). Vitamin D synthesis by kittens. *Vet. Clin. Nutr.* 3 (3): 88–92.

59 Morris, J.G. and Earle, K.E. (1999). Growing kittens require less dietary calcium than current allowances. *J. Nutr.* 129: 1698–1704.

60 Morris, J.G., Earle, K.E., and Anderson, P.A. (1999). Plasma 25-hydroxyvitamin D in growing kittens is related to dietary intake of cholecalciferol. *J. Nutr.* 129: 909–912.

61 Reiter, A.M.. (2004). The role of calciotropic factors in the etiology of feline odontoclastic resorptive lesions (FORL). Dissertation, University of Veterinary Medicine Vienna, Vienna, Austria.

62 Bell, C.M. and Soukup, J.W. (2015). Histologic, clinical, and radiologic findings of alveolar bone expansion and osteomyelitis of the jaws in cats. *Vet. Path.* 52: 910–918.

63 Lewis, J.R., Okuda, A., Shofer, F.S. et al. (2008). Significant association between tooth extrusion and tooth resorption in domestic cats. *J. Vet. Dent.* 25: 86–95.

64 Booij-Vrieling, H.E., Ferbus, D., Tryfonidou, M.A. et al. (2010). Increased vitamin D-driven signalling and expression of the vitamin D receptor, MSX2, and RANKL in tooth resorption in cats. *Euro. J. Oral. Sci.* 118: 39–46.

65 Girard, N., Servet, E., Hennet, P., and Biourge, V. (2010). Tooth resorption and vitamin D3 status in cats fed premium dry diets. *J. Vet. Dent.* 27: 142–147.

66 DeLaurier, A., Jackson, B., Ingham, K. et al. (2002). Biochemical markers of bone turnover in the domestic cat: relationships with age and feline osteoclastic resorptive lesions. *J. Nutr.* 132: 1742S–1744S.

67 Booij-Vrieling, H.E., de Vries, T.J., Schoenmaker, T. et al. (2012). Osteoclast progenitors from cats with and without tooth resorption respond differently to 1,25-dihydroxyvitamin D and interleukin-6. *Res. Vet. Sci.* 92: 311–316.

68 Verstraete, F.J., Kass, P.H., and Terpak, C.H. (1998). Diagnostic value of full-mouth radiography in cats. *Am. J. Vet. Res.* 59: 692–695.

69 Lüps, P. (1976). *Gebiß- und Zahnvariationen an einer Serie von 257 Hauskatzen (Felis silvestris f. catus L., 1758).*, vol. 34(11, 155–165. Dresden: Zoologische Abhandlungen Museum für Tierkunde.

70 Verstraete, F.J.M., Aarde van, R.J., Nieuwoudt, B.A. et al. (1996). The dental pathology of feral cats on Marion Island, part II: periodontitis, external odontoclastic resorption lesions and mandibular thickening. *J. Comp. Pathol.* 115: 283–297.

71 Aghashani, A., Kim, A.S., Kass, P.H., and Verstraete, F.J. (2016). Dental pathology of the California bobcat (*Lynx rufus californicus*). *J. Comp. Pathol.* 154: 329–340.

72 Berger, M., Schawalder, P., Stich, H., and Lussi, A. (1996). Feline dental resorptive lesions in captive and wild leopards and lions. *J. Vet. Dent.* 13: 13–21.

73 Cook, R.A. and Stoller, N.H. (1986). Periodontal status in snow leopards. *J. Am. Vet. Med. Assoc.* 189 (9): 1082–1083.

74 Mendoza, K.A., Manfra Marretta, S., and Klippert, L.S. (2000). Odontoclastic resorptive lesion of a mandibular right first molar in a cougar. *J. Vet. Dent.* 17: 173–176.

75 Pettersson, A. (2010). Tooth resorption in the Swedish Eurasian lynx (*Lynx lynx*). *J. Vet. Dent.* 27: 222–226.

76 Roux, P., Berger, M., Stich, H., and Schawalder, P. (2009). Oral examination and radiographic evaluation of the dentition in wild cats from Namibia. *J. Vet. Dent.* 26: 16–22.

77 Scheels, J.L. (1989). Periodontal disease associated with "feline cervical erosion" resulting in oronasal fistula and osteomyelitis in a Siberian tiger. *J. Vet. Dent.* 6 (3): 24.

78 Coles, S. (1990). The prevalence of buccal cervical root resorptions in Australian cats. *J. Vet. Dent.* 7 (4): 14–16.

79 DeLaurier, A., Boyde, A., Jackson, B. et al. (2009). Identifying early osteoclastic resorptive lesions in feline teeth: a model for understanding the origin of multiple idiopathic root resorption. *J. Periodontal Res.* 44: 248–257.

80 Schlup, D. (1982). Epidemiologische und morphologische Untersuchungen am Katzengebiß. *I. Mitteilung: Epidemiologische Untersuchungen. Kleintierpraxis.* 27: 86–94.

81 Frost, P. and Williams, C.A. (1986). Feline dental disease. *Vet. Clin. North Am. Small Anim. Pract.* 16 (5): 851–873.

82 Roes, F. (1996). Pathogenese, Diagnostik und Therapie bei "neck lesions" der Katze unter Verwendung von Glas-Ionomer-Zementen. Dissertation, Free University of Berlin, Faculty of Veterinary Medicine, Berlin, Germany.

83 Schweighart-Banzhaf, D. and Benz, C. (1997). "Resorptive lesions" bei der Katze. Eine klinische Untersuchung zur Versorgung mit "Dyract®". *Kleintierpraxis.* 42: 97–108.

84 Mihaljevic, S.Y., Kernmaier, A., and Mertens-Jentsch, S. (2012). Radiographic changes associated with tooth resorption type 2 in cats. *J. Vet. Dent.* 29: 20–26.

85 Heaton, M., Wilkinson, J., Gorrel, C. et al. (2004). A rapid screening technique for feline odontoclastic resorptive lesions. *J. Small Anim. Pract.* 45: 598–601.

86 Dobrescu, M.V. (1994). Nekrobazillose der Zähne bei der Katze. *Tierärztliche Umschau* 49: 498–501.

87 Lommer, M.J. and Verstraete, F.J.M. (2001). Radiographic patterns of periodontitis in cats: 147 cases (1998–1999). *J. Am. Vet. Med. Assoc.* 218: 230–234.

88 Pettersson, A. and Mannerfelt, T. (2003). Prevalence of dental resorptive lesions in Swedish cats. *J. Vet. Dent.* 20: 140–142.

89 Remeeus, P.G.K. (1991). Tandhalslaesies bij de kat. *Dier. en. Arts* 7: 223–226.

90 Holmstrom, S.E. (1992). External osteoclastic resorptive lesions. *Feline Practice* 20 (1): 7–11.

91 Lyon, K.F. (1990). Feline dental disease: treatment of subgingival resorption lesions. *J. Vet. Dent.* 7 (1): 13–14.

92 Debowes, L.J. (1994). Odontoclastic resorptive lesions in cats. *Waltham Focus.* 4 (1): 2–8.

93 Harvey, C.E. (1993). Feline dental resorptive lesions. *Sem. Vet. Med. Surg. Small Anim.* 8 (3): 187–196.

94 Legendre, L. (1996). Cervical line lesions: an update. *Can. Vet. J.* 37: 183–184.

95 Lyon, K.F. (1992). Subgingival odontoclastic resorptive lesions. Classification, treatment and results in 58 cats. *Vet. Clin. North Am. Small Anim. Pract.* 22: 1417–1432.

96 Harvey, C.E. and Flax, B.M. (1992). Feline oral-dental radiographic examination and interpretation. *Vet. Clin. North Am. Small Anim. Pract.* 22: 1279–1295.

97 Holmstrom, S.E. (1985). Surgical treatment for osteomyelitis with dental resorption. *Vet. Med.* 80: 48–49.

98 Kapatkin, A.S., Manfra Maretta, S., Patnaik, A.K. et al. (1991). Mandibular swellings in cats: prospective study of 24 cats. *J. Am. Anim. Hosp. Assoc.* 27: 575–580.

99 Lemmons, M. (2013). Clinical feline dental radiography. *Vet. Clin. North Am. Small Anim. Pract.* 43: 533–554.

100 DuPont, G.A. (2005). Radiographic evaluation and treatment of feline dental resorptive lesions. *Vet. Clin. North Am. Small Anim. Pract.* 35: 943–962.

101 Lommer, M.J. and Verstraete, F.J.M. (2000). Prevalence of odontoclastic resorption lesions and periapical radiographic lucencies in cats: 265 cases (1995–1998). *J. Am. Vet. Med. Assoc.* 217: 1866–1869.

102 Lang, L.G., Wilkinson, T.E., White, T.L. et al. (2016). Computed tomography of tooth resorption in cats. *Vet. Rad. Ultrasound.* 57: 467–474.

103 Roza, M.R., Silva, L.A., Barriviera, M. et al. (2011). Cone beam computed tomography and intraoral radiography for diagnosis of dental abnormalities in dogs and cats. *J. Vet. Sci.* 12: 387–392.

104 Vickendey, G. (1981). Klinische und histologische Untersuchungen am gingivoparodontalen Komplex der Katze. Dissertation, University of Hannover, Faculty of Veterinary Medicine, Hannover, Germany.

105 Ohba, S., Kiba, H., Kuwabara, M. et al. (1993). Contact microradiography analysis of feline tooth resorptive lesions. *J. Vet. Med. Sci.* 55: 329–332.

106 Gauthier, O., Boudigues, S., Pilet, P. et al. (2001). Scanning electron microscopic description of cellular activity and mineral changes in feline odontoclastic resorptive lesions. *J. Vet. Dent.* 18: 171–176.

107 Steinberg S. (2002). Histologische Untersuchungen zu Fruehveraenderungen der Felinen Odontoklastischen Resorptiven Laesionen (FORL) an klinisch gesunden Zaehnen. Thesis, Free University of Berlin, Faculty of Veterinary Medicine.

108 Girard, N., Servet, E., Biourge, V., and Hennet, P. (2009). Periodontal health status in a colony of 109 cats. *J. Vet. Dent.* 26: 147–155.

109 Roux, P., Berger, M., Stoffel, M. et al. (2005). Observations of the periodontal ligament and cementum in cats with dental resorptive lesions. *J. Vet. Dent.* 22: 74–85.

110 Eriksen, T., Koch, R., and Nautrup, C.P. (1994). Microradiography of the feline marginal periodontium with a microfocal high-resolution x-ray system. *Scand. J. Dent. Res.* 102: 284–289.

111 Keinath, G. (1997). Tierzahnheilkunde bei Katzen unter besonderer Beruecksichtigung der Aetiologie und Therapie von "Neck-Lesions". Thesis, Munich University, Faculty of Human Medicine.

112 Lyon, K.F. (1990). Feline dental disease - classification and treatment. *Vet. Focus.* 2 (1): 27–29.

113 Dicks, F. and Zöllner, W. (1988). Glas-Ionomer-Zement für einen praktikablen Einsatz in der Tierzahnheilkunde. *Praktischer Tierarzt.* 69 (11): 32–36.

114 Emily, P. (1989). Silver glass ionomer in the treatment of feline neck lesions. *Br. Vet. Dent. Assoc. J.* 2 (April): 2–3.

115 Floyd, M. (1991). External odontoclastic resorptive lesions in cats – another opinion. *J. Vet. Dent.* 8 (2): 22–23.

116 Golden, A.L. and Marretta, S.M. (1989). The use of ESPE Ketac®-Bond Aplicap for the restoration of cervical lesions. *J. Vet. Dent.* 6 (2): 5–7.

117 Mulligan, T.W. (1990). Feline cervical line lesions. *Vet. Med. Report.* 2: 343–349.

118 Zetner, K. and Steurer, I. (1995). Long-term results of restoration of feline resorptive lesions with micro-glass-composite. *J. Vet. Dent.* 12 (1): 15–17.

119 Dorenkamp, B. (1993). Zahnerkrankungen bei Katzen – Klassifizierung und Behandlung. *Biologische Tiermedizin.* 2: 40–45.

120 Anthony, J. (2001). The use of Nd:YAG laser for treatment of feline odontoclastic resorptive lesions. *J. Am. Anim. Hosp. Assoc.* 37 (Jan/Feb): 17–20.

121 Mohn, K.L., Jacks, T.M., Schleim, K.D. et al. (2009). Alendronate binds to tooth root surfaces and inhibits progression of feline tooth resorption: a pilot proof-of-concept study. *J. Vet. Dent.* 26: 74–81.

122 Harvey, C.E. (1991). External odontoclastic resorption lesions in cats – a treatable disease? *J. Vet. Dent.* 8 (1): 16–17.

123 Reiter, A.M. and Soltero-Rivera, M.M. (2014). Applied feline oral anatomy and tooth extraction techniques: an illustrated guide. *J. Feline Med. Surg.* 16: 900–913.

124 Foreest van, A. and tandheelkunde, Z.v.D.V. (1995). (10). Tandhalslaesies bij katten. Etiologie – Klinische diagnostiek – Therapie. *Tijdschrift voor Diergeneeskunde.* 120: 356–360.

125 Johnston, N. (1993). Feline dental disease – the neck lesion. *Br. Vet. Dent. Assoc. J.* 6 (1): 1–4.

126 Eisner, E. (1989). Chronic subgingival tooth erosions in cats. *Vet. Med.* 84 (4): 378–387.

127 Dupont, G. (1995). Crown amputation with intentional root retention for advanced feline resorptive lesions – a clinical study. *J. Vet. Dent.* 12 (1): 9–13.

128 DuPont, G.A. (2002). Crown amputation with intentional root retention for dental resorptive lesions in cats. *J. Vet. Dent.* 19: 107–110.

129 Zetner, K. (1994). Diagnosis, pathogenesis, and treatment of neck lesions in cats. *Vet. Q.* 16 (Suppl 1): 22S–24S.

130 Healey, K.A., Dawson, S., Burrow, R. et al. (2007). Prevalence of feline chronic gingivo-stomatitis in first opinion veterinary practice. *J. Feline Med. Surg.* 9 (5): 373–381.

131 Tenorio, A.P., Franti, C.E., Madewell, B.R., and Pedersen, N.C. (1991). Chronic oral infections of cats and their relationship to persistent oral carriage of feline calici, immunodeficiency or leukaemia virus. *Vet. Immunol. Immunopathol.* 29: 1–14.

132 Addie, D.D., Radford, A., Yam, P.S., and Taylor, D.J. (2003). Cessation of feline calici virus shedding coincident with resolution of chronic gingivostomatitis in a cat. *J. Small Anim. Pract.* 44: 172–176.

133 Dolieslager, S.M.J., Riggio, M.P., Lennon, A. et al. (2011). Identification of bacteria associated with feline chronic gingivostomatitis using culture dependent and culture independent methods. *Vet. Microbiol.* 148 (1): 93–98.

134 Dolieslager, S.M.J., Bennett, D., Johnston, N.W., and Riggio, M.P. (2013). Novel bacterial phylotypes associated with the healthy feline oral cavity and feline chronic gingivostomatitis. *Res. Vet. Sci.* 94 (3): 428–432.

135 Dewhirst, F.E., Klein, E.A., Bennet, M.L. et al. (2015). The feline oral microbiome: a provisional 16S rRNA gene based taxonomy with full-length reference sequences. *Vet. Microbiol.* 175 (2–4): 294–303.

136 Sturgeon, A., Pinder, S.L., Coast, M.C., and Weese, J.S. (2014). Characterisation of the oral microbiotica of healthy cats using next-generation sequencing. *Vet. J.* 201 (2): 223–229.

137 Harley, R., Helps, C.R., Harbour, D.A. et al. (1999). Intra-lesional cytokine mRNA expression in chronic gingivostomatitis in cats. *Clin. Diag. Lab. Immunol.* 6: 471–478.

138 Dolieslager, S.M., Lappin, D.F., Bennett, D. et al. (2013). The influence of oral bacteria on tissue levels of toll-like receptor and cytokine mRNAs in feline chronic gingivostomatitis and oral health. *Vet. Immunol. Immunopathol.* 151 (3–4): 263–274.

139 Anderson, J.G. (2003). Feline Gingivostomatitis complex. *Waltham Forum* 13 (3): 4–10.

140 Zetner, K., Kampfer, P., Lutz, H. et al. (1993). comparative immunological and Virological studies of chronic oral diseases in cats. *Europ. J. Companion Anim. Pract.* 3: 57–61.

141 Anderson, J.G., and Pedersen, N. (1996). Characterization of T-lymphocyte subsets in cats with chronic lymphocytic plasmacytic gingivitis stomatitis complex. In: *10th Annual Veterinary Dental Forum Proceedings*, Houston, Texas.

142 Knowles, J.O., Gaskell, R.M., Gaskell, C.J. et al. (1989). Prevalence of feline calicivirus, feline leukaemia virus and antibodies to FIV in cats with chronic stomatitis. *Vet. Rec.* 124: 336–338.

143 Thompson, R.R., Wilcox, G.E., Clark, W.T., and Jansen, K.L. (1984). Association of calicivirus infection with chronic gingivitis and pharyngitis in cats. *J. Small Anim. Pract.* 25: 201–210.

144 Harbour, D.A., Howard, P.E., and Gaskell, R.M. (1991). Isolation of feline calicivirus and feline herpes virus from domestic cats from 1980 to 1989. *Vet. Rec.* 128: 77–80.

145 Zicola, A., Saegerman, C., Quatpers, D. et al. (2009). Feline herpes virus 1 and feline calici virus infections in a heterogeneous cat population of a rescue shelter. *J. Feline Med. Surg.* 11: 1023–1027.

146 Hennet, P., and Boucrault-Baralon, C. (2005). Relationship between oral Calici virus and Herpes virus carriage and palatoglossitis lesions. In: *Proceedings of 19th Veterinary Dental Forum*, Orlando, FL. 443.

147 Knowles, J.O., McArdle, F., Dawson, S. et al. (1991). Studies on the role of feline calicivirus in chronic stomatitis in cats. *Vet. Microbiol.* 27: 205–219.

148 Johnston, N.W. (2012). An updated approach to chronic feline gingivitis stomatitis syndrome. *Vet. Pract.* 44 (5): 34–38.

149 Johnessee, J. and Huritz, A. (1983). Feline plasma cell gingivitis-pharyngitis. *J. Am. Ani. Hosp. Assoc.* 19: 179.

150 Anderson, J.G., and Pedersen, N. (1996). Clinicopathologic evaluation of lymphocytic plasmacytic gingivitis stomatitis complex in a multicat household. In: *10th Annual Veterinary Dental Forum Proceedings*, Houston, TX, October.

151 Anderson, J.G., Sollecito, T.P., Pringle, G.E. (2004). Histopathologic characterization of feline gingivostomatitis. In: Proceedings of *18th Veterinary Dental Forum*, Fort Worth, TX.

152 Anderson, J.G. (2006). Periodontal and radiographic findings in 100 cases of feline gingivostomatitis. In: *Proceedings of 20th Veterinary Dental Forum*, Portland, OR.

153 Kim, C.G., Lee, S.Y., Kim, J.W., and Park, H.M. (2013). Assessment of dental abnormalities by full mouth radiographs in small breed dogs. *J. Am. Anim. Hosp. Assoc.* 49 (1): 23–30.

154 Hennet, P. (1997). Chronic gingivostomatitis in cats: Long-term follow-up of 30 cases treated by dental extractions. *J. Vet. Dent.* 14: 15–21.

155 Girard, N., and Hennet, P. (2005). Retrospective study of dental extractions for treatment of chronic caudal stomatitis in 60 FCV positive cats. In: *Proceedings of 19th Veterinary Dental Forum*, Orlando, FL. 447.

156 Bellei, E., Dalla, F., Masetti, L. et al. (2008). Surgical therapy in chronic feline gingivostomatitis (FCGS). *Vet. Res. Commun.* 32 (Suppl. 1): S231–S234.

157 Jennings, M.W., Lewis, J.R., Soltero-Rivera, M.M. et al. (2015). Effect of tooth extraction on stomatitis in cats: 95 cases (2000–2013). *J. Am. Vet. Med. Assoc.* 246: 654–660.

158 Hennet, P., Camy, G., Privat, V., and McGahie, D. (2011). Comparative efficacy of a feline recombinant interferon omega in refractory cases of calici positive cats with caudal stomatitis: a randomised, multicentric controlled double blind study of 39 cats. *J. Feline Med. Surg.* 13 (8): 577–587.

159 Gracis, M. (2010). Controlled study using a modified 2 × 2 cross-over design to compare the efficacy of recombinant feline interferon omega and prednisolone in refractory feline chronic gingivostomatitis. In: *Proceedings of 19th European Congress of Veterinary Dentistry*, Nice, France. 192.

160 Arzi, B., Mills-Ko, E., Verstraete, F.J. et al. (2016). Therapeutic efficacy of fresh, autologous mesenchymal stem cells for severe refractory gingivostomatitis in cats. *Stem Cells Transl Med.* 5 (1): 75–86.

161 Sparkes, A.H., Heiene, R., Lascelles, B.D. et al. (2010). ISFM and AAFP consensus guidelines: long-term use of NSAIDs in cats. *J. Feline Med. Surg.* 12 (7): 521–538.

162 Lommer, M.J. (2013). Efficacy of cyclosporine for chronic refractory stomatitis in cats: A randomized, placebo-controlled, double blinded clinical study. *J. Vet. Dent.* 30 (1): 8–17.

163 Lewis, J.R., Tsugawa, A.J., and Reiter, A.M. (2007). Use of CO_2 laser as an adjunctive treatment for caudal stomatitis in a cat. *J. Vet. Dent.* 24 (4): 240–249.

164 Winer, J.N., Arzi, B., and Verstraete, F.J.M. (2016). Feline chronic gingivostomatitis: a systematic review of the literature. *Front Vet. Sci.* 3 (54): doi: 10.3389/fvets.2016.00054.

165 Reed, N. and Gunn-Moore, G. (2012). Nasopharyngeal diseases in cats. *J. Feline Med. Surg.* 14: 317–326.

166 Kudnig, S.T. (2002). Nasopharyngeal polyps in cats. *Clin. Tech. Small Anim. Pract.* 17 (4): 174–177.

167 Veir, J.K., Lappin, M.R., Foley, J.E., and Getzy, D.M. (2002). Feline inflammatory polyps: historical, clinical and PCR findings for feline calici virus and feline herpes virus – 1 in 28 cases. *J. Feline Med. Surg.* 4: 195–199.

168 Greci, V. and Mortellaro, M.C. (2016). Management of otic and nasopharyngeal, and nasal polyps in cats and dogs. *Vet. Clin. Small Anim.* 46: 643–661.

169 Anderson, D.M., Robinson, R.K., and White, R.A.S. (2000). Management of inflammatory polyps in 37 cats. *Vet. Rec.* 147: 684–687.

170 Anders, B.B., Hoelzler, M.G., Scavelli, T.D. et al. (2008). Analysis of auditory and neurologic effects associated with ventral bulla osteotomy for removal of inflammatory polyps of nasopharyngeal masses in cats. *J. Am. Vet. Med. Assoc.* 233: 580–585.

171 Lobprise, H.B. (2012). Oral manifestations of feline viral diseases. In: *Blackwell's Five-Minute Veterinary Consult Clinical Companion: Small Animal Dentistry*, 2e (ed. H.B. Lobprise), 389–396. Ames, IA: Wiley.

172 Barr, M.C. (2016). Feline immunodeficiency virus infection (FIV). In: *Blackwell's Five-Minute Vet Consult: Canine and Feline*, 6e (ed. L.P. Tilley and F.W.K. Smith), 500–501. Ames, IA: Wiley.

173 Werner, A.H. (2016). Eosinophilic granuloma complex. In: *Blackwell's Five-Minute Vet Consult: Canine and Feline*, 6e (ed. L.P. Tilley and F.W.K. Smith), 447–448. Ames, IA.: Wiley.

21

Small Mammal Oral and Dental Diseases

Loïc Legendre

Northwest Veterinary Dental Services Ltd, North Vancouver, British Columbia, Canada

21.1 Introduction

With the growing popularity of some of the "pocket-pets" and rabbits, astute practitioners must be aware of the challenges facing them due to the unique characteristics of rodents' and lagomorphs' oral cavity and dental structures. Being able to recognize normal variations and to assess any changes will help to adequately treat many conditions commonly encountered. Between the two groups, there are similarities and differences, as there are some differences among the various rodents. Where possible, the similarities will be discussed as a whole, while the differences will be pointed out as they are mentioned.

21.2 Patient Oral Assessment

As with any veterinary patient presented, an accurate history will cover the scope of past medical information and include specific items related to oral and dental disease. Any facts on past and present dental problems including treatment, dietary information, and chewing or eating habits can be beneficial. With the owner's assistance, an initial oral assessment can be made in the examination room, but the actual information gathered can vary remarkably depending on the patient's attitude, size, and species. External evidence of swelling, head symmetry, exudate drainage, and rostral malocclusion will be the first signs noted, if present. By gently lifting the lips, the gingivae and mucous membranes can be checked for color, hydration, capillary refill, or any evidence of swelling, discoloration, hemorrhage, ulceration, or recession. Any changes in the teeth, such as fractures, discoloration, plaque, calculus, caries, erosions, malocclusion, mobility, or developmental defects should be recorded. Although sometimes difficult to visualize, the examination should include the palate, floor of the mouth, and all tongue surfaces to check for ulcerations, injuries, tumors, and foreign bodies. Any evidence of epistaxis, halitosis, rhinitis, oral hemorrhage, and masticatory muscle problems should be recorded accurately, along with charting of all oral and dental findings (Figure 21.1) [1]. Charts for most of the common rodent and lagomorph patients are available in the text of Drs. Capello, Gracis, and Lennox [2].

In addition to the information collected during the initial examination and from the history, other oral diagnostics such as biopsies, cultures, transillumination, and radiographs may be utilized. All those will require the patient to be anesthetized or at least sedated. Extraoral radiographic surveys using No. 4 or No. 5 occlusal intraoral dental sensors or films may sometimes be supplemented by the intraoral use of size 0, 1, 2, or specific rodent films, such as modified size 3 film, in sedated patients using the bisecting angle techniques [3] (Figure 21.2). Other data, such as urine, blood, and fecal assays, may not be as helpful as in other species due to the sparseness of significant data to be gathered [4], as well as the difficulty of specimen collection, although urine and feces can sometimes be collected following examination from the table surface.

Complete physical examination of the oral cavity is therefore very important, though at times challenging. Restraint of smaller patients in towels or tubes [5–7], or by carefully grasping a rabbit by the scruff and supporting the hind legs, can help facilitate the assessment [5, 6, 8, 9]. The oral cavity is typically long and narrow, so the rostral portion is the only part readily accessible in the awake patient. Sedation or anesthesia is often necessary for complete examination [7, 9–11], although otoscopes with large cones, small vaginal speculum, and coffee stir sticks are helpful in the conscious patient [12].

Wiggs's Veterinary Dentistry: Principles and Practice, Second Edition. Edited by Heidi B. Lobprise and Johnathon R. (Bert) Dodd.

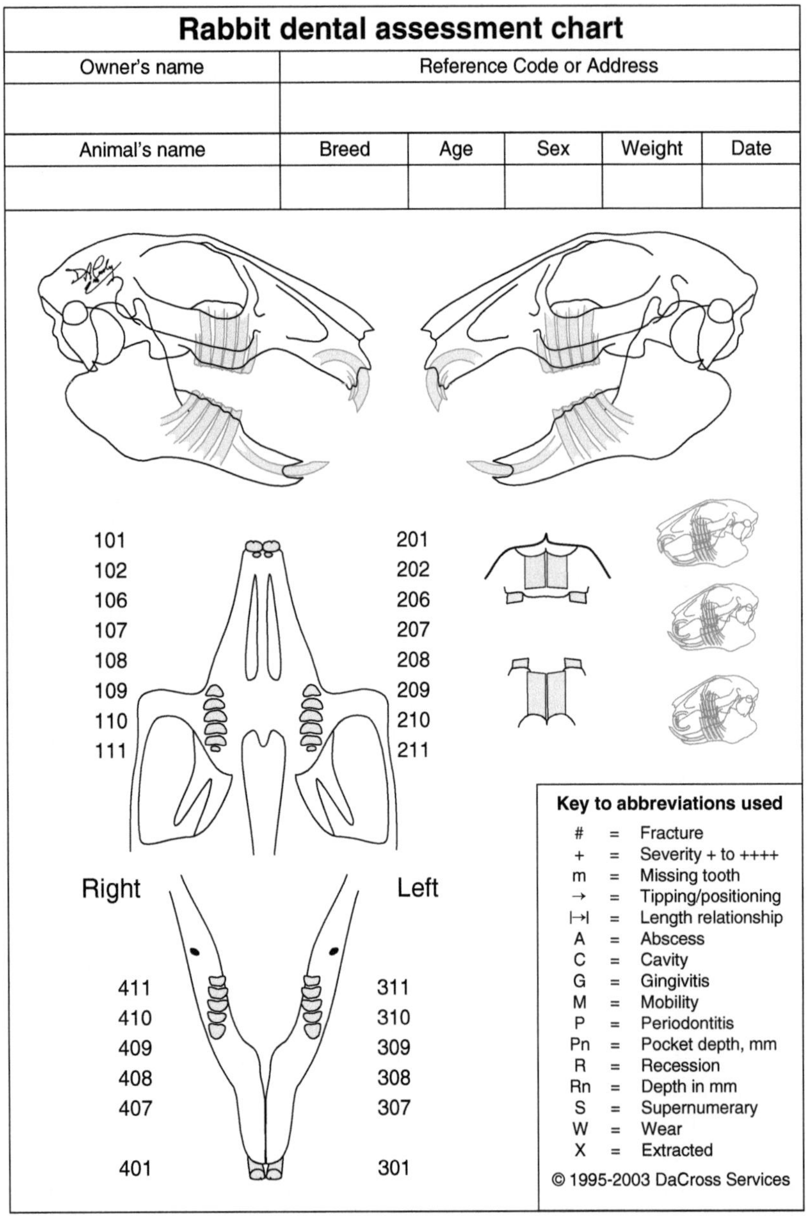

Figure 21.1 Rabbit dental chart. *Source:* Courtesy of David A. Crossley. Reprinted with permission.

21.3 Anesthesia

In rodents, ketamine hydrochloride is probably the most common injectable anesthetic used, although it requires some special considerations. In lagomorphs and other species, there is usually insufficient relaxation of the oral cavity with ketamine alone, so supplements of additional injectable or inhalant anesthesia can be used. Anesthetic depth is best monitored by respiration and jaw tension. Some baseline physiological parameters for a variety of small mammals is presented in Table 21.1 [6, 7, 13].

Care should be taken using injectable agents alone with rabbits because individual reactions to the drugs may be unusual, especially with barbiturates, where there is a very narrow range of safety [4, 5]. Pupil size and corneal or pedal reflexes are too unreliable to be used to monitor the depth of anesthesia, so again jaw tension and respiration should be closely observed [6, 7, 13]. Ketamine hydrochloride, commonly used, can provide a range from sedation to anesthesia at doses from 20 to 50 mg/kg intramuscularly (IM), but with poor muscle relaxation and analgesia [4–7, 10, 11]. There are many drug combinations available today to sedate rabbits and rodents. The author favors a "cocktail" of ketamine 10 mg/kg, alfaxalone 2 mg/kg, dexmedetomidine 10 mg/kg, and midazolam 0.2 mg/kg, all mixed into one syringe and given IM or SQ. The advantage of the mixture is that each drug is used at a low dose, minimizing

Dental procedures

Performed		Required
{ }	Pre-anaesthetic checks	{ }
{ }	General anaesthesia	{ }
{ }	Radiography	{ }
{ }	Occlusal assessment	{ }
{ }	Supra-gingival scaling	{ }
{ }	Subgingival scaling	{ }
{ }	Root planing	{ }
{ }	Polishing	{ }
{ }	Gingival lavage	{ }
{ }	Gingival surgery	{ }
{ }	Extraction	{ }
{ }	Periodontal splinting	{ }
{ }	Crown height reduction	{ }
{ }	Endodontic therapy	{ }
{ }	Restoration	{ }
{ }	Orthodontic treatment	{ }
{ }	Oro-facial surgery	{ }
	Homecare program	{✓}

Assessment by quadrant

(graded +, ++, +++, ++++)

	1 (RU)	2 (LU)	3 (LL)	4 (RL)
Plaque	:	:	:	:
Calculus	:	:	:	:
Gingivitis	:	:	:	:
Periodontitis	:	:	:	:
Occlusion	:	:	:	:
Tooth wear	:	:	:	:

Other comments

Routine Home Dental Care

Herbivores naturally wear their teeth by prolonged chewing. To compensate for this the teeth continue erupting. If they do not have enough natural food the teeth get longer and develop sharp spikes which injure the cheeks and tongue. Chewing exercise is also beneficial as it stimulates natural tooth cleaning and protection mechanisms. In general hard and artificial chewing objects are not a good idea as many animals damage their teeth and gums on them, and swallowed pieces can cause serious problems.

Provide the bulk of the diet as growing grass or hay. Avoid feeding soft sticky foods and never give items containing sugar or oil/fat.

Specific Instructions

Figure 21.1 (Continued)

the chances of harmful side effects. The other advantage of this combination is that dexmedetomidine can be reversed with an equal volume of atipamazole and midazolam can be reversed with flumazenil given at 0.1 mg/kg. The reversal allows the patient to recover quickly and safely. If the patient is somewhat debilitated (which is often the case), a combination of butorphanol 0.2 mg/kg, alfaxalone 2 mg/kg, and midazolam 0.2 mg/kg, all in one syringe, can be given IM or SQ. If needed, one can always top up with more alfaxalone. Monitor the patient carefully as alfaxalone may cause apnea. It is always best to have the patient intubated.

As with most work in the oral cavity, intubation is ideal, but with untrained personnel this can be difficult and even traumatic with the small oral opening and lateral skin folds. Use of topical anesthetics to control laryngospasms should be restricted [13]. Three techniques are available. (i) Blind intubation, where the patient is in the sternal position with its head extended upward. The small uncuffed tube is inserted slowly with the ear of the operator close to the end of the tube. Air movement can be heard; on inspiration the tube is dropped into the entrance of the trachea. This technique is sometimes much easier to describe than to perform. (ii) Stylet guided intubation, where a stiff bendable internal tube guide is inserted into the trachea and the endotracheal tube is slid over the guide (Figure 21.3a,b). This is certainly a versatile technique that does not require lots of extra equipment. (iii) Endoscope guided intubation, where a small (1.9–2.7 mm diameter) rigid endoscope is used to push

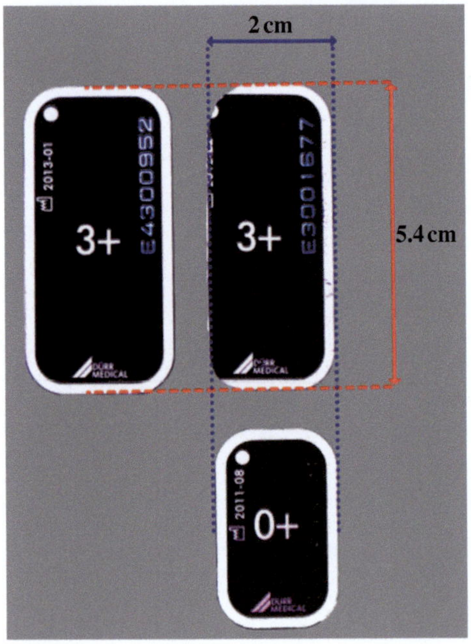

Figure 21.2 Examples of phosphoric sensor plates designed to fit intraorally in rabbits to allow detailed imaging of maxillary and mandibular cheek teeth. With permission of Drs. Regalado and Legendre JVD 2017.

Table 21.1 Baseline physiological data [6, 7, 11, 13].

	Life span mean (years)	Respiration (per minute)	Heart rate (per minute)	Body temperature (Celsius)	PVC (%)	BUN (mg/ dl)
Chinchilla	8–10	40–65	40–100	36.1–37.8	27–54	17–45
Gerbil	2–4	70–120	260–600	38.1–38.4	35–45	17–27
Guinea pig	4–5	42–104	230–380	37.2–39.5	35–45	9.0–31.5
Hamster	1 1/2-3	35–135	250–500	37.0–38.4	45–49.8	12–26
Mouse	1 1/2-3	94–163	325–780	35.5–38.0	35–40	17–28
Rabbit	5–6	32–60	130–325	38.0–39.6	30–50	17–23.5
Rat	2–4	70–115	250–450	35.9–37.5	35–45	15–21

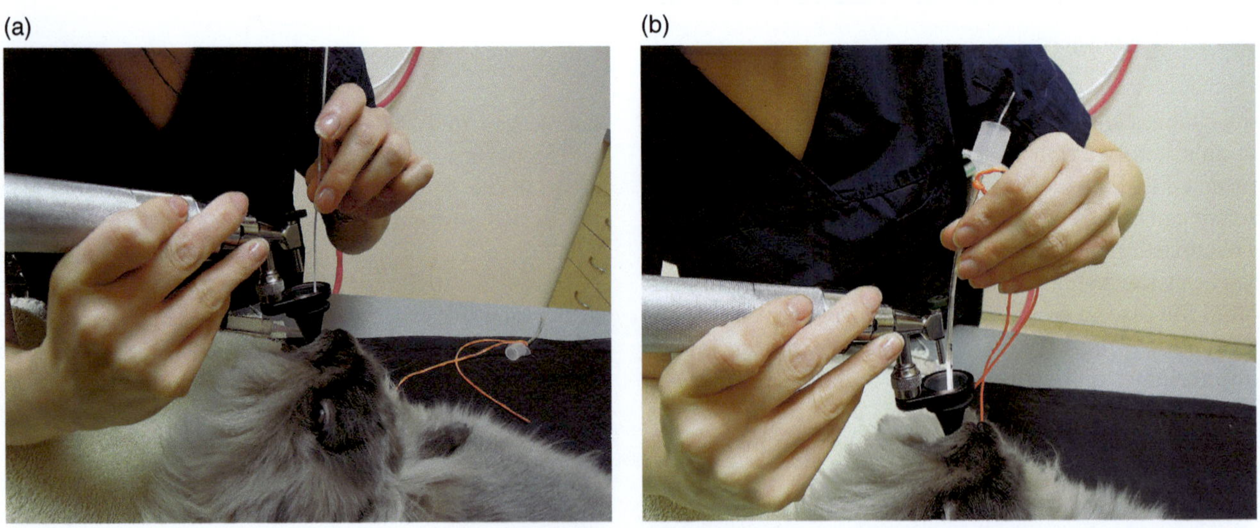

Figure 21.3 (a) Intubation of a rabbit using a stylet guide. The stylet is introduced into the trachea using a large cone otoscope. (b) The endotracheal tube is then slid over the stylet down the trachea and tied into place.

the tongue ventrally, to visualize the tracheal opening, and to serve as a guide for the endotracheal tube. It is the nicest technique but requires an endoscope. A fairly recent paper describes how to intubate GP on their back, using an otoscope cone cut in half lengthwise [14]. For very short procedures where intubation can be avoided, IV induction can be followed by masking with isoflurane or sevoflurane. The induction drugs are then reversed to allow a quick recovery. Respiratory assistance can be provided with a straw or eye dropper placed into the back of the mouth and blowing into the trachea. External cardiac massage with rapid, light digital pressure application to the ribs behind the forelegs can provide some cardiopulmonary resuscitation (CPR) effects.

21.4 Anatomy

Even with excellent techniques of examination and visualization, whether sedated or not, the practitioner must be familiar with the normal anatomy and physiology of the patient being treated. The dentition is a primary reason rodents and lagomorphs were first placed into a similar classification, and later separated [15].

The Latin verb "rodere" means "to gnaw," a reference primarily to the prominent incisors and the fact that most are herbivores, although some rat species are omnivorous [16]. The *Rodentia* order is the largest order of mammals, with a wide variety of species from mice, rats, Guinea pigs, gophers, beavers, chinchillas, nutria, and many more. The *Lagomorpha* order, on the other hand, is quite small, consisting principally of the *Leporidae* family with rabbits, hares, cottontails, and pikas. Of all rodents and lagomorphs, the patients most commonly seen by veterinarians are domestic rabbits, Guinea pigs, and chinchillas, but the occasional "wild" cousin may be of need of dental assistance [17]. Both rodents and lagomorphs have a heterodont dentition, with the varying tooth shapes of incisors, premolars, and molars [17]. Rabbits and hares possess very temporary deciduous teeth (probably non-functional), which place them in a diphyodont classification [18]. The rabbit's deciduous teeth start exfoliating, possibly even before birth, with the tips of the maxillary incisors present at that time, and total replacement by three to five weeks of age [19]. In rodents there has also been a claim that Guinea pigs have deciduous teeth [20], but these may be fetal in nature and non-functional [19]. The question of functionality of these teeth and whether they are fetal or true deciduous teeth appears to be pivotal in the decision of their classification by anatomists. Other variations in both rodent and lagomorph dentition indicate the general lack of in-depth research into the area.

The dental formula of rodents can vary from 2× (I 1/1; C 0/0; P 0/0; M 3/3) = 16 in the *Cricetid* rats to 2× (I 1/1; C 0/0; P 1-2/1; M 3/3) = 20 or 22 in *Sciuridae* squirrels. The presence of four incisors, no cuspids, few to no premolars, 8–12 molars and a large diastema between the incisors and cheek teeth are the common traits (Table 21.2).

The primary difference of the lagomorph dentition is the presence of a total of four maxillary incisors as compared to two in rodents, as well as additional premolars [6, 13]. The most widely accepted dental formula for rabbits is 2× (I 2/1; C 0/0; P 3/2; M 3/3) = 28 (Table 21.3) [5, 21–23]. At least one author notes a possible variation in the number of maxillary molars (either two or three are possible, for a total count of 26–28) [8], which may be due to the last set of molars being exceptionally small and potentially difficult to visualize.

Table 21.2 Dental formulas for rodents [8, 10, 19, 20].

Hamster (*Mesocricetidae*)	2× (I 1/1, C 0/0, P 0/0, M 2–3/2–3) = 12–16
Old World rats and mice (*Muridae*)	2× (I 1/1, C 0/0, P 0/0, M 2–3/2–3) = 12–16
Rats and mice (*Cricetidae*)	2× (I 1/1, C 0/0, P 0/0, M 3/3) = 16
Gerbil (*Merionidae*)	2× (I 1/1, C 0/0, P 0/0, M 3/3) = 16
Guinea pig (*Cavidae*)	2× (I 1/1, C 0/0, P 1/1, M 3/3) = 20
Chinchillas (*Chinchillidae*)	2× (I 1/1, C 0/0, P 1/1, M 3/3) = 20
Capybara (*Hydrochoeridae*)	2× (I 1/1, C 0/0, P 1/1, M 3/3) = 20
Nutria (*Capromyidae*)	2× (I 1/1, C 0/0, P 1/1, M 3/3) = 20
Old World porcupines (*Hystricidae*)	2× (I 1/1, C 0/0, P 1/1, M 3/3) = 20
New World porcupines (*Erethizontidae*)	2× (I 1/1, C 0/0, P 1/1, M 3/3) = 20
Beavers (*Castoridae*)	2× (I 1/1, C 0/0, P 1/1, M 3/3) = 20
Squirrels (*Sciuridae*):	2× (I 1/1, C 0/0, P 1–2/1, M 3/3) = 20–22

Table 21.3 Dental formula for lagomorphs [7, 8, 13, 18, 22].

Pika Permanent teeth	2× (I 2/1, C 0/0, P 3/2, M 2/3) = 26
Rabbits (*Oryctolagidae*) Deciduous teeth	2× (I 2/1, C 0/0, P 3/2, M 0/0) = 16
Rabbits Permanent teeth	2× (I 2/1, C 0/0, P 3/2, M 2–3/3) = 26–28
Hares (*Lepidae*) Deciduous teeth	2× (I 1/0, C 0/0, P 3/2, M 0/0) = 12
Hares Permanent teeth	2× (I 2/1, C 0/0, P 3/2, M 3/3) = 28

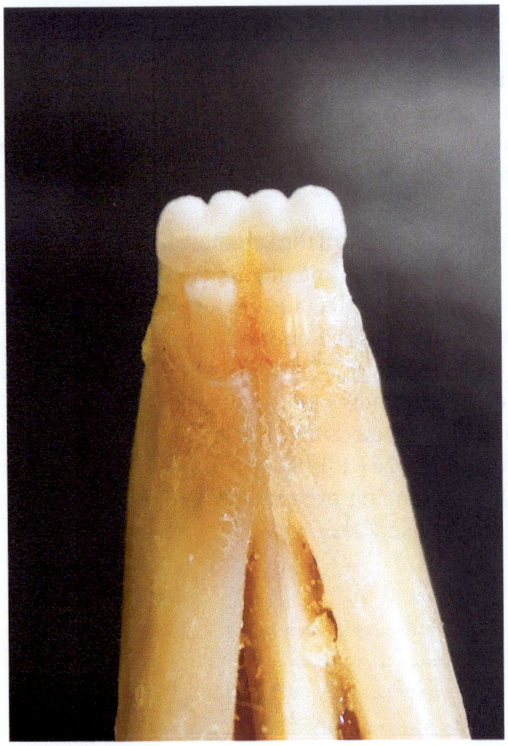

Figure 21.4 Example of duplicidentata (note the peg teeth present in a rabbit maxilla).

The standard single row of maxillary incisors in rodents is known as simplicidentata, or simple dentition [24]. In lagomorphs, the location of the two smaller rudimentary maxillary incisors (peg teeth) [21] directly caudal/palatal to the two large grooved incisors is a double row dentition or duplicidentata (Figure 21.4). The large incisors of both groups are continuously growing and considered to be aradicular hypsodonts, which means long-crowned without a true root structure [25]. The exposed or clinical crown is the supragingival portion, while the reserve crown is subgingival, and combined, they form the anatomical crown. The submerged segment is sometimes called the clinical root, but it is not a true root structure, though using the term open-rooted is acceptable for these teeth. This can be contrasted with equine teeth, which are radicular hypsodonts or rooted, long-crowned teeth, with distinct roots that eventually mature into a closed-root structure [18, 26]. These also have a subgingival reserve crown portion that continues to erupt (not grow) in a coronal direction as the exposed crown is worn away.

All lagomorph cheek teeth and caviomorph rodent (chinchilla, Guinea pig) molars are also aradicular hypsodonts. Most of the other rodents, such as rats, mice, hamsters, and gerbils, have premolars and molars that are brachyodont (short-crowned, closed roots) that do not continuously grow or erupt. With the aradicular hypsodont incisors, these latter individuals have a mixed dental crown classification, as compared to a mixed dentition (both deciduous and permanent counterparts present at the same time).

The continuously growing teeth have some interesting characteristics that fit well with their form and function. To begin with, in the periodontal ligament in rodent teeth (and in developing human teeth), there is an intermediate group of collagen fibers that attach either to the alveolar bone or cementum, not both, with splicing in between. This intermediate plexus differs from the traditional view of ligament fibers running the entire distance from bone to tooth, and may provide a more suitable mechanism by which continually growing or erupting teeth can have extensive tooth movement using this middle zone [27, 28].

Enamel on the incisors of both rodents and lagomorphs is thickest on the facial/labial surfaces, thinning as it extends on to the distal and mesial surfaces, and is nearly non-existent on the lingual aspect, which is covered with softer dentin and some cementum [29]. This configuration of dental hard tissue promotes a wearing pattern that results in a sharp, chisel-like tooth [23]. In the rabbit, the large maxillary incisors grow at a rate of 2.0 mm per week, while the mandibular incisors grow 2.4 mm per week rostromesially. Apparently, there is a faster attrition rate, typically due to dietary influences alone, of the lower incisors to compensate for the difference [21, 22, 30, 31]. Incisor teeth of the chinchilla may grow as much as 6–8 cm per year [32] and are yellow-orange in color, as are most mature rodent incisors.

The position of the most apical portion of incisors may vary, depending on the animal. Rat maxillary incisors extend for two-thirds of the diastema, while the mandibular incisors reach distal to the last molar. The maxillary incisors of hamsters reach to one-half to two-thirds of the diastema (mice up to three-quarters), and are level to or distal to the last molar for the mandibular incisors. Guinea pigs have maxillary incisors that end near the mesial aspect of the first cheek tooth, with their mandibular counterparts traveling lingually and to the level of the second cheek tooth. Chinchilla maxillary incisors reach to one-half of the diastema, and the mandibular incisors to the first or second cheek teeth (Figure 21.5). Lagomorph maxillary incisors extend for one-third of the diastema and the mandibular incisors reach the mesial surface of the first cheek tooth (Figure 21.6).

In rabbits, mastication is typically performed in a lateral, scissor-like fashion due to a horizontal oral mandibular fossa of the TMJ. The mandibular incisor cuts back and forth in between the peg teeth and the larger maxillary incisors [8]. The lateral grinding movement is facilitated in the caudal teeth with a flat occlusal surface and deep transverse enamel folds [31, 33].

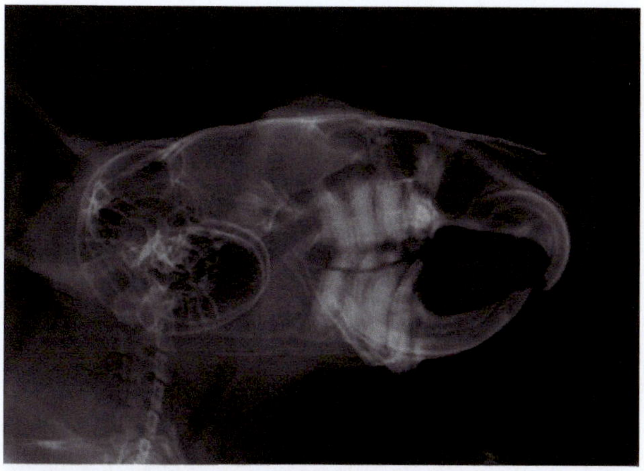

Figure 21.5 Lateral X-ray of a chinchilla skull showing the maxillary incisors reaching one-half of the diastema and the mandibular incisors extending to the third cheek tooth.

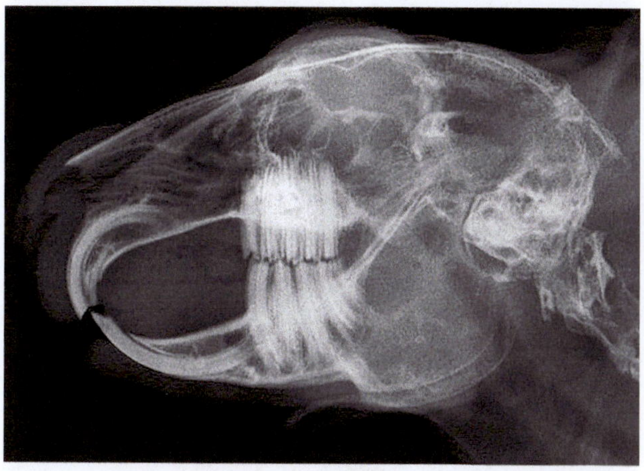

Figure 21.6 Lateral X-ray of a rabbit skull showing the maxillary incisors reaching one-third of the diastema and the mandibular incisor extending to the mesial surface of the first cheek tooth.

Rabbits also differ from caviomorph rodents in that they possess more cheek teeth (six in the maxilla and five in the mandible). The uneven number of cheek teeth in the maxilla and mandible creates a specific occlusion where each cheek tooth from one arcade contacts two cheek teeth from the opposite arcade (Figure 21.7). These points become important when one considers extracting a cheek tooth. Other structures of interest in the oral cavity of rabbits and Guinea pigs is the significant medial folding of skin near the diastema, which separates the rostral mouth from the caudal mouth, thereby permitting separate functions of the incisors and cheek teeth and limits visualization of the oral cavity [4, 8]. Golden hamsters have internal cheek pouches, while some other rodents have external, fur-lined cheek pouches found near the oral opening [34].

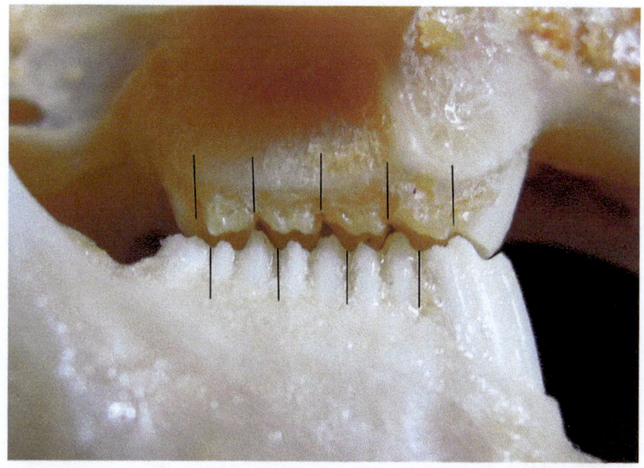

Figure 21.7 A close-up view of a rabbit cheek teeth showing that one tooth touches 2 of the opposite arcades with 6 teeth on the maxilla and 5 on the mandible.

21.5 Malocclusion

With the continually growing nature of lagomorph and rodent incisors (and some molars), it should be readily evident that any disruption in the normal attrition sequence can lead to significant problems with overgrowth [6, 13, 21]. The most common dental problem in rodents [34] and lagomorphs [6, 13, 22, 35] alike is malocclusion. It is also the most common genetic problem in rabbits [11, 22, 36]. These malocclusions are typically classified into atraumatic and traumatic.

21.5.1 Atraumatic

Atraumatic malocclusion results from genetic malpositioning of teeth or dietary causes of insufficient attrition [11, 17, 34]. Rabbits as young as three weeks of age may exhibit mandibular incisors that are level to or even extend labial to their maxillary counterparts [5, 11, 21]. It is typically considered that an autosomal recessive gene for a shortened maxillary diastema is the probable cause [4, 6, 8, 9, 13, 33]. The mechanism of abnormal growth of the dorsal and basal skull bones that give the appearance of a longer mandible [33] may be compared to brachiocephalic conditions in some animals or a Class III malocclusion in man [37]. Dwarf breeds seem to be most affected.

If the teeth continue to grow without proper occlusive wear, the maxillary incisors start to curl or twist in the mouth and at times have been known to penetrate into the skull if left untreated, whereas the mandibular incisors grow into the upper lip and the nostrils [5, 11] (Figure 21.8a,b). Once the incisors are overgrown, the animal cannot eat properly, may drop its food (quidding), traumatize its tongue, and salivate excessively (ptyalism or "slobbers"),

(a) (b)

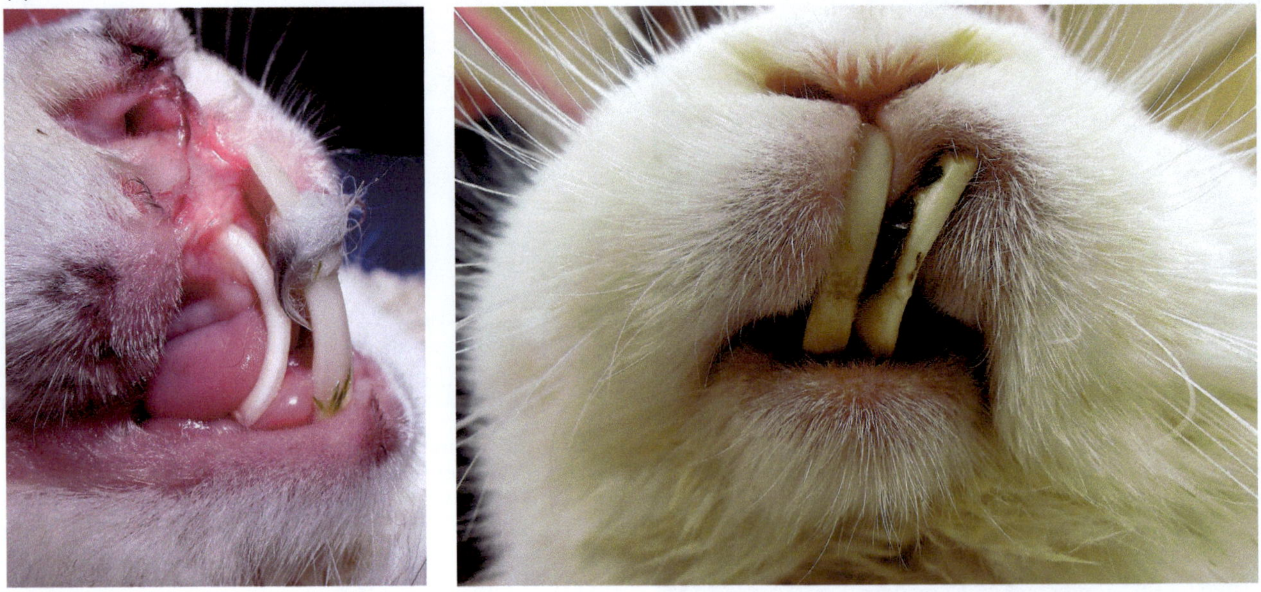

Figure 21.8 (a) The elongated maxillary incisors curl into the oral cavity and if left unchecked can penetrate the palate. (b) The elongated mandibular incisors are less curved and end up labial to the maxillary; unchecked they will grow into the soft tissues of the nose.

(a) (b)

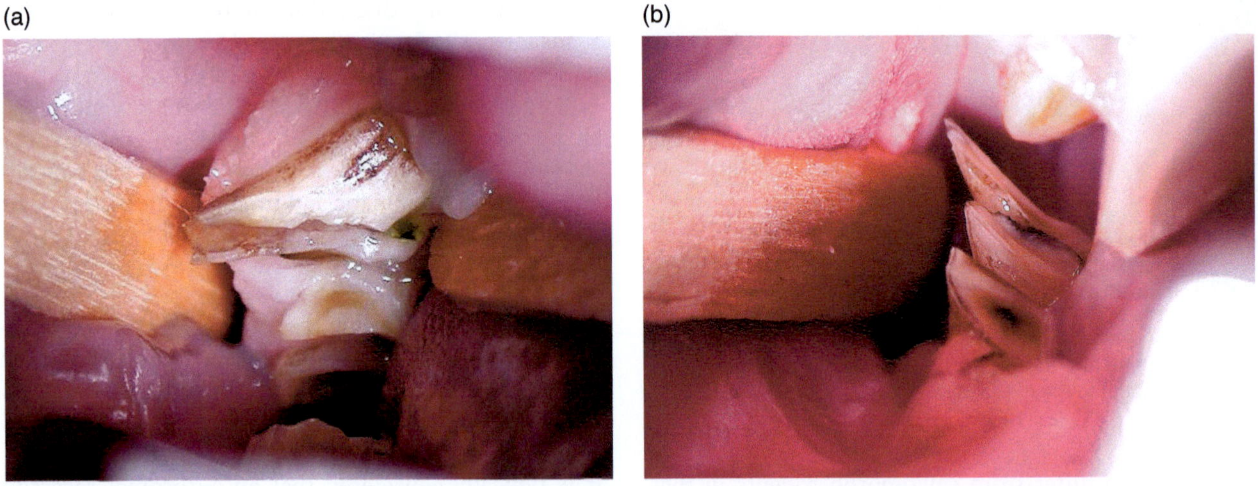

Figure 21.9 (a) With elongation of the rabbit maxillary cheek teeth, there is concurrent formation of buccal spurs that can easily cut into the oral mucosa of the cheeks. (b) Similarly, in the mandible, elongation of the cheek teeth is often accompanied with formation of lingual spurs that can cut into the sides of the tongue.

which can lead to wet dewlap (moist dermatitis) in rabbits [6, 8, 13, 36]. Excessive overgrowth may cause the maxillary incisors to penetrate into the sinuses or ocular sockets. Malocclusion and overgrowth of the incisors with failure to properly close the mouth can further lead to molar overgrowth and malocclusion in rabbits and rodents with aradicular hypsodont cheek teeth [5, 8]. If untreated, maxillary molars may flare outward, lacerating the buccal mucosa, while the mandibular molars overgrow lingually, potentially trapping the tongue either ventrally or dorsally.

If the incisors are normal, by far the most common reason for malocclusion is primary elongation of cheek teeth due to a poor dental diet. In the process of lengthening, the cheek teeth also deviate. The maxillary cheek teeth tip buccally and the mandibular cheek teeth tip lingually. In the rabbit, you can see maxillary buccal spurs cutting into the cheek and mandibular lingual spurs cutting into the tongue (Figure 21.9a,b). The deviation is permanent and even with regular teeth trimmings, the patient will never come back to normal. This condition is now referred to as acquired dental disease (ADD) [38–40].

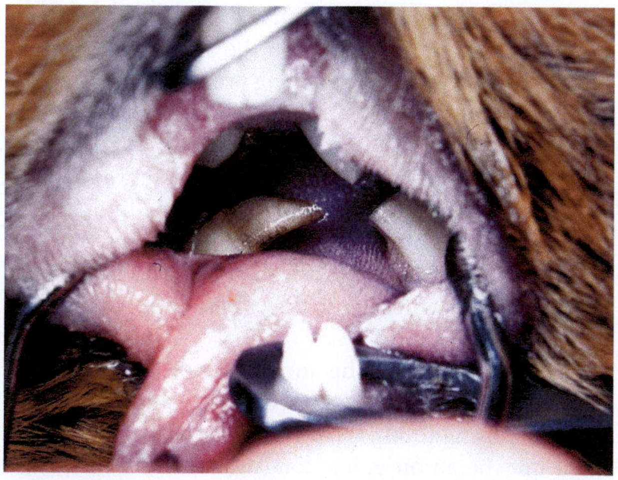

Figure 21.10 In the Guinea pig, because of the angle of the mandibular cheek teeth, elongation creates an arch under which the tongue is trapped. This prevents deglutition and the patient presents unable to swallow.

In the Guinea pig, you see continued curving of the mandibular cheek teeth, forming a bridge and trapping the tongue below (Figure 21.10). Once the tongue is trapped, the patient is unable to swallow. In the chinchilla, molar overgrowth may be exhibited as an apical displacement or impaction while the clinical crowns remain normal. In all three the elongation of the cheek teeth forces the mouth open in a pie wedge shape. This in turn alters the alignment of the incisors; the mandibular incisors being less curved end up occluding labial to the maxillary incisors. You end up with the same presentation (rostral crossbite) as one sees with a brachycephalic patient, the only difference being that in the brachycephalic patient the cheek teeth are normal in length. Primary malocclusion and overgrowth of the cheek teeth have also been known to develop in Guinea pigs due to excessive selenium intake [5]. Whether it is the initial problem or a sequela to other causes, possibly even temporomandibular joint dysplasia, cheek teeth overgrowth is seldom recognized until signs are well advanced, due to the difficulty in routinely examining the teeth. It therefore holds a poor prognosis.

21.5.2 Traumatic

Traumatic malocclusions are a result of tooth overgrowth after the loss or fracture of its opposing counterpart. Loss of proper attrition may lead to many of the same symptoms and problems as in atraumatic malocclusion.

21.5.3 Malocclusion Treatment

The basic rationale behind treatment of malocclusion is adequate crown height control to approximate the wear that would normally be experienced. Crown trimming or reduction must be done on a regular basis (every three to eight weeks) until normal occlusion is reestablished or, in some cases, indefinitely [4, 5, 8, 13, 41, 42]. This is preferably done with the use of a grinding or cutting bur mounted on a straight cone slow-speed handpiece [11, 12, 18, 43]. Treatment consists of first obtaining X-rays to appreciate the severity of the condition. At first the crowns elongate coronally. With increased pressure from one arcade against the other, the crowns start to elongate apically. Coronal growth can be reduced, but apical growth cannot be reduced. If the X-rays show that the apical portions of the crowns have not moved, the prognosis is better than if they have moved. The next part of the treatment is to shorten the crowns back to a normal length in what is referred to as performing an occlusal equilibration. Unfortunately, when the clinical crown elongates, the gingiva moves coronally with it. This has two negative effects: (i) practitioners just "looking" into the mouth report that the visible crowns are normal in length and thus fail to realize the extent of the condition; (ii) reducing the crown down to the gingiva level may not be sufficient to bring the clinical crown back to normal length. To correct those problems always obtain a lateral X-ray and examine the length of the crowns above the bone level, not above the gum level. Always reduce the crowns down to the gingival level and obtain a post-operative X-ray; if the clinical crowns are still too long, advise the owner that a second treatment will be necessary in about three weeks. This interval is long enough to allow the gums to recede naturally and without pain. Reducing the crowns below the level of the gingiva is very painful and results in anorexia on the part of the patient. Remember that the occlusal table in the rabbit and chinchilla is nearly horizontal whereas in the Guinea pig it is at a 40° slant in a form of a "V" [44] (Figure 21.11).

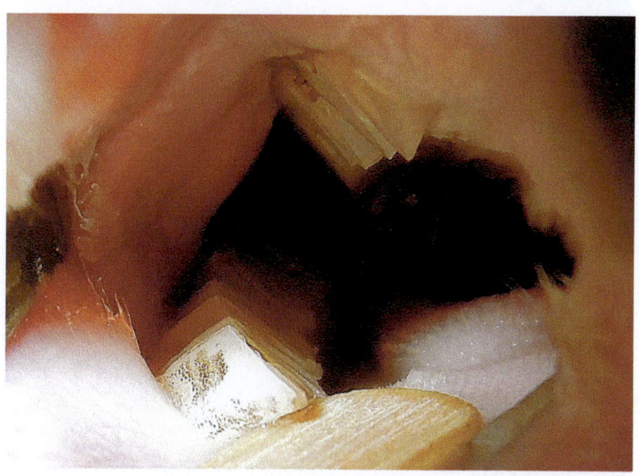

Figure 21.11 The occlusal table of the Guinea pig is naturally set at a 30° angle from dorsobuccal to ventrolingual. This angle needs to be respected when reducing the crowns to maintain proper function.

The incisors should be trimmed only after the cheek teeth have been appropriately reduced. A tongue depressor held behind the incisors can help protect soft tissue and allow stabilization for more accurate odontoplasty, shaping the incisor into a chisel configuration that is closer to normal [45]. Use of nail trimmers, tooth nippers, and bone rongeurs are strongly discouraged, and may even be considered negligent treatment due to potential tooth fractures and cracks that could lead to infection [7, 10]. The tool of choice is a cutting bur or a diamond bur mounted on a high-speed handpiece (Figure 21.12). If a pulp is exposed by crown reduction, it can be treated like a tooth fractured by trauma after cleansing. A calcium hydroxide paste/base, straight calcium hydroxide powder, mineral trioxide aggregate (MTA) powder, or one of the newer MTA light cured pastes should be placed to cap the pulp, preferentially stimulating the pulp to form a reparative dentinal bridge. The site should be closed with an intermediate filling material such as a glass ionomer to approximate the wear the tooth should experience [45]. Crown reduction of the opposing tooth will be necessary until the damaged crown grows to a correct length, barring the possibility of a pulp–capping failure [46–48]. Overgrown cheek teeth benefit from regular crown reduction. This procedure, even though more difficult, is essential. A long shank grinding, cutting, or even diamond bur mounted on the straight slow-speed handpiece is helpful for reducing premolars and molars, but care should be taken to avoid excess trauma to the tongue, palate, and buccal mucosa [45]. Stir sticks become essential to accomplishing that task. One can also use a bur guard; however, the author finds that it restricts access and vision too much. Grinding burs are safer than cutting burs as they abrade but do not rip soft tissues. On the other hand, they are slightly slower than the cutting burs [12].

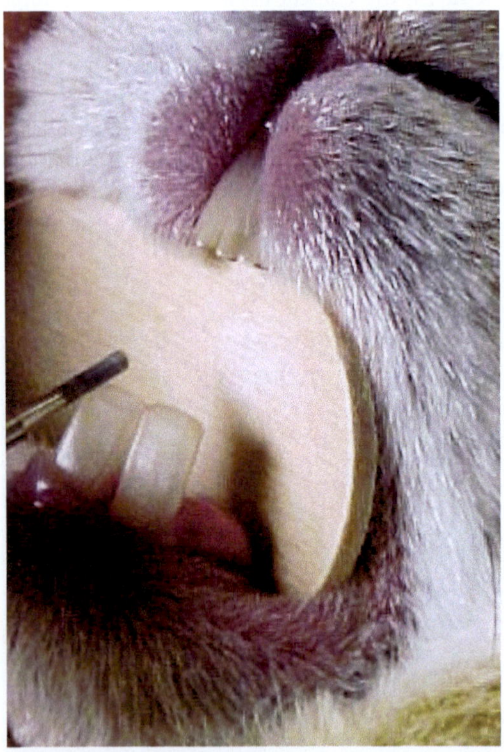

Figure 21.12 When cutting incisors, the tool of choice is a cutting or a diamond bur mounted on a high-speed handpiece. Note the use to the tongue depressor used to protect the soft tissues during the procedure.

Whether involving the incisors and/or the molars, with a malocclusion or loss of a tooth causing overgrowth of the opposing tooth, the owner must realize that treatment may be an on-going, long-term commitment. If a tooth is lost entirely to trauma or has extensive infection that is unresponsive to conservative therapy and antibiotics, extraction of the remaining structure and possibly of the opposing tooth may be chosen over the need for regular crown reduction. If the condition is an inherited malocclusion problem, genetic counseling and culling of all affected animals should be considered [5]. Patients with poor systemic health (contraindicated for frequent anesthetics), refractory cases, or wild animals that should be released might be candidates for euthanasia as a humane alternative.

In other cases involving abnormalities in the diet, such as hypovitaminosis C in Guinea pigs, excess selenium, or inadequate materials for dental exercise, initial treatment with crown reduction will help. Rectification of the diet should be sufficient to reduce or eliminate the need for frequent occlusal equilibration. Unfortunately, changing diet is easier said than done.

21.5.3.1 Extraction – Cheek Teeth

Another alternative that will also provide a permanent solution is extraction. The location of the tooth, type of tooth (hypsodont or brachyodont) and general patient health determine the advisability of extractions. Some individuals are in an extremely poor condition at the time of presentation and antibiotics, anti-inflammatories, fluids, force feeding, and nursing care may be used in order to improve general health prior to anesthetic stress. Location of the tooth becomes important to accessibility. Incisors have good accessibility, while many cheek teeth do not. Occasionally buccotomies must be performed, in some species, for visibility and accessibility, but food impactions, healing problems, and scars may result. Close attention to locations of vascular, neural, and other structures must also be considered.

Closed rooted cheek teeth (brachyodont), such as those in the rat, can be extracted with some care utilizing an intraoral approach, in most cases using bent 18–23 gauge needles as elevators. In the mouse, gerbil, and hamster the brachyodont cheek teeth are extremely small and difficult to properly remove, unless already highly mobile. Broken roots can seldom be addressed without inducing excessive oral trauma in very limited spaces. With extraction, some migration of adjacent teeth and slight supereruption of opposing teeth no longer in satisfactory occlusal contact may occur. These seldom result in serious problems.

Open-rooted cheek teeth (aradicular hypsodont), such as in the Guinea pig, chinchilla, and rabbit, do present a challenge for extraction. Since these are continually growing teeth, extraction may lead to overgrowth of opposing teeth no longer in proper occlusal contact and thus to posterior malocclusions. This results in the need for routine odontoplasty/occlusal equilibration for crown control of the posterior teeth at three to eight week intervals, or for additional extractions. If one extracts one cheek tooth in the middle of the occlusal table, one finds that the extensive chewing motion allows the opposite tooth to be worn against the teeth adjacent to the one just extracted. Thus, it is not compulsory to extract the opposing tooth every time. I prefer to wait several weeks before extracting the opposite tooth, to find out whether it is necessary or not. An intraoral approach requires finesse and the appropriate tools, but with practice it becomes the least complicated of the techniques. The use of a cheek tooth luxator is essential. The teeth are square with two sides running rostrocaudal and two sides running linguo-buccal. The luxator possesses two blades, one in line with the handle and one at 90° to the handle. The blade in line with the handle is introduced on the lingual and buccal surfaces of the teeth, whereas the blade at 90° to the handle is introduced on the mesial and distal surfaces of the teeth. Once in the periodontal ligament space, the blade is pushed apically and rocked back and forth to cut the ligament fibers [49]. Once the elevator is well lodged, pressure is applied against the axis of the tooth and maintained for at least 30 seconds. That time is necessary to fatigue the ligament fibers and loosen the tooth. The process is repeated on all four sides of the tooth. The tooth should be loose enough to be grasped with a pair of cheek teeth extractors, which have short parallel tips designed to fit in the tight spaces offered by our patients. The tooth is pushed apically and rotated slightly. This action is designed to destroy the germinal tissues apical to the reserve crown. If those tissues are left behind intact, the tooth will grow back in 8–12 weeks. The tooth is finally pulled coronally. It is sometimes necessary to cut it into sections to extirpate it from the oral cavity. Usually it can be tipped and moved into the buccal space. Once out, the apical part should be examined to ascertain whether the germinal tissues are present. The alveolus is flushed, the gingiva is elevated on the lingual and buccal sides. It is then sutured closed with a 5-0 absorbable monofilament suture [50].

Buccotomies have their own associated problems: they are a surgical procedure andthere is a risk of cutting through nerves and vessels, they are painful, and the incisions often break down. With the mandible, an extraoral approach through the bone covering the apices is another option. A simple incision is made over the bony enlargement or abscess site. The specific location is best determined with radiographs and a knowledge of the apical anatomy. Guinea pigs commonly have three normal alveolar juga, or bone elevations, that may mimic an abnormality and can be palpated on the ventral surface of the mandible, representing the apical border of the first and last two cheek teeth. The cortical plate can generally be curetted open with a periosteal elevator or a high-speed dental bur. The impacted or infected teeth can be extracted many times through this access site. In some cases, teeth will need to be repelled into the mouth from the access with a large endodontic plugger or other devices. If a cystic lesion is encountered it must be thoroughly curetted. If the tooth is ankylosed, the apical crown and the germinal tissues may be removed and the reserve crown left in [45]. Good closure can be difficult, especially for the intraoral side of the defect. When possible, loosen the attached gingiva with a small periosteal elevator on either side of the defect and suture it closed with size 5-0 absorbable suture material [45].

21.5.3.2 Packing the Abscess

The bony defect may be packed with the appropriate osteogenic material. When dealing with an abscess, do not suture the external access, but instead marsupialize it and pack the defect with an antibiotic slurry. Evaluate the defect two weeks later; if the area is totally clean, let it granulate in. If there is still purulent discharge, curette the area and fill with a different antibiotic mixture. Evaluate again two weeks later [51]. The incision may stay open for up to eight weeks.

Rabbits and rodents are subject to many drug toxicities. Several antibiotics, used systemically, will cause a severe colitis associated with overgrowth of *Clostridium* spp. [7]. Antibiotics such as lincomycin [52] or clindamycin [53] are contraindicated in rabbits, and ampicillin, erythromycin, and products containing procaine are to be used with care. A penicillin G-benzathine injectable suspension, on the other hand, has been used extensively to treat syphilitic rabbits and has been found to be quite safe. Nevertheless, given systemically, it does not reach very high serum levels and does not penetrate abscess walls very efficiently. To bypass this problem, products placed locally in the abscess cavity have been tried with various successes.

Methylmethacrylate beads impregnated with antibiotics such as amikacin, vancomycin, tobramycin, gentamycin, metronidazole, and cetiofur have been fabricated and placed into abscess cavities [54]. They certainly work but they have a few disadvantages: they are sutured in and require a second surgery to remove them. They are fabricated by a compounding pharmacy and thus may take some time to be available, they can be expensive to make, and finally they may be too big for some of our patients. For all the above reasons, the author prefers to avoid their use.

Products have been placed directly into the abscess cavity in the form of powder, slurry, in a plastic carrier, or even in the form of solution using soaked gauzes. Among the advantages are lower cost, no preparation needed, and no closing of the wound and thus no reopening. Products used are: ampicillin powder mixed with saline solution to form a slurry, clindamycin powder mixed with saline solution, tetracycline powder mixed with saline solution, doxycycline solution soaked into gauze, minocycline microbeads packed in directly, and doxycycline hyclate mixed into a plastic carrier [51]. Calcium hydroxide as powder mixed with saline solution has also been used [55], but that compound can cause a superficial necrosis of the tissues it is in contact with [56]. In some cases the zone of necrosis can be substantial, causing some authors to warn against the use of calcium hydroxide. This author has not witnessed any unacceptable necrosis while using this product.

Patients function very well with an open defect on their faces. The hardest part, for the owners, seems to be the prevention of the closure of the defect. As far as what antibiotic order is used, doxycycline hyclate mixed in a plastic carrier is often the first because the mixture is ideal to plug an odd-shaped defect. After that the choice is yours. The order makes little difference to the outcome. No matter which slurry one uses, the local concentration of the antibiotic reaches a thousand-fold of what would be attainable if given systemically. At those concentrations, the antibiotic sterilizes the area without systemic side effects. The important step is to ensure that the granulation tissues lining the defect are healthy before suturing it closed or letting it close by second intention.

21.5.3.3 Extraction – Incisors

The continually growing incisors (aradicular hypsodont) of most rabbits, Guinea pigs, and rats are generally not difficult to extract [45, 57]. The smaller incisors of the mouse and hamster are more of a challenge. In all, the use of a curved incisor luxator (Crossley) greatly facilitates the process. If only some of the incisors are extracted, additional overgrowth, migration, and malocclusion in the rostral teeth are not uncommon. Routine odontoplasty may become necessary for these new problems. For this reason, it may be best to extract all of the incisors at the same time. Many of these species have prehensile lips and only slight, if any, changes in food textures may be required. This is typically not suitable for wild herbivores that are to be placed back into a natural wild habitat, because of their great reliance on the incisors to obtain food (tree bark, etc.), in constructing habitats, and in self-defense.

In rabbits, the oral cavity should be cleaned and disinfected with an oral chlorhexidine solution. Both pre- and post-surgical radiographs should be obtained for complicated or time-consuming extractions. This provides pre-operative knowledge of complicating factors such as reserved crown fractures and weak mandibular support structures (predisposed to fracture). The next step in extraction is the severing of the epithelial attachment. A no.15 C surgical blade, a small sharp periosteal, or a dental elevator can be used for this purpose. The blade is inserted into the gingival sulcus until it meets with the resistance of the alveolar crestal bone. The intrasulcular incision is extended around the entire tooth, thus releasing the epithelial attachment. Actual elevation and removal of the tooth can be performed using a Crossley incisor luxator, a refined 301 apical elevator, an EX-15 (Cislak Manufacturing, Burbank, IL), an EX-16 (Cislak Manufacturing, Burbank, IL), inner curved and outer curved 1.3 mm luxators (Cislak Manufacturing, Burbank, IL), an injection needle (20 or 18 gauge), and a small pair of extracting forceps [45, 50]. Elevators should be sharpened and shaped on a regular basis specifically for small herbivore use.

The luxator is used to open the space between the tooth and alveolar bone crest, in order to break the periodontal ligament fibers. The mesial ligament attachment typically is the most difficult to break down. The instrument is placed against the periodontal ligament and used in a slight twisting movement parallel to the reserved crown while being pressed apically. The angulation of the EX-15, EX-16 elevators as well as the curved 1.3 mm luxators make them useful on the facial and lingual aspects of the tooth as they conform to the tooth's natural curvature. The Crossley incisor luxator conforms to the mesial and distal surfaces of the incisors. The process is repeated around the circumference of the tooth until the reserved crown becomes loose and can be easily removed with small extracting forceps. The extracting forceps should not be used to attempt forcible extractions, as this can result in fractures of the tooth or supporting bone. Before pulling, the tooth is pushed apically instead. This is accomplished to try to destroy the germinal tissues and to prevent the tooth from growing back.

An alternative method is the use of syringe needles in the place of elevators. The needle is inserted beside the tooth and pressed apically with a light twisting force.

Extreme care should be observed when pressing the needle apically as it can easily penetrate hard and soft tissues and cause serious damage to any structure encountered. In rabbits, 18 and 20 gauge needles work well for most teeth. In rodents, because of the greater size variability, the needle must be selected to fit the incisor, typically 27, 25, 23, or 20 gauge. Owing to tooth curvature, pre-bending of the needles is possible due to their soft nature but is not ordinarily necessary. The smaller rodents, such as the mouse, are more of a challenge because of the delicacy of teeth and bone. It is very easy, especially in the maxilla, for the needle to penetrate through bone and to contact with underlying structures. For these a 27 gauge half-inch (0.4 mm × 12 mm) needle and gentle manipulation is required.

Once the tooth is removed, the socket is cleaned and curetted of debris or granulation tissue. Bony prominences and spicules are reduced with a bur, curette, or rongeurs. If infected, the sockets should be left open for drainage, unless hemorrhage is a problem. In these cases, clean the socket well, flush with saline, fill with tetracycline ophthalmic ointment or other antibiotic slurry, and close the suture with absorbable suture material. Antibiotics are recommended if active infection was detected. The patient should be rechecked in approximately 10 days to 2 weeks to inspect the healing process. Most return to eating quickly after surgery in a matter of hours, but occasionally some individuals with sore mouths need encouragement or force feeding. Analgesics are recommended in those situations. A liquid diet of fruit or vegetable juice, such as carrot or apple, or commercial slurry diets, can be fed with an eye dropper or tuberculin syringe. Blunt-end feeding tubes are available to fit most rodents and lagomorphs, but care should be exerted in their use not to injure the animal or inject material into the respiratory system. The owner will need to observe if the patient has problems with any specific dietary materials and, if needed, either reduce its size or remove them from the diet, but this is not commonly required.

Should reserve crown tips be broken off within the alveolus, the tooth may grow back in four to eight weeks, necessitating a second attempt at extraction at that time. Periodically the remaining portion may not grow back properly but becomes a focus of chronic infection requiring additional attention. In some cases, it may even become trapped within the mandible. These may require further surgery. Should radiographs at the initial surgery indicate that material is still present, every attempt should be made with a fine elevator to remove this material. The reserve crown of these teeth is hollow with an open apex that has a thin soft structure. At extraction, occasionally soft tissue on the root tip may be present, representing granulation from infection, or the enamel epithelial organ and Hertwig's epithelial root sheath (Figures 21.13a,b). In a chronically infected mandibular incisor retained reserve crown structure that is non-responsive to normal attempts at extraction, surgical intervention may be required. Radiographs should be used to pinpoint the location as there is great variation as to the apical location within the lagomorphs and rodents. An incision is made along the ventral border of the mandible and reflected facially and coronally. Commonly, alterations in normal bone structure will be observed at the pathological site, indicating appropriate access. If not, rely on radiographs for access selection. In many cases the bony structure will be soft from disease and can be carved away with the sharp spoon excavator or bone curette; otherwise a no. 2 or no. 4 round bur or a

(a) (b)

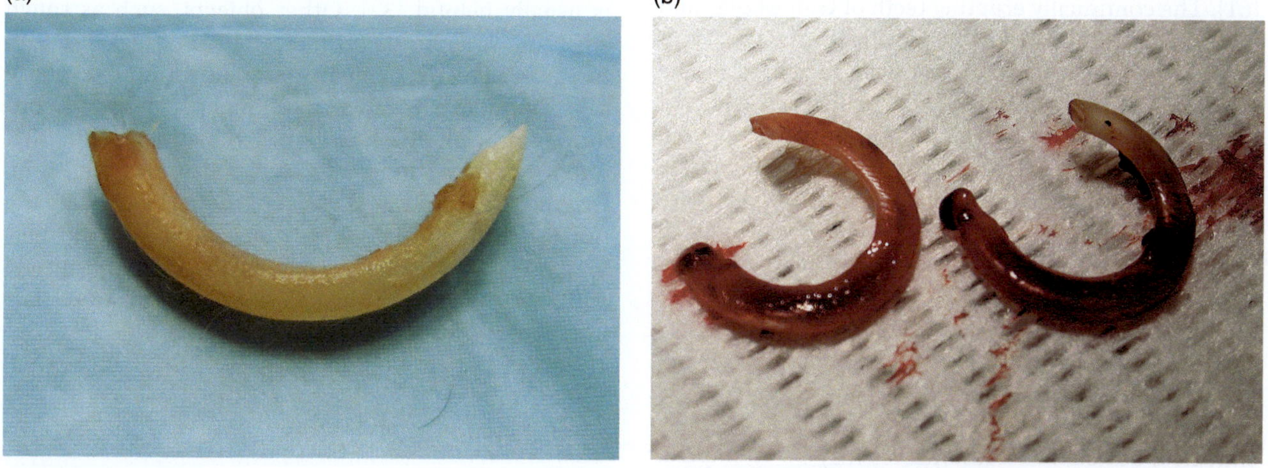

Figures 21.13 (a) Maxillary incisor of a rabbit that came out without the accompanying germinal tissues. There is thus a great chance that this tooth will grow back in several weeks. (b) Maxillary incisors of a rat with the accompanying germinal tissues, ensuring that these teeth are permanently removed.

diamond bur can be used to make access. Use copious water flow with burs to prevent thermal damage to adjacent hard tissues. Once the reserve crown is exposed, remove the fragments and thoroughly curette the lesion. An orthodontic wire can be used as a cleaning rod to be passed through the apical exposure location and exit the normal eruption site to push reserved crown and debris out when necessary. Fill the site with tetracycline ophthalmic ointment and suture closed using 5-0 monofilament absorbable suture material. In more severe cases the area is marzupialized and left open to granulate.

21.6 Other Dental Disease

Besides malocclusion and overgrowth there are a few other dental problems lagomorphs and rodents may experience. Minor trauma to or fractures of the teeth that do not involve the pulp may be handled by smoothing the roughened fracture edges and sealing the exposed dentinal surfaces. Occasionally, odontoplasty of the opposing tooth may be needed until the injured tooth grows back to a more correct height.

In the rat, it is rare to see naturally occurring carious lesions due to the influences of its normal diet, oral pH, and microflora. Since the shape of molars in rats and hamsters somewhat approximates that of humans, they are often used in caries research [58, 59]. Since hamsters' mouths can be opened to nearly 180°, regular inspections for caries and plaque research are facilitated. Advantages for using Syrian hamsters include their usual acceptance of cariogenic diet and typical ease in bacterial colonization, but the potential for developing pit and fissure caries is relatively low [59, 60]. Smooth surface caries is a disadvantage also encountered in gerbils, in addition to their low water consumption that affects oral hydration [61]. The continually erupting teeth of Guinea pigs and rabbits make them unsuitable for most caries studies.

While caries-like lesions have been described in the rabbit [62], these are possibly hypocalcified areas that are most likely sequela of insults during tooth formation, such as fever, dietary deficiencies, trauma, and infection. If minor, treatment is usually unnecessary as these lesions will eventually be lost as the tooth continues to grow. If extensive or involved the caries should be removed and a temporary filling material used to restore the teeth, if needed. Any permanent material that may not wear adequately or produce toxic byproducts if ingested and should be avoided.

Carious lesions in brachyodont teeth are usually extracted, but standard restoratives may be attempted. Glass ionomers are commonly used in smooth surface restorations and on occlusal surfaces; although there is a lack of wearability, it may still be the best alternative [63].

21.7 Periodontal Disease and Stomatitis

Primary periodontal disease is relatively uncommon in rodents and lagomorphs, although it can be induced in laboratory rats with the introduction of *Actinomyces viscosus* [64]. A spontaneous form of the disease, with plaque and calculus accumulation, has been found in gerbils fed a special commercial laboratory diet [65]. Periodontal disease can also be reproduced experimentally in rabbits [66], and even hamsters have been used as models for disease transmission [67]. None of these have been considered very significant clinically, although, if found, can be treated like periodontal disease in other species with a complete prophylaxis, including polishing. Since intubation is usually difficult, hand scaling or use of a sonic scaler without water flow would minimize the chances of the patient aspirating liquids or the aerosolized spray. Chlorhexidine solution can also be used to help control plaque accumulation and treat periodontal disease, as has been shown in the rat [59].

The majority of cases of inflammation in the oral cavity are secondary to non-periodontal causes, such as cheek pouch impaction in the hamster causing a stomatitis [5, 44]. Removal of the impacted material should be followed by application of an antibiotic ointment or solution in the area.

Hypovitaminosis C or scurry in Guinea pigs can cause some serious oral problems such as gingival hemorrhage, periodontal disease, and loose teeth that can become maloccluded [10]. Treatment with the feeding of vitamin C-rich fruits and vegetables should accompany correction of the diet, including replacing outdated foodstuffs. Anorectic animals may require tube feeding, fluids, antibiotics, and vitamin C supplements.

Overgrown teeth due to malocclusions can also cause irritation to the oral cavity, and crown reduction is usually helpful [32]. Other objects, such as rough edges on water bottle tubes, feeders, or cages, can lead to abrasions with gingivitis, stomatitis, and excessive salivation. Thus, ptyalism in rabbits may lead to a condition known as "wet dewlap", a moist dermatitis that often occurs secondary to causes listed above [4, 5]. In chinchillas it is diagnosed as "slobbers." Treating the initial problem usually must be accompanied by clipping the moist area and treating with an appropriate antibiotic, as there may be an associated *Pseudomonas* infection [8].

21.8 Other Oral Diseases

Sialoacryoadenitis as a coronavirus infection in rats may affect the salivary glands, causing swellings under the mandibular and around the neck [6]. Although it is usually self-limiting, it may spread within a colony, and if keratoconjunctivitis is experienced, ophthalmic ointments may be used. The salivary gland virus, *Cytomegalovirus*, in Guinea pigs that infects the salivary gland's ductal epithelium seldom causes overt clinical signs [68].

Viral oral papillomatosis in rabbits is usually seen as fixed or pedunculated white growths, usually under the tongue, but sometimes on the gingiva [6, 13, 69–71]. Animals with malocclusions that result in abraded epithelial surfaces may be predisposed to the infection [21], which is spread by direct contact, but it often recedes spontaneously [13]. This disease is different from Shope Papilloma in the rabbit, which has a potential to transform into malignant squamous cell carcinoma [72–75].

Fusobacterium necrophorum found in unsanitary conditions can cause necrobacillosis or Schmorl's disease, with progressive ulceration of the skin and swelling of subcutaneous tissues in the facial, cervical, and oral regions. If abscesses develop at the angle of the mandible, they should be drained and debrided and the patient treated with the appropriate antibiotics [13]. Bacteremias and transmission to humans are possible, so these animals should be handled carefully [6].

Other abscesses could be present due to periodontal or endodontic disease and should be treated accordingly. Enlargements associated with the oral cavity other than abscesses may be due to impacted teeth resulting from malocclusion trauma or eruption problems. Cysts that are encountered may be treated surgically and thoroughly debrided, while any abnormal mass suspected of being a tumor should always be biopsied.

There are even systemic diseases that will show oral signs, such as lip ulceration in the venereal disease spirochetosis (*Treponema cuniculi*) in rabbits [13]. In 6–12 week-old rabbits, tooth grinding may be a common sign of pain when experiencing the profuse diarrhea of mucoid enteropathy.

No matter what the signs or symptoms, there are many things the general practitioner can successfully treat in lagomorphs and rodents as it pertains to the oral cavity. Knowing the basic problems that might be encountered and becoming familiar with available treatments can offer your patients the best care possible.

21.9 Antibiotics, Anti-inflammatories, and Fluids Treatment

Extreme care must be used in the selection of antibiotics and medications as lagomorphs and rodents have sensitivities and toxicities to many drugs. The most commonplace antibiotics used in rabbit medicine are the penicillins, with benzathene procaine penicillin combination at 0.25 cc per patient less than 2 kg IM, SQ every other day, or 0.25 cc per patient more than 2 kg, IM, SQ every other day. In severe infections, the dosage can be increased to every day. For rabbits or rodents tetracycline has been used at 30–100 mg/kg divided doses, TID orally or 400–1000 mg/l of drinking water [6, 11, 13, 41, 42]. Forty milliliters (40 ml) of sulfamerazine 12.5% solution in a gallon of drinking water for a 0.15% solution has been recommended for both rabbits and rodents [11]. In the rabbit, hamster, and Guinea pig, almost any antibiotic has the potential to cause a fatal colitis due to potent *Clostridium* toxins, making chloramphenicol the drug of choice in this situation or other enteropathies because of its effectiveness against *Clostridium* species [76, 77]. Chloramphenicol succinate in the rabbit at 50 mg/kg TID, SQ or IV [13] and in the Guinea pig at 10–30 mg/kg SQ, BID has been used [5]. Chloramphenicol palmitate has been administered orally at the rate of 50 mg/kg TID for hamsters and Guinea pigs, and 200 mg/kg TID for mice and rats [11]. Lincomycin is contraindicated in rabbits, and ampicillin, erythromycin, and procaine-containing products are to be used with caution [41]. Trimethoprim with sulfa at the dosage of 30–50 mg/kg SID to BID either SQ or PO is a good general antibiotic for rabbits, gerbils, mice, rats, hamsters, and Guinea pigs [11]. Enrofloxacin at the rate of 5 mg/kg BID PO or 2.5 mg/kg BID SQ has been useful in the rabbit for more serious cases.

Although mice, rats, and gerbils do not typically develop the fatal Gram-negative enterotoxemias from antibiotics such as is seen in hamsters, Guinea pigs, and rabbits, they are well known for direct toxic effects of some antibiotics. Mice often have antibiotic toxicity problems, even in low doses with streptomycin and procaine [76]. Mongolian gerbils are highly sensitive to the streptomycins, with dihydrostreptomycin having a direct toxic effect that results in death within a matter of hours [78]. Other antimicrobials are of use in the rabbit, depending on specific pathogens; several excellent texts on rabbit medicine are available, with extensive drug information [6, 13, 41, 42].

Anti-inflammatories, analgesics, and fluids are required for various procedures. In the mouse and rat 1 mg SQ can be used for dexamethasone [13]. In the rabbit the dose varies greatly from 0.6 to 6.6 mg/kg SQ or IV depending on the severity of the condition being treated [11, 79]. Meloxicam is a good anti-inflammatory drug and is used at 0.5 mg/kg SID for three to five days post-op. Buprenorphine has recently become the analgesic of choice given PO or SQ at 0.01–0.02 mg/kg q 12 hours and also for three to five days post-op.

21.10 Rodent and Lagomorph Coprophagy

In the rabbit, one idiosyncrasy associated with the oral cavity that might concern some owners is coprophagy. This is a form of refection that is natural in many lagomorphs and rodents, making them pseudo-ruminants, as they ingest their own feces for re-digestion [41]. Rabbits begin this activity around day 20 of age, approximately three to five days after they begin eating solid food and maternal feces [13]. The cecotrophs, which are about a third of the total fecal output, contain more water, minerals, and B vitamins than dry feces produced during the day [13]. These animals usually eat these mucus-bound clusters at night and early morning hours as part of their natural circadian activity [80].

This behavior can cause a dilemma in evaluation of research data dealing with the teeth and oral cavity. While drugs can be given by gastric intubation or parenteral administration it must be realized that unabsorbed drugs, their metabolites, modified intestinal bacterial flora, and altered contents of the normal excreta may subject the teeth, oral cavity, and associated structures to covert direct exposure to these components [23]. The use of wire-bottom caging aids in reduction of this potential complication, by allowing some of the cecotrophs to fall through the floor and out of the animal's reach. Unfortunately, many of the animals ingest them directly from the anus [80]. This dilemma should be taken into consideration any time medications are administered.

21.11 Ferrets

Ferrets are one of the only small mammals that are not rabbits or rodents. They belong to the order Carnivora and the family *Mustelidae* and are part of the weasel family. Their dental formula is I 2/2, C 1/1, P 3/3, M 1/2 and they possess two sets of dentition [81]. They have been extensively used in periodontology and endodontolgy studies [82–84]. Oral examination in a conscious patient can be challenging as they are very active and hard to restrain. Anesthesia is similar to what is done in cats. They do suffer from rostral crossbite, especially with the second incisors [81]. They do get periodontitis in a comparable manner to what is seen in our other carnivorous patients. They are most commonly presented for complicated crown fractures of the maxillary canine teeth. These fractures lead to pulpitis, pulp necrosis, and periapical infection or even destruction of the apex of the affected tooth, as is seen in cats. Treatment consists of endodontic therapy or extraction. The extraction technique is identical to what is done in cats [81] and the endodontic treatment is covered in Chapter 15 – Basic Endodontic Therapy.

References

1 Crossley, D.A. (1993). Dental chart for rabbits. *J. Vet. Dent.* 10 (3): 13.

2 Capello, V., Gracis, M., and Lennox, A.M. (2005). *Rabbit and Rodent Dentistry Handbook*. Lake Worth, FL: Zoological Education Network.

3 Regalaldo, A.M. and Legendre, L.F. (2017). Full mouth intraoral radiographic survey in rabbits. *J. Vet. Dent.* 34 (1).

4 Harkness, J.E. (1987). Rabbit husbandry and medicine. *Veterinary Clinics of North America –Small Animal Practice*; Exotic Pet Medicine. Philadelphia, PA; WB Saunders. 17 (5): 1091.

5 Williams, C.S.F. (1976). *Practical Guide to Laboratory Animals*. St. Louis, MO: CV Mosby Co.

6 Holmes, D.D. (1984). *Clinical Laboratory Animal Medicine, An Introduction*. Ames, IA: The Iowa State University Press.

7 Lobprise, H.B. and Wiggs, R.B. (1991). Dental and oral disease in lagomorphs. *J. Vet. Dent.* 8 (2): 11.

8 Brooks, D.L. (1986). Rabbits, hares and pikas (*Lagomorpha*). In: *Zoo and Wild Animal Medicine*, 2e (ed. M.E. Fowler). Philadelphia, PA: WB Saunders.

9 Williams, C.S.F. (1979). Guinea pigs and rabbits. *Veterinary Clinics of North America, Small Animal Practice*; Non-Domestic Pet Medicine. Philadelphia, PA: WB Saunders Co.

10 Wiggs, R.B. and Lobprise, H.B. (1990). Dental disease in rodents. *J. Vet. Dent.* 7 (3): 6.

11 Jacobson, E.R. and Kollias, G.V. Jr. (1988). *Exotic Animals*. New York: Churchill Livingstone.

12 Legendre, L.F.J. (2011). Oral examination and occlusal equilibration in rodents and lagomorphs. *J. Vet. Dent.* 28 (1): 52–57.

13 Harkness, J.E. and Wagner, J.E. (1983). *The Biology and Medicine of Rabbits and Rodents*, 2e. Philadelphia, PA: Lea & Febiger.

14 Nambiar, M.P., Gordon, R.K., Moran, T.S. et al. (2007). A simple method for accurate endotracheal placement of an intubation tube in Guinea pigs to assess lung injury following chemical exposure. *Toxicol. Mech. Methods.* 17: 385–392.

15 Craigie, E.H. (1948). *Bensley's Practical Anatomy of the Rabbit*, 8e. Toronto: University of Toronto Press.

16 Braithwaite, R.W. (1979). Natural selection in *Rattus* molars. *J. Zoology.* 189: 545–548.
17 Wiggs, R.B. (1990). Fractured maxillary incisors in a beaver. *J. Vet. Dent.* 7 (2): 21.
18 Kronfeld, R. (1937). *Dental Histology and Comparative Dental Anatomy*. Philadelphia, PA: Lea & Febiger.
19 Habermehl, K.H. (1975). Die Altersbestimmung bei Haus- u. Labortieren, 2. Aufl Vlg Paul Parvey, Berlin u. Hamburg.
20 Keil, A. (1949). Uber die Frage des naturlichen Vorkommens und der experimentellen Erzeugung echter Zahnkaries bei Tieren. *DZZ.* 4; S. 694.
21 Weisbroth, S.H. et al. (1973). *The Biology of the Laboratory Rabbit*. New York: Academic Press.
22 Craigie, E.H. (1973). *Laboratory Guide to the Anatomy of the Rabbit*, 2e. Toronto: University of Toronto Press.
23 Navia, J.M. (1977). *Animal Models in Dental Research*. The University of Alabama Press.
24 Shipp, A.D. and Fahrenkrug, P. (1992). *Practitioners' Guide to Veterinary Dentistry*. This Hills, CA: Shipp's Labs Pub.
25 Wiggs, R.B. and Lobprise, H.B. (1995). Oral diagnosis in pet rodents and lagomorphs. In: *Manual of Small Animal Dentistry* (ed. D.D. Crossley and S. Penman), 74–83. Gloucestershire, UK: BSAVA.
26 Kraus, B.S. et al. (1969). *The Study of the Masticatory System Dental Anatomy and Occlusion*. Baltimore, MD: MA Williams and Wilkins Co.
27 Allen, D.L. et al. (1974). *Periodontics for the Dental Hygienist*, 2e. Philadelphia, PA: Lea & Febige.
28 Sicher, H. and Bhaskar, S.N. (1972). *Orban's Oral Histology and Embryology*. St. Louis. MO: CV Mosby, Co.
29 Crossley, DA. (1967). Oral biology and disorders of lagomorphs *Vet Clin Exot Anim* 6: 629–659.
30 Shadle, A.R. (1936). The attrition and extrusive growth of the four major incisor teeth of domestic rabbits. *J. Mammal.* 17: 15.
31 Weisbroth, S.H. and Ehrman, L. (1967). Malocclusion in the rabbit: a model for the study of the development, pathology and inheritance of malocclusion. *J. Hered.* 58: 245.
32 Eisenmenger, E. and Zetner, K. (1985). *Veterinary Dentistry*. Philadelphia, PA: WB Saunders.
33 Fox, R.R. and Crary, D.D. (1971). Mandibular prognathism in the rabbit: genetic studies. *J. Hered.* 62: 23.
34 Clark, J.D. and Olfert, E.D. (1981). Rodents (*Rodentia*). In: *Zoo and Wild Animal Medicine*, 2e (ed. M.E. Fowler). Philadelphia, PA: WB Saunders Co.
35 Zeman, W.V. and Fielder, F.G. (1969). Dental malocclusion and overgrowth in rabbits. *J. Amer. Vet. Med. Assoc.* 155: 1115.
36 Russell, R.J. et al. (1981). *A Guide to Diagnosis, Treatment and Husbandry of Pet Rabbits and Rodents*. Lenexa, KS: Veterinary Medicine Publishing Co.
37 Neopola, S.R. (1969). The intrinsic and extrinsic factors influencing the growth and development of the jaws: hereditary and functional matrix. *Amer. J. Orthodont.* 55: 499.
38 Donnelly, T.M. and Vella, D. (2016). The mouth of pet rabbits. In: Capello V, ed. *Vet Clin of N Am: Exotic Anim Practice* 19 (3): 737–756.
39 Legendre, L.F. (2016). Anatomy and disorders of the oral cavity of the Guinea pig. In: Capello V, ed. *Vet Clin of N Am: Exotic Anim Practice* 19 (3): 825–842.
40 Mans, C. and Jekl, V. (2016). Anatomy and disorders of the oral cavity of chinchillas and degus. In: Capello V, ed. *Vet Clin of N Am: Exotic Anim Practice* 19 (3): 843–870.
41 Robinson, P.T. (1986). Dentistry in zoo animals. In: *Zoo and Wild Animal Medicine*, 2e (ed. M.E. Fowler). Philadelphia, PA: WB Saunders Co.
42 Crossley, D.A. (1994). Extraction of rabbit incisor teeth. Abstract.
43 Wiggs, R.B. (1988). Extraction, pulpectomy, pulpotomy or blunting of macaque canine teeth. *J. Vet. Dent.* 5 (1): 7.
44 Böhmer, E. (2015). *Dentistry in Rabbit and Rodents*, 32. Chichester, UK: Wiley.
45 Wiggs, R.B. and Lobprise, H.B. (1995). Prevention and treatment of dental problems in rodents and lagomorphs. In: *Manual of Small Animal Dentistry* (ed. D.D. Crossley and S. Penman), 94–90. Gloucestershire, UK: BSAVA.
46 Kostlin, R. and Schebitz, H. (1980). Zur endodontischen behandlung der zahnfractur beim hund. *Kleinter Prox.* 25: 187.
47 Burns, R.B. and Hinshaw, K. (1989). Dentoalveolar abscess with sequestra in a geriatric porcupine. *J. Vet. Dent.* 6 (3): 28.
48 Wiggs, R.B. (1990). Pulpotomy failure in a Rhesus monkey. *J. Vet. Dent.* 7 (1): 15.
49 Capello, V. (2016). Intraoral treatment of dental disease in pet rabbits. In: Capello V, ed. *Vet Clin of N Am: Exotic Anim Practice* 19 (3): 783–798.
50 Legendre, L.F.J. (2012). Rodent and lagomorphs tooth extraction. *J. Vet. Dent.* 29 (3): 204–209.
51 Legendre, L.F.J. (2011). Treatment of oral abscesses in rodents and lagomorphs. *J. Vet. Dent.* 28 (1): 30–33.
52 Maiers, J.D. and Mason, S.J. (1984). Lincomycin – associated enterocolitis in rabbits. *J. Am. Vet. Med. Assoc.* 185 (6): 670–671.
53 Borriello, P.S. and Carman, R.J. (1983). Association of Iota like toxin and *Clostridium spiriformes* with both spontaneous and antibiotics-associated diarrhea and colitis in rabbits. *J. Clin. Microbiol.* 414–418.

54 Seligson, D., Mehta, S., Voos, K. et al. (1992). The use of antibiotic-impregnated polymethylmethacrylate beads to prevent the evolution of localized infection. *J. Orthop. Trauma* 6 (4): 401–406.
55 Remeus, P.G.K. and Verbeek, M. (1995). The use of calcium hydroxide in the treatment of abscesses in the cheek of the rabbit resulting from dental periapical disorder. *J. Vet. Dent.* 12: 19–22.
56 Crossley, D. (2003). Oral biology and disorders of Lagomorphs. *Vet. Clin. North Am. Exot. Anim. Pract.* 6 (3): 629–659.
57 Brown, S.A. (1993). Incisor removal in the rabbit. In: *Technical North American Veterinary Conference 1993 Proceedings*. 791.
58 Goodman, L. and Gilman, A. (1996). *The Pharmacological Basis of Theraputics*, 3e. New York: The Macmillan Co.
59 Shrestha, B.M., et al. (1984). Inoculation and pre-weaning conditioning effects on rat caries. In: Hefferren, JJ, ed. Proceedings of Sixth Conference on Foods, Nutrition and Dental Health. Chicago, IL: American Dental Association Health Foundation.
60 Fitzgerald, R.L. and Keyes, P.H. (1960). Demonstration of the etiologic role of Streptococci in experimental caries in the hamster. *J. Am. Dent. Assoc.* 61: 9.
61 Mundorff, S.A. (1988). Dental decay research in animals. *Lab Animal* 17: 19.
62 Hu, C.K. and Greene, H.S.N. (1935). A lethal acromegalic mutation in the rabbit. *Science* 81: 25.
63 Holmstrom, S.E. and Gammon, R.L. (1988). Glass ionomers. *J. Vet. Dent.* 5 (4): 34.
64 Baer, P.N. (1968). Use of laboratory animals for calculus studies. *Ann. NY Acad. Sci.* 153: 230.
65 Moskow, V.S. et al. (1968). Spontaneous periodontal disease in the Mongolian gerbil. *J. Periodontal Res.* 3: 59.
66 Horodyski, B. and Slowik, T. (1966). Radiograph of periodontal disease in humans and experimental periodontal disease in rabbits. *Czas Stomat.* 19 (11): 1191.
67 Jordan, H.V. and Eye, P.H. (1964). Aerobic, gram-positive, filamentory bacteria as etiological agents of experimental periodontal disease in hamsters. *Arch. of Oral Biol.* 9: 401.
68 Van Hoosier, G.L. Jr. and Robinette, L.R. (1976). Viral and chlamydial diseases. In: *The Biology of the Guinea Pig* (ed. J.E. Wagner and P.F. Manning). New York: Academic Press.
69 Kidd, K.G. and Parsons, R.J. (1936). Tissue affinity of Shope papilloma virus. *Proc. Soc. Exp. Biol. Med.* 35: 438.
70 Parsons, R.J. and Kidd, J.G. (1936). A virus causing oral papillomatosis in rabbits. *Proc. Soc. Exp. Biol. Med.* 35: 441.
71 Parsons, R.J. and Kidd, J.G. (1943). Oral papillomatosis of rabbits: a virus disease. *J. Exp. Med.* 77: 233.
72 Shope, R.E. (1933). Infectious papillomatosis of rabbits (with note on histopathology by E.W. Hurst). *J. Exp. Med.* 58: 607.
73 Shope, R.E. (1936). A change in rabbit fibroma virus suggesting mutation. II. Behavior of the variant virus in cottontail rabbits. *J. Exp. Med.* 63: 173.
74 Shope, R.E. (1937). Immunization of rabbits to infectious papillomatosis. *J. Exp. Med.* 65: 219.
75 Rous, P. and Beard, J.W. (1934). A virus-induced mammalian growth with the characters of a tumor (the Shope rabbit papilloma). I. Growth on implantation within favorable host. *J. Exp. Med.* 60: 701.
76 Jacoby, R.O. and Fox, J.G. Biology and Diseases of Mice. In: *Laboratory Animal Medicine*. (ed. F.G. Fox, G.J. Cohen and F.M. Loew). New York: Academic Press: 31–89.
77 Gutta, G.N. et al. (1983). Susceptibility of *Clostridia* from farm animals to twenty-one antimicrobial agents, including some used for growth promotion. *Antimicrob. Chemther.* 12: 347.
78 Wightman, S.R. et al. (1980). Dihydrostreptomycin toxicity in the Mongolian gerbil, *Meriones unguiculatus*. *Lab. Anim. Sci.* 30: 71.
79 Schuekman, S.M. (1977). Individual care and treatment of rabbits, mice rats, Guinea pigs, hamsters and gerbils. In: *Current Veterinary Therapy*, vol. VI (ed. R.W. Kirk). Philadelphia, PA: WB Saunders.
80 Hornicke, H. and Batsch, F. (1977). Coecotrophy in rabbits – A circadian function. *J. Mammal* 58: 240.
81 Eroshin, V.V. et al. (2011). Oral examination in rescued ferrets: clinical findings. *J. Vet. Dent.* 28 (1): 8–15.
82 Struillou, X., Boutigny, H., Soueidan, A., and Layrolle, P. (2010). Experimental animal models in periodontology: a review. *Open Dent. J.* 29 (4): 37–47.
83 Bladwoski, M., Kotowicz-Gears, A., and Wojtkiewicz, J. (2011). Restoration of fractured canines in ferrets after one-step root canal treatment. *Pol. J. Vet. Sci.* 14 (1): 137–139.
84 Dickens, S.H. et al. (2010). Preclincal effectiveness of a novel pulp capping material. *J. Endod.* 36 (7): 1222–1225.

22

Exotic Animals Oral and Dental Diseases

Roberto Fecchio[1], Marco Antonio Gioso[2], and Kristin Bannon[3]

[1] Safari Co. – Zoo and Exotic Animals Dental Consultant, São Paulo/SP, Brazil
[2] Laboratório de Odontologia Comparada da FMVZ, University of São Paulo, São Paulo, Brazil
[3] Veterinary Dentistry and Oral Surgery of New Mexico, LLC, Algodones, NM, USA

22.1 Introduction

The application of veterinary dentistry is a fairly recent endeavor in Zoo and Exotic Animal Medicine. Despite the emergence of zoos during the nineteenth century, the first scientific publications about dental treatments in wild patients were not available until the 1970s [1–3]. The knowledge of anatomy, physiology, nutrition, and animal behavior can increase the well-being and longevity of animals in captivity [1, 4]. The examination of the oral cavity to detect and correct early problems must be part of an overall evaluation program of animal health [1, 5]. Animal conditioning for examination has been increasingly used (Figure 22.1), but a detailed evaluation of the oral cavity can only be performed when the animal is chemically restrained [5–7] and therefore should be part of every physical examination performed when the animal is anesthetized for other procedures [5, 6, 8]. In addition, chemical restraint provides greater protection to both the animal and the professionals involved.

However, detection of oral lesions in captive animals often occurs only after the clinical signs of diseases such as anorexia, weight loss, drooling, changes on holding and chewing food, pain, and discomfort are noted. As the severity of the oral disease progresses, changes in attitude, breeding behavior, food selection in the diet, oronasal discharge, bumps, and malodor can be identified [1, 5, 7, 8].

Although some diseases are more prevalent, it is important that the examination of the oral cavity assess both hard tissues: tooth and bone (presence of calculus, caries, fracture, mobility, and demineralization), and the soft tissues: lip, tongue, gums, palate, cheeks, and pharynx (swelling, bleeding, ulceration, and coloring) [1].

Preventing oral health problems preserves the efficiency of the digestive processes, contributing to the maintenance of general health, and by improving their reproductive abilities, increasing their life expectancy and substantially improving the quality of animal life [1, 5, 7].

22.2 Teeth Classification

The wide variety of dentition found among wild animals is closely linked to the evolutionary and adaptive aspects of each species. Therefore, the teeth have different functions such as holding and chewing food, social and sexual interaction, dimorphism, defense and predation, locomotion, phonation, inoculation of venom, as working tools, and instruments for body cleaning [1, 7].

The classification of the various sets of teeth of animals is based on their morphophysiological aspects (see Chapter 1 – Oral Anatomy and Physiology).

Anelodont. Animals whose teeth have limited growth and a clear line dividing the crown and root (cementoenamel junction). These teeth undergo rhizogenesis (root development) during which the dental apex forms after full longitudinal tooth development. The neurovascular supply is maintained through a foramen or multiple foramina formed into a delta. This group can be divided into hypsodont (radicular) and brachyodont, described below. Among the anelodonts are carnivores, primates, and some herbivores [3, 5, 9].

Brachyodont. A tooth in which the longitudinal length of the crown is smaller than the root and the entire root portion is inside the alveolar bone. The crowns are fully covered with enamel that extends down to the neck of the tooth. Cementum is only found below the gingival margin. The families Felidae, Canidae, Ursidae, and the Primates are included in this group [3, 5, 9].

Wiggs's Veterinary Dentistry: Principles and Practice, Second Edition. Edited by Heidi B. Lobprise and Johnathon R. (Bert) Dodd.

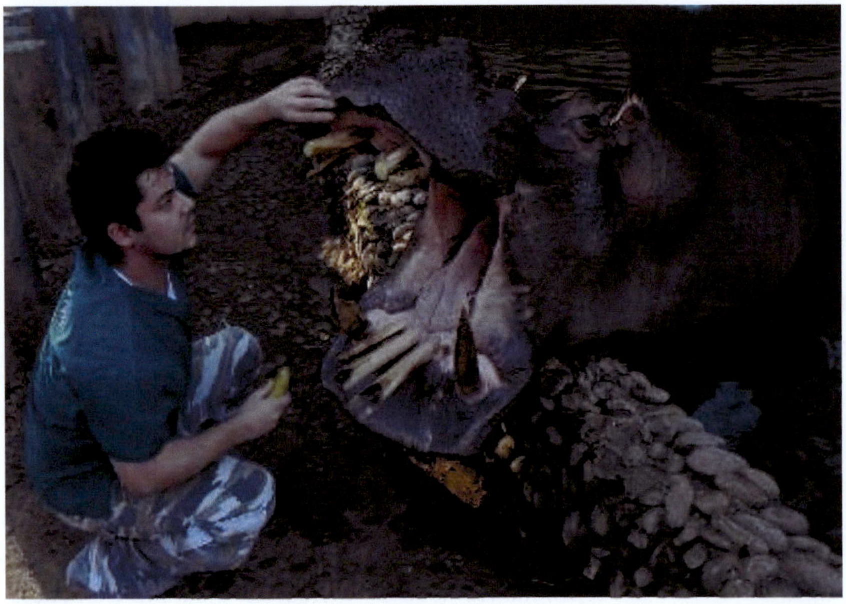

Figure 22.1 Conditioning for restraint aids in examinations.

Hypsodont. A tooth in which the longitudinal length of the crown is greater than the root. Enamel extends below the gingiva margin. This category includes the radicular hypsodont tooth (true root) and aradicular hyposodont tooth (open-rooted) [3, 5, 9].

Radicular Hypsodont (subdivision of Hypsodont). Dentition with true roots, sometimes called "closed rooted" teeth. These teeth erupt throughout life, but eventually develop a true closed apex and the subgingival reserve crown is eventually exposed and placed into occlusion. Anatomically, there is an observed clinical crown (extra-alveolar), reserve crown (intra-alveolar), and root. Examples belonging to this category are the premolars and molars of equines (zebras, horses) and bovines [3, 5, 9]. The crown/root ratio varies according to family. The equidae have long reserve crowns when young, while the bovidae and camelidae have relatively shorter crowns. The occlusal surface has a pattern interspersed with enamel, cementum, and dentin in different proportions, which maintains the surface texture, and have infundibulas or multilobed molars.

Aradicular Hypsodont (subdivision of Hypsodont). Dentition which continually grows throughout the life of the animal with no development of true roots, sometimes called "open rooted" or "open apex." Previously known as "Elodont." As the teeth are worn down, new crown becomes exposed from the continuously growing teeth (such as the incisors of rodents and incisors and cheek teeth of lagomorphs) [3, 5, 9]. While the submerged segment of the crown is sometimes referred to as the "clinical root," it is not a true root structure. The shape of the elodont pulp facilitates a rich blood supply to the pulp tissue and a high activity within the odontoblastic layer sustains continuous growth and often allows for repair to take place on exposure of the pulp chambers. The aradicular hypsodont species groups can be further divided according to the location of these teeth:

- All teeth such as lagomorphs (rabbits and hares), caviomorph rodents (chinchillas, guinea pigs), and wombat.
- Only anterior teeth (the premolars and molars are anelodont) such as miomorph rodents (rats, mice, and squirrels), elephants, and hippopotamus.
- Only posterior teeth such as aardvark and sloths.

Heterodont. Animals whose teeth have different morphology, according to appearance, function, and situation; these teeth are typically divided into incisors, canines, premolars, and molars [3, 5, 9]. The dental eruption can be grouped where the teeth erupt laterally (carnivores, primates, herbivores, and ruminants) or sequentially (molar teeth of elephants and kangaroos), where the teeth erupt horizontally.

Homodont. Animals whose teeth are morphologically similar throughout the mouth. Considered the most primitive type of dentition. Examples of animals belonging to this group are dolphins, crocodiles, alligators, and sharks [3, 5, 9] (Figure 22.2).

Monophyodont. A subdivision of Homodonts without tooth replacement after loss of the first set. This is the typical pattern found in whales and dolphins [3, 5, 9] (Figure 22.3).

Polyphyodont. A subdivision of Homodonts with constant tooth substitutions through life. In this group, dental replacement can occur vertically (crocodiles and snakes) or horizontally (sharks) [3, 5, 9]. They are

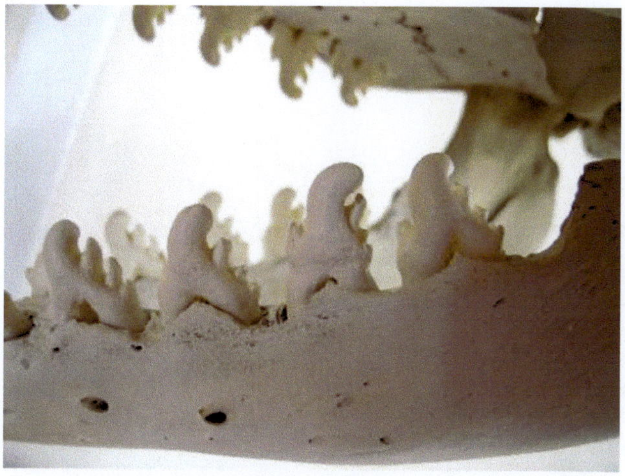

Figure 22.2 Homodont dentition (seal).

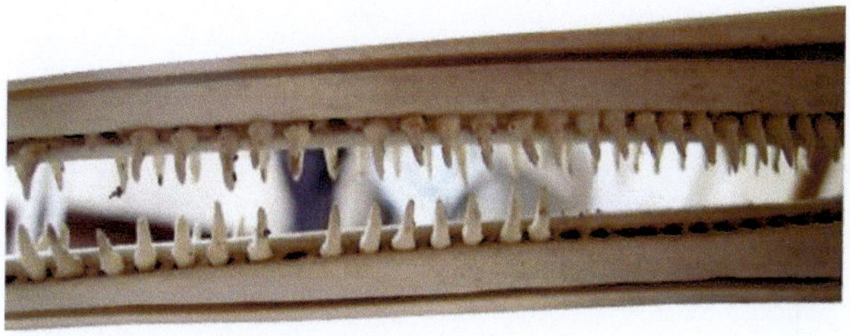

Figure 22.3 Monophyodont dentition (dolphin).

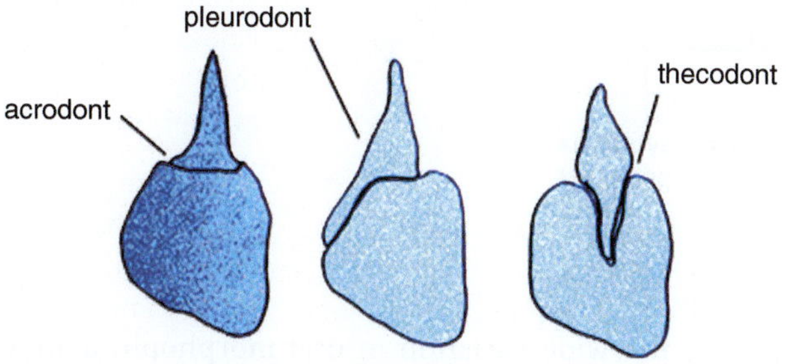

Figure 22.4 Tooth attachment categories.

usually classified according to type and position of attachment (Figure 22.4):

- *Pleurodont.* Have an eroded lingual side and are attached to a higher sided labial wall, such as snakes and lizards.
- *Acrodont.* Found in lizards such as water dragons and chameleons, which have teeth attached to the crest of the bone.
- *Thecodont.* The teeth are embedded in a deep bony socket but, unlike in mammals (that also have a thecodont dentition with teeth in alveoli), there is no periodontal ligament. This type is restricted only to crocodiles.

Lophodont. Each molar consists of intricate folding of enamel and dentin with a ridge or crest complex of dentine lamellae covered by enamel, with cementum among the ridges. The cusps are joined to form ridges or lophs. This anatomical pattern of teeth allows grinding of a variety of native plants during chewing.

Table 22.1, proposed by Kertesz [9], illustrates many of the classification terms described above, with some terminology updated. Although it does not describe all types of teeth, it is very useful for clinical and treatment purposes for most animals.

22.3 Indication for Dental Treatment

The main difficulty of a clinical oral examination in zoo and exotic patients is the detailed inspection. Suspicion of oral diseases is typically based on clinical and behavioral changes [1], such as:

- Aggressive behavior (caused by pain)
- Rubbing the head against objects and friction of the legs/paws on the face
- Changes in drinking or eating behavior
- Acute reactions after food/water ingestion
- Dysphagia or anorexia
- Progressive weight loss
- Change in selection of food items (softer)
- Undigested food in feces
- Oral bleeding.

The most common clinical signs are:

- Head asymmetries
- Abnormal salivation
- Nasal, ocular, dental, or oral discharge
- Malocclusion
- Excessive dental growth.

The characteristic movements of lips, tongue, teeth, and cheeks during mastication of each species should be considered. The veterinarian should understand the differences between species and research individual information with handlers and other professionals who have more intimate contact with particular wild species as necessary [1]. Some of the captive zoo and exotic animals carry a risk of zoonotic diseases. Any clinical examination on these animals requires the use of personal protective equipment (PPE) such as cap, mask, goggles, and gloves.

Oral diseases of wild animals have varied etiologies and have been classified by the American Association of Zoo Veterinarians (AAZV) into four categories: (1) developmental and congenital defects, (2) maxillofacial trauma, (3) periodontal disease, and (4) dental trauma.

Table 22.1 Animal dental classification.

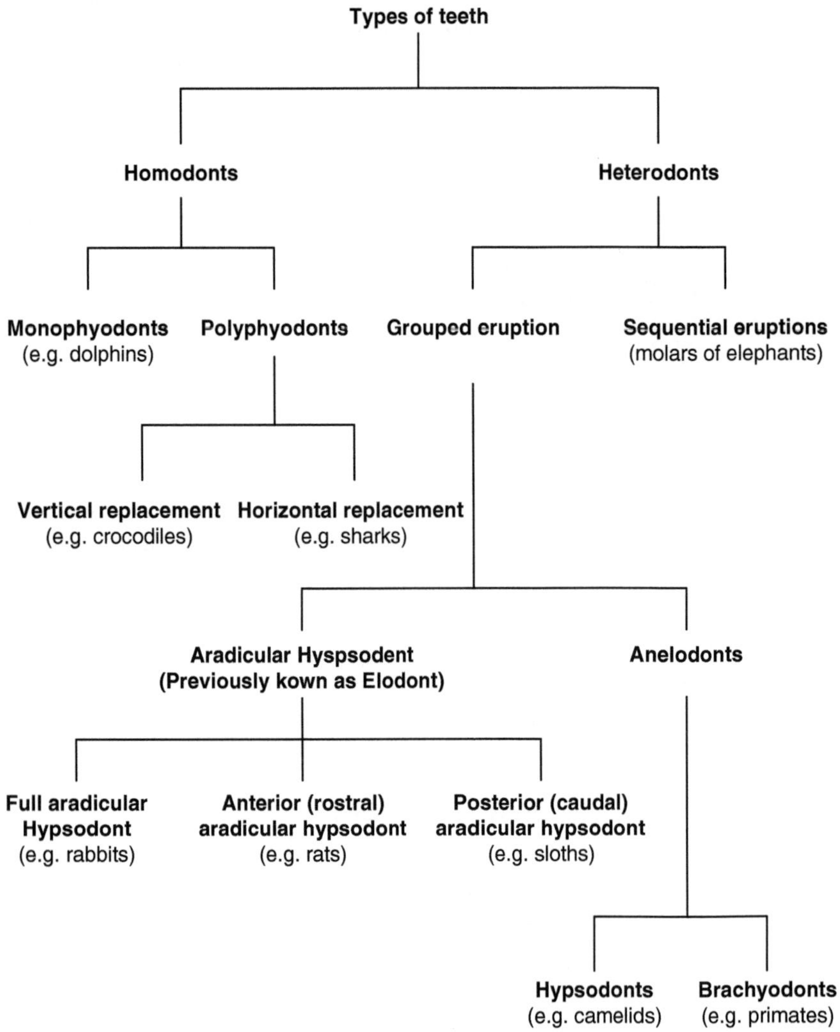

Source: Adapted from reference [9] with updated terminology.

Oral disease results from a wide variety of circumstances and the clinical appearance of the disease process may vary considerably within a single species, and can vary enormously from one species to another. This text will cover the categories, in order of relative importance, of different exotic animal populations.

22.4 Mammals

22.4.1 Primates

Different countries have a large diversity of fauna and flora. Brazil, for instance, has the largest number of species of primates in the world [10]. They are animals that, in most families, have a dental anatomy similar to humans [11]. Dental procedures in primates have many challenges, such as the wide variation in oral morphophysiology and associated zoonoses, and therefore require appropriate knowledge, training, equipment, rapidness, and accuracy.

Due to the evolving proximity between humans and other primates, zoonotic diseases are of fundamental importance to be taken into account during the approach, especially during physical examination and dental treatment when there are released aerosols with the action of the dental handpieces and ultrasound.

The major oral diseases found in primates are as follows.

22.4.1.1 Periodontal Disease

Periodontal disease is the most prevalent disease in captive primates, affecting up to 57% of primates in captivity [12]. Localized periodontal disease is common in all species of primates, but generalized disease has a higher prevalence in the genus *Ateles* (spider monkeys) [5, 7]. Elderly animals seem to be more predisposed to periodontal disease and usually have more advanced degrees of disease. The difference between the diet offered in captivity and what the animal has access to in the wild seems to predispose to plaque buildup and, consequently, to periodontal disease in captive animals [1, 11].

The pathophysiology of periodontal disease in primates is similar to that observed in humans. Dental anatomical similarities indicate similar predisposing factors, mainly due to the absence of interdental spaces (diastema). Proper treatment of periodontal disease in wild animals include supra and subgingival calculus removal and polishing of the entire tooth surface, and antibiotics as indicated [13].

22.4.1.2 Endodontic Disorders

Endodontic disease is highly prevalent among oral lesions, reaching a prevalence of 14% in capuchin monkeys (*Cebus apella*) in captivity [12]. The most common causes of pulp exposure in primates are accidental fractures and the deliberate amputation of the crowns of canine teeth (iatrogenic) [5, 7, 13, 14].

Bacterial invasion of the exposed pulp causes periapical bone loss, infection, and eventually infraorbital (upper) or mandibular (lower) fistula [5, 7, 11]. Similar to treatment of domestic species, endodontic diseases need treatment. Depending on the severity and duration of the lesion, tooth extraction may become the best option, while an endodontic procedure is always an option. Both procedures may require antibiotics [4, 11, 14, 15].

The endodontic treatment technique in primates is analogous to domestic animals. However, primates have a single apical foramen as in humans, not in the form of delta, as in carnivores [15]. The presence of a single apical foramen requires a slightly modified endodontic technique for appropriate cleaning, filing, and obturation of the canal.

22.4.1.3 Caries

By definition, caries is the demineralization of enamel, dentin, or cementum by the action of bacteria and their acid metabolites [5, 11, 13]. Typically the process occurs due to the acid production of bacteria adhered to the teeth in an oral low pH (below 5.5). Caries often occurs in primates kept as pets, in which a poor diet creates conditions conducive to the growth of cariogenic bacteria, such as *Streptococcus mutans*. Further research is required in order to establish the influence of the immune system for each species on the formation of carious lesions.

Several factors may contribute to the onset of caries in primates, such as dental fractures, dental malocclusion or crowding, abnormal dental anatomy (fossae, enamel scars, deep enamel sulcus), acidic oral pH, and inadequate diets (with high levels of carbohydrates) [12, 13].

Similar to caries in domestic species, treatment consists of debridement of necrotic tissue and restoration of the cleaned defect with materials such as glass ionomer and composite resins. In more advanced cases with pulp involvement, treatment involves endodontic therapy of the tooth or extraction [13].

Carious lesions are not commonly identified. In one study of 85 lemurs (*Lemur* sp.), only two had lesions [11] and in a study of 42 monkeys (*Cebus apella*), none had visible caries [12].

22.4.1.4 Occlusal Abnormalities

Occlusal abnormalities are often associated with a greater number of teeth than normal (supranumerary). The excess number of teeth is rarely more than one tooth for each dental arcade [12, 16].

In primates, the teeth most affected by crowding are the premolars. The prevalence of malocclusion in primates in the wild is above 40% and in captivity this percentage can double [16, 17] (Figure 22.5).

In captivity, nutritional disorders can aggravate the incidence of deformities. Insufficient bone growth results in teeth assuming similar positions to those of other teeth, causing serious irregularities. Spencer points to a relationship between the root surface and the amount of chewing force, in which primates eating harder food items would have greater root surface, probably due to the influence of the anteroposterior force that occurs during mastication.

22.4.2 Carnivores

Dental principles in carnivores are based on those used in dogs and cats, although wild animal morphophysiology and dentition functions differ in comparison to domestic animals. Oral diseases are among the most prevalent diseases in captive carnivores and should be part of all management programs on these species [1]. The major oral diseases found in carnivores are the following.

22.4.2.1 Periodontal Disease

Periodontal disease is the most prevalent oral disease in carnivores [1, 5, 7, 18–21]. Like in domestic animals, the growth and the multiplication of microorganisms in dental plaque are determining factors for the initiation and development of periodontal disease. However, some factors may predispose to periodontal disease, such as poor diet, dental and periodontal abnormalities, immune disorders, malocclusion, persistence of deciduous teeth, and some systemic diseases [1, 5, 7, 22].

Recent studies indicate an important relationship between the consistency of the diet and the formation of plaque.

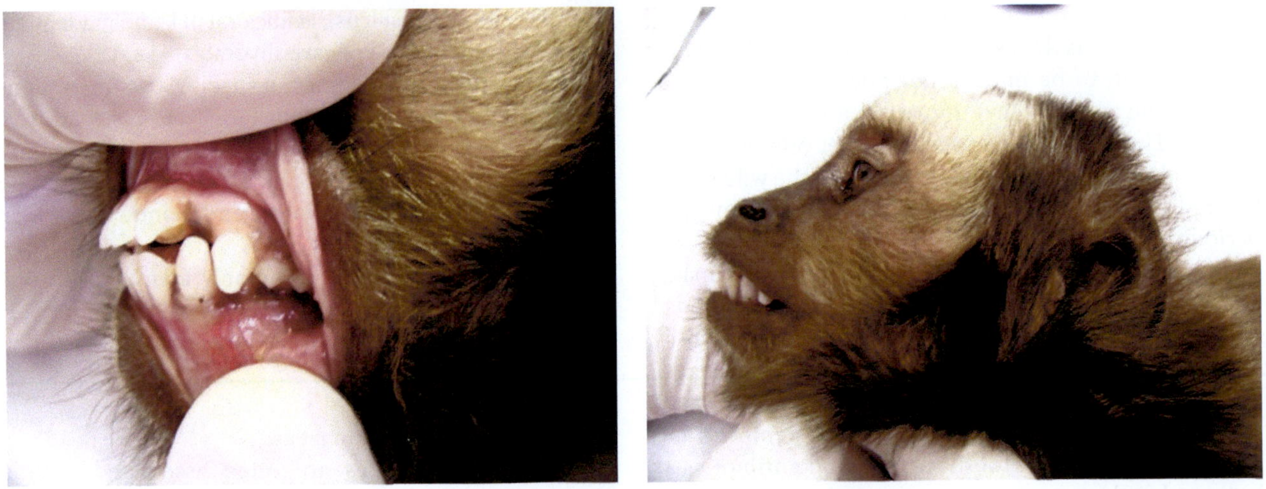

Figure 22.5 Monkey (*Cebus* sp.) with a maxillary incisor malocclusion and subsequent skull deformity.

Artificial and soft diets generally do not have the same composition as the natural foraging and free-range diets (bones, ligaments, joints, etc.). They also require little masticatory exercise, contributing to the formation of gingivitis and plaque, which organizes as a colony and can mineralize to form dental calculus and potentially cause damage to the periodontal tissues [22].

In more advanced cases, there may be involvement of all periodontal tissues and eventual exfoliation of the tooth. Prevention of periodontal disease is obtained by correcting the diet and regular clinical assessment and treatment.

In addition to local infection, microorganisms can reach the bloodstream through gingival bleeding and may contribute to diseases such as glomerulonephritis, arthritis, endocarditis, and meningitis. The death of a black bear (*Ursus americanus*) has been reported due to bacterial endocarditis caused by *Staphylococcus aureus*, with infection of other organs, for which the oral cavity may have been the primary focus of infection [23].

One study [24] was designed to evaluate the major diseases of the oral cavity related to periodontal disease in *Panthera onca* in captivity as well as free-ranging animals, in order to determine if environmental conditions could influence oral health. It used a sample of 42 ($N = 42$) jaguars (*Panthera onca*) from 18 institutions in captivity in São Paulo and four ($N = 4$) free-ranging jaguars (*Panthera onca*), captured in the wetlands of Mato Grosso do Sul, Pantanal. The results of clinical signs that lead to periodontal disease were as follows for the animals in captivity: plaque (7%), gingivitis (50%), dental calculus (100%), furcation exposure (14.2%), periodontal pockets (33.3%), and gingival recession (14.2%).

The clinical signs are basically the same as those found in domestic animals and the proper treatment for periodontal disease in non-domestic animals includes mainly removal of subgingival and supragingival calculus, polishing all tooth surfaces, and antibiotics [1, 4, 13].

22.4.2.2 Dental Trauma and Endodontic Disease

Along with periodontal disease, dental injuries are highly prevalent in wild carnivores, mainly in captive animals [1, 5, 7, 15].

Dental traumas are differentiated by their characteristics and intensity. Attrition is the constant wear between two or more teeth, erosion is destruction of the tooth structure by chemical agents, and abrasion is the destruction of tooth structures from objects. The tooth surface is capable of supporting certain physiological limits of abrasion, attrition, and erosion. If teeth have dysplasia due to injuries or malocclusion, this limit can be overcome and structural damage to the teeth can be seen. This can also occur in fights or frequent contact with hard objects and enclosure fences. This problem is common in large felines and in other carnivores with aggressive habits due to chewing on the steel bars or concrete structures in the enclosures. The tooth surface is capable of supporting certain physiologically limited friction. If this limit is exceeded by malocclusion, injury, or repetition, excessive wear of the teeth occurs that can progress to fracture. In addition to the dental issues, this syndrome is usually associated with behavioral disorders, characterizing situations of stress in animals kept in captivity. When wear occurs slowly, the odontoblasts are capable of producing tertiary dentin in order to repair the tooth and protect the pulp [15]. In a paper on marsupials, it was reported that the genus *Didelphis* suffers premature wear of the teeth in the wild due to their predatory habits [25].

More intense trauma can also cause tooth fractures, may involve different structures, and are classified in different degrees [26, 27]:

Enamel fracture – Fractures involving enamel
Uncomplicated crown fracture – Fracture of enamel and dentin
Complicated crown fracture – Fracture with pulp exposure
Traumatic tooth loss
Root fracture.

In cases of pulp exposure or indirect endodontic involvement, there is contamination by pathogenic microorganisms, which can migrate to the root apex and cause a periapical infection [26, 27]. As a result of this infection, mandibular or maxillary fistulae can be observed.

One study from Brazil [24] reported that 73.07% of the captive population of jaguars (*Panthera onca*) and 58.33% of the population of pumas (*Puma concolor*) were affected by dental fractures. The predisposing factor to these lesions appears to be traumatic wear of the teeth. Iatrogenic fractures can occur when attempting to physically restrain animals not sedated or in early stages of sedation, while they are still responsive to external stimuli.

In some dental fractures, the pulp chamber of the crown was exposed or compromised (42.3% in *P. onca* and 12.5% in *P. concolor*), which often evolves into pulp necrosis (95% in *P. onca*). The most affected teeth are the canines, with cusp fractures: 31.57% in *P. onca* and 71% in *P. concolor*.

Treatment involves endodontics and restorations, as well as prosthodontics and maxillofacial surgery [15, 28, 29]. However, in some cases, extraction is necessary due to extensive periapical alveolar destruction.

22.4.2.3 Caries

Carnivores are virtually free of caries. It has the same pathophysiology seen in primates, but its prevalence is much lower in carnivores. This is due to the non-cariogenic factors presented by carnivores such as diets with lower carbohydrate content, dental anatomy (large spaces between the teeth and occlusal surface in the form of cusps, reducing food impaction), and higher salivary pH [30].

Caries may cause intense pain and can lead to anorexia, especially if it reaches the dentin–pulp complex. Animals living in human areas tend to have more dental caries due to a higher intake of carbohydrates and sweets in their diet. Clinically, demineralization of dental structures by the action of acid metabolites produced by bacteria is observed (Figure 22.6). These should be distinguished from tooth resorptive lesions.

The treatment is similar to primates, with debridement of necrotic tissue and restoration of the carious lesion using materials of glass ionomer or composites. In more advanced cases with dental pulp involvement, root canal or extraction is necessary.

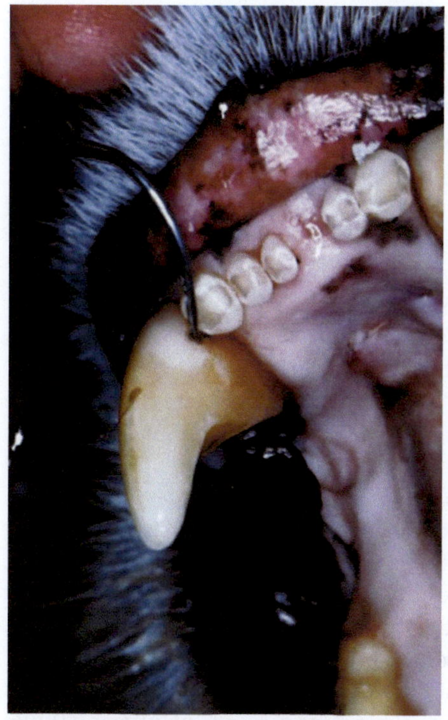

Figure 22.6 Use of dental explorer to show caries in the left lower canine of a lion (*Panthera leo*). *Source:* Photo: Luiz João Rossi Jr.

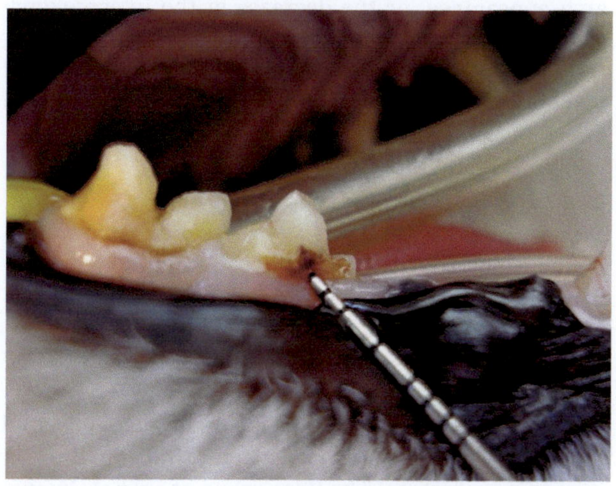

Figure 22.7 Resorptive lesion in the cervical area of a premolar in a Brazilian wild cat (*Leopardus tigrinus*).

22.4.2.4 Resorptive Lesions

Resorptive lesions are common in domestic cats [31] and are also reported in captive and wild animals [20, 32], with only a few studies in these species [33]. There are reports involving lions, leopards [32], jaguars, pumas, ocelots [5], and wild cats [20] (Figure 22.7).

Clinically and radiographically, the resorption appears to destroy the dental structures and can compromise enamel and dentin. While the first visible indications are usually near the gingival margin of the tooth, often root involvement has preceded this detection.

The etiology is still unknown and the main clinical signs are pain and discomfort during eating food or drinking water (especially cold) and anorexia. In the early stages of the disease, restoration with glass ionomer or composite resin was once considered, but extraction is now indicated in most cases [20, 31–33].

22.4.2.5 Occlusal Abnormalities

Amand and Tinkelman [16] describe malocclusion in some species of mammals, affirming that these abnormalities develop in a particular way for different species. The types of malocclusion seen in domestic animals are similar to those seen in wild animals. Captive animals may show these abnormalities due to stress, changes in nutrition, diet texture, trauma, periodontal disease, or resulting from abnormal behavior during mating. Insufficient bone growth results in normal teeth assuming different positions, and the overgrowth tends to shift the teeth, producing, in some cases, extreme irregularities.

A Brazilian study [24] observed that 47.61% of jaguars (*Panthera onca*, $N = 42$) and 5.55% of pumas (*Puma concolor*, $N = 36$) evaluated in captivity in the state of São Paulo showed this deformity. The malocclusion findings related mainly to displacement of incisors, presenting an arch appearance, or the decrease in the interproximal space in the region of the premolars and molars, allowing the accumulation of food debris or plaque. In the wild felines, consequences and treatment of malocclusions are not well described.

22.4.2.6 Other Conditions

Various oral diseases such as oronasal communication (fistula) and neoplasia are also observed in captive carnivores, but are infrequent and rarely reported [34–36].

22.4.3 Herbivores

Dental morphophysiology and pathophysiology of oral lesions in wild herbivores are generally similar to those in domestic herbivores. The large group of animals known as ungulates is divided into those animals that have an odd number of toes (perissodactyl) and those with an even number (artiodactyls). Among the artiodactyls, there are the antelope, deer, and camels. Perissodactyls includes species such as tapirs, rhinos, and horses. Tapirs have 42–44 teeth (2× (3/3 1/1 3–4/3 3/3)) and are lophodont (with transverse grooves of the occlusal surface); rhinos may have 24–34 teeth (2× (0–1/0–1 0/0–1 3–4/3–4 3/3)) and are hypsodonts (crown longer than the root). The exotic equine animals (e.g., zebra, wild Przewalski horse) have the same dental formulas as their domestic counterparts [37]. There are many articles published in equine dentistry and most of the techniques described can be modified to be used in the treatment of exotic ungulates [37].

In general, the skull and teeth vary widely within the group of artiodactyls, but most do not have front teeth. Pigs are true omnivores and their ancestors originally had 44 teeth (heterodont) with a dental formula of 2× (3/3 1/1 4/4 3/3). Currently, some genres have fewer teeth. Regardless of gender, the upper canine teeth are typically hollow and grow continuously. In most species, the canine teeth curve and form a tusk [8, 36]. The miniature pigs maintained as pets may have occlusal deformities due to genetic changes with the species and thus deserve more attention.

Camelids generally have between 30 and 34 teeth, but may have up to 38 teeth. The canines and premolar teeth are hooked, and the lateral incisors are similar to canines. When camels still show primary teeth, they contain three upper incisors, but with the eruption of permanent teeth, only the third pair of upper incisors is present. The lower incisors erupt continuously (hypsodont teeth) and can present "overgrowth" in cases of incorrect wear. Ruminants (most artiodactyls) do not have the upper incisors and the lateral lower incisors are canine shaped. All members of this group are herbivores and chew through lateral and rostrocaudal movement of the mandible [8, 37].

The detection of dental abnormalities in ungulates is not easy because most species show no external signs until the disease has progressed significantly. Frequent behavioral changes, such as lethargy, weight loss, and anorexia are observed. Dental abnormalities commonly cause changes in the animal's ability to grasp and chew food. Certain food items can be dropped, hypersalivation may be evident, or chewing time can be increased [37]. Anesthesia is necessary in most cases for a detailed dental examination in these species, particularly considering the typically small mouth opening.

One of the most common dental abnormalities is infundibular necrosis (alveolitis and mandibular osteomyelitis, known as "lumpy jaw"). Other anomalies include dental malocclusion, dental overgrowth, neoplasia, trauma, and periodontal disease.

22.4.3.1 Infundibular Necrosis

Infundibular necrosis is a chronic process of alveolitis and osteomyelitis manifested through facial swelling and discharge in the affected tooth area, sometimes accompanied by fistulae. The pathogens involved are often *Fusobacterium necrophorum*, *Bacteroides* spp., *Peptostreptococcus* spp., and *Actinomyces* spp. [8]. In the United States, the captive species most affected by this disease are the red kangaroos (*Megaleia rufa*) and the Pronghorn antelope (*Antilocapra American*). Many animals

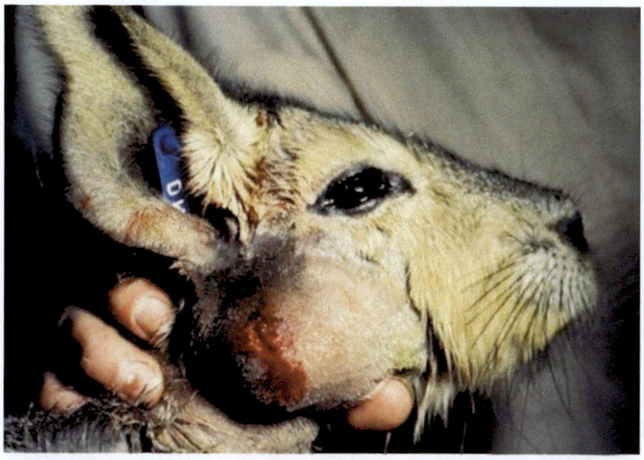

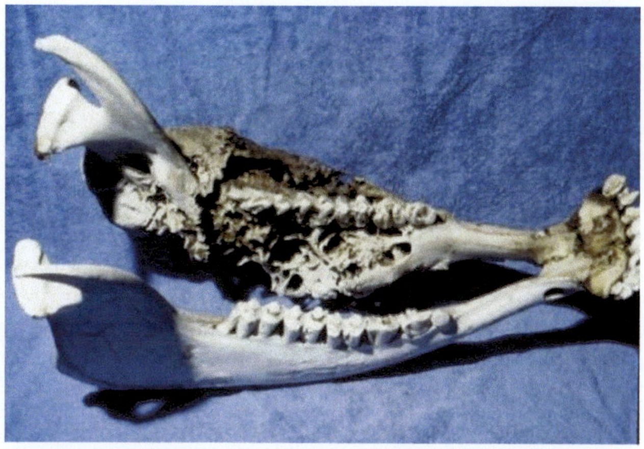

Figure 22.8 Clinical and anatomical aspect of chronic osteomyelitis infundibular necrosis in kangaroo. *Source:* Photo: Peter Emily.

compromised by this infection (67%) end up being euthanized or will die as a direct result of the disease. The clinical signs and symptoms include [5]:

- Drooling and dysphagia
- Maxillary and mandibular swelling
- Weight loss
- Bone lysis and formation of exostosis
- Destruction of periodontal ligament.

Progression of this disease leads to osteomyelitis of the affected region (maxilla or mandible), dental exfoliation, and formation of fistulae (Figure 22.8). Due to this entry pathway of pathogens, the patient can develop septicemia, with involvement of the central nervous system (encephalitis) and visceral abscess formation [1].

The diagnosis can be facilitated by oblique radiographs of the dental arch, giving preference to the use of intraoral dental films.

Extraction and manual debridement is still the treatment of choice for most dental abscesses. Depending on the species affected, surgical access can be difficult. It may be necessary to perform a buccotomy (incision through the facial skin), similar to that performed in horses.

22.4.3.2 Malocclusion and Dental Overgrowth

Malocclusion can be caused by tooth fractures or periodontal disease, resulting in overgrowth of the teeth [38] (Figure 22.9). The formation of sharp edges on the teeth (hooks, beaks, and ramps) results in ulcerations on the cheek and lingual mucosa. Clinical signs include anorexia, "locking" of the teeth during chewing, drooling, accumulation of food in the oral cavity, and weight loss. Diagnosis is based on observation of the animal and physical examination with sedation. The treatment is the same as described in the horse section.

Genetic changes may predispose to occlusal changes, as commonly seen in miniature pigs.

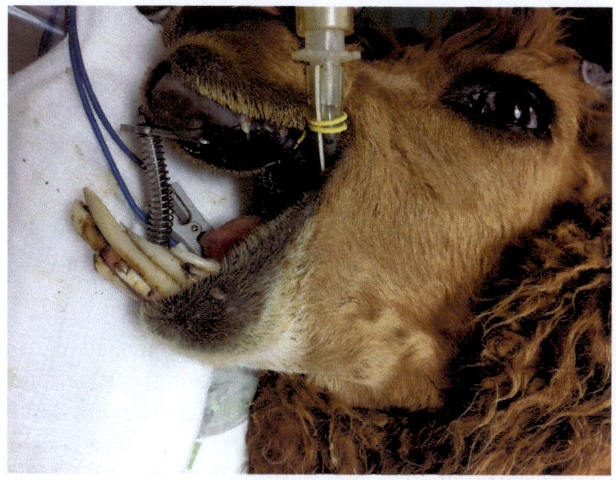

Figure 22.9 Dental overgrowth of lower incisors in llama (*Lama glama*).

22.4.3.3 Trauma

Maxillofacial injuries are common in captive ungulates because these species are easily frightened and tend to attempt escape from human approach or unknown sound stimuli. In distress, animals may throw themselves against enclosure walls, gates, and screens.

Treatment depends on the extent of the injury. "Degloving" injuries of the soft tissue over the rostral area of the mandible are best treated conservatively. In cases of minor laceration, the healing process can occur by second intention with good results [39]. However, mandibular or maxillary fractures may also occur, which would require surgical repair.

22.4.3.4 Neoplasia

A wide variety of malignancies have been reported in wild animals in captivity, but most reports are isolated clinical cases [36, 40–42]. Among the reported tumors, the most common sites are the skin and subcutaneous tissue (including cutaneous mast cell tumors, basal cell epithelioma, duct mammary carcinoma, and subcutaneous fibrosarcoma) and the digestive system (including gastric carcinoma, malignant lymphoma of the biliary tract and two cases of adenocarcinomas of the gallbladder) [43].

22.4.3.5 Periodontal Disease

Periodontitis and dentoalveolar abscesses are rarely described in wild herbivores, perhaps because they are more resistant to disease or poorly diagnosed by technicians and professionals. The apparent cause is related to mineral depletion in food, causing the teeth to have mobility, and accumulation of food in the gingival sulcus and periapical region. Clinical signs are the presence of dental calculus, gingival recession, gingivitis, the presence of partially digested food in feces, anorexia, halitosis, chronic weight loss, and increased salivation.

Tapirs may have physiological periodontal degeneration during the primary dental exfoliation at around 27 months of age, because the permanent teeth are significantly larger than the primary teeth. Treatment includes periodontal scaling and polishing, extractions, diet correction, and administration of antibiotics and analgesics [38].

22.4.4 Mega Vertebrates

Dentistry in mega vertebrates is still a great challenge to the veterinarian. Elephants, hippos, and giraffes are the most susceptible to oral lesions and require more attention. Because the main difficulty is conducting a general physical examination, and specifically a dental examination, it is essential to address behavioral conditioning to approach to the handling and performance of minimally invasive procedures. Conditioning avoids or minimizes the need for sedation and anesthesia except for complex and difficult to perform procedures. Note that it is necessary to use potent opioid drugs such as etorphine or carfentanil to be able to safely immobilize these species with a small volume. These drugs should be reversed after the procedures are performed.

The dentition of elephants is unique among mammals. The dental formula is: 2× (1/1 0/0 0/0 6/6) = 28. The incisors are aradicular hypsodont and the molars change five times with horizontal sequential eruption throughout the animal's life. The molars wear as a set. When the predecessors wear out, the roots are reabsorbed and a successor set erupts [44] (Figure 22.10).

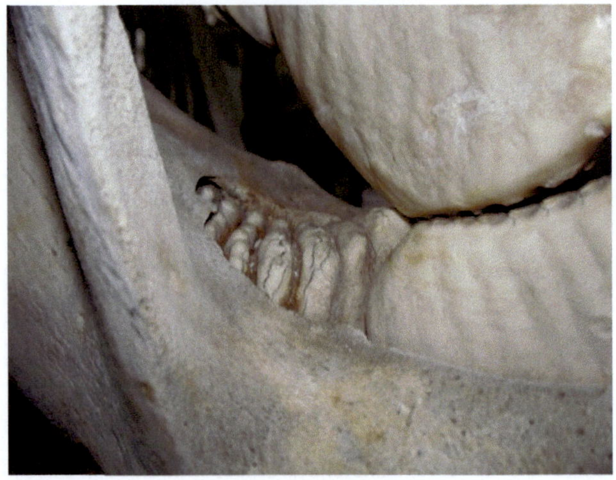

Figure 22.10 African elephant skull (*Loxodonta africana*), with horizontal exchange of dental molar teeth.

Each molar consists of a ridge or crest complex of dentine lamellae covered by dentin enamel, with cementum among the ridges, known as lophodont teeth. This anatomical pattern of teeth allows grinding of a variety of native plants during chewing. It is possible to differentiate the living species of elephants through the conformation of molar teeth [45]. Indian elephants (*Elephas maximus* – including extinct relatives) have a certain parallelism between the lamellae of the occlusal surface of the teeth. In African elephants (*Loxodonta africana*), the lamellae show a curvature in the central line region of the teeth, which can fuse and form the image of a diamond on the occlusal surface (Figure 22.11).

In African elephants, the sixth and last molar erupts at around 26–30 years old. After the last molar is in occlusion, the accuracy in estimating age decreases. Estimators adopt the criterion that when teeth show wear and a reduction of the clinical crown, the individual is at around 45–49 years of age [44].

The tusk of an elephant is a lateral maxillary incisor, composed of dentin, pulp, and enamel. Deciduous tusks are present at birth and during the first year of life, and are covered by enamel. They are exchanged for permanent tusks at approximately one year of age. These teeth are curved and are usually directed forward and below the head, tending to angle up to the midline (Figure 22.12). These teeth may show sexual dimorphism

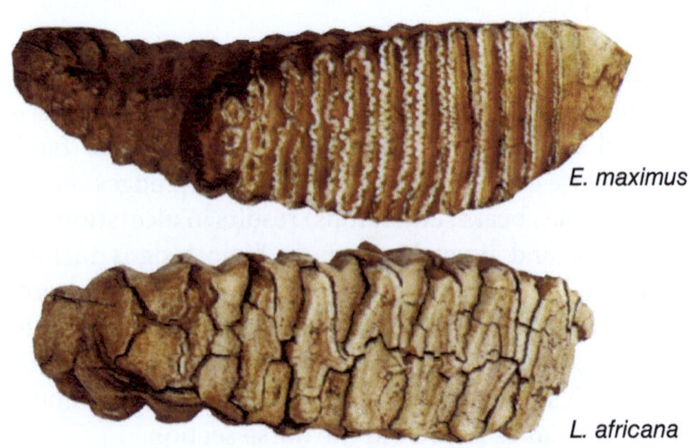

Figure 22.11 Comparison of the occlusal surface of Indian (*Elephas maximus*) and African elephant (*Loxodonta Africana*) molar teeth.

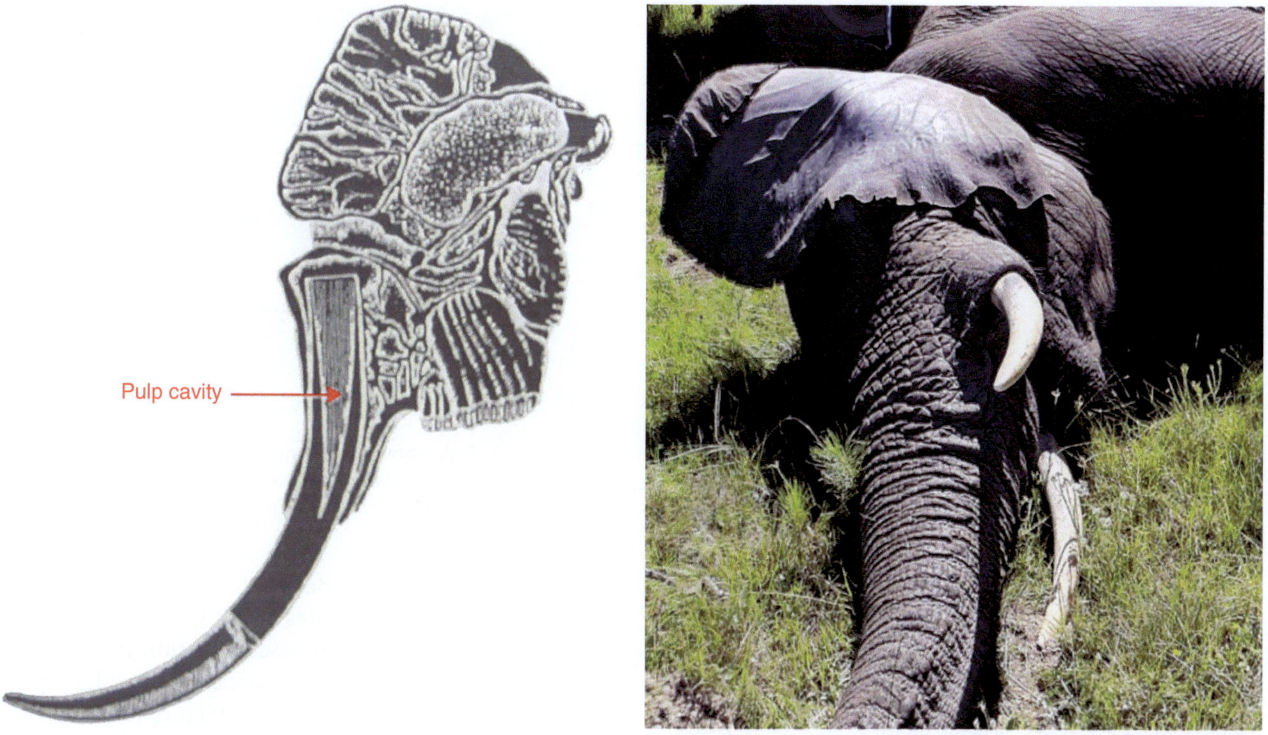

Figure 22.12 Illustration of the skull (left image) and the general appearance of African elephant incisors under general anesthesia (right image).

between individuals, and males present with more developed tusks [44, 45].

Hippos (*Hippopotamus amphibius*) are considered "amphibian mammals," because they live most of the time under water, emerging at night to graze on the banks of rivers and lakes. This behavior is also observed in animals in captivity. Their lower incisor teeth are blunt, long, and separated by a diastema. The upper incisors are smaller. The canines (upper and lower) are large tusks, more than 50 cm long in certain individuals, coated with a thin layer of enamel [44] (Figure 22.13). The incisors and canines are aradicular hypsodont teeth with a constant average growth of 0.42 mm per month [46]. During wear the teeth are naturally sharpened, representing important offensive and defensive tools. The premolars and molars in hippos have large and simple cusps like those seen in horses [45].

Giraffes (*Giraffa camelopardalis*) have a long prehensile tongue that grasps food. Leaves form the basis of their diet, which are carefully selected and processed in the ruminant digestive tract. Their teeth are like most ruminants, with the presence of rough enamel and the dental formula is: 2× (0/3 0/1 3/3 3/3) = 32.

22.4.4.1 Trauma and Injury

As observed in other wild species, mega vertebrates live in constant disputes over territory, social position, sexual partners, and food, among others. These situations predispose the animals to oral and facial trauma. This is exacerbated in situations of mishandling and accidents, such as falls in the enclosure ditches.

Lacerating injuries are common, especially in disputes between males and inexperienced young animals trying to mate with adult females. In hippos, the lacerating wounds can be easily contaminated once animals submerge in the same water tank in which they defecate. Egg infestation by insects and myiasis are also possible complications. The treatment for lacerations is typically the use of systemic and topical antibiotics, and wound treatment by second intention healing.

Intense trauma and falls can lead to tooth fracture, especially in elephant tusks. A study of 60 zoos in the United States revealed that 31% of animals showed dental fractures (N = 379) [44]. Small fractures can be restored with composite or acrylic resins, but fractures with pulp exposure require endodontic treatment [47].

As observed in wild carnivores, the stereotypical behavior generated by chronic stress can have dental consequences when the animals have the habit of biting on hard objects or on the enclosure, which can lead to pulp exposure (Figure 22.14).

22.4.4.2 Dental Overgrowth

Abnormal dental growth in mega vertebrates generally occurs because of problems in the opposing tooth, causing malocclusion and improper wear. In hippos, the

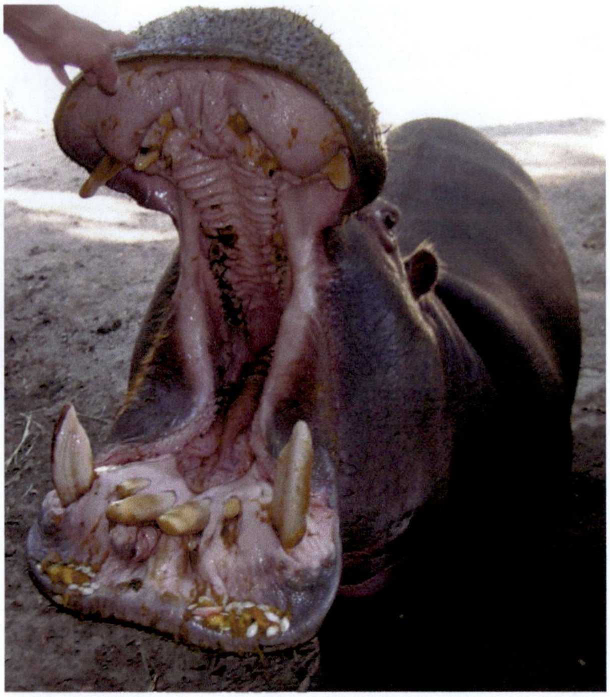

Figure 22.13 Clinical view of hippo teeth.

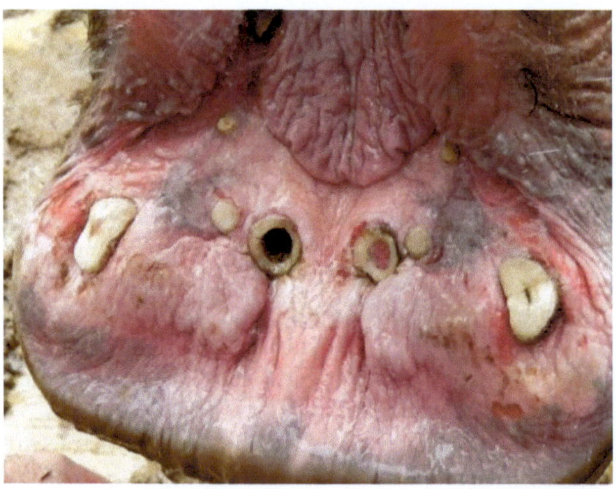

Figure 22.14 Dental wear in incisors and canines of a hippo, with pulp exposure of the central incisors.

lower canines occlude against the upper ones and wear between them keeps the anatomical shape of the clinical crown. Occlusal changes between these teeth can cause dental overgrowth and labial lesions. This creates pain, anorexia, and weight loss [44].

Treatment for tooth overgrowth is similar for other species with continuously growing teeth. Conditioned animals may allow crown reduction, but most of the time, sedation or anesthesia is necessary.

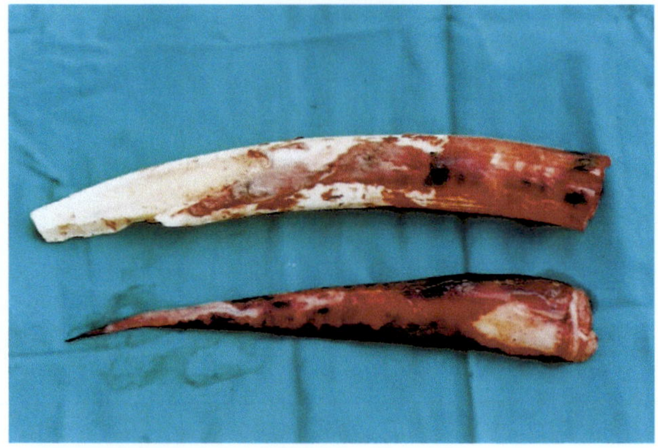

Figure 22.15 Tusk (above) and dental pulp (below) of young African elephant (*Loxodonta africana*). Note the large pulp to tooth ratio. *Source:* Photo: Marcelo Campos Malta.

22.4.4.3 Endodontic Disorders

The tusks of mega vertebrates have a large proportion of dental pulp with significant vascularization and an open apex. Thus, these teeth can often deal better with pulpitis than the teeth of domestic animals (Figure 22.15). However, in cases of pulp exposure, pulpitis can turn to necrosis and produce an alveolar abscess and bacteremia. Clinically, anorexia, weight loss, pain, aggressive behavior, and even death can be observed [44, 47–50].

The treatment for pulp exposure due to tooth fracture usually requires partial pulpectomy [47, 48]. Ideally, no more than the coronal two-thirds of the pulp should be removed, maintaining the pulp within the reserve crown in contact with the alveolar bone.

After partial removal of pulp, the dental canal should be irrigated thoroughly with saline or another biocompatible topical solution. Then the channel must be filled with a dental cement (obturation). An ideal cement is antibacterial, biocompatible, and capable of stimulating tertiary dentin bridge production, which will seal and isolate the pulp in the remaining third of the crown. Literature reports the use of zinc oxide and eugenol for this purpose, but more recently, the most commonly used products are calcium hydroxide [44, 47] or mineral trioxide aggregate (MTA).

The partial pulpectomy is completed by dental restoration, which can be performed using composite or acrylic resins. The ideal restoration should offer a good seal, prevent early wear, and allow the functional use of the tooth. One commonly used option is the self-polymerizing acrylic resin without exothermic reaction, such as bis-acrylic (ProTemp 3M®). The loss of the restorative material and ongoing abnormal and traumatic behaviors are the main causes of failure in endodontic treatment of these animals. In such cases, extraction is typically required [44].

The indications for extraction of tusks varies, but are often associated with complicated fractures and unsuccessful

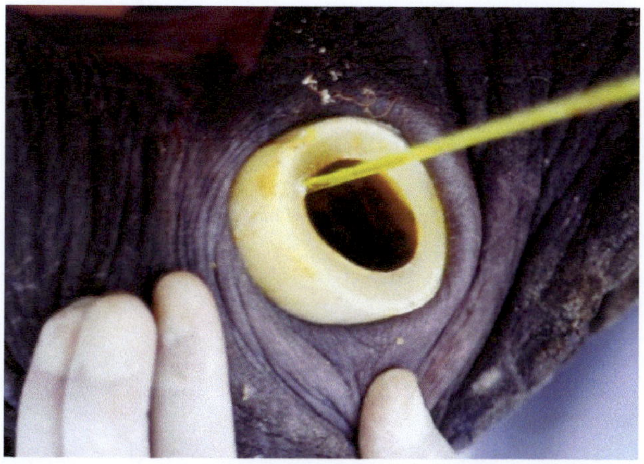

Figure 22.16 Longitudinal section performed in elephant tusk. *Source:* Photo: Marcelo Campos Malta.

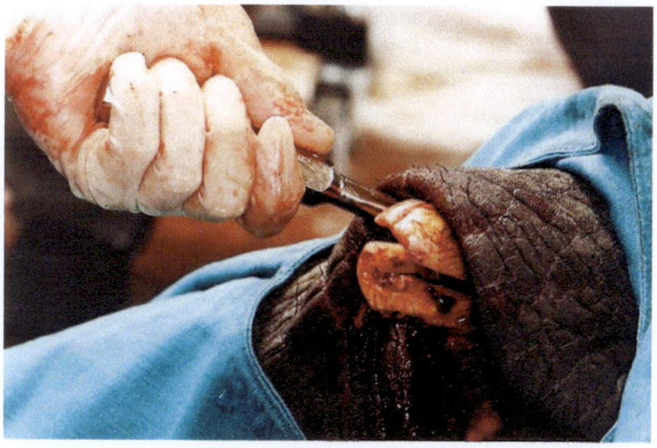

Figure 22.17 Use of chisel to luxate dental fragments in elephant tusk. *Source:* Photo: Marcelo Campos Malta.

endodontic treatments. The standard surgical extraction by the alveolar approach can be used, but tends to be very traumatic [44]. The currently recommended technique is "internal collapse," which is based on sectioning the tooth into four longitudinal sections (Figure 22.16). A chisel is then used to extend the cuts longitudinally. Each fragment is separated from the alveolar wall and dislodged into the central root canal space to facilitate removal (Figure 22.17).

Each piece should then be gently removed to complete tooth extraction (Figure 22.18). Finally, the empty socket must be curetted and thoroughly cleaned. Because these teeth are continuously growing (aradicular hypsodont), the apical curettage should remove or destroy any remaining germinal tissue.

22.4.4.4 Oral Malformations

Tumors in the oral cavity of mega vertebrates are uncommon. Odontomas in African elephants have been reported and one elephant was euthanized due to the presence of an oral tumor incompatible with life [44]. Impacted teeth, malocclusion, and failures of dental eruption and growth can generate bone torus, gingival hyperplasia, and peripheral odontogenic tumors.

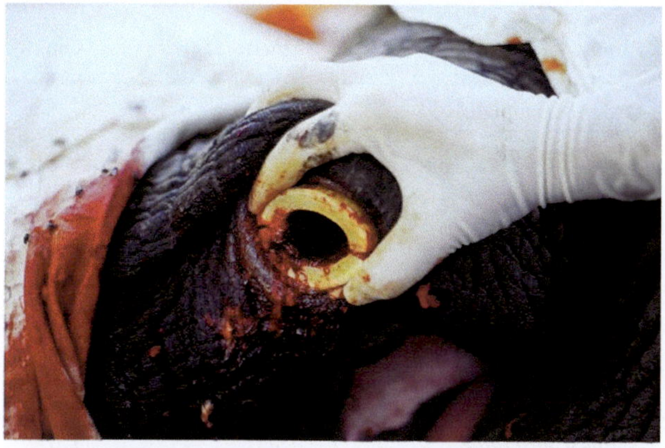

Figure 22.18 Tusk extraction fragments and verification of complete extraction in elephant. *Source:* Photo: Marcelo Campos Malta.

22.5 Dental Formulas and Eruption Tables

See Tables 22.2–22.5.

Table 22.2 Deciduous tooth eruption time in Felidae (in days).

Tooth	Lions	Tigers	Leopards	Puma	Jaguar
First incisor	22–24	12–20	22–26	14–17	15–17
Second incisor	25–29	20–24	26–27	17–20	20–25
Third incisor	33–39	28–29	32–33	23–28	20–32
Canine	31–32	31–34	28–30	28–29	29–35
second premolar	117–152				60–62
Third premolar	60–65	55–59	45–47	40–42	
Fourth premolar	48–85	52–64	40–69	37–47	

Source: Taken from reference [8].

Table 22.3 Deciduous and permanent teeth eruption time in Lynx (bobcat) (*Linx rufus*) (in days).

Teeth	Eruption begins	Eruption complete
Deciduous	11–14	40–60
Permanent		
Incisors	130	160
Canines		150
Maxillary		210
Mandibular		240

Source: Taken from reference [8].

Table 22.4 Deciduous and permanent teeth eruption time in Pacas (*Agouti paca*) (in months of life).

Tooth	Deciduous	Permanent
Incisor		0 – born erupted
Premolars – mandibular	22–24	27–30
Premolars – maxillary	23–24	27–30
First molar		0 – born erupted
Second molar		4
Third molar		14

Source: Taken from reference [51].

Table 22.5 Dental formulae tables.

Family	Incisors	Canines	Premolars	Molars	Total
Order Marsupialia					
Didelphidae	5/4	1/1	3/3	4/4	2× = 50
Dasyuridae	4/3	1/1	3/3	4/4	2× = 46
Mymecobiidae	4/3	1/1	3/3	5–6 / 5–6	2× = 50–54
Notoryctidae	3–4 / 3	1/1	2/3	4/4	2× = 42–44
Caenolestidae	4 / 3–4	1/1	3/3	4/4	2× = 46–48
Phalangeridae	2–3 / 2–3	1/0	1–3 / 1–3	3–4 / 3–4	2× = 28–40
Tarcsipedidae	2/1	1/0	1/0	3/3	2× = 22
Phascolarctidae	3/1	1/0	1/1	4/4	2× = 30
Vombatidae	1/1	0/0	1/1	4/4	2× = 24
Macropodidae	3/1	0–1 / 0	2/2	4/4	2× = 32–34
Peramelidae	4–5 / 3	1/1	3/3	4/4	46–48
Order Insectivora					
Suborder Lipotyphla					
Erifaceidae	2–3 / 3	1/1	3–4 / 2–4	3/3	2× = 36–44
Chrysochloridae	3/3	1/1	3/3	3/3	2× = 40
Talpidae	2/3	1/1	3/3	2–4 / 2–3	2× = 34–40
Solenodontidae	3/3	1/1	3/3	3/3	2× = 40
Potamogalidae	2/3	1/1	3/3	3/3	2× = 38
Soricidae	3 / 1–2	1 / 0–1	1–3 / 1	3/3	2× = 26–32
Suborder Menotyphla					
Macroscelididae	1–3 / 3	1/1	4/4	2 / 2–3	2× = 36–42
Tupaiidae	2/3	1/1	3/3	3/3	2× = 38
Order Chiroptera					
Suborder Megachiroptera					
Pteropodidae	1–2 / 0–2	1/1	3/3	1–2 / 2–3	2× = 24–34
Suborder Microchiroptera					
Rhinfopomatidae	1/2	1/1	1/2	3/3	2× = 28
Craseonycteridae	1/2	1/1	1/2	3/3	2× = 28
Emballonuridae	1–2 / 2–3	1/1	2/2	3/3	2× = 30–34

Table 22.5 (Continued)

Family	Incisors	Canines	Premolars	Molars	Total
Noctilionidae	2/1	1/1	1/2	3/3	2x = 28
Nycteridae	2/3	1/1	1/2	3/3	2x = 32
Megadermatidae	0/2	1/1	1–2 / 2	3/3	2x = 28–32
Rhinfolophidae	1/2	1/1	1–2 / 2–3	3/3	2x = 28–32
Molossidae	2/2	1/1	2/2	3/3	2x = 34
Desmodontidae	1–2 / 2	1/1	1–2 / 2–3	0–2 / 0–2	2x = 20–26
Natalidae	2/3	1/1	3/3	3/3	2x = 38
Furipteridae	2/3	1/1	2/3	3/3	2x = 36
Myzopodidae	2/3	1/1	3/3	3/3	2x = 38
Vespertilionidae	1–2 / 2–3	1/1	1–3 / 2–3	3/3	2x = 28–38
Mystacinfidae	1/1	1/1	2/2	3/3	2x = 28
Molossidae	1 / 1–3	1/1	1–2 / 2	3/3	2x = 26–32
Order Primates					
Suborder Prosimi					
Lemuridae	0–2 / 2	1/1	3/3	3/3	2x = 32–36
Lorisidae	1–2 / 2	1/1	3/3	3/3	2x = 34–36
Daubentonidae	1/1	0–1 / 0	1/0	3/3	2x = 18–20
Tracsiidae	2/1	1/1	3/3	3/3	2x = 34
Suborder Anthropoidae					
Cebidae	2/2	1/1	3/3	3/3	2x = 36
Callitrichidae	2/2	1/1	3/3	2/2	2x = 32
Callimiconidae	2/2	1/1	3/3	3/3	2x = 36
Cercopithecidae	2/2	1/1	3/3	2/2	2x = 32
Pongidae	2/2	1/1	2/2	3/3	2x = 32
Hominidae	2/2	1/1	2/2	3/3	2x = 32
Order Xenarthra					
Bradypodidae	0/0	0/0	5 / 4–5	0/0	2x = 18–20
Dasypodidae	0/0	0/0	0/0	7–25 / 7–25	2x = 28–100
Myrmecophagidae	0/0	0/0	0/0	0/0	2x = 0
Order Tubilidentata					
Orycteropodidae	0/0	0/0	2/2	3/3	2x = 20
Order Lagomorpha					
Ochotonidae	2/1	0/0	3/2	2/3	2x = 26
Leporidae	2/1	0/0	3/2	2–3 / 3	2x = 26–28
Order Rodentia					
Aplodontidae	1/1	0/0	2/1	3/3	2x = 22
Castoridae	1/1	0/0	1/1	3/3	2x = 20
Sciridae	1/1	0/0	1–2 / 1	3/3	2x = 20–22
Anomalurudae	1/1	0/0	1/1	3/3	2x = 20
Pedetidae	1/1	0/0	1/1	3/3	2x = 20
Muridae	1/1	0/0	0/0	2–3 / 2–3	2x = 12–16
Gliridae	1/1	0/0	1/1	3/3	2x = 20

(Continued)

Table 22.5 (Continued)

Family	Incisors	Canines	Premolars	Molars	Total
Platacanthomyidae	1/1	0/0	0/0	3/3	2x = 16
Selevinfiidae	1/1	0/0	0/0	3/3	2x = 16
Rhizomydae	1/1	0/0	0/0	3/3	2x = 16
Erethizontidae	1/1	0/0	1/1	3/3	2x = 20
Caviidae	1/1	0/0	1/1	3/3	2x = 20
Hydrochoeridae	1/1	0/0	1/1	3/3	2x = 20
Dinfomydae	1/1	0/0	1/1	3/3	2x = 20
Dasyproctidae	1/1	0/0	1/1	3/3	2x = 20
Cuniculidae	1/1	0/0	1/1	3/3	2x = 20
Chinchillidae	1/1	0/0	1/1	3/3	2x = 20
Capromyidae	1/1	0/0	1/1	3/3	2x = 20
Ctenodactylidae	1/1	0/0	1–2 / 1–2	3/3	2x = 20–24
Echimyidae	1/1	0/0	1/1	3/3	2x = 20
Zapodidae	1/1	0/0	0–1 / 0	3/3	2x = 16–18
Dipodidae	1/1	0/0	0–1 / 0	3/3	2 x = 16–18
Heteromyidae	1/1	0/0	1/1	3/3	2x = 20
Geomyidae	1/1	0/0	1/1	3/3	2x = 20
Spalacidae	1/1	0/0	0/0	3/3	2x = 16
Abrocomidae	1/1	0/0	1/1	3/3	2x = 20
Thryonomyidae	1/1	0/0	1/1	3/3	2x = 20
Petromyidae	1/1	0/0	1/1	3/3	2x = 20
Bathyergida	1/1	0/0	2–3 / 2–3	0–3 / 0–3	2x = 12–28
Hystricidae	1/1	0/0	1/1	3/3	2x = 20
Octodontidae	1/1	0/0	1/1	3/3	2 = 20
Order Carnivora					
Canidae	3/3	1/1	4/4	1–4 / 2–5	2x = 38–50
Ursidae	3/3	1/1	4/4	2/3	2x = 42
Procynidae	3/3	1/1	3–4 / 3–4	2 / 2–4	2x = 36–40
Felidae	3/3	1/1	2–3 / 2	1/1	2x = 28–30
Mustelidae	3 / 2–3	1/1	2–4 / 2–4	1 / 1–2	2x = 30–38
Viverridae	3/3	1/1	3–4 / 3–4	1–2 / 1–2	2x = 32–40
Hyaenidae	3/3	1/1	3–4 / 1–3	0–1 / 1–2	2x = 26–34
Ailuropodidae	3/3	1/1	2–3 / 3	3/3	2x = 38–40
Order Pinnipedia					
Otarciidae	3/2	1/1	4/4	1–3 / 1	2x = 34–38
Phocidae	2–3 / 1–2	1/1	4/4	0–2 / 0–2	2x = 26–36
Odobenidae	1–2 / 0	1/1	3–4 / 3–4	0/0	2x = 18–24
Order Probocidae					
Elephantidae	1/0	0/0	3/3	3/3	2x = 26
Order Hiracoidea					
Procaviidae	1/2	0/0	4/4	3/3	2x = 34

Table 22.5 (Continued)

Family	Incisors	Canines	Premolars	Molars	Total
Order Sirinia					
Trichechidae	0/0	0/0	0/0	6/6	2× = 24
Order Perissodactyla					
Equidae	3/3	0–1 / 0–1	3–4 / 3	3/3	2× = 36–42
Tapiridae	3/3	1/1	4/4	3/3	2× = 44
Rhinfocerotidae	0–2 / 0–1	0 / 0–1	3–4 / 3–4	3/3	2× = 24–34
Order Artiodactyla					
Suborder Suiformes					
Suidae	1–3 / 3	1/1	2–4 / 2–4	3/3	2× = 34–44
Tayssuidae	2/3	1/1	3/3	3/3	2× = 38
Hippopotamidae	2–3 / 1–3	1/1	4/4	3/3	2× = 38–42
Suborder Tylopoda					
Camelidae	1/3	1/01	2–3 / 2–3	3/3	2× = 30–34
Suborder Ruminantia					
Tragulidae	0/3	1/1	3/3	3/3	2× = 34
Cervidae	0/3	0–1 / 1	3/3	3/3	2× = 32–34
Giraffidae	0/3	0/1	3/3	3/3	2× = 32
Bovidae	0/3	0/1	3 / 2–3	3/3	2× = 30–32

References

1 Fecchio, R.S., Rossi, J.L. Jr., Ferro, D.G., and Gioso, M.A. (2009). Medicina preventiva aplicada à odontologia em animais selvagens. *Nosso Clínico* 12: 44–52.

2 San Roman, F. (1999). *Atlas de Odontologia de Pequenos Animais*. Manole: São Paulo, Brazil.

3 Peyer, B. (1968). *Comparative Odontology*. Chicago, IL: University of Chicago Press.

4 Foreest, A.W.V. (1986). Veterinary dentistry in zoo and wild animals. In: *(ed.), Zoo and Wild Animals Medicine* (ed. E.M. Fowler). Philadelphia, PA: W.B. Saunders Co.

5 Pachaly, J.R. and Gioso, M.A. (2001). Oral cavity. In: *Biology, Medicine, and Surgery of South American Wild Animals* (ed. M.E. Fowler and Z.S. Cubas), 457–463. Ames, IA: Iowa State University Press.

6 Harvey, C.E. (1985). *Veterinary Dentistry*, 289–308. Philadelphia. PA: WB Saunders Co.

7 Pachley, J.R. (1997). Noções de Odonto-estomatologia aplicada aos animais selvagens (Notions of dental-stomatology applied to wild animals). Apostila da disciplina do curso ministrado no Zoológico de São Paulo (Handout of the course of the São Paulo Zoo).

8 Wiggs, R.B. and Lobprise, H.B. (1997). Exotic animal oral disease and dentistry. In: *Veterinary Dentistry. Principles and Practice*. New York: Lippincott- Raven.

9 Kertesz, P.A. (1993). *A Colour Atlas of Veterinary Dentistry and Oral Surgery*. Aylesbury, UK: Wolfe Publishing.

10 Auricchio, P. (1995). *Primatas do Brasil*, vol. 168. São Paulo, Brazil: Terra Brasilis.

11 Amand, W.B. and Tinkelman, C.L. (1985). Oral disease in captive wild animals. In: *Veterinary Dentistry* (ed. C.E.(e. Harvey), 289–308. Philadelphia, PA: WB Saunders Co.

12 Fecchio, R.S., Gomes, M.S., and Gioso, M.A. (2006). Prevalence of oral diseases in capuchin monkey (Cebus apella) captives in the state of São Paulo, Brazil. In: *20th Annual Veterinary Dental Forum*. Portland, OR.

13 Robinson, P.T. (1986). Dentistry in zoo animals. In: *Zoo and Wildlife Animal Medicine*, 2e (ed. M.E. Fowler). Philadelphia, PA: WB Saunders Co.

14 Gioso, M.A., and Fecchio, R.S., Ferreira J (2005). Lesão dental iatrogênica causada por "desarme dental" em Chimpanzé (Pan troglodytes). In *X Congresso e XV Encontro da Associação Brasileira de Veterinários de Animais Selvagens – ABRAVAS*, São Pedro, Brazil.

15 Leon-Roman, M.A. and Rossi, J.L. Jr. (2014). Endodontia. In: *Tratado de Animais Selvagens* (ed. Z.S. Cubas, S. JCR and J.L. (e.) Catao-Dias). São Paulo, Brazil: Roca.

16 Amand, A.B. and Tinkelman, C.L. (1997). Preventive medicine. In: *Wild Mammals in Captivity- Principles and Techniques*, vol. 1997 (ed. D.G. Kleiman, M.E. Allen, K.V. Thompson and S. Lumpkin), 16–24. Chicago, IL: University of Chicago Press.

17 Spencer, M.A. (2003). Tooth-root form and function in platyrrhine seed-eaters. *Am. J. Phys. Anthropol.* 122 (4): 325–335.

18 Fecchio, R.S., Gomes, M.S., Coutino, A, and Sobrihno, C.B. (2005). Doença periodontal grave em cachorro do mato vinagre (Speothos venaticus). In: *IX Congresso e XIV Encontro da Associação Brasileira de Veterinários de Animais Selvagens*, São José do Rio Preto, Brazil.

19 Fecchio, R.S., Gomes, M.S., Rossi, J.L. Jr., and Gioso MA. (2006). Dental problems in Bush Dogs (Speothos venaticus) in Brazil. In: *31st World Small Congress*. Prague, Czech Republic.

20 Fecchio, R.S., Prazeres, R.F., Gioso, M.A., and Carvahlo, V.G.G. (2010). Prevalence of oral diseases in oncilla (*Leopardus pardalis*) captive in Brazil. *Eur. Vet. Dent. Congr.*

21 Correa, S.H.R., Pachally, J.R., Catao Dias, J.L., and Guimaraes, M.A.B.V (2005). Prevalência de lesões orais em pequenos felinos neotropicais na FPZSP. In: *IX Congresso e XIV Encontro da Associação Brasileira de Veterinários de Animais Selvagens*, São José do Rio Preto, Brazil.

22 Fagan DA. The pathogenesis of dental disease in carniores. In: *Meeting of the American Association of Zoo Veterinarians*, Washington, DC, 1980.

23 McBurney, S., Veitch, A.M., and Daoust, P.Y. (2000). Bacterial valvular endocarditis in a black bear from Labrador. *J. Wildl. Dis.* 36 (4): 788–791.

24 Rossi, J.L. Jr. and Gioso, M.A. (2003). Prevalência de maloclusão em *Panthera onca* e *Puma concolor* mantidas em cativeiro no Estado de São Paulo. *Braz. J. Vet. Res. Anim. Sci.* 40 (2): 155–160.

25 Aguiar, M.S. (1998). Patologias no aparelho mastigatório em Didelphis albiventris e Didelphis marsupialis (Marsupialia, Didelphimorphia, Didelphidae) do Sul do Brasil. Dissertação de Mestrado. Pontifícia Universidade Católica do Rio Grande do Sul, Brazil.

26 Foreest, A.V. and Roeters, J. (1997). Restorative dental treatments of abraded canine teeth in a Sumatran tiger (*Panthera tigris sumatrae*). *J. Vet. Dent.* 14 (4): 131–136.

27 Brinkman, R.J. and Williams, R.V. (1975). Root canal and capping on a whitehanded Gibbon. *J. Zoo Anim. Méd.* 6: 26.

28 Fecchio, R.S., Prazeres, R.F, and Dias Neto, R. et al. (2013). Apicectomia em dente canino de tigre de bengala (Pantera tigris tigris). In: *XVI Congresso e XXII Encontro – ABRAVAS*. Salvador/BA.

29 Fecchio, R.S., Bastos, R.R., Coutihno, A. et al. (2014). Adaptação de coroa metálica pré-fabricada em dente canino de onça parda (Puma concolor) - relato de caso. *Rev. Clín. Vet. (São Paulo).* XIX: 82–90.

30 Gioso, M.A. (1997). Afecções Periodontais. *Cadernos Técnicos. Esc. Vet. UFMG.* 20: 71–80.

31 Gioso, M.A. (1999). Prevalence of F.O.R.L. in Brazil. In: *6th World Veterinary Dental Congress*, Hobart, Tasmania, Australia.

32 Berger, M., Schawalder, P., Stich, H., and Lussi, A. (1996). Feline dental resorptive lesions in captive and wild leopards and lions. *J. Vet. Dent.* 13 (1): 13–21.

33 Zetner, K. (1992). The influence of dry food and the development of feline neck lesions. *J. Vet. Dent.* 9 (4): 4–6.

34 Gioso, M.A, Fecchio, R.S., and Rossi, J.L. Jr. (2009) Palatal cleft repair in a lion (Panthera leo). In: *World Small Animal Veterinary Association Congress*, São Paulo, Brazil. 251–251.

35 Fecchio, R.S., Gomes, M.S., and Lopes, F.M. (2009). Fibromatous epulis oral in tiger (Panthera tigris) – Case report. In: *World Small Animal Veterinary Association Congress*. São Paulo, Brazil. 58–59.

36 Sykes, J.M. 4th, Garner, M.M., Greer, L.L. et al. (2007). Oral eosinophilic granulomas in tigers (*Panthera tigris*): a collection of 16 cases. *J. Zoo Wildl. Med.* 38 (2): 300–308.

37 Knightly, F. and Emily, P. (2003). Oral disorders of exotic ungulates. In: Oral Biology, Dental and Beak Disorders. *Vet. Clin. Exotic Anim.* 6: 565–570.

38 Wallach, J.D. and Boever, B.J. (1983). *Diseases of Exotic Animals*. Philadelphia, PA: WB Saunders Co.

39 Reichard, T. and Heinrichs, P. (1989). Natural healing of a laceration to the frenulum and associated soft tissue in the lower lip of a nyala. Zoo Animal Dentistry Abstracts. *J. Vet. Dent.* 6 (3).

40 Douglass, E.M. (1979). Lymphosarcoma and blockage of the biliary duct in an African lion (*Panthera leo*). *Vet. Med. Small Anim. Clin.* 74: 1637.

41 Gillette, D.M., Acland, H.M., and Klein, L. (1978). Ductular mammary carcinoma in a lioness. *J. Am. Vet. Assoc.* 173 (9): 1099–1102.

42 Marker, L., Munson, L., Basson, P.A., and Quackenbush, S. (2003). Multicentric T-cell lymphoma associated with feline leukemia virus infection in a captive Namibian cheetah (*Acinonyx jubatus*). *J. Wildl. Dis.* 39: 690–695.

43 Dorso, L., Risi, S., Triau, S. et al. (2008). High-grade mucoepidermoid carcinoma of the mandibular salivary gland in a lion (*Panthera leo*). *Vet. Pathol.* 45: 104–108.

44 Steenkamp, G. (2003). Oral biology and disorders of tusked mammals. In: Oral biology, dental and beak disorders. *Vet. Clin. Exotic Anim.* 6: 565–570.

45 Hillson, S. (1996). *Teeth*, 77–81. London, UK: Cambridge University Press.

46 Fecchio, R.S. (2013). Megavertebrates dentistry. In: *Congreso Veterinario de Leon*. Leon, México.

47 Malta, M.C., Teixeira da Costa, M.E.L., and Coelho CM.(2000). Pulpotomia nas presas de um elefante africano (Loxodonta africana). In: *XXIV Congresso da Sociedade de Zoológicos do Brasil e V Encontro Internacional de Zoológicos*, Belo Horizonte, Brazil.

48 Miles, A.E. (1972). Healed injuries of elephant tusks. *Br. Dent. J.* 133: 395–400.

49 Von Metnitz, J. (1903). Osteodentine, vasodentine and abscess cavities in dentine. *Q. Circ.* 289–304.

50 Humphreys, H.F. (1926). Particulars relating to the broken tusk of wild Indian elephant. *Br. Dent. J.* 47: 1400–1401.

51 Oliveira, F.S., and Canola, J.C. (2005). Erupção dental em pacas criadas em cativeiro (Agouti paca, Linnaeus, 1766). In: *IX Congresso e XIV Encontro da Associação Brasileira de Veterinários de Animais Selvagens*, São José do Rio Preto, Brazil.

Index

Wiggs's Veterinary Dentistry: Principles and Practice, Second Edition. Edited by Heidi B. Lobprise and Johnathon R. (Bert) Dodd.

C

d

e

n

u